CANCER CHEMOPREVENTION

CANCER DRUG DISCOVERY AND DEVELOPMENT

BEVERLY A. TEICHER, SERIES EDITOR

CANCER CHEMOPREVENTION

VOLUME 2: STRATEGIES FOR CANCER CHEMOPREVENTION

Edited by

GARY J. KELLOFF, MD
ERNEST T. HAWK, MD, MPH

National Institutes of Health
Rockville, MD

CAROLINE C. SIGMAN, PhD

CCS Associates
Mountain View, CA

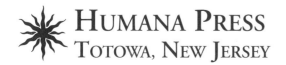 HUMANA PRESS
TOTOWA, NEW JERSEY

© 2005 Humana Press Inc.
999 Riverview Drive, Suite 208
Totowa, New Jersey 07512

www.humanapress.com

Production Editor: Mark J. Breaugh

Cover design by Patricia F. Cleary

This publication is printed on acid-free paper. ⊚
ANSI Z39.48-1984 (American National Standards Institute)
Permanence of Paper for Printed Library Materials

For additional copies, pricing for bulk purchases, and/or information about other Humana titles, contact Humana at the above address or at any of the following numbers: Tel.:973-256-1699; Fax: 973-256-8341; Email: humanapr.com; or visit our Website: http://humanapress.com

Printed in the United States of America.   10 9 8 7 6 5 4 3 2 1

eISBN:1-59259-768-8

Library of Congress Cataloging-in-Publication Data

Cancer chemoprevention / edited by Gary J. Kelloff, Ernest T. Hawk, Caroline C. Sigman.
     p. ; cm. -- (Cancer drug discovery and development)
 Includes bibliographical references and index.
 ISBN 1-58829-077-8 (v. 2 : alk. paper)
 1. Cancer--Chemoprevention.
 [DNLM: 1. Anticarcinogenic Agents--therapeutic use. 2. Neoplasms--prevention & con-
trol. 3. Chemoprevention--methods. QZ 267 C2144 2004] I. Kelloff, Gary. II. Hawk,
Ernest T. III. Sigman, Caroline C. IV. Series.
 RC268.15.C3612 2004
 616.99'4061--dc22
                                                              2004000342

PREFACE

Despite significant advances in cancer treatment and early detection, overall cancer incidence has increased, cancer-associated morbidity is considerable, and overall cancer survival has remained relatively flat over the past several decades *(1,2)*. However, new technology allowing exploration of signal transduction pathways, identification of cancer-associated genes, and imaging of tissue architecture and molecular and cellular function is increasing our understanding of carcinogenesis and cancer progression. This knowledge is moving the focus of cancer therapeutics, including cancer preventive treatments, to drugs that take advantage of cellular control mechanisms to selectively suppress cancer progression.

Carcinogenesis is now visualized as a multifocal, multipath process of genetic progression occurring over a long time period and resulting in increasing loss of cellular controls. This process provides promising opportunities for chemoprevention, which involves using drugs, biologics, or nutrients to inhibit, delay, or reverse neoplastic progression at any time before the onset of invasive disease. Remarkable progress has been made in developing chemoprevention strategies, started by research on mechanisms of chemopreventive drugs and assays for evaluating these drugs in animal models *(3–6)*, and led in the clinic by early studies on prevention of head and neck carcinogenesis *(7,8)*.

Progressive disorganization provides a strong rationale for early intervention in carcinogenesis when mutations are fewer, even before tissue-level phenotypic changes are evident. However, the long latency also presents a significant challenge for prevention and treatment of early cancer *(9,10)*. That is, cancer incidence reduction studies in subjects at relatively low risk may require thousands of subjects and many years to obtain significant and definitive results. The successful trial of tamoxifen as a chemopreventive for breast cancer illustrates the vast resources required for a primary prevention study, even when the cohort is well defined and the drug effect is already well characterized. This trial was carried out in women who at a minimum had a relative risk for breast cancer equivalent to a 60-year old *(11)*. Six thousand six hundred (6600) treated women and an equivalent number of control subjects were required to achieve a significant ($p < 0.05$) treatment effect.

This inherent inefficiency in validating that chemopreventive treatment results in net clinical benefit for the patient (subject) has led to intensive research efforts to develop useful biomarkers. These biomarkers include measures of neoplastic progression, drug effect (or pharmacodynamic markers), and markers that measure prognosis as well as predict responses to specific therapy. All these biomarkers have the potential to greatly augment the development of successful chemoprevention therapies, but two specific types of biomarkers will have the most immediate impact on successful chemopreventive drug development—those that measure the risk of developing invasive life-threatening disease, and those whose modulation can "reasonably predict" clinical benefit and, therefore, serve as surrogate endpoints for later-occurring clinical disease. Thus far, the biomarker that best measures these two phenomena is intraepithelial neoplasia (IEN) because it is a near obligate precursor to cancer. As precancer, it is a very good risk marker for cancer development; and as a recognized disease that is being treated, it has been validated as a surrogate endpoint biomarker *(12–14)*. Since IEN is discussed extensively in many chapters in this volume, the three important features that characterize IEN are presented in some detail below.

IEN is a near obligate precursor to cancer. IEN occurs in most epithelial tissue as moderate to severe dysplasia, is on the causal pathway leading from normal tissue to cancer, and is close in progression to cancer (invasive neoplasia). Genetic progression with loss of cellular control functions is observed as the phenotype gradually changes from normal histology to early dysplasia then to increasingly severe IEN, superficial cancers, and finally invasive disease. For example, in the breast it is estimated that progression from atypical hyperplasia through ductal carcinoma *in situ* (DCIS) to adenocarcinoma requires 10–20 years or more *(15,16)*. Colorectal adenomas may form over a period as long as 5–20 years, and progression from adenoma to colorectal carcinoma usually requires another 5–15 years *(17–20)*. Prostatic intraepithelial neoplasia (PIN) may develop over approximately 20 years. From PIN to early latent cancer may take 10 or more years, and clinically significant carcinoma may not occur until 3–15 years later *(21)*. Progression is marked in target tissues by the appearance of specific molecular and more general genotypic damage associated with increasingly severe dysplastic histology. In many cases, critical early steps include inactivation of tumor suppressors such as APC in colon or BRCA in breast cancers, and activation of oncogenes such as *ras* in colon, lung, and pancreatic cancers. Progression is also influenced by factors specific to the host tissue's environment, such as the action of hormones and cytokines produced in stroma around the developing epithelial tumor and changes in tissue structure. IEN shows these changes and provides a suitable target for treatment intervention because of its phenotypic and genotypic similarities and evolutionary proximity to invasive cancer.

IEN as precancer is a risk marker for cancer. Subjects with IEN, particularly severe IEN, are at significantly higher risk than unaffected populations for developing invasive cancer in the same tissues. Among measurable risk factors, only germline mutations that occur in genetic cancer syndromes confer higher risk. For example and as reviewed previously *(14)*, very strong evidence associates the presence of colorectal adenomas with subsequent development of invasive cancer; increasing risk correlates to type of histological growth pattern (villous > tubulovillous > tubular) and increasing size and severity of dysplasia. PIN as a risk marker for prostate cancer and the characteristics of PIN progression have also been described *(21–24)*. This evidence includes similar cellular morphology and atypia in high-grade PIN (HGPIN) and prostatic adenocarcinoma (cellular atypia observed in HGPIN is virtually indistinguishable from invasive cancer, except that in HGPIN no invasion has occurred). It also includes the spatial and temporal association of HGPIN to prostate cancer, with both being found primarily in the peripheral zone, and much more infrequently in the transition zone. As PIN progresses, the likelihood of damage to the basal cell layer and basement membrane increases. Certain cytoskeletal proteins, secreted proteins, and degree of glycosylation are shared by PIN and cancer, but not by benign prostatic hyperplasia or normal prostate epithelium. The most compelling data on the temporal relationship of PIN and cancer comes from studies showing that patients with HGPIN and no detectable cancer progressed to a 40% incidence of cancer in three years and to approximately 80% incidence in ten years.

IEN is precancer and in its own right is a disease; treatment provides clinical benefit. Because IEN is a near obligate precursor to invasive cancer, it is standard clinical practice to utilize invasive surgical interventions to reduce the burden of IEN, e.g., colon adenomas, oral leukoplakia, cervical IEN (CIN) 2/3, breast DCIS. Therefore, reducing IEN burden is an important and suitable goal for medical (noninvasive) intervention to reduce invasive cancer risk and to reduce surgical morbidity *(14)*. High-risk individuals with established IEN are cohorts for clinical trials to demonstrate the effectiveness of new chemopreventive agents for IEN treatment. Moreover, treatment is needed not only for clinically apparent IEN, but also the entire epithelial sheet at risk of developing IEN ("field cancerization," e.g., ref. *25*), to ensure reduced need for surgical removal of IEN.

These features of IEN explain why it is at present the best surrogate endpoint for invasive cancer, since no serious student of cell biology or pathology questions that the morphologic changes associated with IEN are part of and predict the cancer process, and that the lesions of genetic progression manifest themselves within IEN as cytological abnormalities of neoplasia—increased nuclear size; abnormal nuclear shape; increased nuclear stain uptake; variations in cellular size, shape and stain uptake; increased mitosis; abnormal mitosis; disordered maturation (differentiation) *(26)*. In summary, because of the probability that its presence will lead to cancer, IEN is already accepted as a validated endpoint for measurement of cancer risk reduction by both surgical and drug intervention.

Other promising surrogate endpoint biomarkers— genome/proteome expression profiles. Use (validation) of surrogate endpoint biomarkers that, unlike IEN, are not obviously intrinsic to neoplastic progression mostly fail because of the complexity of neoplasia as well as the need for surrogate endpoint biomarkers to "predict patient benefit with reasonable certainty" *(27)*. The failures result because the disease of cancer is tissue-based, and surrogate endpoint biomarker development has been constrained by naive approaches to modeling the disease and its multipath, multifocal development process with isolated molecular and cellular events. Further, for biomarkers to be useful, techniques to determine them need to be robust and exhaustively validated. When using biomarkers in studies, investigators need to comply strictly with validated methods to assure confidence that what is measured is consistent across studies. Achieving this objective may require extensive efforts such as those used to establish standards for the determination of cholesterol. Criteria for biomarker measurements have been the subject of many reviews (e.g., *12,14,28*), yet much of the lack of progress derives from faulty adherence to these methodologies. Nonetheless, a sound scientific basis now exists to characterize surrogate endpoint biomarkers for developing drugs *(12)*.

The multipath, multifactorial nature of carcinogenesis is predicted by the heterogeneity that can result from processing the human genome. The 30,000 or so human genes contain as many as several hundred thousand allelic variants from single nucleotide gene polymorphisms including splicing variants *(29)*. These variations are compounded another three- to fivefold by posttranslational protein modifications leading to a multitude ($>10^6$) of protein–protein interactions *(30)*. Even if only a small fraction of the genome is critical to cancer, the number of possible molecules and interactions involved is enormous. This level of complexity highlights the uncertainties of using isolated molecular and cellular biomarkers to measure carcinogenesis. Moreover, this complexity is heightened by expected intra-/intersubject and tissue variations.

Nonetheless, increasing understanding of genetic progression in cancer (e.g., *31,32*) and of signal transduction *(33)* in cancer target tissues, and observations of genotypic changes characteristic of selected cancers (e.g., *34,35*) combined with advances in technology for measuring and characterizing changes in gene and protein expression *(30)*, suggest that analyses of such patterns of gene expression have potential for development as surrogate endpoint biomarkers. For example, progress made in gene chip technology suggests that within a few years it will be trivial to measure 6–12 genes defining a genetic progression model *(36)*. As for all surrogate endpoint biomarkers, the feasibility of genome/proteome expression patterns as surrogate endpoint biomarkers will depend on careful evaluation in the context of carcinogenesis. Therefore, the characterization of molecular markers of carcinogenesis and their future development and validation as surrogate endpoint biomarkers will be most effectively done *in situ* within IEN. The further development of genetic progression models will also proceed in this context, as it has from inception. In the not-too-distant future, as understanding of the minimum number of disrupted pathways yielding malignancy grows, patterns of change representing carcinogenesis will be relatively easy to measure. This process will evolve with progress that is being made in understanding and analyzing systems biology. With this understanding will come surrogate endpoint biomarkers in predysplastic tissue (a normal morphologic phenotype); the predictive value of these data will begin to exceed the predictive value of abnormal morphology (IEN). This molecular pathology within IEN lesions, or even prior to appearance of these lesions, will also allow better identification of individuals at risk, improve study efficiency, and provide better quantitative estimation of drug efficacy than effects on IEN alone *(12,14,28)*. These advances in tissue-based biomarkers will be augmented by biomarkers that can be measured non-invasively by molecular imaging, and by functional genomic and proteomic research *(14,28)*.

Net clinical benefit is required. Drug approvals are based on clinical benefit, so the approval of drugs for chemoprevention will depend on some measure of clinical benefit—reduced morbidity, organ preservation, lower cost for surveillance—as well as efficacy against precancers. Because chemopreventive drugs will most likely be administered chronically, they will be expected to demonstrate long-term safety, duration of effect, and minimal drug resistance, or provide alternative strategies to minimize toxicity and maximize efficacy.

Promising Chemopreventive Agents, the companion volume, surveys ongoing efforts to identify drugs, natural products, and other agents that may have potential in cancer chemoprevention. The agents are grouped by pharmacological and/or mechanistic classes and vary widely in terms of stage of development as chemopreventives, ranging from extensively studied groups such as nonsteroidal antiinflammatory drugs (NSAIDs) and antiestrogens to drugs with recently identified potential based on mechanistic activity (e.g., protein kinase inhibitors, histone deacetylase inhibitors, and anti-angiogenesis agents), as well as agents yet to be evaluated in chemoprevention settings (e.g., proteasome and chaperone protein inhibitors). Attention is devoted to food-derived agents (such as tea, curcumin, and soy isoflavones), vitamins, and minerals because of their high promise for prevention in healthy populations.

Provided in this volume, *Strategies for Cancer Chemoprevention,* are guidelines for cancer chemopreventive drug development. Part I is devoted to general strategies and methods for drug discovery, preclinical efficacy, characterization of precancers, safety evaluation, clinical cohorts, and clinical trial design. Part II reviews strategies for and status of chemopreventive agent development at major cancer targets—prostate, breast, colon, lung, head and neck, esophagus, bladder, ovary, endometrium, cervix, skin, liver, and multiple myeloma. Both sections heavily document the characterization and application of reliable biomarkers in chemopreventive drug development.

The first several chapters of Part I consider discovery and preclinical evaluation of new agents. For example, an elegant approach to the challenges of identifying chemopreventive agents in natural products, particularly food plants (e.g., antioxidants, antiinflammatory compounds, and well-defined mixtures) is presented (Chapter 1); this approach addresses factors such as standardization of plant growth and extraction conditions, and considers co-development of a well-defined mixture and its likely active component. The development of preclinical models for evaluating potential chemopreventive agents is particularly important because of the potential for validating surrogate endpoints in animal models where an intermediate biomarker can be evaluated, along with subsequent effects on cancer incidence, and ultimately survival. Chapters in this volume describe well-established carcinogen-induced animal models of carcinogenesis in major cancer targets (Chapter 2), as well as newly defined transgenic and gene knock-in/knock-out mouse models of molecular targets for chemoprevention (Chapter 3), and animal models of genetically inherited cancer susceptibility (Chapter 4).

The importance of precancerous histopathology, particularly IEN, in chemoprevention has been stated. Characteristics and progression of this pathology in most cancer targets are comprehensively reviewed in Chapter 5. The use of computer-assisted image analysis to analyze precancerous tissue in the prostate is described as an example of the potential application of new quantitative imaging techniques to evaluate chemopreventive efficacy in IEN (Chapter 6). As noted before, genome/proteome expression profiles have high potential as surrogate endpoints for carcinogenesis because they correlate with the clinical progression of carcinogenesis. Several chapters in the book assess potential applications of genomics and proteomics to chemoprevention. Uses of genomics databases in discovery of chemopreventive agents and in designing chemopreventive strategies are surveyed (Chapter 7). Surrogate endpoint biomarkers for breast cancer based on functional genomics are described (Chapter 8), as are applications of proteomics in clinical cancer settings (Chapter 9) and interpretation of genome-based data (Chapter 10).

Determining which populations will likely benefit from chemopreventive intervention, particularly those who are asymptomatic, is a significant challenge and an opportunity for chemoprevention. Two approaches are laid out in this volume. One is the construction of multi-factorial models of absolute risk, based primarily on epidemiological statistics (Chapter 11). The second explores the correlation of genetic polymorphisms to cancer susceptibility (Chapter 12). The remaining two chapters in Part I examine some practical aspects of clinical evaluation of chemopreventive agents—i.e., clinical trial design issues (Chapter 13) and subject recruitment (Chapter 14).

For each cancer target organ covered in Part II, one chapter provides an overview of carcinogenesis in the target organ, including cancer and precancer incidences, genetic progression, and risk factors, along with potential opportunities for chemoprevention. Known and promising chemopreventive agents, surrogate endpoints, and clinical trial designs are summarized. For a number of these targets, additional chapters address specific topics that contribute to chemoprevention strategies.

In addition to an overview of strategies for prostate cancer chemoprevention (Chapter 15), a second chapter addresses the controversial topic of using prostate-specific antigen for determining risk and monitoring the progression of prostate cancer (Chapter 16). The overview of breast cancer chemoprevention focuses on defining populations at risk based on evidence of early genetic progression (Chapter 17) and is accompanied by two supplemental chapters. One describes development of ductal lavage as a technique for sampling breast cells in assessment of early neoplasia (Chapter 18), and the second addresses the well-recognized need to control estrogenic activity in suppressing breast carcinogenesis (Chapter 19). Quite possibly, the most significant advances in clinical chemoprevention have been made against colorectal carcinogenesis (Chapter 20) where genetic and histo-pathological progression of early dysplasia to adenoma to

cancer has been well-studied. An additional important preventive strategy in colon is screening for and excision of adenomas (Chapter 21). Chapter 22 provides an overview of lung cancer chemoprevention accompanied by an article on topical delivery as a strategy to allow administration of drugs to lung that may be too toxic for systemic administration (Chapter 23); topical administration is also a promising strategy in other accessible targets such as skin, oral cavity, colon and cervix.

The review of bladder cancer chemoprevention (Chapter 24) focuses on the potential use of chemopreventive drugs to stop the recurrence of superficial bladder cancers; this cohort is at very high risk for recurrence and progression, and a successful chemopreventive intervention could be expected to provide clinical benefit from organ preservation (by delaying or reducing the need for cystectomy). Chapters on the esophagus discuss prevention and delay of progression of Barrett's esophagus, a precursor to adenocarcinoma and an increasing risk factor for esophageal cancer in western populations (Chapter 25), as well as prevention of squamous cell carcinoma (Chapter 27). A third chapter looks at sophisticated new techniques for imaging esophageal dysplasia (Chapter 26). The high rate of second primary tumor formation has been well-documented for the head and neck, which have been studied for more than 20 years as a site for chemoprevention (Chapter 28). Recently, aneuploidy and other biomarkers of genetic progression have been carefully documented as risk and prognostic indicators of head and neck carcinogenesis and potential endpoints for chemoprevention studies (Chapter 29). Incidences of non-melanoma skin cancer are higher by far than any other cancer, and melanoma incidence is increasing (Chapter 30). In addition to oral and topical small molecule drug treatments for prevention and treatment of non-melanoma precursor lesions (actinic keratoses, basal cell nevus syndrome), opportunities exist for novel immunotherapies in skin carcinogenesis and vaccination against melanoma (Chapter 31).

Screening for and surgical removal of suspect CIN is well established, and drugs have shown activity in reducing CIN severity (Chapter 32). Moreover, human papillomavirus infection is strongly associated with onset of cervical cancer, and immunoprevention strategies (both treatment and prophylactic) are under development for populations at risk (Chapter 33). Thus far, chemoprevention strategies in endometrium have not been established; however, remarkable advances have been made in documenting and quantifying carcinogenesis-associated changes in endometrial tissue that provide opportunities for preventive intervention (Chapter 34). In ovary (Chapter 35), pancreas (Chapter 36), liver (Chapter 37), and multiple myeloma (Chapter 38), precancerous lesions that may be targets for chemoprevention are suggested, along with potentially effective chemo-preventive drugs.

The two volumes of *Cancer Chemoprevention* demonstrate that the science of chemoprevention research is solidly established, very active, and offers great promise for lessening the burden of human cancer. Progress in building and understanding genetic/molecular progression models of many human cancers based on seminal work described by Vogelstein and colleagues for the adenoma-carcinoma sequence in colon cancer *(37)* has been substantial and is being enhanced by newer and better animal models. Understanding molecular progression leads to synthesis and discovery of new molecularly targeted agents with high promise of efficacy that, once evaluated for safety, will have an impact on cancer incidence and mortality. The evaluation of drug effect and drug efficacy biomarkers along with better technologies for their measurement is progressing, and the science and utility of surrogate endpoint biomarkers in developing cancer chemopreventive agents against sporadic cancers are solidly established. The issue of validation is a relative one, and IEN is validated for most target organs sufficiently to establish that its prevention/removal provides clinical benefit. With rigorous attention to methodology and to emerging scientific data and new technologies, there is every expectation that new surrogate endpoint biomarkers will now be developed in the context of IEN. These new surrogate endpoint biomarkers will improve the efficiency of clinical chemopreventive agent development, better identify those patients (subjects) who are likely to benefit (or not to benefit), while also opening the door to even earlier identification of individuals at risk (e.g., those with predysplastic molecular lesions that occur prior to IEN). The rapid pace at which systems biology and new technologies are evolving will make surrogate endpoint biomarker science a very productive and exciting area, but will also evoke the need for careful validation of such markers in the context of clinical trials.

Prospects are bright that surrogate endpoint biomarkers will make cancer chemoprevention studies more efficient and informative; however, hard work and exceptional dedication to sound, standardized methods will be required to assure that the application of these efforts in developing chemopreventive drugs is fruitful. The eventual acceptance of surrogate endpoint biomarkers may entail more than scientific rationale. Scientific and regulatory policy changes may also be required (e.g., *38*). It is often observed that candidate surrogate endpoint biomarkers are expressed at higher incidences than the symptomatic clinical disease that they approximate. Such will always be the case when completely unrelated endpoints (other causes of death) do not allow carcinogenesis to go to completion. Based on existing disease models, it is likely that all high-grade IEN-carrying confirmed genetic lesions would end

in cancer if the host lived long enough *(12,32)*. Validation, like causality, is a relative term that only becomes absolute when all variables and elements of a process are known and can be studied quantitatively. It is undesirable and short-sighted to require any data more rigorous than validation based on probabilistic estimates that are consistent with current medical and regulatory practice. Based on existing knowledge, we can assume that IEN and the earlier biomarkers within IEN are on one or more of the possible causal pathways to carcinogenesis. Because they sometimes precede the cancer endpoint by several years, there is potential for interference, diversion, role in other biological processes, etc., that would keep these events from being ideal surrogate endpoint biomarkers. However, intervention to treat or prevent could be shown to provide clinical benefit, much like lipid-lowering in cardiovascular disease and viral load reduction in AIDS *(27,39)*. If interventions show compelling efficacy against surrogate endpoint biomarkers and can be administered safely to populations at risk, it would seem prudent to formulate scientific and regulatory policy changes allowing the use of these biomarkers in evaluating interventions that would lead to more efficient drug approvals to prevent this dread disease.

Gary J. Kelloff, MD
Ernest T. Hawk, MD, MPH
Caroline C. Sigman, PhD

REFERENCES

1. Sporn MB. The war on cancer. Lancet 1996;347:1377–1381.
2. Jemal A, Murray T, Samuels A, et al. Cancer statistics, 2003. CA Cancer J Clin 2003;53:5–26.
3. Sporn MB. Approaches to prevention of epithelial cancer during the preneoplastic period. Cancer Res 1976;36:2699–2702.
4. Wattenberg LW. Chemoprophylaxis of carcino-genesis: a review. Cancer Res 1966;26:1520–1526.
5. Wattenberg LW. Inhibition of chemical carcino-genesis. J Natl Cancer Inst 1978;60:11–18.
6. Wattenberg LW. Chemoprevention of cancer. Cancer Res 1985;45:1–8.
7. Hong WK, Endicott J, Itri LM, et al. 13-cis-Retinoic acid in the treatment of oral leukoplakia. N Engl J Med 1986;315:1501–1505.
8. Hong WK, Lippman SM, Itri LM, et al. Prevention of second primary tumors with isotretinoin in squamous-cell carcinoma of the head and neck. N Engl J Med 1990;323:795–801.
9. Kelloff GJ, Johnson JR, Crowell JA, et al. Approaches to the development and marketing approval of drugs that prevent cancer. Cancer Epidemiol Biomarkers Prev 1995;4:1–10.

10. Hong WK, Sporn MB. Recent advances in chemo-prevention of cancer. Science 1997;278:1073–1077.

11. Fisher B, Costantino JP, Wickerham DL, et al. Tamoxifen for prevention of breast cancer: report of the National Surgical Adjuvant Breast and Bowel Project P-1 Study. J Natl Cancer Inst 1998;90:1371–1388.

12. Kelloff GJ, Sigman CC, Johnson KM, et al. Perspectives on surrogate end points in the development of drugs that reduce the risk of cancer. Cancer Epidemiol Biomarkers Prev 2000;9:127–137.

13. Kelloff GJ. Perspectives on cancer chemoprevention research and drug development. Adv Cancer Res 2000;78:199–334.

14. O'Shaughnessy JA, Kelloff GJ, Gordon GB, et al. Treatment and prevention of intraepithelial neoplasia: an important target for accelerated new agent development. Clin Cancer Res 2002;8:314–346.

15. Frykberg ER, Bland KI. In situ breast carcinoma. Adv Surg 1993;26:29–72.

16. Page DL, Dupont WD, Rogers LW, Rados MS. Atypical hyperplastic lesions of the female breast. A long-term follow-up study. Cancer 1985;55:2698–2708.

17. Muto T, Bussey HJ, Morson BC. The evolution of cancer of the colon and rectum. Cancer 1975;36:2251–2270.

18. Day DW, Morson BC. The adenoma-carcinoma sequence. Major Probl Pathol 1978;10:58–71.

19. Hamilton SR. The adenoma-adenocarcinoma sequence in the large bowel: variations on a theme. J Cell Biochem 1992;16 Suppl G:41–46.

20. A multicenter study of colorectal adenomas. Rationale, objectives, methods and characteristics of the study cohort. The Multicentric Study of Colorectal Adenomas (SMAC) Workgroup. Tumori 1995;81:157–163.

21. Bostwick DG, Brawer MK. Prostatic intra-epithelial neoplasia and early invasion in prostate cancer. Cancer 1987;59:788–794.

22. Lipski BA, Garcia RL, Brawer MK. Prostatic intra-epithelial neoplasia: significance and management. Semin Urol Oncol 1996;14:149–155.

23. Sakr WA, Billis A, Ekman P, et al. Epidemiology of high-grade prostatic intraepithelial neoplasia. Scand J Urol Nephrol Suppl 2000;205:11–18.

24. Foster CS, Bostwick DG, Bonkhoff H, et al. Cellular and molecular pathology of prostate cancer precursors. Scand J Urol Nephrol Suppl 2000;205:19–43.

25. Slaughter DP, Southwick HW, Smekjal W. Field cancerization in oral stratified squamous epithe-lium; clinical implications of multicentric origin. Cancer 1953;6:963–968.

26. Foulds L. Multiple etiologic factors in neoplastic development. Cancer Res 1965;25:1339–1347.

27. Temple RJ. A regulatory authority's opinion about surrogate endpoints. In: Nimmo WS, Tucker GT, eds. Clinical Measurement in Drug Evaluation. New York: John Wiley and Sons, Inc., 1995:1–22.

28. Kelloff GJ, O'Shaughnessy JA, Gordon GB, et al. Counterpoint: because some surrogate end point biomarkers measure the neoplastic process they will have high utility in the development of cancer chemopreventive agents against sporadic cancers. Cancer Epidemiol Biomarkers Prev 2003;12:593–596.

29. Black DL. Protein diversity from alternative splicing: a challenge for bioinformatics and post-genome biology. Cell 2000;103:367–370.

30. Petricoin EF, Zoon KC, Kohn EC, et al. Clinical proteomics: translating benchside promise into bedside reality. Nat Rev Drug Discov 2002;1:683–695.

31. Califano J, van der Riet P, Westra W, et al. Genetic progression model for head and neck cancer: implications for field cancerization. Cancer Res 1996;56:2488–2492.

32. Ilyas M, Straub J, Tomlinson IP, Bodmer WF. Genetic pathways in colorectal and other cancers. Eur J Cancer 1999;35:1986–2002.

33. Hanahan D, Weinberg RA. The hallmarks of cancer. Cell 2000;100:57–70.

34. Sudbo J, Kildal W, Johannessen AC, et al. Gross genomic aberrations in precancers: clinical implications of a long-term follow-up study in oral erythroplakias. J Clin Oncol 2002;20:456–462.

35. Sudbo J, Reith A. Which putatively pre-malignant oral lesions become oral cancers? J Oral Pathol Med 2003;32:63–70.

36. Chen Y, Yakhini Z, Ben Dor A, et al. Analysis of expression patterns: the scope of the problem, the problem of scope. Dis Markers 2001;17:59–65.

37. Vogelstein B, Fearon ER, Hamilton SR, et al. Genetic altera-tions during colorectal-tumor development. N Engl J Med 1988;319:525–532.

38. Metz DC, Alberts DS. Gastrointestinal cancer prevention in the United States: the road ahead. Cancer Epidemiol Biomarkers Prev 2003;12:81–83.

39. Lesko LJ, Atkinson AJ, Jr. Use of biomarkers and surrogate endpoints in drug development and regulatory decision making: criteria, validation, strategies. Annu Rev Pharmacol Toxicol 2001;41:347–366.

CONTENTS

CONTRIBUTORS

STEINAR AAMDAL, MD, PhD • *Department of Clinical Cancer Research, Norwegian Radium Hospital, Oslo, Norway*

JAMES L. ABBRUZZESE, MD • *Gastrointestinal Medical Oncology, University of Texas MD Anderson Cancer Center, Houston, TX*

BULENT AKDUMAN, MD • *Department of Urology, Zonguldak Karaelmas University School of Medicine, Zonguldak, Turkey*

DAVID S. ALBERTS, MD • *Arizona Cancer Center, University of Arizona, Tucson, AZ*

JORGE ALBORES-SAAVEDRA, MD • *Department of Pathology, Louisiana State University Health Sciences Center, New Orleans, LA*

RONALD D. ALVAREZ, MD • *Division of Gynecologic Oncology; Gene Therapy Center; Comprehensive Cancer Center, University of Alabama at Birmingham, Birmingham, AL*

JAN P. A. BAAK, MD, PhD, FRCPath, FIAC(HON), DRHC(ANTWERP) • *Department of Pathology, Central Hospital in Rogaland, Stavanger, Norway; Yader Institute, University of Bergen, Bergen, Norway; Free University, Amsterdam, The Netherlands*

HOWARD BAILEY, MD • *University of Wisconsin Comprehensive Cancer Center and Medical Oncology Section, Department of Medicine, University of Wisconsin Medical School, Madison, WI*

MONICA M. BERTAGNOLLI, MD • *Brigham and Women's Hospital, Dana Farber-Harvard Cancer Center, Boston, MA*

KRISHNA BHAT, PhD • *Department of Molecular and Cellular Oncology, University of Texas MD Anderson Cancer Center, Houston, TX*

MICHAEL J. BIRRER, MD, PhD • *Cell and Cancer Biology Branch, National Cancer Institute, National Institutes of Health, Bethesda, MD*

G. TIM BOWDEN, PhD • *Arizona Cancer Center, University of Arizona, Tucson, AZ*

CURT BURGER, MD, PhD • *Erasmus University Medical Center, Rotterdam, The Netherlands*

PAUL P. CARBONE, MD (DECEASED) • *University of Wisconsin Comprehensive Cancer Center and Medical Oncology Section, Department of Medicine, University of Wisconsin Medical School, Madison, WI*

CHARLES A. COLTMAN JR., MD • *Division of Urology, The Southwest Oncology Group and the San Antonio Cancer Institute, University of Texas Health Science Center at San Antonio, San Antonio, TX*

E. DAVID CRAWFORD, MD • *Section of Urological Oncology, University of Colorado School of Medicine, Denver, CO*

MURIEL CUENDET, PhD • *Department of Medicinal Chemistry and Pharmacognosy, College of Pharmacy, University of Illinois at Chicago, Chicago, IL*

SANFORD M. DAWSEY, MD • *Cancer Prevention Studies Branch, Center for Cancer Research, National Cancer Institute, National Institutes of Health, Bethesda, MD*

SONIA DE ASSIS • *Lombardi Cancer Center, Georgetown University Medical Center, Washington, DC*

ANDREA DECENSI, MD • *Division of Chemoprevention, European Institute of Oncology, Milan, Italy*

LUIGI M. DE LUCA, PhD • *Differentiation Control Section, Laboratory of Cellular Carcinogenesis and Tumor Promotion, National Cancer Institute, National Institutes of Health, Bethesda, MD*

KATHLEEN A. DONOVAN, PhD • *Division of Hematology and Internal Medicine, Mayo Clinic, Rochester, MN*

JANINE G. EINSPAHR, MS • *Arizona Cancer Center, University of Arizona, Tucson, AZ*

ABELARDO ERREJON, MD • *Section of Urological Oncology, University of Colorado School of Medicine, Denver, CO*

CAROL J. FABIAN, MD • *Department of Internal Medicine, University of Kansas Medical Center, Kansas City, KS*

BENT FIANE, MD • *Central Hospital in Rogaland, Stavanger, Norway*

MITCHELL H. GAIL, MD, PhD • *Division of Cancer Epidemiology and Genetics, National Cancer Institute, National Institutes of Health, Bethesda, MD*

GINGER J. GARDNER, MD • *Kelly Gynecologic Oncology Section, The Johns Hopkins Hospital, Baltimore, MD*

JOELL GILLS, PhD • *Cancer Therapeutics Branch, National Cancer Institute, National Institutes of Health, Bethesda, MD*

GREGORY J. GORES, MD • *Division of Gastroenterology and Hepatology, Mayo Clinic College of Medicine, Rochester, MN*

PAUL E. GOSS, MD, PhD, FRCPC, FRCP(UK) • *Princess Margaret Hospital, University Health Network, Toronto, Canada*

JEFFREY GREEN, MD • *Laboratory of Cell Regulation and Carcinogenesis, National Cancer Institutes, National Institutes of Health, Bethesda, MD*

WILLIAM E. GRIZZLE, MD, PhD • *Department of Pathology, University of Alabama at Birmingham, Birmingham, AL*

H. BARTON GROSSMAN, MD • *Department of Urology, University of Texas MD Anderson Cancer Center, Houston, TX*

CLINTON J. GRUBBS, PhD • *Chemoprevention Center; Department of Surgery, University of Alabama Medical School, Birmingham, AL*

SIMONIDA GRUBJESIC, PhD • *Department of Biomedical Engineering, Northwestern University, Evanston, IL*

MARY HAMIELEC, BA • *University of Wisconsin Comprehensive Cancer Center, University of Wisconsin Medical School, Madison, WI*

STANLEY R. HAMILTON, MD • *Division of Pathology and Laboratory Medicine, University of Texas MD Anderson Cancer Center, Houston, TX*

ZIAD HASSOUN, MD • *Centre de Recherche du CHUM, Hôpital Saint Luc, Montreal, Canada*

ERNEST T. HAWK, MD, MPH • *Gastrointestinal and Other Cancers Research Group, Division of Cancer Prevention, National Cancer Institute, National Institutes of Health, Bethesda, MD*

TOVE HELLIESEN, MD • *Department of Pathology, Central Hospital in Rogaland, Stavanger, Norway*

DONALD EARL HENSON, MD • *Department of Pathology, Office of Cancer Prevention and Control, George Washington University Cancer Institute, Washington, DC*

HOWARD HIGLEY, PhD, DABT • *CCS Associates, Mountain View, CA*

WAUN KI HONG, MD • *Division of Cancer Medicine, Department of Thoracic/Head and Neck Medical Oncology, University of Texas MD Anderson Cancer Center, Houston, TX*

BRIAN C. JACOBSON, MD, MPH • *Center for Digestive Disorders, Boston Medical Center, Boston, MA*

FAYE M. JOHNSON, MD, PhD • *Department of Thoracic/Head and Neck Medical Oncology, University of Texas MD Anderson Cancer Center, Houston, TX*

GARY J. KELLOFF, MD • *Biomedical Imaging Program, Division of Cancer Treatment and Diagnosis, National Cancer Institute, National Institutes of Health, Bethesda, MD*

PETER J. KENEMANS, MD, PhD • *VU Medical Center, Amsterdam, The Netherlands*

FADLO R. KHURI, MD • *Winship Cancer Institute, Emory University School of Medicine, Atlanta, GA*

EDWARD S. KIM, MD • *Department of Thoracic/Head and Neck Medical Oncology, University of Texas MD Anderson Cancer Center, Houston, TX*

BRUCE F. KIMLER, PhD • *Department of Radiation Oncology, University of Kansas Medical Center, Kansas City, KS*

A. DOUGLAS KINGHORN, PhD, DSc • *Division of Medicinal Chemistry and Pharmacognosy, College of Pharmacy, The Ohio State University, Columbus, OH*

KJELL-HENNING KJELLEVOLD, MD • *Department of Pathology, Central Hospital in Rogaland, Stavanger, Norway*

JEROME W. KOSMEDER II, PhD • *Ventana Medical Systems Inc., Tucson, AZ*

SERGIO A. LAMPRECHT, PhD • *Strang Cancer Research Laboratory at The Rockefeller University, New York, NY*

DANIEL D. LANTVIT • *Department of Medicinal Chemistry and Pharmacognosy, College of Pharmacy, University of Illinois at Chicago, Chicago, IL*

SANG KOOK LEE, PhD • *College of Pharmacy, Ewha Womans University, Seoul, Korea*

BERNARD LEVIN, MD • *Division of Cancer Prevention, University of Texas MD Anderson Cancer Center, Houston, TX*

PAUL J. LIMBURG, MD, MPH • *Division of Gastroenterology and Hepatology, Mayo Clinic College of Medicine, Rochester, MN*

LANCE A. LIOTTA, MD, PhD • *FDA-NCI Clinical Proteomics Program, Laboratory of Pathology, Center for Cancer Research, National Cancer Institute, National Institutes of Health, Bethesda, MD*

MARTIN LIPKIN, MD • *Strang Cancer Research Laboratory at The Rockefeller University, New York, NY*

SCOTT M. LIPPMAN, MD • *Department of Clinical Cancer Prevention, The University of Texas MD Anderson Cancer Center, Houston, TX*

KJELL LØVSLETT, MD • *Department of Gynecology, Central Hospital in Rogaland, Stavanger, Norway*

DOUGLAS R. LOWY, MD • *Laboratory of Cellular Oncology, Center for Cancer Research, National Cancer Institute, National Institutes of Health, Bethesda, MD*

RONALD A. LUBET, PhD • *Chemopreventive Agent Development Research Group, Division of Cancer Prevention, National Cancer Institute, National Institutes of Health, Bethesda, MD*

JOHN A. LUST, MD, PhD • *Hematology Research; Tumor Biology Program, Mayo Clinic College of Medicine, Rochester, MN*

ANGELO M. DE MARZO, MD, PhD • *Departments of Oncology, Pathology, and Urology, The Johns Hopkins University School of Medicine, Baltimore, MD*

SHAHLA MASOOD, MD • *Department of Pathology, University of Florida Health Science Center at Shands Jacksonville, Jacksonville, FL*

EUGENIA MATA-GREENWOOD, PhD • *Division of Pediatric Research, Northwestern University, Evanston, IL*

MATTHEW S. MAYO, PhD • *Kansas Masonic Cancer Research Institute and Department of Preventive Medicine and Public Health, University of Kansas Medical Center, Kansas City, KS*

DAVID J. MCCONKEY, PhD • *Department of Cancer Biology, University of Texas MD Anderson Cancer Center, Houston, TX*

M. CRAIG MILLER • *Quakertown, PA*

RICHARD C. MOON, PhD • *School of Pharmacy, Purdue University, West Lafayette, IN*

JAMES L. MULSHINE, MD • *Intervention Section, Cell and Cancer Biology Branch, Center for Cancer Research, National Cancer Institute, National Institutes of Health, Bethesda, MD*

GEORGE L. MUTTER, MD • *Brigham and Women's Hospital, Harvard Medical School, Boston, MA*

WILLIAM G. NELSON, MD, PhD • *Departments of Oncology, Pathology, and Urology, The Johns Hopkins University School of Medicine, Baltimore, MD*

JOYCE O'SHAUGHNESSY, MD • *Breast Cancer Research, Baylor Charles A. Sammons Cancer Center, Dallas, TX*

AMIT OZA, MD • *Ontario Cancer Institute, Princess Margaret Hospital, Toronto, Canada*

EUN-JUNG PARK, PhD • *Developmental Therapeutics Program, Tumor Hypoxia Laboratory, SAIC-Frederick Inc., National Cancer Institute at Frederick, Frederick, MD*

HYE-SUNG PARK • *Department of Medicinal Chemistry and Pharmacognosy, College of Pharmacy, University of Illinois at Chicago, Chicago, IL*

ALAN W. PARTIN, MD, PhD • *Department of Urology, Brady Urological Institute, The Johns Hopkins University School of Medicine, Baltimore, MD*

CHARLES M. PEROU, PhD • *Lineberger Comprehensive Cancer Center, Departments of Genetics and of Pathology, University of North Carolina at Chapel Hill, Chapel Hill, NC*

EMANUEL F. PETRICOIN III, PhD • *FDA-NCI Clinical Proteomics Program, Division of Therapeutic Proteins, Center for Biologic Evaluation and Research, Food and Drug Administration, Washington, DC*

JOHN M. PEZZUTO, PhD • *School of Pharmacy, Purdue University, West Lafayette, IN*

JAMES RANGER-MOORE • *Arizona Cancer Center, University of Arizona, Tucson, AZ*

CHANDRAJIT P. RAUT, MD • *Department of Surgical Oncology, University of Texas MD Anderson Cancer Center, Houston, TX*

BRIAN J. REID, MD, PhD • *Divisions of Human Biology and Public Health Sciences, Fred Hutchinson Cancer Research Center, University of Washington, Seattle, WA*

ALBRECHT REITH, MD, PhD, MIAC • *Department of Pathology, Norwegian Radium Hospital, Oslo, Norway*

ELLEN RICHMOND, MS, RN • *Gastrointestinal and Other Cancers Research Group, Division of Cancer Prevention, National Cancer Institute, National Institutes of Health, Bethesda, MD*

GREGORY J. RIGGINS, MD, PhD • *Department of Neurosurgery, Johns Hopkins University School of Medicine, Baltimore, MD*

ANITA L. SABICHI, MD • *Department of Clinical Cancer Prevention, University of Texas MD Anderson Cancer Center, Houston, TX*

JOHN T. SCHILLER, PhD • *Laboratory of Cellular Oncology, Center for Cancer Research, National Cancer Institute, National Institutes of Health, Bethesda, MD*

YU SHEN, PhD • *Department of Biostatistics, University of Texas MD Anderson Cancer Center, Houston, TX*

PETER G. SHIELDS, MD • *Lombardi Cancer Center, Georgetown University Medical Center, Washington, DC*

KAREN SIELAFF, BSN • *University of Wisconsin Comprehensive Cancer Center, University of Wisconsin Medical School, Madison, WI*

CAROLINE C. SIGMAN, PhD • *CCS Associates, Mountain View, CA*

RICHARD SIMON, DSc • *Biometric Research Branch, Division of Cancer Treatment and Diagnosis, National Cancer Institute, National Institutes of Health, Bethesda, MD*

VERNON E. STEELE, PhD, MPH • *Chemopreventive Agent Development Research Group, Division of Cancer Prevention, National Cancer Institute, National Institutes of Health, Bethesda, MD*

ANITA STEINBAKK • *Department of Gynecology, Central Hospital in Ragoland, Stavanger, Norway*

KATHRIN STRASSER-WEIPPL, MD • *First Medical Department with Medical Oncology, Wilhelminen Hospital, Vienna, Austria*

M. SUZANNE STRATTON, PhD • *Arizona Cancer Center, University of Arizona, Tucson, AZ*

STEVEN P. STRATTON, PhD • *Arizona Cancer Center, University of Arizona, Tucson, AZ*

ROBERT L. STRAUSBERG, PhD • *Vice President for Research, The Institute for Genomic Research, Rockville, MD*

ASLE SUDBØ, MSc, PhD • *Department of Physics, Norwegian University of Science and Technology, Trondheim, Norway*

JON SUDBØ, DDS, MD, PhD • *Departments of Medical Oncology and Radiotherapy, Norwegian Radium Hospital, Oslo, Norway*

LULY TADDELE, MD • *Department of Pathology, Central Hospital in Rogaland, Stavanger, Norway*

YINGMEEI TAN, PhD • *Department of Medicinal Chemistry and Pharmacognosy, College of Pharmacy, University of Illinois at Chicago, Chicago, IL*

PHILIP R. TAYLOR, MD, ScD • *Cancer Prevention Studies Branch, Center for Cancer Research, National Cancer Institute, National Institutes of Health, Bethesda, MD*

IAN M. THOMPSON, MD • *Division of Urology, The Southwest Oncology Group and the San Antonio Cancer Institute, University of Texas Health Science Center at San Antonio, San Antonio, TX*

MELISSA A. TROESTER, PhD • *Department of Pathology and Laboratory Medicine, University of North Carolina at Chapel Hill, Chapel Hill, NC*

ASAD UMAR, PhD, DVM • *Gastrointestinal and Other Cancers Research Group, Division of Cancer Prevention, National Cancer Institute, National Institutes of Health, Bethesda, MD*

GISKE URSIN, MD, PhD • *Department of Preventive Medicine, University of Southern California Keck School of Medicine, Los Angeles, Los Angeles, CA; Department of Nutrition, University of Oslo, Oslo, Norway*

JACQUES VAN DAM, MD, PhD • *Division of Gastroenterology and Hepatology, Stanford University Medical Center, Stanford, CA*

BIANCA VAN DIERMEN, MA • *Department of Pathology, Central Hospital in Rogaland, Stavanger, Norway*

PAUL J. VAN DIEST, MD, PhD • *University Medical Center, Utrecht, The Netherlands*

ROBERT W. VELTRI, PhD • *Brady Urological Institute, Department of Urology, The Johns Hopkins University School of Medicine, Baltimore, MD*

RENEE VERHEIJEN, MD, PhD • *Department of Gynecology, VU Medical Center, Amsterdam, The Netherlands*

JAYE L. VINER, MD, MPH • *Gastrointestinal and Other Cancers Research Group, Division of Cancer Prevention, National Cancer Institute, National Institutes of Health, Bethesda, MD*

HEIDI L. WEISS, PhD • *Breast Center, Baylor University, Houston, TX*

MING YOU, MD, PhD • *The Siteman Cancer Center; Division of General Surgery, Washington University School of Medicine, St. Louis, MO*

RONG YU, PhD • *Medical School, The University of Texas Health Science Center at Houston, Houston, TX*

KRISTIN K. ZORN, MD • *Department of Cell and Cancer Biology, Center for Cancer Research, National Cancer Institute, National Institutes of Health, Bethesda, MD*

COLOR PLATES

VALUE-ADDED eBOOK/PDA

This book is accompanied by a value-added CD-ROM that contains an eBook version of the volume you have just purchased. This eBook can be viewed on your computer, and you can synchronize it to your PDA for viewing on your handheld device. The eBook enables you to view this volume on only one computer and PDA. Once the eBook is installed on your computer, you cannot download, install, or e-mail it to another computer; it resides solely with the computer to which it is installed. The license provided is for only one computer. The eBook can only be read using Adobe® Reader® 6.0 software, which is available free from Adobe Systems Incorporated at www.Adobe.com. You may also view the eBook on your PDA using the Adobe® PDA Reader® software that is also available free from Adobe.com.

You must follow a simple procedure when you install the eBook/PDA that will require you to connect to the Humana Press website in order to receive your license. Please read and follow the instructions below:

1. Download and install Adobe® Reader® 6.0 software
   You can obtain a free copy of the Adobe® Reader® 6.0 software at www.adobe.com
   Note: If you already have the Adobe® Reader® 6.0 software installed, you do not need to reinstall it.
2. Launch Adobe® Reader® 6.0 software
3. Install eBook: Insert your eBook CD into your CD-ROM drive
   PC: Click on the "Start" button, then click on "Run"
   At the prompt, type "d:\ebookinstall.pdf" and click "OK"
   Note: If your CD-ROM drive letter is something other than d: change the above command accordingly.
   MAC: Double click on the "eBook CD" that you will see mounted on your desktop.
   Double click "ebookinstall.pdf"
4. Adobe® Reader® 6.0 software will open and you will receive the message
   "This document is protected by Adobe DRM" Click "OK"
   Note: If you have not already activated the Adobe® Reader® 6.0 software, you will be prompted to do so. Simply follow the directions to activate and continue installation.

Your web browser will open and you will be taken to the Humana Press eBook registration page. Follow the instructions on that page to complete installation. You will need the serial number located on the sticker sealing the envelope containing the CD-ROM.

If you require assistance during the installation, or you would like more information regarding your eBook and PDA installation, please refer to the eBookManual.pdf located on your CD. If you need further assistance, contact Humana Press eBook Support by e-mail at ebooksupport@humanapr.com or by phone at 973-256-1699.

*Adobe and Reader are either registered trademarks or trademarks of Adobe Systems Incorporated in the United States and/or other countries.

I CHEMOPREVENTIVE AGENT DEVELOPMENT SCIENCE

1 Characterization of Natural Product Chemopreventive Agents

John M. Pezzuto, PhD, Jerome W. Kosmeder II, PhD, Eun-Jung Park, PhD, Sang Kook Lee, PhD, Muriel Cuendet, PhD, Joell Gills, PhD, Krishna Bhat, PhD, Simonida Grubjesic, PhD, Hye-Sung Park, Eugenia Mata-Greenwood, PhD, YingMeei Tan, PhD, Rong Yu, PhD, Daniel D. Lantvit, and A. Douglas Kinghorn, PhD, DSc

CONTENTS

1. INTRODUCTION

Cancer is a complicated group of diseases characterized by the uncontrolled growth and spread of abnormal cells *(1)*. In 2002, 1,284,900 new cases of cancer were estimated to be diagnosed in the United States (US), and about 555,500 persons were expected to die of cancer, i.e., more than 1500 every day *(2)*. Despite small decreases in overall cancer incidence and mortality rates in the US since the early 1990s, the total number of recorded cancer deaths continues to increase due to an aging and expanding population *(2)*. Furthermore, deaths from certain carcinomas of the lung and bronchus, breast, prostate, and colon and rectum remain high, and 5-yr survival rates for many cancer patients are still very low: for cancers of the brain, 32%; esophagus, 14%; liver, 6%; lung and bronchus, 15%; pancreas, 4%; stomach, 22%; and multiple myeloma, 29% *(2)*. Obviously, cancer remains a formidable public health problem.

A "war on cancer" was proclaimed about 30 yr ago. There was great hope and anticipation of reducing mortality rates for common forms of cancer by half by the year 2000 *(3–6)*. Although this stated goal of the US National Cancer Institute (NCI), National Institutes of Health (NIH), has not been attained, much progress has been made, and basic research has further elucidated mechanisms whereby normal cells and tissues become malignant *(5)*.

From: Cancer Chemoprevention, Volume 2: Strategies for Cancer Chemoprevention
Edited by: G. J. Kelloff, E. T. Hawk, and C. C. Sigman © Humana Press Inc., Totowa, NJ

Cancer is considered the end stage of a chronic disease process characterized by abnormal cell and tissue differentiation *(6)*. This process of carcinogenesis eventually leads to the final outcome of invasive and metastatic cancer. Recent advances in defining cellular and molecular levels of carcinogenesis, along with a growing body of experimental, epidemiological, and clinical trial data, have led to the development of cancer chemoprevention, a relatively new strategy in preventing cancer *(7–10)*. Cancer chemoprevention is defined as the use of synthetic or natural agents to inhibit, retard, or reverse the process of carcinogenesis *(7–11)*.

Invasive cancer derives from complex interactions of exogenous (environmental) and/or endogenous (e.g., genetic, hormonal, and immunological) factors *(5,12,13)*. Carcinogenesis is progressive, and this progression in precancer is characterized by the appearance of specific molecular and more general genotypic damage associated with increasingly severe dysplastic phenotypes *(11)*. The development of this phenomenon may be represented by three stages that often overlap: initiation, promotion, and progression phases *(10)*. Initiation, an irreversible event, begins when normal cells are exposed to a carcinogen and their genomic DNA undergoes damage that remains unrepaired or misrepaired *(10)*. Promotion, an expansion of the damaged cells, leads to the appearance of benign tumors. Progression, an irreversible process, produces a new clone of tumor cells with increased proliferative capacity, invasiveness, and metastatic potential *(10)*. Transitions between successive stages are believed to be enhanced or suppressed by various factors *(5)*.

Most human cancers seem to be potentially preventable because of controllable or removable causative exogenous factors, such as cigarette smoking, dietary factors, environmental and occupational chemicals, lifestyle and socioeconomic factors, radiation, and specific microorganisms *(5,13)*. These exogenous factors offer the most likely opportunities for interventions targeted to primary prevention—that is, elimination of or avoiding exposure to these environmental factors *(10)*. In addition, however, as a serious and practical approach to the control of cancer, cancer chemoprevention can play an integral role in the overall strategy geared toward reducing the incidence of cancer *(3,6,8,14)*.

Cancer chemopreventive agents, based on their individual underlying mechanisms of action, may be classified into three categories: inhibitors of carcinogen formation, blocking (antiinitiation) agents, and suppressing (antiproliferation/antiprogression) agents *(8,10,15–17)*. Many inhibitors of carcinogen formation, such as ascorbic acid *(18)*, phenols (caffeic acid and ferulic acid) *(19)*, sulfhydryl compounds (*N*-acetyl-L-cysteine) *(20)*, and amino acids (proline and thioproline) *(21)*, act to prevent formation of nitrosamines from secondary amines and nitrite in an acidic environment *(16)*.

Chemoprevention strategies address four goals: inhibition of carcinogens, logical intervention for persons at genetic risk, treatment of precancerous lesions, and translation of leads from dietary epidemiology to intervention strategies *(22)*. Rational and successful implementation of chemopreventive strategies relies intrinsically on tests for efficacy and mechanistic assays, as well as availability of promising chemopreventive agents, reliable intermediate biomarkers, and appropriate clinical cohorts to discover safe and effective drugs for primary and secondary prevention of human cancers *(23)*. Established in the early 1980s, the NCI's Chemoprevention Program has since evaluated more than 1000 potential chemopreventive agents or agent combinations, including more than 40 compounds in about 100 clinical trials *(24)*. Included among a number of plant-derived natural products in this group of potential cancer chemopreventive agents are *S*-allyl-L-cysteine, curcumin, epigallocatechin gallate, genistein, lycopene, perillyl alcohol, and a mixture of soy isoflavones, all of dietary origin *(24)*. This program generally begins by identifying candidate agents through in vitro bioassay screening, epidemiology, and other scientific efforts *(13,15)*. Once potential leads have been identified, mechanistic evaluations through additional in vitro and ex vivo assays are important to assess efficacy, and for planning further tests in animal models to design regimens for clinical testing and use *(17,25,26)*. Agents judged to have potential as human cancer chemopreventive agents are subjected to preclinical toxicology and pharmacokinetic studies *(27)*, followed by Phase I clinical safety and pharmacokinetic trials *(28)*. The most successful agents subsequently progress to clinical chemoprevention trials *(23,26)*.

A competitive cancer chemoprevention program titled "Natural Inhibitors of Carcinogenesis" (P01 CA48112) has been supported since 1991 by NCI. The overall theme, and botanical, biological, chemical, biostatistical, and administrative aspects of this program have been summarized previously *(29–33)*. Currently, we provide an update and additional representatives of diverse classes of plant secondary metabolites associated with biological activity in preliminary in vitro assays, with some of these having been subjected to evaluation in a mouse mammary organ culture model *(34,35)* used as a secondary discriminator to prioritize our leads. Several of these compounds have either significant structural interest or exhibit considerable promise for further development as cancer chemopreventive agents through evaluation in full-term inhibition studies with laboratory animals. Below is a brief outline of our current *modus operandi* in this research program.

Using the resources of the University of Illinois Field Station, the herbarium of the Field Museum of Natural History, Chicago, as well as field collection and commercial sources, sufficient quantities and numbers of plant materials have been procured for investigation in our research program on natural inhibitors of carcinogenesis. Priority in plant material selection, based in part on information contained in the NAPRALERT computer database *(36)*, has been accorded to edible plants, as well as species with reported biological activity relating to cancer chemoprevention, plants with no history of toxicity, and finally plants that had previously been poorly investigated from a phytochemical perspective. A small amount (300 g–1 kg) of each dried plant sample is collected for preliminary investigation.

Crude nonpolar and polar extracts, prepared from each plant obtained, are evaluated for their potential chemopreventive activity using a battery of about 10 short-term in vitro bioassays *(30,32,33)*. Based on the results of these bioassays, selected extracts are further evaluated in an ex vivo mouse mammary organ culture model, as mentioned above. In this assay, test materials are evaluated for their ability to inhibit 7,12-dimethylbenz(*a*)anthracene (DMBA)-induced preneoplastic lesions *(34,35)*. A battery of in vitro bioassays has been developed to monitor inhibition of tumorigenesis at the various stages. For initiation, antimutagenic activity *(37,38)*, antioxidant activity *(38,39)*, and induction of NAD(P)H:quinone reductase (QR) activity *(40,41)* are assayed. For promotion, inhibition of activities such as phorbol ester-induced ornithine decarboxylase (ODC) activity *(42,43)*, cyclooxygenase activity *(44–46)*, phorbol dibutyrate receptor binding *(47)*, and transformation of JB6 mouse epidermal cells *(48)* are assayed. For progression, induction of human leukemia cell differentiation *(49,50)*, inhibition of aromatase activity *(51)*, antiestrogenic and estrogenic effects *(52,53)*, and inhibition of estrone sulfatase activity *(54)* are assayed. Additional examples of leads with significant activities in several of these initial in vitro test systems will be provided later in this review.

In the next stage, plant extracts showing potency and/or selectivity in the in vitro bioassay models are selected for bioassay-guided fractionation to uncover their active principles. Active initial extracts are subjected to solvent partitioning, and chromatography (gravity-, flash-) over standard chromatographic materials, with final purification typically effected by semipreparative high-performance liquid chromatography (HPLC). Active isolates in the aforementioned bioassays are characterized by the usual physical, spectral, and chromatographic measurements, and every effort is made to obtain unambiguous nuclear magnetic resonance (NMR) assignments for each compound of interest through the use of combinations of conventional one- and two-dimensional NMR methods. We have increasingly used Mosher ester methodology to determine absolute stereochemistry of secondary alcohols (e.g., *41,55*), and recently a simplified method has been developed in our laboratory to prepare Mosher esters directly in NMR tubes, thus obviating the need to purify these derivatives chromatographically *(56)*. In addition, we have capability to perform small-molecule X-ray crystallography (e.g., *56,57*), and some success has been achieved with the use of a liquid chromatography-mass spectroscopy (LC-MS) dereplication method, which has, for example, been applied to the analysis of various antioxidants *(39)* and flavonoids *(58)*.

Pure active compounds are then evaluated in all the in vitro bioassays, and selected compounds are further processed for evaluation in the mouse mammary organ culture (MMOC) model *(34,35)*. On rare occasions, a compound may be rated as active in this ex vivo system even though no significant preliminary in vitro activity is observed *(59)*. Finally, the in vivo cancer chemopreventive activity of highly promising pure plant constituents is evaluated in animal full-term tumorigenesis models, including the two-stage mouse skin model using DMBA as an initiator and 12-*O*-tetradecanoylphorbol-13-acetate (TPA) as a promoter, and the rat mammary carcinogenesis model with *N*-methyl-*N*-nitrosourea (MNU) or DMBA as a carcinogen *(60,61)*. Additional in vivo models are used as required.

2. PHASE 2 ENZYME INDUCTION

Carcinogenesis is a complex and protracted multistage process, yet the entire course can be initiated by a single event wherein a cellular macromolecule is damaged by an endogenous or exogenous agent. Strategies for protecting cells from these initiating events include decreasing metabolic enzymes responsible for generating reactive species (phase 1 enzymes) while increasing phase 2 enzymes that can deactivate radicals and electrophiles known to intercede in normal cellular processes. Important defenses against electrophile toxicity are provided in the family of phase 2 enzymes, such as glutathione (GSH) *S*-transferases (GSTs) and UDP-glucuronosyltransferases, which catalyze GSH-electrophile or glucuronyl-electrophile conjugates, respectively. Reduction of electrophilic quinones by NAD(P)H:quinone reductase (QR) is another important detoxification pathway, which converts quinones to hydroquinones and reduces oxidative cycling *(62)*. Although phase 1 induction and functionalization of xenobiotics may be required for complete detoxification by the action of phase 2 enzymes, phase 1 enzyme elevation may also be considered a potential cancer risk factor for activation of procarcinogens to reactive species *(63)*. Therefore, an agent that induces phase 2 enzymes selectively would theoretically appear to be a better protector than selective induction of both phase 1 and 2 enzymes. Monofunctional induction of phase 2 enzymes appears to be caused by disrupting the cytoplasmic complex between the actin-bound protein Keap1 and the transcription factor Nrf2, thereby releasing Nrf2 to migrate to the nucleus where it activates the antioxidant response element (ARE) of phase 2 genes and accelerates transcription *(64)*. Alternately, a compound may induce phase 2 enzymes bifunctionally through activation of the aryl hydrocarbon (Ah) receptor-xenobiotic response element (XRE) pathway *(65)*.

QR elevation with in vitro and in vivo systems has been shown to correlate with induction of other protective phase 2 enzymes and provides a reasonable biomarker for the potential chemoprotective effect of test agents against cancer initiation *(66)*. The murine hepatoma cell line Hepa 1c1c7 contains easily measurable inducible QR that provides a reliable, high-throughput system for detecting inducers of phase 2 enzymes *(67)*. This assay can also be used to determine if an agent induces phase 2 enzymes only (monofunctional) or both phase 1 and 2 enzymes (bifunctional). This is accomplished by comparing the induction capability of a compound in wild-type Hepa 1c1c7 cells with that observed in two mutant cell lines designated TAOc1 and BP^{r}c1, which are defective in a functional Ah receptor or unable to translocate the receptor-ligand complex to the nucleus, respectively *(68)*. Compounds that have similar inducing ability in the wild-type and mutant Hepa lines are considered monofunctional inducers. Activity is expressed by the concentration to double (CD) or quadruple (CQ) QR activity over basal

levels, and toxicity is expressed as the concentration to kill 50% (IC$_{50}$) of the cells. A chemoprotective index (CI = IC$_{50}$/CD) can be expressed to provide a measure of the in vitro therapeutic index of a particular drug candidate.

A variety of natural inducers of phase 2 enzymes have been described, including a number of flavonoids, indoles, isothiocyanates, and dithiolthiones *(69,70)*. Our program has identified a number of natural and synthetic monofunctional and bifunctional inducers of phase 2 enzymes (Table 1, Fig. 1). We have employed a series of methods to further investigate induction patterns and protein and RNA expression, using Western and Northern blotting techniques, RT-PCR, and transient and stable transfection of cells with ARE and XRE reporter genes.

Extracts of an edible fruit from *Physalis philadelphica* Lam. (Solanaceae), commonly called the tomatillo, induced QR equally well in the wild-type Hepa 1c1c7 and mutant cell lines. Tomatillo, used in a variety of Latin American foods, such as enchiladas and salsa verde, are also included in North American sauces and relishes. The active principles were determined to be from a steroidal class of compounds designated withanolides *(71)*. Three withanolides were shown to have potent activity in QR induction, including two known compounds, withaphysacarpin (**1** in Fig. 1) and 24,25-dihydrowithanolide D (**2**, CD = 0.70 μ*M*), as well as a novel substance, 2,3-dihydro-3-methoxywithaphysacarpin (**3**, CD = 7.8 μ*M*) *(72)*. Subsequent analysis of an additional 37 withanolides isolated from a variety of species from Solanaceae revealed 16 withanolides with CD values below 1 μ*M* *(73)*. Of those 16 withanolides, only six exhibited a CI above 10: withaphysalin G (**4**, CD = 0.51 μ*M*), withaphysalin H (**5**, CD = 0.52 μ*M*), withaphysalin J (**6**, CD = 0.39 μ*M*), jaborosalactone P (**7**, CD = 0.75 μ*M*), jaborosalactone 1 (**8**, CD = 0.28 μ*M*), and trechonolide A (**9**, CD = 0.27 μ*M*). Large-scale isolation of selected withanolides from *P. philadelphica* has provided sufficient amounts to begin preliminary animal testing.

The whole flowering and fruiting parts of the medicinal plant *Tephrosia purpurea* were shown to have several moderate to strongly QR active compounds *(41,74)*. Isolation of 7,4′-dihydroxy-3′,5′-dimethoxy-isoflavone (**10**), (+)-tephropurpurin (**11**), (+)-purpurin (**12**), pongamol (**13**), lanceolatin B (**14**), (−)-maackiain (**15**), (−)-3-hydroxy-4-methoxy-8,9-methylenedioxypterocarpan (**16**), and (−)-medicarpin (**17**) were the result of activity-guided fractionation with QR. The chalcone (+)-tephropurpurin (CD = 0.15 μ*M*, IC$_{50}$ = 13.4 μ*M*, CI = 89) exhibited a QR value nearly three times higher

Table 1
Quinone Reductase Inducing Ability of Natural and Synthetic Compounds

	Compound	CD^a (μM)	IC_{50}^b (μM)	CI^c
1	withaphysacarpin	0.43	4.8	11
2	24,25-dihydrowithanolide D	0.70	5.5	8
3	2,3-dihydro-3-methoxywithaphysacarpin	7.8	46.9	6
4	withaphysalin G	0.51	9.8	19
5	withaphysalin H	0.52	5.2	10
6	withaphysalin J	0.39	11	28
7	jaborosalactone P	0.75	42.7	57
8	jaborosalactone 1	0.28	8.1	29
9	trechonolide A	0.27	7.7	29
10	7,4′-dihydroxy-3′,5′-dimethoxyisoflavone	17.2	63.7	4
11	(+)-tephropurpurin	0.15	13.4	89
12	(+)-purpurin	5.6	50.7	9
13	pongamol	6.1	18.7	3
14	lanceolatin B	22.9	76.3	3
15	(−)-maackiain	8.8	70.4	8
16	(−)-3-hydroxy-4-methoxy-8,9-methylenedioxypterocarpan	14.7	63.7	4
17	(−)-medicarpin	13.7	74	5
18	brassinin	4.0	ND	ND
19	cyclobrassinin	1.2	ND	ND
20	spirobrassinin	7.9	ND	ND
21	N-ethyl-2,3-dihydrobrassinin	0.13	ND	ND
22	S-selenomethylbrassinin	0.5	ND	ND
23	sulforamate	0.26	34.9	134
24	oxomate	0.96	67	70
25	4′-iodoflavone	0.01	>165	>17,000
26	4′-bromoflavone	0.01	>165	>17,000
27	4′-chloroflavone	0.02	>78	>5000
28	4′-trifluoromethylflavone	0.03	90	3000
29	2′-hydroxy-2-methoxychalcone	0.31	17	55
30	2′-hydroxy-2,6-dimethoxychalcone	0.53	14	26
31	2′-hydroxy-2-methylchalcone	0.67	36	54
32	2′-hydroxy-2-nitrochalcone	0.30	11	37
	sulforaphane^d	0.23	9.9	42

^{a} Concentration to double QR activity in Hepa 1c1c7 cells.

^{b} Concentration to inhibit Hepa 1c1c7 cell growth by 50%.

^{c} Chemoprevention Index (IC_{50}/CD).

^{d} QR assay positive control.

than sulforaphane (CD = 0.23 μM, IC_{50} = 9.9 μM, CI = 42), but with similar toxicity.

Cruciferous vegetables (such as Brussels sprouts, cauliflower, and Chinese cabbage) provided the indole dithiocarbamate brassinin (**18**) and several natural and synthetic analogs, which were shown to induce QR and GST activities with in vitro and in vivo models (75,76). Of 27 brassinin derivatives tested, cyclobrassinin (**19**,

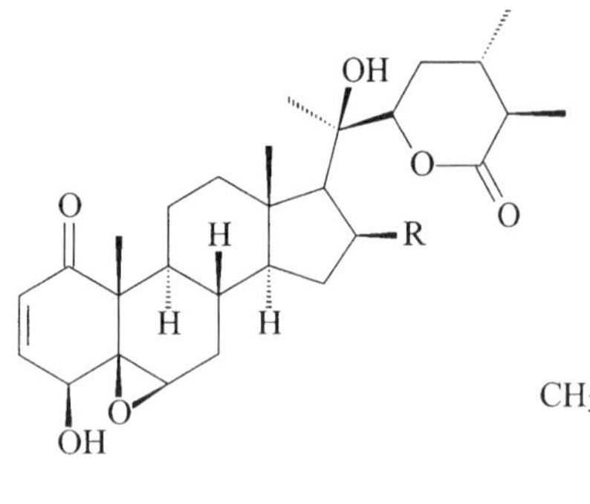

1: R=OH
2: R=H

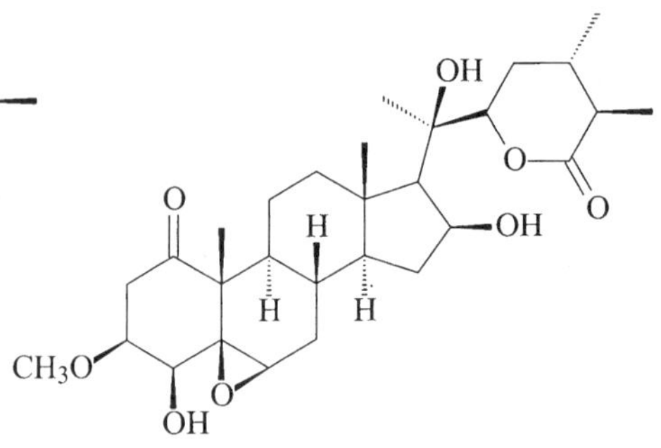

3

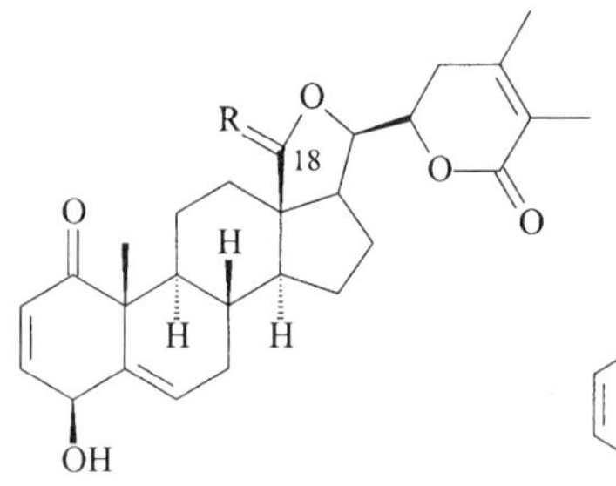

4: R=H, OH (18R/S)
5: R=H, OCH₃ (18R)
6: R=O

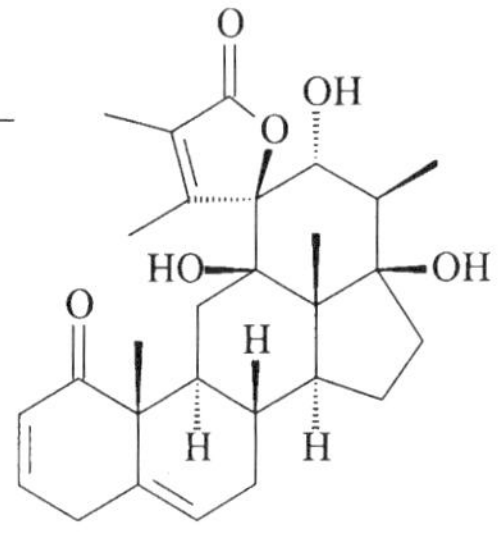

7

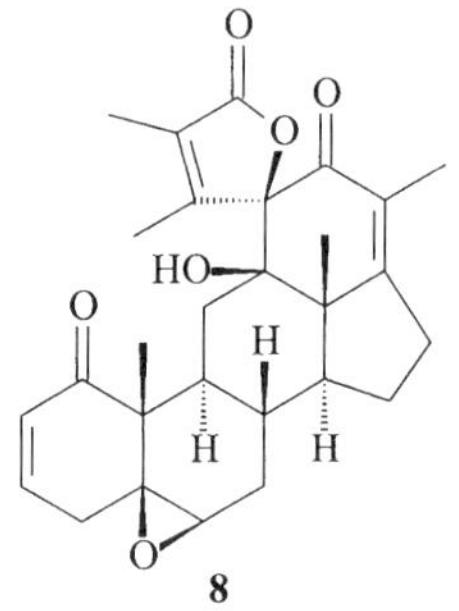

8

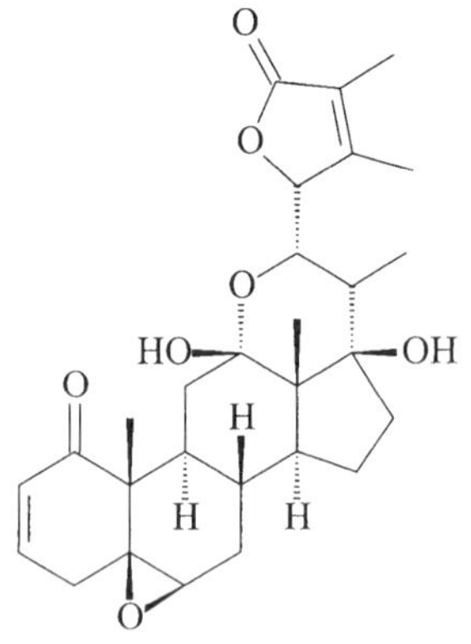

9

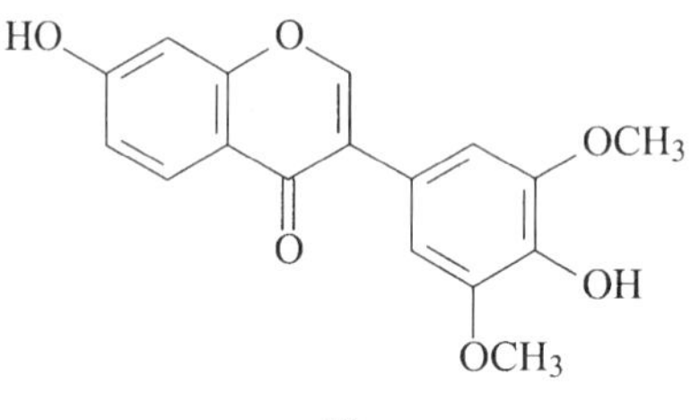

10

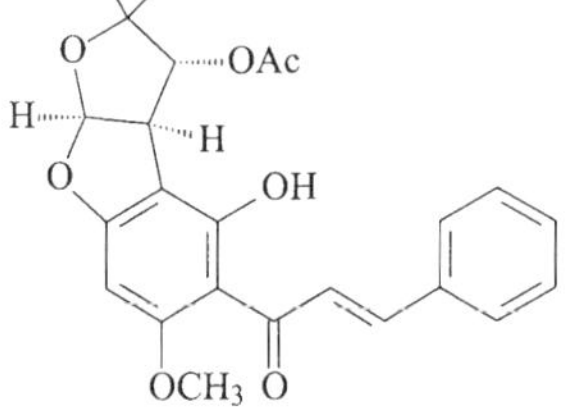

11

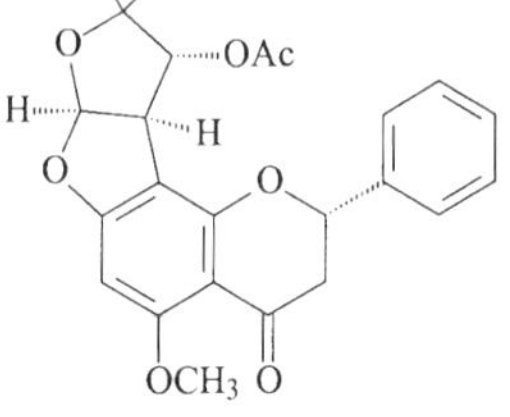

12

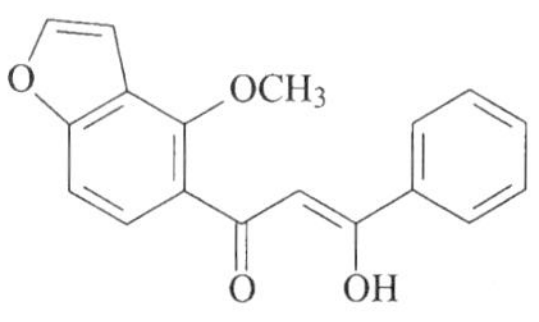

13

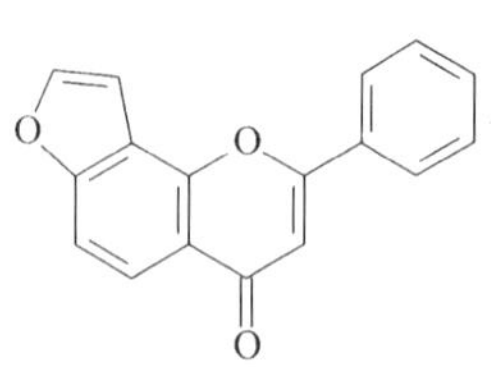

14

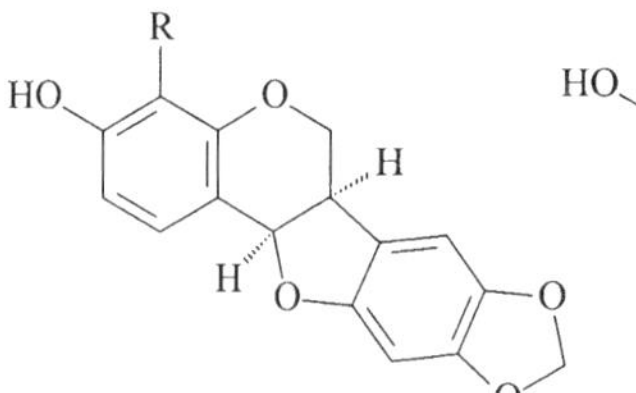

15: R=H
16: R=OCH₃

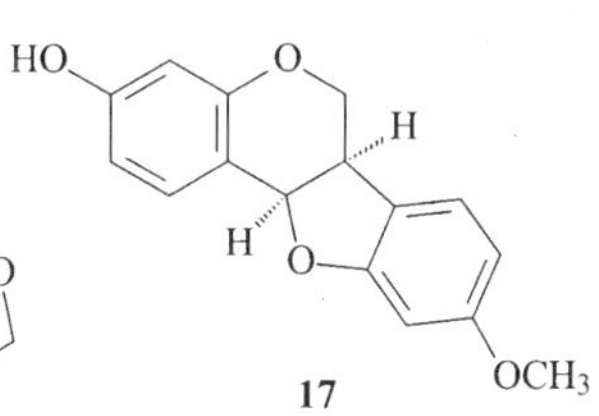

17

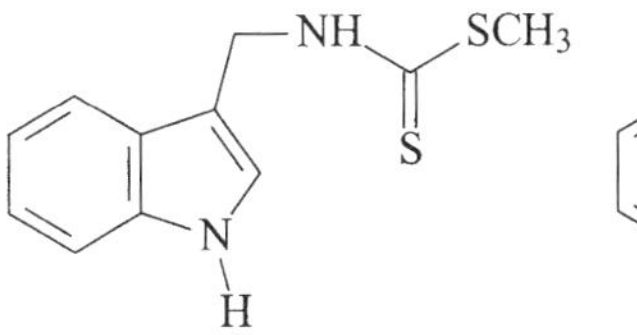

18

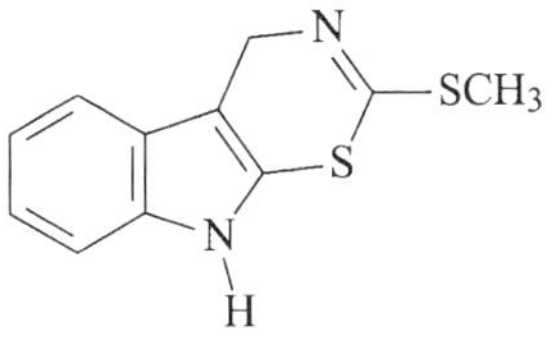

19

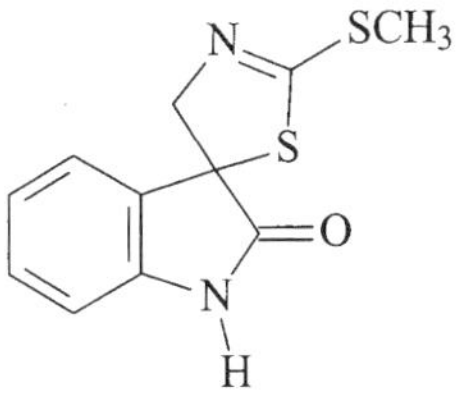

20

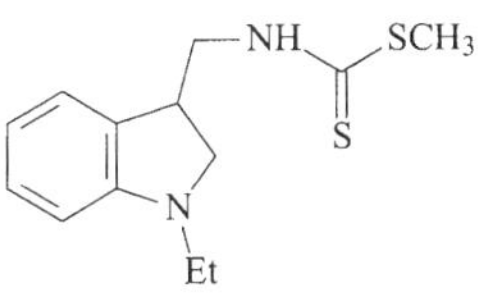

21

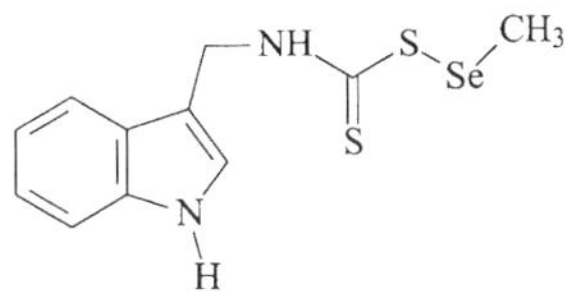

22

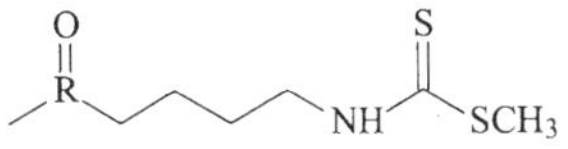

23: R=S
24: R=C

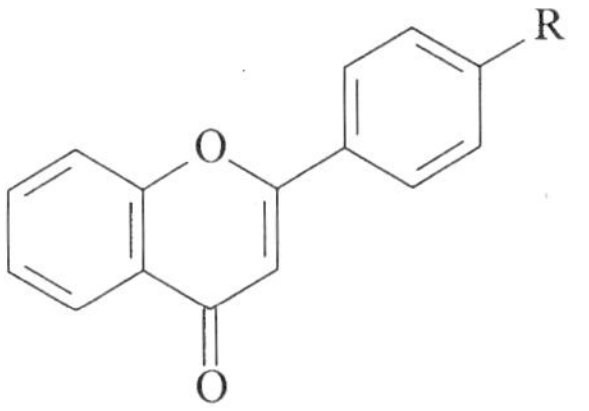

25: R=I
26: R=Br
27: R=Cl
28: R=CF_3

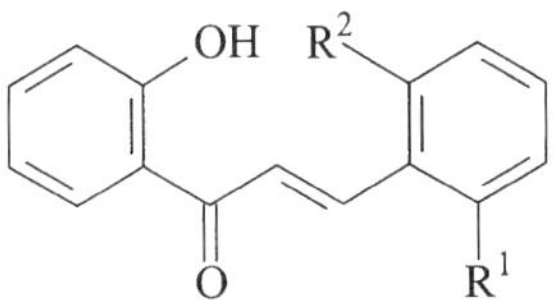

29: R^1=OCH_3, R^2=H
30: R^1=OCH_3, R^2=OCH_3
31: R^1=CH_3, R^2=H
32: R^1=NO_2, R^2=H

Fig. 1. Active leads identified through utilization of the quinone reductase assay.

CD = 1.2 μ*M*), spirobrassinin (**20**, CD = 7.9 μ*M*), *N*-ethyl-2,3-dihydrobrassinin (**21**, CD = 0.13 μ*M*), and *S*-selenomethylbrassinin (**22**, CD = 0.5 μ*M*), were most active. Brassinin and derivatives were not active QR inducers in the mutant cell lines; therefore, the indole class of compounds are likely to be bifunctional in nature.

Sulforaphane, an isothiocyanate isolated from broccoli, has potent monofunctional phase 2 enzyme-inducing activity *(77)*. A novel analog, sulforamate (**23**), was designed using the predicted methyl dithiocarbamate product of myrosinase-induced decomposition of the sulforaphane glucosinolate precursor glucoraphanin *(78)*. Sulforamate exhibited similar potency to sulforaphane (CD = 0.26 vs 0.23 μ*M*), but three times less toxicity (IC_{50} = 34.9 vs 9.9 μ*M*). Sulforamate also increased GSH levels twofold in Hepa 1c1c7 and H4IIE rat hepatoma cells and was shown to interact with the ARE of QR and GST Ya without involvement of XRE. However, difficulty in synthesizing either sulforaphane or sulforamate has precluded their development. Therefore, a more synthetically accessible analog was devised. Oxomate (**24**) is a keto-analog to sulforamate and is substantially easier to produce in multikilogram quantities. Oxomate (CD = 0.96 μ*M*) has weaker QR activity compared to sulforaphane and sulforamate in vitro, but toxicity is also substantially reduced (IC_{50} = 67 μ*M*). Oxomate, sulforamate, and sulforaphane have shown similar dose-response patterns for inhibiting DMBA-induced lesions in MMOC, and significant inhibition of DMBA-induced mammary carcinogenesis in Sprague-Dawley rats has been demonstrated *(79)*. Additionally, oxomate significantly reduced tumor multiplicity in DMBA-induced female Sprague-Dawley rats fed at 3% in the diet.

Many flavonoids from a variety of plants have shown moderate QR-inducing capability; however, a systematic analysis of structural characteristics responsible for this activity has not been undertaken. A variety of B-ring substituted 2′-hydroxychalcones and their related flavanones and flavones were examined for QR-inducing activity in cultured Hepa 1c1c7 cells; more than 10 compounds exhibited CD values less than 1 μ*M* with CI values more than 50. The most potent compounds

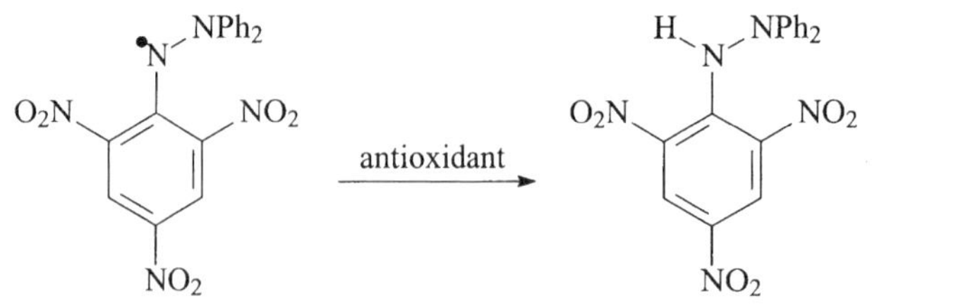

Fig. 2. Antioxidant assay employing DPPH.

were *para*-substituted flavones (**25–28**), followed by several *ortho*-substituted chalcones (**29–32**). 4′-Bromoflavone (**26**, 4′BF) was selected for further development, as it showed potent inducing capability (CD = 10 nM) without toxicity in Hepa 1c1c7 or H4IIE cells (IC$_{50}$ >100 μM) to give a CI above 10,000. Additionally, a simple synthesis of 4′BF was devised that allowed cost-effective scale-up of multikilograms of high-purity material. 4′BF was shown to reduce mammary tumor incidence from 89.5 to 30 and 20% in the 2 and 4 g 4′BF/kg diet groups of DMBA-induced female Sprague-Dawley rats, and reduced tumor multiplicity from 2.63 to 0.65 and 0.20, respectively (*40*).

Use of the QR assay has consistently provided excellent leads, many of which have shown good activity in animal carcinogenesis models and are being considered for preclinical toxicology.

3. ANTIOXIDANTS

Free radicals, species with one or more unpaired electrons, are produced in normal or pathological cell metabolism by ionizing radiation or through transition metal-mediated molecular interactions. In biological systems, reactive oxygen species (ROS) formed by free radical processes are involved in both initiation and promotion of carcinogenesis (*80*). Hydroxyl radicals, superoxide anions, and hydrogen peroxide are associated with initiation of carcinogenesis by causing heritable DNA damage through mutation of DNA or alteration of DNA repair enzymes (*81*). Oxygen radicals and related species may also be involved in tumor promotion by signaling expression of protooncogenes and other growth factors (*82*).

As biological systems have co-evolved with aerobic metabolism to counteract damage from ROS, a strategy of enhancing endogenous antioxidant defense systems with dietary or pharmaceutical agents is a reasonable approach (*83,84*). Several assay systems have been developed to discover potentially active compounds from synthetic and natural sources (*39*). It is important to note that a potential antioxidant lead must be evaluated in more than one antioxidant assay due to variability in the different test systems (*85*).

One assay system is based on the ability of a potential antioxidant to scavenge the stable radical of 1,1-diphenyl-2-picrylhydrazyl (DPPH), producing 1,1-diphenyl-2-picrylhydrazine (Fig. 2). The nitrogen radical of DPPH imparts a deep violet color at 517 nm in solution; this absorbance can be monitored to determine a sample's effectiveness in quenching free radicals. Although this assay has the advantage of high-throughput capability to quickly screen libraries of candidates for potential antioxidant activity, it is based on quenching a nitrogen radical and may yield a high number of false positives. Potential lead compounds from this assay should be confirmed with additional test systems, such as those described below.

A second assay system involves measuring superoxide anion inhibition in TPA-induced cultured HL-60 cells. HL-60 cells can be induced to differentiate with dimethylsulfoxide (DMSO) to give characteristics similar to neutrophils, and stimulation with TPA generates dose-dependent quantities of superoxide anion (*86,87*). Using cytochrome c as a monitor, the inhibitory effects of test samples can be determined.

A third antioxidant assay uses the xanthine/xanthine oxidase system, where superoxide anion scavenging capacity and inhibition of xanthine oxidase is measured by monitoring formation of uric acid at 295 nm (Fig. 3). Xanthine oxidase (XOD) is an enzyme that catalyzes hypoxanthine to xanthine and uric acid in the presence of molecular oxygen to yield superoxide anion. Inhibition of XOD or quenching of superoxide anion results in dose-dependent reduction of uric acid production.

Using the DPPH assay as a primary screen and validating potential leads with the HL-60/TPA and/or XOD

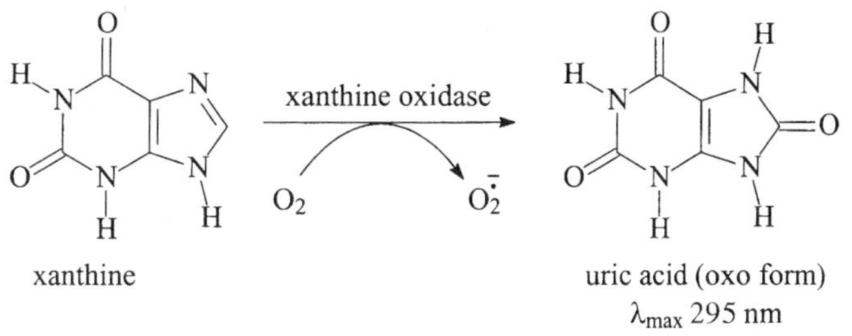

Fig. 3. Antioxidant assay employing xanthine.

systems, a variety of naturally occurring compounds were identified as potential antioxidants (summarized in Table 2). A variety of flavonoids from *Chorizanthe diffusa* Benth. (Polygonaceae) (**33–37**, Fig. 4) were shown to have moderate antioxidant activity in both DPPH and HL-60 antioxidant assays *(38,39).* An extract of *Mezoneuron cucullatum* Roxb. (Leguminosae) yielded two stilbenes, resveratrol (**38**) and piceatannol (**39**), that were active in the HL-60 antioxidant assay; the flavone apigenin (**40**) and chalcone isoliquiritigenin (**41**) exhibited potent activity in the XOD assay *(39).* Scirpusin A (**42**), also from *M. cucullatum*, showed only moderate activity in either of the DPPH and XOD assays. *Cerbera manghas* L. (Apocynaceae) produced olivil (**43**), (−)-carinol (**44**), and (+)-cycloolivil (**45**) as moderately active compounds in the DPPH assay *(53).* Two flavonol glucosides (**46,47**) from *Daphniphyllum calycinum* Benth. (Daphniphyllaceae) *(88),* and an epicatechin (**48**) from *Antirhea acutata* (DC.) Urb. (Rubiaceae) *(89),* were isolated using the DPPH assay, with **48** showing activity in the cytochrome c reduction assay as well. An ornamental shrub, "smoke tree" or *Continus coggygria* Scop. (Anacardiaceae), yielded gallic acid and gallic acid esters, the aurones sulfuretin (**49**) and sulfurein (**50**), and the biaurone disulfuretin (**51**). The Malaysian island shrub *Gyrinops walla* Gaertn. (Thymelaeaceae) yielded mangiferin (**52**) through bioassay-guided fractionation with the DPPH assay *(90).*

4. CYCLOOXYGENASE INHIBITION

The involvement of prostaglandins (PGs) and other eicosanoids in the development of human cancer has been known for more than two decades *(91).* Importantly, an increase in PG synthesis may influence tumor growth in human beings and experimental animals *(92);* numerous studies have illustrated the effect of PG synthesis on carcinogen metabolism, tumor cell proliferation, and metastatic potential *(93,94).* As a result, inhibition of PG synthesis has been examined as a means of preventing tumor development *(94,95).* Two major observations demonstrate the role of PGs in cancer genesis: inhibition of PG synthesis hinders tumor development in animal models and in some human cancers *(93),* and a direct relationship between the levels of PG synthesized and cancer incidence in both humans and animal models. Moreover, members of the arachidonic acid (AA) metabolizing enzyme family seem to play a significant role in carcinogenesis, since modulation of these pathways results in suppression of tumor growth *(96).*

PGs produced by cyclooxygenases (COXs) are represented by a large series of compounds that mainly enhance cancer development and progression, acting as carcinogens or tumor promoters with profound effects on carcinogenesis *(97).* Most malignant human tumors have a prolonged period of pathological development during which they pass through several preneoplastic and premalignant stages. This situation affords the opportunity of interrupting or reversing tumorigenesis at an early stage *(22,98).* Thus, the ability to regulate the COX pathway provides a reasonable opportunity for cancer chemoprevention.

Metabolites of AA, e.g., PGs, prostacyclins, and thromboxanes, are produced in many tissues and facilitate a diverse group of physiological and pathophysiological responses. For example, these bioactive lipids are potent mediators of several signal transduction pathways that modulate cellular adhesion, growth, and differentiation *(99).*

Cleaved from membrane phospholipids by phospholipases, AA can then be metabolized by the COX pathway to produce PGs (Fig. 5). COX, also known as PGH-synthase, is the rate-limiting enzyme in the metabolic conversion of AA to PGs and related eicosanoids. AA is converted to PGH_2 through the action of COX, which exhibits two distinct catalytic activities, cyclooxygenase and peroxidase *(100).* Subsequently, PGH_2 is converted by cell-specific synthases to products such as PGE_2, $PGF_{2\alpha}$, PGI_2, or thromboxanes *(101).*

Table 2
Antioxidant Activity of Plant Natural Products

Compound		DPPH[a] (µg/mL)	HL-60[b] (µg/mL)	XOD[c] (µg/mL)
33	quercetin	15.0	9.3	ND[d]
34	5,8,3′,4′-tetrahydroxy-3,7′-dimethoxyflavone	29.8	>50	ND[d]
35	5,7,3′,4′-tetrahydroxy-3-methoxyflavone	39.2	25.7	ND[d]
36	5,8,3′,4′,5′-pentahydroxy-3,7-dimethoxyflavone	10.4	21.6	ND[d]
37	3″-O-acetylquercitrin	12.0	18.4	ND[d]
38	resveratrol	94.6	6.2	59.1
39	piceatannol	68.4	3.4	10.9
40	apigenin	>200	>20	2.4
41	isoliquiritigenin	>200	>20	8.6
42	scirpusin A	78.0	>20	38.5
43	olivil	37.5	ND[d]	ND[d]
44	(−)-carinol	15.8	ND[d]	ND[d]
45	(+)-cycloolivil	27.5	ND[d]	ND[d]
46	5,6,7,4′-tetrahydroxyflavonol-3-O-rutinoside	43.2	ND[d]	ND[d]
47	kaempferol 3-O-neohesperidoside	79.6	ND[d]	ND[d]
48	8-[1-(3,4-dihydroxyphenyl)-3-methoxy-3-oxopropyl]epicatechin	29.1[e]	ND[d]	ND[d]
49	sulfuretin	18.7	ND[d]	ND[d]
50	sulfurein	16.1	ND[d]	ND[d]
51	disulfuretin	9.7	ND[d]	ND[d]
52	mangiferin	20.1	ND[d]	ND[d]
	gallic acid[f]	3.6	ND[d]	ND[d]

[a]ED$_{50}$ of DPPH (1,1-diphenyl-2-picrylhydrazyl) radical scavenging.

[b]IC$_{50}$ of TPA-induced free radical formation in cultured HL-60 cells.

[c]IC$_{50}$ of XOD (xanthine/xanthine oxidase) activity.

[d]Not determined.

[e]ED$_{50}$ in µM.

[f]Positive control standard.

Two COX isoforms, COX-1 and COX-2, are known. COX-1 is constitutively expressed in many tissues (101,102); PGs produced by COX-1 are thought to mediate housekeeping functions such as cytoprotection of the gastric mucosa, regulation of renal blood flow, and platelet aggregation (103–105). In contrast to COX-1, the isoform COX-2 is not generally detected in most tissues (106). However, COX-2 is an inducible enzyme expressed in response to pro-inflammatory agents, including cytokines, endotoxins, growth factors, tumor promoters, and mitogens (107). COX-2 is expressed in a few specialized tissues such as brain, testes, and macula densa of the kidney, in the apparent absence of any induction process.

Since COX plays an important role in cancer development, we have tested more than 2000 plant extracts for inhibition of COX-1 and COX-2. The assay is based on measurement of PGE$_2$ produced in the COX reaction via an enzyme immunoassay (Fig. 6). The effect of test compounds on COX activity is determined by measuring PGE$_2$ production. Reaction mixtures are prepared in 100 mM Tris-HCl buffer, pH 8.0, containing 1 µM heme, 500 µM phenol, 300 µM epinephrine, sufficient amounts of COX-1 or COX-2 to generate 150 ng of PGE$_2$/mL, and various concentrations of test samples. The reaction is initiated by adding AA (final concentration, 10 µM) and incubating for 10 min at room temperature (final volume, 200 µL). Reactions

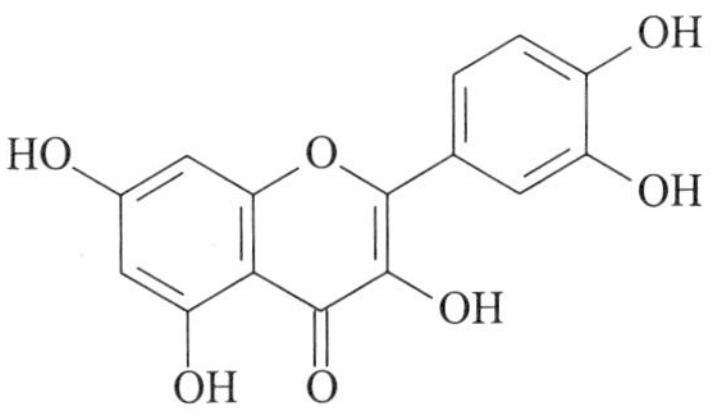

33

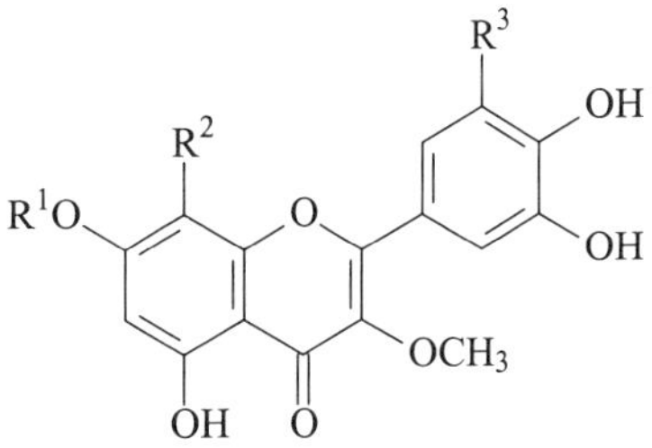

34: R¹= CH₃, R²= OH, R³=H
35: R¹= H, R²= H, R³=H
36: R¹= CH₃, R²= OH, R³=OH

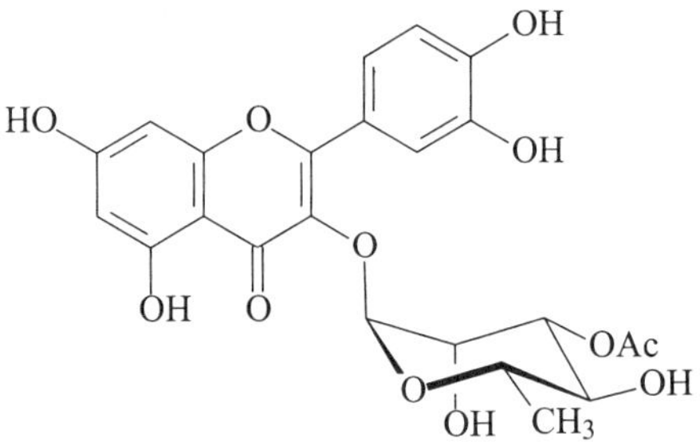

37

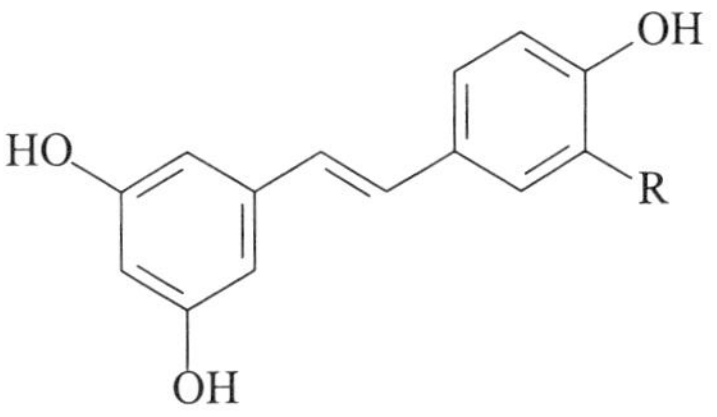

38: R= H
39: R= OH

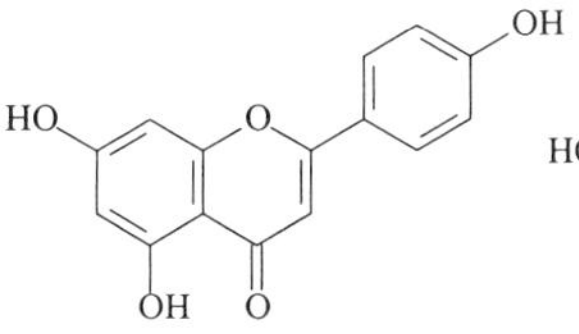

40

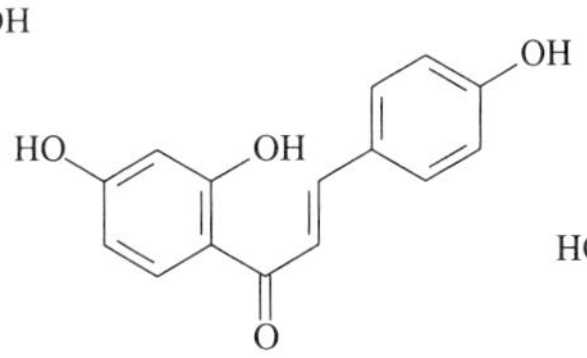

41

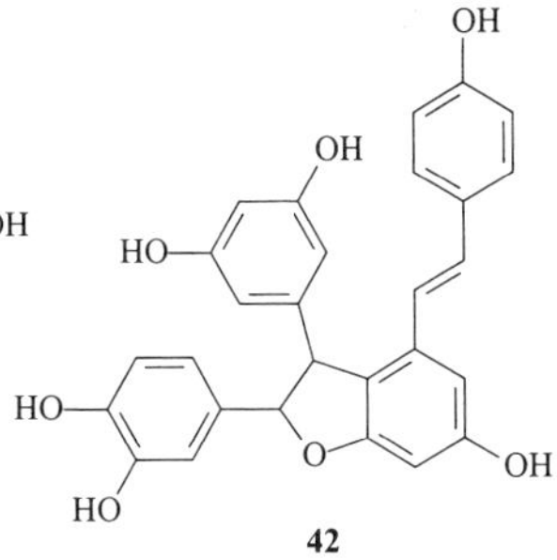

42

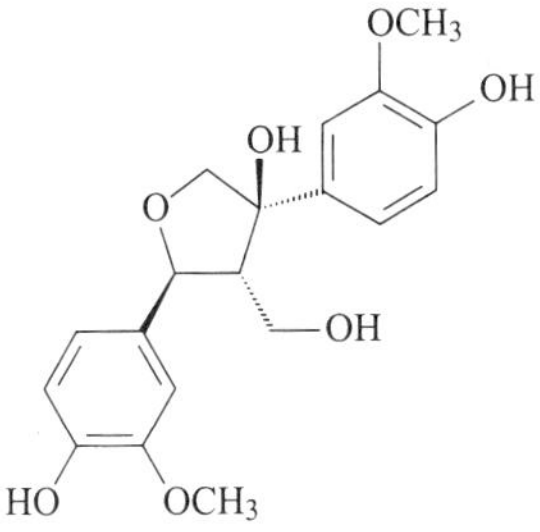

43

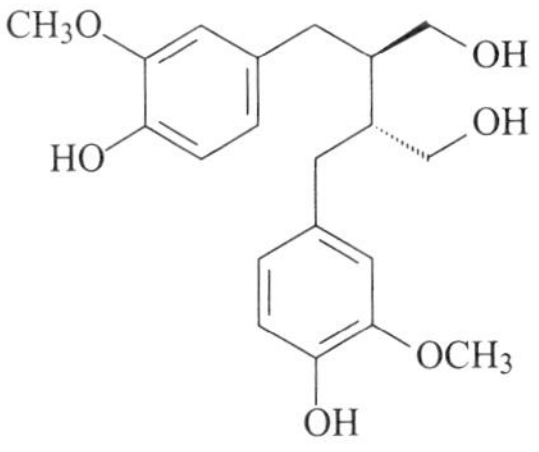

44

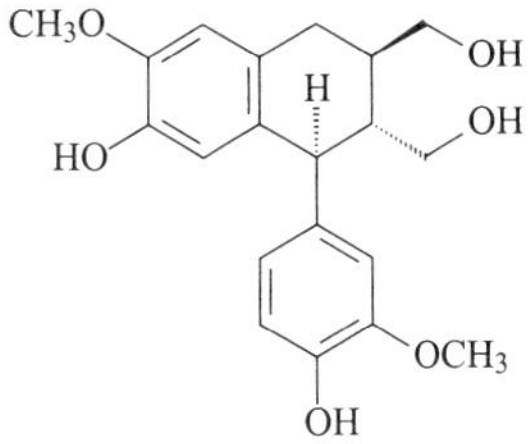

45

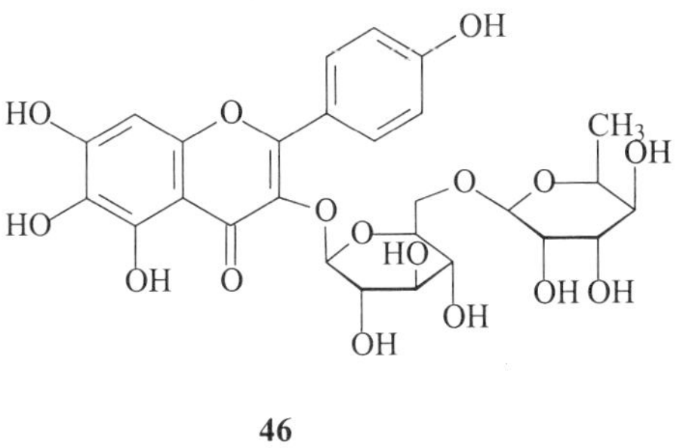

46

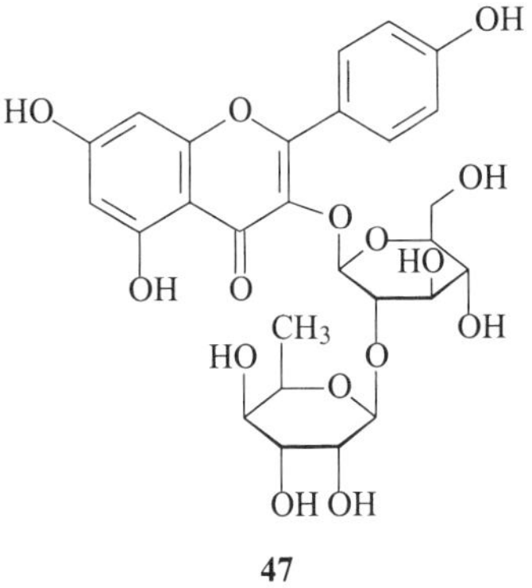

47

Fig. 4. Antioxidant lead compounds (*continued*).

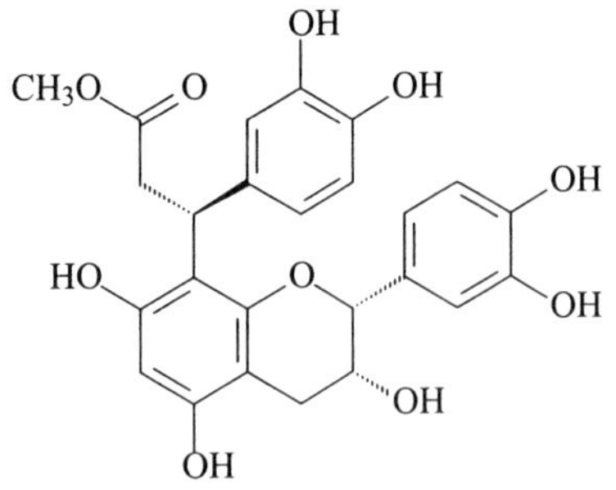

Fig. 4. (Cont.) Antioxidant lead compounds.

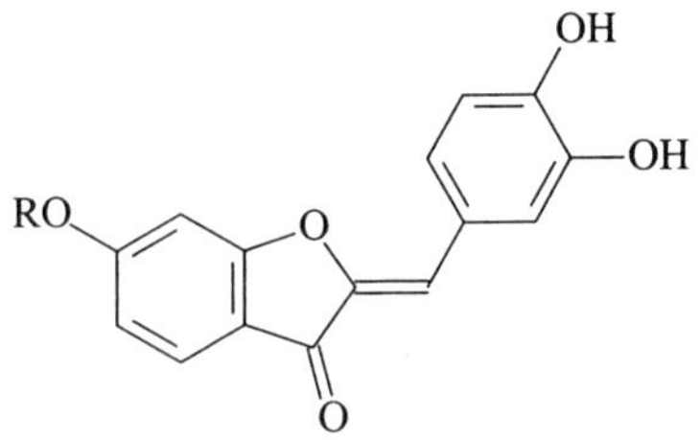

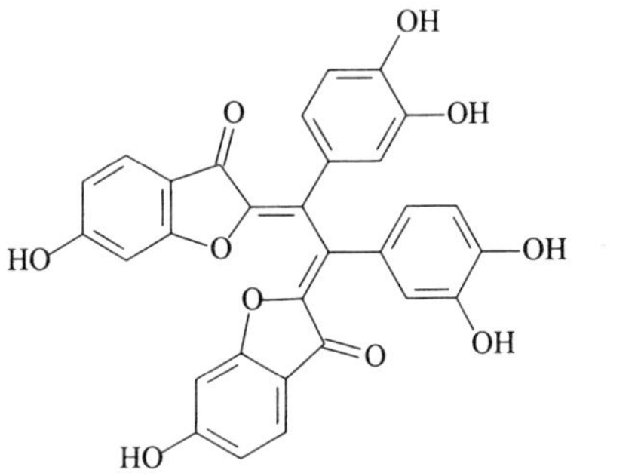

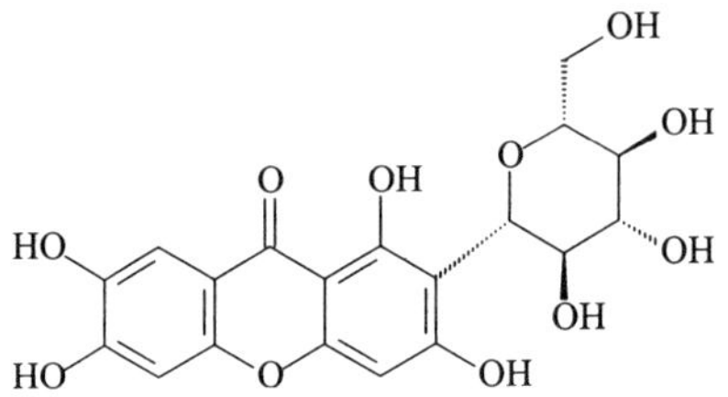

are terminated by adding 20 µL of the reaction mixture to 180 µL of 27.8 µM indomethacin, and PGE$_2$ is quantitated by an ELISA method. Samples are diluted to the desired concentration with 100 mM potassium phosphate buffer (pH 7.4) containing 2.34% NaCl, 0.1% bovine serum albumin, 0.01% sodium azide, and 0.9 mM Na$_4$EDTA. Following transfer to a 96-well plate (Nunc-Immuno Plate Maxisorp, Rochester, NY; Fisher, Itasca, IL) coated with a goat anti-mouse IgG (Jackson Immuno Research Laboratories, West Grove, PA), the tracer (PGE$_2$-acetylcholinesterase, Cayman Chemical, Ann Arbor, MI) and primary antibody (mouse anti-PGE$_2$, Monsanto, St. Louis, MO) are added. Plates are then incubated at room temperature overnight, reaction mixtures are removed, and wells are washed with a solution of 10 mM potassium phosphate buffer (pH 7.4) containing 0.01% sodium azide and 0.05% Tween-20. Ellman's reagent (200 µL) is added to each well and the plate is incubated at 37°C for 3–5 h, until the control wells yield an OD = 0.5–1.0 at 412 nm. A standard curve with PGE$_2$ (Cayman Chemical) is generated on the same plate, which is used to quantify the PGE$_2$ levels produced in the presence of test samples. Results are expressed as a percentage, relative to control (solvent-treated) samples, and dose-response curves are constructed to determine IC$_{50}$ values.

Approximately 80 of more than 2000 plant extracts inhibited COX-2 activity by more than 70% at a concentration of 10 µg/mL, whereas the same extracts showed weak or no activity against COX-1. Some of the active extracts were fractionated using the biological assay to guide the activity *(33,45,46,60,108–117)*, and some active compounds were isolated (Fig. 7). Results are summarized in Table 3.

Resveratrol (**38**) and a host of stilbenoids (**54–60**) were isolated from a variety of plant sources and assessed for COX inhibitory and chemopreventive activity *(45,46,60,108–115)*. Resveratrol is a phytoalexin generated in response to fungal infections or injury *(116)* and can be found in a variety of dietary sources, most notably grape skins, *Vitis vinifera* L. (Vitaceae) and red wine. The stilbenoids oxyresveratrol (**54**), pterostilbene (**55**), isorhapontigenin (**56**), prenylated resveratrol (**57**), prenylated oxyresveratrol (**58**), dihydroxyprenylated resveratrol (**59**), and aiphanol (**60**) were isolated from the seeds of a Peruvian plant, *Aiphanes aculeata* Willd. (Arecaceae), the bark of an Indonesian evergreen tree, *Artocarpus dadah* Miq. (Moraceae), or grape cell cultures of *V. vinifera* *(113–115)*. Most of the stilbenoids were selective for COX-1 inhibition, including the benzofurans moracin M (**61**) and prenylated moracin M (**62**) from *A. dadah*

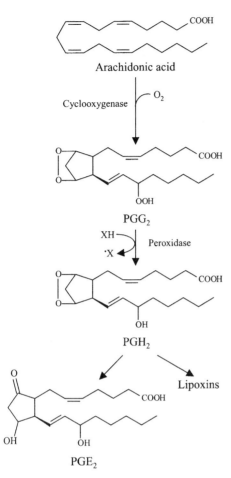

Fig. 5. Overview of the metabolism of eicosanoids. COX metabolites of AA include PGs, prostacyclin, and thromboxanes. COXs catalyze the sequential formation of PGG_2 and PGH_2. PGH_2 is enzymatically and nonenzymatically converted to various bioactive products, including $PGF_{2\alpha}$, PGE_2, and PGI_2 (prostacyclin). PGH_2 can also be metabolized to thromboxane A_2 and B_2.

(115). Two cycloartanes (**63,64**) from the previously uncharacterized Puerto Rican plant *Antirhea acutata* (DC.) Urb. (Rubiaceae) were shown to have moderately selective inhibitory activity against COX-2 *(89).* Work is ongoing with additional plant extracts.

The future discovery of natural or synthetic inhibitors of COX-2 from complex mixtures continues with the need for more rapid identification and isolation of active principles. One method that shows promise for accelerating the discovery process is use of ultrafiltration with LC/MS *(117).* In this assay, an active plant extract or combinatorial library can be incubated with human recombinant COX-2 enzyme in an ultrafiltration chamber. Inactive compounds are then washed off the protein, followed by denaturing the COX-2 and eluting any compounds onto LC/MS for identification by HRMS and tandem MS. Subsequent isolation of the active compounds using their LC profile can produce significant quantities of material for identification by standard analytical techniques (i.e., NMR) and confirmation of activity in the COX in vitro assay.

5. ORNITHINE DECARBOXYLASE INHIBITION

Polyamines, multivalent cations found largely in association with RNA and DNA, are essential for cell proliferation and differentiation. ODC, which catalyzes the first and rate-limiting step in the polyamine biosynthesis pathway *(118,119),* is a highly regulated enzyme that responds to growth-promoting stimuli. It is thought to play a role in the tumor-promotion stage of carcinogenesis, based on observing that ODC activity increases in response to tumor promoters *(120)* and finding that polyamine levels have increased in a variety of both human and rodent neoplastic tissues *(121).* Further, ODC has been shown to play a role in transformation *(122–124)* and to correlate with metastatic potential *(125,126).* α-Difluoromethylornithine (DFMO), an inhibitor of ODC, has been effective in essentially all animal models studied *(121)* and has recently been the subject of clinical trials for skin, Barrett's esophagus, colon, breast, prostate, and cervical cancer *(127).* For these reasons, we initiated a search for natural inhibitors of tumor promoter-stimulated ODC activity. To assess the inhibitory activity of plant extracts, we used TPA to induce ODC activity in ME308 mouse epidermal cells; enzyme activity was measured by quantifying CO_2 released from L-(1-^{14}C) ornithine *(128).* We tested more than 800 plant extracts and used bioassay-guided fractionation to obtain several compounds that inhibited ODC activity in vitro (Table 4, Fig. 8).

Rotenoids and flavonoids (**65–71**) from the African plant *Mundulea sericea* Willd. (Leguminosae) were shown to have potent activity by transcriptional regulation of ODC *(129,130).* Most potent were the rotenoids deguelin (**65**), tephrosin (**66**), (13*R*)-hydroxydeguelin (**67**), and (13*R*)-hydroxytephrosin (**68**); the isoflavones munetone (**69**) and mundulone (**70**); and mundulinol, a flavanol (**71**). Deguelin was further studied and found to be active in the two-stage mouse skin carcinogenesis and MNU rat mammary model tumor models *(42).* Mechanistic studies revealed that deguelin affects TPA-induced transcriptional increase of the ODC gene. Deguelin was also found to inhibit TPA-independent c-*myc*-induced ODC activity in BALB/c c-MycER cells. Rotenoids are known to affect mitochondrial oxidative phosphorylation. Therefore, deguelin and

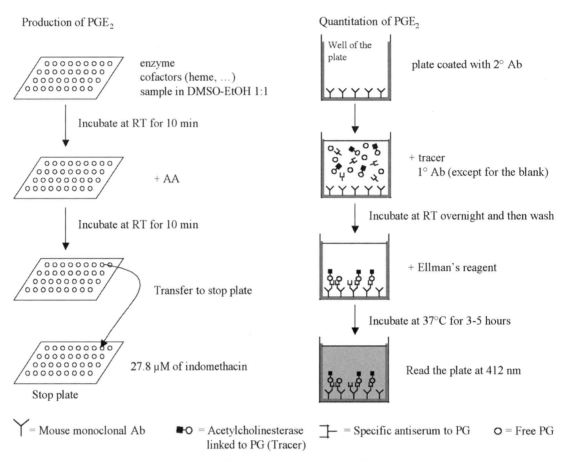

Production of PGE$_2$

enzyme
cofactors (heme, ...)
sample in DMSO-EtOH 1:1

Incubate at RT for 10 min

+ AA

Incubate at RT for 10 min

Transfer to stop plate

27.8 µM of indomethacin

Stop plate

Quantitation of PGE$_2$

Well of the plate

plate coated with 2° Ab

+ tracer
1° Ab (except for the blank)

Incubate at RT overnight and then wash

+ Ellman's reagent

Incubate at 37°C for 3-5 hours

Read the plate at 412 nm

Y = Mouse monoclonal Ab   ▪O = Acetylcholinesterase   ⌐ = Specific antiserum to PG   O = Free PG
                                linked to PG (Tracer)

Fig. 6. Determination of COX activity by measuring PGE$_2$ production.

tephrosin were tested and found to inhibit NADH dehydrogenase activity *(130)*. It is possible that a disturbance of cellular ATP may be the mechanism through which rotenoids influence tumor promoter-induced signaling mechanisms.

Thuja occidentalis L. (Cupressaceae), white cedar, yielded three pimarane diterpenes: (+)-7-oxo-13-*epi*-pimara-14,15-dien-18-oic acid (**72**), (+)-7-oxo-13-*epi*-pimara-8,15-dien-18-oic acid (**73**), and (+)-isopimaric acid (**74**); and three lignans: (1*S*,2*S*,3*R*)-(+)-isopicrodeoxypodophyllotoxin (**75**), (−)-deoxypodophyllotoxin (**76**), and (−)-deoxypodorhizone (**77**); all were shown to have strong inhibitory activity against TPA-induced ODC activity *(43)*. Flavonoids zapotin (**78**) and 5,6,2′-trimethoxyflavone (**79**) from the seeds of the edible fruit of *Casimiroa edulis* Llave et Lex. (Rutaceae) exhibited moderate activity *(131)*.

6. ANTIESTROGENIC AGENTS

Interest in estrogen analogs and antagonists has increased tremendously over the last decade. The

clinical usefulness of the antiestrogen tamoxifen to treat breast cancer and to provide possible chemopreventive effects in women at high risk of developing breast cancer has led to an extensive search for additional antiestrogens *(132,133)*. Also, recent concerns over environmental estrogens and their possible link to increased incidence of breast cancer *(134,135)* and male infertility *(136)* has led to studies concerning their molecular mechanisms of actions. In general, it is important to establish the estrogenic agonism or antagonism of these compounds of interest.

Historically, determination of estrogenic activity or inhibition has been ascertained by in vivo rodent studies, interactions with the isolated estrogen receptor (ER), or activation of reporter proteins in genetically altered cells. The Ishikawa cell line is a unique tool among these assays. The Ishikawa cell line is a stable human endometrial carcinoma displaying an estrogen-inducible alkaline phosphatase *(137–139)* that can be employed for rapid determination of both estrogen and antiestrogen activity. Chief advantages of the Ishikawa system over in vivo studies for screening activity, as with other

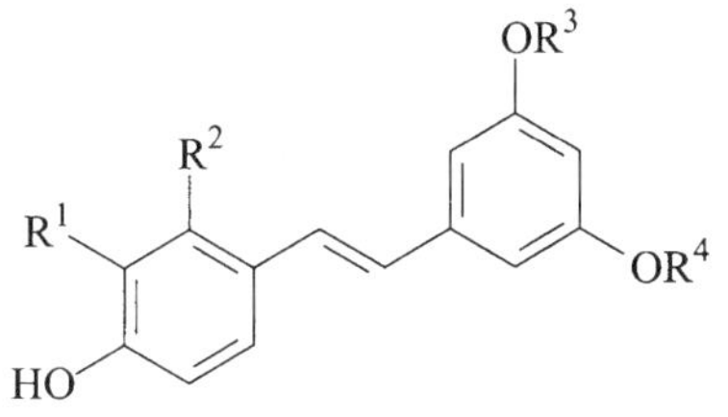

54: R^1=R^3=R^4= H, R^2= OH
55: R^1=R^2= H, R^3=R^4= CH$_3$
56: R^1= OCH$_3$, R^2=R^3=R^4= H

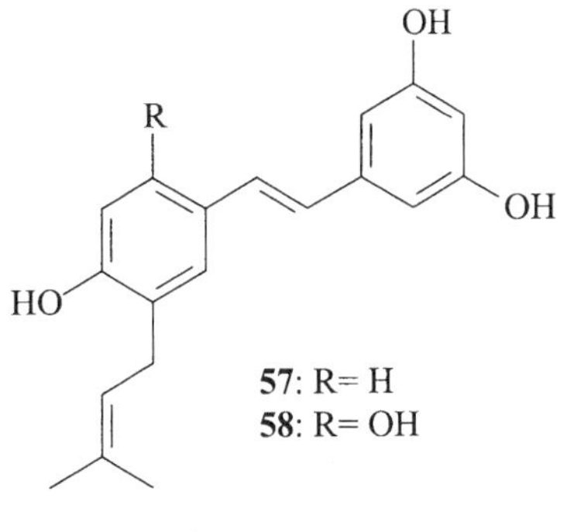

57: R= H
58: R= OH

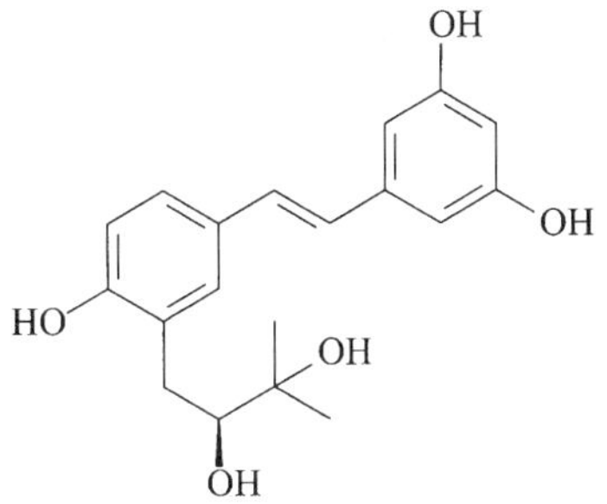

59

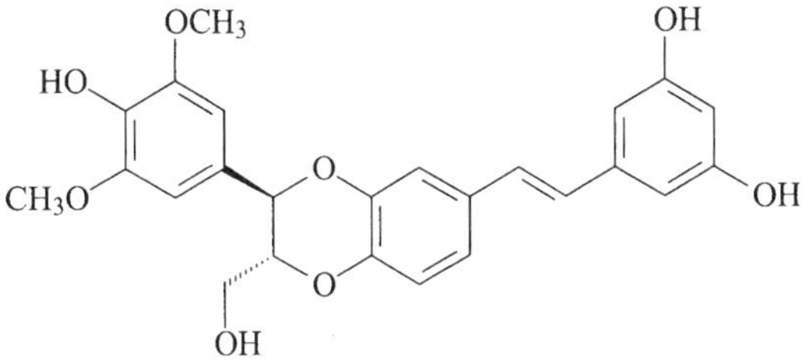

60

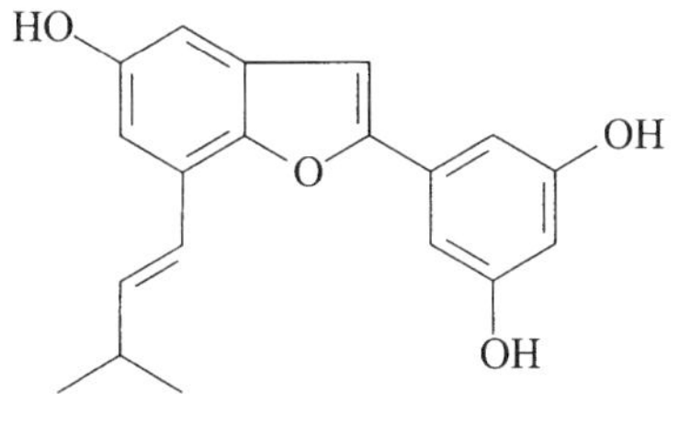

61

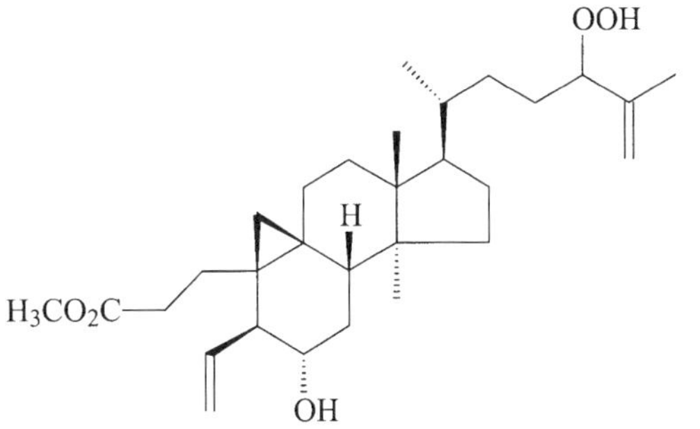

62

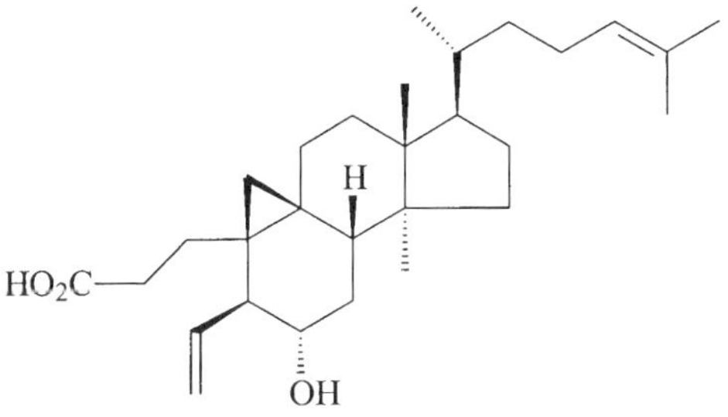

63

Fig. 7. Natural product inhibitors of cyclooxygenases 1 and 2.

in vitro assays, are reduced requirements in time, personnel, and money. Using isolated receptors has the advantage of rapidity, but resulting data do not indicate whether a compound that interacts with the receptor mimics or inhibits subsequent biological response. Genetically altered yeasts have been used as an integral component of several elegant studies, such as denoting estrogenic synergism of various pesticides that are individually innocuous *(140)*, but as a general assay system, Ishikawa has some distinctions that make it superior. The first involves the entire aspect of human genetics. Genetically altered yeasts possess a reporter gene that is ligated to a known estrogen-responsive element; this system fails to measure any interactions that compounds may have with other promoters or repressors of estrogen-sensitive gene activation. Second, the yeast system does

Table 3
Inhibitory Activity of Isolates Against COX-1 and -2

	Compound	COX-1 IC_{50} (μM)	COX-2 IC_{50} (μM)
38	resveratrol	1.1	1.3
54	oxyresveratrol	1.4	109.0
55	pterostilbene	19.8	83.9
56	isorhapontigenin	1.5	6.2
57	3-(γ,γ-dimethylallyl)resveratrol	0.61	9.5
58	5-(γ,γ-dimethylallyl)oxyresveratrol	4.1	36.7
59	3-(2,3-dihydroxy-3-methylbutyl)resveratrol	0.48	13.9
60	aiphanol	1.9	9.9
61	moracin M	0.5	22.3
62	3-(γ,γ-dimethylpropenyl) moracin M	4.9	31.8
63	(6S)-hydroxy-(24ξ)-hydroperoxy-29-*nor*-3,4-*seco*-cycloart-4,25-dien-3-oic acid methyl ester	45.7	18.4
64	(6S)-hydroxy-29-*nor*-3,4-*seco*-cycloart-4,24-dien-3-oic acid	43.7	4.7

not mimic human metabolism of the test compounds, and this may have a strong influence on activity. Also, the Ishikawa assay reveals potential cytotoxic activity of test substances. We have instituted the Ishikawa assay system to assess estrogenic and antiestrogenic activity of plant extracts and pure compounds, and it has proven to be reliable and stable.

Resveratrol (**38**) was shown previously to be a superagonist in MCF-7 cells transfected with an estrogen response element-luciferase reporter gene (EREluc); however, further independent analysis failed to reproduce this effect *(141–144)*. Subsequently, resveratrol was shown to be only weakly estrogenic compared to estrogen in numerous cell lines and animal models *(142–144)*. The antiestrogenic effect of resveratrol, however, has been demonstrated in MCF-7, T47D, LY2, and S30 breast cancer cell lines; it prevented preneoplastic formation in DMBA-induced cultured BALB/c mouse mammary organ glands *(143)*. Additionally, resveratrol protected Sprague-Dawley rats from MMU-induced mammary carcinogenesis *(144)*. In general, resveratrol exerts mixed estrogen agonist/antagonist activities in several cultured mammary cancer cells lines; however, in the presence of estrogen, resveratrol clearly functions as an antiestrogen.

Several steroidal alkaloids were isolated from a native American ornamental plant, *Pachysandra procumbens* Michx. (Buxaceae), based on their antiestrogen binding site (AEBS) and antiestrogenic effect

in cultured Ishikawa cells *(54)*. Four novel compounds, (+)-(20S)-20-(dimethylamino)-3-(3′α-isopropyl)-lactam-5α-pregn-2-en-4-one (**80**), (+)-(20S)-20-(dimethylamino)-16α-hydroxy-3-(3′α-isopropyl)-lactam-5α-pregn-2-en-4-one (**81**), (+)-(20S)-3-(benzoylamino)-20-(dimethylamino)-5α-pregn-2-en-4β-yl acetate (**82**), and (+)-(20S)-2α-hydroxy-20-(dimethylamino)-3β-phthalimido-5α-pregnan-4β-yl acetate (**83**), and five known compounds, (−)-pachyaximine A (**84**), (+)-spiropachysine (**85**), (+)-axillaridine A (**86**), (+)-epipachysamine D (**87**), and (+)-pachysamine B (**88**), were shown to potentiate significant antiestrogenic activity mediated by tamoxifen in Ishikawa cells (Table 5, Fig. 9).

Three cardenolides, (−)-14-hydroxy-3β-(3-O-methyl-6-deoxy-α-L-rhamnosyl)-11α,12α-epoxy-(5β,14β,17βH)-card-20(22)-enolide (**89**), (−)-14-hydroxy-3β-(3-O-methyl-6-deoxy-α-L-glucopyranosyl)-11α,12α-epoxy-(5β,14β,17βH)-card-20(22)-enolide (**90**), and (−)-17β-neriifolin (**91**), were isolated from the roots of a Fijian tree, *Cerbera manghas* L. (Apocynaceae), using bioassay-guided fractionation with the Ishikawa antiestrogenic assay. The antiestrogenic activity of these cardiac glycosides may be due to their structural similarity to estradiol and interaction with the ER *(53,145–147)*.

7. AROMATASE INHIBITION

Estrogens are involved in the development of numerous hormone-related disorders, most notably hormone-dependent carcinomas such as those associated with

Table 4
Ornithine Decarboxylase Inhibitory Activity
of Plant Natural Products

	Compound	ODC^a IC_{50} (μM)
65	deguelin	0.001
66	tephrosin	0.005
67	(13R)-hydroxydeguelin	0.01
68	(13R)-hydroxytephrosin	0.05
69	munetone	0.11
70	mundulone	0.07
71	mundulinol	0.008
72	(+)-7-oxo-13-epi-pimara-14,15-dien-18-oic acid	0.50
73	(+)-7-oxo-13-epi-pimara-8,15-dien-18-oic acid	0.98
74	(+)-isopimaric acid	0.86
75	(1S,2S,3R)-(+)-isopicrodeoxypodophyllotoxin	0.55
76	(−)-deoxypodophyllotoxin	0.08
77	(−)-deoxypodorhizone	6.5
78	zapotin	0.58
79	5,6,2′-trimethoxyflavone	0.96

^{a}IC_{50} of TPA-induced ODC in cultured ME308 cells.

breast and endometrial cancers *(148)*. Approximately one-third of all breast cancers are hormone (estrogen) dependent. The role of estrogen in breast cancer development increases with age, two-thirds of postmenopausal cases are hormone-dependent and can be targeted with endocrine therapy. Though a variety of different treatment options is currently available, breast cancer remains one of the leading causes of death among women *(49)*. The American Cancer Society estimates that in 2002, 203,500 women in the US were diagnosed with breast cancer, and 39,600 women died from this disease *(150)*. Therefore, the development of new therapeutic modalities for prevention and treatment of breast cancer remains a high priority.

Estrogen deprivation is one strategy frequently used for treatment of hormone-dependent tumors. A decrease in estrogen levels can be achieved by blocking ERs with antiestrogens, also known as selective estrogen receptor modulators (SERMs), or by reducing estrogen production by inhibiting aromatase, the key enzyme in estrogen biosynthesis *(151)*. Aromatase is a cytochrome P450 enzyme complex (CYP19) that catalyzes the last, rate-limiting step in estrogen biosynthesis, and is responsible for the conversion of androgens to estrogens, i.e., estradiol (**92**) from testosterone (**93**), and estrone (**94**) from androstenedione (**95**) (Fig. 10). The aromatase complex is associated with the endoplasmatic reticulum and consists of a specific cytochrome P450 heme protein and a flavoprotein NADPH cytochrome P450 reductase *(152)*. This enzyme complex is unique in steroid biosynthesis due to its ability to mediate three separate steps. Three moles of molecular oxygen are consumed, and three moles of NADPH are required to convert one mole of C_{19} androgen to C_{18} estrogen. The first step involves hydroxylation of the C_{19} methyl group (**96**), followed by the second oxidation step to give 19-oxo-steroid (**97**). This is subsequently transformed to C_{18} estrogen in the third oxidative step, resulting in elimination of formic acid and aromatization of ring A. While it has generally been accepted that the first two steps are two sequential P450 oxidations, the mechanism of the aromatization step remains to be elucidated.

Aromatase has been identified in a variety of tissues in both males and females. In men, aromatase activity is associated with muscle, adipose tissue, and testis *(152)*. Aromatase has been also identified in several areas of the brain, including the hypothalamus, amygdala, and hippocampus *(153)*. In premenopausal women, granulosa cells of ovarian follicles are the main source of aromatase. During pregnancy, aromatase is expressed in high levels in the placenta. The enzyme is also present in liver, muscle, and fat, where estrogen is produced extragonadally by aromatization of adrenal androgens. In postmenopausal women, adipose tissue is considered the main site of aromatase expression, and breast tissue of elderly women was found to have several-fold higher estrogen levels than those in plasma *(154)*. In vitro experiments have demonstrated aromatase activity in breast tissue *(155,156)*, and it was further shown that approximately 60% of breast tumors express aromatase *(157)*.

Aromatase is a reasonable target for inhibition since it catalyzes the last in a series of steps in steroid biosynthesis of estrone and estradiol. As a member of a P450 family, aromatase shares common features with other enzymes in the class. In this regard, the selectivity of aromatase inhibitors is an important issue due to the widespread presence of P450 systems in mammals; nonselective inhibition could cause serious side effects.

Aromatase inhibitors have been developed primarily to treat breast cancer in postmenopausal woman. However, these agents have been also recognized as potential chemopreventive agents and several studies

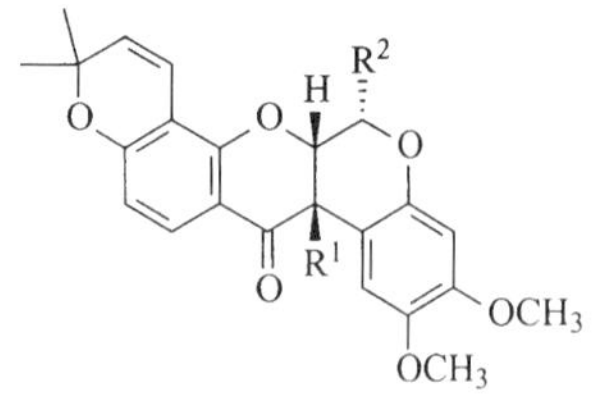

65: R^1 = H, R^2 = H
66: R^1 = OH, R^2 = H
67: R^1 = H, R^2 = OH
68: R^1 = OH, R^2 = OH

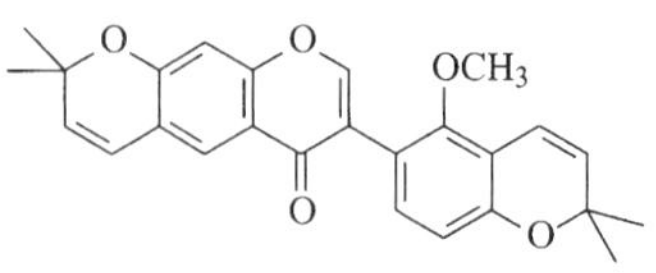

69

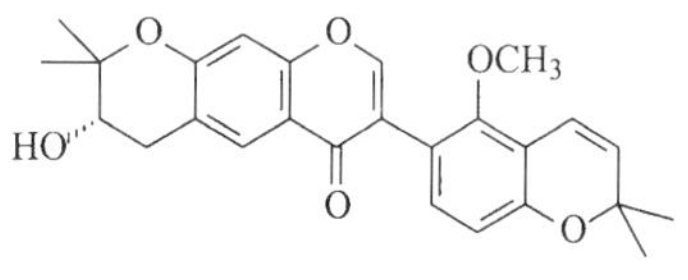

70

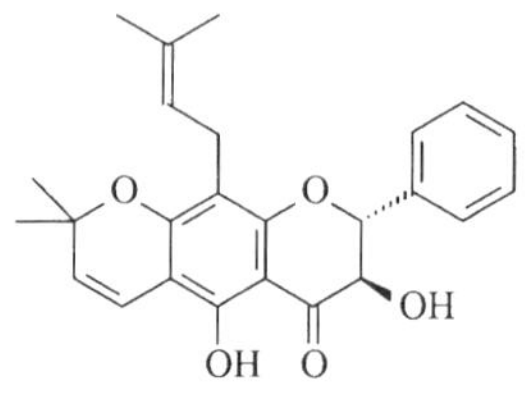

71

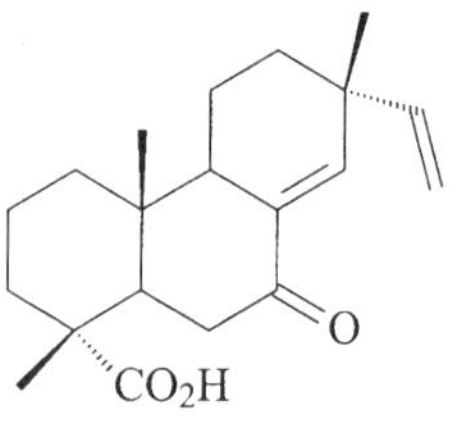

72

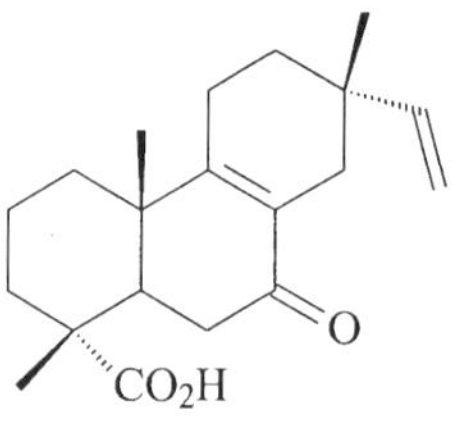

73

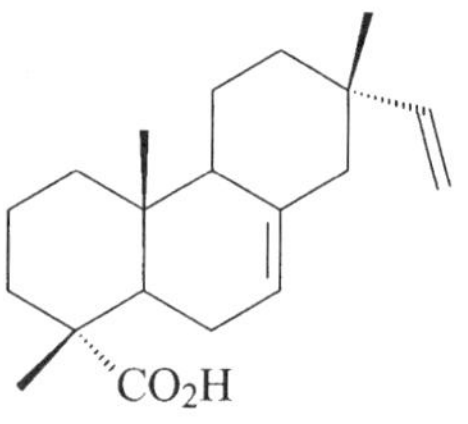

74

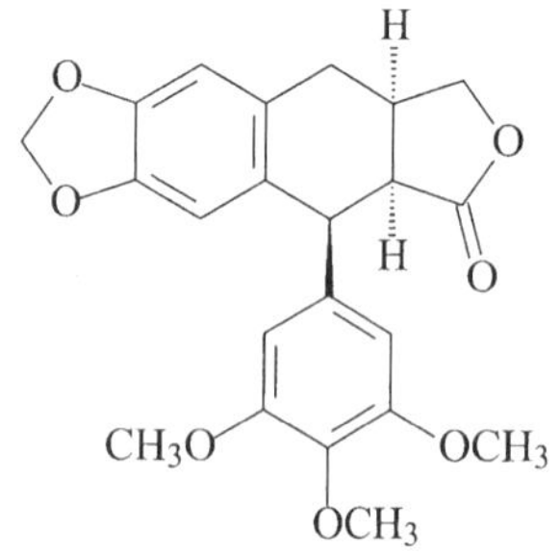

75

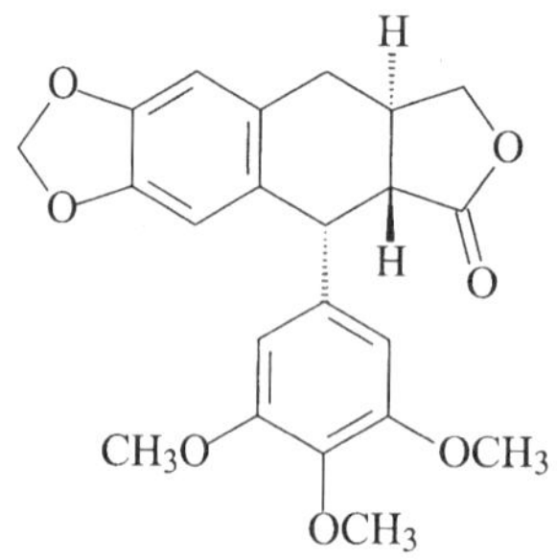

76

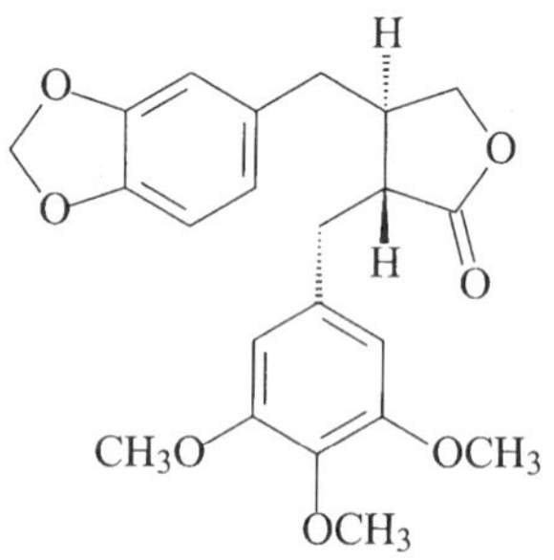

77

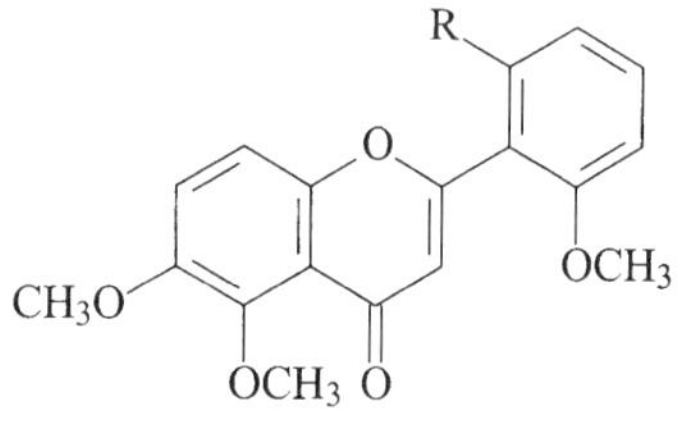

78: R= OCH$_3$
79: R = H

Fig. 8. Inhibitors of ornithine decarboxylase.

have proven their chemopreventive efficacy in animal models *(158–160)*. Aromatase inhibitors have an increasingly important role in breast cancer prevention, and their evaluation in clinical settings is imminent *(161–164)*. Since chemopreventive agents are generally intended for prolonged use in healthy or relatively healthy subjects who have a high risk of developing cancer, even minor side effects can be a major drawback. It is known that total estrogen deprivation may cause adverse side effects in bone and the cardiovascular

Table 5
Antiestrogenic Activity of Plant Natural Products

	Compound	IA^a ED_{50} (μM)	$AEBS^b$ IC_{50} (μM)
38	*trans*-resveratrol	2.3	ND^c
80	(+)-(20S)-20-(dimethylamino)-3-(3'α-isopropyl)-lactam-5α-pregn-2-en-4-one	0.11	2.8
81	(+)-(20S)-20-(dimethylamino)-16α-hydroxy-3-(3'α-isopropyl)-lactam-5α-pregn-2-en-4-one	0.11	3.5
82	(+)-(20S)-3-(benzoylamino)-20-(dimethylamino)-5α-pregn-2-en-4β-yl acetate	0.035	0.6
83	(+)-(20S)-2α-hydroxy-20-(dimethylamino)-3β-phthalimido-5α-pregnan-4β-yl acetate	ND^c	6.8
84	(−)-pachyaximine A	0.07	0.4
85	(+)-spiropachysine	0.19	7.4
86	(+)-axillaridine A	0.16	8.0
87	(+)-epipachysamine D	ND^c	>20
88	(+)-pachysamine B	0.037	0.6
89	(−)-14-hydroxy-3β-(3-*O*-methyl-6-deoxy-α-L-rhamnosyl)-11α,12α-epoxy-(5β,14β,17βH)-card-20(22)-enolide	0.0077	ND^c
90	(−)-14-hydroxy-3β-(3-*O*-methyl-6-deoxy-α-L-glucopyranosyl)-11α,12α-epoxy-(5β,14β,17βH)-card-20(22)-enolide	0.015	ND^c
91	(−)-17β-neriifolin	0.17	ND^c

[a]Concentration required to reduce estradiol-mediated induction of alkaline phosphatase by 50% in cultured Ishikawa cells.

[b]Test agent concentration that inhibited [^{3}H]tamoxifen binding at the antiestrogen binding site.

[c]Not determined.

system. Notably, however, chemopreventive effects can be achieved with lower doses of therapeutic agents relative to drugs for chemotherapy *(160)*, so better therapeutic indices may be achieved.

Known aromatase inhibitors can be classified as steroidal and nonsteroidal compounds based on their structure. All nonsteroidal compounds have a nitrogen atom that coordinates to the heme iron of cytochrome P450. However, a number of reports have shown that plant-derived and synthetic flavonoids are moderate inhibitors of aromatase *(51,165,166)*. Since our research is largely focused on plant-derived, potential chemopreventive leads, we have employed bioactivity-guided fractionations of plant extracts to search for inhibitors of aromatase.

To assess aromatase inhibition, a tritiated water-release in vitro assay is used *(167–169)*. This method has some advantages, but it is not a high-throughput assay. A modified assay based on the fluorescent-based high-throughput screening system from BD Biosciences (San Jose, CA) is employed to identify aromatase inhibitors from natural products *(170)*. Aromatase inhibition is quantified by measuring the fluorescent intensity of fluorescein (**98**), the hydrolysis product of dibenzylfluorescein (**99**, DBF) by aromatase (Fig. 11). In brief, the test substance is pre-incubated with the NADPH regenerating system before the enzyme and substrate mixture are added. Then, the reaction mixture is incubated for 30 min to allow aromatase to generate the product, and quenched with 2 N NaOH. After the reaction is terminated, a 2-h incubation enhances the noise/background ratio and fluorescence is measured at 485 nm (excitation) and 530 nm (emission).

Using this method, 1273 plant extracts were tested. Extracts were dissolved in DMSO; the final DMSO concentration was fixed at 0.5%, a concentration found to have no significant effect on the aromatase reaction. Among 1273 plant extracts, 30 were found to have

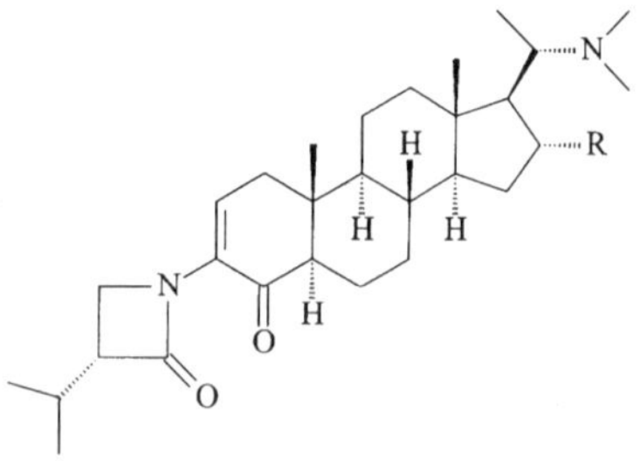

80: R = H
81: R = OH

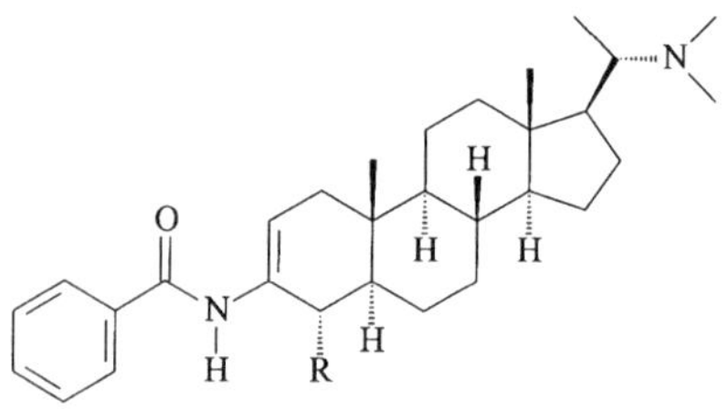

82: R = OAc
86: R = ═O

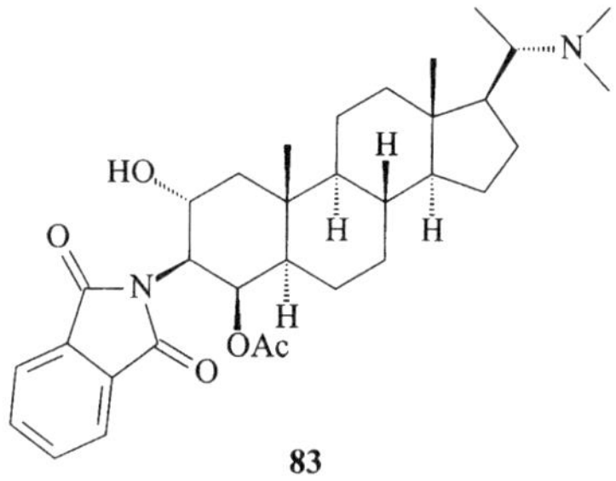

83

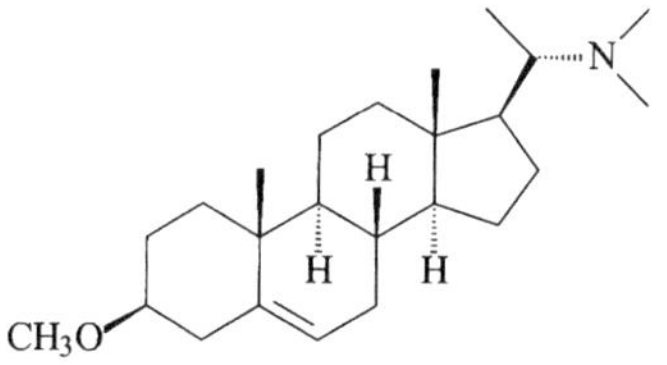

84

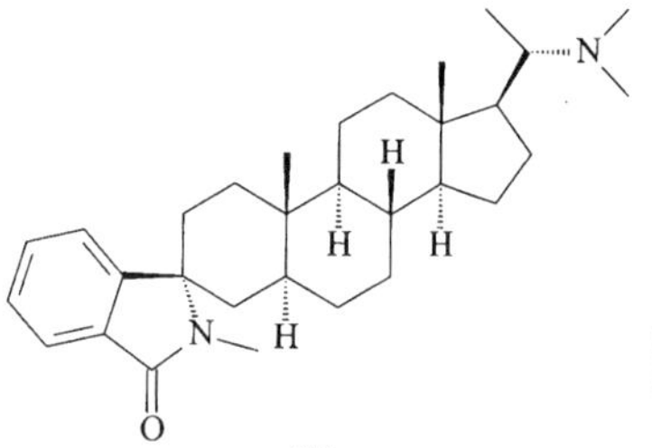

85

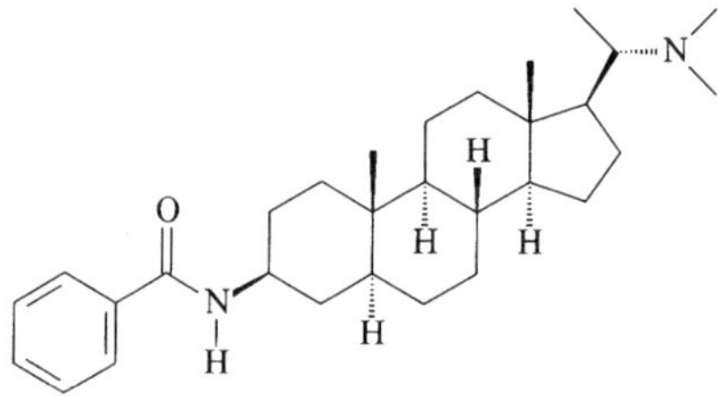

87

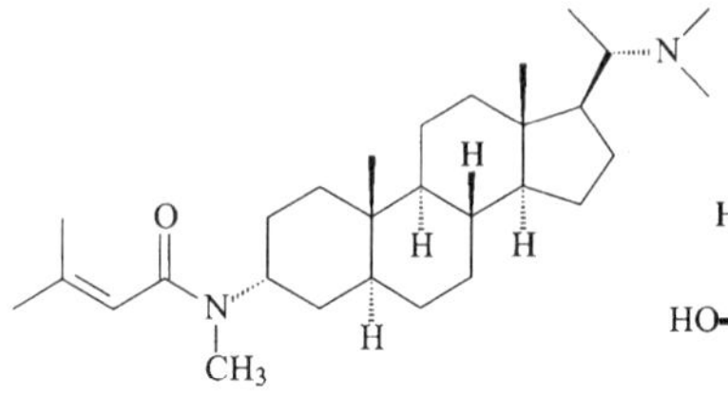

88

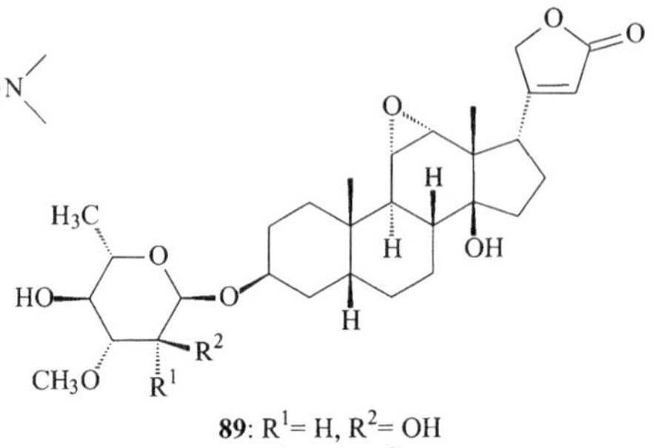

89: R¹= H, R²= OH
90: R¹= OH, R²= H

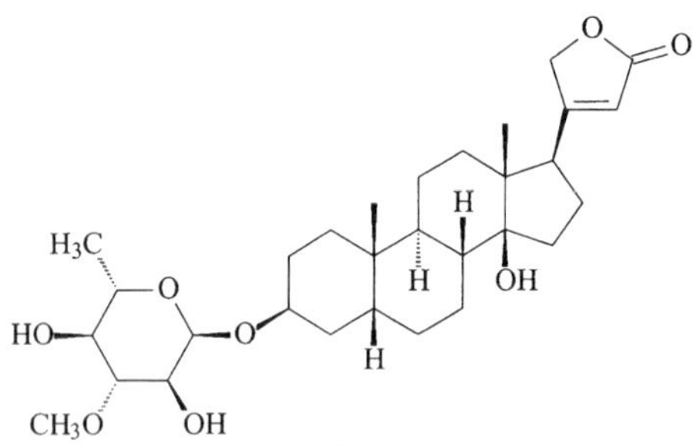

91

Fig. 9. Antiestrogenic compounds from plants.

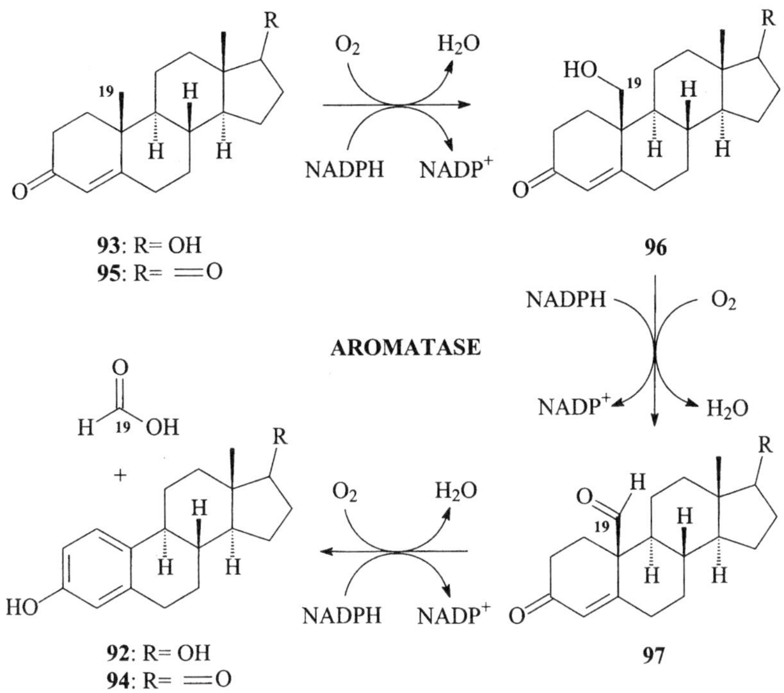

Fig. 10. Estrone and estradiol biosynthesis mediated by aromatase.

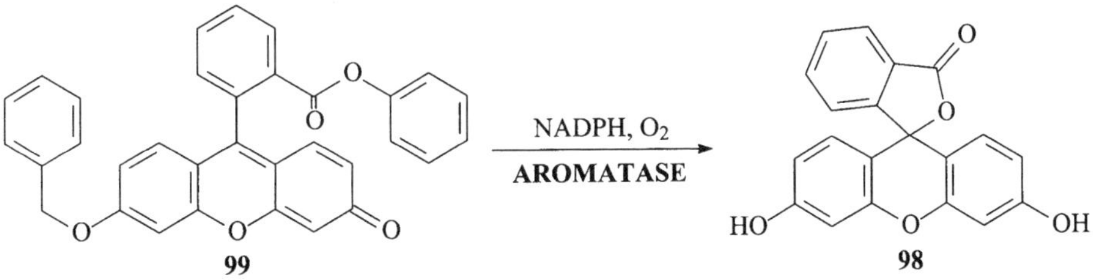

Fig. 11. Fluorescent-based aromatase assay. Conversion of dibenzylfluorescein to fluorescein by aromatase (CYP19).

90% or greater inhibitory activity; bioassay-guided fractionation is in progress to isolate potential antiaromatase compounds (Fig. 12).

Using the ^3H_2O release assay, a variety of flavonoids were shown to be moderate to potent inhibitors of CYP19 (Table 6, Fig. 13). A small library of commercially available, naturally occurring flavonoids was screened for aromatase activity. Four flavones, apigenin (**100**), chrysin (**101**), 7,8-dihydroxyflavone (**102**), and 5,7,3′,4′-tetrahydroxyflavone (**103**), and two flavanones, hesperetin (**104**) and naringin (**105**), exhibited moderate inhibitory activity *(51)*. Eight flavonoids with inhibitory activity below 5 μM were discovered from the paper mulberry tree, *Broussonetia papyrifera* (L.) L'Hér. ex Vent. (Moraceae) *(171)*. Two known flavonols, broussoflavonol F (**106**) and isolicoflavonol (**107**); four flavanones, (2S)-abyssinone II (**108**), (2S)-5,7,2′,4′-tetrahydroxyflavanone (**109**), (2S)-euchrenone

A7 (**110**), and novel (2S)-2′,4′-dihydroxy-2″-(1-hydroxy-1-methylethyl)dihydrofuro[2,3-h]flavanone (**111**); and two chalcones, 2,4,2′,4′-tetrahydroxy-3-prenylchalcone (**112**) and novel 3′-[γ-hydroxymethyl-(E)- γ-methylallyl]-2,4,2′,4′-tetrahydroxychalcone-11′-O-coumarate (**113**), were isolated by bioassay-guided fractionation from the ethyl acetate extract of *B. papyrifera*. Compounds **107, 108, 111**, and **113** were selected by the NCI RAPID program for further in vivo evaluation.

8. DIFFERENTIATION-INDUCING AGENTS

Differentiation-inducing agents have been shown to suppress cancer cell self-renewal selectively from normal stem cell renewal by inducing terminal differentiation followed by apoptosis. For example, reduction or elimination of leukemic stem cell self-renewal, together with restoration of responsiveness to homeostatic control, has been proven in acute promyelocytic

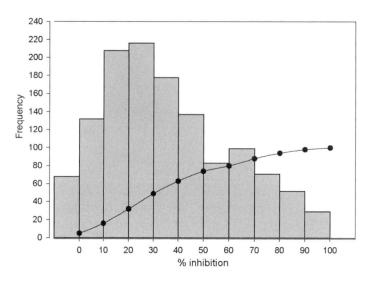

Fig 12. Active plant extracts from fluorescent-based aromatase inhibition assay.

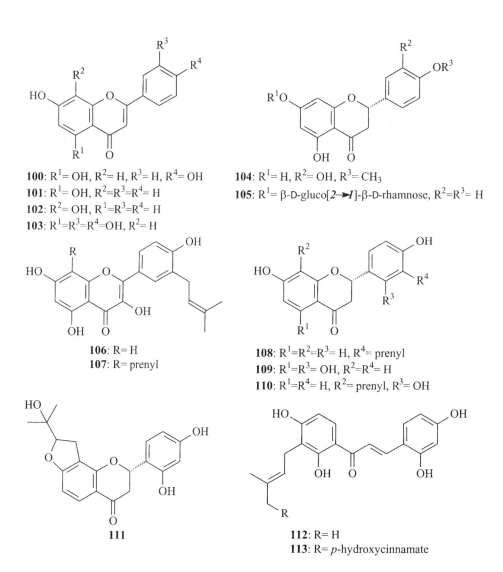

100: R^1= OH, R^2= H, R^3= H, R^4= OH
101: R^1= OH, R^2=R^3=R^4= H
102: R^2= OH, R^1=R^3=R^4= H
103: R^1=R^3=R^4=OH, R^2= H

104: R^1= H, R^2= OH, R^3= CH$_3$
105: R^1= β-D-gluco[2→1]-β-D-rhamnose, R^2=R^3= H

106: R= H
107: R= prenyl

108: R^1=R^2=R^3= H, R^4= prenyl
109: R^1=R^3= OH, R^2=R^4= H
110: R^1=R^4= H, R^2= prenyl, R^3= OH

111

112: R= H
113: R= p-hydroxycinnamate

Fig. 13. Aromatase inhibitors from bioassay-guided fractionation.

Table 6
Natural Product Aromatase Inhibitors

Compound	Aromatase[a] IC_{50} (μM)
100 apigenin	3.3
101 chrysin	4.3
102 7,8-dihydroxyflavone	8.7
103 3',4',5,7-tetrahydroxyflavone	11.5
104 hesperetin	3.3
105 naringin	3.1
106 broussoflavonol F	9.7
107 isolicoflavonol	0.1
108 (2S)-abyssinone II	0.4
109 (2S)-5,7,2',4'-tetrahydroxyflavanone	2.2
110 (2S)-euchrenone A7	3.4
111 (2S)-2',4'-dihydroxy-2''-(1-hydroxy-1-methylethyl) dihydrofuro [2,3-h]flavanone	0.1
112 2,4,2',4'-tetrahydroxy-3'-prenylchalcone	4.6
113 3'-[γ-hydroxymethyl-(E)-γ-methylallyl]-2,4,2',4'-tetrahydroxychalcone-11'-O-coumarate	0.5

[a]Concentration to inhibit 50% of ^3H_2O release from [1,2-^3H]androstenedione by aromatase (CYP19).

leukemia (APL) treated with all-*trans*-retinoic acid (ATRA) *(172,173)*. Clinical studies on APL patients showed complete remissions following treatment with ATRA. Moreover, it has been proven that mature functioning granulocytes originate from a leukemic clone and that the leukemic DNA polymorphic pattern may persist years after remission *(174)*. Differentiation therapy has also shown encouraging results in the treatment of some solid tumors such as prostate cancer *(175)*.

In addition, inducers of terminal differentiation, such as the retinoid and deltanoid (vitamin D_3 derivatives) class of compounds, have shown promising chemopreventive activity as suppressing agents that act during the promotion-progression stages of carcinogenesis *(176)*. These agents have shown promising chemopreventive activity in clinical trials. In particular, the natural retinoids ATRA and 13-*cis*-retinoic acid (13-cRA) have shown efficacy as cancer chemopreventive agents for lung and head/neck cancers *(177–179)*. Although toxicity has hampered the development of these agents as primary chemopreventive agents, novel structural

analogs with high affinity for specific nuclear receptors and highly selective chemopreventive activity, have been developed *(97)*.

The HL-60 cell line, established from the peripheral blood of a patient with APL, is a valuable tool for research on myeloid maturation at the cellular and molecular level *(180)*. In addition, this cell model system has been used to monitor biological activity of large numbers of samples to discover new agents that induce cellular differentiation *(30)*. This cell line can be induced to differentiate into the granulocytic, monocytic/macrophagic, or eosinophilic pathways of cellular development. At the molecular level, this cell line is atypical for APL in that it does not possess the t(15,17) translocation that results in the PML/RARα chimeric protein. In addition, c-*myc* is amplified (i.e., 2–20 extra copies), while p53 is highly deleted, and N-*ras* is mutated *(180)*. Induction of differentiation along the monocytic lineage in the HL-60 cell line is characterized by a decrease in myeloperoxidase, an increase in nonspecific esterase (NSE), downregulation of transferring receptors and insulin receptors, upregulation of chemotactic and complement receptors, and increased plastic adherence *(181–183)*. Induction of differentiation along the granulocytic lineage is characterized by increased specific esterase expression (SE) and morphological changes of lobulated nucleated banded cells *(180,184)*. In addition, mature HL-60 cells display some functional changes characteristic of polymorphonuclear cells and monocytes/macrophages, such as chemotaxis, superoxide generation (evidenced by NBT-reduction ability), and phagocytosis *(185,186)*. Finally, the desired biological effect consists of induction of terminal differentiation that is characterized by irreversible cell-growth arrest followed by postmitotic death.

The HL-60 cell differentiation/proliferation assay is performed using a 4-d incubation protocol *(187)*. In brief, cells in log phase (approx 10^6 cells/mL) are diluted to 10^5 cells/mL and preincubated overnight (18 h) in 24-well plates to allow cell growth recovery. Then, samples dissolved in DMSO are added, keeping the final DMSO concentration at 0.1% (v/v). Control cultures are treated with the same concentration of DMSO. After 4-d of incubation, the cells are analyzed to determine the percentage of cells undergoing maturation as determined by three markers of differentiation: NBT reduction, presence of NSE, or SE enzymes. Concomitantly, the effect on viability and proliferation of HL-60 cells is determined.

Some of the most active inducers of HL-60 cell differentiation have come from the quassinoid class and

Table 7
Natural Product Differentiation Compounds

Compound		TDR^a (μM)	NBT^b (μM)	NSE^c (μM)
114	brusatol	0.07	0.07	ND^d
115	bruceantin	0.04	0.02	ND^d
116	bruceine D	ND^d	$43.1\%^e$	ND^d
117	peninsularinone	0.009	0.019	ND^d
118	quassimarin	0.06	0.09	ND^d
119	glaucarubolone analog	0.009	0.009	ND^d
120	glaucarubolone analog	0.011	0.017	ND^d
121	glaucarubolone analog	0.04	0.025	ND^d
122	glaucarubolone analog	0.04	0.05	ND^d
123	glaucarubolone analog	0.07	0.09	ND^d
124	glaucarubolone analog	0.075	0.055	ND^d
125	glaucarubolone	0.4	1.3	ND^d
126	tithofolinolide	ND^d	ND^d	$37.4\%^e$
127	3β-acetoxy-8β-isobutyryloxyreynosin	ND^d	ND^d	$33.9\%^e$
128	4α,10α-dihydroxy-3-oxo-8β-isobutyryloxyguaia-11(13)-en-12,6α-olide	ND^d	ND^d	$32.4\%^e$
78	zapotin (5,6,2′,6′-tetramethoxyflavone)	ND^d	0.5	ND^d
79	5,6,2′-trimethoxyflavone	ND^d	4.0	ND^d
129	genistein	$44\%^e$	$42\%^e$	9.6
130	dibenzyltrisulfide	ND^d	8.5	ND^d
131	1-benzyldisulfanyl-2-ethanol	ND^d	1.0	ND^d
132	desmethylrocaglamide	ND^d	0.02	ND^d
	all-trans-retinoic acid	ND^d	0.45	ND^d

[a]IC_{50} of [^{3}H]thymidine incorporation.

[b]ED_{50} of nitrobluetetrazolium reduction activity.

[c]ED_{50} of nonspecific esterase activity.

[d]Not determined.

[e]Percent inhibition or differentiation at 4 µg/mL test agent concentration.

have activities in the nanomolar range (Table 7, Fig. 14). Brusatol (114), bruceantin (115), and bruceine D (116) came from the seeds of the Chinese herbal plant "Ya-dan-zi" or *Brucea javanica* (L.) Merr. (Simaroubaceae) *(50,57,188)*. The mechanism has been further investigated *(189)*. Another quassinoid, peninsularinone (117), was obtained as a natural product from *Castela peninsularis* (Simaroubaceae) *(190)*, while others, quassimarin (118) and analogs 119–124, were synthesized from glaucarubolone (125) obtained from *Castela polyandra* (Simaroubaceae) *(191–193)*.

Sesquiterpenoids from *Tithonia diversifolia* (Hemsl.) A. Gray (Asteraceae), a perennial shrub native to Mexico, were shown to have moderate differentiating activity. The

sesquiterpene lactones tithofolinolide (126), 3β-acetoxy-8β-isobutyryloxyreynosin (127), and 4α,10α-dihydroxy-3-oxo-8β-isobutyryloxyguaia-11(13)-en-12,6α-olide (128) were isolated by bioassay-guided fractionation using NSE as a marker of differentiating activity *(194)*.

Flavonoids have also shown differentiation activity in HL-60 cells. Two flavones, zapotin (78) and 5,6,2′-trimethoxyflavone (79), were isolated from the seeds of the edible fruit zapote blanco of *Casimiroa edulis* Llave et Lex. (Rutaceae) *(33,49,133)*. Additionally, the soy isoflavone genistein (129), a human dietary constituent, was found to have significant differentiating activity *(70)*.

Sulfides dibenzyltrisulfide (130) and 1-benzyldisulfanyl-2-ethanol (131) from *Petiveria alliacea* L.

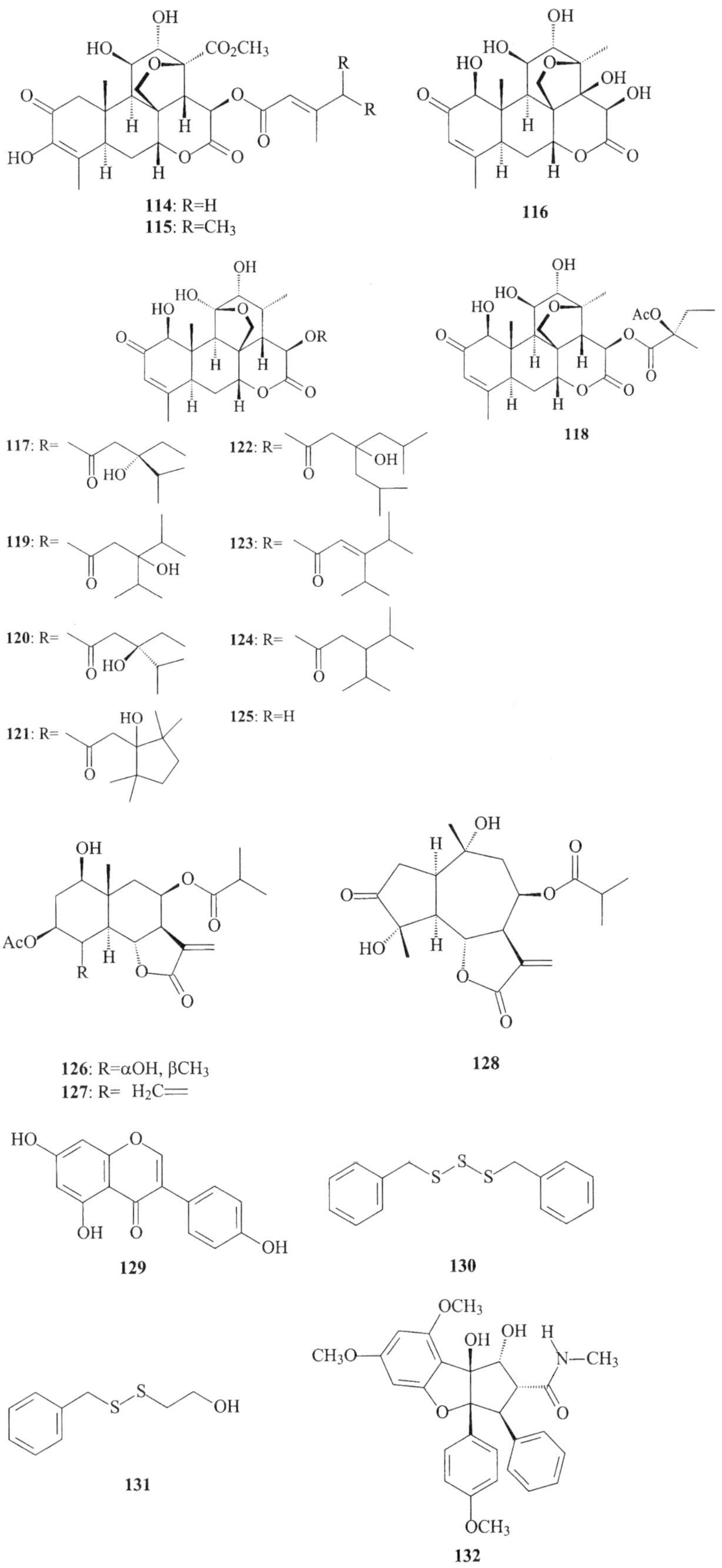

114: R=H
115: R=CH₃

116

117: R=

122: R=

119: R=

123: R=

120: R=

124: R=

121: R=

125: R=H

118

126: R=αOH, βCH₃
127: R= H₂C=

128

129

130

131

132

Fig. 14. Differentiation agents from plant natural products.

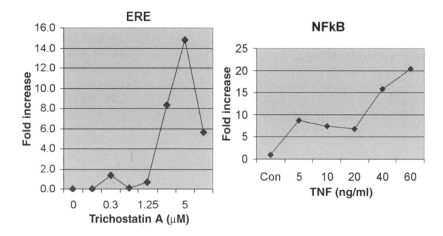

Fig. 15. Examples of positive controls for NFκB-luc and ERE-luc assay systems.

(Phytolaccaceae) were shown to be moderate to strong inducers of differentiation; however, their cytotoxicity precluded further study *(70)*. Bioassay-guided fractionation of *Aglaia ponapensis* Kaneh. (Meliaceae) led to isolation of desmethylrocaglamide (**132**), a lignan that selectively inhibits protein synthesis in human lung carcinoma cell line Lu1 *(70)*.

9. REPORTER ASSAYS LUCIFERASE

Firefly luciferase is a commonly used genetic reporter in cell biology to study regulation of gene expression, such as receptor activity, protein-protein interactions, and intracellular signal transduction *(195)*. Stable transfection of cells using plasmids engineered to contain different upstream promoters of the luciferase gene provides a powerful tool to understand molecular mechanisms of novel anticancer natural products. Promoters are chosen based on their established relationships to the carcinogenic process, i.e., nuclear factor κB (NFκB) *(196)*. The principle of this assay relies on the ability of the natural product to turn on a particular promoter, for example NFκB, artificially constructed upstream of the luciferase gene. Once the promoter is triggered, it leads to transcription and eventually translation of the luciferase protein. Luciferase activity is easily measured using a luminometer and commercially available luciferase substrate. The amount of luciferase protein produced reflects the level of cellular regulation of the natural product on the particular promoter.

For this method, DNA of the desired promoter is sequenced and inserted into a vector containing cDNA encoding luciferase. The vector construct is then cotransfected with a different vector bearing an antibiotic-resistant property into mammalian cells. The resulting cell line possesses the vector construct and has simultaneously been conferred resistance against a specific antibiotic, such as ampicillin. A continuous process using selection pressure exerted by the particular antibiotic over a period of time results in a stably transfected cell line.

Extracts from natural products are added to the stably transfected cells and grown in 96-well plates for a fixed incubation time period. At the end of the incubation period, cells are washed and lysed. Using luciferase substrate, luciferase activity can then be measured with the aid of a luminometer. Assay response is compared to both negative and positive controls to ensure the integrity of the luciferase signal from the stably transfected luciferase construct (Fig. 15). Approximately 250 plant extracts were screened using an antioxidant response element-luciferase construct (ARE-luc) and 5% showed responses of 10-fold or greater (Fig. 16).

10. CANCER CHEMOPREVENTION LEAD DEVELOPMENT

Once a lead compound has been identified through an in vitro screen, a variety of steps are necessary to validate and assess potential cancer chemopreventive activity. One of the most significant hurdles for development of drug leads is to obtain sufficient quantities of pure material to properly evaluate the agent in a variety of animal efficacy trials. Other factors that can have a negative impact on lead development are cost of procurement and animal testing, issues of formulation and stability, poor adsorption, distribution, metabolism, and excretion (ADME) properties, and toxicity from acute or chronic dosing.

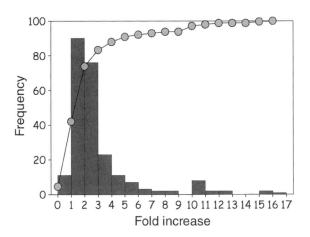

Fig. 16. Screening of plant extracts (8 μg/mL) with HepG2 cells stably transfected with ARE-luc construct.

Numerous experimental carcinogenesis models are reported for evaluating chemopreventive agents *(197)*. The ideal model requires that cancers developing as a result of carcinogen insult are target-organ-specific, but otherwise, the carcinogen should not have adverse effects in the animals. Descriptions of the most commonly used models are summarized elsewhere *(198)*. Studies described here were conducted using three well-established carcinogenesis models: the DMBA-induced and TPA-promoted (two-stage) skin carcinogenesis model in mice *(76,129)*, the DMBA, MNU-induced rat mammary carcinogenesis model *(40,197)*, and the benzo(*a*)pyrene-induced lung tumor model in mice. These models have been used rigorously by numerous investigators and have resulted in consistent and reproducible results. Chemoprevention studies for in vivo carcinogenesis were generally carried out at a dose corresponding to 80% of the maximum tolerated dose (MTD) (highest dose with no apparent toxicity).

As summarized in Table 8, nine agents resulting from this project are considered promising leads for further development. Three of these—brassinin, deguelin, and resveratrol—were evaluated for efficacy in skin and mammary carcinogenesis studies. Brassinin is an indole dithiocarbamate from Chinese cabbage *(76)*. We evaluated effects on DMBA-induced mammary carcinogenesis in Sprague-Dawley rats. Results showed that a 4-wk intragastric treatment with brassinin beginning 3 wk prior to DMBA through 1 wk post-DMBA treatment reduced tumor incidence from 87% in the control to 52% in the treatment group, i.e., a 40% reduction in incidence. Number of tumors was reduced from four tumors per rat to one tumor per rat,

respectively. Numerous analogs of brassinin and flavones have been synthesized as modulators of QR activity. Among these agents, including chloro-, bromo-, and methyl-derivatives, as well as various chalcones, 4'-BF was found to exhibit extremely potent induction of QR activity. We further evaluated 4'-BF in the DMBA-induced mammary carcinogenesis model. The compound was given at 2 and 4 g/kg of diet for 2 wk (−1 to +1 wk in relation to DMBA treatment), and remarkable suppression of both tumor incidence and multiplicity was observed. Incidence was reduced from 94% in the control to 35% and 20% in low- and high-dose groups, respectively. Tumors per rat were reduced from the control level of 2.6 to 0.65 and 0.20, respectively, at the two dose levels tested. There was no effect on body weight due to this treatment *(40)*.

Deguelin, another new chemopreventive agent identified in our program, is a rotenoid from the African plant *Mundulea sericea (129)*. It was found to be a potent inhibitor of ODC activity and inhibited carcinogen-induced mammary lesions in the MMOC assay. In the two-stage skin carcinogenesis model, deguelin remarkably suppressed induction of papillomas from 75% in control mice to 10% in the low-dose (33 μg) treatment group, and complete suppression (no tumors in any mice) was observed with 330 μg of topical deguelin *(42)*. Since deguelin is an analog of rotenone, which is toxic and used as a pesticide, it was essential to compare the mode of action of these two agents. Unlike rotenone, deguelin did not mediate its effects by tubulin polymerization and therefore its action is microtubule-independent. It was also observed that deguelin reduced the steady-state level of mRNA for c-*fos* protooncogene, which could contribute to the transcription of ODC gene via c-*fos/jun* (AP1) complex. We also showed that in c-*myc* ER cells expressing c-*myc*-ER fusion protein, activation of TPA-independent ODC activity was suppressed *(42)*. The efficacy of deguelin was also determined in the MNU-induced rat mammary carcinogenesis model. There was no effect on tumor incidence. However, multiplicity was reduced from 6.8 tumors per rat to 3.2 tumors per rat in the high-deguelin-dose group *(61)*. More recently, we have found deguelin to be effective against human melanoma growth in athymic mice and in experimental colon carcinogenesis (unpublished).

Resveratrol is present in grapes, red wine, and peanuts. As shown in Table 2, we originally noted activity with an extract of *Cassia quinquangulata*, a plant collected in Peru, using cyclooxygenase as a molecular target. The active principle, resveratrol,

Table 8
Selective Chemopreventive Agents Identified From Natural Products

Plant/Source	Compounds	Targets	Efficacy	Carcinogenesis
Brucea javanica	Brusatol	Differentiation (HL-60)	Active	HL-60
Casimiroa edulis	Zapotin	Differentiation (HL-60) apoptosis	Active	Colon
Cassia quinquangulata	Resveratrol	COX inhibition	Active	Skin, mammary, colon, prostate
Mundulea sericea	Deguelin	Ornithine decarboxylase	Active	Skin, mammary colon, melanoma
Brassica spp.	Brassinin	Quinone reductase	Active	Skin, mammary
Physalis philadelphica	Withanolide	Quinone reductase	Active	To be determined
Broussonetia papyrifera	Abyssinone II (RAPID)	Aromatase	Not active	To be determined
Synthetic	4′-Bromoflavone (RAPID)	Quinone reductase	Active	Mammary
Synthetic	Oxomate	Quinone reductase	Active	Mammary

inhibited cyclooxygenase and suppressed development of carcinogen-induced mammary lesion formation significantly, indicating potential to function as a chemopreventive agent. Consistent with this, topical application of 1 to 25 μmol inhibited incidence and multiplicity of papillomas in the two-stage skin carcinogenesis model in a dose-related manner *(60)*. As recently reviewed *(112)*, a large number of chemopreventive studies have now been performed with resveratrol, and the compound demonstrates a plethora of relevant activities. For example, resveratrol was found active against the growth of LNCaP prostate cancer cells, and 4-d treatment reduced intracellular levels of prostate-specific antigen (PSA) by 80% without effecting expression of androgen receptors *(199)*. More recently, we showed that resveratrol was effective in inhibiting multiplicity of MNU-induced mammary carcinogenesis. It was also observed that, in the absence of estrogen, resveratrol functions as an agonist of estrogen function. However, in the presence of estrogen, resveratrol functions as an antiestrogen *(143)*.

In addition to the chemopreventive agents described here, over the past several years, a variety of potentially important chemopreventive agents have been identified using bioactivity-guided fractionation *(31,33)*, and numerous structural analogs have been synthesized. For example, sulforaphane from broccoli was identified as a potent inducer of QR by Talalay and co-workers *(200)*. Since then, more efficacious analogs have been synthesized. Hybrid molecules of brassinin and sulforaphane, such as oxomate and sulforamate, were synthesized and evaluated in our laboratories with in vitro and in vivo models. Both sulforamate and oxomate are less toxic than sulforaphane at effective doses *(78)*. These agents inhibited development of preneoplastic lesions in MMOC and chemically induced mammary carcinogenesis. In murine Hepa1c1c7 cells, sulforamate induced GSH by twofold, and enhanced QR activity at a transcriptional level *(78)*.

Prior to clinical trials, it is mandatory to determine toxicity profiles for chemopreventive agents in at least two mammalian species. Initial preclinical toxicity experiments are usually carried out as 28-d gavage studies using rats and dogs as models under good laboratory practice (GLP) guidelines. Animals are treated with four increasing dose levels for 28 d. Rats and dogs are observed at least once a day. Complete clinical pathology and necropsy are conducted at the end of the study. Tissue sections are examined for possible toxicity. However, more extensive chronic preclinical toxicity studies are needed for chemoprevention studies. These studies should provide a complete toxicity profile for the compound at four dose levels in two species, which is a requirement for clinical trials for anticancer drugs. If the agent appears to be safe at all dose levels with no toxicity, then it may move forward to clinical trials. Among the agents developed in our laboratories, 4′-BF and resveratrol are being evaluated in rats and dogs for dose-tolerance studies. It is expected that once the preclinical toxicity studies are completed, these agents will be further evaluated in clinical trials.

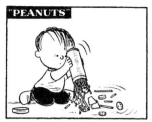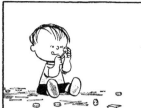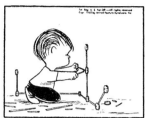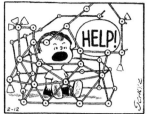

Fig. 17. Linus, a character from the cartoon strip Peanuts, illustrates the sequential development of and verbal response to an avoidable dilemma. As described in the text, some analogies can be drawn between the events depicted in this cartoon and the cancer problem. In sum, interference with the acts or processes leading to the dilemma are vastly superior to allowing the disaster to occur followed by attempts for correction that are unlikely to succeed. Peanuts reprinted by permission of United Feature Syndicate, Inc.

11. CONCLUSIONS

Many essential characteristics of cancer chemoprevention have been described by a working group of the American Association for Cancer Research (AACR) *(5)*. Throughout the course of history, it has been recognized that disease prevention is highly preferable to disease treatment. In the recent past, two therapeutic options have been approved by the FDA for prevention of cancer: tamoxifen (Novadex®) to prevent breast cancer, and celecoxib (Celebrex®) to treat colorectal cancer precursors in patients with familial adenomatous polyposis. These agents may not be perfect, and second- or subsequent-generation derivatives may provide greater long-term efficacy or reduced side effects, especially as related to breast cancer. Nonetheless, if health professionals are conscientious in administering these drugs, we should witness the greatest decrease in cancer incidence since the notable decline achieved as a result of cigarette smoking cessation. The importance of these breakthroughs must be emphasized and applauded, and individuals at risk for developing these cancers should take full advantage of these opportunities.

On the other hand, it is generally recognized that the lifetime probability for an individual to develop some form of cancer is in the range of 50–70%. Some etiological factors such as cigarette smoking are now obvious. However, as eloquently illustrated by the parody shown in Fig. 17, individuals may be naïve. When the consequences of careless acts are finally recognized, it is very difficult to implement palliative action. Conversely, the etiology of some major cancers, such as breast and prostate cancers, remains largely unknown. Therefore, irrespective of how cautious we become, a majority of the general population can be considered at risk and suitable subjects for cancer chemo-

prevention. The logistics of dealing with the general population are extremely complex, but it may be relevant to note that the administration of multiple vitamin tablets on a daily basis has been reasonably well accepted. In a similar manner, a formulation could be constructed that contains multiple cancer chemopreventive agents. Safety is of utmost concern, but this is an achievable goal.

Studies conducted in our laboratories focus on natural product cancer chemopreventive agents, some of which are found in the diet. The discoveries are frequently novel and subject to lead optimization studies through semi-synthesis and establishment of target-based structure-activity relationships. In this way, new pharmaceutical agents may be developed, requiring full regulatory scrutiny. Alternatively, since some of the lead molecules are actually found in the human diet, administration through the diet may be viewed as a convenient method for providing the general population with effective cancer chemopreventive agents. A problem associated with this approach is that low levels of agents often occur in natural dietary materials, so actual effectiveness may be questionable. Natural selection of dietary components containing higher levels of chemopreventive agents may be one method to circumvent this problem, but bioengineering of plants would be more direct. However, genetic modification of edible plant materials is not currently receiving public support. This could undoubtedly change at some point in the future, but as poignantly stated by Max Planck, "An important scientific innovation rarely makes its way by gradually winning over and converting its opponents: it rarely happens that Saul becomes Paul. What does happen is that its opponents gradually die out and that the growing generation is familiarized with the idea from the beginning" *(201)*.

Finally, chemopreventive and chemotherapeutic agents have been traditionally considered as different classes of compounds. While this is true to a certain extent, there is no clear boundary where the function of a chemopreventive agent ends and that of a therapeutic agent begins. Therefore, it may be useful to evaluate the effectiveness of nontoxic chemopreventive agents as possible chemotherapeutic agents.

ACKNOWLEDGMENTS

"Natural Inhibitors of Carcinogenesis" is supported by the National Cancer Institute under the auspices of program project grant P01 CA48112. The authors gratefully acknowledge this support and the contributions of the numerous investigators and collaborators who participate in the project.

REFERENCES

1. Pratt WB, Ruddon RW, Ensminger WD, Maybaum J. *The Anticancer Drugs.* Oxford University Press, Oxford, 1994.
2. Jemal A, Thomas A, Murray T, Thun M. Cancer statistics, 2002. *CA Cancer J Clin* 2002;52:23–47.
3. Sporn MB. The war on cancer. *Lancet* 1996;347:1377–1381.
4. Pezzuto JM. Plant-derived anticancer agents. *Biochem Pharmacol* 1997;53:121–133.
5. Alberts DS, Colvin GM, Conney AH, et al. Prevention of cancer in the next millennium. Report of the Chemoprevention Working Group to the American Association for Cancer Research. *Cancer Res* 1999;59:4743–4758.
6. Sporn MB, Suh N. Chemoprevention of cancer. *Carcinogenesis* 2000;21:525–530.
7. Sporn MB, Dunlop NM, Newton DL, Smith JM. Prevention of chemical carcinogenesis by vitamin A and its synthetic analogs (retinoids). *Fed Proc* 1976;35:1332–1338.
8. Wattenberg L. Chemoprevention of cancer. *Cancer Res* 1985;45:1–8.
9. Kelloff GJ, Boone CW, Steele VE, et al. Inhibition of chemical carcinogens. In *Chemical Induction of Cancer.* Arcos JC, ed. Birkauser, Basel, 1995; pp.73–122.
10. Surh YJ. Molecular mechanisms of chemopreventive effects of selected dietary and medicinal phenolic substances. *Mutat Res* 1999;428:305–327.
11. Kelloff GJ, Sigman CC, Greenwald P. Cancer chemoprevention: progress and promise. *Eur J Cancer* 1999;35:1755–1762.
12. Harris CC. Chemical and physical carcinogenesis: advances and perspectives for the 1990s. *Cancer Res* 1991;51(Suppl):5023S–5044S.
13. Greenwald P, Kelloff GJ, Burch-Whitman C, Kramer BS. Chemoprevention. *CA Cancer J Clin* 1995;45:31–49.
14. Stoner GD, Morse MA, Kelloff GJ. Perspectives in cancer chemoprevention. *Environ Health Perspect* 1997;105 (Suppl):945–954.
15. Boone CW, Kelloff GJ, Malone WE. Identification of candidate cancer chemopreventive agents and their evaluation in animal models and human clinical trials: a review. *Cancer Res* 1990;50:2–9.
16. Morse MA, Stoner GD. Cancer chemoprevention: principles and prospects. *Carcinogenesis* 1993;4:1737–1746.
17. Kelloff GJ. Perspectives on cancer chemoprevention research and drug development. *Adv Cancer Res* 1999;78: 199–334.
18. Mirvish SS. Ascorbic acid inhibition of *N*-nitroso compound formation in chemical, food, and biological systems. In *Inhibition of Tumor Induction and Development.* Zedeck MS, Lipkin M, eds. Plenum, New York, 1981; pp. 101–126.
19. Kuenzig W, Chau J, Norkus E, et al. Caffeic and ferulic acid as blockers of nitrosamine formation. *Carcinogenesis* 1984;5: 309–313.
20. Shenoy NR, Choughuley ASU. Inhibitory effect of diet related sulphydryl compounds on the formation of carcinogenic nitrosamines. *Cancer Lett* 1992;65:227–232.
21. Wakabayashi K, Nagao M, Sugimura T. Prevention of formation of carcinogens in food. Heterocyclic amines, lipophilic ascorbic acid, and thioproline: ubiquitous carcinogens and practical anticarcinogenic substances. In *Cancer Chemoprevention.* Wattenberg L, Lipkin M, Boone CW, Kelloff GJ, eds. CRC Press, Boca Raton, 1992; pp. 311–325.
22. Kelloff GJ, Hawk ET, Karp JE, et al. Progress in clinical chemoprevention. *Semin Oncol* 1997;24:241–252.
23. Kelloff GJ, Crowell JA, Hawk ET, et al. Strategy and planning for chemopreventive drug development: clinical development plans II. *J Cell Biochem* 1996;26(Suppl):54–71.
24. Kelloff GJ, Crowell JA, Steele VE, et al. Progress in cancer chemoprevention. *Ann NY Acad Sci* 1999;889:1–13.
25. Kelloff GJ, Boone CW, Malone WF, Steele VE. Recent results in preclinical and clinical drug development of chemopreventive agents at the National Cancer Institute. In *Cancer Chemoprevention.* Wattenberg L, Lipkin M, Boone CW, eds. CRC Press, Boca Raton, 1992; pp. 41–56.
26. Kelloff GJ, Boone CW, Crowell JA, et al. New agents for cancer chemoprevention. *J Cell Biochem* 1996;26(Suppl): 1–28.
27. Udeani GO, Zhao GM, Shin YG, et al. Pharmacokinetics of deguelin, a cancer chemopreventive agent in rats. *Cancer Chemother Pharmacol* 2001;47:263–268.
28. Kelloff GJ, Johnson JR, Crowell JA, et al. Approaches to development and marketing approval of drugs that prevent cancer. *Cancer Epidemiol Biomarkers Prev* 1995;4:1–10.
29. Pezzuto JM. Cancer chemopreventive agents: from plant materials to clinical intervention trials. In *Human Medicinal Agents from Plants* (Symposium Series No. 534). Kinghorn AD, Balandrin MF, eds. American Chemical Society Books, Washington, DC, 1993; pp. 205–217.
30. Pezzuto JM. Natural product cancer chemopreventive agents. In *Recent Advances in Phytochemistry* (Vol. 29): *Phytochemistry of Medicinal Plants.* Arnason JT, Mata R, Romeo JT, eds. Plenum, New York, 1995; pp. 19–44.
31. Kinghorn AD, Fong HHS, Farnsworth NR, et al. Cancer chemopreventive agents discovered by activity-guided fractionation: a review. *Curr Org Chem* 1998;2:597–612.
32. Pezzuto JM, Angerhofer CK, Mehdi H. In vitro models of human disease states. *Stud Nat Prod Chem* 1998;20:507–560.
33. Pezzuto JM, Song LL, Lee SK, et al. Bioassay methods useful for activity-guided isolation of natural product cancer chemopreventive agents. In *Chemistry, Biological and Pharmacological Properties of Medicinal Plants from the Americas.* Hostettmann K, Gupta MP, Marston A, eds. Harwood Academic Publishers, Chur, Switzerland, 1998; pp. 81–110.
34. Mehta RG, Moon RC. Characterization of effective chemopreventive agents in mammary gland in vitro using an initiation-promotion protocol. *Anticancer Res* 1991;11:593–596.
35. Mehta RG, Bhat KPL, Hawthorne ME, et al. Induction of atypical ductal hyperplasia in mouse mammary gland organ culture. *J Natl Cancer Inst* 2001;93:1103–1106.

36. Loub WD, Farnsworth NR, Soejarto DD, Quinn ML. NAPRALERT: computer handling of natural product research data. *J Chem Inf Comput Sci* 1985;25:99–103.

37. Shamon LA, Pezzuto JM. Assessment of antimutagenic activity with *Salmonella typhimurium* strain TM677. *Methods Cell Sci* 1997;19:57–62.

38. Chung HS, Chang LC, Lee SK, et al. Flavonoid constituents of *Chorizanthe diffusa* with potential cancer chemopreventive activity. *J Agric Food Chem* 1999;47:36–41.

39. Lee SK, Mbwambo ZH, Chung H-S, et al. Evaluation of the antioxidant potential of natural products. *Comb Chem High Throughput Screen* 1998;1:23–34.

40. Song LL, Kosmeder JW II, Lee SK, et al. Cancer chemopreventive activity mediated by 4′-bromoflavone, a potent inducer of phase II detoxification enzymes. *Cancer Res* 1999;59:578–585.

41. Chang LC, Chávez D, Song LL, et al. Absolute configuration of novel bioactive flavonoids from *Tephrosia purpurea*. *Org Lett* 2000;2:515–518.

42. Gerhäuser C, Lee SK, Kosmeder J, et al. Regulation of ornithine decarboxylase induction by deguelin, a natural product cancer chemopreventive agent. *Cancer Res* 1997;57:3429–3435.

43. Chang LC, Song LL, Park EJ, et al. Bioactive constituents of *Thuja occidentalis*. *J Nat Prod* 2000;63:1235–1238.

44. Jang M, Pezzuto JM. Assessment of cyclooxygenase inhibitors using in vitro assay systems. *Methods Cell Sci* 1997;19:25–31.

45. Waffo-Teguo P, Lee D, Cuendet M, et al. Two new stilbene dimer glucosides from grape (*Vitis vinifera*) cell cultures. *J Nat Prod* 2001;64:136–138.

46. Lee D, Cuendet M, Schunke Vigo J, et al. A novel cyclooxygenase-inhibitory stilbenolignan from the seeds of *Aiphanes aculeata*. Org Lett 2001;3:2169–2171.

47. Mbwambo ZH, Lee SK, Mshiu EN, et al. Constituents from the stem wood of *Euphorbia quinquecostata* with phorbol dibutyrate receptor-binding inhibitory activity. *J Nat Prod* 1996;59:1051–1055.

48. El-Sayed KA, Hamann MT, Waddling CA, et al. Structurally novel bioconversion products of the marine natural product sarcophine effectively inhibit JB6 cell transformation. *J Org Chem* 1998;63:7449–7455.

49. Mata-Greenwood E, Ito A, Westenburg H, et al. Discovery of novel inducers of cellular differentiation using HL-60 promyelocytic cells. *Anticancer Res* 2001;21:1763–1770.

50. Mata-Greenwood E, Daeuble JF, Grieco PA, et al. Novel esters of glaucarubolone as inducers of terminal differentiation of promyelocytic HL-60 cells and inhibitors of 7,12-dimethylbenz[*a*]anthracene-induced preneoplastic lesion formation in mouse mammary organ culture. *J Nat Prod* 2001;64:1509–1513.

51. Jeong H-J, Shin YG, Kim IH, Pezzuto JM. Inhibition of aromatase activity by flavonoids. *Arch Pharm Res* 1999;22:309–312.

52. Pisha E, Pezzuto JM. Cell-based assay for the determination of estrogenic and anti-estrogenic activity. *Methods Cell Sci* 1997;19:37–43.

53. Chang LC, Gills JJ, Bhat KPL, et al. Activity-guided isolation of constituents of *Cerbera manghas* with antiproliferative and antiestrogenic activities. *Bioorg Med Chem Lett* 2000;10:2431–2434.

54. Chang LC, Bhat KPL, Fong HHS, et al. Novel bioactive steroidal alkaloids from *Pachysandra procumbens*. *Tetrahedron* 2000;56:3133–3138.

55. Chang LC, Chávez D, Gills JJ, et al. Rubiasins A-C, new anthracene derivatives from the roots and stems of *Rubia cordifolia*. *Tetrahedron Lett* 2000;41:7157–7162.

56. Su B-N, Park EJ, Mbwambo ZH, et al. New chemical constituents of *Euphorbia quinquecostata* and absolute configuration assignment by a convenient Mosher ester procedure carried out in NMR tubes. *J Nat Prod* 2002;65:1278–1282.

57. Su B-N, Chang LC, Park EJ, et al. Bioactive constituents of the seeds of *Brucea javanica*. *Planta Med* 2002;68:730–733.

58. Constant HL, Slowing K, Graham JG, et al. A general method for the dereplication of flavonoid glycosides utilising HPLC/MS analysis. *Phytochem Anal* 1997;8:176–180.

59. Gu J-Q, Park EJ, Luyengi L, et al. Constituents of *Eugenia sandwicensis* with potential cancer chemopreventive activity. *Phytochemistry* 2001;58:121–127.

60. Jang M, Cai L, Udeani GO, et al. Cancer chemopreventive activity of resveratrol, a natural product derived from grapes. *Science* 1997;275:218–220.

61. Udeani GO, Gerhäuser C, Thomas CF, et al. Cancer chemopreventive activity mediated by deguelin, a naturally occurring rotenoid. *Cancer Res* 1997;57:3424–3428.

62. Prochaska HJ, Talalay P. Role of NAD(P)H:quinone reductase in protection against the toxicities of quinones and related agents. In *Oxidative Stress. Oxidants and Antioxidants.* Sies H., ed. Academic Press, London, 1991; pp. 195–211.

63. Yang CS, Smith TJ, Hong JY. Cytochrome P-450 enzymes as targets for chemoprevention against chemical carcinogenesis and toxicity: opportunities and limitations. *Cancer Res* 1994;54:1982s–1986s.

64. Dinkova-Kostova AT, Holtzclaw WD, Cole RN, et al. Direct evidence that sulfhydryl groups of Keap1 are the sensors regulating induction of phase 2 enzymes that protect against carcinogens and oxidants. *Proc Natl Acad Sci USA* 2002;99:11908–11913.

65. Sogawa K, Fujii-Kuriyama Y. Ah receptor, a novel ligand-activated transcription factor. *J Biochem* (Tokyo) 1997;122:1075–1079.

66. Talalay P. Chemical protection against cancer by induction of electrophile detoxication (Phase 2) enzymes. In *Cellular Targets for Chemoprevention.* Steele V, ed. Boca CRC Press, Raton, 1992; pp. 193–205.

67. Prochaska HJ, Santamaria AB. Direct measurement of NAD(P)H:quinone reductase from cells cultured in microtiter wells: a screening assay for anticarcinogenic enzyme inducers. *Anal Biochem* 1988;169:328–336.

68. De Long MJ, Santamaria AB, Talalay P. Role of cytochrome P1-450 in the induction of NAD(P)H:quinone reductase in a murine hepatoma cell line and its mutants. *Carcinogenesis*1987;8:1549–1553.

69. Steinmetz KA, Potter JD. Vegetables, fruit, and cancer prevention: a review. *J Am Diet Assoc* 1996;96:1027–1039.

70. Lee SK, Song L, Mata-Greenwood E, et al. Modulation of in vitro biomarkers of the carcinogenic process by chemopreventive agents. *Anticancer Res* 1999;19:35–44.

71. Ray AB, Gupta M. Withasteroids, a growing group of naturally occurring steroidal lactones. *Fortschr Chem Org Naturst* 1994;63:1–106.

72. Kennelly EJ, Gerhäuser C, Song LL, et al. Induction of quinone reductase by withanolides isolated from *Physallis philadelphica* (tomatillos). *J Agric Food Chem* 1997;45:3771–3777.

73. Misico RI, Song LL, Veleiro AS, et al. Induction of quinone reductase by withanolides. *J Nat Prod* 2002;65:677–680.

74. Chang LC, Gerhäuser C, Song L, et al. Activity-guided isolation of constituents of *Tephrosia purpurea* with the potential to induce the phase 2 enzyme, quinone reductase. *J Nat Prod* 1997;60:869–873.

75. Mehta RG, Liu J, Constantinou A, et al. Structure-activity relationships of brassinin in preventing the development of carcinogen-induced mammary lesions in organ culture. *Anticancer Res* 1994;14:1209–1213.

76. Mehta RG, Liu J, Constantinou A, et al. Cancer chemopreventive activity of brassinin, a phytoalexin from cabbage. *Carcinogenesis* 1995;16:399–404.

77. Zhang Y, Talalay P, Cho CG, Posner GH. A major inducer of anticarcinogenic protective enzymes from broccoli: isolation and elucidation of structure. *Proc Natl Acad Sci USA* 1992;89:2399–2403.

78. Gerhäuser C, You M, Liu J, et al. Cancer chemopreventive potential of sulforamate, a novel analogue of sulforaphane that induces phase 2 drug-metabolizing enzymes. *Cancer Res* 1997;57:272–278.

79. Kosmeder JW, Song, LS Park, EJ et al. Cancer chemopreventive activity of oxomate, a monofunctional inducer of phase 2 detoxification enzymes. Abstracts of Papers, 224th National Meeting of the American Chemical Society, Boston, MA, August 18–22, 2002; American Chemical Society: Washington, DC; MEDI 98.

80. Pezzuto JM, Park EJ. Autoxidation and antioxidants. In *Encyclopedia of Pharmaceutical Technology*, 2nd ed., vol. 1. Swarbrick J, Boylan JC, eds. Marcel Dekker, New York, 2002; pp. 97–113.

81. Gromadzinska J, Wasowicz W. The role of reactive oxygen species in the development of malignancies. *Int J Occup Med Environ Health* 2000;13:233–245.

82. Kensler TW, Egner PA, Taffe BG, Trush MA. Role of free radicals in tumor promotion and progression. *Prog Clin Biol Res* 1989;298:233–248.

83. Janssen YM, Van Houten B, Borm PJ, Mossman BT. Cell and tissue responses to oxidative damage. *Lab Invest* 1993;69: 261–274.

84. Afaq F, Adhami VM, Ahmad N, Mukhtar H. Botanical antioxidants for chemoprevention of photocarcinogenesis. *Front Biosci* 2002;7:d784–792.

85. Schlesier K, Harwat M, Bohm V, Bitsch R. Assessment of antioxidant activity by using different in vitro methods. *Free Radic Res* 2002;36:177–187.

86. Newburger PE, Chovaniec ME, Greenberger JS, Cohen HJ. Functional changes in human leukemic cell line HL-60. A model for myeloid differentiation. *J Cell Biol* 1979;82:315–322.

87. Ahmed N, Williams JF, Weidemann MJ. The human promyelocytic HL60 cell line: a model of myeloid cell differentiation using dimethylsulphoxide, phorbol ester and butyrate. *Biochem Int* 1991;23:591–602.

88. Gamez EJ, Luyengi L, Lee SK, et al. Antioxidant flavonoid glycosides from *Daphniphyllum calycinum*. *J Nat Prod* 1998;61:706–708.

89. Lee D, Park EJ, Cuendet M, et al. Cyclooxygenase-inhibitory and antioxidant constituents of the aerial parts of *Antirhea acutata*. *Bioorg Med Chem Lett* 2001;11:1565–1568.

90. Westenburg HE, Lee KJ, Lee SK, et al. Activity-guided isolation of antioxidative constituents of *Cotinus coggygria*. *J Nat Prod* 2000;63:1696–1698.

91. Jaffe BM. Prostaglandins and cancer: an update. *Prostaglandins* 1974;6:453–461.

92. Marnett LJ. Aspirin and the potential role of prostaglandins in colon cancer. *Cancer Res* 1992;52:5575–5589.

93. Levy GN. Prostaglandin H synthases, nonsteroidal anti-inflammatory drugs, and colon cancer. *FASEB J* 1997;11: 234–247.

94. Marnett LJ. Prostaglandin synthase-mediated metabolism of carcinogens and a potential role for peroxyl radicals as reactive intermediates. *Environ Health Perspect* 1990;88:5–12.

95. Earashi M, Noguchi M, Kinoshita K, Tanaka M. Effects of eicosanoid synthesis inhibitors on the in vitro growth and prostaglandin E and leukotriene B secretion of a human breast cancer cell line. *Oncology* 1995;52:150–155.

96. Lupulescu A. Prostaglandins, their inhibitors and cancer. *Environ Health Perspect* 1990;88:5–12.

97. Hong WK, Sporn MB. Recent advances in chemoprevention of cancer. *Science* 1997;278:1073–1077.

98. Xie WL, Robertson DL, Simmons DL. Mitogen-inducible prostaglandin G/H synthase: a target for non-steroidal anti-inflammatory drugs. *Drug Dev Res* 1992;25:245–265.

99. Smith WL, Garavito RM, DeWitt DL. Prostaglandin endoperoxide H synthases (cyclooxygenases)-1 and -2. *J Biol Chem* 1996;271:33157–33160.

100. Simmons D, Xie W, Chipman JG, Evett GE. Multiple cyclooxygenases: cloning of a mitogen-inducible form. In *Prostaglandin, Leukotrienes, Lipoxins and PAF*. Bailey JM, ed. Plenum, New York, 1991; pp. 67–78.

101. O'Neill GP, Ford-Hutchinson AW. Expression of mRNA for cyclooxygenase-1 and cyclooxygenase-2 in human tissues. *FEBS Lett* 1993;330:156–160.

102. Dewitt DL, Smith WL. Primary structure of prostaglandin G/H synthase from sheep vesicular gland determined from the complementary DNA sequence. *Proc Natl Acad Sci USA* 1988;85:1412–1416.

103. Merlie JP, Fagan D, Mudd J, Needleman P. Isolation and characterization of the complementary DNA for sheep seminal vesicle prostaglandin endoperoxide synthase (cyclooxygenase). *J Biol Chem* 1988;263:3550–3553.

104. Funk CD, Funk LB, Kennedy ME, et al. Human platelet/erythroleukemia cell prostaglandin G/H synthase: cDNA cloning, expression, and gene chromosomal assignment. *FASEB J* 1991;5:2304–2312.

105. Jouzeau JY, Terlain B, Abid A, et al. Cyclo-oxygenase isoenzymes. How recent findings affect thinking about nonsteroidal anti-inflammatory drugs. *Drugs* 1997;53:563–582.

106. O'Banion MK, Winn VD, Young DA. cDNA cloning and functional activity of a glucocorticoid-regulated inflammatory cyclooxygenase. *Proc Natl Acad Sci USA* 1992;89: 4888–4892.

107. Smith WL, Meade EA, DeWitt DL. Interactions of PGH synthase isozymes-1 and -2 with NSAIDs. *Ann N Y Acad Sci* 1994;744:50–57.

108. Subbaramaiah K, Chung WJ, Michaluart P, et al. Resveratrol inhibits cyclooxygenase-2 transcription and activity in phorbol ester-treated human mammary epithelial cells. *J Biol Chem* 1998;273:21875–21882.

109. Jang M, Pezzuto JM. Cancer chemopreventive activity of resveratrol. *Drugs Exp Clin Res* 1999;25:65–77.

110. Jang M, Pezzuto JM. Effects of resveratrol on 12-*O*-tetradecanoylphorbol-13-acetate-induced oxidative events and gene expression in mouse skin. *Cancer Lett* 1998;134:81–89.

111. Bhat KP, Pezzuto JM. Cancer chemopreventive activity of resveratrol. *Ann N Y Acad Sci* 2002;957:210–229.

112. Bhat KPL, Kosmeder JW II, Pezzuto JM. Biological effects of resveratrol. *Antioxid Redox Signal* 2001;3:1041–1064.

113. Rimando AM, Cuendet M, Desmarchelier C, et al. Cancer chemopreventive and antioxidant activities of pterostilbene, a naturally occurring analogue of resveratrol. *J Agric Food Chem* 2002;50:3453–3457.

114. Waffo-Teguo P, Hawthorne ME, Cuendet M, et al. Potential cancer-chemopreventive activities of wine stilbenoids and flavans extracted from grape (*Vitis vinifera*) cell cultures. *Nutr Cancer* 2001;40:173–179.

115. Su BN, Cuendet M, Hawthorne ME, et al. Constituents of the bark and twigs of *Artocarpus dadah* with cyclooxygenase inhibitory activity. *J Nat Prod* 2002;65:163–169.

116. Langcake P, Pryce RJ. The production of resveratrol by *Vitis vinifera* and other members of the Vitaceae as a response to infection or injury. *Physiol Plant Pathol* 1976;9:77–86.

117. Nikolic D, Habibi-Goudarzi S, Corley DG, et al. Evaluation of cyclooxygenase-2 inhibitors using pulsed ultrafiltration mass spectrometry. *Anal Chem* 2000;72:3853–3859.

118. Coffino P. Regulation of cellular polyamines by antizyme. *Nat Rev Mol Cell Biol* 2001;2:188–194.

119. McCann PP, Pegg AE. Ornithine decarboxylase as an enzyme target for therapy. *Pharmacol Ther* 1992;54:195–215.

120. Verma AK. Ornithine decarboxylase, a possible target for human cancer prevention. In *Cellular and Molecular Targets for Chemoprevention*. Steele VE, ed. CRC Press, Boca Raton, 1992; pp.373–389.

121. Verma AK. Inhibition of tumor promotion by DL-alpha-difluoromethylornithine, a specific irreversible inhibitor of ornithine decarboxylase. *Basic Life Sci* 1990;52:195–204.

122. Hurta RA. Altered ornithine decarboxylase and *S*-adenosylmethionine decarboxylase expression and regulation in mouse fibroblasts transformed with oncogenes or constitutively active mitogen-activated protein (MAP) kinase kinase. *Mol Cell Biochem* 2000;215:81–92.

123. Shantz LM, Pegg AE. Ornithine decarboxylase induction in transformation by H-Ras and RhoA. *Cancer Res* 1998;58: 2748–2753.

124. Peralta Soler A, Gilliard G, Megosh L, et al. Polyamines regulate expression of the neoplastic phenotype in mouse skin. *Cancer Res* 1998;58:1654–1659.

125. Kubota S, Kiyosawa H, Nomura Y, et al. Ornithine decarboxylase overexpression in mouse 10T1/2 fibroblasts: cellular transformation and invasion. *J Natl Cancer Inst* 1997;89: 567–571.

126. Hardin MS, Mader R, Hurta RA. K-FGF mediated transformation and induction of metastatic potential involves altered ornithine decarboxylase and *S*-adenosylmethionine decarboxylase expression—role in cellular invasion. *Mol Cell Biochem* 2002;233:49–56.

127. Meyskens FL Jr, Gerner EW. Development of difluoromethylornithine (DFMO) as a chemoprevention agent. *Clin Cancer Res* 1999;5:945–951.

128. Lee SK, Pezzuto JM. Evaluation of the potential of cancer chemopreventive activity mediated by inhibition of 12-*O*-tetradecanoyl phorbol 13-acetate-induced ornithine decarboxylase activity. *Arch Pharm Res* 1999;22:559–564.

129. Gerhäuser C, Mar W, Lee SK, et al. Rotenoids mediate potent cancer chemopreventive activity through transcriptional regulation of ornithine decarboxylase. *Nat Med* 1995;1: 260–266.

130. Lee SK, Luyengi L, Gerhäuser C, et al. Inhibitory effect of munetone, an isoflavonoid, on 12-*O*-tetradecanoylphorbol-13-acetate-induced ornithine decarboxylase activity. *Cancer Lett* 1999;136:59–65.

131. Ito A, Shamon LA, Yu B, et al. Antimutagenic constituents of *Casimiroa edulis* with potential cancer chemopreventive activity. *J Agric Food Chem* 1998;46:3509–3516.

132. Clemons M, Danson S, Howell A. Tamoxifen ("Nolvadex"): a review. Antitumour treatment. *Cancer Treat Rev* 2002;28: 165–180.

133. Clamp A, Danson S, Clemons M. Hormonal risk factors for breast cancer: identification, chemoprevention, and other intervention strategies. *Lancet Oncol* 2002;3:611–619.

134. Wolff MS, Toniolo PG, Lee EW, et al. Blood levels of organochlorine residues and risk of breast cancer. *J Natl Cancer Inst* 1993;85:648–652.

135. Bradlow HL, Davis DL, Lin G, et al. Effects of pesticides on the ratio of 16α/2-hydroxyestrone: a biologic marker of breast cancer risk. *Environ Health Perspect* 1995;103S: 147–150.

136. Jensen TK, Toppari J, Keiding N, Skakkebaek NE. Do environmental estrogens contribute to the decline in male reproductive health? *Clin Chem* 1995;41:1896–1901.

137. Littlefield BA, Gurpide E, Markiewicz L, et al. A simple and sensitive microtiter plate estrogen bioassay based on stimulation of alkaline phosphatase in Ishikawa cells: estrogenic action of Δ^5 adrenal steroids. *Endocrinology* 1990;127:2757–2762.

138. Holinka CF, Hata H, Kuramoto H, Gurpide E. Effects of steroid hormones and antisteroids on alkaline phosphatase activity in human endometrial cancer cells (Ishikawa line). *Cancer Res* 1986;46:2771–2774.

139. Albert JL, Sundstrom SA, Lyttle CR. Estrogen regulation of placental alkaline phosphatase gene expression in a human endometrial adenocarcinoma cell line. *Cancer Res* 1990;50: 3306–3310.

140. Arnold SF, Klotz DM, Collins BM, et al. Synergistic activation of estrogen receptor with combinations of environmental chemicals. *Science* 1996;272:1489–1492.

141. Gehm BD, McAndrews JM, Chien PY, Jameson JL. Resveratrol, a polyphenolic compound found in grapes and wine, is an agonist for the estrogen receptor. *Proc Natl Acad Sci USA* 1997;94:14138–14143.

142. Ashby J, Tinwell H, Pennie W, et al. Partial and weak oestrogenicity of the red wine constituent resveratrol: consideration of its superagonist activity in MCF-7 cells and its suggested cardiovascular protective effects. *J Appl Toxicol* 1999;19:39–45.

143. Bhat KP, Lantvit D, Christov K, et al. Estrogenic and antiestrogenic properties of resveratrol in mammary tumor models. *Cancer Res* 2001;61:7456–7463.

144. Bhat KP, Pezzuto JM. Resveratrol exhibits cytostatic and antiestrogenic properties with human endometrial adenocarcinoma (Ishikawa) cells. *Cancer Res* 2001;61:6137–6144.

145. Dmitrieva RI, Doris PA. Cardiotonic steroids: potential endogenous sodium pump ligands with diverse function. *Exp Biol Med (Maywood)* 2002;227:561–569.

146. Stenkvist B. Cardenolides and cancer. *Anticancer Drugs* 2001;12:635–638.

147. Stenkvist B. Is digitalis a therapy for breast carcinoma? *Oncol Rep* 1999;6:493–496.

148. Brodie A, Njar VCO. Aromatase inhibitors in advanced breast cancer: mechanism of action and clinical implications. *J Steroid Biochem Mol Biol* 1998;66:1–10.

149. Murray R. Role of anti-aromatase agents in postmenopausal advanced breast cancer. *Cancer Chemother Pharmacol* 2001;48:259–265.

150. American Cancer Society. *Facts and figures*, 2002. http://www.cancer.org/downloads/STT/CancerFacts&Figures 2002TM.pdf. Accessed on 11/29/02.

151. Brodie A, Njar VCO. Comprehensive pharmacology and clinical efficacy of aromatase inhibitors. *Drugs* 1999;58:233–255.

152. Recanatini M, Cavalli A, Valenti P. Nonsteroidal aromatase inhibitors: recent advances. *Med Res Rev* 2002;22:282–304.

153. Lephart ED. A review of brain aromatase cytochrome P450. *Brain Res Rev* 1996;22:1–26.

154. Brodie A, Long B. Aromatase inhibition and inactivation. *Clin Cancer Res* 2001;7:S4343–S4349.

155. Brodie A, Long B, Lu Q. Aromatase expression in the human breast. *Breast Cancer Res Treat* 1998;53:S85–S91.

156. Santen RJ, Martel J, Hoagland M, et al. Demonstration of aromatase activity and its regulation in breast tumor and benign breast fibroblast. *Breast Cancer Res Treat* 1998;53:S93–S99.

157. Brodie AMH, Lu Q, Long B. Aromatase and COX-2 expression in human breast cancer. *J Steroid Biochem* 2001;607:1–7.

158. Lubet RA, Steele VE, Casebolt TL, et al. Chemopreventive effects of the aromatase inhibitors vorozole (R-83842) and 4-hydroxyandrostenedione in the methylnitrosourea (MNU)-induced mammary tumor model in Sprague-Dawley rats. *Carcinogenesis* 1994;15:2775–2780.

159. Gunson DE, Steele RE, Chau RY. Prevention of spontaneous tumours in female rats by fadrozole hydrochloride, an aromatase inhibitor. *Br J Cancer* 1995;72:72–75.

160. Kelloff GJ, Lubet RA, Lieberman R, et al. Aromatase inhibitors as potential cancer chemopreventives. *Cancer Epidemiol Biomark Prev* 1998;7:65–78.

161. Lonning PE, Kragh LE, Erikstein B, et al. 2001;7: S4423–S4428.

162. Goss PE, Strasser K. Chemoprevention with aromatase inhibitors-trial strategies. *J Steroid Biochem Mol Biol* 2001;79:143–149.

163. Fabian CJ, Kimler BF. Beyond tamoxifen: new endpoints for breast cancer chemoprevention, new drugs for breast cancer prevention. *Ann NY Acad Sci* 2001;952:44–59.

164. Goss P. Anti-aromatase agents in the treatment and prevention of breast cancer. *Cancer Control* 2002;9:2–8.

165. Seralini G, Moslemi S. Aromatase inhibitors: past, present and future. *Mol Cell Endocrinol* 2001;178:117–131.

166. Pouget C, Fagnere C, Basly JP, et al. Synthesis and aromatase inhibitory activity of flavanones. *Pharm Res* 2002;19:286–291.

167. Thompson EA Jr, Siiteri PK. Utilization of oxygen and reduced nicotinamide adenine dinucleotide phosphate by human placental microsomes during aromatization of androstenedione. *J Biol Chem* 1974;249:5364–5372.

168. Reed KC, Ohno S. Kinetic properties of human placental aromatase. Application of an assay measuring [^{3}H]$_2$O release from 1β,2β-[^{3}H]-androgens. *J Biol Chem* 1976;251:1625–1631.

169. Rabe T, Rabe D, Runncbaum B. New aromatase assay and its application for inhibitory studies of aminoglutethimide on microsomes of human term placenta. *J Steroid Biochem* 1982;17:305–309.

170. Stresser DM, Turner SD, McNamara J, et al. A high-throughput screen to identify inhibitors of aromatase (CYP19). *Anal Biochem* 2000;284:427–430.

171. Lee D, Bhat KP, Fong HHS, et al. Aromatase inhibitors from *Broussonetia papyrifera*. *J Nat Prod* 2001;64:1286–1293.

172. Castaigne S, Chomienne C, Daniel MT, et al. All-*trans* retinoic acid as a differentiation therapy for acute promyelocytic leukemia. I. Clinical results. *Blood* 1990;76:1704–1709.

173. Huang ME, Ye YC, Chen SR, et al. Use of all-*trans* retinoic acid in the treatment of acute promyelocytic leukemia. *Blood* 1988;72:567–572.

174. Fearon ER, Burke PJ, Schiffer CA, et al. Differentiation of leukemia cells to polymorphonuclear leukocytes in patients with acute nonlymphocytic leukemia. *N Engl J Med* 1986;315:15–23.

175. Conley BA, Egorin MJ, Tait N, et al. Phase I study of the orally administered butyrate prodrug, tributyrin, in patients with solid tumors. *Clin Cancer Res* 1998;4:629–634.

176. Kelloff GJ, Boone CW, Steele VE, et al. Mechanistic considerations in chemopreventive drug development. *J Cell Biochem* 1994;20S:1–24.

177. Hong WK, Lippman SM, Itri LM, et al. Prevention of second primary tumors with isotretinoin in squamous-cell carcinoma of the head and neck. *N Engl J Med* 1990;323:795–801.

178. Lippman SM, Benner SE, Hong WK. Retinoid chemoprevention studies in upper aerodigestive tract and lung carcinogenesis. *Cancer Res* 1994;54S:2025–2028.

179. Pastorino U, Infante M, Maioli M, et al. Adjuvant treatment of stage I lung cancer with high-dose vitamin A. *J Clin Oncol* 1993;11:1216–1222.

180. Collins SJ. The HL-60 promyelocytic leukemia cell line: proliferation, differentiation, and cellular oncogene expression. *Blood* 1987;70:1233–1244.

181. Yam LT, Li CY, Crosby WH. Cytochemical identification of monocytes and granulocytes. *Am J Clin Pathol* 1971;55: 283–290.

182. Yamada M, Kurahashi K. Regulation of myeloperoxidase gene expression during differentiation of human myeloid leukemia HL-60 cells. *J Biol Chem* 1984;259:3021–3025.

183. Imaizumi M, Breitman TR. A combination of a T cell-derived lymphokine differentiation-inducing activity and a physiologic concentration of retinoic acid induces HL-60 to differentiate to cells with functional chemotactic receptors. *Blood* 1986;67: 1273–1280.

184. Collins SJ, Ruscetti FW, Gallagher RE, Gallo RC. Terminal differentiation of human promyelocytic leukemia cells induced by dimethyl sulfoxide and other polar compounds. *Proc Natl Acad Sci USA* 1978;75:2458–2462.

185. Collins SJ, Ruscetti FW, Gallagher RE, Gallo RC. Normal functional characteristics of cultured human promyelocytic leukemia cells after induction of differentiation by dimethyl-sulfoxide. *J Exp Med* 1979;149:969–974.

186. Newburger PE, Speier C, Borregaard N, et al. Development of the superoxide-generating system during differentiation of the HL-60 human promyelocytic leukemia cell line. *J Biol Chem* 1984;259:3721–3726.

187. Suh N, Luyengi L, Fong HHS, et al. Discovery of natural product chemopreventive agents utilizing HL-60 cell differentiation as a model. *Anticancer Res* 1995;15:233–240.

188. Luyengi L, Suh N, Fong HHS, et al. A lignan and four terpenoids from *Brucea javanica* that induce differentiation with cultured HL-60 promyelocytic leukemia cells. *Phytochemistry* 1996;43:409–412.

189. Mata-Greenwood E, Cuendet M, Sher D, et al. Brusatol-mediated induction of leukemic cell differentiation and G1 arrest is associated with down-regulation of c-*myc*. *Leukemia* 2002;16:2275–2284.

190. Grieco PA, Moher ED, Seya M, et al. A quassinoid (peninsularinone) and a steroid from *Castela peninsularis*. *Phytochemistry* 1994;37:1451–1454.

191. Moher ED, Grieco PA, Collins JL. (*R*)-(+)- and (*S*)-(−)-5-Ethyl-5-methyl-1,3-dioxolane-2,4-dione reagents for the direct preparation of α-hydroxy-α-methylbutyrate esters: assignment of the absolute configuration of the α-acetoxy-α-methylbutyrate ester side chain of quassimarin via total synthesis. *J Org Chem* 1993;58:3789–3790.

192. Moher ED, Reilly M, Grieco PA, et al. Synthetic studies on quassinoids: transformation of (−)-glaucarubolone into (−)-peninsularinone. In vivo antitumor evaluation of (−)-glaucarubolone, (−)-chaparrinone, and (−)-peninsularone. *J Org Chem* 1998;63:3508–3510.

193. Grieco PA, Vander Roest JM, Piñeiro-Nuñez MM, et al. Polyandrol, a C_{19} quassinoid from *Castela polyandra*. *Phytochemistry* 1995;38:1463–1465.

194. Gu JQ, Gills JJ, Park EJ, et al. Sesquiterpenoids from *Tithonia diversifolia* with potential cancer chemopreventive activity. *J Nat Prod* 2002;65:532–536.

195. Luciferase assay system # TB281, Promega Corporation. Revised 5/2000.

196. Baldwin AS. Control of oncogenesis and cancer therapy resistance by the transcription factor NF-κB. *J Clin Invest* 2001;107:241–246.

197. Mehta RG. Experimental basis for breast cancer. *Eur J Cancer* 2000;36:1275–1282.

198. Moon RC, Mehta RG, Rao KVN. Retinoids in experimental animals. In *The Retinoids: Biology, Chemistry and Medicine*. Sporn MB, Roberts AB, Goodman DS, eds. New York: Raven Press, 1997: pp. 573–595.

199. Hsieh TC, Wu JM. Grape-derived chemopreventive agent resveratrol decreases prostate-specific antigen (PSA) expression in LNCaP cells by an androgen receptor (AR)-independent mechanism. *Anticancer Res* 2000;20:225–228.

200. Zhang Y, Kensler TW, Cho CG, et al. Anticarcinogenic activity of sulforaphane and structurally related isothiocyanates. *Proc Natl Acad Sci USA* 1994;91:3147–3150.

201. Planck M. *The Philosophy of Physics*. New York: WW. Norton & Company, Inc., 1936.

2 Preclinical Animal Models for the Development of Cancer Chemoprevention Drugs

Vernon E. Steele, PhD, MPH, Ronald A. Lubet, PhD, and Richard C. Moon, PhD

CONTENTS

1. INTRODUCTION

Preclinical cell culture and animal efficacy testing models are currently used to identify, assess, and prioritize chemical agents and natural products with the aim of preventing human cancer. If little is known about a potential agent, the first step is a sequential series of short-term in vitro prescreens of mechanistic, biochemical assays. These assays provide quantitative data to help establish an early indication of chemopreventive efficacy and to assist in prioritizing agents for further evaluation in longer-term in vitro transformation bioassays and whole animal models. Promising chemical agents or combinations of agents that work through different inhibitory mechanisms are subsequently tested in well-established chemically induced or spontaneous animal tumor/cancer models, which typically include models of the colon, lung, bladder, mammary, prostate, and skin. These animal bioassays afford a strategic framework for

evaluating agents according to defined criteria, and not only provide evidence of agent efficacy, but also serve to generate valuable dose-response, toxicity, and pharmacokinetic data required prior to Phase I clinical safety testing. Based on preclinical efficacy and toxicity screening studies, only the most successful agents considered to have potential as human chemopreventives will progress into clinical chemoprevention trials.

Six key elements are necessary for the ideal animal model for chemoprevention testing: the animal model should bear relevance to human cancers, not only in terms of specific organ sites but also in producing cancerous lesions of similar pathology; the genetic abnormalities of these lesions should resemble those found in humans; the model should have relevant intermediate lesions that simulate or approximate the human cancer process both histologically and molecularly; the model should be capable of producing a consistent tumor burden of greater than 80% lesions within a reasonable period of time (less

From: Cancer Chemoprevention, Volume 2: Strategies for Cancer Chemoprevention
Edited by: G. J. Kelloff, E. T. Hawk, and C. C. Sigman © Humana Press Inc., Totowa, NJ

Table 1
Animal Models in Current Use for the Screening and Development of Chemopreventive Agents

Organ site	Species	Carcinogen[a]	Endpoint measured
Mammary gland	Rat	MNU	Adenocarcinomas
	Rat	DMBA	Adenocarcinomas and adenomas
Lung	Hamster	DEN	Adenocarcinomas
	Hamster	MNU	Squamous cell carcinomas
	Rat	NNK	Adenomas and squamous cell carcinomas
	Mouse	B[a]P, NNK, vinyl carbamate, DEN, uracil mustard, urethane, cigarette smoke	Adenomas and adenocarcinomas
Colon	Rat	AOM, IQ, PhIP	Aberrant crypts and adeno-carcinomas
Prostate	Rat	MNU	Adenocarcinomas
Bladder	Mouse	OH-BBN	Transitional cell carcinomas
	Rat	OH-BBN	Transitional cell carcinomas
Skin	Mouse	DMBA or UV	Papillomas and squamous cell carcinomas
Ovary	Rat	DMBA	Epithelial and thecal cell carcinomas
	Rat	BOP	Thecal cell carcinomas
Esophagus	Rat	NMBA	Squamous cell carcinomas
Head and neck	Rat	4NQO	Squamous cell carcinomas
	Hamster	DMBA	Squamous cell carcinomas
Pancreas	Hamster	BOP	Ductal carcinomas

[a]Abbreviations: MNU, methylnitrosourea; DMBA, dimethylbenz[a]anthracene; DEN, diethylnitrosamine; NNK, 4-(methylnitrosamino)-1-(3-pyridyl)-1-butanone; B[a]P, benzo[a]pyrene; AOM, azoxymethane; IQ, 2-amino-3-methylimidazo[4,5-f]quinoline; PhIP, 2-amino-1-methyl-6-phenylimidazo[4,5-b]pyridine; OH-BBN, N-butyl-N-(4-hydroxybutyl)nitrosamine; UV, ultraviolet light; BOP, N-nitrobis-(2-oxopropyl)amine; NMBA, N-nitroso-methylbenzylamine; 4-NQO, 4-nitroquinoline-1-oxide.

than 6 mo); the carcinogen or genetic defect used to produce cancer should bear relevance to that encountered by humans; and the predictive values and accuracy of the animal model for human efficacy should be >80% (i.e., agents positive in animal tests are positive in clinical trials and agents negative in animals are negative in clinical trials). While it is generally understood that no current animal model is ideal, research and development of better animal models is ongoing in many laboratories in an increasing variety of organ sites. In this chapter, a review of currently used animal models for chemoprevention efficacy testing will be presented (Table 1).

2. MAMMARY CANCER MODELS

A growing number of animal mammary cancer prevention models are used routinely or currently being developed. Both the 7,12-dimethylbenz[a]anthracene (DMBA)- and methylnitrosourea (MNU)-induced mammary gland carcinogenesis models are routinely used for screening. The 50-d-old rat MNU-induced cancer model is popular because it typically produces 100% incidence of adenocarcinomas within 120–150 d of carcinogen treatment (1). MNU does not require metabolic activation, and therefore cannot detect agents that alter carcinogen metabolism. In this model, 50-d-old Sprague-Dawley female rats are given a single iv injection of 50 mg MNU/kg-bw (pH 5.0). The chemopreventive agent is usually started 1 wk prior to carcinogen treatment and continued until the animals are sacrificed. Tumor multiplicity is typically 4 to 6 per animal and the latency is usually 65–80 d. Agents that are positive in this model are then usually tested in older animals, where the carcinogen is administered to 100–120-d-old animals (2). Mammary glands of older rats are more similar in terms of proliferation rates and differentiation to those of mature women. Incidence and multiplicity of cancers are lower in this case and must be compensated by having more animals per group and experimental times lengthened to 180 d. The cancers produced are hormone-dependent and are usually associated with activated *ras*. This model correctly identified the human cancer-preventive agents tamoxifen and *N*-(4-hydroxy)phenylretinamide *(3–5)*. It should be stated that this model is highly sensitive to weight loss and decreased weight gain over the course of the experiment. For example, acute reductions of body weight gain of 6, 12, or 15% at the time of MNU treatment resulted in decreased mammary cancer multiplicities of 15, 44, and 55% respectively without chemopreventive agent administration *(6,7)*.

The second mammary model commonly used is the DMBA model. Again, 50-d-old rats are given 12 mg of carcinogen ig and tumors arise within 120 d of carcinogen treatment *(8,9)*. These tumors are usually encapsulated adenocarcinomas, adenomas, and fibroadenomas that arise in approx 80–100% of the animals. DMBA is a polycyclic aromatic hydrocarbon and requires activation by the cytochrome P450 enzyme system. Therefore this model can detect agents that modulate the P450 system or detoxify carcinogens via a phase 2 enzyme system (e.g., glutathione-*S*-transferases). Tumor multiplicity is usually in the range of 3–4 per animal, and latency is similar to the MNU model at 65 to 80 d.

Recently, newer transgenic models have become more prevalent. These are covered in a separate chapter by Lubet et al., Chapter 3 in this volume.

3. LUNG CANCER MODELS

Two hamster models, the diethylnitrosamine (DEN) lung and the MNU tracheal model, have been used to evaluate the efficacy of potential chemopreventive agents in inhibiting lung cancer. The DEN model induces lung adenocarcinomas following twice-weekly sc injections of 17.8 mg DEN/kg-bw starting at 7–8 wk of age and continuing for 20 wk *(10)*. This treatment usually produces 90–100% tracheal tumors and 40–50% lung tumors in treated male Syrian golden hamsters. Serial sacrifice studies have shown that these lung tumors arise from pulmonary Clara and endocrine cells, while tracheal tumors arise from the basal cells of the trachea. Chemopreventive agents are usually administered in diet starting 1 wk prior to the first carcinogen treatment and continuing for 180 d.

The primary endpoint is percent reduction of lung tumor incidence. The pathology of these lung tumors resembles small-cell lung cancer with neuroendocrine features. In the MNU hamster tracheal model, 5% MNU in saline is administered once a week for 15 wk by a specially designed catheter that exposes a defined area of the trachea of male Syrian golden hamsters to the carcinogen *(11)*. The chemopreventive agent is supplied in the diet, or more recently by aerosol, for 180 d beginning 1 wk prior to the first carcinogen exposure. Within this time period, 40–50% of the animals acquire tracheal squamous cell carcinomas and chemopreventive efficacy is measured as a reduction in that percentage.

Another lung cancer chemoprevention model uses the tobacco-specific carcinogen 4-(methylnitrosamino)-1-(3-pyridyl)-1-butanone (NNK) to induce lung tumors in rats *(12)*. For this model, male F344 rats are given NNK (1.5 mg/kg-bw) by sc injection three times a week for 21 wk. The assay is terminated at week 98 post-carcinogen exposure; tumor incidence is determined by dividing the number of animals with cancers by the total number of animals treated. Since the tumors are very large, tumor multiplicity is not determined. The majority of animals develop lung adenomas, with fewer adenocarcinomas and occasionally a squamous cell carcinoma. In addition to lung tumors, NNK also induces nasal cavity tumors.

For the past several years, the mouse lung adenoma model has been more frequently used because it is very efficient, consistent, and reliable. Several carcinogens can cause lung adenoma, including benzo[*a*]pyrene (B[*a*]P), NNK, vinyl carbamate, DEN, uracil mustard, and urethane. In the B[*a*]P model, female Strain A/J mice at 15 wk of age are given either a single i.p. dose of 100 mg B[*a*]P/kg-bw or three ig gavages of 2 mg B[*a*]P in 0.2 mL vegetable oil with 3–4 d between dosings. The animals are then held for about 16 wk for development of pulmonary adenomas. Typically, 8–10 adenomas arise per animal with 100% incidence. In this model, the chemopreventive agent can be given either in the diet or by aerosol administration. Aerosol administration has major advantages over diet for agents with known toxicity to gastrointestinal organs and poor metabolic profiles (i.e., they are rapidly metabolized and excreted). For example, striking results have been observed by administering budesonide, a glucocorticoid, by aerosol for very short periods of time *(13,14)*. With most carcinogens (B[*a*]P, NNK, etc.) a small percentage (<10%) of adenomas eventually become carcinomas after a period of 1 yr or more.

The protocol for the NNK Strain A/J mouse model calls for female mice 6 wk of age *(15)* to be given a single dose of 10µm NNK in saline by i.p. injection. Typically 6–8 adenomas per animal develop within the 16-wk bioassay with 100% incidence. At 52 wk, adenocarcinoma incidence is about 70–80% with a multiplicity of 15–17 tumors (mostly solid alveolar adenomas plus a few adenocarcinomas) per animal. In this model, *N*-acetyl-*l*-cysteine and β-carotene had no effect on cancer incidence or multiplicity resulting from exposing respiratory epithelium to a tobacco smoke carcinogen, a result that positively correlates with that found in human studies *(16)*.

Vinyl carbamate was given to 8–9-wk-old Strain A mice by a single i.p. injection of 60mg/kg-bw in 0.2 mL saline. At 24 wk, there are typically 20–30 lung tumors per animal and about 12% are carcinomas; at 1 yr there are about 30% carcinomas *(17)*. This model, with its high tumor multiplicity and capability to produce significant frequencies of carcinomas, is attractive for lung cancer prevention studies.

Recently, tobacco smoke has been used to induce lung adenomas in the Strain A mouse model *(18)*. This animal model is important because it mimics the cancer induction process in humans by a complex mixture of chemical carcinogens and promoting agents. Strain A mice are exposed to cigarette smoke by inhalation of tobacco smoke for 5 mo followed by a 4-mo smoke-free recovery period. Both benign and malignant lung tumors are produced by this model. The tumor incidence of control animals is about 30%, while the tumor incidence in smoke-exposed animals is about 80% *(19)*.

4. COLON CANCER MODELS

The azoxymethane (AOM)-induced aberrant rat colon crypt model has become a primary whole-animal screening assay for potential chemopreventive agents due to its short time course, low cost, and requirement for only a small amount of test agent. Aberrant colon crypts are single and multiple colonic crypts containing cells exhibiting dysplasia *(20–23)*. The aberrant crypts are induced in 8-wk-old F344 rats by two injections of 15 mg AOM/kg-bw 1 wk apart. Protocols A and B are used. Under Protocol A, animals are fed the test agent diet from 1 wk before the first AOM injection to 3 wk after the first injection, for a total of 4 wk. Protocol B was designed to test the effects of the chemopreventive agent on the post-initiation phase of colon carcinogenesis. Rats receive the chemopreventive agent from 4 to 8

wk after the first AOM exposure. The AOM rat colon tumor model treats the animals similarly initially, but holds these animals on the chemopreventive agent diet until about 40 wk post-carcinogen, when cancer incidence is approx 70% and multiplicity is 1–2 tumors per animal. Both benign and malignant tumors are found at sacrifice. In the mouse model, methoxyacetyl-methane acetate, the ultimate carcinogenic metabolite of AOM, is given by ip injection (20 mg/kg-bw) once a week for 4 wk. Colon tumors appear within 38 wk after dosing *(24)*. Celecoxib, a COX-2-specific inhibitor recently approved to prevent polyps in humans, was positive in the AOM rat colon tumor model using both early and late interventions *(25)*. Other carcinogens used in primarily rat models are 2-amino-3-methylimidazo [4,5-*f*]quinoline (IQ) and 2-amino-1-methyl-6-phenylimidazo[4,5-*b*]pyridine (PhIP) *(26)*. Other animal models for colon cancer are discussed in Chapter 4 in this book by Lipkin et al.

5. PROSTATE CANCER MODELS

The MNU Bosland model, named after its developer, is a rat model that develops a high incidence of dorsolateral prostate cancer *(27)*. Male Wistar-Unilever rats are treated with 50 mg of cyproterone acetate at 8–9 wk of age, then receive daily injections of 100 mg testosterone propionate/kg-bw for 3 d. Sixty hours after the first testosterone dose, rats receive a single iv injection of MNU. Two weeks later, each rat is implanted sc with two silastic tubes containing 40 mg of crystalline testosterone. These tubes are replaced after 6 mo. The rats are sacrificed at 13 mo after the MNU injection, and the prostates are examined histologically for microscopic and macroscopic tumors in each area of the prostate and associated tissues. Typically 60–80% of the rats develop carcinomas in the dorsolateral prostate within the 13-mo time frame. It is possible to define the site of origin for small lesions (hyperplasia, carcinoma *in situ*, and small carcinomas). However, for large lesions it is often impossible to determine where the tumor originated. In this model, adenocarcinomas are malignant but rarely metastasize to distant sites.

The Lobund rat model has been used by many investigators to study prostate cancer and its prevention *(28)*. Similarly to the experimental protocol above, MNU is injected once i.v.; one wk later, testosterone pellets are implanted onto the animals' backs. The animals are sacrificed 427 d later when 25% have tumors of the accessory sex organs. Recently, however, histopathological analysis of the tumors found that cancers of the dorso-lateral prostate are the least frequent and at later stages are overgrown by cancers from other glands, such as the seminal vesicle *(29)*.

6. BLADDER CANCER MODELS

The *N*-butyl-*N*-(4-hydroxylbutyl)nitrosamine (OH-BBN)-induced mouse and rat bladder cancer models have been in use for many years with inherent advantages and disadvantages. In mice, bladder tumors induced by OH-BBN typically are transitional cell carcinomas, morphologically similar to those found in human bladder cancer *(30)*. These cancers are highly invasive and aggressive in nature. Intragastric administration of 7.5 mg OH-BBN over an 8-wk period to 50-d-old male DBF mice (C57BL/6 X DBS/2F$_1$) typically results in a 40–60% tumor incidence at 6–8 mo post-carcinogen with an average multiplicity of 0.5–0.7 tumors/mouse. A twice-weekly carcinogen treatment for 8 wk to female F344 rats results in similar transitional cell carcinomas at 8 mo, but the tumors are more papillary and slowly growing. In the rat, incidence of premaligant lesions (hyperplasias and papillomas) is near 100%, and cancer incidence is roughly 60%. Nonsteroidal antiinflammatory drugs (NSAIDs) are profoundly effective in inhibiting bladder cancer in these animal models *(31)*; recently the COX-2 inhibitor celecoxib caused a greater than 90% reduction in bladder cancers in both mice and rats *(32)*. The drug development process for the chemopreventive agents 2-difluoromethylornithine (DFMO) and oltipraz, using animal models for bladder cancer inhibition, has been reviewed *(33,34)*.

7. SKIN CANCER MODELS

Compounds effective in preventing skin carcinogenesis have typically been identified in the classical two-stage DMBA-12-*O*-tetradecanoylphorbol-13-acetate (TPA) mouse skin cancer model *(35,36)*. Both CD-1 and SENCAR mice are highly susceptible to skin tumor induction by a single DMBA dose and multiple doses of TPA applied topically over a 20-wk period. Skin papillomas appear as early as 6 wk post-carcinogen treatment, eventually progressing to squamous cell carcinomas by 18 wk *(37)*. Other carcinogens, most notably B[*a*]P, have also been used in this model to induce skin cancers *(38)*. More recently, a UV mouse skin model is gaining in use for testing chemopreventive agents due to its high relevance to the etiology of human skin cancer. Skh hairless mice are given multiple exposures to UV

irradiation over a 24-wk period and develop skin lesions in approx 30 wk. Chemopreventive test agents are either administered in the diet or applied topically to the skin. Using this protocol, 100% of the mice develop skin tumors by 34–36 wk and have tumor multiplicities of about four tumors per animal *(39)*. A number of NSAIDs and green tea polyphenols have proven effective in this model *(40,41)*.

8. OVARIAN CANCER MODELS

There is no established animal model for ovarian cancer chemoprevention studies. A potential model employs surgical implantation of thread soaked in DMBA into ovaries of Wistar-Furth rats at 7–8 wk of age *(42)*. Sterile silk thread immersed in melted DMBA allows about 200 μg DMBA to be adsorbed to the thread, which is then passed twice through the left ovary of the rats. This model appears promising due to finding that about half of the cancers are epithelial in nature, while the other half are granulosa/thecal tumors. The frequency of tumors is near 80% at 300 d post-carcinogen exposure. More than half of the cancers are poorly differentiated adenocarcinomas and the balance are mainly thecal/granulosa cell tumors (Dr. Keith Crist, Medical College of Ohio, unpublished results).

A second model currently under development also involves a carcinogen, *N*-nitrobis-(2-oxopropyl)amine (BOP), administered to Lewis rats (modified from *43,44*). At 8 and 14 d of age, the female rats are injected sc with 0.8 mg of BOP, and at 45 d of age the animals are put onto diets containing chemopreventive agents. The study typically is terminated when the animals are about 8 mo old. The cancers produced are predominately granulosa/thecal tumors (Dr. Clinton Grubbs, University of Alabama, Birmingham, unpublished results). However, only about 10% of all human ovarian cancers are granulosa/thecal in nature.

9. ESOPHAGUS CANCER MODELS

Esophageal cancers can be induced in rats by the administration of *N*-nitroso-*N*-methylbenzylamine (NMBA). Studies conducted in China indicate that *N*-nitro compounds and their precursors are possible etiological factors in human esophageal cancers *(45)*. In this model, male F344 rats are given NMBA (0.5 mg/kg-bw) by sc injection three times a week for 5 wk *(46)*. The use of this model for chemoprevention studies has recently been reviewed by leaders in its development *(47)*. The chemopreventive agents are given either in diet or in drinking water for the full 25 wk of the experiment.

Then the animals are sacrificed and the esophagi removed and cut longitudinally, fixed in neutral buffered formalin, and examined under a dissecting microscope. This model is one of the first to use computerized image morphometry to validate the modulation of very early changes only recognized by the computer against the inhibition of the cancer endpoint (48).

More recently, an esophageal anastomoses model has been developed that parallels acid reflux disease in human Barrett's esophagus (49,50).

10. HEAD AND NECK CANCER MODELS

Tumors of the head and neck are relatively common epithelial tumors in humans. Typically, tumors of this origin are associated with exposure to tobacco smoke. Cancer induction in rat tongue by 4-nitroquinoline-1-oxide (4NQO) has become a model for chemoprevention studies of head and neck cancer (51,52). Oral lesions produced in rats by 4NQO are similar to human lesions since many are ulcerated and endophytic tongue lesions (53). At 5 wk of age, rats begin exposure to 4NQO in their drinking water (20 ppm) and continue for a period of 10 wk. Chemopreventive agent administration, usually in the diet, begins 2 wk after the end of 4NQO treatment and continues for an additional 22 wk. Oral tissues are histologically examined for evidence of hyperplasia, dysplasia, and cancer. There are reports that these cancers can be prevented by garlic (54).

The DMBA-induced Syrian hamster cheek pouch cancer model is another widely accepted model of oral cancer (55,56). Carcinogenesis protocols with DMBA induce premalignant changes and squamous cell carcinomas that closely resemble human lesions (57,58). Cheek pouches of 6-wk-old noninbred Syrian hamsters are exposed topically to 0.5% DMBA in mineral oil three times a week for 14 wk. The hamster cheek pouch is an anatomically easily accessible pocket that can be readily everted for local carcinogen/preventive agent treatment and macroscopic follow-up. An advantageous and unique feature of this cheek pouch model is the possibility of timed-sequence follow-up of the evolution of intraepithelial neoplasia after DMBA treatment by simply everting the cheek pouch and visually monitoring or biopsying tissue for measurement of the endpoints. Macroscopic/molecular biochemical endpoints can eventually be correlated with histopathological studies of biopsy samples. Thus the cheek pouch tissue is amenable to using a variety of sampling techniques.

11. PANCREAS CANCER MODEL

Human pancreatic cancer has an extremely low 1-yr survival rate and current therapies are usually ineffective. One animal model being used to screen agents with potential cancer preventive activity is the hamster BOP model (59,60). Pancreatic tumors induced in Syrian hamsters resemble human pancreatic cancer in many aspects. In response to BOP, these rodents develop pancreatic ductal (ductular) carcinomas. In this model, male Syrian golden hamsters are injected sc with BOP in normal saline three times at weekly intervals. The test chemopreventive agents are administered in the diet beginning 2 wk after the last BOP exposure. Typically, a 48-wk period following the last carcinogen exposure is needed to develop sufficient tumors in the pancreas. The pancreases are histologically sectioned and scored for hyperplasias, dysplasias, and cancers.

12. CONCLUSIONS

Preclinical animal models have been used extensively in efficacy testing of potential chemopreventive agents (61–64). Standardized statistical methodology has been proposed to evaluate data from most of these animal model experiments based on the various endpoints (65). Clearly, there is much room for improving current animal models to reflect the etiology and progression of the human cancer process. There is also a need to develop animal models for testing cancer preventive agents in other organs, including brain, kidney, cervix, and lymphatic cancers. Validation of animal models for predicting efficacy of agents in human clinical trials will await further human data on positive and negative chemopreventive agents. To date, accuracy has been remarkably high, with positive correlations for tamoxifen and 4-HPR for breast cancer and aspirin and celecoxib for colon cancer, and negative correlation for β-carotene for lung cancer.

REFERENCES

1. Moon RC, Mehta RG. Chemoprevention of experimental carcinogenesis in animals. *Prev Med* 1989;18:576–591.
2. Moon RC, Kelloff GJ, Detrisac CJ, et al. Chemoprevention of MNU-induced mammary tumors in the mature rat by 4-HPR and tamoxifen. *Anticancer Res* 1992;12(4):1147–1153.
3. Gottardis MM, Jordan VC. Antitumor actions of keoxifene and tamoxifen in the *N*-nitrosomethylurea-induced rat mammary carcinoma model. *Cancer Res* 1987;47:4020–4024.
4. McCormick DL, Mehta RG, Thompson CA, et al. Enhanced inhibition of mammary carcinogenesis by combined treatment with *N*-(4-hydroxyphenyl)retinamide and ovariectomy. *Cancer Res* 1982;42:508–512.

5. Moon RC, Steele VE, Kelloff GJ, et al. Chemoprevention of MNU-induced mammary tumorigenesis by hormone modifying agents: toremifene, RU 16117, tamoxifen, aminoglutethimide and progesterone. *Anticancer Res* 1994;14:889–894.

6. Rodriguez-Burford C, Lubet RA, Eto I, et al. Effect of reduced body weight gain on the evaluation of chemopreventive agents in the methylnitrosourea (MNU)-induced mammary cancer model. *Carcinogenesis* 1999;20(1): 71–76.

7. Rodriguez-Burford C, Lubet RA, Steele VE, et al. Effects of acute and chronic body weight gain reductions in the evaluation of agents for efficacy in mammary cancer prevention. *Oncol Rep* 2001;8(2):373–379.

8. Moon RC, Grubbs CJ, Sporn MB. Inhibition of 7,12-dimethylbenz(*a*)anthracene-induced mammary carcinogenesis by retinyl acetate. *Cancer Res* 1976;36:2626–2630.

9. Grubbs CJ, Steele VE, Casebolt T, et al. Chemoprevention of chemically induced mammary carcinogenesis by indole-3-carbinol. *Anticancer Res* 1995;15:709–716.

10. Moon RC, Rao KVN, Detrisac CJ, Kelloff GJ. Hamster lung cancer model of carcinogenesis and chemoprevention. *Adv Exp Med Biol* 1992;320:55–61.

11. Moon RC, Rao KV, Detrisac CJ, et al. Chemoprevention of respiratory tract neoplasia in the hamster by oltipraz, alone and in combination. *Int J Oncol* 1994;4:661–667.

12. Hecht SS, Chen CB, Ohmori T, Hoffmann D. Comparative carcinogenicity in F344 rats of the tobacco-specific nitrosamines, *N*′-nitrosonornicotine and 4-(*N*-methyl-*N*-nitrosamino)-1-(3-pyridyl)-1-butanone. *Cancer Res* 1980;40(2):298–302.

13. Wattenberg LW, Wiedmann TS, Estensen RD, et al. Chemoprevention of pulmonary carcinogenesis by aerosolized budesonide in female A/J mice. *Cancer Res* 1997;57(24): 5489–5492.

14. Wattenberg LW, Wiedmann TS, Estensen RD, et al. Chemoprevention of pulmonary carcinogenesis by brief exposures to aerosolized budesonide or beclomethasone dipropionate and by the combination of aerosolized budesonide and dietary *myo*-inositol. *Carcinogenesis* 2000;21:179–182.

15. Castonguay A, Pepin P, Stoner GD. Lung tumorigenicity of NNK given orally to A/J mice: its application to chemopreventive efficacy studies. *Exp Lung Res* 1991;17:485–499.

16. Conway CC, Jiao D, Kelloff GJ, et al. Chemopreventive potential of fumaric acid, *N*-acetyl-*l*-cysteine, *N*-(4-hydroxyphenyl) retinamide, and β-carotene for tobacco nitrosamine induced lung tumors in A/J mice. *Cancer Lett* 1998;24(1):85–93.

17. Gunning WT, Kramer PM, Lubet RA, et al. Chemoprevention of vinyl carbamate-induced lung tumors in strain A mice. *Exp Lung Res* 2000;26(8):757–772.

18. Witschi H, Espiritu I, Maronphot R, et al. The carcinogenic potential of the gas phase of environmental tobacco smoke. *Carcinogenesis* 1997;18:2035–2032.

19. Witschi H, Espiritu I, Uyeminami D. Chemoprevention of tobacco smoke-induced lung tumors in A/J strain mice with dietary *myo*-inositol and dexamethasone. *Carcinogenesis* 1999;20(7):1375–1378.

20. Bird RP. Role of aberrant crypt foci in understanding the pathogenesis of colon cancer. *Cancer Lett* 1995;93(1): 55–71.

21. Pereira MA, Barnes LH, Rassman VL, et al. Use of azoxymethane-induced foci of aberrant crypts in rat colon to identify potential cancer chemopreventive agents. *Carcinogenesis* 1994;15(5):1049–1054.

22. Wargovich, MJ, Harris C, Chen C, et al. Growth kinetics and chemoprevention of aberrant crypts in the rat colon. *J Cell Biochem Suppl* 1992;16G:51–54.

23. Wargovich MJ, Chen CD, Jimenez A, et al. Aberrant crypts as a biomarker of colon cancer: evaluation of potential chemopreventive agents in the rat. *Cancer Epidemiol Biomarkers Prev* 1996;5:355–360.

24. Reddy BS, Maeura Y. Dose-response studies of the effect of dietary butylated hydroxyanisole on colon carcinogenesis induced by methylazoxymethanol acetate in female CF1 mice. *J Natl Cancer Inst* 1984;72(5):1181–1187.

25. Reddy BS, Hirose Y, Rao CV, et al. Chemoprevention of colon cancer by specific cyclooxygenase-2 inhibitor, celecoxib, administered during different stages of carcinogenesis. *Cancer Res* 2000;60:293–297.

26. Andreassen A, Mollersen L, Vikse R, et al. One dose of 2-amino-1-methyl-6-phenylimidazo[4,5-*b*]pyridine (PhIP) or 2-amino-3-methylimidazo[4,5-*f*]quinoline (IQ) induces tumours in Min/+ mice by truncation mutations or LOH in the Apc gene. *Mutat Res* 2002;517(1–2):157–166.

27. Bosland MC, Prinsen MK, Kroes R. Adenocarcinomas of the prostate induced by *N*-nitroso-*N*-methylurea in rats pretreated with cyproterone acetate and testosterone. *Cancer Lett* 1983;18(1):69–78.

28. Pollard M, Luckert PH. Production of autochthonous prostate cancer in Lobund-Wistar rats by treatments with *N*-nitroso-*N*-methylurea and testosterone. *J Natl Cancer Inst* 1986;77:583–587.

29. Slaytor MV, Anzano MA, Kadomatsu K, et al. Histogenesis of induced prostate and seminal vesicle carcinoma in Lobund-Wistar rats: a system for histologically scoring and grading. *Cancer Res* 1994;54:1440–1445.

30. Becci PJ, Thompson HJ, Strum JM, et al. *N*-butyl-*N*-(4-hydroxybutyl)nitrosamine-induced urinary bladder cancer in C57BL/6 X DBA/2F1 mice as a useful model for study of chemoprevention of cancer with retinoids. *Cancer Res* 1981;41:927–932.

31. Moon RC, Kelloff GJ, Detrisac CJ, et al. Chemoprevention of OH-BBN-induced bladder cancer in mice by piroxicam. *Carcinogenesis* 1993;14(7):1487–1489.

32. Grubbs CJ, Lubet RA, Koki AT, et al. Celecoxib inhibits *N*-butyl-*N*-(4-hydroxybutyl)-nitrosamine-induced urinary bladder cancer in male B6D2F1 mice and female F344 rats. *Cancer Res* 2000;60:5599–5602.

33. Kelloff GJ, Boone CW, Malone WF, et al. Development of chemopreventive agents for bladder cancer. *J Cell Biochem Suppl* 1992;16I:1–12.

34. Moon RC, Kelloff GJ, Detrisac CJ, et al. Chemoprevention of OH-BBN-induced bladder cancer in mice by oltipraz, alone and in combination with 4-HPR and DFMO. *Anticancer Res* 1994;14:5–11.

35. McCormick DL, Moon RC. Antipromotional activity of dietary *N*-(4-hydroxyphenyl)retinamide in two-stage skin tumorigenesis in CD-1 and SENCAR mice. *Cancer Lett* 1986;31:133–138.

36. Warren BS, Slaga TJ. Mechanisms of inhibition of tumor progression. *Basic Life Sci* 1993;61:279–289.

37. DiGiovanni J. Multistage carcinogenesis in mouse skin. *Pharmacol Ther* 1992;54:63–128.

38. Poel WE. Effect of carcinogen dosage and duration of exposure on skin-tumor induction in mice. *J Natl Cancer Inst* 1959;22:19–43.

39. Burke KE, Clive J, Combs GF, et al. Effects of topical and oral Vitamin E on pigmentation and skin cancer induced by ultraviolet irradiation in Skh:2 hairless mice. *Nutr Cancer* 2000;38(1):87–97.

40. Fischer SM, Lo HH, Gordon GB, et al. Chemopreventive activity of celecoxib, a specific cyclooxygenase-2 inhibitor, and indomethacin against ultraviolet light-induced skin carcinogenesis. *Mol Carcinog* 1999;25(4):231–240.

41. Lu YP, Lou YR, Lin Y, et al. Inhibitory effects of orally administered green tea, black tea, and caffeine on skin carcinogenesis in mice previously treated with ultraviolet B light (high-risk mice): relationship to decreased tissue fat. *Cancer Res* 2001;61(13):5002–5009.

42. Nishida T, Sugiyama T, Kataoka A, et al. Histologic characterization of rat ovarian carcinoma induced by intraovarian insertion of a 7,12-dimethylbenz[*a*]anthracene-coated suture: common epithelial tumors of the ovary in rats? *Cancer* 1998;83(5):965–970.

43. Pour PM. Transplacental induction of gonadal tumors in rats by a nitrosamine. *Cancer Res* 1986;46:4135–4138.

44. Pour PM, Redding TW, Paz-Bouza JI, Schally AV. Treatment of experimental ovarian carcinoma with monthly injection of the agonist D-Trp-6-LH-RH: a preliminary report. *Cancer Lett* 1988;41:105–110.

45. Yang CS. Research on esophageal cancer in China: a review. *Cancer Res* 1980;40:2633–2644.

46. Lijinsky W, Saavedra JE, Reuber MD, Singer SS. Esophageal carcinogenesis in F344 rats by nitrosomethylamines substituted in the ethyl group. *J Natl Cancer Inst* 1982;68:681–684.

47. Stoner GD, Gupta A. Etiology and chemoprevention of esophageal squamous cell carcinoma. *Carcinogenesis* 2001;22(11):1737–1146.

48. Boone CW, Stoner GD, Bacus JV, et al. Chemoprevention with theaflavins of rat esophageal intraepithelial neoplasia quantitatively monitored by image tile analysis. *Cancer Epidemiol Biomarkers Prev* 2000;9(11):1149–1154.

49. Chen X, Yang G-Y, Bondoc WD, et al. An esophagogastro-duodenal anastomosis model for esophageal adenocarcinogenesis in rats and enhancement by iron overload. *Carcinogenesis* 1999;20:1801–1807.

50. Chen X, Yang CS. Esophageal adenocarcinoma: a review and perspectives on the mechanism of carcinogenesis and chemoprevention. *Carcinogenesis* 2001;22:1119–1129.

51. Ohne M, Omori K, Kobayashi A, et al. Induction of squamous cell carcinoma in the oral cavity of rats by oral administration of 4-nitroquinoline-1-oxide (4NQO) in drinking water. A preliminary report. *Bull Tokyo Dent Coll* 1981;22(2):85–98.

52. Ohne M, Satoh T, Yamada S, Takai H. Experimental tongue carcinoma of rats induced by oral administration of 4-nitroquinoline 1-oxide (4NQO) in drinking water. *Oral Surg Oral Med Oral Pathol* 1985;59(6):600–607.

53. Gerson SJ. Oral cancer. Review. *Crit Rev Oral Biol Med* 1990;1(3):153–166.

54. Balasenthil S, Ramachandran CR, Nagini S. Prevention of 4-nitroquinoline 1-oxide-induced rat tongue carcinogenesis by garlic. *Fitoterapia*. 2001;72(5):524–531.

55. Salley JJ. Experimental carcinogenesis in the cheek pouch of the Syrian hamster. *J Dent Res* 1954;33:253–262.

56. Gimenez-Conti I. The hamster cheek pouch carcinogenesis model. *Acta Odontol Latinoam* 1993;7(1):3–12.

57. Morris L. Factors influencing experimental carcinogenesis in the hamster cheek pouch. *J Dent Res* 1961;40:3–15.

58. Santis H, Shklar G, Chauncey C. Histochemistry of experimentally induced leukoplakia and carcinoma of the hamster buccal pouch. *Oral Surg Oral Med Oral Pathol* 1964;17:207–218.

59. Pour PM, Salmasi SZ, Runge RG. Selective induction of pancreatic ductular tumors by single doses of *N*-nitrosobis(2-oxopropyl)amine in Syrian golden hamsters. *Cancer Lett* 1978:4(6):317–323.

60. Pour PM, Runge RG, Birt D, et al. Current knowledge of pancreatic carcinogenesis in the hamster and its relevance to the human disease. *Cancer* 1981;47(6 Suppl):1573–1589.

61. Boone CW, Steele VE, Kelloff GJ. Screening for chemopreventive (anticarcinogenic) compounds in rodents. *Mutat Res* 1992;267(2):251–255.

62. Steele VE, Boone CW, Kelloff GJ. Strategies for development of chemopreventive agents. *Comments Toxicol* 1993;4(5):427–436.

63. Kelloff GJ, Boone CW, Malone W, Steele VE. Recent results in preclinical and clinical drug development of chemopreventive agents at the National Cancer Institute. *Basic Life Sci* 1993;61:373–386.

64. Steele VE, Moon RC, Lubet RA, et al. Preclinical efficacy evaluation of potential chemopreventive agents in animal carcinogenesis models: methods and results from the NCI Chemoprevention Drug Development Program. *J Cell Biochem Suppl* 1994;20:32–54.

65. Freedman LS, Midthune DC, Brown CC, et al. Statistical analysis of animal cancer chemoprevention experiments. *Biometrics* 1993;49(1):259–268.

3   Potential Use of Transgenic Mice in Chemoprevention Studies

Ronald A. Lubet, PhD, Jeffrey Green, MD,
Vernon E. Steele, PhD, MPH, and Ming You, MD, PhD

CONTENTS

1. WHAT IS A TRANSGENIC ONCOMOUSE AND WHY WOULD I WANT ONE?

An oncomouse is a transgenic mouse in which the germline has been manipulated to overexpress certain genes or to delete certain genes so that the resulting mice will be more susceptible to developing cancer. For example, if a mutated copy of the epidermal growth factor receptor (EGFR)2/*neu* oncogene is placed on an murine mammary tumorvirus (MMTV) promoter (which is preferentially expressed in mammary epithelial cells), the resulting mice develop mammary tumors *(1)*. In addition, if specific genes are knocked out—e.g., p53 in the germline of the mouse—the resulting animals will preferentially develop certain forms of cancer *(2)*. Many of the earlier knockout models entailed knockout of the gene during embryogenesis and in all tissues. More sophisticated methods currently available allow knockout (or expression) of genes in very specific target cells *(3)* and at specific times during development. Furthermore, by crossbreeding transgenic mice, one may be able to make highly specific compound mice that are a more nearly "ideal" model of human cancer *(4)*.

Electronic searching of cancer websites using the search terms "transgenic mice" and "cancer" shows more than 3000 hits, roughly 1000 of which were published since the year 2000. This attests to the great interest in and potential of transgenic models in delving into many of the most basic questions related to cancer.

2. POTENTIAL USES OF ANIMAL MODELS IN CHEMOPREVENTION

In at least three areas in the field of chemoprevention, animal models may have great potential: developing surrogate endpoint biomarkers (SEBs), developing markers of early detection, and screening for potential chemopreventive agents. The third area will be the primary focus of this short review, but we will briefly discuss the other two areas.

2.1. SEBs

Animal models may be particularly useful in developing modulatable endpoint (surrogate) biomarkers. In fact, large trials employing tumor incidence as the primary endpoint, such as the trial of tamoxifen in prevention of breast cancer *(5)* that examined 12,000 women for a period of roughly 5 yr, cannot, because of their great cost and duration, be employed to examine a wide range of possible chemopreventive agents. Rather, agents are likely

From: Cancer Chemoprevention, Volume 2: Strategies for Cancer Chemoprevention
Edited by: G. J. Kelloff, E. T. Hawk, and C. C. Sigman © Humana Press Inc., Totowa, NJ

to be screened for potential human efficacy in Phase II trials using populations at relatively high risk and employing SEBs, biological parameters (histologic, biochemical, radiologic) whose expression is altered by a chemopreventive agent. The alteration in SEB expression should parallel the effect of the chemopreventive agent on the primary endpoint, cancer incidence.

One potential set of SEBs could be histopathologic biomarkers, e.g., blocking formation of and/or reversing dysplasia. Studies in humans show that surgical removal of colon polyps profoundly decreases the incidence of colon cancer *(6)*. Similarly, epidemiologic studies show that nonsteroidal antiinflammatory drugs (NSAIDs, e.g., aspirin, ibuprofen, piroxicam) prevent the formation of colon adenomas and colon carcinomas and decrease the rate of colon cancer mortality in a similar manner. These results support the use of blocking the formation of new adenomas or reversing the existence of dysplastic adenomas as an acceptable SEB for a colon cancer chemoprevention trial. Unfortunately for preinvasive lesions of many other organ sites, e.g., ductal carcinoma *in situ* (DCIS) in the breast or prostatic intraepithelial neoplasia (PIN) in the prostate, such clear associations have not been shown. Support from animal studies may be required to help establish such a rationale.

In the area of biochemical surrogates, animal experiments showed that decreasing aflatoxin B_1 (AFB_1)-induced macromolecular damage (DNA and protein adducts) caused strong decreases in AFB_1-induced carcinogenesis, providing the rationale for examining the same endpoints in human chemoprevention trials of both oltipraz and chlorophyllin *(7,8)*. The advantage of examining these SEBs in animal models is that one can follow animals to an invasive cancer endpoint. The potential use of animals in the development of surrogates is particularly important because most agents employed in human cancer prevention trials will have undergone similar successful testing in animal trials in the same organ.

2.2. Early Detection

A second use of animal models may be helping to discover and potentially optimize markers of early detection. Animal models in which preinvasive lesions and cancers develop in a routine and predictable manner allow samples to be taken at multiple time points to determine whether specific endpoints (histopathologic, biochemical, genetic, or imaging) may be able to predict or detect invasive cancer prior to gross observation. Certain early detection markers may simultaneously prove useful as SEBs.

2.3. Screening for Chemopreventive Agents

The third and perhaps most obvious use for animal models is to screen for potential chemopreventive agents. Relevant models can be used to determine the efficacy of potential chemopreventive agents, at what point during tumor progression an agent is effective, and whether limited exposure to a given chemopreventive agent might be effective.

3. WHAT IS AN 'IDEAL' TRANSGENIC ANIMAL MODEL?

A variety of criteria contribute to an "ideal" model. Tumors should have a **histopathology** similar to the human disease *(9)*. **Oncogenes or knockout genes** that drive the model should parallel changes that are observed in the human disease; optimally, these over-expressed oncogenes or knocked-out genes should be altered early in progression of the human disease. Models should **respond to known effective therapeutic or chemopreventive agents**. Models should also **respond to known modifiers**—e.g., hormonal stimulation, diet—in the predicted manner. Cancers in the model should **metastasize** to the correct location (i.e., similar to human cancers). Certain additional criteria that may turn out to be of the greatest importance in validating a model, e.g., similarities of **altered gene expression** (RNA or protein) and **genetic alterations** (mutations, deletions, amplifications, recombinations) that are similar to those of their human counterparts, are still at relatively early stages in development *(10)*. However, these comparisons are likely to become routine in the next few years. Transgenic mice can be created that will develop virtually any type of cancer. However, models that **incorporate known etiologic agents**, e.g., tobacco smoke or AFB_1 to enhance tumorigenesis, may be useful particularly if screening for agents that block the early initiation stages of carcinogenesis.

Which of these criteria is most important may depend on the specific objective of the study. For example, although the development of metastasis at the proper site is of paramount importance in developing therapies for metastatic cancer, it may be less important when screening for agents that will prevent cancer.

3.1. Ideal Animal Models and Human Cancer

Certain forms of cancer (breast, lung) may be particularly difficult to model and may require several types of transgenic mice for a given tumor type. Human breast cancer is apparently multiple diseases, as defined by genome analysis *(11,12)*. Roughly two-thirds of these cancers are estrogen-receptor (ER)α positive, and although there may be subcategories within this group, most are responsive to hormonal therapies. However, the one-third of breast cancers that are ER-negative are apparently driven by at least three discrete mechanisms. One mechanism involves amplification and overexpression of *neu*, a second is related to mutations in the BRCA1 gene, and a third set may have a different cell of origin, specifically basal cell instead of luminal cell. Although it may ultimately be shown that one or two agents can effectively "prevent" these various "diseases," at this time specific preventive approaches may have to be developed for each subset. In fact, the monoclonal antibody Herceptin® is effective only against tumors that highly overexpress *neu (13)*. Thus, it is unreasonable to expect any single animal model of breast cancer to simultaneously model this variety of diseases.

In the following section, we have outlined a limited number of transgenic/mutant models, most of which have been employed in chemoprevention studies. These include models of prostate, breast, lung, and cervical cancers. The final section examines the use of transgenic models bearing an alteration in the p53 tumor suppressor oncogene, which may be relevant to cancer in a wide variety of organs.

4. POTENTIAL PROBLEMS ASSOCIATED WITH TRANSGENIC MODELS IN CHEMOPREVENTION STUDIES

The relevance to human disease is probably the primary criterion for employing any particular animal model. However, there are problems that may be unique to the use of transgenics in chemoprevention studies.

4.1. Alteration in Promoter Expression

If an agent blocks the expression of the oncogene by blocking expression of the promoter, decreased cancer incidence may be observed for a "trivial" reason. For example, flutamide, initially reported to strongly decrease tumorigencsis in the transgenic adenocarcinoma of the mouse prostate (TRAMP) model, has subsequently been shown to severely decrease expression of the probasin promoter *(14,15)*, a not-unexpected result since the probasin promoter has multiple androgen-responsive elements *(16)*. In this case, although a decrease in tumorigenesis was described, the primary effect may have been that flutamide decreased expression of the probasin promoter and thus its associated oncogene. It may be relatively easy to determine if an agent highly effective in blocking tumorigenesis strongly affects the expression of the promoter. However, if the effects of an agent are modest, it may be difficult to clearly differentiate effects on expression of the promoter and its linked oncogene vs. direct effect on tumor cells.

4.2. Use of Complex Transgenic Mouse Models

A compound transgenic mouse with a heterozygous mutation of the adenomatous polyposis coli (APC) gene and homozygous knockout of the DNA repair gene MSH2 has been employed for studying intestinal cancer *(17)*. Since mice with MSH-2 gene knockout or APC mutation are not routinely bred in the homozygous state, this model crosses mice that have a mutant APC gene and heterozygous MSH-2 knockout gene. From such a cross, only one of eight mice will have the correct genotype. If 50% of the mice develop tumors and 25 tumors are needed in the control group, this requires breeding and genotyping 400 progeny per group. A study employing controls and two doses of an agent requires a huge breeding and genotyping effort. These logistical questions are raised for any studies employing relatively complex compound transgenics, e.g., tissue-specific knockouts combined with a second transgene.

5. TRANSGENIC MOUSE MODELS OF MAJOR EPITHELIAL CANCER SITES

5.1. Prostate Models

Substantial efforts have been made in the development of transgenic models for prostate cancer. There are two major problems with these models. First, the rodent prostate does not appear to be anatomically comparable to the human prostate. While the rodent prostate can be defined into ventral, anterior, and dorsal lateral lobes, no similar distinction can be observed in humans. In contrast, the human prostate is separated into peripheral and transition zones. Second, a wide variety of genetic changes are associated with prostate cancer, as demonstrated by loss of heterozygosity. However, one or two genetic changes or mutations associated with the preponderance of prostate cancer that occur early in the progression of the disease have not been defined. Therefore, it is not obvious which potential genes would be the primary candidates for creating an "ideal" transgenic model of prostate cancer.

The two main categories of transgenic mice developed for prostate cancer have used either relatively strong viral oncogenes, e.g., SV-40 T antigen, or a relatively heterogenous group of potential oncogenic transgenes, including overexpression of insulin-like growth factor (IGF)-1 or c-*myc*, knockout of PTEN, and germline or conditional knockout of the homeobox transcription factor nkx3.1.

At least two models employ T antigen to produce tumors in the prostate. The so-called TRAMP model *(18)* places T antigen on a minimal probasin promoter; the C3(1) mouse places large T antigen on the C3(1) promoter *(19)*, which codes for a sex hormone binding protein expressed in the prostate. Interestingly, lesion histopathology in these models is similar to human disease. The TRAMP model results in highly malignant tumors in almost 100% of the animals; these tend to metastasize to multiple organs, although not to bone (a primary site of human prostate cancer metastases). Both transgenic models tend to show limited dependence on hormones (orchiectomy has limited effects). Viral SV-40 T antigen affects the widest variety of oncogenes and tumor suppressor genes, including *Rb*, p53, *akt*, etc. Another major viral oncogene model, designated LADY, employs the probasin promoter with large T antigen alone *(20)*. However, though the two SV-40 T antigen models develop tumors quite rapidly, most human prostate cancers develop quite slowly; also, at least at the stage of invasive cancer, both LADY and TRAMP tend to express neuroendocrine markers. Such markers are infrequently associated with human prostate cancer, which certainly raises the question of whether the cell of origin is similar.

Due in major part to its availability, the TRAMP model has been employed in a wide variety of chemoprevention studies. Two antihormonal agents, the antiandrogen flutamide *(14)* and the antiestrogen toremifene *(15)*, have been reported as effective in this model. Interestingly, the flutamide results were contradicted in a more recent paper by the same group detailing their findings that the anticarcinogenic effects reported in their initial paper may have been due to flutamide profoundly decreasing expression of the probasin promoter, resulting in decreased expression of T antigen, and not by directly reducing prostate tumorigenesis. At least two groups have reported preventive efficacy from nonhormonal agents in this model. Wechter et al. showed that *R*-flurbiprofen *(21)* was effective, while Gupta and coworkers demonstrated significant efficacy with 2-difluoromethylornithine (DFMO), a specific suicide inhibitor of ornithine decarboxylase (ODC) *(22)*, and green tea polyphenols *(23)*.

The more eclectic group of other prostate models include a model in which the keratin 5 promoter drives

IGF-1 *(24)*; a model in which the homeobox transcription factor nfk1.3 has been knocked out either in the germline or, more recently, conditionally in the prostate *(25,26)*; and a compound model involving knockout of PTEN plus nfk3.1. All three of these are relatively recent models, having been reported only since 1999. There is some discussion at this time whether these models by themselves develop invasive cancers or tend to stop at higher levels of dysplasia or PIN.

As these models are relatively recent, it is not surprising that their use for therapy or prevention has been limited. Preliminary results with the IGF-1 model have shown that a number of dietary interventions appear to be relatively ineffective in blocking the formation of lesions in this model (Dr. John DiGiovanni, University of Texas M. D. Anderson Cancer Center, unpublished results).

5.2. Breast Cancer Models

At least two significant problems are associated with developing transgenic models of mammary cancer. The first is the purely practical. A mammary-specific transgenic model must employ a promoter that is expressed in mammary epithelial cells. The two primary promoters are MMTV-long terminal repeat (LTR) or whey acidic protein (WAP). Both these promoters are optimally expressed only after an animal has undergone pregnancy and lactation. This has a practical impact on how studies can be performed, and has the slightly disconcerting aspect that pregnancy, which inhibits most breast cancer in humans, is required to achieve tumorigenesis in the model. Second, one or two clearly defined genes that undergo consistent and early mutation in the preponderance of both sporadic and familial breast cancers are lacking, although individuals with germline mutations in BRCA1, BRCA2, or p53 develop breast cancer at a very high rate.

Despite this lack of one or two obvious candidate oncogenes for breast cancer, a wide variety of transgenic models of breast cancer exist. Certain of these models have employed potent oncogenes derived from viruses such as SV-40 T antigen, Polyoma T antigen, or a variety of mutated forms of the *ras* oncogenes (H, N, or Ki) *(28)*. In addition, a number of models employing genes known to exhibit altered expression in human breast cancer have been employed, e.g., cyclin D1, cyclin E, *wnt*-1, and a variety of models based on overexpression of the *neu* oncogene. One of the most intriguing transgenic models recently described found that mice that overexpress cyclooxygenase (COX)-2 in the mammary gland develop invasive mammary cancer that eventually metastasizes *(29)*. This transgenic mouse model may tell us about the role of COX-2 in mammary cancer and might serve as a model for screening chemopreventive agents as well. One would think that a pure COX-2 inhibitor would be highly effective, but given that COX-2 is the specific oncogene driving this model, this might be considered a trivial experiment.

We will initially discuss two models, not necessarily because they are the two "best" models, but because they have been used in various prevention studies. Amplification or overexpression of the nonmutated *neu* gene appears to be associated with a significant number of human breast cancers, roughly 20%, and is observed relatively early during carcinogenesis, having routinely been observed at the preinvasive stage of ductal carcinoma. Overexpression of the normal *neu* oncogene in animals may not be sufficient for cancer to occur. However, the use of a mutated *neu* oncogene has proven to be a profoundly effective oncogenic transgene in both mice and rats *(1,28,30)*. Although it has recently been shown that a transgene highly expressing nonmutated *neu* may develop solitary tumors, it appears that the preponderance of the palpable tumors that develop have acquired mutated *neu*. These *neu*-expressing models have been the primary focus of a variety of studies examining the ability of vaccines directed against the *neu* oncogene to prevent breast cancer *(31)*. In fact, a number of these immunizations have been able to overcome the tolerance that one might expect in such a transgenic animal and have achieved preventive efficacy and, even more recently, therapeutic efficacy. An immunization approach would be particularly appealing as a preventive strategy. More recently, a limited number of chemoprevention studies of retinoids employing this model have shown at least some promise *(32,33)*.

The C31 SV-40 T antigen model develops multiple invasive, hormonally nonresponsive mammary tumors. A number of agents have demonstrated efficacy in this model, including 9-*cis*-retinoic acid (a RAR/RXR receptor pan-agonist) *(34)*, dehydroepiandrosterone (DHEA), a steroid precursor to both androgens and estrogens that alters the hormonal milieu, and DFMO *(35)*. All three agents showed moderate efficacy in this model. Interestingly, though DFMO had a limited effect on preinvasive lesion development, it had a much more striking effect on cancers, implying that most of DFMO's effects may occur in later stages of tumor development. This is an example of using animal models to examine at what stage during tumor development an agent is

effective. This model has also undergone preliminary use in examining the effects of immunologic interventions, specifically a combination of interleukins 2 and 12, and has demonstrated strong efficacy *(36)*.

One interesting transgenic model of breast cancer employs BRCA conditional knockouts. The first model knocked out the BRCA1 gene in the breast. In this case, the CRE recombinase gne gene that specifically cuts out a portion of the BRCA1 gene has been attached to an MMTV promoter. When an animal goes through pregnancy, exon 11 of the BRCA1 gene, which previously had LOX_1 sites inserted flanking it, is specifically cut out in the breast epithlelia at high frequency *(3)*. The resulting model appears to have a variable histopathology similar to that observed in humans and appears to display a variety of genetic changes, including alterations in the p53 gene, which are similarly associated with the preponderance of breast cancers in women with BRCA1 mutations. The palpable tumors that arise in this model are ERα-negative, as are the preponderance of human BRCA1 tumors. This approach of conditional or tissue-specific knockout is likely to prove applicable to a variety of tumor-related genes that cannot be knocked out in the germline because of the embryotoxic effects of such a genotype *(3)*. Initial studies in these mice have demonstrated that early ovariectomy delays the formation of tumors despite the fact that the majority of advanced tumors are ERα-negative *(37)*. The breeding requirements of this model—CRE MMTV, LOXed BRCA1 gene, knockout of at least a copy of p53—are relatively complex, and it is difficult to imagine routine screening for effective chemopreventive agents in such a model. A similar tissue-specific knockout model for BRCA2, the other major hereditary form of breast cancer in humans, has recently been reported *(38)*.

5.3. Lung Cancer Models

Though it is the most common cause of cancer death in both men and women, lung cancer has a relative dearth of animal models, in part because, despite a high incidence of genetic alterations in human lung cancer (e.g., p53, *Rb*, *p16*, *FHIT*, Ki-*ras*,etc.), there is no clear-cut early genetic mutation comparable to that observed in colon cancer. Furthermore, unlike cancers in the colon, breast, kidney, and so on, there are no striking examples of lung cancer families. However, the high incidence of lung cancer in male Li-Fraumeni individuals who smoke certainly indirectly argues that p53 is a strong susceptibility gene for lung cancer. Employing a mouse strain with a dominant negative p53 mutation in conjunction with organotropic carcinogens to induce lung adenomas in A/J × FVB F1 mice *(39)*, we found the chemopreventive agents dexamethasone and green tea both equally effective in mice with or without the p53 mutation. Interestingly, the A/J mouse itself, at least when dealing with adenomas of the lung, functions as a spontaneously occurring mutant mouse. Although a variety of susceptibility genes are observed in A/J mice with regards to lung adenoma formation, the most striking susceptibility gene relates to a profound sensitivity of the Ki-*ras* gene of the A/J mouse mutations induced by a wide variety of carcinogens *(40)*. Thus in F_1 crosses between A/J and certain other mouse strains, the resulting chemically induced adenomas demonstrate mutations in the Ki-*ras* gene of the A/J parental allele and not in the allele from the other parent. This is particularly interesting since Ki-*ras* is a major oncogene in human lung adenomas as well. A major limitation of modeling lung cancer in rodents has not been possible to use the primary environmental inducer of lung cancer (cigarette smoke) in animal models. However, recent results by Witschi et al. *(41)*, more recently confirmed by D'Agostini et al. *(42)*, imply that this is at least possible, albeit technically difficult.

In addition to the p53 model, a number of studies have examined employing SV-40 T antigen as a oncogenic transgene, in which SV-40 T antigen has been placed under the control of a surfactant promoter *(43)*. Although it is obviously not a cause of human lung cancer, using SV-40 T antigen in lung models nevertheless seems rational, since changes in both p53 and *Rb* commonly appear in various types of lung cancer. At present, these SV-40 models do not appear to have been routinely used to determine efficacy of chemopreventive agents.

Three interesting lung cancer transgenics have been reported in the last few years; two involve use of mice driven by Ki-*ras* mutations. In the first model, investigators accomplished a knock in of mutated Ki-*ras (44)*. In the second model, investigators have achieved expression of the mutated Ki-*ras* oncogene in the lung *(45)*. Similar to the A/J mouse, these models develop mostly adenomas and adenocarcinomas driven by Ki-*ras* mutations. One of the most striking aspects of the second model *(45)* is that when expression of the mutated Ki-*ras* is turned off, even for a few days, rapid regression is obtained of even fairly large lesions that histologically appear to be carcinomas. Most recently, a transgenic model of small-cell lung cancer (SCLC) has

been reported in which the *Rb* gene has been knocked out in the lung. The resulting tumors appear histologically typical of SCLC and have expressed certain of the neuroendocrine markers typical of SCLC *(45a)*. Finally, a squamous cell model of lung cancer in mice has been reported *(45b)*.

5.4. Human Papilloma Virus (HPV)-Related Model of Cervical and Skin Cancer

HPV appears to be the primary determinant of cervical cancer, which, although readily treatable when identified early, kills roughly 200,000 women annually in the third world. HPV also appears to be associated with almost all cases of anal cancer and with a significant percentage of cancers of the larynx and squamous cell skin carcinomas that arise in transplant patients. No clear animal model for HPV infection and cancer exists, because HPV does not infect rodent cells. Approximately 8 yr ago, a transgenic model was developed in which the E6 and E7 proteins of HPV 16 were placed under the control of the keratin 14 promoter *(46)*. The resulting transgenic mice developed skin cancers (ear and chest) and anal dysplasia; female mice stimulated with exogenous estrogen developed cervical cancer.

Initial studies in this model found that DFMO strongly inhibited the development of skin cancers when administered at start of weaning *(47)*. Interestingly, treatment of mice with preexisting skin lesions resulted in reversal of most lesions within a 6-wk period. These chemopreventive effects correlated with the effects of DFMO on levels of functional ODC activity in the lesions. Studies with this agent in female mice administered exogenous estrogen showed that DFMO decreased the incidence of cervical cancer by roughly 50% (Dr. Jeffrey Arbeit, University of California, San Francisco). In contrast to the results in skin, late administration of DFMO did not significantly affect the incidence of cervical cancer. Jin et al. have used this model to determine the effects of indole-3-carbinol, which showed moderate levels of chemopreventive efficacy *(48)*.

6. MICE BEARING ALTERATIONS IN THE P53 TUMOR SUPPRESSOR GENE

p53 is perhaps the most commonly mutated tumor suppressor gene in human beings, altered in a high percentage of epithelial cancers, including those of the lung, colon, breast, ovary, bladder, head and neck, and skin (squamous cell carcinoma or basal cell cancer). p53 is mutated in a variety of nonepithelial cell cancers as well. In contrast, it is infrequently altered in most spontaneous or chemically induced cancer in rodents, with the exception of UV-induced skin cancers. When p53 is knocked out or mutated in mice, a variety of cancers occurs, most commonly lymphomas and soft-tissue sarcomas. Although the latter are observed in humans with germline mutations in p53 (Li-Fraumeni syndrome), a number of common epithelial cancers are associated with the syndrome, specifically breast cancer in women and lung cancer in male smokers with Li-Fraumeni genotype. In contrast, breast and lung cancer have not typically been observed in mice with an altered p53 genotype. Hursting and colleagues (49) have employed heterozygous or homozygous p53 knockout mice to examine the chemopreventive effects of various agents, including DHEA, fluasterone (a fluorinated analog of DHEA), and vitamin E. A number of these agents were effective in altering survival and cancer incidence. However, these studies have primarily involved examining the effects of agents on nonepithelial cancers such as lymphomas or osteosarcomas.

A second type of model employing a dominant negative mutation in the p53 gene has also been developed (39,50,51). This model results in mice containing normal p53 alleles in addition to three copies of the dominant negative p53 gene under the control of its endogenous promoter. This model, like the p53 knockouts, results in a high incidence of lymphomas, some osteosarcomas, and a low but significant incidence of lung cancers. Interestingly, the knockout p53, in either the heterozygous or homozygous state, as well as mice containing the dominant negative p53 mutation, have proven susceptible to a wide variety of chemical carcinogens. Employing these specific strains of mice and organ-specific chemical carcinogens, it has been possible to generate cancers in situ containing this most common of human tumor suppressor mutations. Because mutations in p53 often decrease the susceptibility of tumors to various therapies, the presence of tumors with mutations in p53 may have an advantage in examining potential new therapies. Interestingly, certain forms of chemically induced cancers appear to be particularly susceptible to this altered p53 status. Thus, administering a variety of lung carcinogens (benzo(a)pyrene, 4-(methylnitrosamino)-1-(3-pyridyl)-1-butanone,

vinylcarbamate) to mice with dominant negative p53 greatly increased the numbers of lung lesions (39). Treatment with 1,2-dimethylhydrazine, expected to be a colon-specific carcinogen, greatly increased the incidence of lung cancer, liver cancer, and uterine sarcomas in mice with a dominant negative p53 mutation when compared to p53 wild-type litter mates (51a). In contrast, the presence of the dominant negative p53 only modestly increased the incidence of colon cancers and failed to increase the number of bladder cancers induced by nitrosamines (50).

Lung studies employing this model showed that the chemopreventive efficacy of dexamethasone and green tea in lung are independent of p53 status. Recent studies have examined the efficacy of farnesyltransferase inhibitors or an herbal mixture in these mice (51a,51b). Studies in mice administered 1,2-dimethylhydrazine demonstrated that the NSAID piroxicam was effective in preventing colon cancer in p53 mutant or wild-type mice, but failed to inhibit the induction of uterine sarcomas, lung cancer, or hepatomas. This demonstrates the organ specificity of most chemopreventive agents.

In addition, mice with a knockout of p53 have been employed to generate compound transgenic mice with heightened tumorigenic response. This procedure has been used to increase the breast cancer incidence in BRCA1 knockout mice (4) and the incidence of desmoid lesions in mice with APC mutations (52). An additional model with specific expression of mutated p53 in mammary glands has been reported (53). In this model, MMTV promoter was used to cause expression of the mutated p53. Interestingly, these mice did not develop spontaneous mammary tumors but were highly susceptible to induction of mammary tumors by 7,12-dimethylbenz[a]anthracene.

In summary, transgenic mice would appear to have great potential in the field of chemoprevention, both in screening for potential prevention agents as well as in identifying modulatable markers. Nevertheless, potential problems—modulation of expression of the promoter controlling the transgene and complex genotypes involving multiple matings—may make it difficult to employ these models. Finally, experiments employing specific inhibitors of the transgene, e.g., EGFR inhibitors in a model driven by an EGFR transgene, may not be terribly informative about human tumors, which have a constellation of changes in addition to EGFR overexpression.

REFERENCES

1. Muller W, Sinn E, Pattengale PK, et al. Single-step induction of mammary adenocarcinoma in transgenic mice bearing the activated c-*neu* oncogene. *Cell* 1988;54:105–115.

2. Donehower LA. The p53-deficient mouse: a model for basic and applied cancer studies. *Semin Cancer Biol* 1996;7:269–278.

3. Deng CX, Brodie SG. Knockout models and mammary tumorigenesis. *Semin Cancer Biol* 2001;11:387–394.

4. Xu X, Wagner KU, Larson D, et al. Conditional mutation of BRCA1 in mammary epithelial cells results in blunted ductal morphogenesis and tumour formation. *Nat Genet* 1999;22:37–43.

5. Fisher B, Constantino JP, Wickerham DL, et al. Tamoxifen for prevention of breast cancer: report of the National Surgical Adjuvant Breast and Bowel Project P-1 study. *J Natl Cancer Inst* 1998;90:1371–1388.

6. Umar A, Viner J, Hawk E. The future of colon cancer prevention. *Ann NY Acad Sci* 2001;952:88–108.

7. Wang JS, Huang T, Su J, et al. Hepatocellular carcinoma and alflatoxin exposure in Zhuqing Village, Fusui County, People's Republic of China. *Cancer Epidemiol Biomarkers Prev* 2001;10: 143–146.

8. Egner PA, Wang JB, Zhu YR, et al. Chlorophyllin intervention reduces aflatoxin-DNA adducts in individuals at high risk for liver cancer. *Proc Natl Acad Sci USA* 2001;98:14601–14606.

9. Cardiff RD, Anver MR, Gusterson BA, et al. The mammary pathology of genetically engineered mice: the consensus report and recommendations from the Annapolis meeting. *Oncogene* 2000;19:968–988.

10. Desai KV, Xiao N, Wang W, et al. Initiating oncogenic event determines gene-expression patterns of human breast cancer models. *Proc Natl Acad Sci USA* 2002;14:6967–6972.

11. Perou CM, Sorlie T, Eisen MB, et al. Molecular portraits of human breast tumours. *Nature* 2000;406:747–752.

12. van't Veer LJ, Dai H, van de Vijver MJ, et al. Gene expression profiling predicts clinical outcome of breast cancer. *Nature* 2002;415:530–536.

13. Piccart-Gephart MJ. Herceptin: the future in adjuvant breast cancer therapy. *Anticancer Drugs* 2001;4:S27–S33.

14. Raghow S, Hooshdaran MZ, Katiyar S, Steiner MS. Toremifene prevents prostate cancer in the transgenic adenocarcinoma of the mouse prostate model. *Cancer Res* 2002;62:1370–1376.

15. Raghow S, Kuliyev E, Steakley M, et al. Efficacious chemoprevention of primary prostate cancer by flutamide in an autochthonous transgenic model. *Cancer Res* 2000;60: 4093–4097.

16. Zhang J, Thomas TZ, Kasper S, Matusik RJ. A small composite probasin promoter confers high levels of prostate-specific gene expression through regulation by androgens and glucocorticoids in vitro and in vivo. *Endocrinology* 2000;141:4698–4710.

17. Lal G, Ash C, Hay K, et al. Suppression of intestinal polyps in MSH-2 deficient and non- MSH-2 deficient multiple intestinal neoplasia mice by a specific cyclooxygenase-2 inhibitor and by a dual cyclooxygenase-1/2 inhibitor. *Cancer Res* 2001;61:6131–6136.

18. Greenberg NM, De Mayo F, Finegold MJ, et al. Prostate cancer in a transgenic mouse. *Proc Natl Acad Sci USA* 1995;92:3439–3443.

19. Maroulakou IG, Avner M, Garrett L, Green J. Prostate and mammary adenocarcinoma in transgenic mice carrying a rat C3(1) simian virus 40 large tumor antigen fusion gene. *Proc Natl Acad Sci USA* 1994;91:11236–11240.

20. Masumori N, Thomas TZ, Chaurand P, et al. A probasin-large T antigen transgenic mouse line develops prostate adenocarcinoma and neuroendocrine carcinoma with metastatic potential. *Cancer Res* 2001;61:2239–2249.

21. Wechter WJ, Leipold. DD, Murray ED Jr, et al. E-7869 (R-flurbiprofen) inhibits progression of prostate cancer in the TRAMP mouse. *Cancer Res* 2000;60:2203–2208.

22. Gupta S, Ahmad N, Maregno SR, et al. Chemoprevention of prostate carcinogenesis by alpha-difluoromethylornithine in TRAMP mice. *Cancer Res* 2000;60:5125–5133.

23. Gupta S, Hastak K, Ahmad N, et al. Inhibition of prostate carcinogenesis in TRAMP mice by oral infusion of green tea polyphenols. *Proc Natl Acad Sci USA* 2001;98:10350–10355.

24. DiGiovanni J, Kiguchi K, Frijhoff A, et al. Deregulated expression of insulin-like growth factor 1 in prostate epithelium leads to neoplasia in transgenic mice. *Proc Natl Acad Sci USA* 2000;28:3455–3460.

25. Abdulkadir SA, Magee JA, Peters TJ, et al. Conditional loss of Nkx3.1 in adult mice induces prostatic intraepithelial neoplasia. *Mol Cell Biol* 2002;22:1495–1503.

26. Bhatia-Gaur R, Donjacour AA, Sciavolino PJ, et al. Roles for Nkx3.1 in prostate development and cancer. *Genes Dev* 1999;13:966–977.

27. Kim MJ, Cardiff RD, Desai N, et al. Cooperativity of Nkx3.1 and PTEN loss of function in a mouse model of prostate carcinogenesis. *Proc Natl Acad Sci USA* 2002;99:2884–2889.

28. Cardiff RD, Bern HA, Faulkin LJ, et al. Contributions of mouse biology to breast cancer research. *Comp Med* 2002;52:12–31.

29. Liu CH, Chang SH, Narko K, et al. Overexpression of cyclooxygenase-2 is sufficient to induce tumorigenesis in transgenic mice. *J Biol Chem* 2001;276:18,563–18,569.

30. Wang B, Kennan WS, Yasukawa-Barnes J, et al. Difference in the response of neu and ras oncogene-induced rat mammary carcinomas to early and late ovariectomy. *Cancer Res* 1992;52:4102–4105.

31. Pupa SM, Invernizzi AM, Forti S, et al. Prevention of spontaneous *neu*-expressing mammary tumor development in mice transgenic for rat proto-*neu* by DNA vaccination. *Gene Ther* 2001;8:75–79.

32. Rao GN, Ney E, Herbert RA. Effect of retinoid analogues on mammary cancer in transgenic mice with c-*neu* breast cancer oncogene. *Breast Cancer Res Treat* 1998;48:265–271.

33. Wu K, Zhang Y, Celestino J, et al. The RXR selective retinoid, LGD1069, prevents tumor development in MMTV-*erb*B2 transgenic mice. *Cancer Res* 2002;62:6376–6380.

34. Wu K, Kim HT, Rodriguez JL, et al. Suppression of mammary tumorigenesis in transgenic mice by the RXR-selective retinoid, LGD1069. *Cancer Epidemiol Biomarkers Prev* 2002;11:467–474.

35. Green JE, Shibata MA, Shibata E, et al. 2-Difluromethyl-ornithine and dehydroepiandrosterone inhibit mammary tumor progression but not mammary or prostate tumor initiation in C3(1)/SV40 T/t-antigen transgenic mice. *Cancer Res* 2001;61:7449–7455.

36. Yokoyama Y, Green JE, Sukhatme VP, Ramakrishnan S. Effects of endostatin on spontaneous tumorigenesis of mammary adenocarcinoma in a transgenic mouse model. *Cancer Res* 2000;60:4362–4365.

37. Bachelier R, Li C, Xu X, et al. Decreased mammary tumor incidence in conditional BRCA1 mutant mice after bilateral oophorectomy. *Proc Am Assoc Cancer Res* 2002;43:512, abst. no. 2542.

38. Jonkers J, Meuwissen R, van der Gulden H, et al. Synergistic tumor suppressor activity of BRCA2 and p53 in a conditional mouse model for breast cancer. *Nat Genet* 2001;29: 418–425.

39. Zhang Z, Liu Q, Lantry LE, et al. A germ-line p53 mutation accelerates pulmonary tumorigenesis: p53-independent efficacy of chemopreventive agents green tea or dexamethasone/myo-inisitol and chemotherapeutic agents taxol or adriamycin. *Cancer Res* 2000;60:901–907.

40. You M, Wang Y, Stoner G, et al. Parental bias of Ki-Ras oncogenes detected in lung tumors from mouse hybrids. *Proc Natl Acad Sci USA* 1992;89:5804–5808.

41. Witschi H, Uyeminami D, Moran D, Espiritu I. Chemopreven-tion of tobacco-smoke lung carcinogenesis in mice after cessation of smoke exposure. *Carcinogenesis* 2000;21: 977–982.

42. DeFlora S, Balansky RM, D'Agostini F, et al. Molecular alternations and lung tumors in p53 mutant mice exposed to cigarette smoke. *Cancer Res* 2003;63:793–800.

43. Wikenheiser KA, Whitsett JA. Tumor progression and cellular differentiation of pulmonary adenocarcinomas in SV40 large T antigen transgenic mice. *Am J Respir Cell Mol Biol* 1997;16:713–723.

44. Jackson EL, Willis N, Mercer K, et al. Analysis of lung tumor initiation and progression using conditional expression of oncogenic K-*ras*. *Genes Dev* 2001;15:3243–3248.

45. Fisher GH, Wellen SL, Klimstra D, et al. Induction and apoptotic regression of lung adenocarcinomas by regulation of a K-Ras transgene in the presence or absence of tumor suppressor genes. *Genes Dev* 2001;15:3249–3262.

45a. Meuwissen R, Linn SC, Linnoila I, et al. Induction of small cell lung cancer in mice by somatic inactivation of both p53 and RB1 in a conditional mouse model. *Cancer Cell* 2003;4:181–189.

45b. Wang Y, Zhang Z, Yan Y, et al. A chemically induced model for squamous cell carcinoma of the lung in mice: histopathology and strain susceptibility. *Cancer Res* 2004; 64:1647–1654.

46. Arbeit JM, Munger K, Howley PM, Hanahan D. Progressive squamous epithelial neoplasia in K14-human papillomavirus type 16 transgenic mice. *J Virol* 1994;68:4358–4368.

47. Arbeit JM, Riley RR, Huey B, et al. Difluoromethyl-ornithine chemoprevention of epidermal carcinogenesis in K14-HPV16 transgenic mice. *Cancer Res* 1999;59: 3610–3620.

48. Jin L, Qi M, Chen DZ, et al. Indole-3-carbinol prevents cervical cancer in human papilloma virus type 16 (HPV 16) transgenic mice. *Cancer Res* 1999;59:3391–3397.

49. Hursting SD, Perkins SN, Donehower LA, Davis BJ. Cancer prevention studies in p53- deficient mice. *Toxicol Pathol* 2001;29:137–141.

50. Lubet RA, Zhang Z, Wiseman RW, You M. Use of p53 transgenic mice in the development of cancer models for multiple purposes. *Exp Lung Res* 2000;26:581–593.

51. Zhang Z, Li J, Lantry LE, et al. p53 Transgenic mice are highly susceptible to 1,2-dimethylhydrazine-induced uterine sarcomas. *Cancer Res* 2002;62:3024–3029.

51a. Zhang Z, Wang Y, Yao R, et al. Cancer chemopreventive activity of a mixture of Chinese herbs in mouse lung tumor models. *Oncogen* 2004;23:3841–3850

51b. Zhang Z, Wang Y, Lantry LE, et al. Farnesyltransferase inhibitors are potent lung cancer chemopreventive agents. *Oncogene* 2003;22:6257–6265.

52. Halberg RB, Katzung D, Hoff P, et al. Tumorigenesis in the multiple intestinal neoplasia mouse: redundancy of negative regulators and specificity of modifiers. *Proc Natl Acad Sci USA* 2000;97:3461–3466.

53. Li B, Murphy KL, Laucirica R, et al. A transgenic mouse model for mammary carcinogenesis. Oncogene 1998;16:997–1007.

4 Modeling Human Colorectal Cancer in Mice for Chemoprevention Studies

Martin Lipkin, MD, and Sergio A. Lamprecht, PhD

CONTENTS

1. INTRODUCTION

New approaches to chemoprevention studies have evolved from a better understanding of the genetics and molecular biology of cancer. Previous research has focused on human cancer cell lines and xenografts of human cancer cells in immunologically compromised mice. Though these experimental approaches have provided much information on cancer cells, they have precluded any insight into the intricate cross-talk between transformed cells and the host in vivo (1,2).

Mice that exhibit a high degree of genetic similarity with the human genome have provided versatile models of human neoplasia. Current available techniques include inducing germline mutations in mice, thus silencing tumor suppressor genes, or inducing overexpression of oncogenes, known to be altered in the human disease (3–10).

A DNA segment carrying a selected mutated mouse exon transferred into a totipotent mouse egg may successfully replace the targeted exon of the normal gene by homologous recombination. The resulting mouse is aptly designated "knockout" for the targeted gene. This procedure is now being widely used to dissect the function of a large number of mammalian genes (3–10) and it is amply exploited to generate mouse models of human intestinal neoplasia (11–13) for chemoprevention studies (14,15).

Several procedures have been developed to generate mice expressing a mutant gene in a tissue-specific manner to provide models of human sporadic cancer arising from somatic mutations (16,17).

Embryonic mortality of mice homozygous for a specific gene mutation often limits the usefulness of a mouse model under scrutiny. Heterozygous mice or interbreeding mutant mice can circumvent this difficulty, permitting assessment of potential cooperative actions of different genetic lesions known to be involved in the development and progression of human tumorigenesis. Chemoprention interventions during the multistep process of colonic carcinogenesis, which is characterized by the sequential acquisition of gene mutations (18,19), are now being studied in mice with a single mutation and in mutant compound mice harboring complex genotypes.

This review is focused primarily on the use of mutant mice to elucidate the cellular and molecular basis of intestinal tumorigenesis and chemoprevention. Also discussed is the use of the normal mouse, without targeted mutations or exposure to carcinogens, as a valid and versatile model to assess promoting or chemopreventive actions of agents in intestinal tumorigenesis.

2. MOUSE MUTANT MODELS

2.1. Apc Mutant Mice

A widely used rodent model for colorectal carcinogenesis is the multiple intestinal neoplasia (Min) mouse which closely resembles familial adenomatous polyposis (FAP), a human autosomal dominant defect with predisposition to colorectal cancer associated with

From: Cancer Chemoprevention, Volume 2: Strategies for Cancer Chemoprevention
Edited by: G. J. Kelloff, E. T. Hawk, and C. C. Sigman © Humana Press Inc., Totowa, NJ

mutations of the adenomatous polyposis coli (APC) gene *(18,19)*. In the genetic model of colonic adenoma-to-carcinoma progression characterized by the acquisition of sequential mutations *(18,19)*, APC gene alterations are the earliest required to initiate tumorigenesis; the expression of wild-type APC gene is lost in 80% of early colonic adenomas *(18,19)*.

The APC gene product is a salient example of a multifunctional, pleiotropic protein. The APC polypeptide controls a vast number of key functions related to the ordered growth of intestinal cells including: (i) the steady state levels of β-catenin and its degradation by the ubiquitin-proteasome pathway, thus preventing the formation of the transcriptionally active β-catenin/Tcfs complex which leads to inappropriate activation of several genes, including c-myc, cyclin D1, matrilysin and survivin; (ii) maintenance of apoptosis; (iii) cell cycle progression, and (iv) maintenance of chromosomal stability, thus safeguarding the fidelity of chromosomal segregation *(20–26)*.

The Min mouse, the first *Apc* mutant mouse was generated by germline random chemical mutagenesis that introduced a chain-terminating mutation at codon 850 in the *Apc* gene of embryonic stem (ES) cells *(27–29)*. In early embryonic development, ES cells are totipotent and therefore serve as progenitors for all cell lineages ultimately found in adult tissues. While *Apc* null ($Apc^{-/-}$) Min mice die *in utero*, *Apc* heterozygous ($Apc^{Min/+}$) Min mice are born normally, develop a large number of multifocal small polyps of the upper gastrointestinal tract but very few colonic tumors and have a reduced average lifespan of 120 days.

As human APC mutations are clustered in the last and largest exon 15, Fodde et al. *(30)* produced *Apc* mutant mice carrying a targeted mutation in ES cells resulting in a chain-terminating mutation in *Apc* codon 1638. In this mouse line, gene targeting inserted a neomycin expression cassette at the position corresponding to codon 1638 of the *Apc* gene. This mutation resulted in an unstable 182kDa truncated protein. *Apc* 1638 null mice die *in utero*. Apc $1638^{N/+}$ are viable and develop multiple gastrointestinal lesions including adenomas *(31)*. The Apc $1638^{N/+}$ mouse develops tumors more slowly than the Min mouse and exhibit a longer survival time; however, the incidence of intestinal tumors is considerably lower than that observed in mice with the Min phenotype.

A third mutant allele of *Apc*, designed $Apc^{\Delta716}$ has been generated *(32)*. Mice heterozygous for this mutation produce a truncated protein of approximately 80kDa and develop a large number of gastrointestinal adenomas; homozygosity for the $Apc^{\Delta716}$ mutation results in embryonic mortality. Sasai et al. *(33)* used gene targeting to produce a mutant mouse designated $Apc^{\Delta474}$, with a mutation immediately after the exon 10 of the wild *Apc* gene, resulting in a truncated protein. All mice bearing this modified *Apc* genotype developed a large number of intestinal tumors.

Cyclin D1, a gene downregulated by wild type APC, codes for a protein playing a pivotal role in the G1⇒S phase transition of the cell cycle *(34)*. Following APC mutations, upregulation of the cyclin D1 gene represents an important target of free β-catenin mediated—colonic tumorigenesis *(35)*. Of note, cyclin D1 is overexpressed in both human familial and sporadic colorectal adenomas and carcinomas *(36–41)*. Shinozaki et al. *(42)* reported that cyclin D1 was expressed in the nucleus of all tumors in *Apc* $1638^{N/+}$ mice; this expression exhibited a characteristic punctate-cytoplasmic pattern. To examine further the role of cyclin D1 during intestinal carcinogenesis, Wilding et al. *(43)* generated Min mice that, after interbreeding with cyclin D1 knockouts, were rendered nullizygous for cyclin D1. Notwithstanding the absence of cyclin D1, intestinal tumors developed in mutant compound mice ($Apc^{Min/+}$ cyclin $D1^{-/-}$), though in smaller number when compared with Min mice harboring the *Apc* mutation. The investigators suggest that cyclin D1 is not essential for intestinal tumorigenesis and that the wild-type cyclin D1 gene may act as a modifier gene (*see* Section 2.3.), an interesting view consonant with findings that humans who show an earlier onset of hereditary colorectal cancer have a common polymorphysm in the cyclin D1 gene *(44)*.

Additional studies in mice based on germ-line targeting methodology indicate that the *Tcf-1* transcription factor does not necessarily cooperate with free β-catenin in its oncogenic action. Thus, *Tcf-1* null mice develop mammary and colonic carcinomas *(45)*; furthermore, when crossed with $Apc^{Min/+}$ mice, the mutant compound mice exhibited a marked decrease in intestinal polyp formation. In contrast to the prevailing view, these findings suggest that the *Tcf-1* transcription factor may be able to act as feedback repressor of the Wnt–β-catenin signalling pathway.

The p21$^{WAF1/cip1}$ gene, a downstream effector of p53, is an inhibitor of cyclin-dependent kinase activity *(46)*. In its absence, colon tumor cancer cells do not arrest in the G1 phase of the cell cycle and continue to proliferate *(47,48)*. Elimination of both alleles of the

$P21^{WAF1/cip1}$ gene markedly increased the frequency and size of intestinal tumors in mice bearing the *Apc* 1638 N genotype *(49)*.

2.2. Mutant Mice for DNA Mismatch Repair Genes

DNA repair involves an important group of tumor suppressor genes. Mutations in these genes are responsible for human hereditary nonpolyposis colon cancer (HNPCC), *(50,51)*. HNPCC patients are prone to develop multiple epithelial malignancies, including colon cancer. This predisposition to neoplasia results from loss or alteration of enzymes that repair DNA base mismatches *(50,51)*. The primary function of mismatched repair (MMR) proteins is to proofread newly synthesized DNA and identify and correct polymerase errors introduced during DNA replication, such as slippage, which are relatively frequent in short DNA microsatellite repeats *(50,51)*. The MMR enzymes excise misincorporated bases and replace them with the correct ones. Mutations in these genes lead to a replication error phenotype that manifests in microsatellite instability (MSI). HNPCC patients harbor germline mutations in several genes, including MSH2 and MLH1 involved in critical DNA repair functions. *(50,51)*.

The molecular biology and function of several genes coding for MMR proteins have been studied in mutant mice *(12,52)*. An increased DNA mutation rate has been detected in intestinal tissues of *Mlh1* and *Pms*2 homozygous mutant mice *(12,52–53)*; *Pms2* mutants develop only lymphomas and sarcomas, despite the increased mutation rate in intestinal cells *(12,54)*. *Msh2*-null mice are viable, fertile and develop normally but exhibit a reduced lifespan, development of T cell lymphomas, skin tumors and late-onset adenocarcinoma of the small intestine *(12,55,56)*. In a *Tap*$^{-/-}$ background, where CD8+ T cells are missing gastrointestinal and skin tumors develop *(12,57)*; expression of the *Apc* protein in these mice appears to be lost in adenomatous cells. Of note, induction in *Msh2*$^{-/-}$ mice of chronic inflammation-a condition associated with colorectal cancer-resulted in adenoma and adenocarcinoma formation in the large intestine *(58)*.

Loss of *Mlh1* or *Msh2* also accelerates the development of intestinal tumors in Min mice *(59)*. Similar to *Msh2* mice, *Pms2*$^{-/-}$*Apc*$^{Min/+}$double mutant mice give rise to an increased number of intestinal adenomas as compared with *Apc*$^{Min/+}$ mice *(60)*, further implicating impaired DNA mismatch repair activity as an important determinant of intestinal carcinogenesis.

Edelmann et al. *(61)* examined in detail the predisposition of *Mlh1* mutant mice to gastrointestinal tumor development, lymphomas and a number of other tumor types. When the *Apc* 1638 N mutation was crossed into the *Mlh1* mutant background, the mice showed a marked increase in gastrointestinal tumors. The increased tumor multiplicity in the double mutant mice was associated with somatic mutations in the wild-type *Apc* allele; gastrointestinal tumors were adenomas and adenocarcinomas.

A mouse with a null mutation in the *Msh3* gene was generated by Edelmann et al. *(62)*. Mice harboring this mutation develop gastrointestinal tumors or lymphomas at a late age. An additional MMR gene, *Msh6*, has been described; *Mlh6*$^{-/-}$ mice develop both gastrointestinal and lymphoid tumors *(63)*. When the *Msh3*$^{-/-}$ and the *Msh6*$^{-/-}$ mutations were combined, the tumor predisposition phenotype was indistinguishable from *Msh2*$^{-/-}$ or *Mlh1*$^{-/-}$ *(62)*.

Kuraguchi et al. *(64)* have shown that the loss of *Msh1* alone was sufficient to cause a strong predisposition to intestinal tumors in *Apc* 1638$^{N/+}$ mice. While *Msh-3* deficient *Apc* 1638$^{N/+}$ mice showed no difference in survival and tumor multiplicity compared to mice with the *Apc* 1638 N phenotype, *Apc* 1638 $^{N/+}$ mice defective in *Msh6* exhibited reduced survival and a marked increase in intestinal tumor multiplicity *(65)*. The additional loss of *Msh3* in *Apc* $^{1638N/+}$ *Msh6*$^{-/-}$ mice further contributed to enhanced intestinal polyp multiplicity and increased mortality at a younger age; the increase in tumor formation was associated with a high incidence of truncation mutations in the wild-type *Apc* allele.

Flap endonuclease (*Fen1*), an enzyme involved in processing Okazaki fragments in lagging DNA strand synthesis, also contributes to DNA repair *(66)*. Using gene knockout methodology, Kucherlapati et al. *(67)* generated *Fen1* null mice. Mice homozygous for the *Fen1* mutation were not viable. While *Fen1* heterozygous mice appeared to be normal, double heterozygous (*Fen1*$^{+/-}$*Apc*1638$^{N/+}$) mice exhibited a reduced median survival and an increased number of adenocarcinomas with the MSI phenotype. Since one allele of wild type *Fen1* gene was retained in tumor cells, *Fen1* haploinsufficiency appears to be sufficient for rapid tumor development.

2.3. Modifier Genes

Individuals respond differently not only to genetic changes leading to tumor initiation/progression but also to treatment of neoplasia. Such phenotypic changes of

Mendelian traits have been attributed to environmental influences, polymorphysm of tumor suppressor genes, and to tumor modifier genes which in the presence of a defined genetic background ultimately determine the tumor phenotype *(68)*.

Extensive research has focused on genetic loci that might modify the cancer susceptibility phenotype in Min mice; findings led to the identification of a locus designated modifier of Min (*Mom1*) *(69)*. The *Mom1* gene encodes a secretory phospholipase A2 gene (Pla2s) and introduction of the wild-type Pla2s gene into a mouse germline alters the cancer susceptibility phenotype of the Min mouse *(70,71)*. Additional dominant modifier loci that markedly influence polyp burden in Min mice have been recently described *(72)*.

2.4. Transforming Growth Factor β Receptor–SMAD Pathway

TGFβ is a potent inhibitor of epithelial cell growth *in vitro* and in vivo *(73)*. This cytokine binds to specific receptors and conveys its information to the cell nucleus via SMAD proteins *(73,74)*. Following phosphorylation on their carboxyl terminus, SMAD proteins, predominantly SMAD 2 and SMAD 3, interact with a common mediator, SMAD 4, and translocate to the nucleus to act as transcription factors regulating the expression of a large array of genes *(73,74)*.

Mutations at TGFβ receptor levels and within the TGFβ pathways have been found in various human tumors, including colorectal cancer *(75)*: these tumors exhibit the MIS phenotype.

Recently, mutant *Smad* genes have provided much information pertaining to the functional relationship between the TGFβ-*Smad* pathway and intestinal carcinogenesis. Mice harboring heterozygous deletions within TGFβI or TGFβII receptors, or within *Smad* 2 or *Smad* 4 genes, do not develop tumors *(76–79)*. Homozygous mutant *Smad* 4 mice are not viable *(79)*. When Smad 4 heterozygotes were crossed with *Apc*$^{\Delta716}$ mice, the double compound mutant mice produced not only adenomas, as in *Apc* 1638$^{N/+}$ mice, but also invasive adenocarcinomas *(79)*. Hamamoto et al. *(80)* generated compound heterozygous mice which have both *Apc* and *Smad* 2 mutations on the same chromosome in the cis-configuration; this genotype accelerates malignant progression of intestinal tumors.

A peculiar phenotype was obtained in mice produced by targeting *Smad* gene 3 *(81)*. *Smad 3*$^{-/-}$ mice are viable and fertile , but develop metastatic colorectal adenocarcinomas between 1 and 6 months of age. Interestingly, the *Apc* gene was not lost in these tumors and appeared

to be expressed in tumor cells. These investigators have also examined the role of the genetic background in these mice in tumor formation and reported that the median survival and tumor incidence varied between different mouse strains

To date, however, SMAD 3 mutations have not been detected in human colonic cancer, notwithstanding that LOH in chromosome 15q, where SMAD 3 is located, has been observed in a subset of colonic tumors *(82)*. SMAD 2 and SMAD 3 proteins exhibit more than 90% homology in primary structure composition; in biochemical studies in vitro they were shown to have similar roles downstream the TGFβ receptors. It is thus possible that the loss of one SMAD protein is compensated for by the presence of the other one *(83)*.

2.5. Other Mutant Mouse Models

Mice have been generated with mutations in the cdx gene. The caudal-related Cdx-2 gene encodes a transcription factor included in the homeobox family that plays an essential role for development and homeostasis of the intestinal epithelium *(84,85)*. *Cdx-2*$^{+/-}$ mice are viable but develop hamartomatous polyps in the ileum and colon that are characterized by gastric heteroplasia *(86,87)*.

Sasaki et al. *(88)* generated mice that carry a mutation in the P110γ catalytic subunit of phosphoinositide-3-OH kinase γ (PI-3-Kγ). This lipid kinase regulates key cellular responses, including proliferation, differentiation and apoptosis *(89,90)*. P110 γ null mice were viable but exhibited an increased incidence of premature death associated with development of colonic tumors at all stages of transformation. No tumors of the small intestine were found. The expression of *Apc, p21*, and *Smad* proteins was apparently normal. Interestingly, the anti-apoptotic protein *Bcl-2* was found to be upregulated in all tumors. These results indicate that the catalytic activity of PI-3-Kγ impedes colorectal cancer and that a possible contributory mechanism for colonic tumorigenesis in P110γ null mice involves disruption of the apoptosis pathway.

The gastrointestinal tract is lined with a layer of mucus comprised of high molecular weight, heavily glycosylated proteins called mucins *(91)*. Changes in glycosylation patterns and in the level of expression of mucin glycoproteins have been associated with human cancer, including colon cancer *(92)*. Velcich et al. *(93)* generated mice genetically deficient in *Muc2*, the most abundant secreted gastrointestinal mucin, by targeted inactivation of the *Muc2* gene. *Muc 2*$^{-/-}$ mice displayed aberrant intestinal crypt morphology, altered cell maturation and migration rate. These mice frequently developed small-intestine adenomas that progressed to invasive adenocarcinoma and rectal tumors. These findings indicate that a decrease in mucin formation plays an important contributory role in intestinal carcinogenesis.

2.6. Conditional Mutant Mice

Notwithstanding the vast amount of information on initiation and progression to progression to cancer, a limitation of the knockout mouse methodology is that every cell in every tissue has lost the targeted gene and therefore these models do not closely mimic human sporadic cancer arising in specific tissues from somatic mutations.

To obviate this severe difficulty and target genetic lesions in a tissue specific-manner, conditional gene mutation strategies have been developed (17). One procedure used is the Cre-lox system (17) affording the deletion of the targeted DNA segment in a selected tissue.

A conditional mouse tumor suppressor gene designed Apc 580S has been generated (94). Cre recombinase expression in the colon resulted in deletion of exon 14 of the Apc gene resulting in a protein truncated at aa 580. Homozygous mice produced numerous polyps in the large intestine; about 50% of these tumors progressed to invasive adenocarcinomas

3. PRECLINICAL STUDIES FOR CHEMOPREVENTION OF COLORECTAL CANCER

In the previous section, many new mouse models available for chemoprevention studies were reviewed. In this section we examine specific dietary components: fats, vitamin D, calcium, and folate ,along with selected non-steroidal antinflammatory drugs (NSAIDs) as chemopreventive agents in mouse models of human intestinal cancer. Several comprehensive reviews have recently been published pertaining to the general topic of chemopreventive agents in preclinical studies (95,96).

3.1. Nutritional Interventions

The development of intestinal lesions in Apc-mutant mice has been modified with dietary intervention. Wasan et al. (97) demonstrated that dietary fat influences the polyp phenotype in the Min mouse, and a high fat-diet increased intestinal and colonic tumor formation in these mice. In another study (98), Apc$^{\Delta 716}$ knockout

mice were fed either a high-fat (and low fiber) high—risk diet or a low-fat (and higher fiber) low-risk diet; the mice maintained on the low-risk diet had few polyps in the small intestine and in the colon.

We first showed (15,99) in Apc 1638$^{N/+}$ mice that both benign and malignant intestinal polyps were significantly increased by feeding Western-style diets (WDs). WDs used in these studies were modified standard AIN-76A diet with decreased calcium, vitamin D$_3$ and increased fat content at nutrient-density levels similar to those consumed by individuals in some segments of Western populations. A salient finding was that intestinal lesions were decreased by lowering fat content and increasing dietary calcium and vitamin D$_3$ (15,100)

Yang et al. (49) reported that target inactivation in Apc1638 $^{N/+}$ of both alleles of the gene that encodes the cyclin kinase inhibitor p21$^{WAF1/cip1}$ gene, resulted in an increase in the frequency and size of intestinal tumors in mice. Of note, these mice produced more and larger intestinal tumors and exhibited a significant decrease in survival time when maintained on WD.

Short-term treatments of normal mice with a WD induced colonic hyperproliferation and hyperplasia (15,101,102). Long-term studies fed WDs to normal mice for two years, essentially for their entire life span (103). Hyperproliferation and hyperplasia developed, followed by other changes in the colon, including whole crypt dysplasias similar to those seen in the human colon in diseases that increase the risk of colon cancer. It is noteworthy that cell proliferation and hyperplasia were also observed in mammary glands and pancreas (104–107). A salient finding was that adding dietary calcium and vitamin D$_3$ significantly suppressed WD-induced hyperproliferaton of epithelial cells in these tissues (15).

A number of studies have also investigated the effects of dietary intervention with folate and/or other nutrients involved in methyl transfer reactions on the development and progression of intestinal tumors in mice bearing germline mutations in genes known to be mutated in the human disease.

Song et al. (108) using the Min mouse model of colorectal tumorigenesis have shown that dietary folate supplemented for 3 mo interfered with the development of ileal polyps and colonic aberrant crypt foci. Surprisingly, animals kept on a folate-deficient diet for a more prolonged period of time exibited a markedly lower number of ileal polyps compared with those on control and folate-supplemented diets.

Pursuing further this study, these investigators (109) examined the effect of dietary folate intake in Min mice with a null mutation in the *Msh2* gene. As discussed previously, this is one of several mismatch repair genes that contribute to the accurate replication of the genome. Folate supplementation started before establishment of neoplastic foci significantly decreased the number of small intestinal adenomas, colonic preneoplastic lesions and colonic adenomas. In contrast, a moderately deficient diet, initiated after the establishment of intestinal neoplastic lesions, significantly reduced the number of small-intestinal adenomas, but had no effect on colonic aberrant crypt foci and adenomas compared with folate supplementation. Therefore, the developmental stage at which the diet is administered, and modified density of methyl group transfer nutrients, appear to be critical both for their chemopreventive and reported promotional effects during the multistep process of colorectal carcinogenesis.

We have reported *(110)* that intestinal tumors were induced in the absence of a chemical carcinogen or targeted mutation in normal mice, when fed a Western-style diet where folic acid, methionine and choline were reduced in the diet to nutrient-levels approximating these consumed by segments of Western populations. The tumors produced without gene targeting procedures or administration of carcinogens, included tubovillus and tubular adenomas, an early invasive carcinoma and were mainly located in the large intestine.

It is noteworthy that the earliest WDs induced proliferative, hyperplastic and dysplastic abnormalities in normal colonic epithelium, but not colonic adenomas or adenocarcinomas whereas the colonic lesions induced by a modified WD *(110)* low in methyl donor groups progressed further to more advanced neoplasms, indicating a central role of dietary methyl groups in inhibiting colorectal carcinogenesis *(111–113)*.

Cumulatively, these results indicate that components of WDs, such as polyunsaturated n-6 fatty acids, promote intestinal carcinogenesis and that dietary deficiency of critical micronutrients like vitamin D, Ca^{2+}, and folate have a determing role in modifying intestinal carcinogenesis. The cellular and molecular modes of actions of these nutrients in modulating colorectal tumorigenesis have been recently analyzed in detail *(113,114)*.

3.2. Pharmacological Interventions

The importance of cyclooxygenase (COX)-2 in intestinal tumorigenesis was show in a seminal paper by Oshima and coworkers *(115)* who reported that double knockout mice lacking both *Apc* function and COX-2 activity displayed a marked reduction in the number and size of intestinal polyps. These results

were confirmed using homologous disruption in Min mice of *Ptgs-1* or *Ptgs-2*, the genes coding for COX-1 or COX-2, respectively *(116)*.

NSAIDs such as sulindac or second-generation derivatives inhibit COX-2 activity *(117)*. Several studies have shown that prolonged treatment of *Apc* knock-out mice with COX inhibitors or other pharmacological agents altering prostaglandin synthesis inhibit intestinal polyposis. For example, sulindac markedly suppressed tumor formation when added to the drinking water provided to $Apc^{Min/+}$ mice *(118–121)*. Yang et al. *(122)* have reported that sulindac treatment resulted in induction of the cyclin-dependent kinase inhibitor $p21^{WAF1/cip1}$. In *Apc* 1638 N heterozygous mice, targeted inactivation of *p21* increased tumor formation in a gene-dose-dependent manner; but inactivation of p21 completely eliminated the ability of sulindac to both inhibit mitotic activity in the duodenal mucosa and *Apc*-initiated tumor formation. Thus, p21 seems to be essential for the molecular mechanism of sulindac in inhibiting intestinal tumorigenesis. Selective NSAIDs COX-2 inhibitors have also been shown to decrease polyp number and size in Min mice, $Apc^{\Delta716}$ and $Apc^{\Delta474}$ mice *(33,123–125)*.

Findings suggesting that sulindac and other NSAIDs have a chemopreventive action in mouse models of intestinal carcinogenesis remain controversial. Thus, Lal et al. *(126)* reported that sulindac added to standard diet was effective in inhibiting the development of small-bowel polyps in double mutant $Apc^{Min/+}$ $Msh2^{-/-}$ mice but had no effect on large bowel polyps. Yang et al. *(127)* have recently carried out a detailed study of the effects of sulindac on tumorigenesis in the Min mouse. These investigators provided convincing evidence that, while sulindac decreased the number of tumors in the small intestine, it also increased tumor incidence and number in Min mice fed the standard AIN-76 diet al.one. These tumors were mostly adenocarcinomas and flat adenomas. A number of possibilities can be proposed here for these controversial findings, including genetic differences in small and large-bowel cells, variations in the stromal cell make-up in small and large bowel neoplasms, and physiological differences in drug delivery within various regions of the small and large intestine.

The utility of mouse mutant models of intestinal tumorigenesis in analyzing action drug actions was underscored by studies using Min mice fed a standard diet supplemented with PPAR-γ synthetic agonists, such as the thiazolidinendione troglitazone (TGZ) *(128,129)*, previously extensively used for the treatment of type 2 diabetes. PPAR-γ is a nuclear receptor that acts as transcription factor conveying instructive signals from polyunsaturated fatty acids and prostanoid derivatives of arachidonic acid into changes in the expression of specific genes *(130,131)*.

The results show that dietary TGZ promoted colonic polyps in *Apc*$^{Min/+}$ mice. We have extended these findings using double heterozygous *Mlh1/Apc* 1638 N mice and normal C57BL/6J mice fed a standard AIN-76A diet, *(132,133)* and observed that not only does TGZ enhance carcinogenesis in the large intestine of mutant mice predisposed to intestinal carcinogenesis, TGZ also induces colonic tumors in normal mice without gene targeting or carcinogen administration. These findings indicate that pre-existing mutational events are not necessary for colonic tumor formation by activated PPAR-γ in vivo, and are consistent with the view that PPARγ activation may provide a molecular link between a high-fat diet and increased risk of colorectal cancer.

4. CONCLUSIONS AND FUTURE PROSPECTS

Genetically-engineered mice are providing vast information pertaining to intestinal tumor initiation and progression. In addition to permitting the study of known genes and comparing their genetic changes and tumor phenotype pattern with the human disease (e.g., FAP and HNPCC) these murine models have led to identification of new genes playing a determining role in intestinal tumorigenesis: *Mom*-1 is a typical case in point. Further studies in mice of tumor-modifier genes that control phenotypes of intestinal tumors should provide important insights into human individual genetic susceptibility to intestinal neoplasia.

The studies of mouse models as preclinical models of human intestinal cancer have provided invaluable information on the chemopreventive action of nutrients and pharmacological drugs. They have also been very useful in testing the efficacy of combinatorial chemoprevention of intestinal tumors, as shown by Torrance et al. *(134)* who examined inhibition of intestinal tumorigenesis in Min mice using both sulindac and a selective epidermal growth factor receptor tyrosine kinase inhibitor. Most interesting regarding nutritional modulation of cancer has been the recurring finding that the normal mouse without gene-targeting or administration of carcinogen serves as a valid and versatile model to assess the importance of nutrients in initiating, promoting, or preventing intestinal carcinogenesis *(15,101,103,110)*.

Mice bear many similarities to humans but there are notable differences that limit the extent to which human cancer can be faithfully modeled in these rodents *(9,135)*. For instance, when designing chemopreventive protocols, however, much attention should be focused on possible differences between mice and humans in metabolizing experimental drugs. Most conspicuous is the difference between telomere size and telomerase expression in mice and humans; this topic has been extensively investigated *(136)*. Hann and Balmain *(9)* have recently presented in detail the criteria for the "ideal" mouse model faithfully recapitulating the human disease. Therefore, notwithstanding the wide progress in understanding the genetic and molecular basis of intestinal tumorigenesis in genetically-compromised mice and their importance in testing putative chemopreventive agents, a key question to be addressed is: How valid are mutant mouse models in recapitulating human colorectal cancer?

An important comparison would appear to be the positive relationship observed in mutant *Apc* and *Mlh* mice in response to increased or decreased dietary intake of calcium and vitamin D_3. Here, decreased or increased tumor development in the mouse models and humans is seen paralleling human epidemiological and experimental evidence *(100)*. Examinations of intestinal adenomas from *Apc* knockout mice for mutations in other genes responsible for human colonic carcinogenesis have shown that the only consistent alteration found is the loss of the remaining wild type *Apc* gene copy. Intestinal tumors were examined for K-*ras* and *p53* mutations but no mutations were found (137). These results indicate that a mutation of the *Apc* gene is sufficient for *Apc* heterologous cells in the intestinal flat mucosa to grow into polyps. We have recently critically discussed *(138)* the robust evidence that genetic changes in APC are sufficient for an aberrant daughter clone in the colonic mucosa to gradually divide and expand into microadenomas.

One may argue that the inability of *Apc* knockout mice to acquire additional mutations for the formation of carcinomas from adenomas is due to early mortality caused by bleeding and severe anemia. Some evidence for this possibility is provided by studies using *Apc* mutant mice that, by interbreeding with appropriate mouse knockout mutants, have acquired genetic lesions found in humans that foster the progression of adenomas into carcinomas. Various examples have been provided in this review; the increased development of intestinal adenomas in *Apc*$^{Min/+}$ *p53*$^{-/-}$ mice *(139)* is an additional salient case in point.

Why are colonic adenomas so rare in *Apc* knockout mice fed standard diets, whereas small intestinal adenomas are consistently found? There is not a ready answer to this puzzling question. Yamada et al. *(140)* reported that *Apc*^{Min/+} mice develop colonic microadenomatous lesions which have lost the remaining *Apc* allele, indicating that, in contrast with the small intestine, loss of the wild type *Apc* gene is not sufficient for tumor development in the colon. An intriguing possibility is that colonic transformed cells stringently need to recruit their normal neighbor cells (stromal, myofibroblasts endothelial cells) to serve as "active collaborators in their neoplastic agenda" *(1)* and to provide growth-promoting signals *(1,141–143)*. Is a crucial dialogue between these heterotypic cells not possible in the colon of the *Apc*-mutant mouse since *all* cells of this mouse carry the germ-line induced targeted mutation, and therefore transformed colonic cells are not exposed to a normal cellular microenvironment? The rapid adenoma and adenocarcinoma formation by conditional targeting of the *Apc* gene in colonic epithelial cells *(94)*, a procedure that spares neighboring normal cells, is consonant with this view.

The possibilities for generation of more sophisticated mouse models of human cancer, including intestinal cancer, are manifold. Incisive reviews on this subject have been published *(9,144–147)*. Janssen et al. *(148)* have generated a transgenic mouse that expresses K-*ras*^{V12G}, a frequent oncogenic mutation in human colonic tumors, in epithelial cells of the small and large intestine. More than 80% of these transgenic mice showed intestinal lesions ranging from aberrant crypt foci to invasive adenocarcinoma. Expression of the K-*ras* oncogene caused activation of the MAP kinase cascade signaling pathway. Interestingly, no inactivating mutations of *Apc* were found in these mice.

We believe that engineering of mutant mice with combination of mutated tumor suppression genes and oncogenes will provide powerful models for identifying synergistic effects of specific mutations in colonic tumorigenesis and for testing putative chemopreventive agents.

New procedures are available not only to unravel the cellular and molecular basis of intestinal carcinogenesis in the mouse but also to monitor closely the chemopreventive effects of drugs and nutrients. Molecular profiling of mouse tumors have been fostered by several new genome-wide analytical tools, including spectral karyotyping, comparative genomic hybridization, array-based-gene-expression analysis and proteomics *(149–151)*. Most exciting are methodologies such as bioluminiscence, which provides in vivo tumor imaging that specifically marks tumor cells *(152,153)*. These procedures will not only greatly facilitate accurate measurement of tumor development and growth but also will afford invaluable information on the effectiveness of putative chemoprevention agents in the living mouse.

ACKNOWLEDGMENTS

Studies described in this chapter were supported by awards U0I-CA84301, ES11040, U54-cA100926, and NOI-CN25121, from the National Cancer Institute, USPH, NIH.

REFERENCES

1. Hanahan D, Weinberg RA. The hallmarks of cancer. *Cell* 2000;100:57–70.
2. Klausner RD. Studying cancer in the mouse. *Oncogene* 1999;18:5249–5252.
3. Kreidberg JA, Natoli TA. Animal models for tumor suppressor genes. In *Tumor Suppressor Genes in Human Cancer*. Fisher DE, ed. Humana Press, Totowa, NJ, 2001; pp. 1–28.
4. Ghebranious N, Donehower LA. Mouse models in tumor suppression. *Oncogene* 1998;17:3385–3400.
5. Macleod KF, Jacks T. Insights into cancer from transgenic mouse models. *J Pathol* 1999;187:43–60.
6. Iredale JP. Gene knockouts demystified. *J Clin Pathol Mol Pathol* 1999;52:111–116.
7. Wu X, Pandolfi PP. Mouse models for multistep tumorigenesis. *Trends Cell Biol* 2001;11:S2–S9.
8. Hakem R, Mak TW. Animal models of tumor-suppressor genes. *Annu Rev Genet* 2001;35:209–241.
9. Hann B, Balmain A. Building 'validated' mouse models of human cancer. *Curr Opin Cell Biol* 2001;13:778–784.
10. Herzig M, Christofori G. Recent advances in cancer research: mouse models of tumorigenesis. *Biochim Biophys Acta* 2002;1602:97–113.
11. Fodde R, Smits R. Disease model: familial adenomatous polyposis. *Trends Mol Med* 2001;7:369–373.
12. Heyer J, Yang K, Lipkin M, et al. Mouse models for colorectal cancer. *Oncogene* 1999;18:5325–5233.
13. Kucherlapati R, Lin DP, Edelmann W. Mouse models for human familial adenomatous polyposis. *Seminar Cancer Biol* 2001;11:219–225.
14. Bertagnolli MM. APC and intestinal carcinogenesis: insights from animal models. *Ann NY Acad Sci* 1999;889:32–44.
15. Lipkin M, Yang K, Edelmann W, et al. Preclinical mouse models for cancer chemoprevention studies. *Ann NY Acad Sci* 2001;889:14–19.
16. Meuwissen R, Jonkers J, Berns A. Mouse models for sporadic cancer. *Exp Cell Res* 2001;264:100–110.
17. Jonkers J, Berns A. Conditional mouse models of sporadic cancer. *Nature Rev Cancer* 2002;2:251–265.
18. Fearon ER, Gruber SB. Molecular abnormalities in colon and rectal cancer. In *The Molecular Basis of Cancer*. Medelson J, Howeley PM, Israel MA, Liotta LA, eds. Saunders, Philadelphia, 2001; pp. 289–312.

19. Kinzler KW, Vogelstein B. Colorectal tumors. In *The Genetic Basis of Human Cancer*. Vogelstein B, Kinzler KW, eds. McGraw-Hill, NewYork, 2002; pp. 583–612.

20. Goss KH, Groden J. Biology of the adenomatous polyposis coli tumor suppressor. *J Clin Oncol* 2000;18:1967–1979.

21. Van Es JH, Giles RH, Clevers HC. The many faces of the tumor suppressor gene APC. *Exp Cell Res* 2001;264: 126–134.

22. Sieber OM, Tomlinson IP, Lamlun H. The adenomatous polyposis coli (APC) tumor suppressor-genetics, function and disease. *Mol Med Today* 2000;6:462–469.

23. Fearnhead NS, Britton MP, Bodmer WF. The ABC of APC. *Hum Mol Genet* 2001;10:721–733.

24. Kaplan KB, Burds AA, Swedlow JR, et al. A role of the adenomatous polyposis coli protein in chromosome segregation. *Nat Cell Biol* 2001;3:429–432.

25. Fodde R, Kuipers J, Rosenberg C, et al. Mutations in the APC tumour suppressor gene cause chromosomal instability. *Nat Cell Biol* 2001;3:433–438.

26. Zhang T, Otevrel T, Gao Z, et al. Evidence that APC regulates survivin expression: a possible mechanism contributing to the stem cell origin of colon cancer. *Cancer Res* 2001; 61:8664–8667.

27. Moser AR, Pitot HC, Dove WF. A dominant mutation that predisposes to multiple intestinal neoplasia in the mouse. *Science* 1990;247:322–324.

28. Shoemaker AR, Gould KA, Luongo C, et al. Studies of neoplasia in the Min mouse. *Biochim Biophys Acta* 1997;1332: F25–F48.

29. Bilger A, Shoemaker AR, Gould KA, Dove WF. Manipulation of the mouse germline in the study of Min-induced neoplasia. *Seminar Cancer Biol* 1996;7:249–260.

30. Fodde R, Edelmann W, Yang K, et al. A targeted chain-termination mutation in the mouse Apc gene results in multiple intestinal tumors. *Proc Natl Acad Sci USA* 1994;91: 8969–8973.

31. Yang K, Edelmann W, Fan K, et al. A mouse model of human familial adenomatous polyposis. *J Exp Zool* 1997;277: 245–254.

32. Oshima M, Oshima H, Kitagawa K, et al. Loss of Apc heterozygosity and abnormal tissue binding in nascent intestinal polyps in mice carrying a truncated Apc gene. *Proc Natl Acad Sci USA* 1995;92:4482–4486.

33. Sasai H, Masaki M, Wakitani K. Suppression of polypogenesis in a new mouse strain with a truncated $Apc^{\Delta 474}$ by a novel COX-2 inhibitor, JTE-522. *Carcinogenesis* 2000;21: 953–958.

34. Sherr, CJ. D-type cyclins. *Trends Biochem Sci* 1995;20: 187–190.

35. Tetsu O, McCormick F. β-catenin regulates expression of cyclin D1 in colon carcinoma cells. *Nature* 1999;398: 422–426.

36. Sutter T, Doi S, Carnevale KA, et al. Expression of cyclins D1 and E in human colon adenocarcinomas. *J Med* 1997;28: 285–309.

37. Arber N, Hibshoosh H, Moss SF, et al. Increased expression of cyclin D1 is an early event in multistage colorectal carcinogenesis. *Gastroenterology* 1996;110:669–674.

38. Zhang T, Nanney LB, Luongo C, et al. Concurrent overexpression of cyclin D1 and cyclin-dependent kinase 4 (Cdk4) in intestinal adenomas from multiple intestinal neoplasia (Min) mice and human familial adenomatous polyposis patients. *Cancer Res* 1997;57:169–175.

39. Ciaparrone M, Yamamoto H, Yao Y, et al. Localization and expression of p27KIP1 in multistage colorectal carcinogenesis. *Cancer Res* 1998;58:114–122.

40. Bartkova J, Lukas J, Strauss M, Bartek J. The PRAD1/cyclin D1 oncogene product accumulates aberrantly in a subset of colorectal carcinomas. *Int J Cancer* 1994; 58:568–573.

41. Bartkova J, Lukas J, Strauss M, Bartek J. Cyclin D1 oncoprotein aberrantly accumulates in malignancies of diverse histogenesis. *Oncogene* 1995;10:775–778.

42. Shinozaki H, Yang K, Fan K, et al. Cyclin D1 expression in the intestinal mucosa and tumors of Apc1638N mice. *Anticancer Res* 2003;23:2217–2226.

43. Wilding J, Straub J, Bee J, et al. Cyclin D1 is not an essential target of β-catenin signaling during intestinal tumorigenesis, but it may act as a modifier of disease severity in multiple intestinal neoplasia (Min) mice. *Cancer Res* 2002; 62:4562–4565.

44. Kong S, Amos CI, Luthra R, et al. Effects of cyclin D1 polymorphism on age of onset of hereditary nonpolyposis colorectal cancer. *Cancer Res* 2000;60:249–252.

45. Roose J, Huls G, van Beest M et al. Synergy between tumor suppressor and the β-catenin-Tcf4 target *Tcf1*. *Science* 1999; 285:1923–1926.

46. Harper JW, Adami GR, Wei N, et al. The p21 Cdk-interacting protein Cip1 is a potent inhibitor of G_1 cyclin-dependent kinases. *Cell* 1993;75:805–816.

47. Waldman T, Kinzler KW, Vogelstein B. p21 is necessary for the p53-mediated G_1 arrest in human cancer cells. *Cancer Res* 1995;55:5187–5190.

48. Waldman T, Lengauer C, Kinzler KW, Vogelstein B. Uncoupling of S phase and mitosis induced by anticancer agents in cells lacking *p21*. *Nature* 1996;381:713–716.

49. Yang WC, Mathew J, Velcich A, et al. Targeted inactivation of the $p21^{WAF1/cip1}$ gene enhances *Apc*-initiated tumor formation and the tumor-promoting activity of a Western-style high-risk diet by altering cell maturation in the intestinal mucosa. *Cancer Res* 2001;61:565–569.

50. Boland RC. Hereditary nonpolyposis colorectal cancer (HNPCC). In *The Genetic Basis of Human Cancer*, 2nd ed. Vogelstein B, Kinzler KW, eds. McGraw-Hill, New York, 2002; pp. 307–321.

51. Fearon ER. Cancers of the gastrointestinal tract. In *Cancer: Principles & Practice of Oncology*, 6th ed. DeVita VT, Hellman S, Rosenberg SA, eds. Lippincott Williams & Wilkins, Philadelphia, 2001; pp. 1037–1051.

52. Andrew SE, Glazer PM, Jirik FR. Mutagenesis and tumor development in DNA mismatch repair-deficient mice. In *DNA Alterations in Cancer*. Ehrlich M, ed. Eaton Publishing, Natick, MA, 2000; pp. 177–189.

53. Andrew SE, McKinnon M, Cheng BS, et al. Tissues of MSH2-deficient mice demonstrate hypermutability on exposure to a DNA methylating agent. *Proc Natl Acad Sci USA* 1998;95:1126–1130.

54. Narayanan L, Fritzell JA, Baker SM, et al. Elevated levels of mutation in multiple tissues of mice deficient in the DNA mismatch repair gene Pms2. *Proc Natl Acad Sci USA* 1997; 94:3122–3127.

55. Reitmair AH, Schmits R, Ewel A, et al. MSH2 deficient mice are viable and susceptible to lymphoid tumous. *Nat Genet* 1995;11:64–70.

56. Reitmar AH, Redston M, Cai JC, et al. Spontaneous intestinal carcinomas and skin neoplasms in Msh-2 deficient mice. *Cancer Res* 1996;56:3842–3849.

57. de Wind N, Dekker M, van Rossum A, et al. Mouse models for hereditary nonpolyposis colorectal cancer. *Cancer Res* 1998; 58:248–255.

58. Kohonen-Corish MR, Daniel JJ, te Riele H, et al. Susceptibility of *Msh2*-deficient mice to inflammation-associated colorectal tumors. *Cancer Res* 2002;62:2092–2097.

59. Reitmar AH, Cai JC, Bjerknes M, et al. MSH2 deficiency contributes to accelerated APC-mediated intestinal tumorigenesis. *Cancer Res* 1996;56:2922–2926.

60. Baker SM, Harris AC, Tsao JL, et al. Enhanced intestinal adenomatous polyp formation in Pms2 –/– Min mice. *Cancer Res* 1998;58:1087–1089.

61. Edelmann W, Yang K, Kuraguchi M, et al. Tumorigenesis in *Mlh1* and *Mlh1/Apc1638N* mutant mice. *Cancer Res* 1999; 59:1301–1307.

62. Edelmann W, Umar A, Yang K, et al. The DNA mismatch repair genes *Msh3* and *Msh6* cooperate in intestinal tumor suppression. *Cancer Res* 2000;60:803–807.

63. Edelmann W, Yang K, Umar A, et al. Mutation in the mismatch repair gene *Msh6* causes cancer susceptibility. *Cell* 1997;91:467–477.

64. Kuraguchi M, Edelmann W, Yang K, et al. Tumor-associated *Apc* mutations in *Mlh1*$^{-/-}$ *Apc*^{1638N} mice reveal a mutational signature of Mlh1 deficiency. *Oncogene* 2000;19: 5755–5763.

65. Kuraguchi M, Yang K, Wong E, et al. The distinct spectra of tumor-associated *Apc* mutations in mismatch repair deficient *Apc*^{1638N} mice define the roles of MSH3 and MSH6 in DNA repair and intestinal tumorigenesis. *Cancer Res* 2001;61: 7934–7942.

66. Lieber M. The Fen-1 family of structure-specific nucleases in eukaryotic DNA replication, recombination and repair. *Bioessays* 1997;19: 223–240.

67. Kucherlapati M, Yang K, Kuraguchi M, et al. Haplo-insufficiency of flap endonuclease (*Fen1*) leads to rapid tumor progression. *Proc Natl Acad Sci USA* 2002;99:9924–9929.

68. Balmain A. Cancer as a complex genetic trait: tumor susceptibility in humans and mouse models. *Cell* 2002;108: 145–152.

69. Dietrich WF, Lander ES, Smith JS, et al. Genetic identification of *Mom*-1, a major modifier locus affecting *Min*-induced intestinal neoplasia in the mouse. *Cell* 1993;75:631–639.

70. MacPhee M, Chepenik KP, Liddell RA, et al. The secretory phospholipase A2 gene is a candidate for the *Mom1* locus, a major modifier of *Apc* ^{Min} - induced intestinal neoplasia. *Cell* 1995;81:957–966.

71. Cormier RT, Hong KH, Halberg RB, et al. Secretory phospholipase *Pla2g2a* confers resistance to intestinal tumorigenesis. *Nat Gene* 1997;17:88–91.

72. Koratkart R, Pequignot E, Hauck WW, Siracusa LD. The CAST/Ei strain confers significant protection against *Apc*^{Min} intestinal polyps, independent of the resistant modifier of Min 1 (*Mom1′*) locus. *Cancer Res* 2002;62:5413–5417.

73. Wakefield LM, Roberts AB. TGF-β signaling: positive and negative effects on tumorigenesis. *Curr Opin Genet Dev* 2002;12:22–29.

74. Moustakas A. Smad signaling network. *J Cell Sci* 2002; 115:3355–3356.

75. Kim SJ, Im YH, Markowitz SD, Bang YJ. Molecular mechanisms of inactivation of TGF-β receptors during carcinogenesis. *Cytokine Growth Factor Rev* 2000;11: 159–168.

76. Oshima M, Oshima H, Taketo MM. TGF-β receptor type II deficiency results in defects of yolk sac hematopoiesis and vasculogenesis. *Dev Biol* 1996;179:297–302.

77. Sirard C, de la Pompa JL, Elia A, et al. The tumor suppressor gene *Smad4/Dpc4* is required for gastrulation and later for

78. anterior development of the mouse embryo. *Genes Dev* 1998;12:107–119.

78. Waldrip WR, Bikoff EK, Hoodless PA, et al. Smad2 signaling in extraembryonic tissues determines anterior-posterior polarity of the early mouse embryo. *Cell* 1998;92: 797–808.

79. Takaku K, Oshima M, Miyoshi H, et al. Intestinal tumorigenesis in compound mutant mice of both *Dpc4* (*Smad4*) and *Apc* genes. *Cell* 1998;92:645–656.

80. Hamamoto T, Beppu H, Okada H, et al. Compound disruption of *Smad2* accelerates malignant progression of intestinal tumors in *Apc* knockout mice. *Cancer Res* 2002;62: 5955–5961.

81. Zhu Y, Richardson JA, Parada LF, Graff JM. *Smad3* mutant mice develop metastatic colorectal cancer. *Cell* 1998;94: 703–714.

82. Wick W, Peterson I, Schmutzler R, et al. Evidence for a novel tumor suppressor gene on chromosome 15 associated with progression to a metastatic stage in breast cancer. *Oncogene* 1996;12:973–978.

83. Zhang Y, Feng X, Derynck R. Receptor-associated Mad homologues synergize as effector of TGF-β response. *Nature* 1996;383:168–172.

84. Freund JN, Domon-Dell C, Kedinger M, Duluc I. The Cdx-1 and Cdx-2 homeobox genes in the intestine. *Biochem Cell Biol* 1998;76:957–969.

85. Beck F, Chawengsaksophak K, Waring P, et al. Reprogramming of intestinal cell differentiation and intercalary regeneration in Cdx2 mutant mice. *Proc Natl Acad Sci USA* 1999;96: 7318–7323.

86. Tamai Y, Nakajima R, Ishikawa T, et al. Colonic hamartoma development by anomalous duplication in Cdx2 knockout mice. *Cancer Res* 1999;59:2965–2970.

87. Silberg DG, Sullivan J, Kahn E, et al. Cdx2 ectopic expression induces gastric intestinal metaplasia in transgenic mice. *Gastroenterology* 2002;122:689–696.

88. Sasaki T, Irie-Sasaki J, Horie Y, et al. Colorectal carcinomas in mice lacking the catalytic subunit of PI(3)Kγ. *Nature* 2000;406:897–902.

89. Toker A, Cantley LC. Signaling through the lipid products of phosphoinositide-3-OH kinase. *Nature* 1997;387:673–676.

90. Leevers SJ, Vanhaesebroeck B, Waterfield MD. Signalling through phophoinositide 3-kinases: the lipids take centre stage. *Curr Opin Cell Biol* 1999;11:219–225.

91. Gendler SJ, Spicer AP. Epithelial mucin genes. *Annu Rev Physiol* 1995;57:607–634.

92. Kim YS, Gum JR, Brockhausen I. Mucin glycoproteins in neoplasia. *Glycoconj J* 1996;13:693–707.

93. Velcich A, Yang WC, Heyer J, et al. Colorectal cancer in mice genetically deficient in the mucin Muc2. *Science* 2002;295:1726–1729.

94. Shibata H, Toyama K, Shioya H, et al. Rapid colorectal adenoma formation initiated by conditional targeting of the *Apc* gene. *Science* 1997;278;120–123.

95. Kelloff GJ, Crowell JA, Steele VE, et al. Progress in cancer chemoprevention. *Ann NY Acad Sci* 1999;889:1–13.

96. Kelloff GJ. Perspectives on cancer chemoprevention research and drug development. *Adv Cancer Res* 2000;78: 199–334.

97. Wasan HS, Novelli M, Bee J, Bodmer WF. Dietary fat influences on polyp phenotype in multiple intestinal neoplasia mice. *Proc Natl Acad Sci USA* 1997;94:3308–3313.

98. Hioki K, Shivapurkar N, Oshima H, et al. Suppression of intestinal polyp development by low-fat and high-fiber diet

in *Apc*^{Δ716} knockout mice. *Carcinogenesis* 1997;18: 1863–1865.

99. Yang K, Edelmann W, Fan K, et al. Dietary modulation of carcinoma development in a mouse model for human familial adenomatous polyposis. *Cancer Res* 1998;58: 5713–5717.

100. Yang K, Fan K, Shinozaki H, et al. Increasing dietary calcium and vitamin D in mouse models of intestinal carcinogenesis. *Frontiers in Cancer Prevention Res,* 2002, p. 92.

101. Newmark HL, Lipkin M, Maheswari N. Colonic hyperplasia and hyperproliferation induced by a nutritional stress diet with four components of Western-style diet. *J Natl Cancer Inst* 1990;82:491–496.

102. Newmark HL, Lipkin M, Maheswari N. Colonic hyperproliferation induced in rats and mice by nutritional stress diets containing four components of a human Western-style diet (series 2). *Am J Clin Nutr* 1991;54:209s–214s.

103. Risio M, Lipkin M, Newmark H, et al. Apoptosis, cell replication, and Western-style diet-induced tumorigenesis in mouse colon. *Cancer Res* 1996;56:4910–4916.

104. Khan N, Yang K, Newmark H, et al. Mammary ductal epithelial cell hyperproliferation and hyperplasia induced by a nutritional stress diet containing four components of a Western-style diet. *Carcinogenesis* 1994;15:2645–2648.

105. Xue L, Newmark H, Yang K, Lipkin M. Model of mouse mammary gland hyperproliferation and hyperplasia induced by a Western-style diet. *Nutr Cancer* 1996;26:281-287.

106. Xue L, Yang K, Newmark H, Lipkin M. Induced hyperproliferation in epithelial cells of mouse prostate by a Western-style diet. *Carcinogenesis* 1997;18:995–999.

107. Xue L, Lipkin M, Newmark H, Wang J. Influence of dietary calcium and vitamin D on diet-induced epithelial cell hyperproliferation in mice. *J Natl Cancer Inst* 1999;91: 176–181.

108. Song J, Sohn KJ, Medline A, et al. Chemopreventive effects of dietary folate on intestinal polyps in *Apc*^{+/−} *Msh2*^{−/−} mice. *Cancer Res* 2000;60:3191–3199.

109. Song J, Medline M, Mason JB, et al. Effects of dietary folate on intestinal tumorigenesis in the *Apc*^{min} mouse. *Cancer Res* 2000;60:5434–5440.

110. Newmark HL, Yang K, Lipkin M, et al. A Western-style diet induces benign and malignant neoplasms in the colon of normal C57B1/6 mice. *Carcinogenesis* 2001;22:1871–1875.

111. Choi SW, Mason JB. Folate and carcinogenesis: an integrated scheme. *J Nutr* 2000;130:129–132.

112. Choi SW, Mason JB. Folate status: effects on pathways of colorectal carcinogenesis. *J Nutr* 2002;132:2413S–2418S.

113. Lamprecht SA, Lipkin M. Cellular mechanisms of calcium and vitamin D in the inhibition of colorectal carcinogenesis. *Ann NY Acad Sci* 2001;952:73–87.

114. Lamprecht SA, Lipkin M. Chemoprevention of colon cancer by calcium, vitamin D and folate: molecular mechanisms. *Nat Rev Cancer* 2003;3:601–614.

115. Oshima M, Dinchuk JE, Kargman SL, et al. Suppression of intestinal polyposis in *Apc*^{Δ716} knockout mice by inhibition of cyclooxygenase 2 (COX-2). *Cell* 1996;87:803–809.

116. Chulada PC, Thompson MB, Mahler J, et al. Genetic disruption of *Ptgs-1*, as well as of *Ptgs-2*, reduces intestinal tumorigenesis in *Min* mice. *Cancer Res* 2000;60:4705–4708.

117. Gupta RA, DuBois RN. Colorectal cancer prevention and treatment by inhibition of cyclooxygenase-2. *Nat Rev Cancer* 2001;1:11–21.

118. Bolbol SK, Dannenberg AJ, Chadburn A, et al. Cyclooxygenase-2 overexpression and tumor formation are blocked by sulindac in a murine model of familial adenomatous polyposis. *Cancer Res* 1996;56:2556–2560.

119. Beazer-Barclay Y, Levy DB, Moser R, et al. Sulindac suppresses tumorigenesis in the Min mouse. *Carcinogenesis* 1996;17:1757–1760.

120. Mahmoud NN, Boolbol SK, Dannenberg AJ, et al. The sulfide metabolite of sulindac prevents tumors and restores enterocyte apoptosis in a murine model of familial adenomatous polyposis. *Carcinogenesis* 1998;19:87–91.

121. Mahmoud NN, Bilinski RT, Churchill MR, et al. Genotype-phenotype correlation in murine *Apc* mutation: differences in enterocyte migration and response to sulindac. *Cancer Res* 1999;59:353–359.

122. Yang WC, Velcich A, Mariadason J, et al. *p21*^{WAF1/cip1} is an important determinant of intestinal cell response to sulindac *in vitro* and *in vivo*. *Cancer Res* 2001;61:6297–6302.

123. Jacoby RF, Siebert K, Cole CE, et al. The cyclooxygenase-2 inhibitor celecoxib is a potent preventive and therapeutic agent in the Min mouse model of adenomatous polyposis. *Cancer Res* 2000;60:5040–5044.

124. Oshima M, Murai N, Kargman S, et al. Chemoprevention of intestinal polyposis in the *Apc*^{Δ716} mouse by rofecoxib, a specific cyclooxygenase-2 inhibitor. *Cancer Res* 2001;61: 1733–1740.

125. Sunayama K, Konno H, Nakamura T, et al. The role of cyclooxygenase-2 (COX-2) in two different morphological stages of intestinal polyps in *Apc*^{Δ474} knockout mice. *Carcinogenesis* 2002;23:1351–1359.

126. Lal G, Ash C, Hay K, et al. Suppression of intestinal polyps in Msh2-deficient and non-Msh2-deficient multiple intestinal neoplasia mice by a specific cyclooxygenase-2 inhibitor and by a dual cyclooxygenase-1/2 inhibitor. *Cancer Res* 2001;61: 6131–6136.

127. Yang K, Fan K, Kurihara N, et al. Regional response leading to tumorigenesis after sulindac in small and large intestine of mice with *Apc* mutations. *Carcinogenesis* 2003;24:605–611.

128. Lefebvre A-M, Chen I, Desreumaux P, et al. Activation of the peroxisome proliferator-activated receptor γ promotes the development of colon tumors in C57BL/6J-APC^{Min}/+ mice. *Nat Med* 1998;4:1053–1057.

129. Saez E, Tontonoz P, Nelson MC, et al. Activators of the nuclear receptor PPAR-γ enhance colon polyp formation. *Nat Med* 1998;4:1058–1061.

130. Berger J, Moller DE. The mechanisms of action of PPARs. *Annu Rev Med* 2002;53:409–435.

131. Fajas L, Debril M-B, Auwerx J. Peroxisome proliferator-activated receptor-gamma: from adipogenesis to carcinogenesis. *J Mol Endocrinol* 2001;27:1–9.

132. Yang K, Lamprecht SA, Fan K, et al. Troglitazone increases tumorigenesis in the colon of mice with Mlh1/Apc mutations. *Anticancer Res* 2001;21:1577, abst. no. 47.

133. Yang K, Fan K, Lamprecht SA, et al. Troglitazone induces colonic tumors in normal C57BL/6 mice and increases colonic tumors in *Ml/APC* mutant mice. *Proc Am Assoc Cancer Res* 2003;44:285 (abstr).

134. Torrance CJ, Jackson PE, Montgomery E, et al. Combinatorial chemoprevention of intestinal neoplasms. *Nat Med* 2000;6: 1024–1028.

135. Balmain A, Harris CC. Carcinogenesis in mouse and human cells: parallels and paradoxes. *Carcinogenesis* 2000;21:371–377.

136. Rudolph KI, Millard M, Bosenberg MW, DePinho RA. Telomere dysfunction and evolution of intestinal carcinoma in mice and humans. *Nature Gen* 2001;28:155–159.

137. Smits R, Kartheuser A, Jagmohan-Changur S, et al. Loss of *Apc* and the entire chromosome 18 but absence of mutations at the *Ras* and *Tp53* genes in intestinal tumors from *Apc*1638N, a mouse model for *Apc*-driven carcinogenesis. *Carcinogenesis* 1997;18:321–327.

138. Lamprecht SA, Lipkin M. Migrating colonic crypt epithelial cells: primary targets for transformation. *Carcinogenesis* 2002;23:1777–1780.

139. Halberg RB, Katzung DS, Hoff PD, et al. Tumorigenesis in the multiple intestinal neoplasia mouse: redundancy of negative regulators and specificity of modifiers. *Proc Natl Acad Sci USA* 2000;97:3461–3466.

140. Yamada Y, Hata K, Hirose Y, et al. Microadenomatous lesions involving loss of *Apc* heterozygosity in the colon of adult *Apc^{Min/+}* mice. *Cancer Res* 2002;62:6367–6370.

141. Kinzler KW, Vogelstein B. Landscaping the cancer terrain. *Science* 1998;280:1036–1037.

142. Olumi AF, Grossfeld GD, Hayward SW, et al. Carcinoma-associated fibroblasts direct tumor progression of initiated human prostatic epithelium. *Cancer Res* 1999;59: 5002–5011.

143. Skobe M, Fusenig NE. Tumorigenic conversion of immortal human keratinocytes through stromal cell activation. *Proc Natl Acad Sci USA* 1998;95:1050–1055.

144. Jackson-Grusby L. Modeling cancer in mice. *Oncogene* 2002;21:5504–5514.

145. Van Dyke T, Jacks T. Cancer modeling in the modern era: progress and challenges. *Cell* 2002;108:135–144.

146. Tuveson DA, Jacks T. Technologically advanced cancer modeling in mice. *Curr Opin Genet Dev* 2002;12:105–110.

147. Bullard DC, Weaver CT. Cutting-edge technology IV. Genomic engineering for studies of the gastrointestinal tract in mice. *Am J Physiol Gastrointest Liver Physiol* 2002; 283:G1232–G1237.

148. Janssen K-P, El Marjo F, Pinto D, et al. Targeted expression of oncogenic K-*ras* in intestinal epithelium causes spontaneous tumorigenesis in mice. *Gastroenterology* 2002; 123:492–504.

149. Wigle DA, Rossant J, Jurisica I. Minireview: mining mouse microarray data. *Genome Bio* 2001;2:1019.1–1019.4.

150. Bates MD, Erwin CR, Sanford LP, et al. Novel genes and functional relationships in the adult mouse gastrointestinal tract identified by microarray analysis. *Gastroenterology* 2002;122:1467–1492.

151. Minowa T, Ohtsuka S, Hasai H, Kamada M. Proteomic analysis of the small intestine and colon epithelia of adenomatous polyposis coli gene-mutant mice by two-dimensional gel electrophoresis. *Electrophoresis* 2000;21: 1782–1786.

152. Edinger M, Cao Y-A, Hornig YS, et al. Advancing animal models of neoplasia through in vivo bioluminescence imaging. *Eur J Cancer* 2002;38:2128–2136.

153. Lewis JS, Achilefu S, Garbow JR, et al. Small animal imaging current technology and perspectives for oncological imaging. *Eur J Cancer* 2002;38:2173–2188.

5 Pathology of Incipient Neoplasia

Donald Earl Henson, MD, and Jorge Albores-Saavedra, MD

CONTENTS

1. INTRODUCTION

Our knowledge of the pathology of malignant tumors is based largely on invasive forms of cancer. Less is known about early or preclinical stages of tumor development. However, many of the morphologic and molecular abnormalities found in malignant tumors also exist in precursor or incipient lesions. New laboratory techniques, such as microdissection and polymerase chain reaction (PCR), have stimulated interest in early cancer development and events that precede invasion.

Incipient neoplasia, encompassing morphologic changes associated with early neoplastic development, does not imply that invasive cancer is the final outcome. Rather it refers to well-defined histologic lesions with increased probability or risk for invasive cancer (1). Incipient lesions, therefore, are morphologic risk factors for invasive cancer, and for this reason can serve as surrogate endpoints or therapeutic targets for chemoprevention (2).

To expedite chemopreventive agent development, a Task Force of the American Association of Cancer Research recently recommended focusing research on precancerous lesions (2). However, as part of agent development, we must consider histological types, rates of progression, molecular alterations, age of onset, heterogeneity, multifocal origin, and other biological properties, as well as the changing terminology of these lesions and the influence of these variables on clinical trial results and interpretation.

2. TERMINOLOGY

The terminology of incipient lesions has changed through the years. Of necessity, the terminology has conveyed a mixture of diagnostic, prognostic, and etiologic significance. Other terms for incipient neoplasia have included atypical hyperplasia; mild, moderate, or severe dysplasia; epithelial atypia; high grade intraepithelial lesion; carcinoma *in situ* (CIS); intramucosal carcinoma; *in situ* melanoma; borderline tumor; grade one-half carcinoma; intraepithelial neoplasia; and minimal cancer. These terms have been used in different locations to indicate early neoplastic transformation, uncertain biological potential, or both. The diagnostic terms actinic keratosis (AK) and arsenal keratosis, on the other hand, reflect the etiology of these cutaneous *in situ* carcinomas.

Additional definitions of incipient lesions are based on markers associated with early neoplastic development. These can include changes in DNA sequences, oncogene amplification, DNA aneuploidy, heterogeneity, accumulated genetic damage, and others (3). A useful marker, whether genetic alteration or

From: Cancer Chemoprevention, Volume 2: Strategies for Cancer Chemoprevention
Edited by: G. J. Kelloff, E. T. Hawk, and C. C. Sigman © Humana Press Inc., Totowa, NJ

abnormal protein, should have a low prevalence in nondysplastic lesions and increase with the severity of dysplasia. The highest frequency of the marker would be found in cases of severe dysplasia and CIS. However, an ideal marker should be unrelated to morphology. It should occur in high prevalence in all lesions destined to progress regardless of morphology, but occur in low prevalence in lesions that will not progress regardless of morphology. DNA cytometric aneuploidy corresponding to chromosomal aneuploidy is accepted as a marker for preneoplasia regardless of morphology *(4)*.

Finally, pathologists often designate incipient epithelial lesions by the inclusive term intraepithelial neoplasia, which is now recommended by the World Health Organization (WHO). For some sites, i.e., prostate and cervix, this terminology is standard (prostatic intraepithelial neoplasia, PIN, and cervical intraepithelial neoplasia, CIN). Unless the diagnosis is qualified by mild, moderate, severe, or another modifier, the inclusive term will not provide information about the risk of progression, which is an important parameter useful to clinicians and investigators.

3. DIFFERENCES FROM INVASIVE CANCER

Incipient lesions are biologically different from invasive cancers. As risk factors, they can be considered separate entities, each with its own morphological features and natural history. They differ from invasive cancers in prevalence, presentation, treatment, management, development, and molecular profiles. They may arise sporadically or be genetically determined. Some are associated with specific predisposing factors. Since it is often difficult to predict their biological behavior from morphologic observations alone, most incipient lesions are treated as potentially malignant. The light microscopic interpretation can give both false-positive results (overestimation of malignant potential) and false-negative results (underestimation of malignant potential).

3.1. Age

Incipient lesions arise at a younger age than do invasive cancers, which has implications for chemoprevention. The peak age at which most sporadic tumors arise is on average around 10 yr earlier than the peak age of invasive cancers. These differences in peak age depend on anatomic site and histologic type. Progression of breast cancer from atypical hyperplasia to carcinoma may require 10–20 yr *(5,6)*. Thus progression is a relatively

slow process at a population level, although individual patients vary a great deal. However, genetically determined cancers tend to occur at a younger age, often during childhood, adolescence, or early adult life. Genetically determined C-cell hyperplasia and medullary microcarcinoma of the thyroid are often detected in children *(7)*. In familial adenomatous polyposis (FAP), adenomas appear at a mean age of 25 yr, cancer at 39 yr, and death from cancer at 42 yr.

3.2. Location

Incipient lesions are found primarily on epithelial surfaces, such as skin, cervix, gastrointestinal tract, esophagus, respiratory mucosa, urinary bladder, and breast. In contrast to epithelium, the concept of incipient neoplasia is not well defined for mesenchymal and lymphoid tissues, primarily because these tissues lack a basement membrane and their tumors are invasive from inception. However, progress has been made with some precursor lesions in these sites, such as follicular hyperplasia in the stomach that may progress to malignant lymphoma when associated with *Helicobacter pylori* infection *(8)*. Lymphoid hyperplasia associated with autoimmune diseases, viral infections, or immunodeficiency syndromes may also lead to malignant lymphoma. Follicular lymphoma *in situ* has been defined as involvement of single or scattered follicles within an otherwise normal lymph node *(9)*.

3.3. Size

In general, incipient epithelial lesions are relatively small, occupying only the mucosal surface, and by definition not extending below the basement membrane. They may be flat or papillary. Often they are only microscopic in size and not recognized on gross examination. However, these lesions can reach unusually large sizes by growing along the epithelial surface. *In situ* lesions in the breast, for instance, can measure 5 cm in diameter as they wind their way through the mammary ducts. Flat urothelial CIS of the urinary bladder may extend into the prostate and seminal vesicles. Adenomas in the colon often measure 5 cm in size. Mucinous cystic neoplasms of the pancreas of low malignant potential (borderline) are quite large but show only dysplastic and *in situ* changes along the surface epithelium.

3.4. Frequency

Epithelial incipient lesions are more common than corresponding invasive cancers. Sporadic colonic adenomas are far more prevalent than corresponding adenocarcinomas. Postmortem studies have revealed that 25–50% of the population will have single or multiple adenomas in the large intestine by age 70 *(10,11)*. In FAP, for instance, the colon contains hundreds of adenomas, but only one, or at the most several, will evolve into invasive cancer during the lifetime of the patient. In the skin, dysplastic and congenital nevi are more common than malignant melanomas, and AKs are more prevalent than squamous cell carcinomas (SCCs). The vast majority of incipient lesions, therefore, do not progress to invasive cancer.

3.5. Multicentricity

Incipient lesions are often multicentric and may cover wide areas of a mucosal surface. Even a single microscopic lesion may indicate the existence of others nearby *(12)*. In the lungs of smokers, for example, these lesions are often multiple, involve more than one bronchus, and occur bilaterally. When these lesions are multiple, they are usually seen in various stages of development, which suggests that they do not arise at the same time or progress at the same rate. Incipient lesions may also coexist with invasive tumors in adjacent organs. Pancreatic intraepithelial neoplasia is a multicentric lesion that often coexists with ampullary carcinoma, suggesting a field effect similar to that documented for urothelial carcinomas of the urinary bladder *(13)*. Lobular breast CIS is usually multicentric and frequently bilateral. Familial C-cell hyperplasia (medullary CIS) of the thyroid is nearly always bilateral *(7)*.

3.6. Preceding Conditions and Non-Neoplastic Lesions

Preexisting conditions, including inflammatory diseases and immunologic disorders, may give rise to incipient lesions. For instance, chronic inflammatory conditions, such as reflux esophagitis, ulcerative colitis, and primary sclerosing cholangitis, may induce dysplastic lesions and incipient neoplasms. Benign tumors, such as colonic adenomas, which by definition are accompanied by dysplastic changes, may progress to CIS and intramucosal carcinoma. Proliferative lesions such as chronic lymphedema can give rise to incipient lymphangiosarcomas. Immunodeficiency states may be associated with lymphoproliferative disorders and smooth muscle neoplasms. Non-neoplastic lesions such as fibrous dysplasia and Paget's disease of the bone may give rise to osteogenic sarcomas. While malignant transformation in non-neoplastic conditions is unusual, a variety of conditions are associated with malignant transformation *(14,15)*. Thus, the concept of incipient neoplasia becomes very broad when benign conditions occasionally serve as a source of cancer.

3.7. Genetic Independence

Multiple lesions arising in a whole area of tissue are often independent, because they have different genetic alterations *(16)*. Genetic independence has been extensively studied in the lung *(17,18)*. This independence may complicate chemoprevention research, since different genetic alterations may indicate multiple pathways for malignant transformation, and it may not be possible to block all pathways with one or two agents.

3.8. Genetic Abnormalities

It is assumed that progression is driven by continued genetic instability, that is, an increased rate of unrepaired DNA damage with the formation of abnormal genomic variants *(19,20)*. However, evidence shows that genetic instability occurs early in the neoplastic process, before morphologic changes are visible. Genetic changes have been found in normal-appearing lung mucosa and head and neck epithelium of smokers *(18,21)*. In the lung, genetic changes occurring in normal-appearing epithelium have resembled those seen in SCCs *(18)*. Similarly, genetic alterations have been found in colonic mucosa that shows no morphologic evidence of neoplastic transformation *(22)*.

Mutations have also been observed in early incipient lesions. K-*ras* mutations, found in more than 80% of invasive pancreatic carcinomas, have also been detected in hyperplastic and atypical hyperplastic lesions and CIS arising in the pancreatic ducts *(23,24)*. Genetic changes, especially 16p loss, have been found in cases of atypical breast hyperplasia *(25)*. Genetic alterations have also been found in precancerous lesions of the lung, especially loss of heterozygosity (LOH) on chromosome 3 and mutations in p53 *(26,27)*.

3.9. Heterogeneity

As a consequence of genetic instability, a tumor develops increasingly different subpopulations that reflect heterogeneity and clonal evolution. Heterogeneity can be viewed as distinct subpopulations with differing selective growth advantage under different conditions within the host *(28)*. Incipient lesions are heterogeneous morphologically, genetically, and cytologically, as evidenced by nuclear pleomorphism and variations in size and shape of individual cells. Preinvasive lesions are also heterogeneous when it comes to progression, as lesions of similar histology do not progress at the same rate. Invasive forms of cancer are also heterogeneous morphologically, which has long been recognized by pathologists. This heterogeneity occurs not only in similar tumors from different patients (intertumor heterogeneity), but also within the same tumor from a single patient (intratumor heterogeneity). Two or three different cell types may be present in the same tumor as determined by light microscopy, histochemistry, and immunohistochemistry.

Incipient lesions are heterogeneous genetically. Genetic alterations occur in dysplastic lesions that are not found in the synchronous invasive cancer (29). Variable genetic changes occur during progression of incipient lesions to invasive cancer in different patients even though these lesions are morphologically similar (interneoplastic heterogeneity). Heterogeneity is also seen when different mutations are found in the same gene of lesions that morphologically progress from one into another. For example, different p53 mutations were found in the adenomatous and carcinomatous components of colonic adenomas containing early cancer (30).

In theory, heterogeneity may affect the response of tissues to chemoprevention interventions. Because of heterogeneity, chemopreventive agents may not affect all subpopulations within a precursor lesion. A variable response to chemoprevention has been observed clinically. Tamoxifen, for instance, is more effective in preventing estrogen receptor (ER)+ breast cancer than ER− tumors.

3.10. Neoplastic Progression

3.10.1. PREDICTORS OF PROGRESSION

Along with diagnosis, estimating risk of progression is most useful clinically. Currently, estimates depend primarily on morphologic variation. In the future, molecular genetic changes may supplement histologic observations, allowing improved predictions of tumor response to treatment.

Dysplasia is the *sine qua non* of incipient neoplasia. High-grade dysplasia is generally considered an irreversible change that is truly neoplastic and the morphologic forerunner of most malignant epithelial tumors. Clinically, a diagnosis of high-grade, severe, or grade III dysplasia usually indicates persistence of the lesion or eventual progression in a high proportion of untreated patients.

Incipient epithelial lesions often follow a morphologic sequence from hyperplasia or metaplasia through dysplasia to CIS and subsequent invasion. Lesions most advanced along the sequence are likely to progress most rapidly. However, there is morphologic evidence that not all lesions follow the sequence; some may even reverse direction. In the stomach, for example, endocrine cell hyperplasia occurring in the gastric mucosa of pernicious anemia patients is reversible if the trophic stimulus that results from G cell hyperplasia in the antrum is removed (31). In the lung, incipient lesions along the bronchi may regress if an individual quits smoking.

Metaplasia presages cancer in some sites, because it seems to make tissues more susceptible to malignant transformation. An acquired condition, metaplasia is the physiologic transformation of one type of differentiated tissue into another, usually in response to chronic irritation. Often considered a phenotypic reactive change, metaplasia always develops before cancer. Intestinal metaplasia of the stomach, for example, often precedes invasive carcinoma. In some sites, e.g., Barrett's esophagus, metaplasia is considered a premalignant lesion. Mutations showing intestinal metaplasia have been found in non-neoplastic stomach mucosa (32). Metaplasia may even influence the type of invasive cancer. Intestinal metaplasia in the gallbladder is thought to give rise to intestinal-type carcinomas, and in the cervix, squamous metaplasia gives rise to SCCs.

3.10.2. RATES OF PROGRESSION

Incipient lesions progress to invasive cancer at variable rates that correlate with the severity of pathologic changes. These rates of progression are difficult to estimate from single biopsy specimens or cell samples, as they may vary with age, sex, ethnicity, hormonal status, and other factors. Changes in diagnostic criteria and terminology may also affect analysis of progression. In some patients, lesions require years to progress, whereas in others only a short time is needed. Incipient lesions of the pancreas may require many years, 29 in one case, to progress (33,34). Progression of colonic adenomas to carcinoma varies from 5 to 15 yr (35).

Clearly, longer progression times create wider windows of opportunity to interrupt the process. However, in designing chemoprevention protocols, sample size must take into account regression and progression rates of incipient lesions and estimated response to treatment. Finally, it is possible that faster progression creates greater carcinogenic stimulus, making it more difficult to prevent subsequent invasion with chemopreventive interventions.

4. MIMICKERS

Mimickers include reparative changes that resemble incipient lesions and incipient lesions that are actually part of an invasive cancer. In many organs, inflammation and mucosal ulceration are followed by regeneration of the epithelium. Regenerating epithelial cells often show large vesicular nuclei with prominent nucleoli and increased mitotic activity. As a result, reactive cells can be confused with dysplastic and malignant cells, which in turn may distort intervention results and even lead to unnecessary treatment. This is especially true in the esophagus, biliary tree, stomach, and colon. On the other hand, many invasive carcinomas can spread along epithelial-lined structures above the basement membrane, simulating *in situ* lesions. For example, invasive carcinoma of the pancreas may extend along normal ducts and simulate high-grade intraepithelial neoplasia *(36)*.

5. GENETICALLY DETERMINED INCIPIENT LESIONS

The development of genetic tests for germline mutations has revolutionized prevention of some hereditary cancers. An example is C-cell hyperplasia or medullary thyroid CIS associated with the MEN II syndromes and familial medullary carcinoma. These cancers can be excised by surgery before they develop because genetic tests provide an early diagnosis.

Neoplastic C-cell hyperplasia (medullary CIS) is the precursor of invasive medullary thyroid carcinoma. C-cell hyperplasia in MEN IIa is monoclonal, genetically heterogeneous, and shows downregulated apoptosis, supporting its neoplastic nature *(37)*. Neoplastic C-cell hyperplasia may be the only pathological finding in children with familial medullary carcinoma or the MEN IIa or MEN IIb syndrome. It can be diagnosed in asymptomatic children or adolescents with MEN II syndrome by detecting germline mutations in the Ret proto-oncogene using an inexpensive, highly sensitive, and specific nonradioactive genetic test that can be performed on peripheral blood. Patients with a positive genetic assay, even those without a positive pentagastrin stimulation test or with normal calcitonin levels, should undergo surgical treatment (total thyroidectomy) *(7)*.

Neoplastic C-cell hyperplasia is nearly always bilateral and shows focal, diffuse, and nodular growth patterns. In focal hyperplasia, only some follicles are surrounded by calcitonin-positive C-cells, which compress and push the follicular cells upward. The diffuse form of C-cell hyperplasia is characterized by follicles with a ring-like lining of C-cells. In nodular hyperplasia, follicles are obliterated, with formation of C-cell nodules surrounded by an intact basal lamina. The intrafollicular C-cells are mildly to moderately atypical, recognizable with conventional histological stains, and similar to those of invasive medullary carcinoma *(38)*.

Many germline-determined tumors are multicentric, involving more than one organ. For instance, FAP usually involves most of the colon, the ampulla of Vater, and less frequently, the small intestine and pancreas. MEN IIa syndrome involves bilateral C-cell hyperplasia or medullary thyroid carcinoma, bilateral adrenal medullary hyperplasia or pheochromocytomas, and parathyroid hyperplasia. Hereditary nonpolyposis colorectal cancer (HNPCC) syndrome involves the colon and frequently the endometrium, and Li-Fraumeni syndrome affects soft tissues and mammary glands.

6. EFFECTS OF CHEMOPREVENTIVE AGENTS ON HISTOPATHOLOGY

Chemopreventive agents may affect the morphology of incipient lesions, which may influence the interpretation of interventions if intraepithelial neoplasia is the endpoint or target of chemoprevention. Moreover, any change in morphology may also change our ability to detect or image these lesions. Agents may inhibit development of incipient lesions, in which case invasive cancers should not develop. Some agents may cause established lesions to regress completely and permanently along with eliminating all genetic changes (phenotypic and genotypic regression). Other agents may cause temporary regression, but the lesion may regrow and acquire an entirely different morphology than initially observed (phenotypic divergence). Some agents may produce morphologic changes in lesions; though still present, they can no longer be histologically identified with certainty because of genetic changes. Moreover, lesions may regress morphologically (phenotypic regression) but persist genetically, eventually evolving into cancer because of continuing genetic instability, without passing through the usual histologic precancerous stages.

Alternatively, some chemopreventive agents may not eliminate or prevent the lesion, but may reduce the risk of progression by preventing additional genetic changes (genetic stability). If histologic regression does

Table 1
Classification of Precancerous Lesions and Conditions
of the Oral Mucosa *(153)*

Precancerous Lesions
  Leukoplakia
     Homogeneous leukoplakia
     Nodular leukoplakia
     Speckled leukoplakia
     Proliferative verrucous leukoplakia
  Erythroplakia
Precancerous Conditions
  Oral submucous fibrosis
  Actinic keratosis
  Lichen planus
  Sideropenic dysphagia
  Discoid lupus erythematosus

not occur after chemopreventive intervention, it seems safe to assume that the genetic abnormalities will remain even though the lesion does not progress.

7. PATHOLOGY OF SPECIFIC ANATOMIC SITES

7.1. Upper Aerodigestive Tract

Incipient lesions can arise in any anatomically defined region of the upper aerodigestive tract (UADT). For the most part, these lesions develop from squamous epithelium that lines the tract and gives rise to different types of SCCs. Nasopharynx and sinonasal passages, on the other hand, are lined primarily with pseudostratified ciliated epithelium. Preinvasive lesions and invasive tumors arising in the UADT and lower respiratory tract are often multiple, appearing either synchronously or metachronously. For this reason, the mucosa lining the UADT and bronchial epithelium is regarded as a field of growth for tumor development. The larynx is the most common UADT site for incipient lesions and invasive tumors. The UADT is an important site for chemoprevention research because of the relatively high frequency of metachronously occurring tumors. Lesions in the UADT are consistently associated with cigarette smoking and/or chronic alcohol intake. Microscopically, the most common lesions include hyperkeratosis, dysplasia, and CIS (Table 1) *(39)*.

7.1.1. HYPERKERATOSIS

Most commonly seen in the buccal mucosa, alveolar ridge, hard palate, dorsal surface of the tongue, and laryngeal glottis, hyperkeratosis is characterized by an increase of surface keratin and thickening of the underlying epithelium. Clinically, these lesions are usually described as leukoplakia, but a more precise diagnosis should depend on biopsy. The extent of surface keratin seen clinically does not indicate underlying cellular changes. Oral leukoplakia has some advantage for chemopreventive interventions, as these lesions can be visualized clinically and are the most common precancerous lesions in the oral cavity. However, the rate of progression to invasive carcinoma is unpredictable. Erythroplakia, which is less common than leukoplakia, is often considered an intraepithelial neoplasm.

7.1.2. SQUAMOUS CELL DYSPLASIA

Dysplastic lesions are similar to those seen in other sites that give rise to SCCs, such as the lung and cervix *(40)*. However, UADT lesions are more likely to accumulate surface keratin in response to injury, imparting a white color. As with most dysplastic lesions, major maturation abnormalities in the epithelium become more pronounced with progression *(41)*. Squamous intraepithelial neoplasia (SIN, grades I–III) is occasionally used as a synonym for dysplasia.

7.1.3. OTHER LESIONS

The UADT is susceptible to other uncommon premalignant lesions with an uncertain rate of progression. They include Schneiderian (sinonasal tract) papillomas, occasionally associated with carcinoma; laryngeal papillomatosis, associated with human papillomavirus infection; and keratizing or adult papillomas. Laryngeal papillomatosis, often found in adolescents, is more apt to undergo malignant transformation after radiotherapy. Papillomas found in adults rarely if ever undergo malignant transformation. Nasopharyngeal carcinoma, the most common tumor of the nasopharynx, accounts for 85% of malignant tumors in this region and does not have a histologically defined precursor lesion.

7.1.4. PROGRESSION

While severe dysplasia indicates a very high risk for progression, the grading of dysplasia is not always proportional to the risk for transformation. It has been estimated that 3% of oral lesions and 4–7% of laryngeal lesions classified as mild dysplasia by light microscopy will progress *(42,43)*. Overall, the rate of progression of dysplasia is roughly 20%. Progression of CIS to invasive carcinoma varies for different regions in the UADT. Published figures indicate that 11–50% of lesions in the oral cavity progress and in the larynx from 3–25% progress *(44,45)*, although figures as high as 90% have appeared. Estimating progression is not possible on clinical examination alone, since the underlying pathology is unknown. Because of morbidity often associated with treatment, a variety of diagnostic methods have been evaluated to assess the potential for progression, including proliferation markers that usually correspond to histologic grade, DNA ploidy, p53, and cytogenetics. For the most part, these are still investigational, although ploidy analysis may prove more accurate in predicting progression than histologic grading *(46)*.

The histopathological growth pattern also provides an estimate of progression in some cases. Proliferative verrucous leukoplakia, an especially aggressive form of leukoplakia, has a high rate of progression to invasive carcinoma *(47)*. Histologically, the lesion has broad pushing borders extending downward into the underlying stroma, producing a verrucous-type SCC during early invasion. As clinicopathological entities, these lesions should be treated aggressively.

As already noted, genetic alterations have been found in normal-appearing UADT epithelium in smokers. *(21)* Because of the broad field effect, UADT may serve as a surrogate anatomic site for evaluating genetic alterations in anatomic regions contiguous with the UADT but not as accessible, such as bronchial epithelium and esophagus.

7.2. Lung

Unlike two of the four major types of lung cancer, large-cell and small-cell carcinoma, SCC and peripheral adenocarcinoma are preceded by defined precursor lesions. In general, preinvasive squamous cell lesions are found in the bronchial epithelium and precursor lesions for adenocarcinomas occur in the outlying pulmonary parenchyma. Bronchial lesions are usually uncovered during endoscopy for suspected cancer, while lesions arising in peripheral lung fields are more likely to be detected by spiral computed tomography (CT).

Multiple incipient lesions in different stages of develop-ment characteristically co-occur in the bronchial epithelium, especially in heavy smokers. The most significant of these in WHO classification include squamous cell metaplasia, squamous cell dysplasia, and CIS *(48–51)*. Other lesions, including goblet cell hyperplasia and basal cell hyperplasia, are thought to have a very low risk for progression. Basal cell or stem cell hyperplasia is considered one of the earliest morphologic steps required for malignant transformation. As with other epithelial tumors, invasive lung cancers are preceded by multiple incipient lesions progressing through sequential stages of development. However, the extent to which these lesions precede each other in time

is largely conjectural. Genetic evidence indicates that these multiple lesions arise independently *(17)*. Bronchial hyperplasia and squamous metaplasia are relatively common along the airways of smokers, while dysplasia and CIS are usually more common in smokers with cancer.

7.2.1. SQUAMOUS CELL METAPLASIA

The bronchial epithelium is susceptible to squamous cell metaplasia, in which mature squamous cells producing keratin and connected by intercellular bridges replace normal pseudostratified and ciliated respiratory epithelium. In contrast to dysplasia, there is no cellular atypia. Often associated with chronic irritation, in this case exposure to cigarette smoke, metaplasia is thought to predispose the epithelium to malignant transformation. Metaplasia is reversible, although it can evolve into dysplasia if the irritation persists.

7.2.2. SQUAMOUS CELL DYPLASIA

Squamous cell dysplasia is subcategorized as mild, moderate, or severe. In general, these lesions are characterized by increasing cellular atypia, nuclear enlargement, pleomorphism, hyperchromasia, and eventually loss of differentiation. An estimated 11% of moderate dysplastic lesions and 19–46% of severe dysplastic lesions will progress to invasive carcinoma as determined by sputum cytology *(52–54)*. Since most cigarette smoke impinges directly on the carina, incidence of dysplasia tends to be high around this anatomic divide.

7.2.3. CIS

In CIS, the full thickness of bronchial epithelium is replaced by squamous cells with the cytological features of cancer (Fig. 1A). The cells become hyperchromatic and pleomorphic, and exhibit loss of stratification and orientation. The nucleoli are enlarged and the nuclei irregular in shape.

Presence of CIS may indicate additional lesions within the bronchial epithelium, including invasive cancer or subsequent development of invasive cancer. Clinical observations show that slightly more than 50% of *in situ* lesions detected by bronchoscopic examination will progress within 6 mo *(55)*. Three months after diagnosis, 11–22% are likely to progress *(55,56)*. In contrast to some dysplastic lesions, CIS will not regress.

Perhaps it should be emphasized that invasion is occasionally difficult to assess in small bronchial biopsy specimens. On the other hand, microinvasive SCC is often an incidental finding (Fig. 1B). Further, adenocarcinomas are less likely to be detected by sputum cytology than by bronchial washes. These tumors

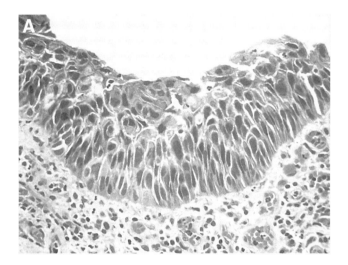

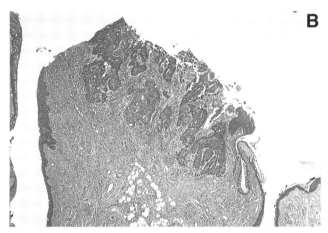

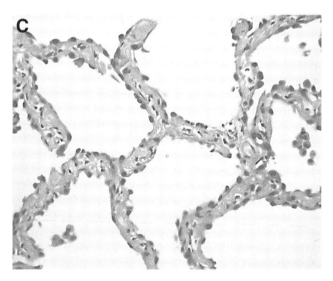

Fig. 1. (A) Squamous cell CIS of bronchus. The respiratory epithelium is replaced by neoplastic squamous cells. **(B)** Microinvasive squamous carcinoma of bronchus. Nests of malignant squamous cells infiltrate the subepithelial connective tissue. **(C)** Atypical adenomatous hyperplasia. The hyperplastic pneumocytes show mild to moderate atypia. (Courtesy of Dr. Masayaki, Noguchi, Japan.)

are primarily found in the peripheral lung compartment, and malignant cells from adenocarcinomas are less likely to desquamate than malignant cells from squamous carcinomas.

7.2.4. PROGRESSION

Progression of dysplastic lesions and CIS to invasive cancer correlates with a series of morphologic and genetic changes. In the bronchi, abnormal vascular patterns are found in dysplastic and metaplastic lesions that may indicate impending invasion *(57,58)*. Increased numbers of capillaries reflecting angiogenic activity often extend into these lesions that have been identified as high risk by LOH at chromosome 3p and by an increase in proliferative rate *(58)*. Molecularly, a series of progressive antigenic and genetic changes that accompany morphologic progression (Table 2) have been observed in preinvasive lesions within the airways *(59)*. Bronchial dysplastic lesions showing p53 overexpression have a greater risk for progression than similar lesions without overexpression *(60)*.

7.2.5. ATYPICAL ADENOMATOUS HYPERPLASIA

Small adenomatous peripheral lesions have long been noted, especially in pulmonary resections for carcinoma. They are usually multiple, millimeters in size, and found in the peripheral fields often at a distance from central tumors. Originally described with a variety of terms *(49)*, these lesions are now uniformly designated as atypical adenomatous hyperplasia (AAH) of the lung. They have been noted in 5–20% of pulmonary resection specimens, depending on the extent of search and diagnostic criteria. More benign-appearing forms are often designated as alveolar cell hyperplasia, considered primarily a reactive lesion and not a preneoplastic change.

AAH has been associated with adenocarcinomas, especially the nonmucinous bronchioloalveolar type. Evidence for this association is based on their frequent co-occurrence with cancer, molecular biology, immunohistochemical observations, and morphometric studies. Interestingly, these lesions are more common in lungs resected for adenocarcinoma or large cell undifferentiated carcinoma than for SCC *(61,62)*.

Histologically, the involved alveoli and respiratory epithelium of the distal bronchioles are lined by atypical cuboidal to low columnar cells, more accurately type II pneumocytes (Fig. 1C). Atypia is usually more pronounced in larger lesions. Lesions are not well demarcated; their periphery usually blends in with surrounding normal lung. The alveolar septae are thickened

Table 2
Various Changes Occurring With Progression From Normal Bronchial Mucosa
to Invasive Carcinoma in Central Bronchial Carcinogenesis (51)

	Normal epithelium	Squamous metaplasia	Low-grade dysplasia	High-grade dysplasia	CIS	Invasive carcinoma
Hyperproliferation	+	++	++	++	+++	+++
3p LOH	+	+	++	++	+++	+++
9p LOH	+	+	++	++	+++	+++
p53 overexpression	+	+	++	++	+++	+++
Rb expression	+	++	++	++	++	++
Cyclin D1 overexpression		+	+	++	++	
Telomerase overexpression		+	+	+	+	+++
Bcl-2 overexpression			+	+	++	++
Aneuploidy			+	++	++	+++
p53 mutation				+		++
p16 loss			+		++	
FHIT loss				+	++	+++
13q and 17p LOH				+	+++	+++
5p and 5q LOH						+

and often contain lymphocytes. For the most part, atypical cells are noninvasive with respect to the alveolar septae. Mitotic figures are rarely seen.

Differentiating AAH from early adenocarcinoma may be difficult. Consequently, chemoprevention trial results may be difficult to interpret because of the uncertain nature of the target lesions. As yet, no reliable markers or patterns of marker expression have been found to separate the lesions. AAH may act as an adenoma in the adenoma-carcinoma sequence. Radiologic

Table 3
Various Morphological, Morphometric, Immunohistochemical, and Molecular
Biological Findings in AAH and Adenocarcinoma (51)

	Low-grade AAH	High-grade AAH	Adenocarcinoma including BAC[a]
Cellularity and atypia	+	++	+++
Mean nuclear area	+	++	+++
Nuclear DNA content	+	++	++
Aneuploidy	+	++	++
AgNOR count	+	++	+++
CEA[a], p450, ApoA expression	+	++	++
P53 expression	+	++	+++
K-ras mutation	–/+	+	++
C-erb-B2 expression		+	++
Loss of Rb and p16			+
3p, 7p, 17p/q LOH		+	++
Blood group antigen expression	+++	+	+
Cyclin D1 overexpression	+++	++	+

[a]BAC, bronchioloalveolar cell carcinoma; CEA, carcinoembryonic antigen.

evaluation of AAH is often difficult because of their small size, location, and radiographic similarity to non-neoplastic lesions such as granulomas,.

Molecular changes occurring in AAH are listed in Table 3.

7.2.6. Small-Cell Carcinoma

The cell that gives rise to small-cell carcinoma has not as yet been identified. Most likely, it is a stem cell in the bronchial mucosa that may differentiate in endocrine and exocrine directions. Small-cell carcinomas often show areas of glandular or squamous cell differentiation. Diffuse idiopathic neuroendocrine cell hyperplasia is often thought to be a precursor to small-cell carcinomas because it seems to serve as a precursor to peripheral carcinoid tumors. Idiopathic neuroendocrine cell hyperplasia is relatively common and often associated with chronic inflammation and fibrosis.

7.2.7. Persisting Molecular Abnormalities

Molecular changes occurring in bronchial epithelium seem to be permanent or persist for many years. Molecular alterations similar to those seen in precancerous lesions have been detected in normal and in abnormal epithelium from current and former smokers *(63,64)*.

7.3. Barrett's Esophagus

Barrett's esophagus (BE) is a premalignant lesion characterized by metaplastic replacement of normal squamous epithelium of the distal esophagus with specialized epithelium containing goblet cells. Usually a result of gastric acid reflux, the metaplasia may progress over several years to low-grade dysplasia, high-grade dysplasia, and carcinoma. The lesion, often recognized endoscopically, can extend for several centimeters proximal from the gastroesophageal junction. Goblet cells, needed for diagnosis, can be highlighted by staining histologic sections with alcian blue. The special stain is often used to find cells that have goblet cell-type mucin but do not have full goblet cell morphology.

Histologically, BE consists of two cell types—columnar mucin-producing cells and goblet cells—that line villiform structures. Glands in the lamina propria are also lined with intestinalized columnar and goblet cells. Paneth and endocrine cells may also be present.

In low-grade dysplasia, glands present in the lamina propria are lined with pseudostratified columnar or elongated cells with large hyperchromatic nuclei. These abnormal glands often resemble tubular adenomas of the colon with mild dysplasia. Dysplastic

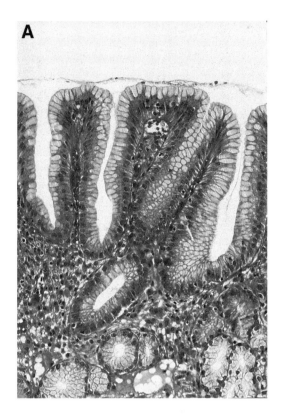

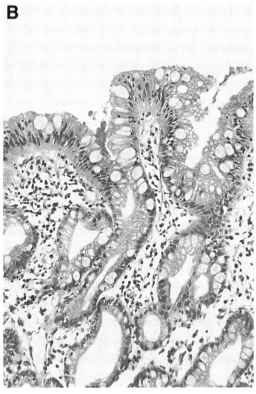

cells usually extend to the surface epithelium. High-grade dysplasia has greater cytologic atypia, both in glands and in surface epithelium, and mitotic activity increases (Fig. 2A–C).

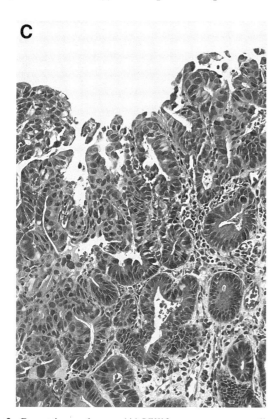

Fig. 2. Barrett's esophagus. (**A**) Villiform structures are lined by tall columnar cells with mucin-containing cytoplasm. (**B**) This villiform structure contains goblet cells intermixed with the tall columnar cells. No dysplasia is seen. (**C**) High-grade dysplasia. The surface epithelium and the glands contain highly atypical cells with large hyperchromatic and overlapping nuclei.

Pathological evaluation is the basis for patient stratification and management. The histologic classification of Barrett's dysplasia is identical to the classification for dysplasia used for inflammatory bowel disease (Table 4). Standard definitions for grades of dysplasia have been published *(65)*.

BE has the potential to progress to invasive cancer, although the frequency of progression is difficult to assess, since disease prevalence is unknown, though reports estimate 22.6 clinically diagnosed cases per 100,000 population. Adenocarcinoma has developed in 20–25% of patients followed for 10 yr, although this percentage has varied in different reports. Progression to invasive cancer is characterized by sequential changes through mild, moderate, and severe dysplasia as seen on endoscopic biopsy.

The risk of progression has been difficult to predict, since current morphologic criteria cannot always separate high-risk from low-risk patients. Furthermore, interpretation of biopsy specimens has not always been consistent because of variation in

Table 4
Classification of Epithelial Dysplasia
in Barrett's Esophagus *(154)*

Negative
   Indefinite for dysplasia
Positive
   Low-grade (mild/moderate dysplasia)
   High-grade (severe dysplasia and CIS)

diagnostic criteria and sampling. About 2–8% of patients with low-grade dysplasia progress to invasive cancer; among patients with high-grade dysplasia, 15% will progress. Overall, risk seems related to duration of disease, severity of dysplasia, length of the Barrett's column, and extent of dysplasia. Focal high-grade dysplasia takes longer to progress than multifocal high-grade changes (Fig. 3) *(66)*.

Presently, the best-documented factors associated with progression are p53 overexpression and DNA ploidy status *(67)*.

7.4. Colon and Rectum

Of all incipient lesions, those arising in the colon and rectum have attracted the greatest interest because of their frequency, growth pattern, and prominent size. These lesions are primarily polyps that include benign tumors, such as several types of adenomas, hyperplastic polyps, and hamartomatous polyps. Flat adenomas, which remain level with the surface mucosa, are also thought to serve as precursors. Histologically, the concepts behind colon cancer are the aberrant crypt focus (ACF)/adenoma-carcinoma sequence, and more recently the hyperplastic polyp-serrated adenoma-carcinoma sequence *(68)* Most colorectal carcinomas arise from preexisting adenomas, usually as a result of a mutation in a single suppressor gene (adenomatous polyposis coli, or APC) in a colonic epithelial stem cell. A smaller number, around 5–15%, arise in the ascending colon from hyperplastic polyps, presumably a result of microsatellite instability (MSI) caused by defective nucleotide mismatch repair.

7.4.1. ABERRANT CRYPT FOCI

ACF formation is considered one of the earliest histologic events in colorectal cancer development *(69)*. Therefore, clusters of these abnormal crypts are potentially the first stage in the ACF-adenoma-carcinoma sequence. The crypts can be identified in vivo through low-magnification endoscopy after methylene blue staining of the mucosa. ACF are larger than normal

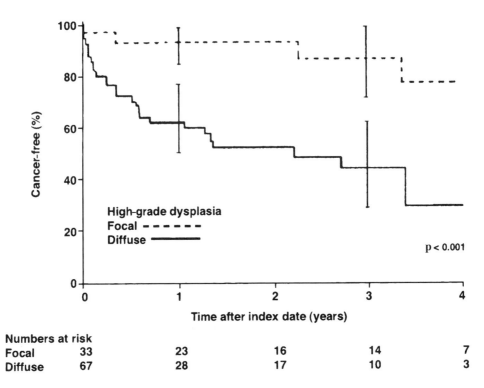

Fig. 3. Kaplan-Meier curves comparing focal and diffuse high-grade dysplasia. The percentage of patients who are cancer free at a given time is shown on the y axis, whereas duration of follow-up from the index date in years is shown on the x axis. Vertical bars indicate 95% confidence intervals. Using the log-rank statistic, the p value is 0.0006. (From ref. *66.*)

crypts, stain more intensely with methylene blue, and have either bulging or concave surfaces. Found throughout the colon and rectum, ACF are more common in the distal colon.

Morphologically, ACF also progress through hyperplastic and dysplastic stages *(70)*. These diverse stages can be found within the same abnormal focus. As these lesions progress to dysplasia, the cell proliferation rate increases and the proliferating compartment expands. Although normal mitotic indices characterize typical ACF, hyperproliferation seems a characteristic of hyperplastic and dysplastic ACF. In normal mucosa, the proliferating compartment is limited to the lower third of the crypt, although in response to injury it may expand temporarily to encompass a greater proportion of the gland. In ACF, the expansion is much greater, often reaching the luminal surface.

Animal experiments have revealed an association between ACF formation and carcinoma. In humans, ACF is thought to progress from adenoma to carcinoma. The prevalence of dysplastic ACF is significantly higher in patients with adenomas or carcinomas than in normal individuals *(71)*. A number of molecular alterations accompany ACF development. In most reports, 69–100% of ACF contain K-*ras* mutations, especially typical and hyperplastic ACF. About 5% of ACF have APC mutations *(72)*. MSI, an indication of loss of

mismatch repair gene function, is occasionally found. The number of ACF increases with age.

7.4.2. HYPERPLASTIC POLYPS

These polyps are characterized histologically by overmaturation and extended cellular differentiation resulting from failure of the normal sloughing process at the mucosal surface. They are probably the most common polypoid lesions found in the colon. Originally not considered precancerous, these lesions have now been found to progress to invasive cancer, especially when large, multiple, and located proximally *(73,68)*. Other risk factors include high-grade dysplasia in the polyp, coincidental adenomas, and first-degree relatives with hyperplastic polyps or colorectal cancer *(74)*.

Serrated adenomas are mixed hyperplastic and adenomatous polyps with potential for malignant transformation similar to that of tubular adenomas *(75)*. Most likely, they have a higher risk for invasion than pure hyperplastic polyps because of the adenomatous component. Studies suggest that nearly 5% of colorectal carcinomas are the result of serrated adenomas *(76)*. Clearly, the vast majority of hyperplastic polyps do not progress to invasive cancer. Molecular studies have revealed genetic changes that are also found in colorectal cancer, including mutations of K-*ras*, TGF RII, and MSI.

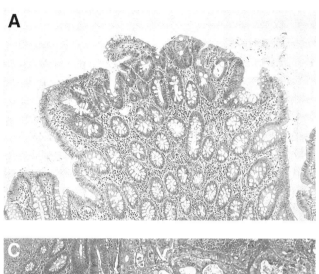

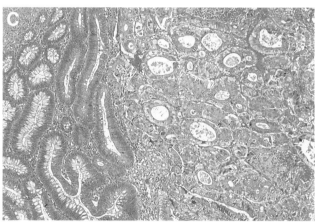

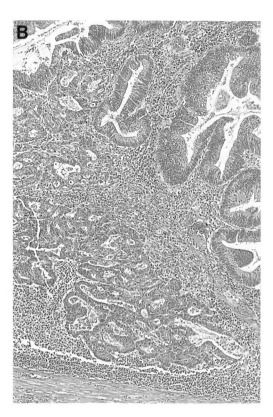

Fig. 4. Tubular adenoma of colon. **(A)** Tiny tubular adenoma in a patient with familial adenomatous polyposis. Although the normal architecture of the mucosa is maintained, some superficial crypts show adenomatous changes that are easily distinguished from the adjacent normal glands. **(B)** Tubular adenoma with intramucosal carcinoma. A cribriform structure is seen in the lamina propria beneath a tubular adenoma. **(C)** Tubular adenoma and infiltrating adenocarcinoma. The adenocarcinoma is composed of closely packed neoplastic glands different from those of the overlying tubulo-villous adenoma.

In all likelihood, these polyps are precursor lesions for colorectal cancers with MSI *(68)*.

7.4.3. ADENOMAS

Adenomas are benign glandular neoplasms arising from the intestinal mucosa and containing dysplastic epithelium. They may be solitary, multiple, sporadic, or hereditary (APC). Histologically, adenomas are classified as tubular (the most common type), villous, or mixed tubulovillous (Fig. 4A). Adenomas are thought to arise from ACF. These polyps can grow to large size, more than 5 cm in diameter.

Adenomas usually progress to invasive carcinomas within 5–15 yr, although their natural history is almost impossible to ascertain (Fig. 4B,C) *(35)*. Nearly all adenomas are resected when found. The chance of finding a carcinoma in an adenoma is 5% *(35)*. Only a small proportion of adenomas appear to progress to cancer; the adenoma to-carcinoma sequence is relatively slow. Factors that favor progression include the size of the tumor, its villous type, high-grade dysplastic changes, and extent of dysplasia within the adenoma. Also, larger adenomas with greater extent of dysplasia increase the likelihood of additional adenomas. While adenomas often serve as targets in chemoprevention studies, the response of serrated adenomas and hyperplastic polyps to chemopreventive agents is unclear. It is also unclear how frequently right-sided serrated adenomas progress to invasive cancer.

7.4.4. POLYPOSIS SYNDROMES

In addition to FAP, other polyposis conditions should be considered in view of potential chemoprevention (Table 5). Two are Peutz-Jeghers syndrome and familial juvenile polyposis syndrome.

Peutz-Jeghers syndrome, considered a premalignant condition, may be sporadic or familial. It is characterized by multiple hamartomatous polyps arising in the intestinal tract, mucocutaneous pigmentation, and an elevated risk for cancer, especially in the stomach, small

Table 5
Hereditary Polyposis Syndromes

Familial adenomatous polyposis
    Adenomatous polyposis coli (APC)
Gardner, Turcot, attenuated (APC)
    Familial juvenile polyposis (SMAD-4)
Hamatomatous polyposis
    Peutz-Jeghers (STK11)
    Cowden's disease (PTEN)
    Ruvalcabe-Mythe-Smith syndrome (PTEN)

bowel, pancreas, colon, and other sites, including unusual gonadal tumors. Those with Peutz-Jeghers syndrome have an estimated 15 times greater risk for nongastrointestinal cancer than the general population *(77)*. Hamartomatous polyps are found most often in the small intestine, stomach, and colon. Grossly, the polyps often resemble adenomas. Histologically, they contain branching, tightly packed glands with minimal supporting stroma containing smooth muscle that extends into the polyp fronds from the muscularis mucosae. Most cancers seem to originate from coexisting adenomas and not necessarily from the hamartomatous polyps. Dysplasia tends to be unusual within the polyps. The germline mutation involves the STK11 gene in about 70% of cases. Some 30–70% of sporadic cases also have STK11 mutations.

Patients with familial juvenile polyposis syndrome have an elevated risk for colorectal cancer that varies from 20% to 70%. Histologically, polyps are characterized by dilated glands and abundant, often inflamed, intervening stroma that lacks smooth muscle. Dysplasia develops in the glandular epithelium of the polyp and is followed by invasive carcinoma. Dysplasia in these polyps is occasionally confused with the mimicker reactive inflammatory atypia because of inflammation often occurring in the stroma. Polyps are most common in the colon and rectum, but they may also occur in the stomach and small intestine. Two genes, SMAD-4 and BMPR1A, have been associated with familial juvenile polyposis. Both genes are involved in the transforming growth factor (TGF)-β transduction pathway and are found in the stroma.

7.4.5. CHRONIC INFLAMMATORY CONDITIONS

Ulcerative colitis, a chronic inflammatory condition, predisposes to carcinoma. The morphologic pathway seems to follow the low-grade dysplasia–high-grade dysplasia–carcinoma route, illustrating that long-standing inflammation can lead to malignant transformation *(78)*. In areas of persisting inflammation, dysplastic changes eventually develop in the colonic mucosa. These changes are usually small and multifocal, but have the potential to progress. Cancer risk is related to disease duration (>10 years), disease extent, early age of onset, and co-occurrence of primary sclerosing cholangitis. The incidence of dysplasia is difficult to estimate, but most studies indicate a 5% incidence after 10 yr and 25% after 20 yr. The cumulative incidence of colorectal cancer ranges from 3% to 43% after 25–35 yr. Dysplastic lesions associated with a mass or polypoid growth are most likely to progress.

p53 mutations have been found in the dysplastic lesions *(79)*. As expected, molecular alterations including p53, APC, *K-ras*, and deleted in colon cancer gene (DCC) mutations have been found in cancers arising in ulcerative colitis *(78)*. Nonetheless, cancer in ulcerative colitis seems to develop along molecular pathways different from those followed in sporadic colorectal cancer *(78)*. In addition, ulcerative colitis may induce endocrine cell hyperplasia that can progress to endocrine neoplasia, such as carcinoid tumors (80).

Crohn's disease, a chronic granulomatous disease of the intestine, also carries an increased risk for cancer when it involves the colon *(81,82)*. Dysplasia in Crohn's is similar to that seen in ulcerative colitis.

7.5. Liver

Cirrhosis and chronic inflammation with regeneration, regardless of cause, have long been recognized as predisposing factors for hepatocellular carcinoma. In the past several years, our concept about premalignant lesions has changed.

Although large-cell hepatic dysplasia was first described as a preneoplastic lesion, it is now considered a senescent change with no malignant potential. Small-cell dysplasia, on the other hand, shows increased proliferative activity and is believed to be a precancerous lesion for liver cancer in humans.

In recent years, most studies have focused on mass lesions that can be detected by imaging techniques in cirrhotic livers. Three nodular lesions have been defined: macroregenerative nodules, adenomatous hyperplasia/low-grade dysplastic nodules, and atypical adenomatous hyperplasia/high-grade dysplastic nodules *(83,84)*. The reported incidence of dysplastic nodules in cirrhotic livers has varied from 14% to 25%. These nodules are found in cirrhosis associated with viral hepatitis B or C and in primary biliary cirrhosis. Macroregenerative nodules are like any other cirrhotic nodule but larger. Adenomatous hyperplasia/ low-grade dysplastic nodules show minor cytologic abnormalities of nuclear shape, size, cellularity, and plate thickness. Steatosis and Mallory bodies may be seen. Adenomatous hyperplasia/high-grade dysplastic nodules are characterized by highly atypical nuclei, significantly increased nucleo-cytoplastmic ratio, basophilia, pseudoglands, nodule-in-nodule formation, and resistance to iron accumulation.

Finding adenomatous hyperplasia/high-grade dysplastic nodules in association with hepatocellular carcinoma has provided circumstantial evidence for the dysplasia-carcinoma sequence. Approximately 40% of high-grade dysplastic nodules progress to hepatocellular carcinoma in months or years.

7.6. Pancreas

Invasive carcinomas of ductal derivation are the most common histologic types originating in the pancreas. Though precursors or incipient phases of these neoplasms have been well characterized in recent years, precursors of invasive carcinomas with acinar or endocrine phenotype are less well known and therefore will not be considered.

Pancreatic intraepithelial neoplasia (PanIN) is the diagnostic term recommended for precursors of ordinary ductal carcinoma (36). Four histologic categories of PanIN are recognized: PanIN IA is defined as flat mucinous hyperplasia; PanIN 1B represents papillary mucinous hyperplasia; PanIN 2 is characterized by papillary hyperplasia with mild to moderate cytologic atypia; and PanIN 3 is similar to CIS, high-grade dysplasia or high-grade atypical ductal hyperplasia (Fig. 5A,B). The stepwise grading system parallels the incremental prevalence of mutational events found in duct lesions, such that genetic alterations in higher grade PanIN approach those found in the infiltrating ductal carcinoma (36).

Most agree that risk of progression for PanIN 1 is minimal. Moreover, progression of PanIN 3 to invasive carcinoma can take a long time—29 yr, in one remarkable example (33). Although PanIN is often encountered in pancreatic tissue adjacent to invasive ductal carcinomas, it is also found in association with intraductal papillary mucinous neoplasms as well as adenomas and carcinomas of the ampulla of Vater, probably reflecting a field effect (13).

Even though mucinous cystic neoplasms of the pancreas are usually large lesions, their lining columnar epithelium may lack cytologic atypia (cystadenoma). Some tumors, however, may be lined by columnar

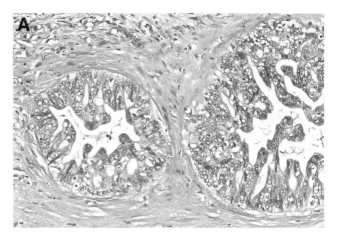
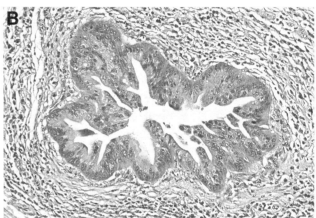

Fig. 5. Pancreatic intraepithelial neoplasia. **(A)** Pancreatic duct with high grade PanIn. Micropapillary structures and early cribriforming are seen. The atypical cells show overlapping nuclei and prominent nucleoli. **(B)** Larger pancreatic duct lined by neoplastic cells, PanIN III.

epithelium showing moderate dysplasia or CIS changes. Despite their large size, these borderline pancreatic mucinous cystic neoplasms are forms of incipient neoplasia; if completely excised, they follow a benign clinical course (85). Since these large cystic neoplasms may harbor small foci of invasive carcinoma, extensive sampling is needed to avoid miscategorization. Mucinous cystadenocarcinomas have a better prognosis than conventional ductal carcinomas of the pancreas (86).

Intraductal papillary mucinous neoplasm, a recently recognized pancreatic tumor, is a distinctive clinicopathological entity. When papillary mucinous carcinomas are entirely intraductal, they behave as CIS and should be regarded as forms of incipient neoplasia. Even invasive papillary mucinous carcinomas follow a more favorable clinical course than conventional ductal carcinomas (87).

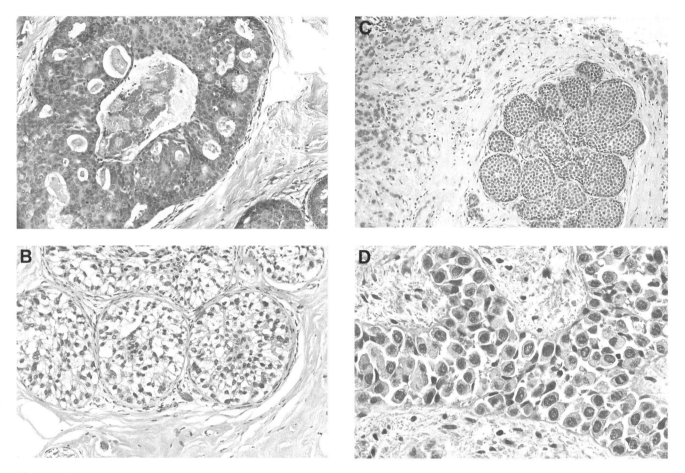

Fig. 6. (**A**) DCIS of the breast with cribriform pattern. Note the bland cytological features. (**B**) DCIS of the breast, solid type, composed of clear cells. (**C**) LCIS and invasive lobular carcinoma. (**D**) Pleomorphic LCIS. The cells are large and lack cohesion.

7.7. Breast

Traditionally based on anatomic origin, preinvasive and invasive carcinomas of the breast have been divided into ductal and lobular types. Ductal carcinoma *in situ* (DCIS) is the precursor of invasive ductal carcinoma, and lobular carcinoma *in situ* (LCIS) represents the preinvasive phase of infiltrating lobular carcinoma and occasionally of ductal carcinoma. In recent years, however, it has become apparent that some *in situ* and invasive breast carcinomas show combined ductal and lobular features.

DCIS incidence has increased dramatically because the disease is usually detected by mammographic calcification. Biologically and morphologically, it is a heterogeneous disease. The cribriform and micropapillary types usually show minimal cytologic atypia and are considered low-grade lesions, while the solid type with comedonecrosis often shows anaplastic features and is classified as high-grade. Incidence of recurrence after lumpectomy is higher with the solid type with comedonecrosis than in cribriform and micropapillary

types (Fig. 6A,B). Moreover, the last two variants take longer to recur than the solid type. Likewise, the rate of progression is much higher and shorter in the solid type with comedonecrosis than in the cribriform and micropapillary types. Depending on histology, size, age, surgical margins, and type of therapy, 6–30% of DCIS lesions will recur as non-invasive or invasive cancers, usually many years after diagnosis (*88,89*). Overall, women with DCIS or LCIS have an 8–10 times greater relative risk of developing invasive breast cancer (*90*).

LCIS is usually an incidental finding in patients biopsied for other lesions. It is usually multifocal and multicentric, and frequently bilateral. For this reason, it is more likely to be associated with invasive cancer in the contralateral breast than DCIS. Morphologically, conventional and pleomorphic variants have been described (Fig. 6C,D). LCIS and DCIS may coexist in the same breast.

Cribriform and micropapillary types of DCIS nearly always express ER, progesterone receptor (PR), and Bcl2, whereas a smaller proportion of DCIS solid type with comedonecrosis express ER and PR. p53 is expressed predominantly by high-grade DCIS but not by low-grade variants *(91)*. C-erbB2 expression has been observed in 0–50% of cribriform and micropapillary DCIS compared to 50–100% of high-grade DCIS *(92)*.

Atypical ductal hyperplasia (ADH), considered the precursor of DCIS, has some morphologic features of cribriform and micropapillary types of CIS. It involves only a portion of a single duct or several ducts, of which the aggregate sectional diameter does not exceed 2 mm. For this reason, some pathologists believe that ADH is a limited form of DCIS. As with DCIS, the frequency of ADH has increased considerably among mammographically screened women. Its immunohistochemical profile is similar to that of low-grade DCIS.

ADH may progress to invasive carcinoma. The absolute risk of a woman with ADH developing invasive breast cancer varies from 5–12% within 8–21 yr of follow-up *(93)*. Expressed as relative risk, women with ADH have a moderate (4–5 times) risk for developing invasive carcinoma *(90)*. The proliferative index seems to be a major factor in estimating risk of invasive cancer *(94)*. At least eight histologic classification systems have been proposed for DCIS *(95)*.

DCIS is considered an obligate precursor of invasive breast cancer. However, unless DCIS can be detected specifically and reliably through imaging or another diagnostic procedure, its role as a surrogate endpoint biomarker will be limited, as invasive cancer may be present microscopically. According to serial mammographic findings, DCIS involves only a single ductal system and grows both toward and away from the nipple at nearly equal rates, about 2.7 mm per yr on average. The rate of growth correlates with histologic grade *(96)*.

7.8. Ovary

Most ovarian tumors arise from the surface epithelium, although our knowledge of the precursor lesions is far from complete. Of a wide variety of ovarian tumors, most common are serous and mucinous cystic epithelial varieties, which account for more than 60% of all ovarian cancers. Other epithelial types include endometrioid, clear cell, Brenner tumor, and cystadenofibroma.

While no well-defined precursor lesions are consistently reported for all ovarian cancers, proliferative and metaplastic changes and cellular atypia are considered putative precursors of serous and mucinous tumors. These changes have been described along the surface epithelium and in its cystic derivatives located in the ovarian cortex *(97–99)*. They have also been reported in women having prophylactic oophorectomy because of high risk due to family history or BRCA mutations, in grossly noninvolved contralateral oophorectomy specimens removed from women with unilateral carcinoma, and in women suspected of having ovarian cancer *(100)*. A number of very small carcinomas accidentally discovered in oophorectomy specimens have also been reported *(101,102)*. Controversy exists regarding the frequency and type of precursor lesions that occur in ovaries of high-risk women. Some observers have reported distinct precancerous changes, while others have not confirmed the results *(103–105)*.

Most serous cystic ovarian cancers are thought to arise from superficial epithelial inclusion cysts located in the ovarian cortex *(102)*. While their origin is uncertain, these microscopic cysts may result from downgrowth of the surface epithelium following ovulation, or more likely from invaginations of surface epithelium into the cortex. The epithelium in these cysts can undergo Müllerian metaplasia, that is, resemble the epithelium in the normal fallopian tube and endometrium. This metaplasia is thought to represent the first morphologic evidence of malignant transformation. Occasionally, these inclusion cysts will also reveal dysplastic changes that represent ovarian intraepithelial neoplasia. Overexpression of p53, a common finding in serous carcinomas, occurs in areas of atypia in cysts associated with ovarian carcinoma *(106)*. Tumor markers such as CA-125 and CA 19-9 are often seen in these cysts by immunohistochemistry. Thus, most ovarian tumors arise within the substance of the ovary, presumably the result of stromal-epithelial interaction *(107)*. Mucinous tumors, on the other hand, may originate from endocervical-type Müllerian metaplasia of either ovarian surface epithelium or cortical inclusion cysts.

Between benign and overt malignant tumors is a group of biologically and morphologically heterogeneous ovarian tumors of low malignant potential (LMP). Often bilateral, they may be found in either serous or mucinous tumors. Histologically, these tumors are characterized by focal epithelial stratification, papillary tufting, atypical-appearing cells, pleomorphism, and increased mitotic activity. While these epithelial changes resemble cancer, invasion of the underlying stroma has not occurred. These tumors as a group have an excellent prognosis with a 5-yr survival rate of 90–100%. Borderline mucinous tumors are more likely to progress to overt cancer than serous tumors.

Indirect evidence, based largely on age distribution and histology, suggests that benign ovarian tumors can serve as precursors for carcinoma *(98)*. The average age for benign tumors is 44 yr; the average age for carcinoma is 56 yr. Occasionally, various combinations of benign, LMP, and invasive changes are found in the same specimen. Transitions have also been observed between benign-appearing epithelium and frank cancer.

Because of a lack of symptoms, preinvasive or early invasive lesions are rarely seen in the ovary. Therefore, prevention studies must depend on cancer incidence in the ovary or validation of markers for incipient lesions. The risk of ovarian cancer is known to increase with the number of ovulatory cycles. Because of possible stromal-epithelial interaction in the pathogenesis of most ovarian tumors, modulation of this interaction may prove effective in prevention.

7.9. Endometrium

There are two morphologic pathways for endometrial carcinoma—atypical hyperplasia for the endometrioid type, and endometrial intraepithelial carcinoma for the serous carcinoma. Molecular genetic changes are also unique for each pathway *(108)*. Accounting for 80%–90% of all uterine cancers, the endometrioid type has been associated with unopposed estrogen stimulation. Serous carcinomas, the most common nonendometrioid type of endometrial carcinoma, tend to be more aggressive and usually occur in older age groups.

Endometrial hyperplasia is classified into typical and atypical, and further subclassified into simple and complex on the basis of glandular density, shape, and distribution. Because of a lack of diagnostic reproducibility, there have been proposals to simply this classification *(109)*. The designation endometrioid neoplasia has been proposed for atypical and complex hyperplastic lesions, which are considered precancerous. The highest rate of progression to invasive cancer occurs with the atypical hyperplasia, ranging from 15% to 40% in different studies. Separation of atypical hyperplasia from well-differentiated endometrioid carcinoma can be difficult. Typical endometrial hyperplasia is a benign lesion almost without risk (<3%) for progressing to cancer. Endometrial incipient lesions often regress.

Serous carcinoma is often associated with endometrial intraepithelial carcinoma, which is considered CIS of the surface glandular epithelium. It is characterized by glandular atrophy, anaplastic nuclei, abnormal mitotic figures, and apoptotic bodies.

Mutation of the p53 suppressor gene is not found in cases of endometrial hyperplasia and only rarely occurs in endometrioid carcinomas. On the other hand, p53

mutations are more common in cases of serous carcinoma. Atypical endometrial hyperplasia shares genetic abnormalities with endometrial carcinoma by comparative genomic hybridization *(110)*.

Women with HNPCC have a higher lifetime risk of endometrial cancer than of colon cancer *(111)*. Moreover, endometrial cancer tends to occur in a younger age group than sporadic endometrial carcinoma.

7.10. Uterine Cervix

Using cytologic examination to detect precursors of invasive SCC of the uterine cervix is responsible for the dramatic reduction in incidence of this tumor in the US. Furthermore, it has been firmly established that human papillomavirus (HPV) infection is associated with development of cervical dysplasia and SCC. HPV genus-specific structural antigens, DNA sequences, or both are found in 90% of cervical dysplasia and CIS cases *(112)*.

7.10.1. Squamous Cell Dysplasia

Of more than 60 known genotypes of HPV, about 20 preferentially infect the squamous epithelium of the genital tract. Types 6 and 11 are almost always associated with lesions of low malignant potential. Types 31, 33, and 35 are associated with lesions of intermediate malignant potential. HPV types 16 and 18 are associated with most cases of severe dysplasia, as well as CIS and invasive SCC.

According to the extent of cytologic atypia, cervical squamous dysplasia is divided into mild (CIN I), moderate (CIN II) and severe (CIN III) (Fig. 7A–C). Applying the Bethesda System to these lesions, mild dysplasia (CIN I) is classified as low-grade squamous intraepithelial lesion (LSIL) and moderate to severe dysplasia and CIS (CIN II and CIN III) as high-grade squamous intraepithelial lesion (HSIL). Atypical cells of undetermined significance (ASCUS) are reserved for borderline cytological changes. The Bethesda system is now widely used for reporting screening results.

In biopsy specimens, increased mitotic activity, immature cell proliferation, incomplete or lack of maturation, nuclear pleomorphism, and clumping of the chromatin characterize dysplasia. Excess proliferation is first seen in basal or reserve cells located along the basement membrane. Dysplasia is considered when abnormal cells occupy less than the full thickness of the cervical epithelium. Full thickness involvement is considered CIS *(113)*. Squamous cell dysplasia is also described histologically as CIN that is divided into the

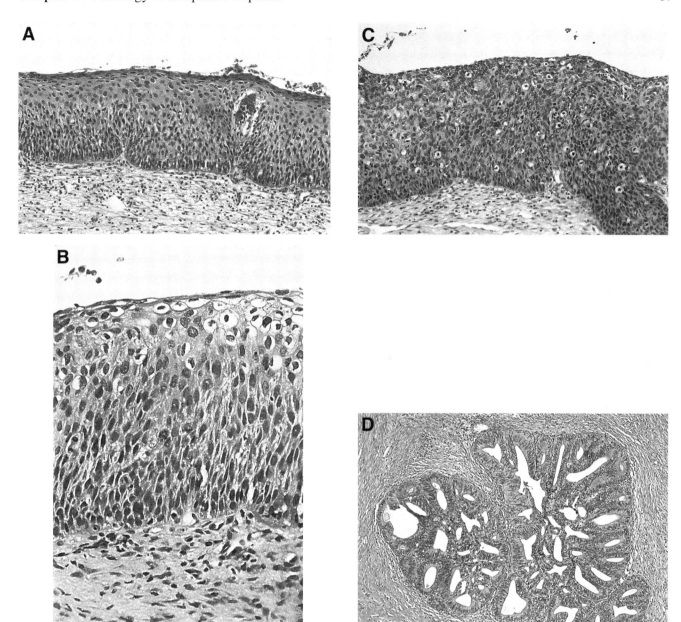

Fig. 7. (**A**) Mild squamous dysplasia (CIN I) of the cervix. Some cells show large nuclei. (**B**) Severe squamous dysplasia (CIN III) with koilocytotic cells. (**C**) Squamous cell CIS (CIN III). (**D**) Adenocarcinoma *in situ* of endocervix, endometrioid type.

three grades discussed above. Koilocytotic atypia, manifested by large cells with prominent cytoplasmic vacuoles and enlarged nuclei, is often a prevalent feature of dysplasia and usually indicates a cytopathic effect of HPV. As in other sites, squamous cell dysplasia is preceded by squamous metaplasia.

7.10.2. ADENOCARCINOMA *IN SITU*

Adenocarcinoma *in situ*, an uncommon but well-defined preinvasive lesion of the endocervical glands, is considered the preinvasive phase of invasive endocervical adenocarcinoma (Fig. 7D) *(113)*. The US has

seen an absolute as well as a relative increase in adenocarcinomas of the endocervix. The relative increase is due to reduction in SCC incidence resulting from widespread screening. In women younger than 35 years of age, the adenocarcinoma rate increased from 1.7 (per million women per year) in 1973–1975 to 3.8 in 1979–1982 *(114)*. In contrast to the high frequency at which squamous dysplasia and squamous cell CIS are identified in cervicovaginal smears, detection of adenocarcinoma *in situ* by cytologic screening is much less common.

Squamous cell dysplasia and CIS of the cervix often coexist with adenocarcinoma *in situ*. This association

Table 6
Follow-Up of 593 Cases of Squamous Intraepithelial Lesions (24 mo) *(118)*

DNA Diagnosis	Histological Follow-up			Cytologic Follow-up	
	CIN I	*CIN II*	*CIN III/CIS*	*Returned to normal*	*No change*
108 diploid	1	2	2	93	10
198 polyploid	5	11	17	133	32
287 aneuploid	6	102	109	0	70
Of 241 LSIL cases, 94 were diploid, 9 aneuploid, and 138 polyploid					
Of 352 HSIL cases, 14 were diploid, 278 aneuploid, and 60 polyploid					

suggests that the same etiologic agent may play a role in malignant transformation of the reserve cell, which is presumed to be the cell of origin for both types of cervical neoplasms. HPV types 16 and 18 were detected by PCR in 15 of 36 cases (42%) of adenocarcinoma *in situ (115)*.

7.10.3. PROGRESSION

While available data vary, reports indicate that most squamous lesions of mild or moderate dysplasia will either regress or persist, whereas those of severe squamous dysplasia or CIS are more apt to progress. Of 894 patients with moderate dysplasia, 54% showed regression, 16% persistence, and 30% progression *(116)*. Progression occurred after a mean follow-up of 51 mo. In contrast, the rate of progression of CIS to invasive cancer ranges from 30%–50%. The latent period for progression, often called transit time, of CIS to invasive carcinoma is 7–10 yr; from CIS to clinically manifest invasive carcinoma is 10–15 yr. Based on a meta-analysis of cytology, 7.1% of ASCUS and 20.8% of LSIL progressed to HSIL. HSIL persisted in 23.4% of cases. Cumulative rates of progression to invasive cancer after 24 mo were 0.3% for ASCUS, 0.2% for LSIL, and 1.4% for HSIL. Rates of regression to a normal Pap smear were 68.2% for ASCUS, 47.4% for LSHIL, and 35% for HSIL *(117)*.

The rate of progression may also depend on the type of HPV infection, age, smoking history, immune status, and other factors. Unfortunately, the biologic behavior of dysplastic lesions, especially less severe lesions, cannot be reliably predicted on the basis of histology alone. An important criterion for estimating progression is the presence of abnormal mitotic figures.

DNA aneuploidy has served as an objective marker for progression or persistence of preinvasive lesions of the cervix (Table 6) *(118)*. Aneuploidy can be demonstrated

with microspectrophotometry after stoichiometric Feulgen staining of the DNA.

7.11. Prostate Gland

The only incipient lesion identified morphologically that carries a proven risk of progression is high-grade PIN, or simply PIN as now recommended. Cases of low-grade PIN are usually not reported by pathologists because of a lack of clinical relevance. It is assumed that nearly all invasive carcinomas in the prostate arise from preexisting PIN, although it has been suggested that some tumors may arise from other putative incipient lesions. Multiple independent foci of PIN in different stages of development are typically found within the prostate, which strongly suggests that a field effect underlies the origin of prostatic neoplasia *(119,120)*. As with tumors arising in other sites, PIN seems to originate from the pluripotent stem cells located in the basal layer of the prostatic glands. PIN, especially when the lesions are multiple, is often associated with a subsequent diagnosis of invasive cancer.

Histologically, PIN usually arises in the peripheral zone of the prostate and is characterized by a proliferation of epithelial cells lining the ducts and acini *(121)*. In high-grade PIN, the cells appear highly atypical, stain more basophilic, show nuclear enlargement, and contain prominent nucleoli, changes that are similar to invasive cancer. For this reason, the glandular structures of PIN are often recognized under low power of the microscope because they stain darker than normal ones (Fig. 8A,B). Mitotic figures are usually not seen. As the cells continue to proliferate, they extend into the glandular lumen leading to intraluminal papillae, which later may fuse and take on a cribriform pattern. Invasion is associated with loss of the continuous basal cell layer and destruction of the basement membrane. In early invassion, neoplastic cells are seen in close proximity to PIN.

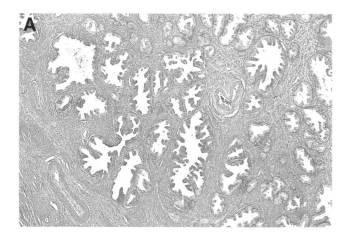

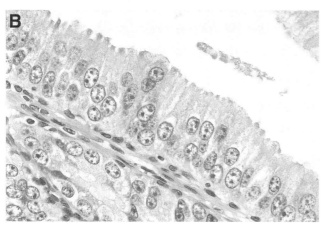

Fig 8. (A) Low power view of PIN. **(B)** Higher magnification of PIN showing neoplastic cells with vesicular nuclei and prominent nucleoli.

Incontrovertible evidence based on clinical, epidemiological, morphologic, cytogenetic, immunohistochemical, morphometric, and molecular genetic observations indicates that high-grade PIN progresses to invasive carcinoma. High-grade PIN has been consistently associated with carcinoma in biopsy and in prostatectomy specimens. In general, high-grade PIN first occurs about 5–10 yr before carcinoma. The thymidine-labeling index of atypical cells is similar to that of poorly differentiated carcinoma and three times greater than simple hyperplasia *(122)*. The DNA content of PIN is intermediate between the DNA content of normal glands and that of carcinomas as determined by quantitative cytometry. Furthermore, the number of aneuploid nuclei increases as the degree of PIN increases *(123,124)*. PIN exhibits many genotypic changes found in prostatic cancer *(125–127)*. An accumulation of consistent chromosomal gains and losses occurs during development and progression of PIN to invasive carcinoma as revealed by comparative genomic hybridization *(128)*.

Atypical PIN cells express PSA and the androgen receptor *(129)*. Consequently, PIN lesions eventually regress under conditions of reduced androgen stimulation. Basal cells, on the other hand, generally lack androgen receptors and do not show regressive changes after androgen deprivation. Apparently basal cells are not stimulated by androgen.

The differential diagnosis of PIN and early prostatic carcinoma may be difficult. A number of histopathological descriptions of these lesions have been published *(130)*. AAH, which has been considered a precursor lesion, is now thought to be a benign lesion that resembles well-differentiated carcinomas.

It has been claimed that quantitative nuclear morphometry is a useful predictor when coupled with other prognostic factors *(131)*.

There is evidence that PIN is preceded by chronic inflammatory lesions described as proliferative inflammatory atrophy (PIA) *(132)*. The lesion is characterized by repeated bouts of inflammation that cause repeated injury to the normal prostatic epithelium. As a consequence, cells proliferate as part of the reparative process. Continued proliferation eventually leads to PIN and carcinoma.

As a surrogate lesion for prostate cancer, PIN leaves much to be desired. The rate of detection of PIN in the general population is low and its clinical significance uncertain, at least in the short term. Studies in screened populations have revealed detection rates of only 1–1.5% *(133)*, although figures as high as 16% have been reported. Furthermore, PIN has a high association with carcinoma. The prevalence of PIN in cases of established carcinoma has been reported as 82%, but in cases without carcinoma, PIN is found in 43% of biopsy specimens *(125,134)*. Even in the presence of multicentric PIN, current biopsy techniques may not sample a coexisting invasive cancer. Finally, according to autopsy surveys, PIN and carcinoma are seen at ages as low as 30–40 yr (Table 7), which has implications for prostate cancer prevention *(135)*.

7.12. Urinary Bladder

Urothelial CIS has two forms. Noninvasive papillary transitional cell carcinoma has a papillary architecture compared with flat urothelial CIS. Both are precursors of invasive urothelial carcinomas. Papillary transitional cell tumors are often divided into four histologic grades. Both forms of CIS are frequently seen adjacent to invasive urothelial carcinomas. It should be emphasized that most of our information about incipient lesions, such as CIS, dysplasia, and atypia, has been

Table 7
Histological Findings Distributed by Age and Race (155)

	Patient Age (yrs)				
	10–19	*20–29*	*30–39*	*40–49*	*Totals (%)*
Histology	PIN				
Low-grade					
Black pts.	0/10 (0)	2/28 (7)	7/32 (22)	11/28 (39)	20/98 (20)
White pts.	0/2 (0)	1/7 (14)	4/23 (17)	6/22 (27)	11/54 (20)
Totals	0/12 (0)	3/35 (9)	11/55 (20)	17/50 (34)	31/152 (20)
High-grade					
Black pts.	0/10 (0)	0/28 (0)	0/32 (0)	3/28 (11)	3/98 (3)
White pts.	0/2 (0)	0/7 (0)	0/23 (0)	2/22 (9)	2/54 (4)
Totals	0/12 (0)	0/35 (0)	0/55 (0)	5/50 (10)	5/152 (3)
Histological					
Black pts.	0/10 (0)	0/28 (0)	8/32 (25)	10/28 (36)	18/98 (18)
White pts.	0/2 (0)	0/7 (0)	7/23 (30)	7/22 (32)	14/54 (26)
Totals	0/12 (0)	0/35 (0)	15/55 (27)	17/50 (34)	32/152 (21)

All values are reported as number of patients/total.

observed in bladders that have already developed non-invasive or invasive carcinoma *(136, 137)*. In the bladder, precursor lesions are usually asymptomatic and therefore do not come to the attention of the patient. However, urothelial dysplasia discovered in the absence of an associated carcinoma is a significant risk for progression to CIS and invasive cancer. From 14%–20% of patients with dysplasia will progress to CIS or invasive cancer within 8–11 yr after diagnosis *(138,139)*.

Flat urothelial CIS not associated with invasive tumors is quite rare. It is multifocal and may involve the entire bladder mucosa, indicating a field effect. It may also coexist with invasive urothelial carcinomas in other segments of the urologic tract. Flat urothelial CIS can rapidly progress to invasive carcinoma, usually in less than 4 yr *(140,141)*. It is impossible, however, to separate *in situ* lesions that will progress from those that will not on morphologic and immunohistochemical grounds. At least two molecular pathways to transitional cell carcinoma (TCC) are involved in progression *(142)*. Deletions of chromosomes 8p12, 11q12, 4p16.3, 9p21, and 14q have recently been postulated to play a role in the progression of *in situ* lesions to invasive bladder cancer. Likewise, overexpression of *c-myc* has been reported in low-grade papillary TCC, while p53 mutations and loss of Rb gene function appear to be frequent events in the evolution of flat urothelial CIS *(143)*.

In most cases of flat transitional cell CIS, the malignant cells involve the full thickness of the surface epithelium (Fig. 9A,B). In the clinging, pagetoid, and lepidic variants, however, only partial involvement of the surface urothelium is seen. Moreover, the umbrella cell layer is maintained in some cases. Flat urothelial CIS may extend into the von Brunn's nests, prostatic ducts, and acini, simulating invasion. In some cases the tumor may extend to the urethra and periurethral glands. Extension into the seminal vesicles and ejaculatory duct epithelium has rarely been reported.

7.13. Skin

Invasive carcinomas of the skin and their *in situ* or incipient phases are the most common forms of human cancer. AK, Bowen's disease, and arsenical and radiation keratosis are all morphologic expressions of CIS with the phenotype of epidermal keratinocytes *(144,145)*. Approximately 5–14% of the adult population in the US develops AK, with a prevalence as high as 26% in high-risk groups *(146)*.

Microscopically, these forms of incipient neoplasia are characterized by atypical epidermal keratinocytes with increased mitotic activity and loss of cell polarity. In some examples, such as AK and radiation keratosis, cytologic abnormalities may not involve the full

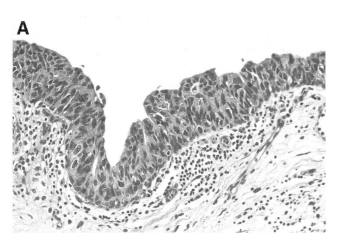
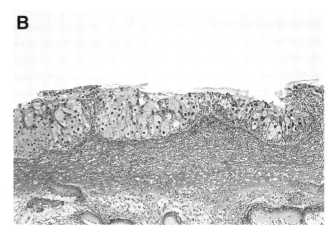

Fig. 9. Transitional cell CIS. **(A)** The normal urothelium is replaced by neoplastic cells showing loss of polarity and hyperchromatic nuclei. **(B)** This urothelial CIS is composed of clear cells.

thickness of the epidermis (Fig. 10). AK, the most common form of cutaneous incipient neoplasia, appears on sun-exposed skin, especially that of white persons chronically exposed to the sun. Bowen's disease is a variant of squamous cell CIS that has been related to ingestion of inorganic arsenic when it occurs on unexposed areas. In anal and vulvar skin, squamous cell CIS appears to be etiologically related to HPV and HIV infections *(147)*. In these anatomical locations, squamous cell CIS may arise from a preexisting condyloma acuminatum, a sexually transmitted disease caused by HPV *(148)*.

Individuals chronically exposed to small amounts of radiation, such as radiotherapists and dentists, have developed cutaneous lesions known as radiation keratosis, a form of incipient squamous neoplasia. Erythroplasia of Queyrat is a squamous cell CIS of the mucosa of the glans penis that appears commonly in

uncircumcised elderly males. If untreated, all types of squamous cell CIS of the skin may invade into the dermis and eventually metastasize *(149)*. The rate of progression, however, varies according to histologic type, extent of cytologic atypia, and anatomic site.

Basal cell carcinoma, the most common histologic type of cutaneous carcinoma, may be superficial, multicentric, and remain attached to the epidermis, thus qualifying as a form of incipient neoplasia.

Extramammary Paget's disease is an *in situ* adenocarcinoma with apocrine differentiation that occurs preferentially in the vulva, followed by the scrotum, perianal region, and axilla *(150)*. Neoplastic cells may be confined to the epidermis but often extend to the skin adnexa. Intraepidermal neoplastic cells usually have clear mucin with cytoplasm that contains carcinoembryonic antigen (CEA) (Fig. 11). Carcinomas with sebaceous and eccrine differentiation that are

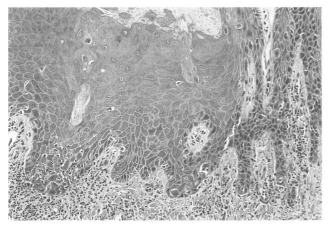

Fig. 10. Actinic keratosis. Hyperplastic variant of AK. The epidermis is thickened and shows atypical keratinocytes more prominent on the right side of the photograph.

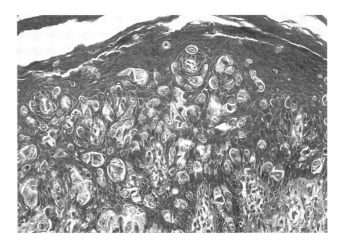

Fig. 11. Extramammary Paget's disease. Large neoplastic clear cells are present at all levels of the epidermis.

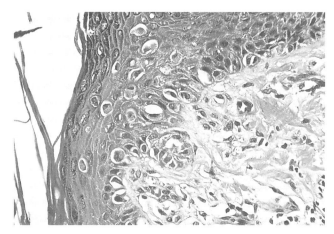

Fig. 12. Melanoma *in situ*. Scattered neoplastic melanocytes are seen in the epidermis.

confined to the epidermis are also considered forms of adenocarcinoma *in situ*. Extramammary Paget's disease usually remains localized for years. Rarely, tumor cells invade the dermis and from there may spread to regional lymph nodes. When sebaceous gland CIS becomes invasive, it behaves as a highly malignant neoplasm capable of metastasizing widely and causing death.

7.14. Melanoma

When neoplastic melanocytes are confined to the epidermis and skin adnexa, the term melanoma *in situ* is applied (Fig. 12) *(151)*. In its early stage, superficial spreading melanoma may be confined to the epidermis and therefore is a form of incipient neoplasia. The invasive superficial spreading melanoma usually coexists with an *in situ* component. Lentigo maligna melanoma, also known as melanotic freckle of Hutchinson, is characterized by an *in situ* phase that over many years evolves into invasive malignant melanoma. Lentigo malignant melanoma occurs on the chronically exposed cutaneous surfaces of the elderly, most commonly on the face, and occasionally on the back, forearms, or legs. Acral lentiginous melanoma preferentially affects hairless skin of the palms and soles as well as the ungual and periungual regions. It appears to be most common among Asians, Hispanics, and African-Americans, for whom the overall incidence of melanoma is low. Acral lentiginous melanoma has an *in situ* phase. When invasive, this type of melanoma is associated with poor prognosis.

The occasional coexistence of nevi and melanoma suggests neoplastic progression. Large congenital nevi have a 10% or more lifetime risk of developing into melanomas and, rarely, sarcomas *(152)*. For this reason, it has been suggested that all congenital nevi regardless of size should be completely excised to prevent development of melanoma.

8. CONCLUSION

The early stages of cancer development offer the best chance of intervening to change the course of the disease without exposing the patient to excessive toxicity. A broad knowledge of the biological properties of incipient neoplasias is essential in order to provide effective therapeutic targets for chemoprevention.

REFERENCES

1. Henson DE, Albores-Saavedra J, eds. *Pathology of Incipient Neoplasia*, 3rd ed. Oxford University Press, New York; 2001.
2. O'Shaughnessy JA, Kelloff GJ, Gordon GB, et al. Treatment and prevention of intraepithelial neoplasia: an important target for accelerated new agent development. *Clin Cancer Res* 2002;8:314–346.
3. Thiberville L, Payne P, Vielkinds J, et al. Evidence of cumulative gene losses with progression of premalignant epithelial lesions to carcinoma of the bronchus. *Cancer Res* 1995;55:5133–5139.
4. Böcking A, Giroud F, Reith A. Consensus report of the European Society for Analytical Cellular Pathology Task Force on standardization of diagnostic DNA image cytometry. *Anal Quant Cytol Histol* 1995;17:1–7.
5. Page DL, Dupont WD, Rogers LW, et al. Atypical hyperplasia lesions of the female breast. A long-term follow-up study. *Cancer* 1985;55:2698–2708.
6. Frykberg ER, Bland KI. *In situ* breast carcinoma. *Adv Surg* 1993;26:29–72.
7. Albores-Saavedra J, Krueger JE. C-cell hyperplasia and medullary microcarcinoma. *Endocrine Pathol* 2001;12:365–377.
8. Isaacson PG. Mucosa-associated lymphoid tissue lymphoma. *Semin Hematol* 1999;36:139–147.
9. Beaty MW, Jaffe E. Lymphoid system. In: *Pathology of Incipient Neoplasia*, 3rd ed. Henson DE, Albores-Saavedra J, eds. Oxford University Press, New York; 2001; pp. 453–455.
10. Rickert RR, Auerbach O, Garfinkel L, et al. Adenomatous lesions of the large bowel: an autopsy survey. *Cancer* 1979;43:1847–1857.
11. Williams AR, Balasooriya BA, Day DW. Polyps and cancer of the large bowel: a necropsy study in Liverpool. *Gut* 1982;23:835–842.
12. Albores-Saavedra J, Henson DE, Klimstra D. Tumors of the gallbladder, extrahepatic bile ducts and ampulla of Vater. *Atlas of Tumor Pathology*, Third Series, Fascicle 27. Armed Forces Institute of Pathology, Washington DC; 2000.
13. Agoff SN, Crispin DA, Bronner MP, et al. Neoplasms of the ampulla of Vater with concurrent pancreatic intraepithelial neoplasia: a histological and molecular study. *Mod Pathol* 2001;14:139–146.

14. Fechner RE, Mills SE. Tumors of bones and joints. *Atlas of Tumor Pathology*, Third Series, Fascicle 8. Armed Forces Institute of Pathology, Washington DC; 1993.

15. Unni KK, Dahlin DC, Premalignant tumors and conditions of bone. *Am J Surg Pathol* 1979;3:47–60.

16. Cheng L, Gu J, Ulbright TM, et al. Precise microdissection of human bladder carcinomas reveals divergent tumor subclones in the same tumor. *Cancer* 2002;94:104–110.

17. Sozzi G, Miozzo M, Pastorino U, et al. Genetic evidence for an independent origin of multiple preneoplastic and neoplastic lung lesions. *Cancer Res* 1995;55:135–140.

18. Boyle JO, Lonardo F, Chang JH, et al. Multiple high-grade bronchial dysplasia and squamous cell carcinoma: concordant and discordant mutations. *Clin Cancer Res* 2001;7: 259–266.

19 Park I-W, Wistuba II, Maitra A, et al. Multiple clonal abnormalities in the bronchial epithelium of patients with lung cancer. *J Natl Cancer Inst* 1999;91:1863–1868.

20. Minna JD, Sekido Y, Fong KM, et al. Molecular biology of lung cancer. In *Cancer; Principles and Practice of Oncology*, 5th ed. DeVita VT Jr, Hellman S, Rosenberg SA, eds. Lippincott-Raven, Philadelphia, 1997: pp. 849–857.

21. Lydiatt WM, Anderson PE, Bazzana T, et al. Molecular support for field cancerization in the head and neck. *Cancer* 1998;82:1376–1380.

22. Fearon ER, Vogelstein B. A genetic model for colorectal tumorigenesis. *Cell* 1990;61:759–767.

23. Sugio K, Molberg K, Albores-Saavedra J, et al. K-ras mutations and allelic loss at 5q and 18q in the development of human pancreatic cancers. *Int J Pancreatol* 1997;21: 205–217.

24. Moskaluk CA, Hruban RH, Kern SE. p16 and K-*ras* gene mutations in the intraductal precursors of human pancreatic adenocarcinoma. *Cancer Res* 1997;57:2140–2143.

25. Gong G, DeVries S, Chew KL, et al. Genetic changes in paired atypical and usual ductal hyperplasia of the breast by comparative genomic hybridization. *Clin Cancer Res* 2001;7:2410–2414.

26. Sundaresan V, Heppell-Parton A, Coleman N, et al. Somatic genetic changes in lung cancer and precancerous lesions. *Ann Oncol* 1995;6S:27–32.

27. Sozzi G, Miozzo M, Donghi R, et al. Deletions of 17p and p53 mutations in preneoplastic lesions of the lung. *Cancer Res* 1992;52:6079–6082.

28. Jotwani G, Misra A, Chattopadhyay P, et al. Genetic heterogeneity and alterations in chromosome 9 loci in a localized region of a functional pituitary adenoma. *Cancer Genet Cytogenet* 2001;125:41–45.

29. Roth MJ, Hu N, Emmert-Buck MR, et al. Genetic progression and heterogeneity associated with the development of esophageal squamous cell carcinoma. *Cancer Res* 2001;61: 4098–4104.

30. Giaretti, W, Macciocu B, Geido E, et al. Intratumor heterogeneity of k-ras and p53 mutations among human colorectal adenomas containing early cancer. *Anal Cell Pathol* 2000;21:49–57.

31. Kern SE, Yardley JH, Lazenby AJ, et al. Reversal by antrectomy of endocrine cell hyperplasia in the gastric body in pernicious anemia: a morphometric study. *Mod Pathol* 1990;3: 561–566.

32. Ochiai A, Yamauchi Y, Hirohashi S. p53 mutations in the non-neoplastic mucosa of the human stomach showing intestinal metaplasia. *Int J Cancer* 1996;69:28–33.

33. Brockie E, Anand A, Albores-Saavedra J. Progression of atypical ductal hyperplasia/carcinoma *in situ* of the pancreas to invasive adenocarcinoma. *Ann Diagn Pathol* 1998;2: 286–292.

34. Brat DJ, Lillemoe KD, Yeo CJ, et al. Progression of intraductal neoplasia to infiltrating adenocarcinoma of the pancreas. *Am J Surg Pathol* 1998;22:163–169.

35. Sherlock P, Winawer SJ. Are there markers for the risk of colorectal cancer? *N Engl J Med* 1984;311:118–119.

36. Hruban RH, Adsay NV, Albores-Saavedra J, et al. Pancreatic intraepithelial neoplasia: a new nomenclature and classification system for pancreatic duct lesions. *Am J Surg Pathol* 2001;25:579–586.

37. Diaz-Cano SJ, de Miguel M, Blanes A, et al. Germline RET634 mutation positive MEN2A-related C-cell hyperplasias have genetic features consistent with intraepithelial neoplasia. *J Clin Endocrinol Metab* 2001;86:3948–3957.

38. Perry A, Molberg K, Albores-Saavedra J. Physiologic versus neoplastic C-cell hyperplasia of the thyroid: separation of distinct histologic and biologic entities. *Cancer* 1996;77: 750–756.

39. Luna MA, Pineda-Daboin K. Upper aerodigestive tract. In *Pathology of Incipient Neoplasia*, 3rd ed. Henson DE, Albores-Saavedra J, eds. Oxford University Press, New York; 2001: pp. 57–85.

40. Lumerman H, Freedman P, Kerpel S. Oral epithelial dysplasia and the development of invasive squamous cell carcinoma. *Oral Surg Oral Med Oral Pathol* 1995;79:321–329.

41. Crissman JD, Zarbo RJ. Dysplasia, *in situ* carcinoma, and progression to invasive squamous cell carcinoma of the upper aerodigestive tract. *Am J Surg Pathol* 1989;13(S):5–16.

42. Bosatra A, Bussani R, Silvestri F. From epithelial dysplasia to squamous carcinoma in the head and neck region: an epidemiological assessment. *Acta Otolaryngol (Stockh)* 1997;527(S):49–51.

43. Gallo A, de Vincentiis M, Rocca CD, et al. Evolution of precancerous laryngeal lesions: a clinicopathologic study with long-term follow-up on 259 patients. *Head Neck* 2001;23: 42–47.

44. Bouquot JE, Kurland LT, Weiland LH. Carcinoma *in situ* of the upper aerodigestive tract. Incidence, time trends, and follow-up in Rochester, Minnesota, 1935–1984. *Cancer* 1988;61:1691–1698.

45. Bouquot JE, Gnepp DR. Laryngeal precancer: a review of the literature, commentary, and comparison with oral leukoplakia. *Head Neck* 1991;13:488–497.

46. Sudbø J, Bryne M, Johannessen AC, et al. Comparison of histological grading and large-scale genomic status (DNA ploidy) as prognostic tools in oral dysplasia. *J Pathol* 2001;194:303–310.

47. Zakrzewska JM, Lopes V, Speight P, et al. Proliferative verrucous leukoplakia; a report of ten cases. *Oral Surg Oral Med Oral Pathol Oral Radiol Endod* 1996;82: 396–401.

48. Vermylen P, Roufosse C, Ninane V, et al. Biology of pulmonary preneoplastic lesions. *Cancer Treat Rev* 1997;23: 241–262.

49. Colby TV, Koss MN, Travis WD. Tumors of the lower respiratory tract. *Atlas of Tumor Pathology*, Third Series, Fascicle 13. Armed Forces Institute of Pathology, Washington DC; 1994.

50. Travis WD, Colby TV, Corrin B, et al. Histological typing of lung and pleural tumours. In *World Health Organization International Histological Classification of Tumours*, XIII, 3rd ed. Springer-Verlag, Berlin;1999.

51. Kerr KM. Pulmonary preinvasive neoplasia. *J Clin Pathol* 2001;54:257–271.

52. Band P, Feldstein M, Saccomanno G. Reversibility of bronchial marked atypia: implication for chemoprevention. *Cancer Detect Prev* 1986;9:157–160.

53. Frost JK, Ball WC Jr, Levin ML, et al. Sputum cytopathology: use and potential in monitoring the workplace environment by screening for biological effects of exposure. *J Occup Med* 1986;28:692–703.

54. Risse EKJ, Vooijs GP, van't Hof MA. Diagnostic significance of "severe dysplasia" in sputum cytology. *Acta Cytol* 1988;32:629–634.

55. Venmans BJW, van Boxem TJM, Smit EF, et al. Outcome of bronchial carcinoma *in situ*. *Chest* 2000;117:1572–1576.

56. Thiberville L, Metayer J, Raspaud C, et al. A prospective, short term follow-up study of 59 severe dysplasias and carcinoma in situ of the bronchus using auto fluorescence endoscopy. *Eur Respir J* 1997;10 (S25):425S.

57. Fisseler-Eckhoff A, Rothstein D, Müller KM. Neovascularization in hyperplastic, metaplastic, and potentially preneoplastic lesions of the bronchial mucosa. *Virchows Arch* 1996;429:95–100.

58. Keith RL, Miller YE, Gemmill RM, et al. Angiogenic squamous dysplasia in bronchi of individuals at high risk for lung cancer. *Clin Cancer Res* 2000;6:1616–1625.

59. Wistuba II, Behrens C, Milchgrub S, et al. Sequential molecular abnormalities are involved in the multistage development of squamous cell lung carcinoma. *Oncogene* 1999;18: 643–650.

60. Ponticiello A, Barra E, Giani U, et al. p53 immunohistochemistry can identify bronchial dysplastic lesions proceeding to lung cancer: a prospective study. *Eur Respir J* 2000;15:547–552.

61. Nakanishi K. Alveolar epithelial hyperplasia and adenocarcinoma of the lung. *Arch Pathol Lab Med* 1990; 114:363–368.

62. Chapman AD, Kerr KM. The association between atypical adenomatous hyperplasia and primary lung cancer. *Brit J Cancer* 2000;83:632–636.

63. Wistuba II, Lam S, Behrens C, et al. Molecular damage in the bronchial epithelium of current and former smokers. *J Natl Cancer Inst* 1997;89:1366–1373.

64. Mao L, Lee JS, Kurie JM, et al. Clonal genetic alterations in the lungs of current and former smokers. *J Natl Cancer Inst* 1997;89:857–862.

65. Reid BJ, Haggitt RC, Rubin CE, et al. Observer variation in the diagnosis of dysplasia in Barrett's esophagus. *Hum Pathol* 1988;19:166–178.

66. Buttar NS, Wang KK, Sebo TJ, et al. Extent of high-grade dysplasia in Barrett's esophagus correlates with risk of adenocarcinoma. *Gastroenterology* 2001;120:1630–1639.

67. Krishnadath KK, Reid BJ, Wang KK. Biomarkers in Barrett esophagus. *Mayo Clin Proc* 2001;76:438–446.

68. Hawkins NJ, Ward RL. Sporadic colorectal cancers with microsatellite instability and their possible origin in hyperplastic polyps and serrated adenomas. *J Natl Cancer Inst* 2001;93:1307–1313.

69. Fenoglio-Preiser CM, Noffsinger A. Aberrant crypt foci: a review. *Toxicol Pathol* 1999;27:632–642.

70. Di Gregorio C, Losi L, Fante R, et al. Histology of aberrant crypt foci in the human colon. *Histopathology* 1997;30: 328–334.

71. Takayama T, Katsuki S, Takahashi Y, et al. Aberrant crypt foci of the colon as precursors of adenoma and cancer. *N Engl J Med* 1998;339:1277–1284.

72. Smith AJ, Stern HS, Penner M, et al. Somatic APC and K-ras codon 12 mutations in aberrant crypt foci from human colons. *Cancer Res* 1994;54:5527–5530.

73. Riddell RH. Large bowel polyps and tumours. In *Gastrointestinal Pathology*. Riddell RH, Lewin K, Weinstein F, eds. Igaku-Shoin Medical Publishers, New York, 1992; pp. 1198–1317.

74. Jass JR. Hyperplastic polyps of the colorectum — innocent or guilty? *Dis Colon Rectum* 2001;44:163–166.

75. Iwabuchi M, Sasano H, Hiwatashi N, et al. Serrated adenoma: a clinicopathological, DNA ploidy, and immunohistochemical study. *Anticancer Res* 2000;20:1141–1147.

76. Mäkinen MJ, George SMC, Jernvall P, et al. Colorectal carcinoma associated with serrated adenoma—prevalence, histological features, and prognosis. *J Pathol* 2001;193: 286–294.

77. Giardiello FM, Brensinger JD, Tersmette AC, et al. Very high risk of cancer in familial Peutz-Jeghers syndrome. *Gastroenterology* 2000;119:1447–1453.

78. Wong NACS, Harrison DJ. Colorectal neoplasia in ulcerative colitis—recent advances. *Histopathology* 2001;39:221–234.

79. Hussain SP, Amstad P, Raja K, et al. Increased p53 mutation load in noncancerous colon tissue from ulcerative colitis: a cancer-prone chronic inflammatory disease. *Cancer Res* 2000;60:3333–3337.

80. Greenstein AJ, Balasubramanian S, Harpaz N, et al. Carcinoid tumor and inflammatory bowel disease: a study of eleven cases and review of the literature *Am J Gastroenterol* 1997;92;682–685.

81. Ekbom A, Helmick C, Zack M, et al. Increased risk of large-bowel cancer in Crohn's disease with colonic involvement. *Lancet* 1990;336:357–359.

82. Rubio CA, Befrits R. Colorectal adenocarcinoma in Crohn's disease: a retrospective histologic study. *Dis Colon Rectum* 1997;40:1072–1078.

83. International Working Group. Terminology of nodular hepatocellular lesions. *Hepatology* 1995;22:983–993.

84. Ishak KG, Goodman ZG, Stocker JJ. Tumors of the liver and intrahepatic bile ducts. *Atlas of Tumor Pathology*, Third Series, Fascicle 31. Armed Forces Institute of Pathology, Washington DC; 2002.

85. Wilentz RE, Albores-Saavedra J, Zahurak M, et al. Pathologic examination accurately predicts prognosis in mucinous cystic neoplasms of the pancreas. *Am J Surg Pathol* 1999;23:1320–1327.

86. Wilentz RE, Albores-Saavedra J, Hruban RH. Mucinous cystic neoplasms of the pancreas. *Semin Diagn Pathol* 2000;17:31–42.

87. Adsay NV, Conlon KC, Zee SY, et al. Intraductal papillary mucinous neoplasms of the pancreas: an analysis of *in situ* and invasive carcinomas in 28 patients. *Cancer* 2002; 94:62–77.

88. Solin LJ, Fourquet A, Vicini FA, et al. Mammographically detected ductal carcinoma *in situ* of the breast treated with breast-conserving surgery and definitive breast irradiation: long term outcome and prognostic significance of patient age and margin status. *Int J Radiat Oncol Biol Phys* 2001;50: 991–1002.

89. Ottesen GL, Graversen HP, Blichert-Toft M, et al. Carcinoma *in situ* of the female breast. 10 Year follow-up results of a prospective nationwide study. *Breast Cancer Res Treat* 2000;62:197–210.

90. Fitzgibbons PL, Henson DE, Hutter RVP. Benign breast changes and the risk for subsequent breast cancer: an update

of the 1985 consensus statement. Cancer Committee of the College of American Pathologists. *Arch Pathol Lab Med* 1998;122:1053–1055.

91. Barnes R, Masood S. Potential value of hormone receptor assay in carcinoma *in situ* of breast. *Am J Clin Pathol* 1990;94:533–537.

92. Barnes D. C-erb-2 amplification in mammary carcinoma. *J Cell Biochem* 1993;176:132–138.

93. Bodian CA, Perzin KH, Lattes R, et al. Prognostic significance of benign proliferative breast disease. *Cancer* 1993;71:3896–3907.

94. Goldstein NS, Murphy T. Intraductal carcinoma associated with invasive carcinoma of the breast: a comparison of the two lesions with implications for intraductal carcinoma classification systems. *Am J Clin Pathol* 1996;106:312–318.

95. Leong ASY, Sormunen RT, Vinyuvat S, et al. Biologic markers in ductal carcinoma *in situ* and concurrent infiltrating carcinoma. a comparison of eight contemporary grading systems. *Am J Clin Pathol* 2001;115:709–718.

96. Thomson JZ, Evans AJ, Pinder SE, et al. Growth pattern of ductal carcinomas in situ (DCIS); a retrospective analysis based on mammographic findings. *Brit J Cancer* 2001;85; 225–227.

97. Scully RE. Pathology of ovarian cancer precursors. *J Cell Biochem* 1995;23(S):208–218.

98. Bell DA, Scully RE. Ovary. In *Pathology of Incipient Neoplasia*, 3rd ed. Henson DE, Albores-Saavedra J, eds. Oxford University Press, New York; 2001: pp. 419–440.

99. Feeley KM, Wells M. Precursor lesions of ovarian epithelial malignancy. *Histopathology* 2001;38:87–95.

100. Resta L, Russo S, Colucci GA, et al. Morphologic precursors of ovarian epithelial tumors. *Obstet Gynecol* 1993;82: 181–186.

101. Scully RE, Young RH, Clement PB. Tumors of the ovary, maldeveloped gonads, fallopian tube and broad ligament. *Atlas of Tumor Pathology*, Third Series, Fascicle 23. Armed Forces Institute of Pathology, Washington DC: 1998.

102. Aoki Y, Kawada N, Tanaka K. Early form of ovarian cancer originating in inclusion cysts: a case report. *J Reprod Med* 2000;45:159–161.

103. Sherman ME, Lee JS, Burks RT, et al. Histopathologic features of ovaries at increased risk for carcinoma: a case-control analysis. *Int J Gynecol Pathol* 1999;18:151–157.

104. Barakat RR, Federici MG, Saigo PE, et al. Absence of premalignant histologic, molecular, or cell biologic alterations in prophylactic oophorectomy specimens from BRCA1 heterozygotes. *Cancer* 2000:89:383–390.

105. Salazar H, Godwin AK, Daly MB, et al. Microscopic benign and invasive malignant neoplasms and a cancer-prone phenotype in prophylactic oophorectomies. *J Natl Cancer Inst* 1996;88:1810–1820.

106. Hutson R, Ramsdale J, Wells M. p53 protein expression in putative precursor lesions of epithelial ovarian cancer. *Histopathology* 1995;27:367–371.

107. Karseladze AI. On the site of origin of epithelial tumors of the ovary. *Eur J Gynaecol Oncol* 2001;22:110–115.

108. Matias-Guiu X, Catasus L, Bussaglia E, et al. Molecular pathology of endometrial hyperplasia and carcinoma. *Hum Pathol* 2001;32:569–577.

109. Dietel M. The histological diagnosis of endometrial hyperplasia. Is there a need to simply? *Virchows Arch* 2001;439: 604–608.

110. Baloglu H, Cannizzaro LA, Jones J, et al. Atypical endometrial hyperplasia shares genomic abnormalities with endometrioid carcinoma by comparative genomic hybridization. *Hum Pathol* 2001;32:615–622.

111. Aarnio A, Sankila R, Pukkala E, et al. Cancer risk in mutation carriers of DNA mismatch-repair genes. *Int J Cancer* 1999;81:214–218.

112. Tase T, Okagaki T, Clark BA, et al. Human papillomavirus DNA in adenocarcinoma *in situ*, microinvasive adenocarcinoma of the uterine cervix, and coexisting cervical squamous intraepithelial neoplasia. *Int J Gynecol Pathol* 1989;8:8–17.

113. Kurman RJ, Norris HJ, Wilkinson E. Tumors of the cervix, vagina, and vulva. *Atlas of Tumor Pathology*, Third Series, Fascicle 4. Armed Forces Institute of Pathology, Washington DC; 1992.

114. Schwartz SM, Weiss NS. Increased incidence of adenocarcinoma of the cervix in young women in the United States. *Am J Epidemiol* 1986;124:1045–1047.

115. Jawaiski RC. Endocervical glandular dysplasia, adenocarcinoma *in situ* and early invasive (microinvasive) adenocarcinoma of the uterine cervix. *Semin Diagn Pathol* 1990;7: 190–204.

116. Nasiell K, Nasiell M, Vaclavinkova V. Behavior of moderate cervical dysplasia during long-term follow-up. *Obstet Gynecol* 1983;61:609–614.

117. Melnikow J, Nuovo J, Willan AR, et al. Natural history of cervical squamous intraepithelial lesions: a meta-analysis. *Obstet Gynecol* 1998;92(Part 2):727–735.

118. Bollmann R, Bollmann M, Henson DE, et al. DNA confirms the utility of the Bethesda System for the classification of Papanicolaou smears. *Cancer Cytopathol* 2001;93: 222–228

119. Troncoso P, Babaian RJ, Ro JY, et al. Prostatic intraepithelial neoplasia and invasive prostatic adenocarcinoma in cystoprostatectomy specimens. *Urology* 1989;34(S):52–56.

120. Qian J, Wollan P, Bostwick DG. The extent and mutlicentricity of high-grade intraepithelial prostatic neoplasia in clinically localized prostatic adenocarcinoma. *Hum Pathol* 1997;28: 143–148.

121. Foster CS, Bostwick DG, Bonkhoff H, et al. Cellular and molecular pathology of prostate cancer precursors. *Scand J Urol Nephrol* 2000;205(S):19–43.

122. Helpap B. The biological significance of atypical hyperplasia of the prostate. *Virchows Arch A Pathol Anat Histol* 1980;387:307–317.

123. Amin MB, Schultz DS, Zarbo RJ, et al. Computerized static DNA ploidy analysis of prostate intraepithelial neoplasia. *Arch Pathol Lab Med* 1993;117:794–798.

124. Montironi R, Scarpelli M, Sisti S, et al. Quantative analysis of prostate intraepithelial neoplasia on tissue sections. *Anal Quant Cytol Histol* 1990;12:366–372.

125. McNeal JE, Bostwick DG. Intraductal dysplasia: a premalignant lesion of the prostate. *Hum Pathol* 1986;17:64–71.

126. Bostwick DG. High grade prostatic intraepithelial neoplasia. The most likely precursor of prostate cancer. *Cancer* 1995;75:1823–1836.

127. Bostwick DG, Pacelli A, Lopez-Beltran A. Molecular biology of prostatic intraepithelial neoplasia. *Prostate* 1996;29: 117–134.

128. Zitzelsberger H, Engert D, Walch A, et al. Chromosomal changes during development and progression of prostate adenocarcinomas. *Br J Cancer* 2001;84:202–208.

129. Van der Kwast TH, Labrie F, Tetu B. Prostatic intraepithelial neoplasia and endocrine manipulation. *Eur Urol* 1999;35: 508–510.

130. Bostwick DG, Montironi R, Sesterhenn IA. Diagnosis of prosta-tic intraepithelial neoplasia. Prostate Working Group/Consensus Report. *Scand J Urol Nephrol* 2000;205(S):3–10.

131. Partin AW, Steinberg GD, Pitcock RV, et al. Use of nuclear morphometry, Gleason histologic scoring, clinical stage, and age to predict disease-free survival among patients with prostate cancer. *Cancer* 1992;70:161–168.

132. De Marzo AM, Putzi MJ, Nelson WG. New concepts in the pathology of prostatic epithelial carcinogenesis. *Urology* 2001;57:103–114.

133. Joedemaeker RF, Kranse R, Rietbergen JB, et al. Evaluation of prostate needle biopsies in a population-based screening; a study: the impact of borderline lesions. *Cancer* 1999;85:145–152.

134. Sakr WA, Partin AW. Histological markers of risk and the role of high-grade prostatic intraepithelial neoplasia. *Urology* 2001;57:115–120.

135. Sakr WA, Haas GP, Cassin BF, et al. The frequency of carci-noma and intraepithelial neoplasia of the prostate in young male patients. *J Urol* 1993;150:379–385.

136. Murphy WM, Beckwith JB, Farrow GM. Tumors of the kid-ney, bladder, and related urinary structures. *Atlas of Tumor Pathology*, Third Series, Fascicle 11. Armed Forces Institute of Pathology, Washington DC; 1994.

137. Murphy WM, Busch C, Algaba F. Intraepithelial lesions of urinary bladder: morphologic considerations. *Scand J Urol Nephrol Suppl* 2000;205:67–81.

138. Zuk RJ, Rogers HS, Martin JE, et al. Clinicopathological importance of primary dysplasia of bladder. *J Clin Pathol* 1988;41:1277–1280.

139. Cheng L, Cheville JC, Neumann RM, et al. Natural history of urothelial dysplasia of the bladder. *Am J Surg Pathol* 1999;23:443–447.

140. Torti FM, Lum BL. Superficial bladder cancer: risk of recur-rence and potential role for interferon therapy. *Cancer* 1987;59(S):613–616.

141. Torti FM, Lum BL, Aston D, et al. Superficial bladder cancer: the primary of grade in the development of invasive disease. *J Clin Oncol* 1987;5:125–130.

142. Spruck CH III, Ohneseit PF, Gonzalez-Zulueta M, et al. Two molecular pathways to transitional cell carcinoma in the bladder. *Cancer Res* 1994;54:784–788.

143. Ayala AG, Ro J, Amin MB, et al. Urinary bladder. In Henson DE, Albores Saavedra J, eds. *Pathology of Incipient Neoplasia*, 3rd ed. Oxford University Press, New York; 2001;pp 489–534.

144. Pinkus H, Mehregan AH. Premalignant skin lesions. *Clin Plast Surg* 1980;7:289–300.

145. Cockerell CJ. Histopathology of incipient intraepidermal squamous cell carcinoma ("actinic keratosis"). *J Am Acad Dermatol* 2000;42 (Part 2):11–17.

146. Dinehart SM. The treatment of actinic keratoses. *J Am Acad Dermatol* 2000;42 (Part 2):25–28.

147. Kiviat NB, Critchlow CW, Holmes KK, et al. Association of anal dysplasia and human papillomavirus with immunosup-pression and HIV infection among homosexual men. *AIDS* 1993;7:43–49.

148. Metcalf AM, Dean T. Risk of dysplasia in anal condyloma. *Surgery* 1995;118;724-726.

149. Dinehart SM, Nelson-Adesokan P, Cockerell C, et al. Metastatic cutaneous squamous cell carcinoma derived from actinic keratosis. *Cancer* 1997;79:920–923.

150. Helwig EB, Graham JH. Anogenital (extramammary) Paget's disease: a clinicopathological study. *Cancer* 1963;16:387–403.

151. Ackerman AB. Malignant melanoma in situ; the flat curable stage of malignant melanoma. *Pathology* 1985;17: 298–300.

152. Hoang M, Sinku P, Albores-Saavedra J. Rhabdomyosarcoma arising in a congenital melanocytic nevus. *Am J Dermatopathol* 2002;24:26–29.

153. Warnakulasuriya S. Histological grading of oral epithelial dysplasia: revisited. *J Pathol* 2001;194:294–297.

154. Riddell RH, Goldman H, Ransohoff DF, et al. Dysplasia in inflammatory bowel disease: standardized classifica-tion with provisional clinical applications. *Hum Pathol* 1983;14:931–968.

155. Sakr WA, Haas GP, Cassin BF, et al. The frequency of carci-noma and intraepithelial neoplasia of the prostate in young male patients. *J Urol* 1993;150:379–385.

6 Quantitative Nuclear Grade

Clinical Applications of the Quantitative Measurement of Nuclear Structure Using Image Analysis

Robert W. Veltri, PhD, Alan W. Partin, MD, PhD, and M. Craig Miller

CONTENTS

INTRODUCTION
GENERAL PRINCIPLES OF QNG
DISCUSSION
REFERENCES

1. INTRODUCTION

Changes in nuclear structure occur in response to normal physiological processes such as cell division, apoptosis, cell differentiation, and senescence, as well as in disease-related processes such as cancer, where they are manifested in response to numerous alterations in gene expression *(1)*. Therefore, the accurate and reproducible measurement of nuclear structure changes can provide important objective information when assessing and managing the pathologic disease process *(2–4)*. Several studies have demonstrated that transformation of a normal cell into a malignant cell requires a series of genetic changes (or hits) *(5–7)* such as mutations, DNA methylation events in promoters or exons, chromosome deletions, insertions, amplifications, and translocations *(7–13)*. Additionally, several classes of well-characterized nuclear organelles (spliceosomes, centrosomes, telomeres, and nucleosomes), gene families (HMGA, SWI/SNF modifiers, RARs, MARs, etc.), and key structural and regulatory proteins (e.g., nuclear matrix proteins, HMG proteins, nuclear histones H1, H2A, H2B, H3, and H4, and SWI/SNF complex) have been identified as being important to maintenance of nuclear chromatin structure and function *(13–27)*. One example in this area involves work on the combinatorial chemistry of the histone tails of the nucleosome's protein core. There is

evidence that acetylation, methylation, phosphorylation, glycosylation, and ubiquination of the histone tail can produce changes in chromatin structure directly related to differential patterns of gene expression *(27)*.

To date, only very select genetic alterations have been assessed and applied clinically with more classically accepted methodology, such as immunoassays, and in some cases, polymerase chain reaction (PCR)-based and fluorescent *in situ* hybridization (FISH) technologies *(28–32)*. A more modern approach that utilizes molecular technology to assess gene expression more globally applies gene chip array technologies, but this is not yet ready for clinical laboratory applications *(33–34)*. These latter sophisticated molecular assessments, though very informative, can be cumbersome, generate complex data, and expensive to perform. Another pathology-based approach employs DNA ploidy with computer-assisted image analysis or cytogenetics as a method of measuring abnormal DNA content, which represents rather large-scale chromosomal alterations (i.e., tetraploidy, aneuploidy, hyperploidy, etc.) that usually reflect late-stage changes of genetic instability in cancer cells *(1,3,35–38)*. Important nuclear morphometry information critical to disease assessment can also be derived from the nuclear images captured from benign, atypical, dysplastic, and malignant cell types normally used for DNA ploidy assessment *(3,37)*.

From: Cancer Chemoprevention, Volume 2: Strategies for Cancer Chemoprevention
Edited by: G. J. Kelloff, E. T. Hawk, and C. C. Sigman © Humana Press Inc., Totowa, NJ

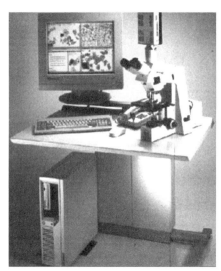

- **Zeiss Axioskop Microscope**
- **3CCD Color Camera**
- **High Resolution (768 × 494)**
- **Square Pixels**
- **~60 Nuclear Morphometric Descriptors**
- **User-Friendly Software**
- **High-Speed/High-Capacity Computer System**
- **Commercially Available and not Cost-Prohibitive**

Fig. 1. Photograph of the AutoCyte™ Imaging system that our laboratories currently employ to perform DNA ploidy and QNG analysis.

Nuclear morphometric descriptors (NMDs) measure subtle alterations in nuclear size, shape, DNA content, and chromatin organization in both intact (i.e., cytology) and cut (i.e., histology) cell nuclei in response to a disease process (malignant or nonmalignant) or treatment for a disease process *(38–46)*. Furthermore, one can use both nonparametric statistical or nonlinear mathematical modeling with neural networks to construct computational solutions employing the NMDs as well as other nuclear biomarkers *(3,46–51)*. Applying nonparametric statistical modeling, or constructing nonlinear models using neural networks (NNs) based on mathematical weighting of input variables, has permitted new approaches to managing complex data derived from such nuclear images, as well as clinical information, to create objective decision-support tools *(3,38,39,41–52)*.

This review will focus on how to perform quantitative nuclear grading (QNG) of tissue or intact cells using NMDs, how to utilize QNG results, and future potential applications of the technology in preventive medicine.

2. GENERAL PRINCIPLES OF QNG

Images of benign, premalignant, and malignant Feulgen-stained nuclei are captured and analyzed from a pathologist-marked slide (~125–150 per area) by an image specialist using a computer-assisted image analysis system with the appropriate DNA ploidy and morphometry software. A system extensively tested by our group is the AutoCyte™ Pathology Workstation with QUIC-DNA v1.201 (TriPath Imaging, Burlington, NC) (Fig. 1) *(31–32)*. This system not only generates DNA ploidy histograms, but also calculates 60 different NMDs, based on equations that utilize single-step analysis of pixel intensity maps, for each of the Feulgen-stained nuclei analyzed, which include 11 nuclear size and shape features, 18 DNA content measurements, 10 non-Markovian and 21 Markovian chromatin texture features (Table 1). The NMDs described in Table 1 are provided in the QUIC-DNA user's manual version 1.201, and are used to calculate nuclear features of size, shape, DNA content, and chromatin texture. The NMDs within a particular class of features demonstrate a great deal of correlation; however, across the various classes of NMDs (e.g., size, shape, DNA content, chromatin texture) there is much less correlation. Therefore, in order to take advantage of the information contained in the 60 NMDs, we utilize the variance of each NMD, which is calculated using all nuclear images captured from each specimen being analyzed (~125–150 cells per specimen). This generates a database containing a variance for each of the 60 NMDs for every case. At this point, a variety of computational methodologies can reduce complexity of information so that only essential feature information required to make specific clinical decisions is used. Fig. 2 shows a schematic depicting how a QNG solution is calculated. We have used such computational methods as modeling with logistic regression (LR) *(4,39–46)* or NN *(47–50)* to determine which NMDs multivariately contributed to a computational solution (QNG) to predict a disease-specific outcome or treatment effect. These approaches can be used to select the most predictive and least redundant NMDs that assist in differentiating two classes of patients; for example, organ-confined from non-organ-confined cancer or

Table 1
Nuclear Morphometric Descriptors (NMDs)

1. Cell class	21. Minimum OD	41. Contrast
2. Perimeter	22. Maximum OD	42. Correlation
3. Area	23. Median OD	43. Difference moment
4. Circular form factor	24. Mean OD	44. Inverse difference moment
5. Diameter equiv. circle	25. SD of OD	45. Sum average
6. Feret X	26. Skewness of OD	46. Sum variance
7. Feret Y	27. Excess of OD	47. Sum entropy
8. Minimum feret	28. DNA ploidy	48. Entropy
9. Maximum feret	29. DNA index	49. Difference variance
10. Area convex hull	30. Transmission	50. Difference entropy
11. Perimeter convex hull	31. Variance	51. Information measure A
12. Excess of gray values	32. Sum average (AC)	52. Information measure B
13. Skewness of gray values	33. Sum entropy (AC)	53. Maximal correlation coefficient
14. SD of gray values	34. Sum variance (AC)	54. Coefficient of variation
15. Mean gray value	35. Cluster shade	55. Peak transition probability
16. Median gray value	36. Cluster prominence	56. Diagonal variance
17. Maximum gray value	37. Diagonal moment (AC)	57. Diagonal moment
18. Minimum gray value	38. Kappa	58. Second diagonal moment
19. Intensity	39. Sum of homogeneity	59. Product moment
20. Integrated OD	40. Angular 2nd moment	60. Triangular symmetry

NMD#	NMD Classes
1–11	Size and shape
12–29	DNA content
30–39	Non-Markovian texture
40–60	Markovian texture

Key: OD, optical density; (AC), AutoCyte version of calculation; SD, standard deviation.

Note: Grain may be viewed as a unit of measurement (in pixels) of the width of an average sized object. The grain values for all of these measurements were set to one (1) pixel.

progressors from nonprogressors. Surely numerous other mathematical approaches or combinations thereof can be used to calculate a patient-specific QNG solution through reducing complexity and/or collapsing the number of variables required within each category of the NMDs to make the disease decisions. The ultimate successful clinical application of QNG relies totally on the design of IRB-approved clinical trials (retrospective or prospective) in terms of selecting the appropriate patient disease criteria of interest, accurate pathologist diagnoses, developing a computational model with a statistically valid patient cohort for training, and testing for reproducibility and robustness. This is followed by validation with patients and controls from a patient cohort from nongeographically limited locations to test the ability of the QNG computer model to classify these unknowns that have never been used for training or testing the model. In the case of LR, these populations are completely separated; however, an NN always divides the patient sample randomly into training, testing, and validation sets at an investigator-selected ratio (for example, 60:30:10) in order to build the most clinically useful computational decision model. In the latter case, large patient samples are required at the onset to provide the best results (48–52). Notably, any significant change in patient demographics of a disease decision computational model (either LR or NN) requires retraining with patients who exemplify the altered demographics.

Analyze specimen using Image Analysis System, generate a DNA ploidy histogram, and save nuclear images for the calculation of the quantitative nuclear grade (QNG)

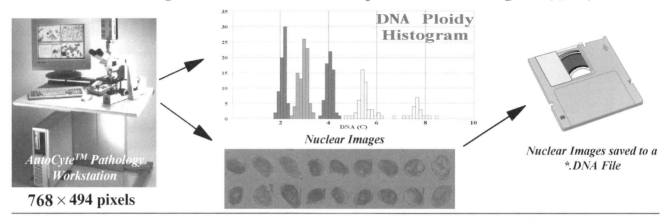

Calculate size, shape, and DNA complexity features for each of the nuclear images saved in the computer files and create the quantitative nuclear grade solution

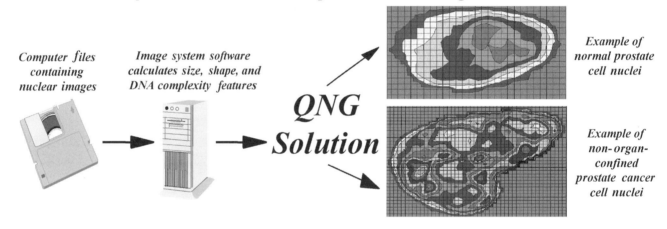

Fig. 2. Schematic diagram of the process used to determine a QNG solution for either cytology or histology specimens. Feulgen-stained nuclei are captured for DNA ploidy analysis using the QUIC-DNA v1.201 program and simultaneously pixel gray level data are collected to measure the 60 nuclear morphometric descriptors (NMDs) seen in Table 1 that are used to calculate QNG solutions.

Figure 3 is a 3D bitmap image of individual normal, atypical, and transitional cell carcinoma (TCC) single nuclei from a bladder cancer patient's urine cytology specimen. It illustrates the complexity of individual pixel gray level intensities and their distribution using 2D and 3D histogram plots of each pixel as well as a smoothed 3D surface plot of the same data. Information on the gray level intensity, as well as frequency and distribution of individual pixels for every nuclear gallery from each case, is used to calculate variance of size, shape, DNA content, and chromatin texture features for 60 NMDs, and ultimately QNG as described below.

2.1. QNG Bladder Cancer Applications

2.1.1. CANCER CELL CLASSIFIER

The process starts by obtaining a consensus opinion from expert cytopathologists as to the actual histopatho-

logic and matching cytopathologic diagnosis of the patient, followed by identification of the specific cells to be collected from patients that meet their visual criteria of classification (i.e., normal, atypical, dysplastic, cancer) (4,39). To illustrate this application, we captured cell nuclei for bladder cytology specimens obtained from voided urine specimens of normal donors, patients with biopsy-proven low-grade TCC (LGTCC), high-grade TCC (HGTCC) and no history of TCC and negative cystoscopic findings, as well as patients with cytological atypia. The specimens were immediately ethanol-fixed (75–100 mL of urine in 50–100 mL of 50% buffered ethyl alcohol) and received in our laboratory 24–48 h after collection. Using a Feulgen-stained primary 25-mm filter (0.5 micron) imprint, two expert cytopathologists selected intact urothelial cell nuclei most representative of normal

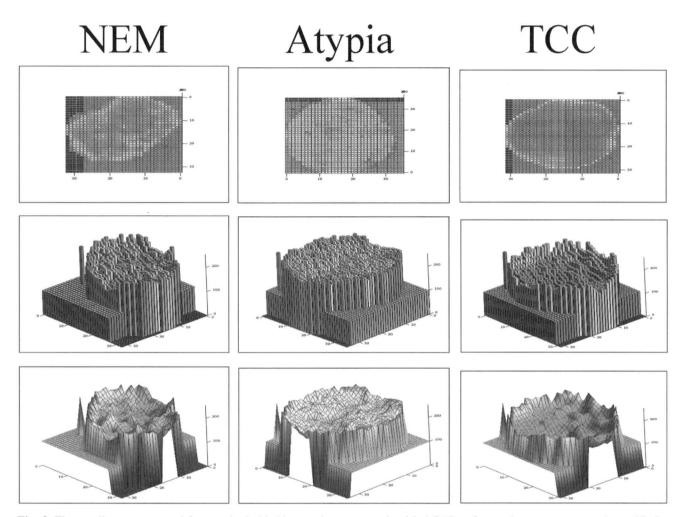

Fig. 3. Three cells were captured from a single bladder cytology case; using MathCAD software they were converted to a 2D flat image and two 3D images, one being an individual pixel map of the intensity of each gray level and the other a smoothed texture map of the same.

(n = 1083 nuclear images from 12 normal donors), atypia (n = 1893 nuclear images from 40 atypia cases), LGTCC (n = 1010 nuclear images from 43 patients), and HGTCC (n = 1000 nuclear images from 51 cases). All images were captured and analyzed using a commercial image analysis system (BD-CIS, San Jose, CA). All data (NMDs) were analyzed with the Stata™ statistical analysis software program (Stata Corporation, College Station, TX). Logistic regression analysis and backwards stepwise variable selection at a stringency of $p_z < 0.05$ was used to univariately select which NMDs contributed to a QNG model solution to accurately classify normal, atypical, or LGTCC cells (Table 2). Table 2 presents the statistics and area under the receiver operator characteristic (AUC-ROC) curves that compare the ability of QNG solutions to differentiate normal vs atypia, atypia vs LGTCC, normal vs LGTCC, and LGTCC vs HGTCC. Such a tool would permit rapid identification of cytology specimens at high risk for containing cancer cells or malignancy-associated changes (MACs) reflective of possibly active TCC. Such a cytology classifier system would save time and money and improve patient care through early detection of autochthonous cancer during patients' monitoring for TCC recurrence.

2.1.2. PATIENT-SPECIFIC CYTOLOGY DISEASE OUTCOME CLASSIFIERS

The objective of this approach is to identify a series of patients with pathologist biopsy-confirmed disease (i.e., normal, atypia, dysplasia, LGTCC) in an age-and/or sex-matched statistically balanced patient cohort. A cytopathologic diagnosis is made by an expert cytopathologist and compared with results obtained using computer-assisted microscopy on the Feulgen-stained urothelial nuclei as described above. Each case accepted for such an IRB-approved study must have a cystoscopy/biopsy-confirmed diagnosis. Next, cells

Table 2
Ability of QNG to Differentiate Normal, Atypical, and TCC Cells From Voided Urines

Diagnostic parameter	Normal vs atypia	Normal vs LGTCC	Normal vs HGTCC	Atypia vs LGTCC	LGTCC vs HGTCC
Cutoff	0.50	0.50	0.45	0.50	0.50
Sensitivity	88%	85%	99%	83%	96%
Specificity	65%	86%	98%	93%	97%
PPV	82%	87%	98%	88%	97%
NPV	74%	84%	99%	90%	96%
AUC-ROC	87%	93%	99%	96%	99%
# NMDs	14	16	12	16	17

are collected and routine cytology staining with Papanicolaou as well as Feulgen stain is performed on two separate monolayer cytopreps. We recently utilized the AutoCyte™ system (Burlington, NC) in collaboration with Dr. Ihor Sawczuk at Columbia University School of Medicine, Department of Urology (Dr. Sawczuk is currently at Hackensack University Medical Center) to detect recurrent BlCa using cytology specimens (both voided urine and bladder washes). A total of 87 prospectively accrued patients being monitored for recurrence of their previously diagnosed bladder cancer were sampled under an IRB-approved protocol with informed consent. We compared the ability of QNG to identify TCC in these two specimen types to that of cytopathology and DNA

ploidy alone (logistic regression stringency levels of $p < 0.20$ and model cutoffs of 0.50). Figures 4 and 5 illustrate AUC-ROC curves as well as sensitivities, specificities, and accuracies of QNG to accomplish this clinical diagnostic objective in comparison to DNA ploidy and cytopathology (data unpublished) in both voided urine and bladder wash specimens, respectively. Clearly, QNG is capable of identifying cancer cases across a spectrum of cytopathology calls with improved sensitivity and specificity. The use of QNG to augment cytopathology would have great clinical value for early detection of active recurrent tumors requiring intervention. Hence, properly trained computational training models populated with appropriate patient controls and cases exemplifying target disease states that require

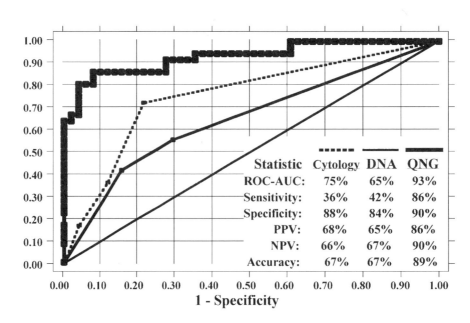

Statistic	Cytology	DNA	QNG
ROC-AUC:	75%	65%	93%
Sensitivity:	36%	42%	86%
Specificity:	88%	84%	90%
PPV:	68%	65%	86%
NPV:	66%	67%	90%
Accuracy:	67%	67%	89%

1 - Specificity

Fig. 4. ROC curves indicate the ability of QNG to detect cancer based on nuclear information captured from urothelial nuclei in voided urine specimens from 87 patients compared to DNA ploidy and cytology alone.

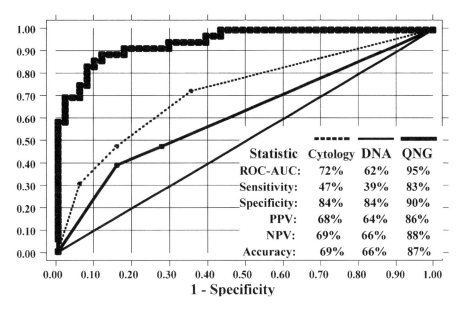

Fig. 5. ROC curves indicate the ability of QNG to detect cancer based on nuclear information captured from urothelial nuclei in bladder wash specimens from 87 patients compared to DNA ploidy and cytology alone.

rapid and definitive identification should benefit from such an image-based patient-specific cell classifier. Once again, the ultimate success or failure of such cancer cell classifiers depends on having expert pathologists select cells and provide an accurate histologic diagnosis of each case that populates the training-testing database, then validating the database with cases that were not included when developing the model, which meet performance specifications indicated for the model.

2.2. QNG Prostate Cancer Applications

2.2.1. PRETREATMENT PATHOLOGIC STAGING

This application requires the same clinical specimen routinely provided to the pathologist for a histologic diagnosis; an additional juxtaposed tissue section is made for Feulgen staining. The most significant areas of the H&E primary stained slide that support the best prognosis decision are marked by a pathologist and confirmed by a second pathologist. QNG has been used by both imaging systems to accomplish this task using prostate biopsies (4). An example using biopsy material involved a prospectively enrolled patient cohort of 255 men between October 1998 and January 2000 (average age = 58.8 ± 6 yr) diagnosed with clinical stage T1c prostate cancer (PCa) who underwent radical prostatectomy (RRP) at a single institution (22). Exclusion criteria included neoadjuvant treatment or medications that could affect the serologic or histologic presentation of PCa. Preoperative sera, biopsy histology slides, clinical information, RRP pathology, and gland weights

were obtained. Biomarkers assessed included total prostate-specific antigen (tPSA), complexed PSA (cPSA), free PSA (fPSA), f/t PSA ratio, cPSA density, and biopsy Gleason score. We calculated a QNG equation and algorithm solution to predict the pathologic stage of clinical stage T1c patients with the Stata™ software program, using backward stepwise logistic regression analysis at a stringency of $p < 0.20$. The results are shown in Table 3 and clearly demonstrate QNG's contribution to making the stage prediction compared to pathology and clinical variables, as well as its multivariate contribution for this prediction using needle-core biopsy-captured information. It is important to note that QNG alone provided superior information that was independent of Gleason score. Some current limitations to consider when using needle core biopsies include compression artifacts introduced by obtaining the needle-core sample and immediately extruding it directly into buffered formalin fixative, inadequate fixation of the needle-core specimen, and inadequate specimen to make a definitive diagnosis. Most of these obstacles can be overcome through modification of tissue sample collection and processing schemas.

A second example used postoperative material from 214 men with a Gleason score of 5.0–7.0 and a clinical stage of T1b–T2c with long-term follow-up of at least 5 yr for patients without biochemical progression. Images were captured with the earlier commercial imaging system (BD-CIS). We constructed multivariate backward stepwise LR models to predict progression

Table 3
Ability to Preoperatively Predict Prostate Cancer Stage in 255 Men With Clinical Stage T1c Disease

Independent variable	p-value	Sensitivity[a]	Specificity[a]	Accuracy[a]	ROC-AUC
Age at biopsy	0.2809	42.9%	65.1%	60.8%	54.6%
Biopsy Gleason score	0.0003	34.7%	89.8%	79.2%	61.9%
Preoperative total PSA (ng/mL)	0.0002	40.8%	77.2%	70.2%	63.7%
Preoperative complexed PSA (ng/mL)	0.0001	42.9%	77.2%	70.6%	65.1%
Complexed PSA density	< 0.0001	46.9%	76.2%	70.6%	67.3%
Quantitative nuclear grade (QNG)	< 0.0001	67.4%	80.6%	78.0%	80.6%
cPSA density + biopsy Gleason	< 0.0001	51.0%	78.2%	72.9%	70.7%
QNG + cPSA density + biopsy Gleason	< 0.0001	73.5%	83.0%	81.2%	82.4%

[a]Cutoff of 0.20 used for logistic regression models to determine sensitivity, specificity, and accuracy values.

(Table 4), and QNG performed to similar specifications as postoperative Gleason score; together, results further improved. We also prepared various NN training models combining postoperative pathology and QNG that performed in the range of ~80–94% and validated in the range of 68–71% (data not shown). Future use of larger patient samples and improved resolution AutoCyte imaging systems should further improve the accuracy of predicting early biochemical recurrence, but this example demonstrates feasibility.

Treatment for cancer, especially solid tumors, often requires removal of the tumor, which then provides tissue for making a complete diagnostic and prognostic pathology report. The availability of this type of specimen affords an opportunity to perform additional testing with immunohistochemistry for established biomarkers and new biomarkers such as QNG. In addition, the development of tissue microarray (TMA) procedures has provided an opportunity to study large patient cohorts with unique biomarkers to assess their clinical utility. Our group recently demonstrated that QNG can be performed on prostate TMAs (unpublished data).

We have recently utilized TMAs of four replicate 0.6-mm tissue spots prepared from the PCa and adjacent benign areas of 24 Japanese and 22 Japanese-American prostate glands removed at radical prostatectomy. The AutoCyte pathology workstation was used to measure QNG. A Feulgen-stained TMA slide was used to cap-

ture benign or malignant epithelial nuclei from each of four replicate spots. A multivariate backward stepwise LR QNG solution was determined, which differentiated either benign or PCa epithelial nuclei components between these two Japanese populations. This model solution had an AUC-ROC of 83% ($p < 0.0001$) and an accuracy of 82% to distinguish benign component nuclear changes in the PCa glands of these two patient samples. Another QNG model was constructed to distinguish nuclear changes in the malignant component of PCa glands of these two patient samples; the AUC-ROC was 84% with 78% accuracy. The ability to distinguish benign from malignant areas in the same glands of each patient group was easily determined by QNG with greater than 90% accuracy (data not shown). In summary, QNG was capable of differentiating nuclear structure changes from benign and malignant epithelial components of native Japanese and Japanese-American prostate glands. QNG may detect variations in nuclear structure between these two patient populations that are possibly attributable to differing patterns of genetic and/or epigenetic events. Though extreme care must be taken in interpreting these preliminary results due to limited sample size and specimen processing issues, the trends demonstrated remain interesting and require confirmation.

Finally, in prostate cancer as well as other types of cancer, it should be possible to identify significant

Table 4
Ability to Predict Prostate Cancer Progression Postoperatively in 214 Men With ≥ 5 yr Follow-Up

Independent variable	p-value	Sensitivity[a]	Specificity[a]	Accuracy[a]	ROC-AUC
DNA ploidy	0.0479	60.7%	53.1%	56.1%	56.9%
Age	0.032	54.8%	57.7%	56.5%	56.9%
Clinical stage	0.1564	45.2%	69.2%	59.8%	57.3%
OC status	0.0203	78.6%	36.2%	52.8%	57.4%
Post-op Gleason score	< 0.0001	66.7%	74.6%	71.5%	73.6%
QNG	< 0.0001	64.3%	78.5%	72.9%	79.2%
QNG + post-op Gleason score	< 0.0001	75.0%	80.0%	78.0%	84.3%

[a]Cutoff of 0.40 used for logistic regression models to determine sensitivity, specificity, and accuracy values.

MACs by capturing cells from normal as well as different abnormal pathological stages, including, for example, high-grade prostatic intraepithelial neoplasia (HGPIN). We captured images of prostate epithelial cells from 35/228 RRP surgical specimens containing normal, HGPIN, and PCa from men who experienced biochemical progression and were being followed for development of distant metastasis and death. Figure 6 illustrates the ability of QNG to distinguish three pathological phenotypes in subsets of RRP specimens from 228 cases, which were marked for areas of normal, HGPIN, and/or cancer. QNG was capable of differentiating these histologic states (e.g., normal, HGPIN, and/or PCa) using the 60 NMDs. The next step is to determine nuclear changes that occur in the non-cancer areas and assess their contribution to making clinical outcome predictions. This work is currently under way using a set of 228 RRP cases that have recurred biochemically, of which a subset of men metastasized and died. We intend to use nuclear structure changes in the benign and malignant areas to help predict those men at risk for rapid progression to metastasis and death.

3. DISCUSSION

One method to assess the relationship between altered nuclear structure and cancer biology is through the use of computer-assisted image analysis of cytological and histological patient material (1–4). The required engineering platform for an image system capable of capturing nuclear images stained for DNA (chromatin), storing them, and subsequently processing the data to derive feature measurements is a computer with a frame grabber, high-resolution camera, microscope with quality optics, and a custom software program to process the data (4). In addition, it is critical that the reproducibility

of the nuclear staining technique be standardized and quality-controlled (4,35,38,51). The imaging hardware platform should be commercially available and sufficiently robust in terms of availability of all necessary components with service support from both software and hardware perspectives. The image capture and processing system must perform well with intact cells captured from both cytologic and histologic specimens, providing erosion algorithms that address overlapping or degenerate cells. Another important characteristic of the imaging system is the number of pixels per unit area as well as its size and shape (small and square), providing sufficient resolution of the nuclear image to be able to conduct sophisticated pixel intensity and distribution analysis of nuclear size, shape, and texture. This feature analysis may be accomplished using a variety of equations, but those that are especially important solve for specific nuclear chromatin texture using Markovian and non-Markovian equations (4,35,38,51). The machine-to-machine technical performance must be stable and the operator-to-operator reproducibility must be high (<10%) when testing the same samples.

In general, normal cell nuclei tend to be round or at least smoothly curved, and DNA chromatin tends to be evenly distributed (40–42). This is not so for cancer cells, which tend to be irregularly shaped with their DNA chromatin distributed in clumped and disordered patterns (4,35,38–42). We have taken advantage of the disparity in size, shape, DNA content, and chromatin structure of cancer, premalignant, and malignancy juxtaposed cells to assess nuclear structure alterations of clinical significance by using the variance of NMDs. Any image analysis technology may be used to generate such a QNG variable; however, it is the "expert patient training set" that ultimately determines the

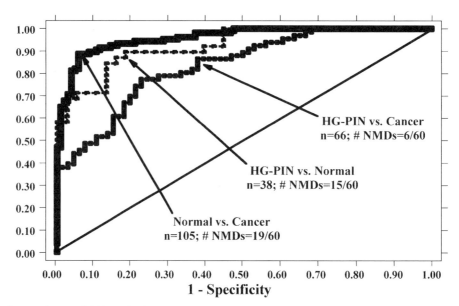

Fig. 6. Tissue slides from subsets of 228 radical prostatectomy patients were marked for normal, HGPIN, and cancer areas by a pathologist, and Feulgen-stained nuclei were captured from each of the areas (i.e., normal, HGPIN, and cancer) using the AutoCyte™ system. The ROC curves illustrate the ability of three QNG solutions (the number of NMDs required for each model noted) to differentiate the three histologic phenotypes on a single radical prostatectomy specimen block.

clinical value and potential applications to predict patient-specific disease outcomes within the validation patient cohorts.

We have provided several clinically relevant examples of past and current studies that clearly illustrate the applications of QNG computational solutions, derived by a variety of computational methods *(4,38,44,45–51)*, to both cytology and histology specimens (those derived from biopsies or radicals). In addition, we have shown how the information collected may be used to classify cells or disease-specific outcomes reliably as verified by validation *(4,44–52)*.

Our results confirm that QNG derived with robust imaging systems provides valuable information that can predict existence of disease through MACs, extent of disease state, biochemical or clinical progression and metastasis, and treatment response. Also, it is quite possible that QNG may be able to eventually replace Gleason score as an objective pathological measurement of disease prognosis. Additionally, we believe that these alterations in nuclear structure, as measured through QNG, are closely related to numerous alterations in gene expression that occur in the premalignancy as well as progression of malignancy *(1,5–28)*. Hence, the QNG variable, especially when it is combined with clinical and pathological patient information, produces computational decision-support tools for making more accurate decisions in patient management. These decisions may involve selection of patients for expectant management clinical decisions, chemoprevention, and timely intervention of first-line chemotherapy and/or adjuvant therapy for recurrence. We also believe that quantitative morphometry may be useful in assessment of new treatments such as those associated with restoration of normal gene expression patterns and cellular functions. Finally, the clinical usefulness of quantitative image technology has been repeatedly demonstrated. It is available using commercially supported hardware and software and should be implemented more routinely in the management of oncology patients.

REFERENCES

1. Stein GS, Berezney R, Getzenberg RH, eds. Nuclear structure and cancer. *J Cell Biochem Suppl* 2000;35:1–157.
2. Bartels PH Computer-generated diagnosis and image analysis: an overview. *Cancer* 1992;69:1636–1638.
3. Palcic B. Nuclear texture: can it be used as a surrogate endpoint biomarker? *J Cell Biochem* 1994;Suppl 19:40–46.
4. Veltri, RW, Partin AW, Miller MC. Quantitative nuclear grade (QNG): a new image analysis-based biomarker of clinically relevant nuclear structure alterations. *J Cell Biochem* 2000;35:151–157.
5. Fearon ER. A genetic basis for multi-step pathway of colorectal tumorigenesis. *Princess Takamatsu Symp* 1991;22:37–48.
6. Vogelstein B, Kinzler KW. The multistep nature of cancer. *Trends Genet* 1993;9:138–141.
7. Knudson AG. Two genetic hits (more or less) to cancer. *Nat Rev Cancer* 2001;1:157–162.

Analyze Specimen Using Image Analysis System, Generate a DNA Ploidy Histogram, and Save Nuclear Images for the Calculation of the Quantitative Nuclear Grade (QNG)

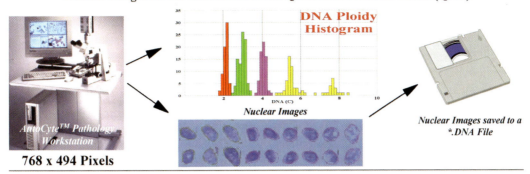

Calculate Size, Shape, and DNA complexity Features for each of the Nuclear Images saved in the Computer Files and Create the Quantitative Nuclear Grade Solution

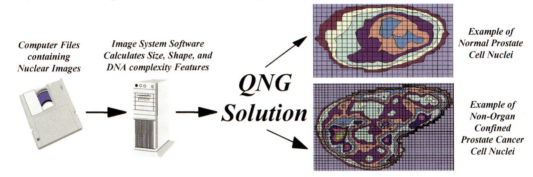

Color Plate 1, Fig. 2. (*see* discussion in Ch. 6 on pp. 98–99 and complete caption on p. 100). Determining a QNG solution for cytology/histology specimens.

NEM   Atypia   TCC

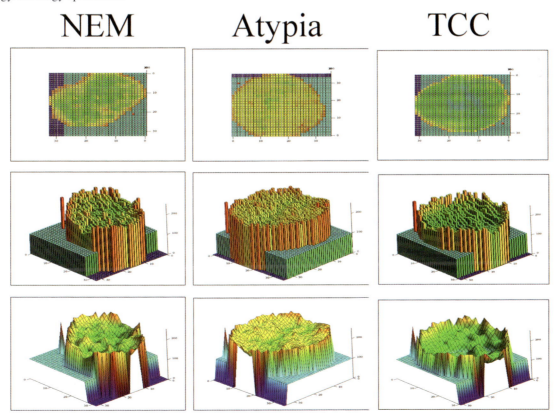

Color Plate 2, Fig. 3. (*see* discussion in Ch 6 on pp. 99–100 and complete caption on p. 101). Three bladder cells converted to 2D/3D images.

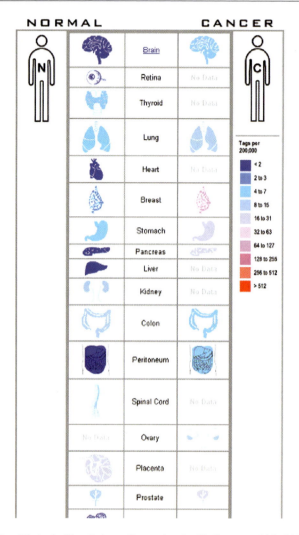

Color Plate 3, Fig. 2. (*see* discussion in Ch 7 on pp. 111–112 and complete caption on p. 112). SAGE Genie Anatomic Viewer display of *erb*B2 gene expression in normal tissue and in tumors.

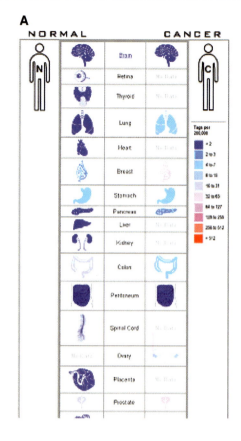

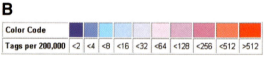

Library	Total Tags in Library	Tags per 200,000	Color Code
SAGE_Breast_metastatic_carcinoma_B_95-260	45087	133	
SAGE_Breast_carcinoma_B_95-259	39364	127	
SAGE_Breast_carcinoma_CL_MCF7control_0h	59877	126	
SAGE_Breast_carcinoma_B_95-347	67070	122	
SAGE_Prostate_carcinoma_B_LN-1	22599	115	
SAGE_Prostate_adenocarcinoma_MD_PR317	64951	95	
SAGE_Breast_carcinoma_B_95-348	60343	92	
SAGE_Prostate_carcinoma_CL_A+	30298	92	
SAGE_Prostate_carcinoma_CL_LNCaP-T	43542	82	
SAGE_Breast_carcinoma_CL_MCF7estradiol_10H	59583	77	
SAGE_Breast_carcinoma_CL_MCF7estradiol_3h	59683	77	
SAGE_Breast_carcinoma_MD_DCIS-2	28719	48	
SAGE_Prostate_adenocarcinoma_CL_LNCaP	22344	35	
SAGE_Ovary_adenocarcinoma_B_OVT-7	53514	26	
SAGE_Colon_normal_B_NC1	49610	24	
SAGE_Colon_normal_B_NC2	48479	24	
SAGE_Prostate_carcinoma_CL_LNCaP_no-DHT	62160	22	
SAGE_Prostate_normal_B_2	64058	21	
SAGE_Breast_carcinoma_MD_DCIS	40783	19	
SAGE_Prostate_carcinoma_B_pool2	66034	15	

Color Plate 3, Fig. 3. (*see* discussion and complete captions in Ch 7 on pp. 112–113). SAGE Genie Anatomic Viewer display of prostate-specific Ets factor expression (**A**) and expression in individual SAGE libraries (**B**).

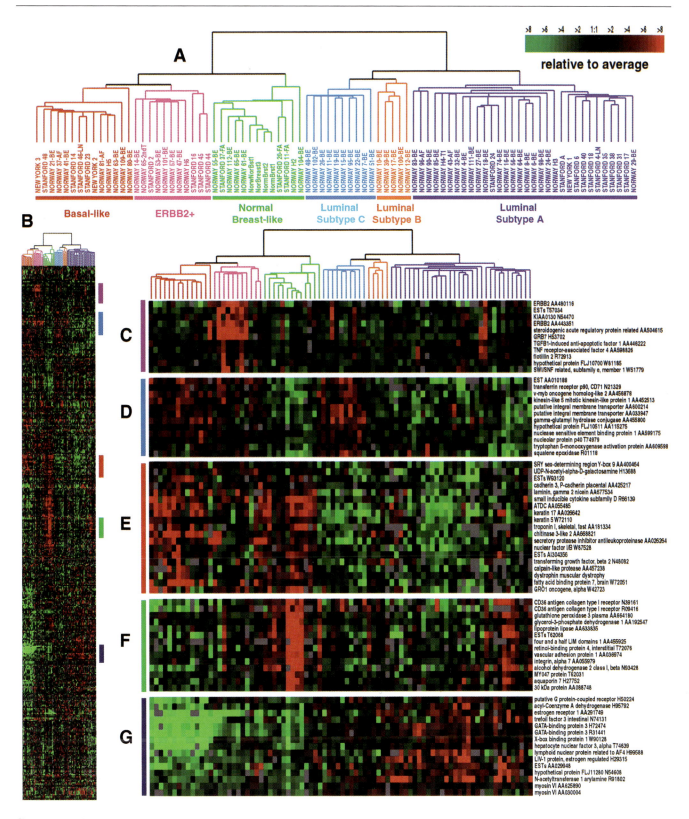

Color Plate 4, Fig. 1. (*see* discussion in Ch. 8 on pp. 117, 119 and complete caption on p. 118). Eighty-five samples analyzed with the 476 "intrinsic" clone set. With permission.

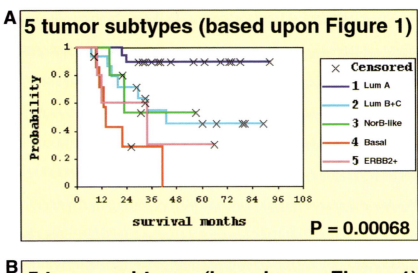

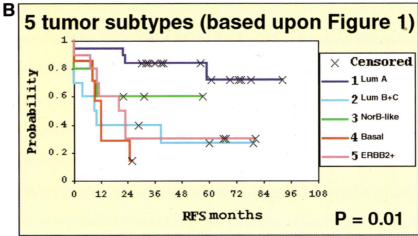

Color Plate 4, Fig. 2. (*see* full caption and discussion in Ch. 8 on p. 119). Fifty-one patients treated using gene expression-based tumor groupings.

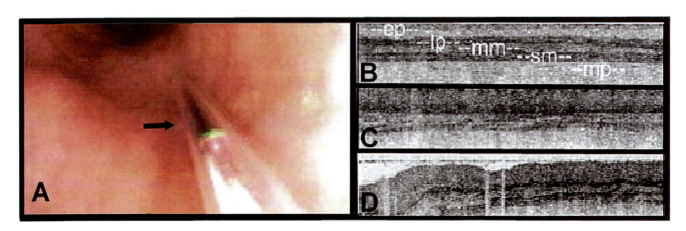

Color Plate 6, Fig. 4. (*see* discussion in Ch. 26 on p. 348 and full caption on p. 349). (**A**) OCT probe in upper endoscopy; (**B–D**) esophageal layers at 10 μm.

8. Rountree MR, Bachman KE, Herman JG, Baylin SB. DNA methylation, chromatin inheritance, and cancer. *Oncogene* 2001;20:3156–3165.

9. Lalani el-N, Laniado ME, Abel PD. Molecular and cellular biology of prostate cancer. *Cancer Metastasis Rev* 1997;16:29–66.

10. Fearon ER. Molecular genetic studies of the adenoma-carcinoma sequence. *Adv Intern Med* 1994;39:123–147.

11. Sidranski D, von Eschenbach A, Tsai YC, et al. Identification of p53 gene mutations in bladder cancers and urine samples. *Science* 1991;252:706–708.

12. Spruck CH, Ohneseit PF, Gonzalez-Zulueta M, et al. Two molecular pathways to transitional cell carcinoma of the bladder. *Cancer Res* 1994;54:784–788.

13. Stein GS, Montecino M, van Wijnen AJ, et al. Nuclear structure-gene interrelationships: implications for aberrant gene expression in cancer. *Cancer Res* 2000;60:2067–2076.

14. Konety BR, Getzenberg RH. Nuclear structural proteins as biomarkers of cancer. *J Cell Biochem* 1999;32:183–191.

15. Holth LT, Chadee DN, Spencer VA, et al. Chromatin, nuclear matrix and cytoskeleton: role of cell structure in neoplastic transformation (review). *Int J Oncol* 1998;13:827–837.

16. Getzenberg RH. Nuclear matrix and regulation of gene expression: tissue specificity. *J Cell Biochem* 1994;55:22–31.

17. Leman ES, Getzenberg RH. Nuclear matrix proteins as biomarkers in prostate cancer. *J Cell Biochem* 2002;86:213–223.

18. Reeves R, Beckerbauer L. HMGI/Y proteins: flexible regulators of transcription and chromatin structure. *Biochim Biophys Acta* 2001;1519:13–29.

19. Sutherland HGE, Mumford GK, Newton K, et al. Large-scale identification of mammalian proteins localized to nuclear sub-compartments. *Hum Mol Genet* 2001;10:1995–2011.

20. Robertson K. DNA methylation and chromatin—unraveling the tangled web. *Oncogene* 2002;21:5361–5379.

21. Jones PA, Takai D. The role of DNA methylation in mammalian epigenetics. *Science* 2001;293:1068–1070.

22. Ehrlich M. DNA methylation in cancer: too much, but also too little. *Oncogene* 2002;12:5400-5413.

23. Berger SL, Felsenfeld G. Chromatin goes global. *Mol Cell* 2001;8:263–268.

24. Davie JR, Samuel SK, Spencer VA, et al. Organization of chromatin in cancer cells: role of signaling pathways. *Biochem Cell Biol* 1999;77:265–275.

25. Klochendler-Yeivin A, Yaniv M. Chromatin modifiers and tumor suppression. *Biochim Biophys Acta* 2001;1551: 1–10.

26. Duensing S, Munger K. Centrosome abnormalities, genomic instability and carcinogenic progression. *Biochim Biophys Acta* 2001;1471:81–88.

27. Jenewein T, Allis CD. Translating the histone code. *Science* 2002;293:1074–1079.

28. Prescott JL, Montie J, Pugh TW, Veltri RW. Clinical sensitivity of p53 mutation detection in matched bladder tumor, bladder wash, and voided urine specimens. *Cancer* 2001;91: 2127–2135.

29. Solkolova IA, Halling KC, Jenkins RB, et al. The development of a multitarget, multicolor fluorescence *in situ* hybridization assay for the detection of urothelial carcinoma in the urine. *J Mol Diag* 2000;2:116–123.

30. Steiner G, Schoenberg MP, Linn JF, et al. Detection of bladder cancer recurrence by microsatellite analysis of urine. *Nat Med* 1997;3:621–624.

31. Cairns P, Sidransky D. Molecular methods for the diagnosis of cancer. *Biochim Biophys Acta* 1999;1423:C11–C18.

32. Sturgeon C. Practice guidelines for tumor marker use in the clinic. *Clin Chem* 2002;48:1151–1159.

33. Macgregor PF, Squire JA. Application of microarrays to analysis of gene expression in cancer. *Clin Chem* 2002;48:1170–1177.

34. Khan J, Bittner ML, Chen Y, et al. DNA microarray technology: the anticipated impact on the study of human disease. *Biochim Biophys Acta* 1999;1423:M17–M28.

35. Bacus JW, Grace LJ. Optical microscope system for standardized cell measurements and analyses. *Appl Opt* 1987;26: 3280–3293.

36. Gibas Z, Gibas L. Cytogenetics of bladder cancer. *Cancer Genet Cytogenet* 1997;95:108–115.

37. Slaton JW, Dinney CPN, Veltri RW, et al. DNA ploidy enhances the cytologic prediction of recurrent transitional cell carcinoma of the bladder. *J Urol* 1997;158: 806–811.

38. Veltri RW, O'Dowd GJ, Orozco R, Miller MC. The role of biopsy pathology, quantitative nuclear morphometry, and biomarkers in the preoperative prediction of prostate cancer staging and prognosis. *Semin Urol Oncol* 1998;16: 106–117.

39. Wojcik EM, Miller MC, O'Dowd GJ, Veltri RW. Value of computer-assisted quantitative nuclear grading in differentiation of normal urothelial cells from low and high grade TCC. *Anal Quant Cytol Histol* 1998;20:69–76.

40. Palcic B, MacAulay C. Malignancy associated changes: can they be employed clinically? In *Compendium on Computerized Cytology and Histology Laboratory*. Weid GL, Bartels PH, Rosenthal DL, Schenck U, eds. Tutorials of Cytology, Chicago; 1994: pp. 157–165.

41. Diamond DA, Berry SJ, Umbricht C, et al. Computerized image analysis of nuclear shape as a prognostic factor for prostatic cancer. *Prostate* 1982;3:321–332.

42. Partin AW, Walsh AC, Pitcock RV, et al: A comparison of nuclear morphometry and Gleason grade as a predictor of prognosis in stage A2 prostate cancer: a critical analysis. *J Urol* 1989;142:1254–1258.

43. Veltri RW, Miller MC, Slaton JW, et al. Computer-assisted quantitative nuclear grading (QNG) can predict bladder cancer recurrence using bladder cancer cytology samples. *J Urol* 1997;157:342.

44. Badalament RA, Miller MC, Peller PA, et al. An algorithm for predicting non-organ confined prostate cancer using the results obtained from sextant core biopsies with PSA level. *J Urol* 1996;156:1375–1380.

45. Veltri RW, Miller MC, Mangold LA et al. Prediction of pathological stage in patients with clinical stage T1c prostate cancer: the new challenge. *J Urol* 2002;68:100–104.

46. Veltri RW, Miller MC, Partin AW, et al. Ability to predict biochemical progression using Gleason score and computer-generated quantitative nuclear grade derived from cancer cell nuclei. *Urology* 1996;48:685–691.

47. Potter SR, Miller MC, Mangold LA, et al. Genetically engineered neural networks for predicting prostate cancer progression after radical prostatectomy. *Urology* 1999;54: 791–795.

48. Reckwitz T, Potter SR, Snow PB, et al. Artificial neural networks in urology: Update 2000. *Prostate Cancer Prostatic Dis* 1999;2:222–226.

49. Veltri RW, Chaudhari M, Miller MC, et al. Comparison of logistic regression and neural net modeling for prediction of prostate cancer pathologic stage. *Clin Chem* 2002;48:1828–1834.

50. Veltri, RW, Miller MC, Partin, AW, et al. Prediction of prostate cancer stage using quantitative biopsy pathology. *Cancer* 2001;91:2322–2328.

51. Veltri RW, Miller MC, An G. Standardization, analytical validation, and quality control of intermediate endpoint biomarkers. *Urology* 2001;57:164–170.

52. Haese A, Chaudhari M, Miller MC, et al. Quantitative biopsy pathology for the prediction of pathologically organ confined prostate cancer: a multiinstitutional validation study. *Cancer* 2003;97:969–978.

7

Enabling Discovery Through Online Cancer Genome Databases and Analytic Tools

Robert L. Strausberg, PhD and Gregory J. Riggins, MD, PhD

CONTENTS

INTRODUCTION
THE NCI CANCER GENOME ANATOMY PROJECT
FUTURE DIRECTIONS IN CANCER GENOMICS
REFERENCES

1. INTRODUCTION

Over the past two decades, our understanding of the complex molecular underpinnings of cancer has increased dramatically. While we know that the genetic events associated with cancer are quite diverse, with much genetic heterogeneity within and among tumors, careful analysis of the complex data has revealed a limited number of common categories of acquired capabilities of cancers *(1)*. As described by Hanahan and Weinberg, these capabilities include insensitivity to antigrowth signals, independence from growth signals, ability to evade apoptosis, unlimited replicative potential, sustained angiogenesis, and the abililty to invade tissue and metastasize. Although the acquisition sequence of each of these capabilities can vary, as can the specific molecular changes that lead to the acquired capability, the notion that there are a limited number of such events, and that they are common to diverse tumors, provides a firm foundation for additional discovery, improved cancer detection, and new intervention strategies.

The first human genome sequence is being finished *(2,3)*, organized cancer genomics efforts are in their early stages, and there is already evidence that careful analysis of genomic changes can provide effective molecular targets for intervention. For example, the discovery that the *erb*B2 gene product is overexpressed in about 25–30% of all breast cancers (usually resulting from amplification of the gene) led to development of a monoclonal antibody-based therapeutic (Herceptin®)

that extends survival time in patients with tumors in which this gene is overexpressed, often resulting from direct amplification of the *erb*B2 gene *(4)*.

The opportunity and challenge of new genome-based molecularly targeted approaches to cancer intervention are also richly illustrated by the events and developmental time frame leading to approval of the tyrosine kinase inhibitor Gleevec™ for treating chronic myelogenous leukemia (CML) *(5–7)*. The discovery process, as summarized by the National Cancer Institute (NCI) (http://newscenter.cancer.gov/ pressreleases/ gleevactimeline .html), started in 1960 with the first description of the abnormal Philadelphia chromosome, present in most CML patients. In 1973, the Philadelphia chromosome was described as a translocation of segments of chromosomes 9 and 22. Almost a decade later (and two decades after the original observation), the *abl* oncogene was identified at the juncture of the 9:22 translocation. In the mid-1980s, a series of biological and biochemical studies validated the protein product as a candidate target for intervention. The first laboratory studies of the candidate, STI571, began in 1993 following a period of candidate drug development, and the first human tests commenced in 1999. Following a remarkably fast clinical trial process, STI571 received FDA approval in 2001 and was subsequently marketed as Gleevec.

The Gleevec development story is remarkable for many reasons. First, it beautifully demonstrates the power of genomics to identify key events in cancer development and progression. Second, validation of the

From: *Cancer Chemoprevention, Volume 2: Strategies for Cancer Chemoprevention*
Edited by: G. J. Kelloff, E. T. Hawk, and C. C. Sigman © Humana Press Inc., Totowa, NJ

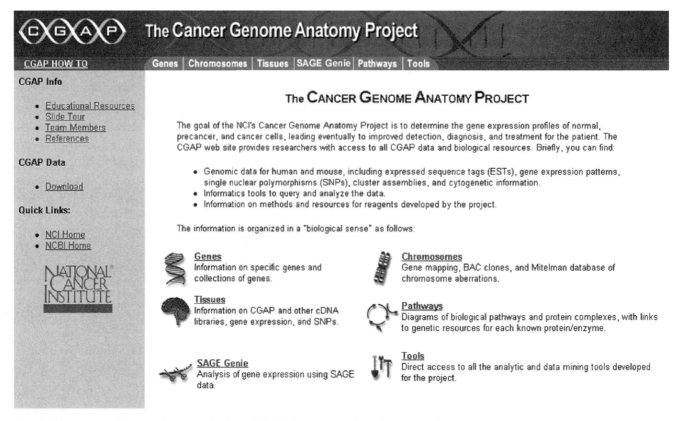

Fig. 1. The Cancer Genome Anatomy Project (CGAP) home page (http://cgap.nci.nih.gov). The home page provides access to all CGAP data as well as analysis tools. Various entry points are provided based on particular scientific interests such as genes, tissues, chromosomes, and pathways. The site also provides information for accessing CGAP reagents and educational tools. A list of CGAP team members is accessible, as are CGAP publications.

abl-proto-oncogene gene product required an elegant series of studies to provide sufficient evidence that this was a target worthy of an expensive drug development program. Third, results suggest that careful attention to discovery and validation of this target then facilitated a remarkably successful drug development process. Unfortunately, the first discovery of the Philadelphia chromosome preceded approval of Gleevec by about 40 yr. The rapidly emerging field of cancer genomics is expected to greatly expedite identification and precise molecular definition of new targets, setting the stage for many new success stories in the development of molecularly targeted cancer therapeutics.

2. THE NCI CANCER GENOME ANATOMY PROJECT

Illustrative of cancer genomics efforts is the NCI's Cancer Genome Anatomy Project (CGAP) *(8)*, established to interface genomics and cancer research through platform information and technological infrastructures. Three component projects, the Tumor Gene Index (TGI)

(9,10), the Cancer Chromosome Aberration Project (cCAP) *(8,11)*, and the Genetic Annotation Initiative (GAI) *(12)*, are linked within CGAP to provide an integrated view of molecular events associated with cancer development and progression. This discussion focuses on certain illustrative aspects of TGI and cCAP. Detailed descriptions of CGAP are available elsewhere *(9,11–13)*. All CGAP data and analysis tools are accessible through the CGAP web site (Fig. 1).

2.1. The CGAP Tumor Gene Index

TGI focuses on identifying and characterizing transcriptional changes as cells progress from normal to cancer. Initially, TGI used a technological approach based on expressed sequence tags (ESTs). In this approach, cDNA libraries are generated from normal tissues and tumors, and several thousand cDNAs from each library are tagged through single-pass sequencing of each cDNA, usually starting from the 3′ end. While the entire cDNA sequence is generally not obtained through this approach, the sequence tag (generally several hundred nucleotides in length) is often sufficient to identify known genes expressed in these tissues and tumors, and also to identify genes not previously known. CGAP has produced more than 1 million ESTs, all of which are deposited in GenBank. The additional value of the EST approach is that a physical cDNA clone is also generated, and these clones are made accessible to the community through a distribution network (http://image.llnl.gov/).

2.2. CGAP Serial Analysis of Gene Expression

More recently, TGI has focused on a different technological approach called serial analysis of gene expression (SAGE) (14,15) for generating sequence-based transcript tags. This approach was chosen for several reasons. Like EST technology, this sequence-based transcript tagging method facilitates development of a public database that can be integrated with other sequence-based data, including human and mouse genome sequences, as well as EST data. Also, SAGE is more cost-effective, as about 30–40 gene tags are obtained from each sequencing reaction, compared with one tag from EST. While SAGE tags are quite short (usually about 10 nucleotides), they are generated at a precise restriction site, thereby enhancing our ability to relate a tag to a specific gene. Moreover, as the human genome sequence becomes complete and public databases become rich in accurate full-length cDNA sequences (16), the value of SAGE data increases as even more precise alignments of tags to genes becomes possible.

The CGAP SAGE Project is an interesting interface of large-scale science and a network of individual laboratories. Many SAGE libraries are produced directly for CGAP. However, in other cases, libraries have been produced in individual laboratories, and CGAP provides high-quality DNA sequencing, submission to the public databases, and development of analysis tools. Through this approach, CGAP has been able to build a biologically rich SAGE database of libraries produced within the context of carefully controlled experiments reflecting the expertise of individual investigators, and designed to evaluate the effects of genetic and environmental changes on the cancer phenotype. A key attraction for participation in this project is the resulting ability to evaluate datasets within the context of not just one experiment, but also the wealth of data produced by the network.

CGAP collaborated with the National Center for Biotechnology Information to build a database called SAGEmap (17,18). As with other CGAP components, informatics tools directly associated with SAGEmap enable in silico experimentation with the SAGE data.

More recently, a new SAGE web tool, SAGE Genie (19), has been developed through a collaboration of the Ludwig Institute for Cancer Research, Duke University, and the NCI. SAGE Genie provides automatic links between gene names and SAGE transcript levels, and accounts for tags resulting from alternative transcript processing and the many potential errors associated with these short tags. Based on this novel tag-to-gene mapping, the Web site visualizes human gene expression analysis in tissues or individual libraries using highly intuitive displays. The SAGE Genie Anatomic Viewer provides a graphic view of transcript expression in the human body, permitting rapid comparisons of expression in normal tissues and tumors. The initial search also provides access to the Digital Northern Tool that provides the transcript copy number for a given gene in each tissue or cell type represented by a SAGE library.

Examples of erbB2 expression analysis are illustrative of how the SAGE Genie tool provides a simple and intuitive view of gene expression data. The erbB2 gene is important to the Herceptin example described previously, as well as known to be overexpressed in prostate tumors. Examining erbB2 gene expression cataloged in the CGAP SAGE libraries and viewed with the SAGE Genie anatomic viewer shows overexpression in breast cancer compared with a normal breast, consistent with previous observations (Fig. 2).

The erbB2 example provides validation for SAGE data based on previous observations. However, most important is employing CGAP SAGE data to discover previously unknown gene expression patterns that might be useful for cancer detection or intervention. Many examples already in the literature demonstrate the utility of CGAP SAGE data to identify potential markers and targets for various types of cancer, such as brain (20), ovarian (21), and breast cancers (22). Moreover, through carefully designed library production and mining of the datasets, CGAP SAGE data have already been useful for studying gene expression changes related to the tumor environment (23,24), including response to hypoxia as well as specific expression in tumor endothelial cells.

Mitas et al. (25) recently described using the CGAP SAGE database to examine global expression of a gene for prostate-specific Ets factor, a transcription factor previously known to be overexpressed in prostate cancer. Through examination of the CGAP SAGE data, it was noted that in addition to being overexpressed in most prostate cancer libraries, this gene is also overexpressed in many CGAP breast cancer

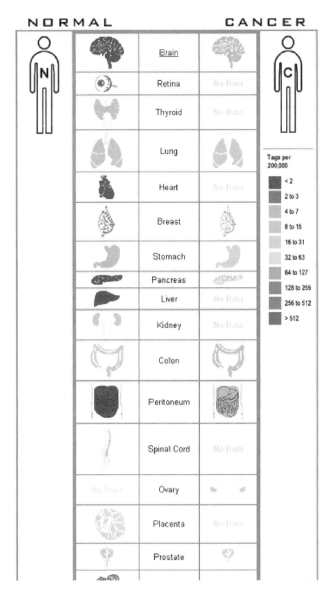

Fig. 2. SAGE Genie Anatomic Viewer display of *erb*B2 gene expression in normal tissues and tumors. Expression of each gene is color-coded based on the number of SAGE tags for that gene per 200,000 total tags. As shown in this figure, the *erb*B2 gene is overexpressed in breast cancer compared with the normal breast.

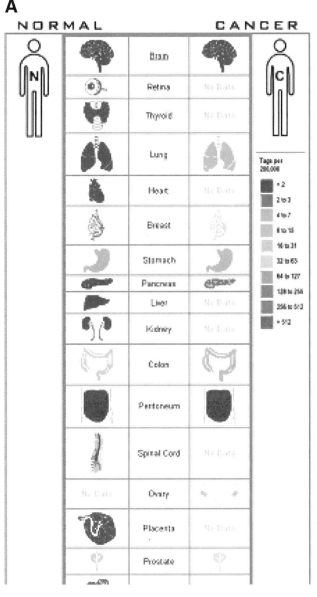

Fig. 3A. SAGE Genie Anatomic Viewer display of prostate-specific Ets factor expression. Note that this "prostate-specific" gene is overexpressed in both prostate and breast tumors.

libraries. While the SAGE Genie tool was not available at the time of this study, the SAGE Genie Anatomic Viewer clearly depicts this result (Fig. 3A), and the associated Virtual Northern tool (Fig. 3B) also shows the high level of expression of this gene in breast and prostate cancer samples. As with all data mining studies of this type, validation studies are required to confirm (and extend) the result. In this case, real-time PCR was performed on lymph nodes containing metastatic breast cancer, confirming that the gene is overexpressed in some breast cancers and

providing evidence that this gene may be a useful marker for detecting metastatic breast cancer.

2.3. The CGAP Cancer Chromosome Aberration Project

The overall goal of cCAP (led by Drs. Ilan Kirsch and Thomas Ried of the NCI) *(11)* is to integrate the cytogenetic and physical (sequence) maps of the human and mouse genomes to facilitate the study of chromosomal aberrations of cancer. A collection of about 1300 BAC clones has been mapped by high-resolution fluorescence

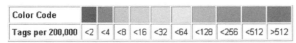

Library	Total Tags in Library	Tags per 200,000	Color Code
SAGE_Breast_metastatic_carcinoma_B_95-260	45087	133	
SAGE_Breast_carcinoma_B_95-259	39364	127	
SAGE_Breast_carcinoma_CL_MCF7control_0h	59877	126	
SAGE_Breast_carcinoma_B_95-347	67070	122	
SAGE_Prostate_carcinoma_B_LN-1	22599	115	
SAGE_Prostate_adenocarcinoma_MD_PR317	64951	95	
SAGE_Breast_carcinoma_B_95-348	60343	92	
SAGE_Prostate_carcinoma_CL_A+	30298	92	
SAGE_Prostate_carcinoma_CL_LNCaP-T	43542	82	
SAGE_Breast_carcinoma_CL_MCF7estradiol_10H	59583	77	
SAGE_Breast_carcinoma_CL_MCF7estradiol_3h	59683	77	
SAGE_Breast_carcinoma_MD_DCIS-2	28719	48	
SAGE_Prostate_adenocarcinoma_CL_LNCaP	22344	35	
SAGE_Ovary_adenocarcinoma_B_OVT-7	53514	26	
SAGE_Colon_normal_B_NC1	49610	24	
SAGE_Colon_normal_B_NC2	48479	24	
SAGE_Prostate_carcinoma_CL_LNCaP_no-DHT	62160	22	
SAGE_Prostate_normal_B_2	64058	21	
SAGE_Breast_carcinoma_MD_DCIS	40783	19	
SAGE_Prostate_carcinoma_B_pool2	66034	15	

Fig. 3B. Expression of the prostate-specific Ets factor in individual SAGE libraries. Shown is a partial display of the SAGE libraries, starting from those with the highest level of expression of this gene as a fraction of the total SAGE tags for that library. The color code is identical to that used for the SAGE Genie Anatomic Viewer.

in situ hybridization (FISH) to prometaphase human cells, at a spacing of 1–2 Mb across the human genome, and linked to cytogenetic landmarks previously defined through G-banding. The mapped set of clones is mostly derived from those clones used to sequence the human genome, thereby allowing for direct correlations of chromosomal bands and the genome sequence.

In addition, cCAP has collaborated with Professor Felix Mitelman of Sweden's Lund University to produce an online version of the cCAP database. This dataset is now freely available to researchers through the CGAP Web site.

cCAP resources provide a rapid means to move from observations of chromosomal aberration to molecular definition of the genomic region. In the Gleevec example described above, a period of about 10 yr was required to define the gene affected by the chromosomal 9:22 translocation. With the close linkage of cytogenetic and

sequence maps of the human genome now afforded through cCAP and other projects *(11,26)*, that process of molecular definition should now be quite rapid. This situation will be even further enhanced as the human genome sequence is completed and a minimum tiling path of BAC clones spanning the entire human genome becomes accessible.

3. FUTURE DIRECTIONS IN CANCER GENOMICS

As illustrated by the Herceptin and Gleevec examples, cancer results from dynamic changes of the human genome that are reflected in expression of transcripts and proteins. While the primary genomic changes in these examples are gene amplification and chromosomal translocation events, it is clear that molecular changes related to the development of cancer have many forms, from point mutations to deletions and amplifications, to chromosomal translocations. Moreover, targets for intervention are often likely to be several steps removed from the primary genetic event. For both Herceptin and Gleevec, proteins are the targets for intervention strategies. However, the most ready means for initial detection in both cases was based on chromosomal changes. In the future, there likely will not be one "best" method for identifying changes that inform detection and intervention in cancer, but rather a multitude of strategies.

Therefore, the interface of genomics and cancer will require functionally integrated databases spanning different molecular areas from genomics (such as point mutations, chromosomal translocations, etc.), to transcriptome analysis and proteomics. While meaningful integration of databases has been and will continue to be challenging, completion of the human genome sequence provides a unique platform to form these functional links. Full integration of datasets based on different technological approaches will mean that cancer researchers will be liberated to think outside the box as they become part of a cancer genomics center without walls. This virtual center (database) will incorporate public data from worldwide efforts and will mean that creative researchers could go beyond their own cancer focus (e.g., prostate or breast cancer) to the more common features of cancer that might lead to development of agents that would serve the needs of a larger population of cancer patients. For example, Gleevec, originally developed for treatment of CML, has potential application to other cancers, such as gastrointestinal stromal tumors *(27)*. Perhaps integrated databases will suggest new examples of interventions that might cross the boundaries of traditional anatomical classification of cancers.

Importantly, integrated databases offer the potential not just to meet the needs of a segment of the cancer research community, but to integrate basic and clinical cancer research as never before possible. For example, NCI has initiated work on a Cancer Molecular Analysis Project *(28)* designed to integrate datasets based on molecular profiles such as gene-based expression patterns; molecular targets, or genes organized by pathway and functional category to permit an overview of different types of changes (such as mutations and gene over- or underexpression); agents molecularly targeted to specific molecular anomalies, pathways, and ontologies; and information on clinical trials of molecularly targeted agents. While this is at an early stage, and represents just one approach to such integration, the vision is one of a functionally integrated database that facilitates information flow not only from basic to clinical research, but also from clinical research to basic. That is, such a database will likely change the current paradigm of one-way flow in which basic research is "translated" to the clinical arena. This will provide a wonderful opportunity for cancer genomics to be a bridge to functionally link and improve communication among all aspects of cancer research, thereby expediting progress in discovery, prevention, detection, and intervention.

REFERENCES

1. Hanahan D, Weinberg RA. The hallmarks of cancer. *Cell* 2000;100:57–70.
2. Lander ES, Linton LM, Birren B, et al. Initial sequencing and analysis of the human genome. *Nature* 2001;409: 860–921.
3. Venter JC, Adams MD, Myers EW, et al. The sequence of the human genome. *Science* 2001;291:1304–1351.
4. Pegram MD, Konecny G, Slamon DJ. The molecular and cellular biology of HER2/neu gene amplification/overexpression and the clinical development of herceptin (trastuzumab) therapy for breast cancer. *Cancer Treat Res* 2000; 103:57–75.
5. Druker BJ. Perspectives on the development of a molecularly targeted agent. *Cancer Cell* 2002;1:31–36.
6. Druker BJ. STI571 (Gleevec) as a paradigm for cancer therapy. *Trends Mol Med* 2002;8:S14–S18.
7. O'Dwyer ME, Druker BJ. STI571: an inhibitor of the BCR-ABL tyrosine kinase for the treatment of chronic myelogenous leukaemia. *Lancet Oncol* 2000;1:207–211.
8. Strausberg RL, Greenhut SF, Grouse LH, et al. In silico analysis of cancer through the Cancer Genome Anatomy Project. *Trends Cell Biol* 2001;11:S66–S71.
9. Riggins GJ, Strausberg RL. Genome and genetic resources from the Cancer Genome Anatomy Project. *Hum Mol Genet* 2001;10:663–667.
10. Strausberg RL, Buetow KH, Emmert-Buck MR, Klausner RD. The cancer genome anatomy project: building an annotated gene index. *Trends Genet* 2000;16:103–106.
11. Kirsch IR, Green ED, Yonescu R, et al. A systematic, high-resolution linkage of the cytogenetic and physical maps of the human genome. *Nat Genet* 2000;24:339–340.
12. Buetow KH, Edmonson M, MacDonald R, et al. High-throughput development and characterization of a genomewide collection of gene-based single nucleotide polymorphism markers by chip-based matrix-assisted laser desorption/ionization time-of-flight mass spectrometry. *Proc Natl Acad Sci USA* 2001;98:581–584.
13. Strausberg RL, Camargo AA, Riggins GJ, et al. An international database and integrated analysis tools for the study of cancer gene expression. *Pharmacogenomics J* 2002;2:156–164.
14. Velculescu VE, Madden SL, Zhang L, et al. Analysis of human transcriptomes. *Nat Genet* 1999;23:387–388.
15. Velculescu VE, Zhang L, Vogelstein B, Kinzler KW. Serial analysis of gene expression. *Science* 1995;270:484–487.
16. Strausberg RL, Feingold EA, Klausner RD, Collins FS. The mammalian gene collection. *Science* 1999;286:455–457.
17. Lash AE, Tolstoshev CM, Wagner L, et al. SAGEmap: a public gene expression resource. *Genome Res* 2000;10:1051–1060.
18. Lal A, Lash AE, Altschul SF, et al. A public database for gene expression in human cancers. *Cancer Res* 1999;59:5403–5407.
19. Boon K, Osorio EC, Greenhut SF, et al. An anatomy of normal and malignant gene expression. *Proc Natl Acad Sci USA* 2002;99:11,287–11,292.
20. Loging WT, Lal A, Siu IM, et al. Identifying potential tumor markers and antigens by database mining and rapid expression screening. *Genome Res* 2000;10:1393–1402.
21. Hough CD, Sherman-Baust CA, Pizer ES, et al. Large-scale serial analysis of gene expression reveals genes differentially expressed in ovarian cancer. *Cancer Res* 2000;60:6281–6287.
22. Porter DA, Krop IE, Nasser S, et al. A SAGE (serial analysis of gene expression) view of breast tumor progression. *Cancer Res* 2001;61:5697–5702.
23. Lal A, Peters H, St Croix B, et al. Transcriptional response to hypoxia in human tumors. *J Natl Cancer Inst* 2001;93: 1337–1343.
24. St Croix B, Rago C, Velculescu V, et al. Genes expressed in human tumor endothelium. *Science* 2000;289:1197–1202.
25. Mitas M, Mikhitarian K, Hoover L, et al. Prostate-Specific Ets (PSE) factor: a novel marker for detection of metastatic breast cancer in axillary lymph nodes. *Br J Cancer* 2002; 86:899–904.
26. Cheung VG, Nowak N, Jang W, et al. Integration of cytogenetic landmarks into the draft sequence of the human genome. *Nature* 2001;409:953–958.
27. Joensuu H, Roberts PJ, Sarlomo-Rikala M, et al. Effect of the tyrosine kinase inhibitor STI571 in a patient with a metastatic gastrointestinal stromal tumor. *N Engl J Med* 2001;344: 1052–1056.
28. Buetow KH, Klausner RD, Fine H, et al. Cancer Molecular Analysis Project: weaving a rich cancer research tapestry. *Cancer Cell* 2002;1:315–318.

8 Functional Genomics for Identifying Surrogate Endpoint Biomarkers in Breast Cancer Chemoprevention

Melissa A. Troester, PhD, and Charles M. Perou, PhD

CONTENTS

INTRODUCTION
BREAST CANCER PREVENTION
GENOMIC PROFILING OF INVASIVE BREAST TUMORS AS A MODEL FOR STUDYING
     EARLY BREAST LESIONS
EXPERIMENTAL DESIGN FOR GENOMIC ANALYSIS IN PHASE II PREVENTION TRIALS
REFERENCES

1. INTRODUCTION

Human tumors have great diversity in morphology and natural history; this is reflected in variations in clinical outcome. Assessment of morphology and a few immunohistochemical markers in tumors have guided treatment of most cancers. By studying gene expression patterns for a large number of genes, morphologically similar tumors can be further subdivided into distinct categories of clinical relevance. Recent studies have applied DNA microarrays to the study of many types of cancer, including breast *(1–6)*, brain *(7,8)*, ovary *(9–11)*, lung *(12–14)*, colon *(15–17)*, kidney *(18)*, prostate *(19–22)*, gastric *(23)*, leukemia *(24–26)*, and lymphoma *(27–29)*. Most of these studies identified clinically relevant tumor subtypes that were believed to represent more homogenous clinical entities. Thus, using cDNA microarrays to characterize variation in tumors could add value to the standard battery of clinical tests.

Invasive breast carcinomas are a particularly heterogeneous category of human tumors where advances in classification, risk assessment, and outcome predictions are needed. Recent studies using DNA microarrays identified new and clinically important subtypes of breast cancer that correspond to differences in clinical outcome *(1–3)*. The genomic "profiling" approach has led to a rapid increase in the number of candidate risk and response biomarkers for invasive human breast tumors; therefore, it is likely that gene expression profiles of early breast lesions will also be valuable. Studying gene expression profiles of early lesions of the breast, such as atypical ductal hyperplasia, lobular carcinoma *in situ*, and ductal carcinoma *in situ*, can identify new biomarkers of risk and response for chemoprevention studies and treatment. In this chapter, we present a model for using genomic profiling to identify targets for chemoprevention in Phase II trials. The basic methodology described here for breast lesions could also be applied to other tissues to identify tissue-specific risk and response biomarkers.

2. BREAST CANCER PREVENTION

A mathematical model developed by Gail and Greene has been used as the standard for predicting risk of breast cancer development on the basis of age, race, age at menarche, parity, family history, and history of breast biopsy *(30)*. This model was employed to determine eligibility for a chemoprevention clinical trial of tamoxifen conducted by the National Surgical Adjuvant Breast Project (NSABP). The NSABP trial P-1 demonstrated that tamoxifen treatment resulted in a statistically significant 50% reduction in breast cancers and a 67%

From: Cancer Chemoprevention, Volume 2: Strategies for Cancer Chemoprevention
Edited by: G. J. Kelloff, E. T. Hawk, and C. C. Sigman © Humana Press Inc., Totowa, NJ

reduction in estrogen receptor (ER)-positive cancers compared to placebo *(31)*. The improved selection of high-risk subjects based on the Gail model is a widely cited explanation for the NSABP study's increased statistical power relative to the Royal Marsden Prevention Trial and the Italian Prevention Trial, neither of which showed statistically significant reductions in breast cancer due to tamoxifen treatment *(32,33)*. While empirically the Gail model allows improved selection of clinical trial participants over other risk assessment models, incorporation of biologically based criteria in clinical trials is desirable. Furthermore, the Gail model has been useful in clinical decision making, but it does not elucidate biological and molecular events that lead to cancer and is not useful in evaluating biological response to chemopreventive interventions *(34)*. Thus, a priority in breast cancer chemoprevention research has been to identify new risk and response biomarkers, termed surrogate endpoint biomarkers (SEBs), for chemoprevention trials *(35,36)*.

SEBs suggested for use in breast chemoprevention studies include mammographic breast density, serum insulin-like growth factor (IGF)-I and its binding protein, IGF-binding protein-3, and serum levels of estradiol and testosterone in postmenopausal women *(37)*. These criteria have offered improvements in the design of clinical studies and in our understanding of the progress of breast cancer. However, while circulating levels of growth factors or hormones have the advantage of being measurable using minimally invasive methods, these markers are only proxies for tissue levels and their causal relationships with tumors or early lesions are not clear. Morphological markers also have demonstrated utility as SEBs; however, morphology can be subjective and is difficult to quantitate at best *(38,39)*. An important study by Fabian et al. *(37)* showed that the short-term risk of developing breast cancer could be predicted in a multivariate analysis that included Gail risk estimates and assessments of atypical hyperplasia, measured using fine-needle aspiration (FNA). Based on their findings, Fabian et al. argued that cytomorphology from FNA should be used to improve the design of cancer chemoprevention studies and used as a SEB to monitor efficacy of potential chemopreventive agents.

The morphologic changes observed in FNA are still likely to represent a wide range of underlying gene expression changes. The study by Fabian et al. examined changes in the expression levels of several specific genes. Expression of epidermal growth factor receptor

(EGFR), ER, p53, and HER2/ERBB2 were significantly associated with atypical hyperplasia, but could not be used to predict development of breast cancer in multivariate analysis *(37)*. These findings were consistent with those of other investigators, indicating that many of the molecular markers previously thought to be expressed only in breast tumors were also sometimes expressed in benign breast tissue. Only when expression of multiple markers in the three-marker set (EGFR, ER, and p53) was considered could statistically sound predictions be made as to which patient was likely to develop cancer. The development of modern genomic analysis tools such as cDNA microarrays allows us the opportunity to simultaneously determine the expression level of thousands of genes at once. These gene expression patterns, commonly known as profiles, can be used to learn more about biological properties of normal and hyperplastic breast tissue, and might also provide a new set of markers that could be used to predict breast cancer risk. For this technology to be successfully used in the prevention setting, small amounts of tissues/cells obtained from FNA must be used to measure gene expression. The feasibility of this approach has been demonstrated in primary breast cancers where cDNA microarrays were performed with tumor material obtained from FNAs *(40)*. The small amounts of starting RNA can also be linearly amplified using a modification of the Eberwine amplification protocol *(41)*. DNA microarrays performed on FNA samples can thus provide insights about the course of breast cancer using a design similar to that used to study invasive breast lesions.

3. GENOMIC PROFILING OF INVASIVE BREAST TUMORS AS A MODEL FOR STUDYING EARLY BREAST LESIONS

Difficulties in predicting which cancers will become invasive and metastatic versus those that will remain localized and indolent is a continuing challenge in the clinical setting. Several molecular biomarkers of breast cancer risk and prognosis are currently in clinical use, most notably ER and progesterone receptor status, HER2/ERBB2 status, and alterations of p53 *(42)*. These classifications are more quantitative and less susceptible to interpretive variance than morphological examinations; however, they provide only limited information about the biology of the tumor and have limited predictive ability, as cited above. Cancer cells are heterogeneous in their gene expression patterns, and a wide range of genes is involved in the control of cell growth, differentiation, and death. Hence, genome-wide expression of tumor patterns may be much more informative than any individual prognostic marker.

For most microarray-based classification studies, once the tumor sample has been assayed on DNA microarrays containing thousands of genes, the complex analysis process can be broken into two steps: gene selection and pattern identification. Perou et al. studied genome-wide expression patterns in 40 breast tumors using cDNA microarrays, with 20 of the tumors being sampled before and after monotherapy *(1)*; for those tumors with two samples, an open surgical biopsy was conducted before treatment, patients were treated with doxorubicin for an average of 16 wk (range 12–23 wk), and finally, the remaining tumor was resected and a second sample taken for analysis (after sample). As step one in the analysis process, a statistical analysis of the before-and-after tumor pairs was performed. This unique analysis searched for a set of genes whose expression pattern was similar within paired samples taken from the same tumor but whose expression varied greatly across different tumors. This list of "intrinsic" genes represented the gene expression signatures inherent to the tumors themselves, rather than those patterns due to differences between samplings.

Next, to search for patterns and other relationships across tumors, hierarchical clustering analysis was conducted using the set of intrinsic genes *(43)*. Hierarchical clustering analysis, as applied to the study of gene expression patterns, has been a valuable method for the identification of coordinately expressed sets of genes within model systems such as yeast *(44–46)* and within human cell lines and tissues *(47–51)*. Briefly, the hierarchical clustering algorithm creates a table where genes on the microarray are grouped together based on similarities in their patterns of expression *(43)*. The same algorithm is used to group experimental samples (i.e., tissue samples) based on their overall similarities. The data are then presented graphically as a colored image with genes along the vertical axis ordered by the clustering algorithm so that those with the most similar expression patterns are placed adjacent to each other. Along the horizontal axis, experimental samples are similarly arranged such that those samples with the most similar overall expression patterns are placed adjacent to each other. The color of each square in this tabular diagram represents the median expression ratio of each gene as determined across the selected set of experimental

samples *(1,48,52)*. Color saturation of each square in the cluster diagram is also directly proportional to the magnitude of the ratio, with the brightest red squares having the highest R/G median ratios (eightfold or greater above the median ratio for that gene), the brightest green squares having the lowest R/G ratio (eightfold or less than the median), black squares indicating the median R/G ratio, and gray squares indicating insufficient data. Finally, next to the genes and above the experimental samples is a cluster diagram-associated dendrogram, whose branching pattern and length of branches is a direct relay of relatedness between the genes or experimental samples.

The study by Perou et al. grouped the majority of ER-positive tumors together into one dendrogram branch shown by immunohistochemical analysis to express luminal epithelial cytokeratins 8/18 *(1)*. In contrast, most ER-negative tumors were grouped into another dendrogram branch that showed at least two distinct subtypes. One ER-negative subtype expressed the basal epithelial cytokeratins 5 and 17, and a second subtype of ER-negative tumor expressed high levels of HER2/ERBB2, an acknowledged marker of clinical outcome. A major finding of this study was the identification of breast basal-like tumors as a new and potentially clinically important subtype of breast cancer. This study also demonstrated the robustness of the analysis tool: molecular portraits of human tumors provided by gene expression data represent the tumor itself and not merely sampling variation.

A more recent study demonstrated that classification of invasive breast tumors based on gene expression patterns can be used as a prognostic marker with respect to overall and relapse-free survival in a set of patients that received uniform therapy *(2)*. Figure 1 illustrates the results of a hierarchical clustering analysis conducted for this study *(2)* that followed up on the findings of Perou et al. *(1)* by expanding the total number of tumors analyzed to 78 breast carcinomas. Using the intrinsic gene set on this expanded group of tumor samples, tumors were once again classified into two main branches based on their gene expression patterns. Again, the two branches corresponded to a group of tumors with low or no ER expression and a group of tumors with moderate to high expression of ER and estrogen-regulated genes. Among the ER-negative tumors, three subgroups were identified: a basal-like subtype (Fig. 1A, red) was characterized by high expression of keratins 5 and 17, an HER2/ERBB2-positive subtype was present and characterized by high expression of genes in

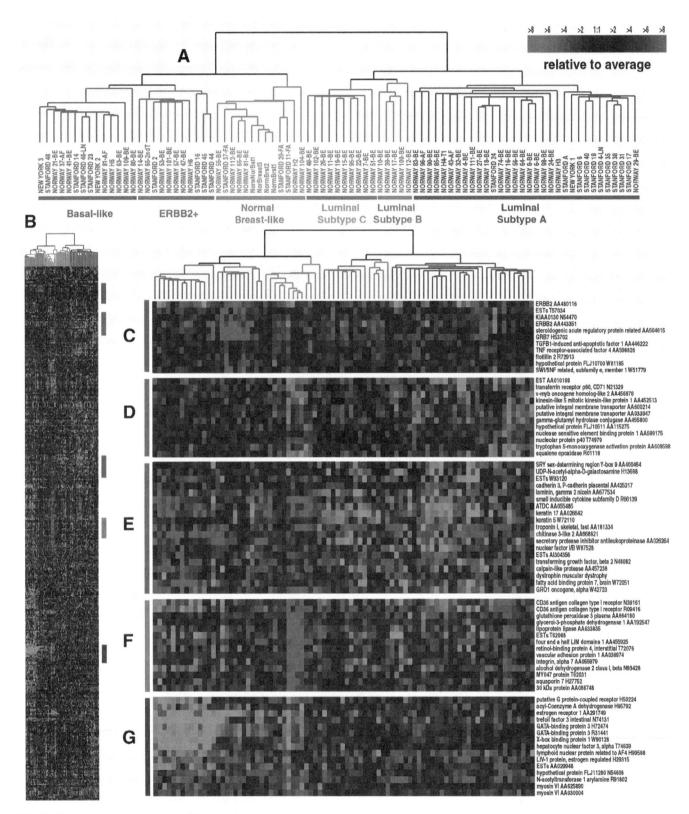

Fig. 1. Gene expression patterns of 85 samples analyzed by hierarchical clustering using the 476 "intrinsic" clone set. (**A**) The tumor specimens were divided into five (or six) subtypes based on differences in gene expression. The cluster dendrogram showing the five (six) subtypes of tumors are colored accordingly: luminal subtype A = dark blue; luminal subtype B = yellow; luminal subtype C = light blue; normal breast-like green; basal-like = red; and HER2/ERBB2+ = pink. (**B**) The full cluster diagram scaled down. The colored bars on the right represent the inserts presented in C–G. (**C**) HER2/ERBB2 amplicon gene set. (**D**) Novel gene set of unknown function. (**E**) Basal epithelial cell gene set. (**F**) Normal breast cluster. (**G**) Luminal epithelial gene cluster containing the estrogen receptor and GATA-binding protein 3 (previously published in [2] and at www.pnas.org).

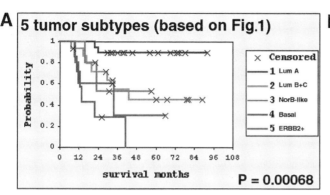 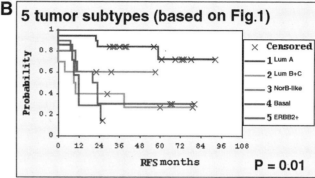

Fig. 2. Kaplan-Meier survival analysis of 51 Norwegian cohort patients, who were uniformly treated in a prospective study, using gene expression-based tumor groupings. **(A)** Overall patient survival and **(B)** relapse-free survival for the five gene expression-defined tumor subtypes based on the classification presented in Fig. 1 (Luminal B and C were considered one group for this analysis) (previously published in [2] and at www.pnas.org).

the HER2 amplicon at 17q22 including HER2 and GRB7 (Fig. 1A, pink), and a third subtype contained normal breast samples. The second branch of tumors comprising the ER-positive group (Fig. 1A, right side) was further divided in this study and showed two, or possibly three, subtypes. One ER-positive subtype comprising 32 tumors (luminal subtype A, Fig. 1, dark blue) showed the highest expression of ERα, GATA binding protein 3, X-box binding protein, hepatocyte nuclear factor 3α, and estrogen-regulated LIV-1. A second subgroup of ER-positive tumors consisted of eight tumors (luminal subtype B/C, Fig. 1, yellow/light blue) and showed moderate expression of these luminal-specific genes.

The five to six different subtypes identified in this study represented clinically distinct subgroups of patients as defined by correlations with clinical parameters (2). This was demonstrated by univariate survival analyses where the subtypes were compared with respect to overall survival and relapse-free survival. Kaplan-Meier curves (Fig. 2) computed from the subtypes presented in Fig. 1 showed a statistically significant difference in overall survival between the groups (p < 0.01). ER-negative basal-like and HER2/ERBB2-positive tumors had the shortest survival and relapse-free times. There was also a difference in outcome for ER-positive tumors classified as luminal subtype A vs luminal subtype B/C, with luminal subtype B/C representing a clinically distinct group of tumors with a poor disease course, particularly with respect to relapse. These profiling results highlight the power of microarray analysis in studying histologically similar tumors and show that gene expression profiling can identify biologically distinct subtypes of tumors with diverse cellular origins that show different clinical outcomes.

4. EXPERIMENTAL DESIGN FOR GENOMIC ANALYSIS IN PHASE II PREVENTION TRIALS

The application of this type of study to characterization of early breast lesions has significant potential to similarly separate groups of patients at high risk of developing breast cancers from those at low risk. The underlying assumption for this approach is that individuals at high risk will have abnormal expression patterns within their normal tissue samples before the appearance of any histologically abnormal cells, and further, that early atypical lesions from high-risk individuals will have different abnormalities than similar lesions from low-risk individuals. The notion that variations exist in normal tissue or tissue with early lesions is a reasonable expectation based on findings from the studies described above, where significant variation was observed in gene expression patterns of normal samples (1,2). In addition, a recent rodent study that conducted a profiling analysis of normal tissues showed that statistically significant variation was observed for 3.3%, 1.9%, and 0.8% of genes studied in mouse liver, kidney, and testis, respectively (53).

Characterization of normal variation in gene expression profiles for high-risk patients is an important first step in incorporating genomic analysis into chemoprevention studies. This type of study could be conducted as part of Phase II prevention trials that use minimally invasive sampling procedures. Figure 3 is an adaptation of a schematic diagram presented in a recent chemoprevention review on the design of a Phase II FNA-based clinical trial for chemopreventive drug evaluation (32). Figure 3 illustrates how genomic analysis could be included in this design. Phase II prevention designs that use FNA to select patients with atypical hyperplasia

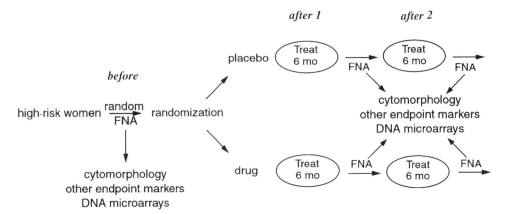

Fig. 3. Schematic diagram of a design for a Phase II chemoprevention trial. High-risk women with FNA evidence of hyperplasia are randomized to placebo or control and treated for 6 mo. FNAs are repeated after 6 mo and 1 yr of treatment. The tissue from each FNA could be used to conduct cytomorphology, immunohistochemistry, and DNA microarrays.

have increased the statistical power to detect changes in clinical outcome with treatment. In our design, previously validated SEBs will be assessed, including morphology and markers such as ER or COX-2. In addition, a DNA microarray will also be performed on each FNA sample at each time point. By conducting genomic analysis on FNA samples before and during treatment, increased statistical power to detect changes in gene expression patterns is conferred. This approach is likely to yield new candidate biomarkers of risk when used in conjunction with "supervised" analyses of microarrays *(3,54)*.

In supervised analyses, sets of genes that correlate with important clinical features can be identified. For example, at the end of a chemoprevention trial, untreated patients (placebo group) could be classified according to whether disease progressed and/or tumors developed. By assigning a supervision parameter to classify patients into two groups, those who developed disease and those who did not develop disease, the data of the "before" therapy samples could be queried to identify expression profiles in those samples that predict who will develop disease. Once these sets of genes are validated as risk biomarkers, they could be used in the clinical setting to identify candidates for chemoprevention treatment or to select individuals for clinical trials.

Even if those who are likely to develop cancer can be reliably predicted, the studies on tamoxifen conducted by the NSABP demonstrated that the phenotype of the developing lesion was an important determinant of the response to therapy. In particular, ER-positive lesions responded to tamoxifen treatment while ER-negative lesions did not *(31)*; these data, along with the data of Perou et al. *(1,2)*, suggest that unique prevention

strategies for ER-negative tumors will also be required. Data sets acquired using the design in Fig. 3 could help to identify those likely to respond to new treatments based on their gene expression patterns. Once patients have been identified as responders or nonresponders in the drug treatment arm, response status could be used as a supervising parameter for analysis of gene expression data. Using this approach, one might be able to identify sets of genes within "before" samples that will predict who will respond and who will not respond. These markers from "before" treatment would be further pursued as biomarkers of response.

The two supervised analysis approaches discussed thus far use the "before" samples to identify important genes that predict disease and response. A commonly used marker of response to chemoprevention is reversion of the lesion to a more normal morphological phenotype. Gene expression analogs of morphological phenotypes could be identified by searching for genes that are expressed differently between atypical and normal "after" therapy samples. Again, gene expression-based evaluations of response have the advantage of being easier to quantitate, and if several markers could be identified that predict response, use of these markers in combination could allow greater specificity in evaluating response than would be offered by more qualitative morphological analyses.

The "after 1" and "after 2" samples collected by FNA could also be useful in identifying mechanistically important genes. Comparisons of "before" and "after" samples will allow identification of genes that may be drug targets. Most chemopreventive drugs have pleiotropic effects, and many of the overlapping pathways these drugs affect may be unknown. Genes whose expression is altered by treatment could be studied in more directed molecular biology experiments to determine their role in mitigating the response to therapy and to identify them as potential targets for the next generation of drugs. Supervised analysis of microarray data obtained in a Phase II FNA-based clinical trial has the potential to improve our understanding of gene expression profiles of breast cancer risk, the biology of early lesions, gene expression pathways involved in progression of early breast cancers, and mechanisms of action of chemopreventive drugs.

Advances in the genomic sciences have allowed us to gain powerful insights into the molecular taxonomy of invasive breast tumors and other tumors that arise from different cellular origins. The intrinsic properties of individual tumors can be captured in molecular profiles that are biologically and clinically meaningful. The application of genomic profiling to the study of other aspects of tumor biology is clearly very promising, with the realm of chemoprevention likely to be the next frontier.

REFERENCES

1. Perou CM, Sorlie T, Eisen MB, et al. Molecular portraits of human breast tumours. *Nature* 2000;406:747–752.
2. Sorlie T, Perou CM, Tibshirani R, et al. Gene expression patterns of breast carcinomas distinguish tumor subclasses with clinical implications. *Proc Natl Acad Sci USA* 2001; 98:10,869–10,874.
3. van' t Veer LJ, Dai H, van de Vijver MJ, et al. Gene expression profiling predicts clinical outcome of breast cancer. *Nature* 2002;415:530–536.
4. West M, Blanchette C, Dressman H, et al. Predicting the clinical status of human breast cancer by using gene expression profiles. *Proc Natl Acad Sci USA* 2001;98:11,462–11,467.
5. Hedenfalk I, Duggan D, Chen Y, et al. Gene-expression profiles in hereditary breast cancer. *N Engl J Med* 2001;344: 539–548.
6. Gruvberger S, Ringner M, Chen Y, et al. Estrogen receptor status in breast cancer is associated with remarkably distinct gene expression patterns. *Cancer Res* 2001;61: 5979–5984.
7. MacDonald TJ, Brown KM, LaFleur B, et al. Expression profiling of medulloblastoma: PDGFRA and the RAS/ MAPK pathway as therapeutic targets for metastatic disease. *Nat Genet* 2001;29:143–152.
8. Pomeroy SL, Tamayo P, Gaasenbeek M, et al. Prediction of central nervous system embryonal tumour outcome based on gene expression. *Nature* 2002;415:436–442.
9. Jazaeri AA, Yee CJ, Sotiriou C, et al. Gene expression profiles of BRCA1-linked, BRCA2-linked, and sporadic ovarian cancers. *J Natl Cancer Inst* 2002;94:990–1000.
10. Welsh JB, Zarrinkar PP, Sapinoso LM, et al. Analysis of gene expression profiles in normal and neoplastic ovarian tissue samples identifies candidate molecular markers of epithelial ovarian cancer. *Proc Natl Acad Sci USA* 2001;98:1176–1181.
11. Wang K, Gan L, Jeffery E, et al. Monitoring gene expression profile changes in ovarian carcinomas using cDNA microarray. *Gene* 1999;229:101–108.
12. Beer DG, Kardia SL, Huang CC, et al. Gene-expression profiles predict survival of patients with lung adenocarcinoma. *Nat Med* 2002;8:816–824.
13. Garber ME, Troyanskaya OG, Schluens K, et al. Diversity of gene expression in adenocarcinoma of the lung. *Proc Natl Acad Sci USA* 2001;98:13,784–13,789.
14. Bhattacharjee A, Richards WG, Staunton J, et al. Classification of human lung carcinomas by mRNA expression profiling reveals distinct adenocarcinoma subclasses. *Proc Natl Acad Sci USA* 2001;98:13,790–13,795.
15. Zou TT, Selaru FM, Xu Y, et al. Application of cDNA microarrays to generate a molecular taxonomy capable of distinguishing between colon cancer and normal colon. *Oncogene* 2002;21:4855–4862.
16. Lin YM, Furukawa Y, Tsunoda T, et al. Molecular diagnosis of colorectal tumors by expression profiles of 50 genes expressed differentially in adenomas and carcinomas. *Oncogene* 2002;21:4120–4128.
17. Alon U, Barkai N, Notterman DA, et al. Broad patterns of gene expression revealed by clustering analysis of tumor and normal colon tissues probed by oligonucleotide arrays. *Proc Natl Acad Sci USA* 1999;96:6745–6750.
18. Takahashi M, Rhodes DR, Furge KA, et al. Gene expression profiling of clear cell renal cell carcinoma: gene identification and prognostic classification. *Proc Natl Acad Sci USA* 2001;98:9754–9759.
19. Singh D, Febbo PG, Ross K, et al. Gene expression correlates of clinical prostate cancer behavior. *Cancer Cell* 2002;1:203–209.
20. LaTulippe E, Satagopan J, Smith A, et al. Comprehensive gene expression analysis of prostate cancer reveals distinct transcriptional programs associated with metastatic disease. *Cancer Res* 2002;62:4499–4506.
21. Welsh JB, Sapinoso LM, Su AI, et al. Analysis of gene expression identifies candidate markers and pharmacological targets in prostate cancer. *Cancer Res* 2001;61:5974–5978.
22. Dhanasekaran SM, Barrette TR, Ghosh D, et al. Delineation of prognostic biomarkers in prostate cancer. *Nature* 2001;412:822–826.
23. Hippo Y, Taniguchi H, Tsutsumi S, et al. Global gene expression analysis of gastric cancer by oligonucleotide microarrays. *Cancer Res* 2002;62:233–240.
24. Yeoh EJ, Ross ME, Shurtleff SA, et al. Classification, subtype discovery, and prediction of outcome in pediatric acute lymphoblastic leukemia by gene expression profiling. *Cancer Cell* 2002;1:133–143.
25. Hofmann WK, de Vos S, Elashoff D, et al. Relation between resistance of Philadelphia-chromosome-positive acute lymphoblastic leukaemia to the tyrosine kinase inhibitor STI571 and gene-expression profiles: a gene-expression study. *Lancet* 2002;359:481–486.
26. Ferrando AA, Neuberg DS, Staunton J, et al. Gene expression signatures define novel oncogenic pathways in T cell acute lymphoblastic leukemia. *Cancer Cell* 2002;1:75–87.
27. Shipp MA, Ross KN, Tamayo P, et al. Diffuse large B-cell lymphoma outcome prediction by gene-expression profiling and supervised machine learning. *Nat Med* 2002;8: 68–74.
28. Rosenwald A, Wright G, Chan WC, et al. The use of molecular profiling to predict survival after chemotherapy for diffuse large-B-cell lymphoma. *N Engl J Med* 2002;346:1937–1947.

29. Alizadeh AA, Eisen MB, Davis RE, et al. Distinct types of diffuse large B-cell lymphoma identified by gene expression profiling [see comments]. *Nature* 2000;403:503–511.

30. Gail MH, Greene MH. Gail model and breast cancer. *Lancet* 2000;355:1017.

31. Fisher B, Costantino JP, Wickerham DL, et al. Tamoxifen for prevention of breast cancer: report of the National Surgical Adjuvant Breast and Bowel Project P-1 Study. *J Natl Cancer Inst* 1998;90:1371–1388.

32. Fabian CJ, Kimler BF. Chemoprevention for high-risk women: tamoxifen and beyond. *Breast J* 2001;7:311–320.

33. Jordan VC, Costa AF. Chemoprevention. In *Diseases of the Breast.* Harris JR, Lippman ME, Morrow M, Osborne CK, eds. Lippincott Williams & Wilkins, Philadelphia, 1999; pp. 265–279.

34. Daly MB, Ross EA. Predicting breast cancer: the search for a model. *J Natl Cancer Inst* 2000;92:1196–1197.

35. Kelloff GJ, Sigman CC, Johnson KM, et al. Perspectives on surrogate end points in the development of drugs that reduce the risk of cancer. *Cancer Epidemiol Biomarkers Prev* 2000;9:127–137.

36. Kelloff GJ, Boone CW, Crowell JA, et al. Risk biomarkers and current strategies for cancer chemoprevention. *J Cell Biochem Suppl* 1996:25:1–14.

37. Fabian CJ, Kimler BF, Zalles CM, et al. Short-term breast cancer prediction by random periareolar fine-needle aspiration cytology and the Gail risk model. *J Natl Cancer Inst* 2000;92:1217–1227.

38. Boone CW, Kelloff GJ, Steele VE. The natural history of intraepithelial neoplasia: relevance to the search for intermediate endpoint biomarkers. *J Cell Biochem Suppl* 1992; 16G:23–26.

39. Boone CW, Kelloff GJ. Endpoint markers for cancer chemoprevention trials derived from the lesion of precancer (intraepithelial neoplasia) measured by computer-assisted quantitative image analysis. *J Cell Biochem Suppl* 2000;34: 67–72.

40. Assersohn L, Gangi L, Zhao Y, et al. The feasibility of using fine needle aspiration from primary breast cancers for cDNA microarray analyses. *Clin Cancer Res* 2002;8: 794–801.

41. Phillips J, Eberwine JH. Antisense RNA amplification: a linear amplification method for analyzing the mRNA population from single living cells. *Methods* 1996;10:283–288.

42. Tavassoli FA, Schnitt SJ. *Pathology of the Breast.* Elsevier, New York, 1992.

43. Eisen MB, Spellman PT, Brown PO, Botstein D. Cluster analysis and display of genome-wide expression patterns. *Proc Natl Acad Sci USA* 1998;95:14,863–14,868.

44. Lyons TJ, Gasch AP, Gaither LA, et al. Genome-wide characterization of the Zap1p zinc-responsive regulon in yeast. *Proc Natl Acad Sci USA* 2000;97:7957–7962.

45. Cho RJ, Mindrinos M, Richards DR, et al. Genome-wide mapping with biallelic markers in *Arabidopsis thaliana. Nat Genet* 1999;23,203–207.

46. Chu S, DeRisi J, Eisen M, et al. The transcriptional program of sporulation in budding yeast. *Science* 1998;282: 699–705.

47. Iyer VR, Eisen MB, Ross DT, et al. The transcriptional program in the response of human fibroblasts to serum. *Science* 1999;283:83–87.

48. Ross DT, Scherf U, Eisen MB, et al. Systematic variation in gene expression patterns in human cancer cell lines. *Nat Genet* 2000;24:227–235.

49. Perou CM, Jeffrey SS, van de Rijn M, et al. Distinctive gene expression patterns in human mammary epithelial cells and breast cancers. *Proc Natl Acad Sci USA* 1999;96: 9212–9217.

50. DeRisi J, Penland L, Brown PO, et al. Use of a cDNA microarray to analyse gene expression patterns in human cancer. *Nat Genet* 1996;14:457–460.

51. Khan J, Simon R, Bittner M, et al. Gene expression profiling of alveolar rhabdomyosarcoma with cDNA microarrays. *Cancer Res* 1998;58:5009–5013.

52. Perou CM, Brown PO, Botstein D. Tumor classification using gene expression patterns from DNA microarrays. In *New Technologies for Life Sciences: A Trends Guide.* Elsevier, New York, 2000; 67–76.

53. Pritchard CC, Hsu L, Delrow J, Nelson PS. Project normal: defining normal variance in mouse gene expression. *Proc Natl Acad Sci USA* 2001;98:13,266–13,271.

54. Ramaswamy S, Tamayo P, Rifkin R, et al. Multiclass cancer diagnosis using tumor gene expression signatures. *Proc Natl Acad Sci USA* 2001;98:15,149–15,154.

9 Clinical Applications of Proteomics

Emanuel F. Petricoin III, PhD and Lance A. Liotta, MD, PhD

CONTENTS

INTRODUCTION

SERUM PROTEOMIC PATTERN DIAGNOSTICS: PREVENTION THROUGH EARLY DETECTION

PATIENT-TAILORED THERAPY: PATHWAY BECOMES TARGET

CONCLUSIONS

REFERENCES

1. INTRODUCTION

The field of molecular medicine is moving beyond genomics to proteomics, which is often viewed as creation of a compendium "master list" of all proteins and their possible post-translational modifications. However, the effort made to elucidate this index is not likely to be rewarded by any real clinical impact, as the function of proteins is closely tied to their cellular, tissue, and physiological context. The ultimate goal of clinical proteomics (the translational subdiscipline of the larger field) is really twofold. First, characterize information flow through protein networks—which are deranged as a cause or consequence of disease processes as they exist, not in cell culture or animal models systems, but in the tissue microenvironment of the host—and how that information content changes during therapeutic intervention; second, develop biomarker profiling technologies to detect disease earlier and treat it more effectively.

A cell's information flow is driven through fluctuating and ever-changing protein pathways and networks (1–6) mediated by protein–protein interactions (Fig. 1), in which proteins transfer information content by modifying a protein-binding partner by, for example, phosphorylation, cleavage, or alteration of its conformation. Our overarching need is to access and visualize the entire interconnecting circuitry of biological processes—both inside and outside a cell—as it forms following a stimulus, and then dissolves after the stimulus ceases. A detailed circuit map of only a subset of key physiological processes such as cell growth and division could have a

profound effect, not only on basic functional biology and understanding of disease mechanisms, but also on the rational design of targeted therapeutics in the clinic.

In a functional sense, cancer is a proteomic disease. Genetic mutations that underpin the disease process provide an information archive to generate mutated proteins that can result in aberrant signaling pathways. This creates a survival advantage for the cell, which can then ignore negative inhibitory signals or perpetually receive a false positive signal.

The realization that cancer is a product of the tissue microenvironment has important implications, shifting the view of therapeutic targets away from individual molecules. As cellular circuitry itself can now be considered the target, it might make more sense to target entire deranged signal pathways inside and outside the cancer cell. Moreover, the tumor-host microenvironment involves enzymatic events and sharing of growth factors, which could be a source for biomarkers that could ultimately be shed into the serum proteome.

2. SERUM PROTEOMIC PATTERN DIAGNOSTICS: PREVENTION THROUGH EARLY DETECTION

Ovarian cancer is a prime example of the clinical dilemma faced when no effective detection biomarker exists in the clinic. More than two-thirds of ovarian cancers are detected at an advanced stage, when cancer has disseminated throughout the peritoneal cavity (7,8). Unfortunately, even then, ovarian cancer rarely produces specific or diagnostic symptoms; as a result,

From: Cancer Chemoprevention, Volume 2: Strategies for Cancer Chemoprevention
Edited by: G. J. Kelloff, E. T. Hawk, and C. C. Sigman © Humana Press Inc., Totowa, NJ

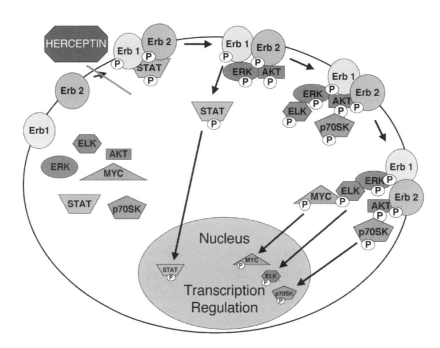

Fig. 1. Protein signal pathways and networks consist of protein complexes that assemble in response to a stimulus. Posttranslational modification (e.g., phosphorylation) allows for specific protein–protein interactions to percolate information within the cell. Sample components of the EGF pathway are shown. This pathway is a target for treatment with Herceptin, an antibody recognizing the ERB2 receptor.

it is not usually treated until it is at an advanced stage when therapeutic intervention has limited success *(9)*. The resulting 5-yr survival rate is 35–40% for surgical and chemotherapeutic intervention of late-stage patients. However, when ovarian cancer is detected while still confined to the ovary (stage I), conventional therapy produces a much higher 5-yr survival rate (95%) *(9–13)*. Critically, simply developing a biomarker to detect ovarian cancer at stage I could have a profound impact on successful treatment of this disease.

An effective, clinically useful biomarker should be measurable in a readily accessible body fluid, such as serum, urine, or saliva. However, until now, the search for cancer-related biomarkers for early disease detection has been a one-at-a-time approach looking for over-expressed proteins shed into the circulation as a consequence of the disease process *(14–17)*. Unfortunately, this approach is slow and time consuming; identifying potentially thousands of intact and cleaved proteins in the human serum proteome could take years to accomplish. Finding one disease-related protein biomarker is like searching for a needle in a haystack, requiring separation and identification of these entities individually.

Serum-based proteomic pattern diagnostics offer a new paradigm for disease detection *(18)*. In this example, the diagnostic endpoint for ovarian cancer detection

was a pattern consisting of many individual proteins that independently were not able to differentiate diseased from healthy individuals. These patterns are reflective of the blood proteome without knowledge of the disease-related proteins. These disease-related differences may be the result of proteins being over-expressed and/or abnormally shed and added to the serum proteome, clipped or modified as a consequence of disease, or subtracted from the proteome due to abnormal activation of proteolytic degradation pathways. Even quaternary effects due to disease-related protein-protein interactions and protein complex formation can modify and subtly change the serum proteome. Since initially reported, this analytical method has been extended to prostate cancer *(19)*; other research groups have confirmed this new paradigm for breast *(20)* and prostate cancer detection *(21)*. Using this method, 1 μL of raw unfractionated serum is analyzed by surface-enhanced laser desorption ionization time-of-flight spectrometry (SELDI-TOF) to create a proteomic signature of the patient's serum (Fig. 2). This serum proteomic fingerprint is composed of thousands of protein ion signatures requiring high-ordered data mining operations for analysis. The two main types of bioinformatics data mining systems are supervised systems that require a training set consisting of a body of data where outcome or classification is known ahead of time, and unsupervised systems. A supervised system might

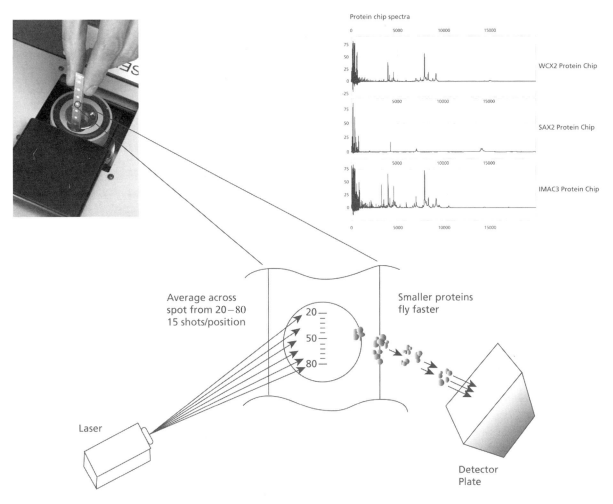

Fig. 2. Surface-enhanced laser desorption and ionization (SELDI) is a type of mass spectroscopy useful in high-throughput proteomic profiling that utilizes chemical matrices for ion-chip separation and analysis. Depending on the type of surface used—weak cation exchange (WCX2), strong anion exchange (SAX2), or immobilized metal affinity chromatography (IMAC)—a subset of the proteins in the sample bind to the surface of the chip. The bound proteins are treated with a matrix-assisted laser desorption/ionization (MALDI) matrix, washed, and dried. The chip, containing multiple patient samples, is inserted into a vacuum chamber, where it is irradiated with a laser. The laser desorbs the adherent proteins, causing them to be launched as ions. The time of flight (TOF) of the ion prior to detection by an electrode is a measure of the mass to charge (M/Z) value of the ion. The ion spectra can be analyzed by computer-assisted bioinformatic tools to classify a subset of the spectra by their characteristic patterns of relative intensity.

include linear regression models, nonlinear feed-forward neural networks (NLFN), and genetic algorithms (GAs) *(22–29)*. Unsupervised systems that cluster or group records without previous knowledge of outcome or classification include K-means nearest-neighbor analysis, Euclidean distance-based nonlinear methods, fuzzy pattern matching methods, and self-organizing mappings (SOMs) *(30–32)*. However, any approach used for data mining has the same difficulty: finding optimal feature sets that withstand continual validation with larger and larger test sets, or in this instance, proteins in a large unbounded information archive that is unknown at this time. A typical SELDI-TOF proteomic profile will have 15,500 to 400,000 data points that

comprise data recordings between 500 and 20,000 M/Z depending on the resolution of the underlying mass spectrometer. Heuristic artificial intelligence (AI)-based systems that learn, adapt, and gain experience over time are uniquely suited for proteomic data analysis because of the huge dimensionality of the proteome itself. In fact, it is possible to generate not just one, but multiple combinations of proteomic patterns from a single mass-spectral training set, each pattern combination readjusting as the models get better in the adaptive mode. This is exactly what has been observed as the expanding ovarian cancer patient sera set has now given rise to multiple pattern combinations that have over 98% sensitivity and specificity.

3. PATIENT-TAILORED THERAPY: PATHWAY BECOMES TARGET

Most current therapeutics are directed at protein targets. Since tissues are a heterogeneous milieu of different interacting cell populations, new technology was needed to analyze pure populations of diseased cells in the tissue section itself. Laser capture microdissection (LCM) enables the experimentalist to procure pure cell populations from heterogeneous tissue sections, under direct microscopic visualization (33). This technology has been applied to discover dozens of potential protein targets (34–42).

However, the marriage of LCM with new proteomic technologies can have significant limitations due to low microdissection throughput and an inadequate amount of relevant sample procured. Discovery platforms, such as 2-D gels, isotope-coded affinity tagging (ICAT), multidimensional liquid chromatography/mass spectroscopy platforms, and multiplexed antibody arrays, require fairly substantial quantities of material—orders of magnitude greater than the quantity procured during a clinical biopsy (43–50). These biopsy specimens may contain only a few hundred cells as the starting point for any proteomic analysis. Specifically, clinical proteomics, or the use of clinical trial material for proteomic analysis, requires development of new technologies that can employ these small amounts of cellular material. Additionally, another limitation of many proteomic technologies is a requirement for denatured proteins. Since denaturation will break apart protein complexes, these methods may not be able to determine cellular circuitry mediated by protein-protein interactions.

Protein microarrays represent the first new technology that can actually profile the state of a signaling pathway target even after the cell is lysed (51–53). In fact, the reverse-phase protein array has shown the unique ability to analyze signaling pathways using small numbers of human tissue cells microdissected from biopsy specimens procured during clinical trials (54) (Fig. 3). Employing this approach, LCM-procured pure cell populations are taken from human biopsy specimens, and a protein lysate is directly spotted onto nitrocellulose slides. Comparing this method with tissue arrays (55) or antibody arrays (56) reveals several unique advantages. First, the reverse phase array uses denatured lysates, defusing antigen retrieval issues that represent a large limitation for tissue arrays. Second, arrays can be composed of nondenatured lysates derived directly from LCM-procured tissue cells, leaving protein-protein, protein-DNA, and/or protein-RNA complexes intact.

Third, each patient sample is arrayed in a miniature dilution curve, providing an internal standard curve; since the analysis gives a measurement within the linear dynamic range of any antibody–analyte interaction, direct quantitative measurements can be ascertained. Last, arrays do not require direct tagging of the protein for detection. This yields a dramatic improvement in reproducibility, sensitivity, and robustness over other techniques.

Reverse-phase arrays can now be used to study key nodes in cellular circuitry and profile the functional state of protein pathways and signaling events within cells contained in biopsy samples. Reverse phase analysis of LCM-procured patient-matched normal epithelial, premalignant, and invasive prostate carcinoma cell study sets revealed that phosphorylation and activation of AKT occurred as a critical early step in cancer progression (54). Thus, inhibition of AKT activity through molecular targeted therapeutics may have a profound impact in treating prostate cancer and preventing progression. Moreover, the arrays can now be manufactured in a sectored array format, where dozens of analytes can be measured simultaneously on one slide, thereby increasing the throughput and facile data analysis. With this technologic leap, we now use reverse-phase arrays in the research clinic by analyzing the phosphorylation status of multiple points within the signaling pathway in cancer cells before and after therapy. This will yield a true picture of the coordination of signaling events as they change and flux in response to targeted therapy.

As each patient's cancer may have a unique complement of pathogenic molecular derangements, a specific therapy may be effective for only a subset of patients who harbor tumors with certain susceptible molecular derangements. A strategy that selects appropriate treatment combinations that best match the individual tumor's molecular profile will likely have a much better success rate at the bedside (57–64). Molecular profiling using gene arrays can classify patient populations according to disease stage or survival outcome (25,65). However, transcript profiling alone provides an incomplete picture, as gene transcript levels may bear absolutely no relationship to the activated or phosphorylated state of the protein. Additionally, gene transcripts provide no direct information about protein–protein interactions and the resultant state of signaling pathways. Patient-tailored therapeutic treatment strategies must include direct proteomic pathway analysis of biopsy material.

Current cancer therapy has been directed at a single molecular target. In the future, we envision targeting an

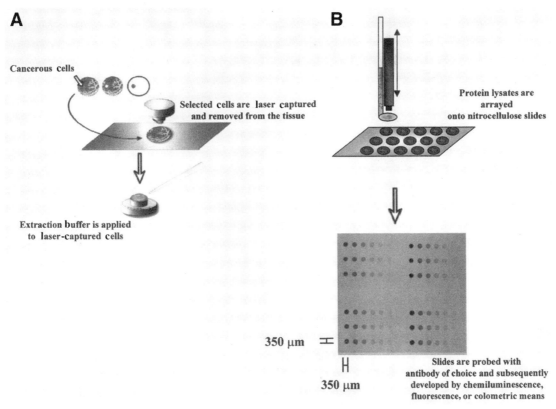

Fig. 3. A new class of protein array, reverse-phase array, immobilizes the cellular lysate sample to be analyzed on a treated slide (e.g., nitrocellulose). Lysates are prepared from cultured cells or microdissected tissues, and arrayed in miniature dilution curves. The analyte molecule contained in the sample is then detected by a separate labeled probe (e.g., antibody) applied to the surface of the array. This array is highly linear, is very sensitive, and requires no labeling of the sample proteins.

entire set of nodes all along the pathogenic signal pathway (Fig. 4) for greater efficacy with reduced toxicity. Proteomic signal pathways consist of an amplification cascade of enzymatic events. Stages of the pathway can be ordered from upstream to downstream events (Figs. 1 and 4).

In order to completely shut down the entire pathway, it is necessary to treat the upstream target at a high drug concentration that blocks the target with a high degree of efficiency. At this high concentration, the drug dose may produce unwanted toxic side effects. Combinatorial therapy, an alternative to single-agent therapy, offers the promise of higher specificity at lower treatment doses *(66–69)*. Patient-tailored therapeutic regimes, using knowledge gained from proteomic pathway profiling, can prescribe a cocktail of inhibitors and antagonists at lower concentrations acting at several points along the the pathway with increased efficacy. This synergism is possible because we can now take advantage of the inherent interdependency of cell signaling networks and use inhibitors that work in series at different points along the pathway. The ultimate output of the pathway is affected by each part of the circuitry flowing together with the others. Thus, molecular profiling allows us to map the cellular circuit to define the optimal set of interconnected drug targets.

4. CONCLUSIONS

Today, the micro- and nano-proteomic technologies being developed, and specifically clinical proteomics, will have direct bedside impact. In the not too distant future, the physician will use these different proteomic tools at multiple steps within disease management and therapeutic intervention. The impact will be felt in critical elements of patient care and management—early detection of disease using proteomic patterns diagnostics, use of proteomic signatures to complement histopathology, individualized selection of therapeutic combinations that best target the patient's entire disease-specific cellular circuitry, and rational redirection of therapy based on changes in the diseased protein network associated with drug resistance and toxicity.

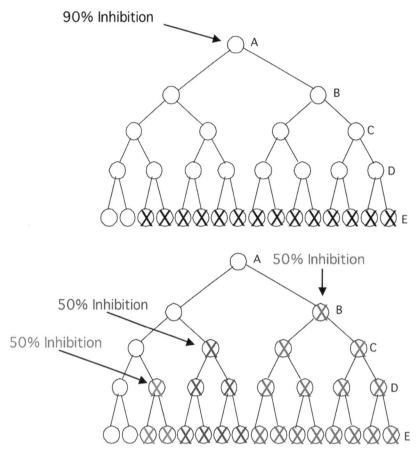

Fig. 4. Combinatorial therapy. A generic signal cascade is depicted. A high dose of the drug is required to target a single upstream node (upper). In contrast, targeting a series of interconnected nodes can achieve the same efficacy with a lower dose of each drug (lower).

REFERENCES

1. Liotta L, Petricoin E. Molecular profiling of human cancer. *Nat Rev Genet* 2000;1:48–56.
2. Ideker T, Thorsson V, Ranish JA, et al. Integrated genomic and proteomic analyses of a systematically perturbed metabolic network. *Science* 2001;292:929–934.
3. Schwikowski B, Uetz P, Fields S. A network of protein-protein interactions in yeast. *Nat Biotechnol* 2000;18:1257–1261.
4. Legrain P, Jestin JL, Schachter V. From the analysis of protein complexes to proteome-wide linkage maps. *Curr Opin Biotechnol* 2000;4:402–407.
5. Blume-Jensen P, Hunter T. Oncogenic kinase signaling. *Nature* 2001;411:355–365.
6. Pawson T. Protein modules and signaling networks. *Nature* 1995;373:573–580.
7. Ozols RF, Rubin SC, Thomas GM, Robboy SJ. Epithelial ovarian cancer. In *Principles and Practice of Gynecologic Oncology*. Hoskins WJ, Perez CA, Young RC, eds. Lippincott Williams & Wilkins, Philadelphia, 2000: pp. 981–1058.
8. Menon V, Jacobs IJ. Tumor markers. In *Principles and Practice of Gynecologic Oncology*. Hoskins WJ, Perez CA, Young RC, eds. Lippincott Williams & Wilkins, Philadelphia, 2000; pp. 165–182.
9. Bast RC, Klug TL, St John E, et al. A radioimmunoassay using a monoclonal antibody to monitor the course of epithelial ovarian cancer. *N Engl J Med* 1983;309:883–887.
10. Menon U, Jacobs IJ. Recent developments in ovarian cancer screening. *Curr Opin Obstet Gynecol* 2000;12:39–42.
11. Jacobs IJ, Skates SJ, MacDonald N, et al. Screening for ovarian cancer: a pilot randomized controlled trial. *Lancet* 1999;353:1207–1210.
12. Cohen LS, Escobar PF, Scharm C, et al. Three-dimensional power Doppler ultrasound improves the diagnostic accuracy for ovarian cancer prediction. *Gynecol Oncol* 2001;82:40–48.
13. Richter R, Schulz-Knappe P, Schrader M, et al. Composition of the peptide fraction in human blood plasma: database of circulating human peptides. *J Chromotogr B Biomed Sci Appl* 1999;726:25–35.
14. Adam BL, Vlahou A, Semmes OJ, Wright GL Jr. Proteomic approaches to biomarker discovery in prostate and bladder cancers. *Proteomics* 2001;1:1264–1270.
15. Carter D, Douglass JF, Cornellison CD, et al. Purification and characterization of the mammaglobin/lipophilin B complex, a promising diagnostic marker for breast cancer. *Biochemistry* 2002;41:6714–6722.
16. Rosty C, Christa L, Kuzdzal S, et al. Identification of hepatocarcinoma-intestine-pancreas/pancreatitis-associated protein I as a biomarker for pancreatic ductal adenocarcinoma by protein biochip technology. *Cancer Res* 2002;62:1868–1875.
17. Xiao Z, Adam BL, Cazares LH, et al. Quantitation of serum prostate-specific membrane antigen by a novel protein biochip immunoassay discriminates benign from malignant prostate disease. *Cancer Res* 2001;61:6029–6033.

18. Petricoin EF, Ardekani AM, Hitt BA, et al. Use of proteomic patterns in serum to identify ovarian cancer. *Lancet* 2002;359:572–577.

19. Petricoin EF 3rd, Ornstein DK, Paweletz CP, et al. Serum proteomic patterns for detection of prostate cancer. *J Natl Cancer Inst* 2002;94:1576–1578.

20. Li J, Zhang Z, Rosenzweig J, et al. Proteomics and bioinformatics approaches for identification of serum biomarkers to detect breast cancer. *Clin Chem* 2002;48:1296–1304.

21. Adam B-L, Qu Y, Davis JW, et al. Serum protein fingerprinting coupled with a pattern-matching algorithm distinguishes prostate cancer from benign prostate hyperplasia and healthy men. *Cancer Res* 2002;62:3609–3614.

22. Ball G, Mian S, Holding F, et al. An integrated approach utilizing artificial neural networks and SELDI mass spectrometry for the classification of human tumours and rapid identification of potential biomarkers. *Bioinformatics* 2002;18:395–404.

23. Ting KL, Lee RC, Chang CL, Guarino AM. The relationship between the mass spectra of drugs and their biological activity—an application of artificial intelligence to chemistry. *Comput Biol Med* 1975;4:301–332.

24. Nicholson JK, Connelly J, Lindon JC, Holmes E. Metabonomics: a platform for studying drug toxicity and gene function. *Nat Rev Drug Disc* 2002;1:153–161.

25. Alizadeh AA, Eisen MB, Davis RE, et al. Distinct types of diffuse large B-cell lymphoma identified by gene expression profiling. *Nature* 2000;403:503–511.

26. Golub TR, Slonim DK, Tamayo P, et al. Molecular classification of cancer: class discovery and class prediction by gene expression monitoring. *Science* 1999;286:531–537.

27. Lindahl D, Palmer J, Edenbrandt L. Myocardial SPET: artificial neural networks describe extent and severity of perfusion defects. *Clin Physiol* 1999;19:497–503.

28. Lapuerta P, L'Italien GJ, Paul S, et al. Neural network assessment of perioperative cardiac risk in vascular surgery patients. *Med Decis Making* 1998;18:70–75.

29. Holland JH, ed. *Adaptation in Natural and Artificial Systems: An Introductory Analysis with Applications to Biology, Control, and Artificial Intelligence*, 3rd ed. MIT Press, Cambridge, MA, 1994.

30. Kohonen T. The self-organizing map. *Proc IEEE* 1990;78:1464–1480.

31. Kohonen. T. Self-organizing formation of topologically correct feature maps. *Biol Cybern* 1982;43:59–69.

32. Tou JT, Gonzalez R. Pattern classification by distance functions. In *Pattern Recognition Principles*. Tou JT, Gonzalez R, eds. Addison Wesley, Reading, MA, 1974, pp. 75–109.

33. Emmert-Buck MR, Bonner RF, Smith PD, et al. Laser capture microdissection. *Science* 1996;274:998–1001.

34. Emmert-Buck MR, Gillespie JW, Paweletz CP, et al. An approach to proteomic analysis of human tumors. *Mol Carcinog* 2000;27:158–165.

35. Craven RA, Totty N, Harnden P, et al. Laser capture microdissection and two-dimensional polyacrylamide gel electrophoresis: evaluation of tissue preparation and sample limitations. *Am J Pathol* 2002;160:815–822.

36. Ornstein DK, Gillespie JW, Paweletz CP, et al. Proteomic analysis of laser capture microdissected human prostate cancer and in vitro prostate cell lines. *Electrophoresis* 2000;21:2235–2242.

37. Wulfkuhle JD, McLean KC, Paweletz CP, et al. New approaches to proteomic analysis of breast cancer. *Proteomics* 2001;1:1205–1215.

38. Jones MB, Krutzsch H, Shu H, et al. Proteomic analysis and identification of new biomarkers and therapeutic targets for invasive ovarian cancer. *Proteomics* 2002;2:76–84.

39. Knezevic V, Leethanakul C, Bichsel VE, et al. Proteomic profiling of the cancer microenvironment by antibody arrays. *Proteomics* 2001;1:1271–1278.

40. Ahram M, Best CJ, Flaig MJ, et al. Proteomic analysis of human prostate cancer. *Mol Carcinog* 2002;33:9–15.

41. Paweletz CP, Gillispie JW, Ornstein DK, et al. Rapid protein display profiling of cancer progression directly from human tissue using a protein biochip. *Drug Dev Res* 2000;49:34–42.

42. Cazares LH, Adam BL, Ward MD, et al. Normal, benign, preneoplastic, and malignant prostate cells have distinct protein expression profiles resolved by surface enhanced laser desorption/ionization mass spectrometry. *Clin Cancer Res* 2002;8:2541–2552.

43. Shen Y, Tolic N, Zhao R, et al. High-throughput proteomics using high-efficiency multiple-capillary liquid chromatography with on-line high-performance ESI FTICR mass spectrometry. *Anal Chem* 2001;73:3011–3021.

44. Li J, Wang C, Kelly JF, et al. Rapid and sensitive separation of trace level protein digests using microfabricated devices coupled to a quadrupole—time-of-flight mass spectrometer. *Electrophoresis* 2000;21:198–210.

45. Gygi SP, Rist B, Gerber SA, et al. Quantitative analysis of complex protein mixtures using isotope coded affinity tags. *Nat Biotechnol* 1999,17:994–999.

46. Washburn MP, Wolters D, Yates JR. Large scale analysis of the yeast proteome by multidimensional protein identification technology. *Nat Biotechnol* 2001,19:242–247.

47. Krutchinsky AN, Kalkum M, Chait BT. Automatic identification of proteins with a MALDI-quadrupole ion trap mass spectrometer. *Anal Chem* 2001;73:5066–5077.

48. Washburn MP, Ulaszek R, Deciu C, et al. Analysis of quantitative proteomic data generated via multidimensional protein identification technology. *Anal Chem* 2002;74:1650–1657.

49. Zhou H, Ranish JA, Watts JD, Aebersold R. Quantitative proteome analysis by solid-phase isotope tagging and mass spectrometry. *Nat Biotechnol* 2002;20:512–515.

50. Zhou G, Li H, DeCamp D, et al. 2D differential in-gel electrophoresis for the identification of human esophageal squamous cell cancer specific protein markers. *Mol Cell Proteomics* 2002;1:117–124.

51. MacBeath G, Schreiber SL. Printing proteins as microarrays for high-throughput function determination. *Science* 2000;289:1760–1763.

52. Kuruvilla FG, Shamji AF, Sternson SM, et al. Dissecting glucose signalling with diversity-oriented synthesis and small-molecule microarrays. *Nature* 2002;416:653–657.

53. Walter G, Bussow K, Lueking A, Glokler J. High-throughput protein arrays: prospects for molecular diagnostics. *Trends Mol Med* 2002;8:250–253.

54. Paweletz CP, Charboneau L, Bichsel VE, et al. Reverse phase protein microarrays which capture disease progression show activation of pro-survival pathways at the cancer invasion front. *Oncogene* 2001;20:1981–1989.

55. Torhorst J, Bucher C, Kononen J, et al. Tissue microarrays for rapid linking of molecular changes to clinical endpoints. *Am J Pathol* 2001;159:2249–2256.

56. Knezevic V, Leethanakul C, Bichsel VE, et al. Proteomic profiling of the cancer microenvironment by antibody arrays. *Proteomics* 2001;1:1271–1278.

57. Liotta LA, Kohn EC, Petricoin EF. Clinical proteomics: personalized molecular medicine. *JAMA* 2001;286:2211–2214.

58. Liotta L, Petricoin E. Molecular profiling of human cancer. *Nat Rev Genet* 2000;1:48–56.

59. Karpati G, Li H, Nalbantoglu J. Molecular therapy for glioblastoma. *Curr Opin Mol Ther* 1999;1:545–552.

60. Brown CK, Kirkwood JM. Targeted therapy for malignant melanoma. *Curr Oncol Rep* 2001 Jul;3(4):344–352.

61. Frankel AE, Sievers EL, Scheinberg DA. Cell surface receptor-targeted therapy of acute myeloid leukemia: a review. *Cancer Biother Radiopharm* 2000;15:459–476.

62. Cheng JD, Rieger PT, von Mehren M, et al. Recent advances in immunotherapy and monoclonal antibody treatment of cancer. *Semin Oncol Nurs* 2000;16:2–12.

63. Gasparini G, Gion M. Molecular-targeted anticancer therapy: challenges related to study design and choice of proper endpoints. *Cancer J Sci Am* 2000;6:117–131.

64. Cimoli G, Bagnasco L, Pescarolo MP, et al. Signaling proteins as innovative targets for antineoplastic therapy: our experience with the signaling protein c-myc. *Tumori* 2001;87:S20–S23.

65. Rosenwald A, Wright G, Chan WC, et al. The use of molecular profiling to predict survival after chemotherapy for diffuse large-B-cell lymphoma. *N Engl J Med* 2002;346:1937–1947.

66. Normanno N, Campiglio M, De LA, et al. Cooperative inhibitory effect of ZD1839 (Iressa) in combination with trastuzumab (Herceptin) on human breast cancer cell growth. *Ann Oncol* 2002;13:65–72.

67. Moasser MM, Basso A, Averbuch SD, Rosen N. The tyrosine kinase inhibitor ZD1839 ("Iressa") inhibits HER2-driven signaling and suppresses the growth of HER2-overexpressing tumor cells. *Cancer Res* 2001;16:7184–7188.

68. Cuello M, Ettenberg SA, Clark AS, et al. Down-regulation of the *erb*B-2 receptor by trastuzumab (Herceptin) enhances tumor necrosis factor-related apoptosis-inducing ligand-mediated apoptosis in breast and ovarian cancer cell lines that overexpress *erb*B-2. *Cancer Res* 2001;61:4892–4900.

69. Vile RG, Chong H. Immunotherapy III: combinatorial molecular immunotherapy—a synthesis and suggestions. *Cancer Metastasis Rev* 1996;15:351–364.

10 Bioinformatics and Whole-Genome Technologies

Richard Simon, DSc

CONTENTS

1. INTRODUCTION

The last half of the 20th century saw dramatic improvements in cancer treatment, including curative treatments for pediatric acute lymphocytic leukemia, Wilms tumor, osteosarcoma, testicular cancer, Hodgkin's disease, diffuse large B cell lymphoma, and other neoplasms. Mortality for breast cancer has been reduced as a result of improvements in chemoprevention, early detection, and therapy. For many other solid tumors, however, progress has been more limited.

This same period also saw a biotechnology revolution. This has provided powerful new reagents, experimental techniques, instruments, and assays that have led to whole genome DNA sequencing and genome-wide RNA transcript quantification. Proteome-wide protein quantification is within view.

Also developed was the randomized clinical trial, which has made medicine a science. Unfortunately, in many cases developments in clinical trial methodology were more powerful and effective than the interventions being evaluated. However, randomized clinical trials protected us from the broad introduction of ineffective and toxic treatments. It also enabled identification of improved treatments and chemoprevention of breast cancer that would not have been possible otherwise.

It is important that the interventions brought to clinical trial in the 21st century have a stronger scientific basis than has been the case to date. Even now, progress in reducing cancer mortality is limited by an inadequate understanding of the molecular basis of these diseases.

The new instrumentation and assays provided by the biotechnology revolution have facilitated creation of extensive biological data resources. Biology is in the process of becoming an information and system science, but obstacles remain in using the data becoming available to create biological knowledge. The following sections will explore some of these obstacles and opportunities in developing genomic-based approaches to cancer prevention research.

2. BIOINFORMATICS

Bioinformatics, an ambiguous term, refers to all aspects of collection, analysis, and integration of biological information. Its components include software engineering, statistical analysis, and algorithm development. Many biologists and organizations are confused about bioinformatics, do not appreciate its diversity, and struggle to determine staff selection or structure for a bioinformatics group. A common misconception is too narrow a focus on software engineering. Software engineers cannot build analysis tools unless they have access to professional advice about data analysis. That advice should generally come from statisticians involved in data analysis and methodology development. A second common misconception about bioinformatics is that it can be effectively structured as a service component that can be purchased. This is certainly not true for the statistical analysis and algorithm development components of bioinformatics. Such a view of bioinformatics reflects a lack of appreciation for the significance of the changing nature of biology. Taking advantage of the

From: Cancer Chemoprevention, Volume 2: Strategies for Cancer Chemoprevention
Edited by: G. J. Kelloff, E. T. Hawk, and C. C. Sigman © Humana Press Inc., Totowa, NJ

revolution taking place in biology requires recognition that statistical and computational scientists working in bioinformatics must be full members of a research team interacting with wet-lab experimentalists on a collaborative basis and conducting self-initiated research on bioinformatics methodology.

Some biologists view bioinformatics as a service activity creating analysis tools for use by experimentalists. Though analysis tools are important, many problems require interdisciplinary collaboration in order to fully understand and utilize the data. This type of collaboration is difficult to achieve in many laboratory environments, but has been successfully accomplished between biostatisticians and clinical investigators in clinical trial research. Interdisciplinary collaboration requires not only mutual respect, but also substantial cross-training of statistical and computational scientists in biology and of biologists in statistical and computational matters. It also requires funding of bioinformatics groups as research groups, interacting with experimentalists and also doing research to extend the methodology of bioinformatics. Understanding the complex interactions among genes and cells requires greater use of mathematical methods, not for quantification, but for elucidating the principles involved. This effort will require an environment that encourages the best minds to get involved in bioinformatics activities. Organizations holding onto outdated views and old hierarchical structures will not be able to take advantage of the opportunities offered in the genomic era.

3. DNA MICROARRAYS

DNA microarrays can be used to quantify the abundance of mRNA transcripts for each gene of the human genome in a sample of cells. Although active research is being done on the assays and methods for data analysis, microarrays are still currently useful and very powerful. For cancer prevention research, DNA microarrays can elucidate the sequence of changes in gene expression that occur as tumors develop, identify molecular targets for preventive strategies, and identify candidate biomarkers for surrogate endpoints in developmental prevention trials.

There are a number of myths prevalent concerning DNA microarrays; some are listed in Table 1. The first is that the greatest challenge in the use of DNA microarrays is management of the large volume of data generated. Though effective data management is essential, it can be accomplished using established principles of software engineering. An increasing number of commercial and

Table 1
Microarray Myths

The greatest challenge is managing the mass of microarray data
Pattern recognition is the appropriate paradigm for analyzing microarray data
Cluster analysis is generally useful for analyzing microarray data
Microarray data analysis is about looking for red or green spots
Prepackaged analysis tools are a substitute for collaboration with statistical scientists in complex problems

academic database systems is available for managing microarray data. The more conceptually challenging problem is determining how to design the experiments, analyze the resulting data to obtain reliable information, and combine sources of information to obtain answers to important biological questions.

A second myth is that pattern recognition is the appropriate paradigm for microarray analysis. One view is that unstructured specimens are fed into a pattern recognition algorithm to identify unexpected regularities and provide answers to unasked questions. This view does not provide a prescription for the effective use of microarrays. The microarray is an assay; as when using any assay, experiments and analyses must be carefully planned. Microarrays are generally not used to test gene-specific hypotheses. Gene-specific mechanistic hypotheses can often be better addressed using other, more sensitive, assays. But effective microarray-based research has clear objectives that drive the planning of both experiment and analysis. For example, to identify genes that are disregulated early in oncogenesis, samples of tissue taken early in the development of an invasive cancer are needed. The type and number of samples, as well as the analysis plan, should be determined based on the objectives.

A third myth is that cluster analysis is the generally appropriate method of analyzing microarray data. The microarray is useful for experiments with a wide variety of objectives. Cluster analysis is useful for identifying coexpressed genes and for trying to determine whether a disease is uniform with regard to gene expression, but it is inappropriate for many other objectives. Cluster analysis is not a very powerful approach for comparing expression profiles among predefined classes of samples. For example, one may be interested in finding genes that are differentially expressed between tumor and normal samples. Distance metrics used in cluster analysis are generally global distance metrics based on all genes or on genes that show variability across the set of samples. This metric may not be sensitive to differences in the relatively few genes that discriminate among predefined classes. Cluster analysis is a nonsupervised method, in the sense that it does not utilize information about which sample is in which predefined class. Supervised methods for comparing the classes to determine differentially expressed genes and to build multivariate classifiers based on these genes are generally more powerful for such problems.

The fourth microarray myth listed in Table 1 is that microarray data analysis is about looking for red and green spots. Early use of cDNA microarrays was based on single arrays in which RNA from a collection of wild-type cells was labeled with one fluorescent dye (e.g., Cy3) and hybridized against RNA from a mutated cell type, labeled with a different fluorescent dye (e.g., Cy5). Computer software that performs image analysis of pixel-level data computes two numbers at each pixel location on the slide. One number is intensity of fluorescence when illuminated with laser light of the intensity that causes Cy3 dye to fluoresce, and the other number is the intensity when the slide is illuminated with light that causes Cy5 dye to fluoresce. The relative magnitude of these two numbers can be color-coded and displayed. Usually the color-coding ranges from green to red. The spots in which there is more mRNA from one sample relative to the other will appear either reddish or greenish.

One problem with analysis by color is that it assumes that one can draw conclusions based on analysis of a single microarray, which does not take into account the many sources of variation not represented by looking at a single microarray. This confusion was enhanced by the publication of formulae and "error models" claiming to represent confidence intervals for the red-to-green ratio on a single array. Unfortunately, these confidence intervals do not incorporate many important sources of variability. RNA is easily degradable, and differences in handling the cells or tissues compared on an array can greatly influence the results. The labeling reaction is also a major source of variability and it cannot be properly controlled when analyzing a single array. Not only is substantial variability involved in labeling, but there is also bias. The two labels commonly used, Cy3 and Cy5, have different affinities for DNA and different sensitivities for fluorescence. These relative affinities are gene-dependent and fluorescence bias varies based on the level of expression. One may attempt to control

some of these biases by "normalization" of the data, but normalizations are imperfect and obtaining unbiased results generally requires multiple arrays and, in some cases, dye-swap replication.

Generally, biological variation is the greatest source of variation in microarray studies. If you wish to compare tissue of tumors from a specified tissue to normal tissue of the same type, you need to study multiple tumors and multiple normal tissues. If you do multiple arrays with sub-aliquots of the same specimen of tumor and normal tissue, then you may learn something about relative gene expression in those two RNA samples. You may be able to control for the labeling bias and variation and for hybridization variation, but you won't know whether the differential expression found is the result of differential tissue handling, or whether it applies more generally to tumors and normal tissues of that type. Even for experiments involving cell lines instead of tissues, gene expression can vary seriously with the confluence state at which cells are harvested. As cells start to crowd and compete for nutrients, various pathways get turned on and off. Hence, comparing expression in an RNA sample from one cell line to expression in an RNA sample from a different cell line, we will not know whether the results are more than experimental artifacts unless the experiment is replicated at the biological level of repeating cell growth and harvest. The amount of replication appropriate depends on degree of variability from all sources and is discussed somewhat by Simon et al. (1) along with other aspects of designing microarray experiments. There is value in doing some replication of arrays at a lower level—independently labeled duplicate arrays for the same RNA samples—in order to assure that your experimental technique, instrumentation, and reagents are working properly.

The final myth listed in Table 1 is that software analysis tools substitute for collaboration with professional statistical scientists on major studies using microarrays. Many biologists perform a small number of microarrays in order to get a view of gene expression for planning more definitive experiments using either microarrays or other technologies. It is important that good software analysis tools be available for such use. We have developed BRB-Array Tools (2) as a DNA microarray analysis package for use by biologists. BRB-Array Tools is also intended to educate biologists in good statistical practices for analysis of microarray data. Too few available statisticians are experienced in microarray data analysis; often if falls to biologists to analyze their own data. However, for many experiments, collaboration with professional statisticians experienced in design and analysis of microarray data is very important. Studies involving DNA microarrays are in many ways more complicated than clinical trials or cohort studies. There are many more opportunities to misanalyze data and publish erroneous conclusions. Many signal processing analysis steps require careful examination of the raw data. These include image analysis of pixels, background adjustment, quantification of signal, normalization, combining probe signals on Affymetrix arrays, identification of artifacts, and quality assessment. There are many types of experimental artifacts. There are also many competing methods of analysis, not all of which are equally good. The available software packages cannot be relied on to produce good data automatically for all sets of arrays. Equally complex are issues of data analysis after the signal processing stage, including what analysis methods to use, how to control for multiple comparisons, how to evaluate a multivariate classifier, and how to perform and validate cluster analysis. Some available software packages do not handle these issues effectively or even validly. Many packages overemphasize cluster analysis for problems where it is inappropriate. The Affymetrix software currently available does not even provide for comparison of expression levels of genes in two sets of samples by a standard statistical test. It provides only for comparison of individual samples.

In comparing expression levels of genes in two sets of samples, cognizance must be taken of the multiple comparison issue. If expression levels for two sets of samples for 10,000 genes are compared, 500 false positives statistically significant at the 0.05 level can be expected, even though expression levels are correlated among sets of some of the genes. The correlation affects distribution variance of the number of false positives, but not the expected number. Hence, the conventional 0.05 significance level in comparing expression levels of individual genes is not appropriate. Some investigators select genes differentially expressed between the two classes at the 0.05 level, and then cluster the samples with regard to that gene set. This is an erroneous way of evaluating whether the classes are different with regard to expression profile. Even if two classes do not truly differ with regard to expression profile, on average 500 (out of 10,000) genes will be significant at the 0.05 level and the classes will cluster separately with regard to this set of false positive genes.

One among many methods for controlling the number of false positives is to use a stringent 0.001

threshold for declaring significance. Other methods specifically control the "false discovery rate," the proportion of genes claimed to be differentially expressed between the classes which are false positives. Some methods also take into account the correlation structure of expression level among genes and thereby gain statistical power.

There is substantial interest in developing multivariate classifiers of two or more predefined classes based on gene expression levels. Substantial literature exists on different types of mathematical functions that can be used as classifiers, ranging from linear discriminant functions to neural networks. However, these methods were not developed for problems where the number of candidate predictors vastly exceeds the number of cases (samples). Many methods do not work well in that setting. The key principles in developing an effective multivariate classifier are selecting informative features and avoiding overfitting the data. For contexts where the number of candidate predictors (genes) is an order of magnitude greater than the number of cases, complex methods that have many parameters to be determined from the data, such as neural networks, often perform very poorly *(3)*.

It is essential to obtain an unbiased estimate of the misclassification rate of multivariate classifiers in high-dimensional situations with relatively few cases. Applying the classifier to the same set of cases from which it was developed results in a severely biased estimate of misclassification rate unless a cross-validation (or other bias reduction) procedure is properly used. One simple type of cross-validation is to separate the data into a training set and a validation set before any analysis is performed and to not look at the validation set until a fully specified model is developed on the training set. The fully specified classifier is then applied to the cases of the validation set, without any additional variable selection, fitting of parameter values, or estimating cutoff values. An unbiased estimate of misclassification rate can be obtained in this way.

An alternative approach for some circumstances is algorithmic cross-validation. With algorithmic leave-one-out cross-validation *(4)*, one sample is set aside as a singleton validation set. The classification model is developed from scratch on the training set defined by the remaining samples; this model is used to classify the validation sample that was excluded from the training set. The correctness of that classification is then recorded. This process is repeated *n* times, where *n* is the total number of samples. Each time, a different sample is excluded and a classification model developed from scratch using the same algorithm on the training set consisting of the remaining samples. Leave-one-out cross-validation is often performed incorrectly. "Developed from scratch" means that all variable selection and other steps must be reperformed on each training set. The variables (genes) in the model will change for each training set. No preanalysis that uses the class labels can be performed using the entire data set. Inexperienced data analysts sometimes select the genes using the entire data set, or select the principal components using the entire data set. Then they cross-validate the parameters of the model. This generally gives quite a biased estimate of the misclassification rate.

4. CONCLUSION

Biotechnology has given rise to genomic and important new tools, approaches, and opportunities for understanding the nature of cancers. Such under-standing will lead us to major improvements in reducing cancer mortality through prevention, early detection, and molecularly targeted treatment. However, taking advantage of the opportunities available to us will require a greater appreciation of changes that have taken place and the need for closely interacting with statistical and computational scientists in a setting of collaboration among equal research scientists.

REFERENCES

1. Simon R, Radmacher MD, Dobbin K. Design of studies using DNA microarrays. *Genet Epidemiol* 2002;23:21–36.
2. Simon R, Peng A. BRB-ArrayTools Users Guide. http://linus.nci.nih.gov/BRB-ArrayTools.
3. Dudoit S, Fridlyand J, Speed T. Comparison of discrimination methods for the classification of tumors using gene expression data. *J Am Statistical Assoc* 2002; 97:77–87.
4. Radmacher MD, McShane LM, Simon R. A paradigm for class prediction using gene expression profiles. *J Comput Biol* 2002;9:505–511.

11 Models of Absolute Risk

Uses, Estimation, and Validation

Mitchell H. Gail, MD, PhD

CONTENTS

1. INTRODUCTION: DEFINITION AND USES OF ABSOLUTE RISK

Individualized absolute risk is the probability that a person with defined risk factors who is free of the disease of interest at age a will be observed to develop the disease over the age interval $(a, a + \tau)$. For example, the chance that a 40-yr-old nulliparous white woman who began menstruating at the age of 14, who has had no breast biopsies, and whose mother had breast cancer, will develop breast cancer by the age of 70 can be calculated as 0.116, or 11.6%, using the Gail model for breast cancer risk (1). In this paper, breast cancer will usually be the disease of interest, but the ideas apply to any disease.

It is important to distinguish absolute risk from relative risk, which is the ratio of the age-specific incidence rate in a woman with given risk factors to that in a woman without risk factors. In the previous example, the woman's relative risk is 2.76 compared to a 40-yr-old woman with no risk factors. Relative risk is useful for studying the association between a risk factor and disease; relative risks can be estimated from retrospective evaluation of risk factors in diseased and non-diseased subjects, namely case-control studies (2). Knowing that a woman's relative risk of disease is 2.76, however, does not by itself define the chance that she will develop the disease over a given time interval, namely the absolute risk.

Absolute risk is influenced by several factors. Age is usually one of the most influential factors, as the risk of diseases such as cancer usually increases sharply with age. The duration of the age interval $(a, a + \tau)$ also affects absolute risk, which increases with increasing duration, τ. The woman's individual risk factors influence absolute risk. Finally, the absolute risk of a disease like breast cancer is reduced by the chance of dying of some other disease before breast cancer develops. Each of these factors needs to be taken into account in calculating individualized absolute risk (see subheading 2).

Absolute risk estimates are useful for medical counseling. For example, a 40-year-old woman whose absolute risk of developing breast cancer in the next 5 yr is 0.5% might be advised to undergo routine annual examinations with mammography, whereas a similar woman with a projected 5-yr risk of 5% might consider taking a preventive agent, such as tamoxifen (3) in addition to mammographic surveillance. In making such decisions, one must weigh the various risks and benefits of the proposed intervention. For example, tamoxifen is associated with an increased risk of stroke, pulmonary embolus, deep vein thrombosis, and endometrial cancer (4). A key ingredient for comparing risks and benefits of an intervention such as tamoxifen is an estimate of the absolute risks of the various health outcomes in the presence and absence of the intervention (3). Using such estimates of absolute risk and a

From: Cancer Chemoprevention, Volume 2: Strategies for Cancer Chemoprevention
Edited by: G. J. Kelloff, E. T. Hawk, and C. C. Sigman © Humana Press Inc., Totowa, NJ

categorization of potential adverse events into life-threatening, severe, and other, Gail et al. *(3)* defined categories of women for whom there was good evidence that the benefits of tamoxifen outweighed the risks. Such calculations required absolute risk estimates for each of the potential adverse outcomes.

Absolute risk is also useful in designing prevention trials. If the trial emphasis is on a single endpoint, such as invasive breast cancer, the concept of absolute risk is directly relevant. The power of a survival analysis based on the logrank test to detect a preventive effect in the active intervention arm compared to placebo depends mainly on the total number of events (e.g., invasive breast cancers) that arise during the trial *(5)*. One can estimate the number of events for a given sample size by averaging the risk-factor-specific absolute risks, calculated for trial duration, over the risk factor distribution in the source population, and multiplying the result by the sample size. Conversely, the required sample size can be computed by dividing the required number of events by the average absolute risk.

The design of an intervention study that examines intervention effects on several health outcomes is more complex. For example, Freedman et al. *(6)* proposed various procedures for monitoring the several beneficial and potentially deleterious effects of hormone replacement therapy in the Woman's Health Initiative. Regardless of the procedure chosen, a computation of the absolute risk of each component health outcome is central to understanding the statistical power of such trial designs and to developing procedures for monitoring the trial *(7)*.

2. ESTIMATION OF ABSOLUTE RISK

Follow-up data from a cohort are required to estimate absolute risk. Gail et al. *(1)* studied a cohort of 243,221 white women followed over 5 yr in the Breast Cancer Detection Demonstration Project (BCDDP) to estimate the absolute risk of breast cancer. If risk factors such as family history of breast cancer and age at first live birth had been available for each of these women, one could have cross-classified the women according to such risk factors, and, for each combination of risk factors (including initial age, *a*), estimated the absolute risk of developing breast cancer in the next 5 yr.

This approach was not applicable for three reasons. First, detailed risk factor information was available only on the subset of 2582 women with breast cancer and 3146 women without breast cancer who participated in a nested case-control study within the cohort.

Second, even if detailed risk factor information had been available on all cohort members, data on breast cancer incidence would have been too sparse to yield reliable estimates within many of the risk factor combinations; thus, some modeling of joint effects on relative risk was required. Finally, to make long-term projections of absolute risk with only 5 yr of follow-up, age- and risk-factor-specific risks will be assumed to remain constant over calendar time.

Formula number 5 in reference *(1)* shows how to compute absolute risk in terms of a relative risk function, $r(t)$, a baseline hazard of the disease of interest, $h_1(t)$, and the hazard of mortality from causes of death except the disease of interest, $h_2(t)$. We discuss these quantities next.

2.1. Relative Risk, r(t)

Relative risk, $r(t)$, is the ratio of disease risk at age t for a woman with risk factors $X(t)$ at age t to the risk for a woman whose risk factors are at their lowest ("baseline") level at age t. The relative risk factor in Gail et al. depended on age at menarche, age at first live birth, number of affected first-degree relatives, and number of previous breast biopsies. In projecting risk, it was assumed that these factors remained constant at their values determined at the age $t = a$ of the initial consultation, but, using the same formulas, risk projection could be altered to take changes in these risk factors into account. Relative risk function $r(t)$ can be estimated from cohort data, or more feasibly from case-control studies.

2.2. Baseline Hazard, h₁(t)

The baseline age-specific hazard $h_1(t)$ is the age-specific breast cancer incidence rate for women whose risk factors were all at the lowest (baseline) level. Follow-up data from cohorts yield an estimate of the composite age-specific hazard rate $h_1^*(t)$ that reflects a mixture of women with various risk factor combinations. Gail et al. estimated $h_1(t)$ from $h_1(t) = h_1^*(t)\,[1 - AR(t)]$, where $AR(t)$ is the attributable risk for women aged t. Gail et al. estimated $h_1^*(t)$ from BCDDP follow-up data and $1 - AR(t)$ from BCDDP case-control data *(1)*.

The original model of Gail et al. *(1)* was designed to project all incident breast cancer, including *in situ* breast cancer. Estimating the absolute probability of invasive breast cancer to determine eligibility for the Breast Cancer Prevention Trial (BCPT) *(4)*, Anderson et al. used population-based invasive breast cancer incidence rates from the National Cancer Institute's (NCI) Surveillance, Epidemiology and End Result (SEER) program to estimate $h^*_1(t)$ (8,9). They estimated the corresponding attributable risk needed to compute $h_1(t)$ by combining the relative risk function $r(t)$ from Gail et al. (1) with information on the prevalence of risk factors in the general population in the Cancer and Steroid Hormone Study (10). The resulting "model 2," which was described and studied by Costantino et al. (9), very accurately predicted the numbers of invasive breast cancers actually observed in the BCPT.

The general strategy of estimating relative risk function $r(t)$ from a population-based case-control study and estimating baseline hazard $h_1(t)$ by combining an attributable risk estimate from population-based case-control data with SEER data on age-specific composite incidence, $h^*_1(t)$, is a powerful and practical approach that could be used to develop models to project absolute risk for other cancers, such as colon cancer.

2.3. The Hazard of Mortality From Causes Other Than the Disease of Interest, h2(t)

The third ingredient needed to compute absolute risk is the hazard of mortality, $h_2(t)$, from all causes of death except the disease of interest. Gail et al. (1) obtained $h_2(t)$ from general US mortality rates, and assumed that $h_2(t)$ did not depend on the covariates used to predict breast cancer incidence. In some applications, a risk factor such as a genetic mutation that increases risk for the disease of interest might also influence mortality from other causes. If such effects are known, they can be incorporated into formula number 5 in Gail et al. (1) for computing absolute risk by allowing $h_2(t)$, and the corresponding survival distribution, $S_2(t)$, to depend on covariates.

3. VALIDATING A MODEL FOR PROJECTING ABSOLUTE RISK

Costantino et al. (9) reviewed previous efforts to evaluate the original model of Gail et al. for projecting total breast cancer incidence ("model 1") and the modified model for projecting the risk of invasive breast cancer by Anderson and Redmond ("model 2"). Costantino et al. compared the relative risk function, which is common to both these models, with estimates of this function from independent case-control and cohort study data. The features of relative risk function were quantitatively consistent across studies, with few exceptions. Costantino et al. then assessed how well the observed number of breast cancers (O) agreed with the expected number (E) based on models 1 and 2. A model in which O and E are in good agreement is said to be well calibrated. Using data from the placebo arm of the BCPT, Costantino et al. found a ratio of E/O = 0.84 (95% confidence interval 0.73–0.97) for all breast cancer (model 1) and E/O = 1.03 (95% confidence interval 0.88–1.21) for invasive breast cancer (model 2). Thus, the models are well calibrated, especially model 2 for invasive breast cancer.

Rockhill et al. (11) confirmed the good calibration of these models in a larger set of data from the Nurses Health Study (NHS). However, they raised another important criterion for consideration, namely the discriminatory power of the model. Pointing out that distribution of absolute risk estimates in women in the NHS who ultimately developed breast cancer tended to be only modestly higher than distribution of risk prediction values in women who remained disease-free, they concluded that the ability of the model to discriminate women who will develop breast cancer from those who will not was modest. (The area under the receiver operating curve, AUC-ROC, was estimated as 0.58). Thus, despite these models being well calibrated and therefore useful in weighing risks and benefits, as in tamoxifen use (3), considerable scope remains for improving the sensitivity, specificity, and discriminatory power of this model.

4. IMPROVING MODELS AND OTHER FUTURE DIRECTIONS

One way to improve the discriminatory power of a model is to include more powerful predictors. For example, one might try to incorporate information on mammographic density, on cytology from nipple aspirates, or on genetic mutations to improve the discriminatory power for identifying women who will develop breast cancer. Such an effort to improve discriminatory power is certainly worthwhile. However, an advantage of the current Gail model (1), and of a model based only on a detailed family history of breast cancer by Claus et al. (12), is that they only require interview data. Requiring information on more powerful (and invasive) predictors can restrict the range of application of the models.

Additional information must be obtained on the calibration of available models in various ethnic and racial groups. Work is needed to determine whether the relative risk function in Gail et al. (1), which was derived from white women in the BCDDP, applies to other racial or ethnic groups. The version of model 2 available on the NCI's "Risk Disk" (http://bcra.nci.nih.gov/brc/) includes separate baseline hazard estimates for black women and Hispanic women, but more work is needed to check the calibration of the model in racial and ethnic subgroups. Calibration must be also be checked of models such as those proposed by Claus et al. *(12)* and extensions of that model strongly based on the assumption that familial aggregation of breast cancer is due to an autosomal dominant mutation. Considerable evidence indicates that other factors contribute to such aggregation *(13)*.

Section 2.3. mentions a simple general strategy for estimating the absolute risk of a cancer by combining information on the relative risk function $r(t)$ and the attributable risk from a population-based case-control study with SEER data on age-specific composite incidence, $h^*_1(t)$. Ongoing work to develop a model to project the risk of colon or rectum cancer is based on this approach.

Models for projecting absolute risk to assist in medical decision-making will usually require weighing absolute risks of several health outcomes in the presence and absence of a proposed intervention, as when considering tamoxifen use *(3)* as mentioned in Section 1. An important need in this area is development of individualized models of absolute risk for each of the health endpoints that influence the intervention decision. Epidemiologists and risk modelers will need to take a broad view of the available data resources. In weighing risks and benefits, there is a pressing need to improve data sources for estimating absolute risks for a range of health outcomes.

REFERENCES

1. Gail MH, Brinton LA, Byar DP, et al. Projecting individualized probabilities of developing breast cancer for white females who are being examined annually. *J Natl Cancer Inst* 1989; 81:1879–1886.

2. Cornfield J. A method of estimating comparative rates from clinical data. Applications to cancer of the lung, breast, and cervix. *J Natl Cancer Inst* 1951;11:1269–1275.

3. Gail MH, Costantino JP, Bryant J, et al. Weighing the risks and benefits of tamoxifen treatment for preventing breast cancer. *J Natl Cancer Inst* 1999;91:1829–1846.

4. Fisher B, Costantino JP, Wickerham DL, et al. Tamoxifen for prevention of breast cancer: report of the National Surgical Adjuvant Breast and Bowel Project P-1 Study. *J Natl Cancer Inst* 1998;90:1371–1388.

5. Gail MH. Sample size estimation when time-to-event is the primary endpoint. *Drug Info J* 1994;28:865–877.

6. Freedman L, Anderson G, Kipnis V, et al. Approaches to monitoring the results of long-term disease prevention trials: examples from the Women's Health Initiative. *Control Clin Trials* 1996;17:509–525.

7. Gail MH. The estimation and use of absolute risk for weighing the risks and benefits of selective estrogen receptor modulators for preventing breast cancer. *Ann NY Acad Sci* 2001; 949:286–291.

8. Anderson SJ, Ahnn S, Duff K. NSABP Breast Cancer Prevention Trial risk assessment program 2. NSABP Biostatistical Center Technical Report, August 14, 1992.

9. Costantino JP, Gail MH, Pee D, et al. Validation studies for models projecting the risk of invasive and total breast cancer incidence. *J Natl Cancer Inst* 1999;91:1541–1548.

10. Wingo PA, Ory HW, Layde PM, Lee NC. The evaluation of the data collection process for a multicenter, population-based, case-control design. *Am J Epidemiol* 1988;128: 206–217.

11. Rockhill B, Spiegelman D, Byrne C, et al. Validation of the Gail et al. model of breast cancer risk prediction and implications for chemoprevention. *J Natl Cancer Inst* 2001; 93:358–366.

12. Claus EB, Risch N, Thompson WD. Autosomal dominant inheritance of early-onset breast cancer. Implications for risk prediction. *Cancer* 1994;73:643–651.

13. Claus EB, Schildkraut J, Iversen ES Jr, et al. Effect of BRCA1 and BRCA2 on the association between breast cancer risk and family history. *J Natl Cancer Inst* 1998;90:1824–1829.

12 Genetic Polymorphisms and Risk Assessment for Cancer Chemoprevention

Sonia de Assis and Peter G. Shields, MD

CONTENTS

1. INTRODUCTION

Cancer risk carries wide interindividual variation; only a fraction of the population exposed to a known carcinogen develops cancer. Genetic susceptibility is both inherited and acquired. Genes that affect cancer susceptibility can be found in those controlling behavior, carcinogen metabolism, and cellular response to carcinogen exposure. Genetic traits affect DNA repair, cell cycle control, and immune response. Polymorphic genetic variants are under intense study. It stands to reason that if genetic traits that affect cancer risk can be measured, these traits would also govern responses to cancer prevention strategies such as chemoprevention. Cancer prevention strategies may become more focused if it is possible to identify susceptible subgroups of the population. Thus, incorporating such measures should lead to more rational chemoprevention studies, allowing for smaller sample size and shorter duration. This chapter describes concepts underlying genetic susceptibility and current technology used to assess it, provides specific examples of low-penetrance genes involved in cancer susceptibility, and comments on the implications for cancer prevention.

2. SUSCEPTIBILITY TO CANCER

It has been long recognized that people differ in their susceptibility to cancer. Several decades after the report of scrotal cancer among chimney sweeps, it was observed that not all chimney sweeps exposed to soot were affected *(1)*. This suggests that constitutional factors play a role in cancer development. In many other instances, tumors arise in only a fraction of the population exposed to a known human carcinogen *(2)*. For example, only about 10% of cigarette smokers develop lung cancer in their lifetimes *(3)*. Although it is possible that chance plays a part in the complex process of carcinogenesis, there is evidence that genetic factors interact with environmental exposures to cause cancer *(4,5)*. Variations in the genetic code that lead to alterations in expression, function, or localization of proteins could modify an individual's susceptibility to cancer. It stands to reason that genetic susceptibilities that affect cancer risk will also affect the success of chemopreventive strategies. Also, some chemopreventive agents might prevent risks relating to some gene–environment interactions and not others. Since evidence indicates that cancers such as lung, breast, colon, liver, and leukemia are preventable *(6)*, identifying susceptible subgroups would help focus prevention strategies.

2.1. Genetic Susceptibility to Cancer

Genes with a high penetrance have a large effect on cancer risk, while others with a low penetrance have less of an effect (Table 1). High-penetrance cancer susceptibility genes are associated with very high relative risks, and cause the so-called familial cancer syndromes, where several family members develop cancer,

From: Cancer Chemoprevention, Volume 2: Strategies for Cancer Chemoprevention
Edited by: G. J. Kelloff, E. T. Hawk, and C. C. Sigman © Humana Press Inc., Totowa, NJ

Table 1
Inherited Predisposition—High-Penetrance and Low-Penetrance Genes

Characteristics	High-penetrance genes	Low-penetrance genes
Type of cancer	Familial	Sporadic
Frequency in the population	Rare	Common
Individual risk	High	Low
Environmental effects	Modest	Essential

often at a young age. Mutations in high-penetrance genes are rare and account for a small fraction of cancer incidence. For instance, the combined contribution to overall breast cancer incidence of mutations in *BRCA1* and *BRCA2*, which confer individual risk of around 45–80% by age 70, is less than 5% (7,8).

Low-penetrance genes are associated with more common sporadic cancers. These cancers are caused by environmental exposures, where the risk is modulated by low-penetrance genes (9). These genes affect a greater part of the population and so have a high attributable risk. For example, a predisposing allele present in 20% of the population that confers a relative risk of 2.0 could account for up to 20% of breast cancer incidence (7).

Genetic polymorphism, a trait that occurs in at least 1% of the population, is responsible for the variation in low-penetrance genes. These polymorphic genetic traits can be due to nucleotide base substitutions, deletions (including large parts of genes), insertions, or tandem repeats. Polymorphisms are present throughout the genome, occurring at a frequency of about one in every 500 to 1000 bases. Genes with polymorphic variants might affect the expression or function of a protein, or they might not. For example, polymorphisms in introns (except at splice sites) or those that do not cause amino acid changes would be expected to have no effect. Some polymorphisms result in complete loss of a gene product (10). Several genes known to affect cancer susceptibility include those controlling behavior and cellular functions such as carcinogen metabolism (activation and detoxification), DNA repair, cell cycle, and immune status (10).

The concept of gene-environment interactions is based on the belief that sporadic cancers are due to environmental exposures, and that the genes enable the carcinogen to trigger carcinogenesis. Statistical methods to identify significant interactions might find additive or multiplicative effects. Essentially, these models indicate that while cancer risk increases with increasing exposure, risk might vary depending on the level of exposure. Also, if some protective mechanisms are saturated, different alleles might confer different risks (i.e., an allele might become more important at higher levels of exposures, or an allele at one level could give the opposite effect at higher levels). An example of gene–environment interaction (10) occurs in several studies showing that the effect of genotype is greater for lung and bladder cancer at lower exposures (11,12). The list of environmental exposures linked to cancer includes tobacco smoking, alcohol, diet, ultraviolet and ionizing radiation, occupational toxins, infectious agents, body weight, exercise, reproductive history, and certain medications (13,14).

2.2. Current Technology

Genetic susceptibility to cancer can be assessed by two classes of assays, reflecting either a genotype or phenotype. Genotypic assays determine the sequence variation (polymorphism) in a gene of interest. Phenotypic assays measure variation (result of a genetic polymorphism) in the expression or activity of a particular enzyme (10). Examples of phenotypic expression include the way a cell responds to a carcinogen, the biologically effective dose (15), the penetrance of a genetic trait, the molecular characteristics of a tumor, and behavioral factors. Phenotypes are typically complex genetic traits; relating a single genetic trait to a phenotype might not be possible without considering the other traits. Phenotypes might be affected by acquired traits (i.e., prior exposures might induce protein expression). In a phenotypic assay, enzymatic activity (meaning catalytic activity or levels of the enzyme) is assessed by measuring levels of metabolites in blood or urine after administering probe drugs. Alternatively, enzyme activity can be assessed by measuring carcinogen metabolism in cultured lymphocytes, or by measuring endogenously produced substances such as estrogen and estrogen metabolites (10).

In the genotypic assay, DNA is extracted from blood, exfoliated cells, mucosa, archival tissues, or other sources. Current technologies first amplify a segment of the gene containing a polymorphism of interest using polymerase chain reaction (PCR), although new

Table 2
Examples of Genetic Polymorphisms and Related Cancers

Genes	Cancer
Cytochrome P450s	Lung, breast, colon, liver, ovarian, prostate
NAT2	Bladder, colon, breast
GSTs	Lung, head and neck, prostate
MTHFR	Colon
MS	Colon
COMT	Breast
XRCC1	Lung, head and neck, colon, skin
XPD	Lung

technologies might eliminate this step. The most readily assayed form of genetic sequence variation is the single nucleotide polymorphism (SNP). SNPs can be detected by methods such as restriction fragment length polymorphism, fluorescence probes (quantitative PCR), direct sequencing, oligonucleotide arrays, denaturing high-performance liquid chromatography, and matrix-assisted laser desorption ionization time-of-flight mass spectrometry (MALDI-TOF). Some methods have higher throughput speeds and some are quite costly. Generally, the genotypic assay is the method of choice to assess cancer risk, because DNA is easily obtained from different biological sources and these assays are technically simpler. Moreover, these assays require only small amounts of DNA. However, phenotypic assays may still be preferable in certain instances—for example, when one needs to measure a complex trait.

3. EXAMPLES OF LOW-PENETRANCE GENES INVOLVED IN CANCER SUSCEPTIBILITY

The role of the genetic polymorphisms that contribute to interindividual variation in sporadic cancer risk is receiving widespread attention (Table 2). Many cohort and case-control studies have compared the prevalence of common genetic polymorphism in cancer patients with unaffected controls. To date, gene variants involved in carcinogen metabolism have been the most studied. Genes that influence other aspects of carcinogenesis, such as those involved in DNA synthesis and repair or in the production of sex hormones, are increasingly being studied, as are the genes that affect behavior (e.g., nicotine addiction).

3.1. Carcinogen Metabolism Genes

The biotransformation of a foreign compound or carcinogen is governed by phase 1 and 2 enzymes (Fig. 1). This pathway is intended to convert a toxin (endogenously produced or from an endogenous exposure) to a compound that can be more easily excreted, for example by conjugating to a carrier for excretion in urine or bile. Phase 1 enzymes usually add one or more hydroxyl groups onto a compound molecule, converting it into an electrophilic intermediate that can either bind to a carrier or—because of its reactivity—to DNA or protein. Sometimes this binding to DNA yields carcinogen-DNA adducts that can be promutagenic. Phase 1 enzymes include cytochrome P450s coded by *CYP* genes. Phase 2 or conjugating enzymes eliminate electrophilic intermediates from the body via conjugation to carriers such as glutathione. Several families of phase 2 enzymes include glutathione-*S*-transferases (GSTs), *N*-acetyltransferases (NATs), microsomal epoxide hydrolase, sulfotransferases, and UDP-glucoronosyl-transferases. Polymorphic variants of phase 1 and 2 enzymes may increase or decrease cancer risk depending on the specific enzymatic activity that is being stimulated and the substrate involved *(16)*.

Cytochrome P450, a family of enzymes that catalyze the oxidative metabolism of several endogenous and exogenous chemicals, is expressed differently in various tissues. Thus, this class of enzymes is important to genetic susceptibility, carcinogen metabolism, and metabolism of chemopreventive agents (Fig. 1). Examples are discussed below.

3.1.1. PHASE 1 GENES

Polymorphic variants of *CYP1A1* may be associated with a highly inducible form of the enzyme or enhanced catalytic activity *(17)*. The frequency of these polymorphisms is about 10% in the Caucasian population and 30% in the Japanese population *(11,19)*. Several studies suggest that *CYP1A1* polymorphisms increase cancer in Japanese. This *CYP1A1* variant increases lung cancer in smokers ranging from twofold in heavy smokers to sevenfold in lighter smokers *(19,20)*. Reports also associate *CYP1A1* variants with increased stages of disease and shorter survival for lung cancer patients *(21)*. Furthermore, polymorphisms of *CYP1A1* have been linked with mutations in the p53 tumor suppressor gene *(19)*. However, while most individual Western studies of *CYP1A1* are null, a recent meta-analysis suggested a slight but statistically significant risk (Dr. Paolo G. Toniolo, New York University School of Medicine, unpublished results). Demonstrating

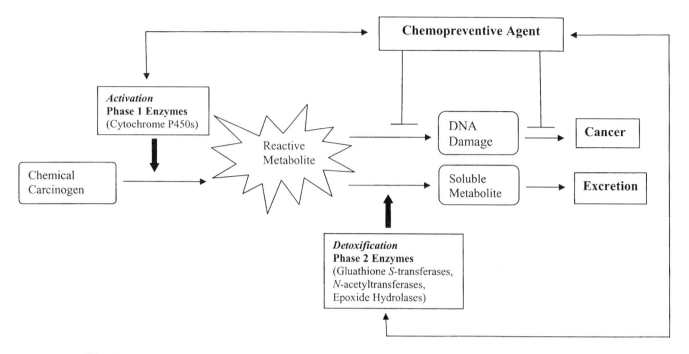

Fig. 1. Carcinogen metabolism by phase 1 and 2 enzymes and interaction with chemopreventive agent.

increased risk in Western populations could be difficult because the *CYP1A1* variant is less common in Europeans and North Americans, thus limiting statistical power, or because different haplotypes among races affect penetrance.

CYP1A2 is involved in the metabolic activation of aromatic and heterocyclic amines. Wide interindividual variations in *CYP1A2* activity have been described *(22)*. To date, no sufficient explanation for phenotypic variability has been found in the genetic sequence, limiting epidemiological studies, but phenotypically the genetic trait might influence the risk of cancers such as colon (in presence of meat consumption) *(23)* and lung (in presence of tobacco smoking) *(22)*. Liver cytochrome P450 enzymes have been shown to metabolize retinol and retinoic acid to polar metabolites, and vitamin A administration has been shown to induce cytochrome P450s in laboratory animals *(24,25)*. Results from intervention trials indicate that supplemental β-carotene enhances lung cancer incidence and mortality in smokers *(26,27)*. Subsequently, it was reported that *CYP1A1* and *CYP1A2* and other P450 genes were activated by high doses of a β-carotene metabolite experimentally administered to rats *(28)*. No studies in humans that address the effect of carotenoids on P450 enzyme activity have been reported, but this might be a factor in paradoxical human findings.

Other P450 enzymes have also been linked to cancer risk. Both *CYP3A3* and *CYP3A4* are polymorphic and have been suggested to modify liver cancer risk in association with exposure to aflatoxin B$_1$, a fungal contaminant of peanuts *(29,16)*. *CYP3A4* polymorphic variant has also been associated with altered metabolism of cancer drugs and increased risk of secondary cancers for leukemia-related treatments *(30)*. Studies have linked the polymorphic variant of *CYP1B1* to ovarian *(31)*, breast *(32)*, lung *(33)*, and prostate cancer incidence *(34)*. A recent study investigating the effects of the chemopreventive resveratrol on a human bronchial epithelial cell line indicates that this agent may exert its chemopreventive activity by inhibiting expression of *CYP1B1 (35)*.

Tamoxifen is widely used to treat breast cancer. It was also recently approved for use as a chemopreventive agent in women at high risk of contracting breast cancer *(36)*. The metabolism of tamoxifen shows considerable interindividual variation, which is probably due to polymorphisms in CYPs, affecting efficacy and toxicity *(37)*. The 4-hydroxylation of tamoxifen is catalyzed by CYP2D6, 2C9, and 3A4 *(37,38)*. The product of this reaction is 100 times more potent than the parent drug. Numerous SNPs, insertions, and deletions decrease or increase activity, especially that of CYP2D6. Because genotypic classification of activity is too difficult, phenotypic assessment of CYP2D6 by such means as administering probe drugs (e.g., dextro methorphan or debrisoquine) more accurately reflects inherited CYP2D6 capacity. Tamoxifen is known to enhance systemic elimination of other drugs and to enhance its own elimination following repeated dosing by inducing drug metabolizing enzymes such as CYP3A4 *(36)*; thus, it can affect acquired traits.

3.1.2. PHASE 2 GENES

GSTs are a family of enzymes that catalyze the conjugation of reduced glutathione to a large number of electrophilic compounds formed by phase 1 enzymes. Because electrophiles can bind to DNA and form adducts that can result in mutations, GSTs play a critical role in maintaining genomic integrity by making fewer reactive electrophiles available for binding to DNA. GSTs are divided into four major classes: α (GSTA), π (GSTP), μ (GSTM), and θ (GSTT) *(39)*. Genetic polymorphisms have been identified in the GSTM, GSTT, and GSTP classes *(40–42)*. Inherited homozygous large deletions result in deficiencies of GSTM1 and GSTT1 activity. Both null genotypes confer a higher risk for several types of cancer, particularly among individuals exposed to sources of carcinogens *(43)*. A *GSTM1* genetic polymorphism has been shown to affect tobacco-related lung cancer risk in Western and Asian populations *(44,45)*. In addition to increasing lung cancer risk in smokers, the *GSTM1*-null genotype also increases risk in nonsmokers exposed to passive smoke *(46)*. The *GSTM1*-null genotype may signal increased risk when combined with *CYP* polymorphisms; for example, lung cancer risk was significantly increased in *GTSM1*-null Japanese individuals who had the *CYP1A1* Msp I genotype *(18)*. A meta-analysis of studies reporting on *GSTM1* and lung cancer risk showed that carriers of the null genotype had a 1.2-fold increased risk among Caucasians and a 1.5-fold increased risk among Asians *(22)*. In addition to lung cancer, the *GSTM1*-null genotype has been reported as a risk factor for head and neck cancers *(47)*. We also know that *GSTM1* can affect the level of DNA adducts in the lung *(48,49)*.

Fourteen studies have examined the *GSTT1* deletion genotype in the risk of head and neck cancer. Six have suggested increased risk; the remaining studies found a weak to moderate association *(47)*. A Japanese study associated this variant with increased chemotherapy toxicity in acute myeloid leukemia patients *(50)*. In another study, the nondeleted variant of *GSTT1* was associated with prostate cancer *(51)*.

The *GSTP1* polymorphism in exon 5 of the gene is associated with a threefold risk of lung cancer in presence of the *GSTM1*-null genotype *(22)*. GSTP1 enzyme is known to be involved in the detoxification of chemotherapeutic agents and is thought to protect against cytotoxic effects of their reactive metabolites. Results from a recent case-control study suggest that inheritance of at least one variant allele of *GSTP1* confers a significantly increased risk of developing acute myeloid leukemia after cytotoxic chemotherapy for other cancers *(52)*.

NATs are enzymes that catalyze detoxification and activation of aryl-aromatic and heterocyclic amine carcinogens, respectively. NAT1 and NAT2 enzymes have been identified in humans; polymorphisms have been found in both *(53)*. The *NAT2* variant, one of the earliest polymorphisms to be described, was first associated with impaired metabolism of isoniazid, a drug used to treat tuberculosis patients *(54)*. Fast or slow acetylators can be determined phenotypically by measuring caffeine metabolites in the urine (this assay also determines CYP1A2 activity), or genotypically by measuring three or four polymorphic sites. The NAT2 slow acetylator occurs in 50–60% of Caucasians and 30–40% of African-Americans *(7)*. The *NAT2* variant has been associated with increased bladder cancer risk, particularly in workers exposed to certain aromatic amines *(53,55)*. Increased risk of breast cancer due to smoking has also been reported in postmenopausal women who are NAT2 slow acetylators *(56–58)*, although some studies have not found this *(59,60)*. Cooking meat at high temperatures causes formation of mutagenic heterocyclic amines. These are metabolically activated by NAT2, and *NAT2* variants are thought to affect the risk of colorectal cancer *(61)* and breast cancer *(62)* by different metabolic activities.

3.2. One-Carbon Metabolism Genes

These genes are involved in a series of biochemical reactions involving the transfer of one-carbon groups, leading to nucleotide synthesis and gene regulation (i.e., methylation). Methylenetetrahydrofolate reductase (MTHFR) and methionine synthase (MS) are enzymes in the one-carbon metabolism pathway; genetic variants have been described for both. Micronutrients such as folic acid and vitamin B_{12} have a great influence on the proper function of this pathway *(63)*.

MTHFR catalyzes the reduction of 5,10-methylenetetrahydrofolate to 5-methyltetrahydrofolate, the methyl donor for methionine synthesis *(64)*. The most common variant of the *MTHFR* gene is a C-T substitution at base pair 677 that causes a substitution of valine for alanine in the enzyme. This single substitution results in lower specific activity and increased thermolability of the enzyme *(65)*. The frequency of the *MTHFR* C677T polymorphism varies among racial and ethnic groups. Analysis of Caucasian and Asian populations typically shows rates of approx 12% for homozygous (TT) and up to 50% for those are heterozygous (CT). African-Americans have a very low incidence of the TT genotype, whereas European Caucasians exhibit substantial variation *(66,67)*. Strong interactive effects have been noted between the *MTHFR* genotype, folate status, and methionine intake. An inverse relationship between the TT *MTHFR* genotype and risk for colorectal cancer has been reported *(68,69)*. The TT genotype was found to be protective for colon cancer, particularly for those with low alcohol and high methionine intakes *(70)*. A plausible explanation for this phenomenon is that reduced activity of the thermolabile MTHFR variant could have a positive effect on nucleotide synthesis by increasing the availability of 5,10-methylenetetrahydrofolate required for normal DNA synthesis and cell division *(64)*. Consistent with this hypothesis, a recent study found that risk of distal colorectal adenomas increased for TT homozygous with low folate status and decreased for those homozygous with high plasma folate *(71)*.

MS catalyzes the conversion of homocysteine to methionine, a precursor to *S*-adenosylmethionine. Vitamin B_{12} is a cofactor for this enzyme. Several polymorphisms in the MS gene have been reported *(72,73)*. The frequency of 2756A-G polymorphism in Caucasians is about 4%. This polymorphism has been associated with lower homocysteine levels and higher folate in a study of middle-aged healthy men in Britain *(74)*. The association of the GG polymorphism and colon cancer risk was investigated in the Physicians' Health Study *(75)*, which found fewer homozygous for the GG variant in the cases than in the controls. The risk was even smaller in persons who drank less than one alcoholic drink per day.

3.3. Steroid Hormone Metabolism Genes

Estrogens, which control activation of genes that affect cell growth and cell proliferation, are known to promote breast carcinogenesis. The biosynthesis and metabolism of estrogen is complex and controlled by several genes. Those involved in the synthesis pathway may affect production and exposure to estrogens. Genes in this pathway include *CYP17* and *CYP19*. Estrogen availability is also affected by metabolic enzymes such as catechol-*O*-methyltransferase (COMT) *(76)*.

CYP17 catalyzes the conversion of pregnolone to 17-hydroxypregnolone. A 1931T-C polymorphism in the promoter region of *CYP17* gene has been described *(77)*. This polymorphism is hypothesized to increase the rate of gene transcription and thus increase the level of endogenous steroid hormone. The homozygous variant for this gene occurs with a frequency of 13% in the population. One study found an increased risk of breast cancer for the *CYP17* polymorphism *(78)*. This finding was not confirmed in three other studies *(79–81)*. In a prostate cancer case control study, white males homozygous for the *CYP17* gene variant with affected first-degree relatives had a significant elevation in risk *(82)*.

CYP19 is an aromatase that catalyzes the formation of estrone in the estrogen biosynthesis pathway. Estrone can be either hydroxylated and catabolized by COMT or converted to estradiol *(76)*. A tetranucleotide (TTTA) repeat polymorphism is present in intron 4 of the *CYP19* gene *(83)*. A possible role for this gene in breast cancer has been suggested in two studies *(83,84)*; both reported an increased risk for carriers of the (TTTA)12 polymorphism. However, others have failed to confirm these results *(85)*. An increased risk of breast cancer for carriers of the rare (TTTA)10 *CYP19* allele also was reported *(83)*. Again, this finding has not been confirmed by others *(85)*.

COMT is one of several phase 2 enzymes involved in the conjugation and inactivation of catechol estrogens *(76)*. A polymorphism in *COMT* leads to an amino acid change (Val158Met) that has been linked to decreased methylation activity and higher levels of catechol estrogens *(86)*. Two studies found a significant breast cancer increase in women carrying the COMT Val158Met polymorphism *(86,87)*. However, one of the studies reported these findings for premenopausal women and the other for postmenopausal women.

3.4. DNA Repair Genes

DNA repair systems correct endogenous- or exogenous-induced DNA damage. These genes have a critical role in protecting the genome from mutations. The efficiency of DNA repair systems can potentially be affected by polymorphisms that alter either enzymatic activity or the ability of a component protein to bind to a necessary protein partner *(88)*. Multiple polymorphisms in DNA repair genes have been identified.

X-ray cross-complementing group 1 protein (XRCC1) is involved in the base excision repair pathway. Recently, three polymorphisms in the coding region of the XRCC1 gene were identified at codon 194 (Arg to Trp), 280 (Arg to His), and 399 (Arg to Gln). These polymorphisms code for nonconservative amino acid changes that could alter XRCC1 function

(89). Individuals with the 399Gln variant have been shown to have higher levels of aflatoxin B_1 adducts and glycophorin A somatic mutations in their erythrocytes *(90)*. In another study, the same variant was associated with higher adduct levels in never-smokers *(91)*. A significant association between the 399Gln allele and lung cancer was found in a case-control study *(92)*. Another study, investigating the association of *XRCC1* polymorphism 399Gln and lung cancer risk in males, associated this variant with higher risk, especially in light cigarette users *(93)*. A case-control study has also demonstrated elevated risk of oropharyngeal squamous cell carcinoma in association with polymorphisms at codon 194 and 399 of *XRCC1*, particularly in current users of tobacco and alcohol *(94)*. These findings were inconsistent with those reported by another study *(95)*. A pilot case-control study of colorectal cancer among Egyptians demonstrated an association between the 199Trp and 399Gln genotypes and disease, especially among carriers living in urban areas *(96)*. The variant 399Gln has also been associated with a lower risk of non-melanoma skin cancer *(97)*.

The *XPD* gene codes for a DNA helicase involved in transcription and nucleotide excision repair. Several polymorphisms in the *XPD* gene have been reported, namely Lys751Gln and Asp312Asn *(89)*. These two genetic variants have been associated with suboptimal DNA repair capacity *(98)*. The 312Asp allele is also associated with attenuated apoptosis *(99)*. A lung cancer case-control study examining the Lys751Gln and Asp312Asn XPD polymorphisms found that both variants were associated with low DNA repair capacity *(98)*. In a case control study of NSCLC, individuals with the 312Asp *XPD* were found to have almost twice the risk of lung cancer *(99)*. Another study reporting on the relationship between DNA damage (DNA adducts) and *XPD* polymorphisms in healthy subjects associated the 751Gln genotype with higher DNA adduct levels in never-smokers *(91)*.

4. IDENTIFICATION OF NEW CANCER SUSCEPTIBILITY GENES

Candidate genes evaluated in previous studies on cancer susceptibility represent a relatively small number of loci, probably accounting for a small subset of actual genes with variants that modulate cancer risk *(2)*. Data from the Human Genome Project is increasing the number of genes considered worthy of study *(100)*. Initiatives such as the National Cancer Institute's Cancer Genome Anatomy Project have already identified more than 50,000 genes and 10,000 variants within these genes *(101)*. It is anticipated that in the near future all genes will be cataloged and their common variants identified.

Identification of new susceptibility genes, however, is still constrained by technical limitations that prevent rapid characterization and interpretation of large numbers of genetic variants. Problems such as the number of assays to be performed, the amount of sample material required, and the cost per individual assay need to be addressed *(102)*. Investigators are currently using several approaches. One is to study candidate genes, usually one at a time. In this case, some investigators limit their studies only to those polymorphisms shown to have a phenotypic effect, while others prefer to assess genotype frequency in an epidemiology study, studying any positive phenotypes. The second approach is to study numerous genes at once, for example using microarray technology, and then mine the data for patterns predicting risk.

Different technical approaches can be used. Of particularly interest is the automated oligonucleotide array technology *(103)*. This technology may be cost-effective for high-throughput polymorphism analysis, since it has the potential to detect thousands of SNPs in parallel. In addition, only small samples are required. Commercially available microarray chips can provide data for about 2000 SNPs. However, this technology is expensive and time consuming, requiring 24 separate PCR amplifications per person, and so is not yet ready for population studies. Another proposed technical approach expands the concept of sequencing by adding fluorescent probes that differ depending on an individual's DNA constitution *(104)*. This assay can be performed in multiplex and also holds the promise of low expense.

5. PERSPECTIVES

Significant data show that genetic susceptibility and gene-environment interaction contribute to cancer risk. A large number of studies have focused on variants of genes involved in carcinogen metabolism and more recently on DNA repair and one-carbon metabolism. Although the biological consequences of polymorphic variation in cell cycle control genes are currently unclear, it is very likely that variants of those genes will have an effect on cancer risk.

Cancer chemopreventive strategies aim to inhibit specific steps in the carcinogenic process before malignant tumors develop. Some chemopreventive agents act by preventing carcinogens from reaching or reacting with critical target sites. Other agents prevent evolution of the neoplastic process in cells already affected by carcinogens. Numerous agents are in various stages of development.

Conceptually, the efficiency of randomized chemoprevention trials would be enhanced by enrolling population subgroups at high risk of developing cancer. Genetic susceptibility data may be a particularly useful tool to identify these subgroups. Different forms of the same genes can result in different dose-response patterns following environmental exposure and affect the degree of cancer risk in the population. Thus, variation in low-penetrance genes may be used as biomarkers in studies of cancer prevention. Selected individuals can then become subjects in appropriate chemoprevention trials. In addition to identifying appropriate cancer cohorts for chemoprevention studies, polymorphic genes could be useful as biomarkers to assess the efficacy of the numerous chemopreventive agents being developed. For instance, modulation of expression and activity of specific enzymes can be used as indicators of an agent's therapeutic effects. Furthermore, genetic polymorphisms affecting the metabolism of chemopreventive agents themselves may be used to adjust the dose administered to each individual.

Incorporation of measures of genetic susceptibility should lead to more rational chemoprevention studies, allowing for smaller samples sizes and shorter duration. Advances in genomics may enable detailed profiling of susceptible subgroups and increased understanding of genetic risk factors with specific carcinogenesis events. A chemoprevention paradigm that includes risk assessment based on genetic variation is both appropriate and timely.

REFERENCES

1. Waldron HA. A brief history of scrotal cancer. *Br J Ind Med* 1983;40:390–401.
2. Rothman N, Wacholder S, Caparoso NE, et al. The use of common genetic polymorphisms to enhance the epidemiologic study of environmental carcinogens. *Biochem Biophys Acta* 2001;1471:c1–c10.
3. Goodman GE. Prevention of lung cancer. *Crit Rev Oncol Hematol* 2000;33:187–197.
4. Harris CC. Interindividual variation among humans in carcinogen metabolism, DNA adduct formation and DNA repair. *Carcinogenesis* 1989;10:1563–1566.
5. Lai C, Shields PG. The role of interindividual variation in human carcinogenesis. *J Nutr* 1999;129:552S–555S.
6. Perera FP. Molecular epidemiology: on the path of prevention? *J Natl Cancer Inst* 2000a;92:602–612.
7. Ponder BAJ. Cancer genetics. *Nature* 2001;411:336–341.
8. Streuwing JP, Hartgre P, Wacholder S, et al. The risk of cancer associated with specific mutations of BRCA1 and BRCA2 among Ashkenazi Jews. *N Engl J Med* 1997;336:1401–1408.
9. Perera FP. Environment and cancer: who are susceptible? *Science* 1997;278:1068–1073.
10. Shields PG, Harris CC. Cancer risk and low-penetrance susceptibility genes in gene-environment interactions. *J Clin Oncol* 2000;18:2309–2315.
11. Nakachi K, Imai K, Hayashi S, Kawajiri K. Polymorphisms of the CYP1A1 and glutathione S-transferase genes associated with susceptibility to lung cancer in relation to cigarette dose in a Japanese population. *Cancer Res* 1993;53:2994–2999.
12. Vineis P, Bartsch H, Caparoso N, et al. Genetically based N-acetyltransferase metabolic polymorphism and low-level environmental exposure to carcinogens. *Nature* 1994;369:154–156.
13. Perera FP, Weinstein IB. Molecular epidemiology: recent advances and future directions. *Carcinogenesis* 2000b;21:517–524.
14. Schairer E, Schoniger E. Lung cancer and tobacco consumption. *Intl J Epidemiol* 2001;30:24–27.
15. Perera FP, Santella RM, Brenner D, et al. Application of biological markers to the study of lung cancer causation and prevention. *IARC Sci Publ* 1988;89:451–459.
16. Rock CL, Lampe JW, Patterson RE. Nutrition, genetics and risks of cancer. *Annu Rev Public Health* 2000;21:47–64.
17. Crofts F, Taioli E, Trachman J, et al. Functional significance of different human CYP1A1 genotypes. *Carcinogenesis* 1994;15:2961–2963.
18. Kihara M, Noda K. Risk of smoking for squamous and small carcinomas of the lung modulated by combinations of CYP1A1 and GSTM1 gene polymorphisms in a Japanese population. *Carcinogenesis* 1995;16:2331–2336.
19. Kawajiri K, Eguchi H, Nakachi K, et al. Association of CYP1A1 germ line polymorphisms with mutations of the p53 gene in lung cancer. *Cancer Res* 1996;56:72–76.
20. Nakachi K, Imai K, Hayashi S, et al. Genetic susceptibility to squamous cell carcinoma of the lung in relation to cigarette smoking dose. *Cancer Res* 1991;51:5177–5180.
21. Okada T, Kawashima K, Fukushi S, et al. Association between a cytochrome P450 CYP1A1 genotype and incidence of lung cancer. *Pharmacogenetics* 1994;4:333–340.
22. Bouchardy C, Benhamou S, Jourenkova N, et al. Metabolic genetic polymorphisms and susceptibility to lung cancer. *Lung Cancer* 2001;32:109–112.
23. Lang NP, Butler MA, Massengill J, et al. Rapid metabolic phenotypes of acetyltransferase and cytochrome P4501A2 and putative exposure to food-borne heterocyclic amines increase the risk for colorectal cancer or polyps. *Cancer Epidemiol Biomarkers Prev* 1994;3:675–682.
24. Raner GM, Vaz AD, Coon MJ. Metabolism of all-*trans*, 9-*cis*, and 13-*cis* isomers of retinal by purified isozymes of microsomal cytochrome P450 and mechanism-based inhibition of retinoid oxidation by citral. *Mol Pharmacol* 1996;49:515–522.
25. Roberts ES, Vaz AD, Coon MJ. Role of isozymes of rabbit microsomal cytochrome P450 in the metabolism of retinoic acid, retinol, and retinal. *Mol Pharmacol* 1992;41:427–433.
26. Albanes D, Heinonen OP, Taylor PR, et al. Alpha-tocopherol and beta-carotene supplements and lung cancer in the alpha-tocopherol, beta carotene cancer prevention study compliance. *J Natl Cancer Inst* 1996;88:1560–1570.

27. Blumberg J, Block G. The alpha-tocopherol beta-carotene cancer prevention study in Finland. *Nutr Rev* 1994;52:242–245.
28. Gradelet S, Leclerc J, Siess MH, Astorg PO. Beta-apo-8′-carotenal, but not beta-carotene, is a strong inducer of liver cytochromes P4501A1 and 1A2 in rat. *Xenobiotica* 1996;26:909–919.
29. McGlynn KA, Rosvold EA, Lustbader ED, et al. Susceptibility to hepatocellular carcinoma is associated with genetic variation in the enzymatic detoxification of aflotoxin B1. *Proc Natl Acad Sci USA* 1995;92:2384–2387.
30. Spareboom A, Nooter K. Does P-glycoprotein play a role in anti-cancer drug pharmacokinetics? *Drug Resist Update* 2000;3:357–363.
31. Goodman MT, McDuffie K, Kolonie LN, et al. Case-control study of ovarian cancer and polymorphisms in genes involved in catecholstrogen formation and metabolism. *Cancer Epidemiol Biomarkers Prev* 2001;10:209–216.
32. Watanabe J, Shimada T, Gillam EM, et al. Association of CYP1B1 genetic polymorphism with incidence of breast and lung cancer. *Pharmacogenetics* 2000;10:25–33.
33. Spivack SD, Hurteau GJ, Reilly AA, et al. CYP1B1 expression in human lung. *Drug Metab Dispos* 2001;29:916–922.
34. Tang YM, Green BL, Chen GF, et al. Human CYP1B1 Leu432Val gene polymorphism: ethnic distribution in African-Americans, Caucasians and Chinese; oestradiol hydroxylase activity; and distribution in prostate cancer cases and controls. *Pharmacogenetics* 2000;10:761–766.
35. Mollerup S, Ovrebo S, Haugen A. Lung carcinogenesis: reveratrol moduates the expression of genes involved in the metabolism of PAH in human bronchial epithelial cells. *Int J Cancer* 2001;92:18–25.
36. Desai PB, Nallani SC, Sane RS, et al. Induction of cytochrome P450 3A4 in primary human hepatocytes and activation of the human pregnane x receptor by tamoxifen and 4-hydroxytamoxifen. *Drug Metab Dispos* 2002;30:608–612.
37. Crewe HK, Ellis SW, Lennard MS, Tucker GT. Variable contribution of cytochrome P450 2D6, 2C9 and 3A4 to the 4-hydroxylation of tamoxifen by human liver microsomes. *Biochem Pharmacol* 1997;53:171–178.
38. Dehal SS, Kupfer D. Cytochrome P-450 3A and 2D6 catalyze ortho hydroxylation of 4-hydroxytamoxifen and 3-hydroxytamoxifen (droloxifene) yielding tamoxifen catechol: involvement of catechols in covalent biding to hepatic proteins. *Drug Metab Dispos* 1999;27:681–688.
39. Mannervik B, Awasthi YC, Board PG, et al. Nomenclature for human glutathione transferases. *Biochem J* 1992;282:305–308.
40. Harries LW, Stubbins MJ, Forman D, et al. Identification of genetic polymorphisms at glutathione *S*-transferase Pi locus and association with susceptibility to bladder, testicular and prostate cancer. *Carcinogenesis* 1997;18:641–644.
41. Pemble SE, Hallier E. Human glutathione *S*-transferase theta (GSTT1): cDNA cloning and the characterization of a genetic polymorphism. *Biochem J* 1994;300:271–276.
42. Seidegard J, Vorachek WR, Pero RW, Pearson WR. Hereditary differences in the expression of the human glutathione transferase activity on trans-stilbene oxide are due to a gene deletion. *Proc Natl Acad Sci USA* 1988;85:7293–7297.
43. Brockmoller J, Cacorbil I, Kerb R, et al. Polymorphisms in xenobiotic conjugation and disease predisposition. *Toxicol Lett* 1998;102:173–183.
44. Rebbeck TR. Molecular epidemiology of the human glutathione *S*-transferase genotypes GSTM1 and GSTT1 in cancer susceptibility. *Cancer Epidemiol Biomarkers Prev* 1997;6:733–743.
45. McWilliams JE, Sanderson BJ, Harris EL, et al. Glutathione-*S*-transferase M1(GSTM1) deficiency and lung cancer risk. *Cancer Epidemiol Biomarkers Prev* 1995;4:589–594.
46. Bennett WP, Alavanja MC, Blomeke B, et al. Environmental tobacco smoke and genetic susceptibility as lung cancer risk factors in never-smoking women. *J Natl Cancer Inst* 1999;91:2009–2014.
47. Geisler SA, Olshan AF. GSTM1, GSTT1, and the risk of squamous cell carcinoma of the head and neck: a mini-HuGE review. *Am J Epidemiol* 2001;154:95–105.
48. Kato S, Bowman ED, Harrington AM, et al. Human lung carcinogen-DNA adduct levels mediated by genetic polymorphisms in vivo. *J Natl Cancer Inst* 1995;87:902–907.
49. Ryberg D, Skaug V, Hewer A, et al. Genotypes of glutathione transferase M1 and P1 and their significance for lung DNA adduct levels and cancer risk. *Carcinogenesis* 1997;18:1285–1289.
50. Naoe T, Tagawa Y, Kiyoi H, et al. Prognostic significance of the null genotype of glutathione *S*-transferase-T1 in patients with acute myeloid leukemia: increased early death after chemotherapy. *Leukemia* 2002;16:203–208.
51. Rebbeck TR, Walker AH, Jaffe JM, et al. Glutathione *S*-transferase-mu (GSTM1) and -theta (GSTT1) genotypes in the etiology of prostate cancer. *Cancer Epidemiol Biomarkers Prev* 1999;8:283–287.
52. Allan JM, Wild PC, Rollinson S, et al. Polymorphism in glutathione *S*-transferase P1 is associated with susceptibility to chemotherapy-induced leukemia. *Proc Natl Acad Sci USA* 2001;98:11,592–11,597.
53. Hein DW, Doll MA, Fretland AJ, et al. Molecular genetics and epidemiology of the NAT1 and NAT2 acetylation polymorphisms. *Cancer Epidemiol Biomarkers Prev* 2000;9:29–42.
54. Hein DW, Omichinski JG, Brewer JA, Weber WW. A unique pharmacogenetic expression of the *N*-acetylation polymorphism in the inbred hamster. *J Pharmacol Exp Ther* 1982;220:8–15.
55. Cartwright RA, Glashan RW, Rogers HJ, et al. Role of *N*-acetyltransferase phenotypes in bladder carcinogenesis: a pharmacogenetic epidemiological approach to bladder cancer. *Lancet* 1982;2:842–845.
56. Ambrosone CB, Freudenheim JL, Graham S, et al. Cigarette smoking, *N*-acetyltransferase 2 genetic polymorphisms, and breast cancer risk. *JAMA* 1996;276:1494–1501.
57. van der Hel OL, Hein DW, Doll M, et al. *N*-acetyltransferase 2 genotype and smoking in relation to breast cancer in the Netherlands. *Proc Am Assoc Cancer Res* 2002;43:851–852, abst. no. 4220.
58. Chang-Claude JC, Kropp S, Bartsch H, Risch A. Active and passive smoking, NAT1*10 and NAT2 genotype and breast cancer risk. *Proc Am Assoc Cancer Res* 2002;43:852, abst. no. 4221.
59. Hunter DJ, Hankinson SE, Hough H, et al. A prospective study of NAT2 acetylation genotype, cigarette smoking, risk of breast cancer. *Carcinogenesis* 1997;18:2127–2132.
60. Millikan RC, Pittman GS, Newman B, et al. Cigarette smoking, *N*-acetyltransferases 1 and 2, and breast cancer risk. *Cancer Epidemiol Biomarkers Prev* 1998;7:371–378.
61. Sinha R, Caparoso N. Diet, genetic susceptibility and human cancer etiology. *J Nutr* 1999;129:556S–559S.

62. Deitz AC, Zheng W, Leff MA, et al. *N*-Acethyltransferase-2 genetic polymorphism, well-done meat intake, and breast cancer risk among postmenopausal women. *Cancer Epidemiol Biomarkers Prev* 2000;9:905–910.

63. Potter JD. Colorectal cancer: molecules and populations. *J Natl Cancer Inst* 1999;91:916–932.

64. Bailey LB, Gregory JF. Polymorphisms of methylenetetrahydrofolate reductase and other enzymes: metabolic significance risks and impact on folate requirement. *J Nutr* 1999;129: 919–922.

65. Frosst P, Blom HJ, Milos R, et al. A candidate genetic risk factor for vascular disease: a common mutation in methylenetetrahydrofolate reductase. *Nat Genet* 1995;10: 111–113.

66. Austin H, Hooper WC, Dilley A, et al. The prevalence of two genetic traits related to venous thrombosis in whites and African-Americans. *Thromb Res* 1997;86:409–415.

67. Gudnason V, Stansbie D, Scott J, et al. C677T (thermolabile alanine/valine) polymorphism in methylenetetrahydrofolate reductase (MTHFR): its frequency and impact on plasma homocysteine concentration in different European populations. *Atherosclerosis* 1998;136:347–354.

68. Chen J, Giovannucci E, Kelsey K, et al. A methylenetetrahydrofolate reductase polymorphism and the risk of colorectal cancer. *Cancer Res* 1996;56:4862–4864.

69. Chen J, Giovannucci E, Hankinson SE, et al. A prospective study of methylenetetrahydrofolate reductase and methionine synthase gene polymorphisms, and risk of colorectal adenoma. *Carcinogenesis* 1998;19:2129–2132.

70. Chen J, Giovanucci E, Hunter DJ. MTHFR polymorphism, methyl-replete diets and the risk of colorectal carcinoma and adenoma among U.S. men and women: an example of gene-environment interactions in colorectal carcinogenesis. *J Nutr* 1999;129:560S–564S.

71. Ma J, Stampfer MJ, Giovannucci E, et al. Methylenetetrahydrofolate reductase polymorphism, dietary interactions, and risk of colorectal cancer. *Cancer Res* 1997;57: 1098–1102.

72. Chen LH, Liu ML, Hwang HY, et al. Human methionine synthase cDNA cloning, gene localization, and expression. *J Biol Chem* 1997;272:3628–3634.

73. van der Put NM, van der Molen EF, Kluijtmans LA, et al. Sequence analysis of the cooling region of human methionine synthase: relevance to hyperhomocysteinaemia in neural-tube defects and vascular disease. *Q J Med* 1997b;90:511–517.

74. Dekou V, Gunadson V, Hawe E, et al. Gene-environment and gene-gene interaction in the determination of plasma homocysteine levels in healthy middle-aged men. *Thromb Haemost* 2001;85:67–74.

75. Ma J, Stampfer MJ, Christensen B, et al. A polymorphism of the methionine synthase gene: association with plasma folate, vitamin B12, homocyst(e)ine, and colorectal cancer risk. *Cancer Epidemiol Biomarkers Prev* 1999;8:825–829.

76. Dunning AM, Healey CS, Pharoah PD, et al. A systematic review of genetic and polymorphisms and breast cancer risk. *Cancer Epidemiol Biomarkers Prev* 1999;8:843–854.

77. Carey AH, Waterworth D, Patel K, et al. Polycystic ovaries and premature male pattern baldness are associated with one allele of the steroid metabolism gene CYP17. *Hum Mol Genet* 1994;3:1873–1876.

78. Feigelson HS, Coetzee GA, Kolonel LN, et al. A polymorphism in the CYP 17 gene increases the risk of breast cancer. *Cancer Res* 1997;57:1063–1065.

79. Dunning AM, Healey CS, Pharoah PD, et al. No association between a polymorphism in the steroid metabolism gene CYP 17 and risk of breast cancer. *Br J Cancer* 1998;77: 2045–2047.

80. Helzlsouer KJ, Huang HY, Strickland PT, et al. Association between CYP 17 polymorphism and the development of breast cancer. *Cancer Epidemiol Biomarkers Prev* 1998;7:945–949.

81. Weston A, Pan CF, Bleiweiss IJ, et al. CYP17 genotype and breast cancer risk. *Cancer Epidemiol Biomarkers Prev* 1998;7:941–944.

82. Stanford JL, Nooman EA, Iwasaki L, et al. A polymorphism in the CYP 17 gene and risk of prostate cancer. *Cancer Epidemiol Biomarkers Prev* 2002;11:243–247.

83. Haiman CA, Hankinson SE, Spiegelman D, et al. A tetranucleotide repeat polymorphism in CYP 19 and breast cancer risk. *Int J Cancer* 2000;87:204–210.

84. Kristensen VN, Andersen TI, Lindblom A, et al. A rare CYP 19 (aromatase) variant may increase the risk of breast cancer. *Pharmacogenetics* 1998;8:43–48.

85. Siegelmann-Danieli N, Buetow KH. Constitutional genetic variation at the human aromatase gene (CYP 19) and breast cancer risk. *Br J Cancer* 1999;79:456–463.

86. Thompson PA, Shields PG, Freudenheim JL, et al. Genetic polymorphisms in catechol-*O*-methyltransferase, menopausal status, and breast cancer risk. *Cancer Res* 1998; 58:2107–2110.

87. Lavigne JA, Helzlsouer KJ, Huang HY, et al. An association between the allele coding for a low activity variant of catechol-*O*-methyltranferase and the risk for breast cancer. *Cancer Res* 1997;57:5493–5497.

88. Miller MC, Mohrenweiser HW, Bell DA. Genetic variability in susceptibility and response to toxicants. *Toxicol Lett* 2001;120:269–280.

89. Shen MR, Jones IM, Mohrenweiser H. Nonconservative amino acid substitution variants exist at polymorphism frequency in DNA repair genes in healthy humans. *Cancer Res* 1998;58:604–608.

90. Lunn RM, Langlois RG, Hsieh LL, et al. XRCC1 polymorphisms: effects on aflatoxin B_1-DNA adducts and glycophorin A variant frequency. *Cancer Res* 1999;59:2557–2561.

91. Matullo G, Palli D, Peluso M, et al. XRCC1, XRCC3, XPD gene polymorphisms, smoking and ^{32}P-DNA adducts in a sample of healthy subjects. *Carcinogenesis* 2001;22: 1437–1445.

92. Divine KK, Gilliland FD, Crowell RE, et al. The XRCC1 399 glutamine allele is a risk factor for adenocarcinoma of the lung. *Mutat Res* 2001;461:273–278.

93. Park JY, Lee SY, Jeon HS, et al. Polymorphism of the DNA repair gene XRCC1 and risk of primary lung cancer. *Cancer Epidemiol Biomarkers Prev* 2002;11:23–27.

94. Sturgis EM, Castillo EJ, Li L, et al. Polymorphisms of DNA repair gene XRCC1 in squamous cell carcinoma of head and neck. *Carcinogenesis* 1999;20:2125–2129.

95. Olshan AF, Watson MA, Weissler MC, Bell DA. XRCC1 polymorphisms and head and neck cancer. *Cancer Lett* 2002;178:181–186.

96. Abdel-Rahman SZ, Soliman AS, Bondy M, et al. Inheritance of the 194Trp and the 399Gln variant alleles of the DNA repair gene XRCC1 are associated with increased risk of early-onset colorectal carcinoma in Egypt. *Cancer Lett* 2000;159:79–86.

97. Nelson HH, Kelsey KT, Mott LA, Karagas MR. The XRCC1 Arg399Gln polymorphism, sunburn and non-melanoma skin

cancer: evidence of gene-environment interaction. *Cancer Res* 2002;62:152–155.

98. Spitz MR, Wu X, Wang Y, et al. Modulation of nucleotide excision repair capacity by XPD polymorphisms in lung cancer patients. *Cancer Res* 2001;61:1354–1357.

99. Butkiewicz D, Rusin M, Enewold L, et al. Genetic polymorphisms in DNA repair genes and risk of lung cancer. *Carcinogenesis* 2001;22:593–597.

100. Fink L, Collins FS. The human genome project: view from the National Institutes of Health. *J Am Med Wom Assoc* 1997;52:4–15.

101. Strausberg RL, Dahl CA, Klausner RD. New opportunities for uncovering the molecular basis of cancer. *Nature Genet* 197;15:415–416.

102. Kwov PY. Approaches to allele frequency determination. *Pharmacogenomics* 2000;1:231–235.

103. Guo Z, Gatterman MS, Hood L, et al. Oligonucleotide arrays for high-throughput SNPs detection in the MHC class I genes: HLA-B as a model system. *Genome Res* 2002;12:447–457.

104. Schaid DJ, Buetow K, Weeks DE, et al. Discovery of cancer susceptibility genes: study designs, analytic approaches, and trends in technology. *J Natl Cancer Inst Monogr* 1999;26:1–16.

13 Design Issues in Prostate Cancer Chemoprevention Trials

Lessons From the Prostate Cancer Prevention Trial

Ian M. Thompson, MD and Charles A. Coltman Jr., MD

CONTENTS

1. INTRODUCTION

The study of potential chemopreventive interventions has increased substantially over the past few years. While there has been a proliferation of reports from epidemiologic observational studies, preclinical studies, and biomarker-based trials, the number of Phase III (randomized, placebo-controlled) trials has remained relatively small because of the large number of subjects required, the long duration of study, and the high cost of these studies.

When Phase III trials are conducted, it is critical that the study design for these trials be carefully planned to take advantage of lessons learned from other studies. In general, there are no perfect trial designs but only relative advantages and disadvantages of such designs. Study leaders should carefully analyze issues regarding these studies, taking into account resources available and the ultimate public health impact of their study, to make a conscious decision regarding each of these design issues.

We have had considerable experience with design and implementation of two large-scale chemoprevention trials that will ultimately enroll more than 50,000 men. These two trials encompass 10 yr of experience from which many useful observations have been made for the development of new chemoprevention studies.

We will use the experience of the Prostate Cancer Prevention Trial (PCPT) to highlight these observations and recommendations.

2. THE PROSTATE CANCER PREVENTION TRIAL—STUDY DESIGN AND HISTORY

A confluence of medical events in 1992 led to an interest in developing a study on the prevention of prostate cancer. These events included the exponential use of prostate-specific antigen (PSA) for prostate cancer screening (and the attendant dramatic increase in rate of disease diagnosis) *(1)*, approval of finasteride (Proscar) for urinary obstructive symptoms *(2)*, the aging US population's dramatic increase in treatment for obstructive urinary symptoms (with the potential that the majority of men may quickly begin taking this medication, and growing evidence that androgen stimulation was linked with prostate cancer risk) *(3)*. Thus, in 1992, a window of opportunity appeared for commencing a study to prevent prostate cancer, a major public health issue. More men were being diagnosed and treated, and an agent with relatively low toxicity that might reduce the risk of prostate cancer was becoming available.

Recognizing this opportunity, the Board of Scientific Advisors for the National Cancer Institute

From: Cancer Chemoprevention, Volume 2: Strategies for Cancer Chemoprevention
Edited by: G. J. Kelloff, E. T. Hawk, and C. C. Sigman © Humana Press Inc., Totowa, NJ

(NCI), Division of Cancer Prevention and Control (now known as the Division of Cancer Prevention, DCP) recommended the development of a study to determine if finasteride could reduce the risk of prostate cancer. A group of investigators from NCI and the Oncology Cooperative Groups were assembled and a variety of design issues were considered.

From the outset, there were a number of major hurdles in study design. Many of these issues can be generalized and will be discussed below. Perhaps the biggest issues were population, endpoint, and management of the "PSA problem." The populations initially considered for enrollment included patients with T1a (A1) disease, various high-risk populations (e.g., African-American men, men with a family history of prostate cancer), or the general population. Due to factors discussed below, the population selected were men over age 55 with no evidence of prostate cancer. The endpoint ultimately selected for the study was biopsy-proven prostate cancer. Most specifically, this endpoint included cancers diagnosed by biopsy over the course of the 7 yr of study, as well as tumors diagnosed at the end of each subject's 7 yr when a prostate biopsy was performed. The sum total of the results of these biopsies in the two arms of the study then were compared between finasteride and placebo study groups.

The final hurdle was potentially the greatest: the "PSA problem." Upon initiation of finasteride in men, PSA falls by 50% on average *(4)*. Elevated PSA is the most common reason for performing a prostate biopsy and obtaining a subsequent diagnosis of prostate cancer. Men receiving finasteride whose PSA is lowered have a decreased likelihood of prostate biopsy and diagnosis of existing disease, which may lead to an erroneous conclusion that prostate cancer incidence was affected. Studies of patients with benign prostatic hyperplasia (BPH) showed an average PSA fall of 50% *(4)*. However, the degree of decrease in other populations was not known and any adjustment that was not absolutely perfect could inject bias into prostate cancer ascertainment. After considering several options, it was decided that an adjusted PSA value would be reported for all participants over the course of the trial. This adjusted value would be monitored by the independent Data and Safety Monitoring Committee (DSMC), and the adjustment periodically reassessed to ensure an equal opportunity for cancer detection in both arms of the study. While the trial was still ongoing, the exact adjustment was known only by the DSMC. However, by enrolling a group of men with a PSA less than 3.0 ng/mL and with a normal digital rectal examination (DRE), it was

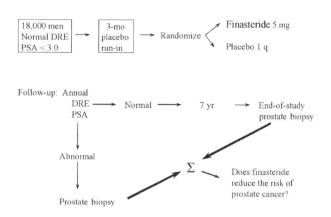

Fig. 1. The Prostate Cancer Prevention Trial.

expected that the majority of prostate cancers would be diagnosed at the 7 yr mark and that this unbiased method of evaluating PSA would preclude bias introduction.

The final design is demonstrated in Fig. 1. As can be seen, the period prevalence of the prostate cancers detected is a sum of those found over the 7 yr of the study as well as those detected at the end-of-study biopsy.

3. DESIGN LESSONS LEARNED FROM THE PCPT—THEIR APPLICATION TO LARGE-SCALE PREVENTION STUDIES

3.1. Biorepository

Many lessons learned over the course of the PCPT might be viewed today as obvious. Unfortunately, what is obvious 10 yr later is not so clear at the time decisions are being made. One lesson was the importance of a biorepository for correlational studies. Because of the key importance of PSA determinations over the course of the trial (small variations from lab to lab could lead to dramatic interinstitutional differences in biopsy rates and cancer detection rates), it was immediately obvious that a central laboratory would be required for PSA determinations. An expensive but reasonable decision was made from the outset that a serum repository would be created. This serum repository was established at Endocrine Sciences, Inc., the laboratory that provided all centralized PSA determinations. Multiple aliquots were stored from each annual blood draw and could be used both for quality-assurance repeat assays (performed prospectively on a regular basis) as well as for future studies of biomarkers, and so on.

Over the course of the trial, it became apparent that additional biologic samples would be of significant importance to correlational studies. One obvious example that affects the primary endpoint of the study, which questioned whether finasteride reduced the risk of prostate cancer, was not apparent at study inception. It now appears that polymorphisms of various androgen pathway genes, including the *SRD5A2* gene that codes for the 5α-reductase enzyme, play a role in prostate cancer risk *(5)*. Specifically for *SRD5A2*, the reported polymorphisms not only have an impact on the response of the receptor to similar levels of androgenic stimulus, but also influence the activity of finasteride, a competitive inhibitor of the enzyme. Thus, based on differences in the gene itself, there is the distinct possibility that different men will experience different effects of finasteride on any preventive activity against prostate cancer.

With the recognition of this and other opportunities that would require genetic material, the Steering Committee of the PCPT took steps to develop a white blood cell biorepository. A considerable period of time was required to navigate the ever-changing seas of consent with regards to such a repository; but ultimately, an amendment to the protocol was published and the repository was established at the NCI facility in Frederick, MD.

3.2. Translational Studies Oversight Committee

From the outset of any large-scale chemoprevention trial, it is strongly encouraged that a committee be established not only to guide but also to encourage translational research. It was a challenging effort to do so within the context of the PCPT because it was expected that these studies were really not possible until the end of the trial. For example, case-control-type studies (e.g., studies that might examine the impact of dietary fat on the risk of prostate cancer), could really not be conducted properly until the study was completed. Issues, such as the fact that the majority of cases were expected at the end of the study, as well as potential unblinding of cases and controls allowing for premature speculation on study outcomes, played an important role in this factor. For this reason, the enthusiasm of investigators with such good ideas was often dampened due to the duration of the trial.

As the end of the study approached, the Executive Committee of the PCPT took the proactive stance of encouraging these translational types of studies. With the support of DCP, an initial solicitation for applications for translational studies has been accomplished with the receipt of a very strong group of such applications. These investigators were assembled for a series of planning meetings to address a number of very complicated issues *prior to* the completion of the study.

Two of the most obvious potential correlational studies of the issues involved the role of polymorphisms of *SRD5A2* and the androgen receptor (AR) on the risk of prostate cancer and the impact of finasteride *(5,6)*.

Four obvious hypotheses related to SRD5A2 and AR polymorphisms are that these are related to prostate cancer risk overall and that they are related to the impact of finasteride. Ideally, at the end of the study, the optimal reporting of the trial's results will include both the conclusions with regard to the primary hypothesis (that finasteride reduces the risk of prostate cancer) as well as the results of these four additional secondary analyses. In order to provide these results in a timely fashion a whole host of tasks are being accomplished in advance. First, the full range of hypotheses must be developed. This requires open-ended thinking and may not include just those related to the primary objective of the study (e.g., related to PCPT, androgen pathway single nucleotide polymorphisms (SNPs), dietary impact, supplement use) but may incorporate other disciplines (e.g., in PCPT, various factors that may affect survival, cardiac disease, or BPH). The second step is to determine how cases and controls will be identified. Ideally, if this effort is prospective, both groups can be identified on an ongoing basis such that upon completion of the trial, their clinical information and specific identifiers of the biologic samples are immediately available. The third step is to determine which of many hypotheses must be tested in the first wave of studies. It may not be possible—either due to resource issues or other considerations—to do all studies at the time the trial is completed. Some translational or correlative studies may be considered at a later time when new scientific methods are perfected or when resources are available. The fourth step requires a determination of what studies are required. An example for this step might be the type of techniques used for polymorphism analysis. The fifth step requires an evaluation of what types of quality control will be required: will the analyses be performed in duplicate? Triplicate? Will they be repeated by another laboratory? Will a sampling QC process be implemented? How will the QC results be folded into the final analysis? Obviously, inherent in making this decision are issues with regard to logistics of sample movement. If, for example, QC requires repeat analysis in a completely different lab, how will specimens be divided and distributed? The sixth step requires a fundamental decision to be made: will analyses be performed in one or multiple laboratories? As, within any given organization, there may be experts on a specific translational technique (e.g., in the PCPT, co-investigators

Table 1
Advantages and Disadvantages of Study Populations for Cancer Prevention Trials

	Advantages	*Disadvantages*
General Population	1. Results generalizable to general population 2. Subgroup analyses possible	1. Larger sample size 2. Longer duration 3. Costly 4. Subgroup analyses may not have sufficient power to have reliable results 5. Recruitment may be imbalanced among risk groups, further reducing ability for secondary analyses
High-Risk Population	1. Smaller sample size 2. Shorter duration 3. Less costly 4. May be used for a scientifically driven intervention	1. Results may not be applicable to general population 2. High-risk population may not be the group that benefits from intervention

who have the abilities to evaluate the presence of SNPs of *SRD5A2*), some form of objective process has been initiated that determines which of these investigators performs the analyses. Such an analysis must be objective and must focus on the good of the trial and meritorious science rather than the preferences of individual investigators. (This step may be the most difficult of all!) Finally, from the outset, our biostatistical colleagues must have intimate involvement in the planning of analyses. Sample sizes, quality control issues, specimen tracking, and types of analyses to be performed must all be determined *ab initio*.

It is easy to see that the logistics of planning for correlational studies of large-scale chemoprevention trials may actually be more difficult than the design and planning of the study itself. However, to extract the greatest benefit of the study for science, this tedious and sometimes unpleasant requirement (upon completion, however, it may be the most scientifically rewarding) is absolutely essential.

3.3. Study Population

A critical issue that must be addressed during the study design phase is that of the population for the chemoprevention study. Various trade-offs that must be weighed are depicted in Table 1. In general, these studies will enroll either a population-based sample of subjects or individuals who meet criteria to realize a specific risk of the disease process. In an ideal world, all prevention studies would be accomplished in the general population. If such were accomplished, it would allow, on the completion of the study and if the study is positive,

a public health recommendation for all individuals at risk. Unfortunately, these types of studies are extremely expensive, require large numbers of subjects, and require many years before results are available, generally due to the relatively low hazard rate of most diseases. Additionally, these general population studies, as they are powered for the primary objective (e.g., does agent *x* prevent cancer *y*), are usually of inadequate size to allow for definitive subgroup analyses. The subgroup with a different risk is sufficiently uncommon that recruitment of these subgroups will be imbalanced when large-scale trials open for accrual. A good example of this is the PCPT. Although it would be ideal to examine the impact of finasteride on the risk of prostate cancer among men with a family history of the disease, only 15% of participants had this risk factor. While this was higher than that in the general population, it is probably insufficient to allow for any conclusions to be drawn with respect to this risk factor.

The PCPT example is illustrative. While there are numerous risk factors for prostate cancer—age, ethnicity, family history, diet, and many others—we decided from the outset that it was desirable to have as generalized a recommendation as possible upon the study's completion. After electing a general population study, however, it was obvious that some sort of selection factors must be chosen. Most important of these was age. In general, when one examines risk of prostate cancer by age, the risk of disease becomes measurable only after age 50 or 55. For this reason, we opted to enroll men age 55 and older. While it would not be unreasonable to have begun the study at an earlier age, every additional 5 yr earlier than this age would actually dramatically increase the study sample size and would probably extend the study beyond 5 additional yr. (The reason for the greater-than-5-yr extension is that with each year, a fraction of patients will drop out, be lost to follow-up, or die.) With unlimited resources, an earlier age limit would be reasonable. A realistic approach to resource availability and a desire to have results within a reasonable period of time led to this 55-and-older age limit. Despite this age limit, the study's results were not expected until 11 yr after the first participant entered the study.

3.4. Selection of Primary Objective and Associated Endpoint

A major decision to be made in the design of all large-scale cancer prevention trials is the primary endpoint and associated primary objective. Again, the PCPT is illustrative of the issues involved in trial design. Options available for prostate cancer included biomarkers, disease incidence, quality-of-life endpoints, metastasis, or survival—either cancer-specific or overall. For each endpoint there are trade-offs.

3.4.1. BIOMARKER ENDPOINTS

Ideally, chemoprevention trials should incorporate validated intermediate or biomarker endpoints whenever possible, because intermediate or biomarker endpoints occur earlier and allow a more rapid (and less expensive) completion of the study. Additionally, there is the possibility that if these intermediate endpoints are reached early, trial participants would be more likely to benefit from the study themselves by incorporating successful preventive measures during their lifetimes. Unfortunately, validated intermediate/biomarker endpoints are few and far between. For prostate cancer, various endpoints that have been suggested include PSA, prostate-specific membrane antigen, other kallekreins, or prostatic intraepithelial neoplasia (PIN) (a putative premalignant lesion) *(7)*. Despite an abundance of evidence linking these endpoints to a risk of prostate cancer, none have been validated. This problem exists for virtually all cancer sites and remains one of the most important opportunities for research. Development of validated markers or the validation of other surrogate endpoints would move forward the science of cancer prevention by decades and substantially reduce the cost of this effort.

3.4.2. DISEASE INCIDENCE ENDPOINTS

One of the most attractive endpoints for cancer prevention trials is probably the most obvious. If an intervention reduces the rate of cancer diagnosis, it would seem to stand to reason that the intervention is worthwhile. There are advantages and disadvantages of this endpoint, however. If it were true that a diagnosis of a given cancer uniformly led to adverse effects for a given patient and if it were known definitively that ascertainment was unaffected by the intervention, such conclusion would probably be correct. Unfortunately, neither is probably correct in most instances. Prostate cancer is certainly the best example for a neoplasm of uncertain biologic impact. There is an ongoing debate currently that calls into question what fraction of tumors detected using PSA and prostate biopsy are of clinical significance *(8)*. Certainly, it is clear that some tumors are insignificant: when a low-grade tumor is detected that occupies a microscopic focus when the entire gland is examined pathologically, and when such a tumor is detected in an older man, the tumor has a potential for *not* leading to morbidity nor causing a survival disadvantage. The ability to identify clinically insignificant tumors currently does not exist.

For reasons that will become apparent below, a process of weighing pros and cons of all endpoints was conducted for the PCPT. Because of the time and resources that would be required for more definitive endpoints (e.g., disease-specific survival, metastatic-free survival, or overall survival), the prevalence endpoint was selected. (The PCPT primary endpoint is the period prevalence of prostate cancer at 7 yr.) Additionally, as it was recognized that a diagnosis of prostate cancer is an occurrence that has clear adverse consequences for a man, it was felt to be an important and meaningful endpoint.

3.4.3. HARD ENDPOINTS—METASTASIS-FREE, DISEASE-SPECIFIC, AND OVERALL SURVIVAL

Each of these endpoints would be almost uniformly acceptable to anyone evaluating the design of a clinical trial. While these are clinically important, they are associated with a variety of disadvantages. All are probably less common than disease incidence and almost always occur later than disease diagnosis. As such, size of the study would have to be increased, along with a longer time of follow-up. Far in excess of 50,000 participants would be required, for example, for a prostate cancer prevention trial that used a survival endpoint. The duration would probably exceed 15 yr.

For prostate cancer, the theoretically ideal endpoint would be overall survival. Thus, if one knew that the prevention intervention being studied improved overall survival, it would probably be defined as "successful" and worthwhile. Unfortunately, while ideal in that regard, there are possible problems with this endpoint.

Table 2
Racial Distribution of Participants in the Prostate Cancer
Prevention Trial

Race	Number Randomized	Percent
Caucasian	17,272	92
African-American	702	4
Other	782	4
Unknown	126	
Total	18,882	

If one thought that there was a possibility that the prevention agent chosen had other effects (for example, if an intervention was selected that reduced the risk of cardiovascular events), there is the intriguing possibility that, because of much greater prevalence of cardiovascular deaths than prostate cancer deaths, a DSMC might find it necessary to close the study when the cardiovascular survival benefit was identified—before the prostate cancer endpoint was reached. Certainly, we could speculate that a variety of potential prostate cancer prevention agents (e.g., reduction in dietary fat, antioxidant supplementation, calcium/vitamin D axis agents) might have this problem if a survival study were conducted.

It is thus apparent that there is no single best endpoint. Investigators must juggle sample size, cost, duration, adherence, advancement of science, and other issues as they determine the optimal endpoint for a specific study.

3.5. Recruitment of Minority and Underserved Populations

It was a goal from the outset of the PCPT to recruit and randomize minority populations into the trial. A Recruitment and Adherence Committee was established with a group of experts to implement steps to achieve these goals. Over the course of the trial, many workshops were conducted to educate investigators and clinical research associates (CRAs) on the importance of minority recruitment and methods to achieve these goals. Additionally, a number of focus groups and small grants were awarded to seek methods to increase minority recruitment. Finally, a Minority Recruitment Manual was published by study investigators to assist individual sites in achieving this goal.

Despite these continuous efforts to recruit and enroll minority men into PCPT, as can be seen from in Table 2, ultimately, 92% of study participants were Caucasian.

From the experience of the trial and our own experience currently during the recruitment to a smaller (10,000-participant) study in San Antonio (the San Antonio Center for Biomarkers of Risk of Prostate Cancer [SABOR]—a Clinical and Epidemiologic Center of the Early Detection Research Network of the NCI), we have a good perspective on what is required for a study to be successful for minority recruitment. (SABOR, by its eighth month of full recruitment, had more than 30% of its participants from minority and underserved populations.)

Table 3 demonstrates the participant population that prevention trials will enroll—as can be seen, they are remarkably well educated. Indeed, their educational level far exceeds that of the general population. The reason is that for an individual to value preventive medicine and desire to participate in an interventional study for this purpose, he or she must be assured of current treatment for medical conditions. Thus, an individual without medical insurance is unlikely to value highly interventions aimed at prevention of disease. Similarly, individuals who live below or near the poverty level are unlikely to similarly value preventive medicine efforts. For them, it is almost certainly a daily struggle just to put bread on the table. The likelihood that they will miss work, pay for a bus trip across town, have a potentially uncomfortable experience (e.g., phlebotomy, physical examinations), and then potentially learn that they have a medical problem when they feel perfectly fine, is unlikely.

The corollary to this observation is that a passive approach to participant recruitment will almost assuredly enroll a population of well-educated, affluent participants. This approach relies on the initial press release and periodic notices or media events. Who reads newspapers? Who responds to preventive medicine updates on the 5 PM news? It is generally the same group of individuals—not the medically underserved.

We have found that the only method to adequately enroll minority populations and the medically underserved requires considerably more effort. It requires that the institution go to the underserved and minority medical institutions, providing clinics where these individuals live and work. Clinics must often be in the evening or on weekends. They must be on bus lines or at centers often frequented by this population. Advocates from the specific population must be recruited. For the SABOR project, we have been exceptionally successful by inclusion of a Community Board of Advisors, including ministers from ethnically diverse congregations as well as public advocates for the underserved and minority populations. These individuals have been instrumental in taking the message to the community.

Table 3
Educational Level of Participants in the Prostate
Cancer Prevention Trial

Highest educational level	Number randomized	Percent
Grade school	258	1
Some high school	553	3
High school graduate	2739	15
Vocational/ training school	846	5
Some college	4603	25
College graduate	3092	16
Postgraduate education	6649	35
Unknown	142	
Total	18,882	

A final observation is key to minority enrollment. The most successful organizations in enrolling minorities to prevention clinical trials are those organizations providing care for this population before the trial began and those organizations that will be there long after the trial is completed. It is understandable how skeptical an underserved population would be of an organization that desires to work with the population only when the organization stands to gain from enrollment into the trial and that disappears after it has taken what it can get. Thus, coordinators of prevention clinical trials should be encouraged to use the track record of institutions for providing care of these underserved and minority populations in the award of status as trial members. These centers are often the most challenged for participant recruitment; they generally are institutions with older facilities, fewer research faculty, little information management infrastructure, and less experience with the conduct of clinical trials. It is for this reason that early and continuous assistance must be provided to these institutions to guarantee their success.

Minority and underserved population recruitment is obviously a complex and challenging process. By adhering to these recommendations and through hard work, however, success can be achieved.

3.6. Importance of Data Management

Because of the sample size required for prevention clinical trials, one of the most challenging aspects of trial activation and oversight is data management. In the PCPT, for example, 2 yr before the trial was expected to end, there were more than 4 million sheets of data in the data archives. In order to assure study success, a well-thought-out plan for data management must be in place before the first participant is enrolled. If this dictum is not adhered to, it will be an extremely unpleasant process to learn that thousands of participants are trying to enroll from hundreds of institutions and that hundreds of CRAs are on the phone to the central office of the study, asking questions, complaining, and wondering if the central office is really competent.

The PCPT relied on data transfer through a fax optical recognition system that allows a document, created in a standard fashion, to be created at the clinical site where the participant is being seen, and then faxed into a central office. In that office, optical recognition programs read the form and populate data fields. A reviewer scans a split screen (one showing the handwritten form and one showing the computer reading of the form), makes edits as required, and then enters the data directly into the database. The advantages are enormous, including a dramatic reduction in storage requirements for data files. For such a system to be effective, data fields must be predetermined and standardized. For the SELECT trial, data entry is completely web-based.

Because of the requirement for source documentation verification during PCPT audits, it was necessary to conduct multiple educational sessions with PCPT CRAs and investigators to ensure that they were aware of the requirement that a source document, containing the information present on the faxed form, be available and maintained at the site for review at subsequent audits.

3.7. Quality-of-Life Measurements

Because of the unique nature of prevention clinical trials, we would contend that the burden of proof is on the investigator to demonstrate why quality-of-life (QOL) measures are not necessary. Recall that participants in these trials are generally healthy and without disease. As such, virtually any intervention with almost any risk of side effects runs the risk of causing a detriment in the individual's QOL. Thus, it will be necessary to compare any benefits from the study's results to any decrement in QOL.

The science of measurement of QOL is complex and beyond the scope of this chapter. However, there are several general concepts that are germane:

• Investigators should consider QOL measures before randomization and several measures over time. There is the distinct possibility that QOL differences may change at different periods—if repeated measures are not performed, the investigators will miss these outcomes.

- Strong consideration should be given to incorporating QOL measures that are both general and disease-specific. General measures include global function, while disease-specific measures, using the PCPT study as an example, might include urinary and sexual function *(9)*.

3.8. Endpoint Review

At the outset of the study, investigators will determine a primary objective (for example, in the PCPT, the reduction of risk of prostate cancer) as well as secondary objectives (again, urinary symptoms, prostate cancer mortality, other cancer rates, etc.). At that time, the investigators should begin the process of establishing endpoint review criteria. While these may appear straightforward, they are not. Let's take the example of the endpoint event of the PCPT—a diagnosis of prostate cancer. By using an end-of-study biopsy, read by a core pathology laboratory, for the majority of participants, we will have a validated endpoint. However, there are innumerable variations on this theme. First is the certainty of diagnosis. If a biopsy is received and read centrally, the endpoint is verified. What happens if the participating institution refuses to forward slides and only sends a pathology report? Does that participant meet the criterion of prostate cancer? What happens if the participant is lost to follow-up and an obituary announces his death due to prostate cancer? What happens if all that is available is a death certificate with its cause of death?

As can be seen, just for the prostate cancer endpoint, there are various levels of certainty regarding the endpoint. These levels of certainty are exaggerated for other endpoints such as cardiac disease, other cancers, and other medical diagnoses. Ideally, at the outset of the study, an endpoints review committee should be established and charged with the development of a set of criteria for categorization of endpoints of importance to the study. Such a committee operates in the PCPT and prospectively determines whether these primary and secondary endpoints are met.

3.9. Flexible Structure

Perhaps most important for a prevention trial is the flexibility of investigators, research associates, and even participants. When one designs a trial in which the final analysis is expected more than a decade after the trial begins, it will not be possible to anticipate all the changes that occur in diagnosis and disease management for the years to come. The DSMC must meet on a regular basis to determine if the essential assumptions of the trial remain valid and whether the study should continue. A group of investigators must be assembled to oversee the conduct of the study; these individuals must be aware of clinical advances in the disease and be able to incorporate changes that maintain the applicability of the study to current practices of medicine.

Over the course of the PCPT, many changes led to the publication of study amendments. They were implemented based on changes in clinical practice, changes in the basic science of prevention and prostatic disease, and recommendations of participating investigators and participants themselves in order to maintain a relevant study for all involved.

3.10. Key-Individual Redundancy

One of the tragic observations directly from the PCPT is the importance of assuring transitions of leadership. The primary endpoint of PCPT is the diagnosis of prostate cancer. In the PCPT, the validation of that diagnosis was made in the Core Pathology Laboratory at the University of Colorado Health Science Center. Dr. Gary Miller, an exceptionally talented individual, was the final authority who established the diagnosis of prostate cancer.

In May 2001, at the height of the period of receipt of end-of-study biopsies, Dr. Miller died at a tragically young age. Immediately after attending his funeral, the leaders of the study as well as NCI representatives met with members of the Core Pathology Laboratory and established a transition leadership. Fortunately, Dr. Scott Lucia, a member of the University of Colorado genitourinary pathology faculty and originally trained years before by Dr. Miller, was on-site and agreed to continue with the trial efforts.

The PCPT was extremely fortunate. If Dr. Lucia had not been available, the study would have been severely crippled. This occurrence illustrates the importance of establishing redundancy of key leadership of these types of studies. History is replete with examples of the importance of this concept. Many historical examples demonstrate how individuals stepped up into leadership positions, achieving the goal of the original leader. Similarly, other examples demonstrate how a lack of such planning led to extraordinary failures *(10)*.

Cancer prevention studies must have a plan for transition of key leadership. Individuals must be identified who will assume and carry on the efforts of study leaders. These individuals must understand the history of the study; they must especially understand the original study assumptions and design as well as the rationale for any amendments over the course of the study. They must have an understanding of the workings of the various executive committees of the study and must be familiar with the other leadership. While such planning should be unnecessary in most cases, its presence will prevent catastrophic failures of the conduct of these trials and is essential when one analyzes the amount of effort required in the conduct of Phase III prevention trials.

3.11. When to Consider the Study Endpoint

In the PCPT, the study hypothesis was that 7 yr of finasteride administration would reduce the risk of prostate cancer. With participant enrollment over a period of 3 yr and with the majority of enrollment occurring during the first year, this meant that when the first man completed his 7 yr of administration, it would be another 3 yr until the results of the study were known. What does this man do during these 3 yr? Does he just stop an agent that he has been taking for 7 yr? Does he request unblinding and then take it anyway? To address this issue, the study organizers developed a short-term extension that would continue individuals on follow-up between the time of the first end-of-study biopsy and the last biopsy. During this period, individuals are offered annual follow-up examinations but do not take study drug (as the initial hypothesis was that 7 yr of administration would reduce the risk of disease).

A better method of developing the study endpoint is to enroll participants until the sample size is obtained and then to continue individuals on treatment until a difference in the primary objective is observed (or is not observed). This requires periodic and regular review of the study by the DSMC. Thus, when the study results are obtained, all participants go off-study and the study is completed.

Of interest, this means that differing lengths of exposure to the study intervention will be present among participants. It allows for some element of dose-effect analyses but these types of analyses may not have sufficient power for a reliable conclusion to be reached.

3.12. Consider a Plan for Providing Intervention to Participants on Completion of Study

If a prevention trial proves to be positive and cancer risk is reduced, the study's executive committee should consider developing a plan for provision of the study agent free to participants at the end of the study, depending on the type of agent and other design issues. For studies that use, for example, nutritional supplements or trace elements (e.g., vitamin E or selenium) that have a very low risk of side effects and that are available over the counter, the appropriateness or need of providing the agent at the end of the study may be less than if the agent is finasteride. In the PCPT, for example, many participants have written that they feel that they should receive the study drug for life if the study proves to be positive. At the very least, the study's organizers should address this issue at the time of initial design.

4. CONCLUSION

It can be readily seen that the design and activation of large-scale cancer prevention trials is an extremely complex process. Not only does the initial design work require attention to detail, but the oversight of the study during its course also requires constant attention to ensure that, when complete, the results not only are accurate but also have an impact on the general population.

REFERENCES

1. Brawer MK. Prostate-specific antigen: current status. *CA Cancer J Clin* 1999;49:264–281.
2. Steers WD. 5alpha-reductase activity in the prostate. *Urology* 2001;58:17–24.
3. Gormley GJ, Brawley O, Thompson I. The potential application of finasteride for chemoprevention of prostate cancer. *Ann NY Acad Sci* 1995;768:163–169.
4. Guess HA, Gormley GJ, Stoner E, Oesterling JE. The effect of finasteride on prostate specific antigen: review of available data. *J Urol* 1996;155:3–9.
5. Makridakis NM, Ross RK, Pike MC, et al. Association of mis-sense substitution in SRD5A2 gene with prostate cancer in African-American and Hispanic men in Los Angeles, USA. *Lancet* 1999;354:975–978.
6. Xue W, Irvine RA, Yu MC, et al. Susceptibility to prostate cancer: interaction between genotypes at the androgen receptor and prostate-specific antigen loci. *Cancer Res* 2000;60: 839–841.
7. Stephan C, Jung K, Lein M, et al. Molecular forms of prostate-specific antigen and human kallikrein 2 as promising tools for early diagnosis of prostate cancer. *Cancer Epidemiol Biomarkers Prev* 2000;9:1133–1147.
8. Prorok PC, Potosky AL, Gohagan JK, Kramer BS. Prostate cancer screening: current issues. *Cancer Treat Res* 1996;86: 93–112.
9. Moinpour CM, Feigl P, Metch B, et al. Quality of life end points in cancer clinical trials: review and recommendations. *J Natl Cancer Inst* 1989;81:485–495.
10. Tuchman BW. The First Salute. A View of the American Revolution. New York: Random House, Inc, 1988.

14 Recruitment Strategies for Cancer Prevention Trials

Paul P. Carbone, MD,* Karen Sielaff, BSN, Mary Hamielec, BA, and Howard Bailey, MD

CONTENTS

1. INTRODUCTION

A prevention trial based on solid preclinical or clinical data may fail without a well-thought-out strategy for recruitment, retention of subjects, and sufficient expenditure of resources. Ruffin and Baron *(1)* point out that less than 10% of subjects identified as eligible for the trials are ultimately recruited. Since prevention trial subjects are well, they may feel that they have little to gain by participating. Concerns over waiting, travel time, costs, and fear of randomization are some of the barriers to recruitment. In addition, failure to recognize the importance of health care providers in recruitment and overly complex trial designs may also delay or inhibit accrual goals. In studies involving hereditary high-risk subjects, participants may not wish to enroll because of fear of loss of employment or loss of insurability.

This chapter summarizes information gained by reviewing the relevant literature as well as providing experience of our own recruitment measures at the University of Wisconsin (UW) in cancer prevention trials. Much has been written about recruitment to cardiovascular prevention and AIDS trials. These trials have a much longer history and the published experiences provide important lessons for cancer prevention trials. A common thematic problem with prevention trials has been a relative lack of recruitment of the elderly, minorities, and the economically disadvantaged. A paucity of information exists as to what the costs of various recruitment strategies are. Ethical issues of using healthy subjects in prevention trials also deserve comment. A common method of identifying subjects has been reviewing hospital charts of individuals who might fit the eligibility criteria for specific trials. Recently new federal regulations, the Health Insurance Portability and Accountability Act (HIPAA), appear to make this form of subject identification more problematic. These regulations and their impact will be discussed.

---

*Deceased.

From: Cancer Chemoprevention, Volume 2: Strategies for Cancer Chemoprevention
Edited by: G. J. Kelloff, E. T. Hawk, and C. C. Sigman © Humana Press Inc., Totowa, NJ

2. RECRUITMENT TO RANDOMIZED CLINICAL TRIALS

Recruitment of subjects represents a key component for successfully completing any clinical trial. The challenge is even more daunting in large-scale Phase III prevention trials. These trials usually involve individuals who do not have diseases but must take medications and undergo examinations and laboratory tests for years. The scope becomes even more challenging when the investigators are attempting to balance gender, race, and socioeconomic status among the subjects. Lovato et al. *(2)* have published a literature review and bibliography of 91 titles on recruitment for controlled clinical trials identified by MEDLINE searches. Rimer has also summarized recruitment, participation, and compliance issues in chemoprevention trials *(3)* that cover important components of cancer prevention trials. In particular, she stresses the role of compliance and how to promote compliance. Prout, in a 1981 review article, stressed three major issues that need to be taken into account in recruitment, using the examples of cardiovascular trials *(4)*. These are problem selection, population selection, and study acceptance. Preparation for recruitment includes building local interest in the participating hospital, visiting local hospitals and medical groups, and informing the general public when feasible. Frequent reassessments are needed to maintain goals, and innovative methods for reviving the campaign need to be put in place. In one of these trials, despite identifying many eligible subjects and receiving doctor consent, only 3% of the total population approached consented to the study and were randomized.

Using a cross-sectional survey of healthy women in a mammography screening center or women with a new diagnosis of breast cancer in oncology clinics, Ellis and colleagues *(5)* surveyed the willingness to participate and attitudes about participation in a randomized clinical trial (RCT). They found that women willing to participate were more knowledgeable about RCT, younger and better educated, and wanted an active role in decision making. Women newly diagnosed with breast cancer were less willing to participate. They seemed to be unwilling to accept the uncertainty of treatment options. Ellis suggests that doctors and the research team need to take the time to explain the trials and the fact that the trial treatments are good therapy.

Tilley and co-workers *(6)* described the details of their randomized trial for treatment of osteoporosis. From a base of 664 screened subjects only 84 (12.6%)

Table 1
Enhancement of Recruitment and Compliance in Randomized Clinical Trials

Major Areas	Approaches
Common recruitment strategies	Advertisements and posters
	TV and radio media
	Direct mail
	Involving community physicians,
	HMOs, practice groups
	Chart reviews
	Tumor registries
	Occupational screening
	Approaching relatives
Compliance promotion	Study reminders to participants
	Reimbursement for extra costs and participation
	Run-in phase
	Improving problem-solving skills of subjects
	Enhancing trust and rapport with study team
Reassessment of goals	Revise plans
	Develop new strategies to overcome barriers

were randomized and 23 (27%) completed the four-year trial. They carefully outlined the barriers, which were very similar to those seen in prevention trials, namely extra costs to the patient, too-rigorous entry criteria, lack of transportation to the sites, too many tests, and poor communication with participants by study staff. Table 1 summarizes results of studies focusing on enhancement of recruitment to RCTs.

3. WHY DO INDIVIDUALS PARTICIPATE IN CLINICAL TRIALS?

Subject motivation is an important component of recruitment (Table 2). Trauth et al. *(7)* have stated, "Although the general public expects and demands that the biomedical community will discover new, safe, and effective approaches to the prevention and treatment of diseases, that same public is not as aware of the important role that public participation plays in the development of medical advances. Yet, it is this population that comprises the potential pool of participants for future treatment and prevention studies." Trauth and colleagues used a telephone survey to measure willingness to participate in a medical research study. Data sets included the respondent's health status, demographic characteristics, attitudes and beliefs about participation, and knowledge

Table 2
Why Individuals Participate in Randomized Clinical Trials

Positive Factors	Negative Factors
Participation related to relevance of study objectives to the subject	Too much time spent in clinics
Altruism	Expense of studies not covered
Anticipation of better treatment or follow-up	Complexity of protocol, tests, and visits
Benefit of treatment	Rigid eligibility rules

about the conduct of medical research. The study indicated that about half of the 469 responders to the survey were willing to participate in research on a new treatment for a specific disease of concern to them, 25% said no, and 29% were undecided. Under some circumstances, such as having cancer, over half of the undecided said they would be willing to participate. Trauth concluded that targeting recruitment efforts to the willing as well as those who are undecided may increase participation.

Hudmon et al. examined the reasons why subjects participated in a Phase I colon cancer chemoprevention trial using a calcium intervention *(8)*. Questionnaires were mailed to trial participants. The study found that the most highly rated trial benefit was the perception of possible benefit for colon cancer prevention. The barrier reported to be the most troublesome was inappropriate or mistaken billing for study visits. Others have noted that two of the perceived benefits include better follow-up and altruism, a sense of helping future generations. Other barriers reported were too much time spent in clinics, and worry about side effects *(9)*. Arnold and colleagues *(10)*, in a lung cancer prevention trial involving smokers, reported that about a third of the participants were involved because they were concerned about developing cancer. Only 15% wanted to participate in a research study as their sole reason.

3.1. Recruitment Problems

Tangrea and coworkers *(11)* reported that the difficulties for cancer prevention trials included patient accrual, adherence, and the behavioral dynamics of physicians with the participants. Attracting racially and ethnically diverse populations to trial participation adds additional problems. Tangrea et al. suggested that investigators should carefully design cancer prevention protocols that minimize complexity, maximize participant

eligibility, and simplify data collection. One way to increase compliance is a run-in phase before randomization. Subjects are asked to take a study medication for one to three months to see if they are compliant, and only those who take more than 80% of their medication are then randomized. This eliminates a significant proportion of the noncompliers.

Another source of problems with recruitment is the loss of participation by too rigid rules for subject exclusion. By trying to restrict eligibility to very high-risk subjects in prevention trials, recruitment becomes more difficult and costly. It also makes results of any such trial less applicable as a public health effort. Britton and colleagues *(12)* reviewed the literature for exclusion criteria in RCTs. Medical reasons for exclusion included a concern for toxicity and the belief that benefit will be small. Scientific reasons included better alternative treatment and excluding those individuals most likely to be lost to follow-up. Some RCTs have blanket exclusions for the elderly, women, and ethnic minorities. RCT research is usually done in universities or teaching centers, resulting in a skewed subject bias (too ill or younger). Participants in treatment trials are usually more severely ill than those who do not participate. In contrast, those who participate in prevention trials are more likely to have a healthy lifestyle than those who decline. Most RCTs fail to document the characteristics of the eligible subjects who elected not to participate. Subjects in RCTs (i.e., eligible and participating) often have different prognostic characteristics from those identified from clinical databases. They are usually younger, more homogeneous, and better educated. Britton et al. state, "Selective participation by teaching centers and sicker patients in treatment RCTs may exaggerate the measured treatment effect. Prevention trials, on the other hand, may underestimate effects as participants have less capacity to benefit."

3.2. Recruitment Experiences in Cardiovascular Trials

Recruitment strategies used in cardiovascular trials are relevant to cancer prevention trials. Two recruitment sources, a random-digit-dial telephone survey and a community media campaign, were used to identify subjects for a primary cardiovascular prevention trial addressing ways to increase physical activity in sedentary men and women smokers *(13)*. Baseline characteristics of 357 randomized men and women aged 50 to 65 yr were compared by recruitment source. There were few differences between recruitment sources for demographic variables. Telephone survey recruitment was particularly successful in recruiting smokers and persons with other cardiovascular risk factors into the trial. The results suggested that the more expensive telephone survey method was useful for locating higher-risk subjects who may especially benefit from increased physical activity but who rarely are recruited through more traditional media campaign approaches. This approach of using telephone follow-up after the initial direct mail proved to be the most successful recruitment strategy used by Rudick et al. *(14)*.

Boles and colleagues raised an important point about recruitment of individuals who are healthy and elderly to primary prevention studies *(15)*. Using their experiences in a cardiovascular prevention trial, they evaluated a comprehensive recruitment strategy using computerized medical database screening, statistical sampling, health plan mailings, and e-mail communication with primary care providers in a well-established research clinic in an effort to enroll healthy elderly individuals in a prevention trial testing aspirin in an HMO population (65 yr or older). Among a random sample of 47,453 eligible patients over age 65, 44% responded to recruitment efforts, but only 3% were enrolled—an overall yield of slightly less than 2%. They then conducted focus groups with 225 randomly selected "eligible refusers" and found that healthy elders were hesitant to give up their choice to use aspirin, unwilling to travel to the research center, and reluctant to risk good health to participate in a study of primary prevention. They pointed out that the elderly-well present logistical recruitment problems.

4. STRATEGIES

Numerous strategies are used to identify subjects and educate the public and physicians to bring attention to prevention trials. These include use of paid and public service announcements in newspapers and television, telephone contact, use of federal agency resources such as the National Cancer Institute's (NCI's) Cancer Information Service, media announcements, focus and forum groups, chart and registry reviews, and identifying potential candidates by approaching living cancer patient relatives (Table 3). Approaching specific populations such as the elderly and minorities also require specific and innovative strategies.

4.1. Radio and Television Advertisements

Most prevention trials involve use of some form of paid or free advertisements and referral from individual doctors. Kaakko and co-workers *(16)* evaluated three

Table 3
Strategies for Recruitment

Strategies	Approaches
Chart review	May have privacy problem
Media	Radio/TV
	Posters/flyers
Mailings	Short vs long letters
	Personal letters or mass mailing
Doctor referrals	Recommendation of practitioners important
	Private practice better than academic centers
	Involvement of HMO and group physician directors
Electoral, drivers registration rolls	
Telephone surveys	Include both the willing and the undecided
Community involvement	Recognized spokesperson, focus groups, churches, clubs
Tumor registries	Sensitivity to privacy issues

strategies in the recruitment of 144 dental injection phobics for a clinical trial evaluating the effectiveness of alprazolam. The recruitment strategies were paid advertising, free publicity, and professional referral. Sixty-three percent (63%) of subjects were enrolled from paid advertising. The authors reported the success of specific forms of advertising: bus advertisements, 27.0%; posters on the UW campus, 20.1%; and newspaper advertisements, 13.2%. Free publicity (e.g., television coverage, word of mouth) yielded 18.8% of enrolled subjects, and referrals from doctors, 14.6% of subjects. The average cost (1996 dollars) of enrolling one subject was $79. Bus and poster advertising attracted more initial contacts and yielded the greatest enrollment. This is one of the rare studies of the costs of recruitment.

Efficacy studies are important for the development of long-term cancer prevention strategies. The Concerned Smoker Study *(10)*, aimed at smokers with at least a 15 pack-year history and bronchial atypia on sputum sampling, used various media sources for recruitment. During the first year of randomization, 905 potential participants expressed interest. Of these, 80 were eventually randomized. With more than 60 participants having completed the study, only one has defaulted and compliance with the study protocol has been high. Participants became aware of the study through the following sources: daily newspaper

36.6%; weekly newspaper 16.2%; television 14.9%; radio 13.8%; community television 1.3%; other sources 13.3%.

4.2. Primary Care Physician Participation

A key factor in encouraging involvement in prevention trials is the recommendation from a primary care physician (PCP). Kinney and colleagues *(17)* evaluated the effects of physician recommendation on enrollment in the Breast Cancer Prevention Trial (BCPT). They surveyed 360 women who were eligible based on increased risk for breast cancer and analyzed behavioral factors that influenced their decision to participate. Less than half of the women *(175)* discussed their decision with a PCP. Physician recommendation was the most important factor that influenced the decision to enroll in the BCPT. Women whose physician advised them to enroll in the trial were 13 times more likely to participate than were women who were advised not to participate.

Wadland and co-workers *(18)* compared the rates of recruitment in a randomized clinical trial for smoking cessation in two primary care practices, a private family practice setting with about 15,000 patients and a six-physician academic medical practice. Enrollment of smokers was 3.3 times greater in the private practice setting than in the academic practice.

McBride and colleagues *(19)* pointed out that prior studies have focused on individual physician recruitment in academic settings. They noted the increased efficiency and utility of other recruitment methods to encourage community practice groups to participate in a preventive services research trial. Primary care practices in four Midwestern states were recruited using different sources for initial mailings (physician lists, practice lists, and a managed care organization's primary care network). Of the 86 eligible practices contacted, 52 (60%) consented to participate. Mailings to individual physicians were the most cumbersome and expensive method and had the lowest response rate. Initial contacts with practice medical directors increased participation rates substantially, and practice recruitment meetings improved both study participation and practice-project communication.

4.3. Mailings as a Recruitment Tool

Gerace and colleagues *(20)* investigated the process of mailing notices to potential subjects requesting participation. They conducted two studies of response rates to specific kinds of mailings for the Women's Health Trial aimed at university employees or women

in the community. The potential participants, 50- to 79-yr-old women, were requested to return an enclosed postcard to learn more about the trial. In the first study, they sent at random either a short or a long message to women who worked at the University of Miami ($N = 862$) or a community cohort from Dade County ($N = 2964$). More university women and the Dade County cohorts responded to the short message than to the long message. This was unexpected, but the authors surmise that the long messages listed details of the intervention, particularly diet restrictions and medication side effects, which women may have used to decide against participating. In a second study, they also examined response rates to two different ways of addressing the mailings, i.e., handwritten envelopes or machine-printed labels. They also evaluated three methods for delivering the short message: formal invitation, business letter with an inside name and address of the recipient, and business letter without the recipient's name and address. Response rates were similar between the methods of addressing envelopes and among the three vehicles used for the message, suggesting that the least costly method of mailing should be used.

Garrett et al. examined different recruitment strategies for the Vitamin E, Cataract and Age-related Maculopathy (VECAT) Study in Australia, a 4-yr, double-blind, placebo-controlled, randomized clinical trial of vitamin E in the prevention of cataract and age-related maculopathy *(21)*. Five recruitment methods were employed: newspaper advertising, radio advertising, approaches to community groups, approaches via general medical practices, and an electoral roll mail-out. Participants (1204) in Melbourne, Australia, were recruited and enrolled within 15 mo (age range: 55–80 yr, mean 66 yr; gender ratio: 57% female, 43% male). The electoral roll mail-out and newspaper advertising were the most efficient methods of recruitment in terms of absolute numbers of participants recruited and cost per participant. Garrett reported the costs of recruitment for the strategies used in his study. These were A $71.53 for using election rolls, A $74.62 for local newspapers, A $241.29 for general practice referrals, A $53.87 for word-of-mouth recruits, A $128.32 for community education approaches, and A $121.09 for radio advertisements. More than 1040 participants of the 1200 recruited came from electoral rolls and newspaper advertisements.

4.4. Telephone Surveys

Another study also looked at telephone survey recruitment. Daly and colleagues *(22)* examined telephone recruitment from an HMO population for a breast cancer prevention trial. A random sample of 203 women aged 50 and older with a family history of breast cancer were contacted. A telephone interview assessed self-perceived risk of breast cancer, willingness to participate, and barriers to participation. Of the 203 names generated from the HMO, 128 (63%) met eligibility criteria and participated in the interview. Forty-five percent (45%) of the eligible women expressed interest in the tamoxifen trial. They concluded that contact by telephone can identify a significant proportion of women who are interested in primary chemoprevention for breast cancer.

4.5. Community Involvement

Evaluation of recruitment strategies is limited for clinical trials conducted in the community setting rather than in hospitals. Turning to the cardiovascular literature, Silagy and co-workers (23) evaluated different recruitment strategies in an Australian community setting as part of a primary prevention trial of low-dose aspirin in elderly persons (aged 70 yr and above). Three techniques were used: recruiting from the electoral roll (by individual invitation using direct mail), local community approach (through retirement villages, local media, elderly community groups), and using general/family medical practice (identifying persons over 70 within a practice and direct mail invitation to participate). The target recruitment of 400 was achieved in 4 mo using the equivalent of 1.5 full-time nurses. General practice recruitment was the most effective method utilized, with a yield of 18.2% at an estimated cost of A $48.36 per recruited participant. The estimated time per recruitment was 13.3 h. This compares with yield rates of 3.4% for the local community approach and 5.7% for the electoral roll, costs per participant of A $42.54 and A $59.37, and hours per randomized subject of 20.4 and 18.1 h, respectively.

4.6. Use of Tumor Registries

Cancer-control investigations in the US rarely use population-based registries as a resource for recruitment (24). A placebo-controlled, double-blind, randomized trial of tamoxifen toxicity was planned for postmenopausal node-negative breast cancer. To achieve the accrual goal of 140 subjects in this single-institution study, Newcomb and co-workers used the Wisconsin Cancer Reporting System (WCRS), a population-based cancer registry. Registry information was used to identify 3585 women who met the study criteria with respect to age, stage, and previous ther-

apy. The status of these women was confirmed using Wisconsin state death records. The names of these women were sent to the primary physician of record with a letter describing the study. The physicians were asked to confirm the status of the subjects and sign letters to the eligible women. Thirty-eight percent (38%) of women who received letters and study information from their physicians contacted the study office about participation. Eighteen months from its initiation, 140 women were entered into the study. This successful use of a population-based cancer registry illustrates an efficient recruitment method that can be modified for other cancer control or prevention trials.

Sugarman and colleagues (25) described the influence of two methods of recruitment from a cancer registry on voluntary and meaningful informed consent. Of 416 women approached to participate, 351 women were recruited by direct contact by research staff; the remaining 65 women were recruited after their physician had sent them an alert letter. There was no difference in the enrollment rate using the two methods. The authors noted that only two or three subjects had concerns regarding confidentiality or felt pressure to participate when physician notification was part of the process.

4.7. Pilot Studies to Improve Recruitment

Many papers have described the importance of doing pilot studies and modulating the recruitment strategy based on pilot studies. The Prostate, Lung, Colorectal, and Ovary (PLCO) study had a total enrollment goal of recruiting almost 150,000 participants at 10 screening centers across the US. All screening centers tested recruitment methodologies during a 1-yr pilot phase (26). The main phase of recruitment was planned to take place over a 3-yr period, though the actual recruitment took 7 yr and required changes in eligibility criteria. One of these changes was to lower the entry age to 55 from 60. Another change was to include women who had had oophorectomies and hysterectomies, because a large number of American women had had concomitant oophorectomies at the time of hysterectomies. A special center was added to enhance recruitment of African Americans. This article points out the need for monitoring recruitment, communication among centers, adaptation of strategies to the local environment, and major increases in financial and public education resources for recruitment.

Development of contingency recruitment plans in cancer chemoprevention research is as important as formulation of the initial plan. Loescher and associates *(27)* found that obtaining recruitment data from early participants in the Chemoprevention Trial of Cervical Dysplasia (CTCD) provided a rationale for a revised plan. The revised recruitment plan consisted of (1) calling and sending letters to community gynecologists in private practice or affiliated with HMOs to explain the study and ask for referrals; (2) continued personal contact by the principal investigator with referring physicians; (3) sending thank-you and follow-up letters to every physician who referred patients to the study; (4) soliciting Pap smear reports from HMOs, if physicians of women with abnormal Papanicolaou smears gave permission to pathologists to release this information; (5) utilizing free media, such as feature articles on the CTCD in local papers, public service announcements, and television spots; (6) continued use of brochures and posters printed for the initial recruitment effort; and (7) continued presentations to local professional physician and nurse groups about the study. The contingency plan has resulted in 100% of the projected accrual, pointing out the importance of getting feedback from the subjects as well as evaluating the recruitment strategies as the study progresses.

5. RECRUITMENT OF MINORITIES AND ELDERLY

The US population has become diversified, with Hispanic and African-Americans comprising significant components and those over 65 becoming an increasing proportion. These populations are not likely to utilize screening tools or participate in clinical trials (Table 4). Several papers have reviewed the problem and have attempted to incorporate solutions for including these populations into prevention trials.

Thornquist and colleagues *(28)* evaluated age and gender participation and adherence rates to protocol in older adults in pilot studies for Carotene and Retinol Efficacy Trial (CARET), a multicenter trial utilizing β-carotene and retinol to prevent lung cancer in smokers. Men and women aged 50–69 who were current or recent former smokers, and men aged 45–74 with occupational exposure to asbestos, were eligible. Thornquist found negligible differences by age in response to recruitment mailings, drop-outs during the enrollment process, or after randomization.

Paskett and co-workers *(29)* identified eight strategies that were important in recruiting African Americans to cancer prevention and control trials: characterizing the

Table 4
Issues Related to Recruitment of Minorities and the Elderly

Issues
Involve members of the target community
Use community hospitals as well as academic centers
Develop culturally sensitive materials
Remove as many cost barriers as possible (transportation, time lost, babysitters, test costs)
Improve staff sensitivity to cultural matters
Involve minority physicians and staff in study
Use of community spokesperson

target population (county population vs hospital patients); involving members of the target population in the process; delivering the message to the target population; giving something back to the population; using a prominent community spokesperson; identifying and removing barriers (costs, transportation, literacy, time lost, babysitting, etc.); improving staff sensitivity; and education of the population of the need for prevention and early detection.

5.1. Barriers to Minority Recruitment

Roberson *(30)* evaluated racial/ethnic participation in clinical trials. Using telephone surveys, African-Americans, Hispanics, and Native Americans in three Buffalo, NY, communities were selected as study subjects. Each of the three groups had cultural factors believed to influence participation. A primary concern was "mistrust of white people" and the feeling of being treated like "guinea pigs." This racial mistrust is echoed in other reports. In a study by Mouton and colleagues *(31)*, African-American women who did not respond to requests to participate were found to have more negative attitudes overall to clinical trials than Caucasian women. The studies showed that about a third of the African-American women felt that the clinical investigators could not be trusted and that they were not going to get better care in a trial. Two-thirds argued that the clinical trials were not ethical. There was also a significant percentage that wanted to be treated by African-American physicians in the trials. They concluded that the major barrier was a lack of trust among African-American women to clinical research. Their recommended solutions were to involve influential African-American community leaders, include African American investigators in trials, and provided better health services for the African-American communities.

Zhu and coworkers *(32)* examined the financial, social, physical, and cognitive factor barriers for older single African-American women as clinical research subjects. Multiple strategies were conducted in 10 public housing complexes in Nashville, TN. Out of 367 eligible women, 325 participated in the study, a rate of 89%. Face-to-face presentation of the study by culturally similar research staff was the most effective recruitment strategy in the higher-education populations. In contrast, telephone recruitment and neighborhood canvassing were the more successful strategies for the working class. Using a local spokesperson to increase the credibility of the study was important. Investigators also stressed good communication and showing compassion and friendliness, making the study more palatable to prospective recruits. Providing small monetary benefits to the women as a token of appreciation also helped.

5.2. Overcoming Barriers

This theme of devising specific strategies for recruitment based on demographics is echoed by the report of Fitzgibbon et al. *(33)*. They analyzed recruitments for two projects; both were part of a nationally funded cardiovascular trial aimed at dietary fat reduction and/or increased exercise among inner-city African-American families or a working-class community. The two populations differed in demographic characteristics. Direct presentation was the most effective recruitment strategy in the inner-city trial. In contrast, telephone recruitment and neighborhood canvassing were more successful strategies in the working-class population trial with a higher socioeconomic status (SES). Although both populations were comparable for cardiovascular disease risks, the differing demographics between the groups made two recruitment strategies necessary.

For the Women's Health Trial Feasibility Study in Minority Populations (WHT:FSMP), Lewis and coworkers *(34)* examined the feasibility of recruiting postmenopausal women from African-American, Hispanic, or low socioeconomic backgrounds into a prevention trial requiring marked reductions in dietary fat. Three centers each successfully randomized 750 women in 18 mo. The three centers contacted 210,000 women of whom 9.2% completed the basic eligibility screens; 65% of these appeared eligible. Overall yield was 11.5%. The greatest source of participants was from mass mailing, followed by items about the study on television and radio, referrals from physicians and other participants, and radio public service announcements.

Recruitment yields were generally similar for the ethnic groups but lower for less-educated participants. The average non-personnel cost for the mass mailings was $124 per randomized participant and $152 for the media campaign.

To enhance the recruitment of African-Americans, several strategies have been undertaken, funded by the NCI. The NCI and the Centers for Disease Control and Prevention *(35)* funded pilot projects to ensure adequate representation of African-Americans in the PLCO cancer screening trial. They include the African-American Men Project, a randomized trial to evaluate the efficacy of three increasingly intensive interventions; the establishment of a minority-focused PLCO trial screening center, a study to identify factors that influenced the decisions, and the psychosocial factors affecting participation and decision making in the PLCO trial. One of these studies, conducted by Outlaw and coworkers *(36)*, attempted to define the barriers and solutions using "a culturally competent lens." They noted that fewer minority discharges were reported in a comprehensive cancer center relative to the racial makeup of the community. Differences in the racial makeup of the physicians and the community contributed to this racial imbalance.

African-American men have a higher prostate cancer risk profile than that of other men in the US. The Prostate Cancer Prevention Trial (PCPT), coordinated by the Southwest Oncology Group (SWOG), is a randomized trial of finasteride vs placebo for preventing prostate cancer in healthy men age 55 yr and older. The study has accrued more than 18,000 subjects, who have a high socioeconomic status, healthy lifestyle behaviors, and better health than the general population *(37)*. African-American men comprised only 4% of the total randomized sample compared to a goal of 8% *(38)*. Several supplemental minority recruitment activities were initiated: minority recruitment presentations at PCPT training seminars at SWOG meetings, distribution of additional minority recruitment materials, engagement of four consultants for minority recruitment, production of a Minority Recruitment Manual, and a small pilot study involving minority outreach recruiters at five PCPT sites. The consultants were helpful in implementing the pilot project and in suggesting and reviewing materials for minority recruitment. The five-site pilot project did not increase either enrollment or randomization of minorities (with a possible exception at one site).

A very successful strategy to recruit African-Americans to oncology trials was reported from

Louisiana State University Medical Center in Shreveport, LA. Holcombe and colleagues *(39)* reported a recruitment strategy that was able to recruit 38% of subjects into treatment and prevention trials in the SWOG. They identified barriers to recruitment to be inadequate time by doctors to explain the study, access to health care, cost, illiteracy, transportation, cultural concerns about clinical research, distrust, informed consent, and noneligibility for studies. They identified possible solutions such as additional support staff, providing indigent care by doctors and hospitals, alternative (nonwritten) consent procedures, community outreach, and simplified consent forms. This paper stresses the importance of knowing the population that is served and understanding and overcoming the barriers.

Using findings from four studies, Brown and coworkers *(40)* examined barriers to the recruitment and retention of minority women to clinical cancer research trials and reviewed effective recruitment strategies. Among the major barriers to recruitment were lack of awareness, lack of transportation, interference with work/family responsibilities, financial costs, negative side effects, and burdensome procedures. Effective recruitment strategies focused on using culturally targeted mass mailings and media presentations based on understanding of the minority community.

6. OTHER BARRIERS TO RECRUITMENT IN PREVENTION TRIALS

Barriers to recruitment include participant issues, physician variables, features of the study design, and characteristics of the health care system in the US. To enhance recruitment, one must understand the barriers that inhibit recruitment.

6.1. Education and Recruitment

Lerman and colleagues *(41)* sought to identify factors that facilitate or hinder participation in a breast cancer health promotion trial that compared breast cancer risk counseling to general health counseling among women ages 35 yr and older who have a family history of breast cancer in at least one first-degree relative Analyses of structured telephone interviews showed that education level was a key determinant in participation. Women with a high school education or less were more likely to participate if they perceived increased personal risk, were employed, had a relative with breast cancer, and were 40–49 yr old. By contrast, among

women with education beyond high school, study participation was higher for women who were married, unemployed, not practicing breast self-examination regularly, and having more relatives with breast cancer. The authors suggested that recruitment strategies needed to be tailored to women's educational levels as well as risk factors.

6.2. Financially Disadvantaged Subject Recruitment

While recruitment of diverse ethnic and racial populations is often considered an important factor in clinical trials, a relationship exists between race and poverty with cancer *(42)*. McCabe et al. mention that poverty is often overlooked and is often integrally entwined with racial factors. The factors that influence recruitment and involvement are access to care, affordability, and acceptability *(43)*. McCabe and associates describe the barriers to participation in clinical trials for the economically disadvantaged as fear and mistrust, cost to the patient, lack of access to the site, and lack of culturally appropriate consent and recruitment materials *(42)*. They describe the approaches needed to recruit low-SES subjects: public presentations of information; developing an advisory committee that includes subject representatives; including minority personnel as clinic staff; assisting in the costs of trials; providing a stipend and travel costs to the participants, off-hours clinics; providing child care and meals, increasing community outreach; and public recognition for involvement. Prevention trials carry an increased burden to the financially disadvantaged subjects (FDS) because they need to be convinced that treatment for remote risk of disease is worthwhile.

6.3. Recruitment Costs

Recruitment costs represent a major portion of the budget for large clinical trials during the initial years of the study. Valanis and coworkers *(44)* monitored recruitment yields of eligible heavy smokers for the CARET at the Portland Study Center. Yields from mailings, measured by response rate, percent of potential participants randomized, and related costs per randomization, ranged from $58 to $169 and varied both by mailing strategy and by targeted population. According to these authors, tracking the recruitment process yielded useful information and allowed adjustment of recruitment approaches and achievement of randomization goals. Other cost-assessment studies were mentioned earlier in this chapter *(16,21,23,34)*.

7. ETHICAL ISSUES

Prevention of malignancy is a relatively new concept in clinical medicine, and little has been written about the ethics of identifying and enrolling eligible subjects in cancer prevention clinical trials. Vogel and Parker *(45)* identified ethical issues raised in the conduct of clinical prevention trials and reviewed ethical considerations that should guide clinical researchers in the design and conduct of this new type of clinical trial. They concluded that the ethics of prevention clinical trials are complicated because prevention lies at the intersection of disease management and health promotion, there are conflicting interests competing in these trials, and multiple values play a role in determining the nature and magnitude of the risks and benefits of cancer prevention. They state that participants in prevention research are individuals who are likely to be healthy. Ethical issues related to these trials (Table 5) are enrollment of healthy individuals (loss of time, expenses of clinic visits, and additional tests), confidentiality in recruitment (insurance or employment discrimination), enrollment of "high-risk" subjects (overly anxious, overassessment of risks), randomization, informed consent, trial monitoring, and competing outcomes and toxicities.

Weed argues that unlike a chemotherapy new agent trial that uses individuals who have failed standard treatments as its recruits, in cancer prevention trials the subjects are not sick *(46)*. He states further that individuals on prevention trials have much to lose and little to gain, the exact opposite of those on chemotherapy studies. Most drugs are not toxicity-free. He then raises the issue of subject compensation for injury for participating in a nontherapeutic trial. He goes on to say that "moral considerations need not focus upon how frequently an injury will occur, rather on...what should be done when an injury occurs." The moral responsibility of the investigator is to minimize the risks. Informed consent or the probability of societal good does not exclude the need for subject compensation for harm. The approach he advocates is paid remedial treatment to bring the subject back to his or her previous state and monetary compensation appropriate to the damage. Unfortunately, few studies, chemotherapy or prevention, are able to offer any kind of compensation.

Tambor and colleagues *(47)* assessed the practical and ethical barriers to conducting RCTs as preventive interventions for breast and ovarian cancers. Eighty-seven *(87)* at-risk women who attended an education

Table 5
Ethical Issues in Prevention Trials

Issues	
Involvement of well individuals	Expense, time, confidentiality, additional tests
Compensation	Injuries, costs of tests, transportation, time
Uncertainty of risk	Causing undue fear, insurability, avoiding misinformation
Data privacy	Safeguards of confidentiality must be in place, access to records, informed consent

and counseling session about BRCA1/2 testing were asked about their willingness to participate in hypothetical research studies for breast and ovarian cancer risk reduction. In addition, 247 Maryland physicians from five specialties completed a mail survey including a question about their likelihood of recommending RCT participation to an at-risk woman. Nineteen percent (19%) of at-risk women reported willingness to participate in a hypothetical RCT of prophylactic mastectomy for breast cancer risk reduction and 17% for ovarian cancer risk reduction. More than half of the women would be willing to participate in nonrandomized trials or registries. Fifty-two percent (52%) of physicians responded that they would be likely to recommend RCT participation to a woman carrying a breast cancer susceptibility mutation. Oncologists were the most likely to recommend an RCT. Tambor et al. also suggest that nonrandomized trials may be a viable alternative to randomized trials for evaluation of preventive interventions using prophylactic surgery for breast and ovarian cancers.

Clinical risk assessment holds great promise for identifying individuals who might benefit from preventive interventions. In the case of breast cancer, statistical models, notably the Gail model, have been developed to assess an individual woman's future risk of developing disease. However, according to Parascandola *(48)*, the estimates derived from these models are subject to substantial uncertainty, and there is controversy over how to translate risk information into prevention and control measures. In light of these uncertainties, ethical concerns have been raised about appropriate use of these models. Potential benefits of individualized risk assessment must be weighed against current limitations of the models and potential harm. The fact that breast cancer is a significant source of anxiety for many women suggests that potential harm from misinformation is substantial. The author concludes that the uncertainties surrounding breast cancer risk assessment warrant caution in the use of such models. When public health officials promise individualized risk information, there is potential for women to place too much importance and trust in these risk estimates. Moreover, use of these models in counseling women about participation in clinical trials should be part of the informed consent process.

"The idea of preventing cancer with a pill sounds attractive to most people," writes Nyrén *(49)*. "Undue fear of cancer—not only among the participants—may be triggered if the information to the public is not formulated with great care. Since prolonged treatment is typically required, the participants' quality of life may become impaired; they may even perceive themselves as already sick." Nyrén adds that "the benefits of the intervention are likely to be small and not noticeable for the individual, who will never know whether he/she would otherwise have developed cancer. But participants who get cancer despite complying with the study protocol will feel disappointment."

8. SUBJECT COMPENSATION

Compensation for injured subjects of medical research in clinical trials is a weighty ethical and moral issue in the UK *(50)*. Guest states that "medical research morally requires compensation on a no-fault basis even where there is proper consent on the part of the research subject." Current patient guidelines of the Association of the British Pharmaceutical Industry make "no legal commitment" to paying compensation for injury to subjects. Guest argues that there is a need for the provision of both adequate insurance and contractual arrangements for payments. He argues that the local review boards should withhold approval of the protocols where such compensation is not clearly spelled out.

In the US, compensation for injury is not mandatory as long as the subject is notified in advance and gives informed written consent *(46)*. Therapeutic trials in the field of oncology regularly serve the dual purpose of expanding existing knowledge and meeting the doctor's obligation to provide medical care. Patient information requirements for consent are strict and include the provision of information about alternative forms of treatment as well as about the absence of health insurance funding and the future funding of further treatment on termination of the study. In the case of clinical trials, inclusion of an insurance contract for the participants is mandatory, and in the case of other therapeutic studies is urgently recommended.

Another issue is the impact of costs to the patient of participating in a chemoprevention trial and the subject remuneration for participation. Hudmon et al. *(8)* noted that remuneration was atypical for prevention trials and that only a third of the subjects indicated that they would participate if they had to pay trial costs for a 16-wk trial of calcium supplements. Three quarters said that they would not pay costs for a 3-yr prevention trial. In many academic institutions, studies done as part of the National Institutes of Health (NIH) grant program can be subsidized by using the federally sponsored General Clinical Research Units.

9. DATA PRIVACY ISSUES

The consent form states that the data will be analyzed and published and any patient identifying characteristics will be cleansed. This assurance of patient privacy has become a federal issue with publication of new standards that may affect subject recruitment and data use. HIPAA created incentives for a public-private partnership to develop and implement standards of uniformity for health care data used in electronic administrative health transactions and standards for the privacy and security of health information *(51)*. The rule states that any identifiable information in any form, whether communicated electronically, on paper, or orally, must not be transmitted. The rule also affords patients the rights to be informed about privacy safeguards and about access to their medical records, and provides patients with a process to correct data in their records *(52)*. One of the most restrictive rules limits medical record searches and use of patient databases. Consent for use of data is restricted to one study and cannot be carried over into another. Melton has stated that this rule, and equally stringent Minnesota state rules, threaten medical record research *(53)*. He speaks on behalf of the Mayo Clinic, which has conducted hundreds of such chart review studies over the years that tie into outcomes data.

Korn *(54)*, in an article that looks at privacy and biomedical research, points out that HIPAA rules restrict access to archival patient materials, especially for genetic information, de-identified medical information, and the need for consent for archived patient materials.

In Phase III prevention trials, subjects will often be normal individuals or those at high risk of developing the disease. Up until now, chart reviews inquiring about the health status of relatives, and mandated public patient registries, have been used to identify subjects. For Phase I and II trials, disease-free cancer patients and or cancer registries have been used to identify subjects. Particularly important have been extensive chart reviews, followed by contacting the patient. HIPAA rules may make it difficult, if not impossible, to utilize these mechanisms to recruit subjects.

10. UNIVERSITY OF WISCONSIN EXPERIENCE

Over the past two decades, UW has enrolled more than 600 subjects in 11 Phase I, II, and III chemoprevention trials using difluoromethylornithine (DFMO), a polyamine inhibitor (55–63). The drug was tested in patients with skin, colon, prostate, bladder, and breast cancer, in patients at risk for these cancers, and in organ transplant recipients. Early studies of drug toxicity, tolerance, and biological activity on human skin tissue were succeeded by more targeted studies of DFMO activity on specific organ tissue such as colorectal, prostate, and bladder.

10.1. Phase I and II Trials

Not unexpectedly, the study with the highest accrual goal also required the longest recruitment period. This Phase II single-site study of the biological activity of DFMO in superficial bladder cancer enrolled 88 subjects in 62 mo. This study was also hampered by the fact that the recruitment was done by study coordinators who had responsibility for many other trials. In a related drug toxicity study performed at seven different NCCTG/ECOG sites, 76 subjects with superficial bladder cancer were enrolled within 22 mo (61). Somewhat surprising was the enrollment of 45 subjects over 15 mo in a Phase II study of DFMO in subjects at risk for colon cancer (58). This was primarily an evaluation of DFMO biologic activity on colorectal tissue where biopsies were taken during two colonoscopies and three flexible sigmoidoscopies over a 12-mo treatment period. In another setting, these highly invasive tests could have been considered a disadvantage. However, in this study they were perceived as state-of-the-art screening procedures provided at no cost to patients known to be at risk for a cancer that is the third highest cancer killer in this country.

In the developing field of cancer prevention, where often the only alternatives to testing of a new chemopreventive agent are lifestyle changes and recommended screening tests, physician bias is rarely a barrier to recruitment. A more likely cause of physician reluctance

to enroll patients is the complex nature of the study (64). Evidence of this was the 49-mo recruitment period required to enroll 45 subjects in a Phase I chemoprevention study of piroxicam and DFMO (57). This two-step protocol involved a 6-mo test to determine a tolerable dose of piroxicam in subjects with a history of skin cancer followed by a 6-mo, three-arm randomized evaluation of treatment (DFMO vs piroxicam vs combination of DFMO/piroxicam) on biological markers in subjects with skin, prostate, colon, and breast cancer or subjects who had a family history of these cancers. While treatment and testing of subjects was not complicated, investigators had to be knowledgeable about changing eligibility criteria and a variety of treatment options.

Another important factor affecting accrual was the priority given by the recruitment staff to accrual for a particular study. In studies with the lowest average monthly accrual rates, nurse recruiters were responsible for patient accrual on multiple research trials. Except for the intergroup bladder study (61), trials with the highest average monthly accrual rates were conducted by staff dedicated to a particular research trial. Overall, length of treatment, number of clinic visits, invasiveness of testing, or randomization to placebo did not affect accrual rates. Free media coverage was accessed via news conferences held by the principal investigator. Recruitment costs were limited to printed brochures, direct mailings, and salaries of the research staff.

10.2. Phase III Trials

Our largest recruitment effort was for a Phase III study comparing a placebo to DFMO in a skin cancer prevention trial (62). A total of 334 subjects with previously treated basal or squamous cell cancer (SCC) were enrolled onto a two-step protocol. Subjects who were 80% compliant with medication during a month-long placebo run-in period were randomized to receive either DFMO at 0.5 gm/m^2/d or placebo for 3–5 yr (average 4 yr of treatment). This double-blind placebo-controlled study began in August 1998 and was completed in the fall of 2003. The primary objective of this study is to determine if subjects on DFMO with a history of nonmelanoma skin cancer will have a decrease in new skin cancers. Secondary objectives are to determine if inhibition of 12-O-tetradecanoylphorbol-13-acetate (TPA)-induced ornithine decarboxylase (ODC) and inhibition of polyamine levels in skin samples of subjects on DFMO will be validated as intermediary markers for DFMO as a chemoprevention agent.

Table 6
Eligibility Criteria for DFMO Phase III Skin Trial

Eligible	Not Eligible
History of basal or squamous cell cancer, Stage 0, 1, 2	Use of hearing aid
Age ≥21 Performance status 0, 1, 2	History of melanoma
Adequate hearing for age ≥4 wk since last chemotherapy or radiation treatment	History of organ transplant Taking prednisone, methotrexate, seizure medication
Signed informed consent	Using Retin-A, Efudex, Accutane, PUVA
Adequate marrow function	Pregnant or nursing

Eligible subjects were those over 21 yr of age with a history of basal or SCC, hearing appropriate for age (based on an objective whisper and finger rubbing test), and laboratory values signifying adequate marrow and organ function (Table 6). Subjects were not eligible if they required a hearing aid, had a history of melanoma or organ transplant, were taking marrow-suppressive, immunosuppressive or anti-seizure medications, were using Retin-A, Efudex, or Accutane, or were pregnant or nursing.

Scheduled study activities included skin examinations by participating investigators every 6 mo; laboratory tests pre-study and at the end of the study; and audiograms prior to randomization, at the end of 1 yr on the drug, at the end of the study, and at any time a subject reported subjective hearing loss. A physical exam was done prior to randomization and at the end of the study. Punch biopsies of non-sun-exposed skin for ODC and polyamine levels were done at randomization, at time of diagnosis of a new nonmelanoma skin cancer, and at the end of 2, 3, and 4 yr on study for a select group of subjects.

All 334 subjects were recruited within a 22-mo period. Initially subjects were recruited from the UW Mohs Surgery Clinic, UW Dermatology Clinic, and the William S. Middleton Memorial Veterans Administration (VA) Hospital Dermatology Clinic. When it was apparent that the rate of accrual was lagging behind schedule at 10 mo into the enrollment period and again at 19 mo, two additional community dermatologists from UW Health-Physicians Plus (a local HMO affiliated with UW) were added as investigators.

Multiple recruitment strategies were utilized, including chart reviews and personal interviews, direct mailings

to potential subjects, and a news conference held by the principal investigator, which received wide local media coverage. Several marketing tools developed prior to study initiation were also used during the recruitment phase.

The most productive strategy was a tedious daily chart review of patients being seen for regularly scheduled clinic appointments followed by personal interview of interested patients. Over 22 mo, approximately 20,000 charts were reviewed for major eligibility criteria, identifying 6000 potential subjects (Table 7). These charts were flagged and the surgeons or nursing staff inquired about patient interest in the study. Ten to 15% of these patients were referred to the research staff. During a personal interview, a thorough explanation was given of the research objectives, treatments being offered, and the schedule of study activities. Eligibility was further assessed and financial considerations were discussed. Successful enrollment via these personal interviews depended, in large part, on having adequate time to provide patient education while conveying a caring attitude. Three hundred subjects (90% of recruited subjects) were enrolled as a result of this process.

When new investigators were added to the study, letters about the study personally signed by the physicians were mailed to potential candidates identified in a physician/diagnosis database. Individuals who were interested in participation were asked to call the research staff. Those who appeared eligible were scheduled to meet with research staff at the time of their next regularly scheduled dermatology appointment. Some letters with a prestamped return post card to indicate interest in the study were sent to patients identified in chart review at the VA Dermatology Clinic. Direct mailings to 786 potential candidates yielded an enrollment of 22 subjects.

A surprisingly low rate of return was experienced when a personal letter from one investigator was sent to 130 area dermatologists inviting referrals for the study. These mailings included a Fast Fact Sheet (protocol

Table 7
Recruitment Strategies for DFMO Skin Trial

Strategy	Subjects Identified	Interviews/Inquiries	Enrolled
Chart review	6000	600	300 (90%)
Letters	786	55	22 (6.5%)
TV news	0	38	12 (3.5%)
MD letters	130	4	0

abridgement) for physicians and a patient brochure. There were four telephone inquiries, but no subjects enrolled as a result of this endeavor.

Sixteen months into the study, after an initial brisk response to recruitment efforts, accrual rates dropped despite evidence that the pool of participants was not exhausted. It was clear that an alternative strategy was needed. Given the NCI report that lack of public awareness and knowledge about cancer trials is the major reason for insufficient accrual, an appeal through the media was warranted. Fortunately, the UW Comprehensive Cancer Center (UWCCC), widely recognized as a research center and very well supported in the community, has an active public relations department that arranged for a news conference given by the principal investigator. In addition to a discussion of the concepts of research, scope of skin cancer, and possibilities for cancer prevention, personal and public appeal was heightened by an interview with a participant in the research study. The news conference was publicized by three local TV stations and in two daily newspapers. The UWCCC Connect Service that screened patients for major eligibility criteria handled the phone inquiries following this media coverage. The research staff contacted potential candidates and arranged for personal interviews and appointments with physician investigators. Twelve of 38 potential candidates were enrolled.

These self-referred subjects provided an opportunity to work jointly with community physicians and insurers not affiliated with UW. Challenges of payment for services and maintaining physician/patient relationships were met with unique solutions. Examinations were provided by investigators without a professional fee and with a minimum clinic charge, acceptable to subjects. A large part of this charge was recouped in the $50 per yr subjects were given as compensation for participating in the study. If questionable lesions were identified on exam and biopsy or surgical procedures were indicated, subjects were sent back to their referring physicians so that insurance coverage of any treatment could be maximized. Good communication between the research staff, investigators, and community physicians is essential to the success of these arrangements. This link with community physicians benefits research by significantly adding to the accrual base and benefits the physicians by providing an opportunity to align with research that provides a foundation for evidence-based practice.

A trifold brochure advertising the study was available in the reception area of all participating clinics,

Table 8
Reasons Given by Subjects
for Participation or Nonparticipation

For participation	Decline participation
Altruism: contribute to medical progress, benefit children, grandchildren	Too much travel
Give back something to the medical system	Dislike of daily treatment schedules
Possible personal benefit	Did not want placebo
Close follow-up skin exams	Cumbersome drug administration
	Expense of travel, visits
	Advised by family against experimental treatment
	Blood donor

from the nursing staff, and was distributed in direct mailings to potential candidates. The focus was patient education about the treatment offered, the activities required during the study, and the possible risks associated with the treatment. Information was given in a question-answer format using easily readable language in large print. In addition, the brochure contained a photograph of one of the investigators that may have been a motivating factor for some patients. A Fast Fact Sheet (abridgement of the protocol) presenting information about the drug, the study schema, and basic eligibility criteria was used as an educational tool for investigators and referring physicians. In addition, visually appealing posters announcing the study were displayed in clinic exam rooms. A letter from surgeons at the UW Mohs Clinic indicating their interest and inviting patients to participate was available in the clinic reception area.

Ultimately, one of 20 potential candidates identified enrolled in the study. This is well within the reported rate of 1:5 to 1:40 in other large cancer treatment and prevention trials. The median age of subjects enrolled was 63 yr and 61% were male, reflecting typical demographics of nonmelanoma skin cancer.

Similar to previous large skin cancer prevention trials *(9)*, the most common reason subjects offered for choosing to participate were a desire to contribute to medical knowledge, to benefit their children and grandchildren, and the provision of close follow-up skin exams (Table 8). Some subjects expressed a desire to repay the system for excellent care they had received in the past and some subjects viewed participation as a chance to derive personal benefit.

Subjects declined participation because of time requirements, dislike of the travel required, unwillingness to take a daily medication, and rejection of the idea of receiving a placebo. The cumbersome method of drug delivery (pouring the liquid drug into a medicine cup, withdrawing the correct dose into a syringe, and diluting it in another liquid, usually grape juice) was too complicated for some individuals. Expense of biannual exams was a consideration for those with limited insurance coverage. As noted in previous reviews of barriers to recruitment, a negative attitude about experimental drugs from friends and family members influenced some potential candidates to decline. Several individuals were regular blood donors at the American Red Cross and chose to continue with this personal contribution rather than join the study. Subsequent to questioning early in the enrollment period, we learned that individuals taking investigational agents cannot donate blood until 30 d after the drug is stopped.

Keys to efficient enrollment were motivated investigators, utilization of multiple recruitment strategies, good communication between the research staff and clinic staff, adequate space resources, and experienced staff. All the investigators had a requisite belief in the important role of research in defining good clinical practice. They understood the scientific rationale behind the study, were willing to propose participation in the study to their patients, and they had a high regard for the principal investigator. While there was no monetary compensation to physicians for successful enrollment, like their patients, they derived some personal satisfaction from knowing they were contributing to medical knowledge and the project provided intellectual stimulation different from their usual clinical practice.

A variety of recruitment strategies were utilized, giving a periodic modest boost to lagging accrual (Table 9). Clearly, daily chart review and personal interviews coinciding with regularly scheduled clinic appointments was the most effective. However, employing other tactics such as direct mailings and media coverage were productive and allowed us to complete enrollment ahead of the projected 2 yr.

Good communication between the research staff and the investigators, the clinic nursing staffs, and the secretarial staff responsible for scheduling appointments was critical. Updating investigators on accrual and progress of the trial acknowledged their important involvement in the study and furthered their interest in enrolling subjects.

Investigators were universally concerned about possible interruptions in their busy clinic schedules and the

Table 9
Keys to Efficient Enrollment

Motivated investigators

Experienced and committed study team

Minimal interruptions of doctors' clinic routine

Good communication with subjects and staff

Multiple recruitment strategies

Adequate space in dermatology clinics for research staff

need for adequate support staff for data management. Space for research activities was negotiated with each clinic. This required some staff flexibility and portability of materials. These accommodations kept interruptions of clinic schedules to a minimum and allowed the research staff the necessary time for personal interviews. The research staff performed all data collection and form completion.

Appropriating funds for an adequate period of protocol development and hiring qualified staff are essential. In this study, the program manager responsible for shepherding the protocol through various approval committees, developing the budget, preparing reports, and overseeing the staff hired a nurse for the full-time position of recruitment and clinical coordination of the study. Experience and commitment are also helpful. Both the program manager and nurse recruiter had long-standing contacts within various groups including the Human Subjects Committee, research administration offices, the UW Hospital Clinical Research Unit, clinical and research labs, and pharmacy. These contacts proved useful in arranging for a smooth flow of events during recruitment and conduct of the trial. Efficient recruitment to this trial and the positive relationships the staff generated with investigators and NCI sponsors reflect an environment that fosters personal commitment and pride in the work being done.

UW was one of 85 institutions enrolling subjects in a DFMO-placebo randomized Phase III trial in superficial bladder cancer. This was a joint NCI/ILEX Oncology Services, Inc. trial, accruing 450 subjects over 33 mo (63). Subjects were treated for 1 yr and followed an additional 3 yr for recurrence. A companion study assessing biological activity of DFMO in urine and bladder washings was conducted in a subset of the UW patients.

The key to successful accrual for this large Phase III study was a close working relationship between the drug company CRAs and institutional research staffs. ILEX Oncology Services, Inc. encouraged investigators to meet accrual goals and sponsored investigator meetings in conjunction with national professional conferences. Paid advertisements were placed in medical journals and media ads were run locally at selected sites. The sponsor also provided reimbursement to subjects for out-of-pocket study expenses. This improved the accessibility and affordability of the trial. One novel approach to promote education and public awareness was the use of a web site for professionals and patients.

The precise impact of these strategies on accrual is unknown. Analysis would likely find that the cost per subject enrolled is considerably higher than in trials sponsored solely by governmental agencies with limited resources. These costs are justified by industry sponsors based on their research goals and stringent time lines imposed on new drug development.

11. SUMMARY

Successful recruitment involves careful planning, monitoring, and restructuring of methods as needed. There is a wealth of published information on how to enhance recruitment and overcome barriers. This chapter summarizes the published data, as well as detailing the experience at UW over the last one-and-a-half decades of cancer prevention trials. The experience of the cardiovascular prevention trials is considered relevant. Appreciating the importance of devising appropriate recruiting strategies for minorities, women, socially disadvantaged, and the elderly are discussed. Ethical issues involved in recruiting subjects, especially the impact of the new HIPAA regulations, are discussed.

REFERENCES

1. Ruffin MT, Baron J. Recruiting subjects in cancer prevention and control studies. *J Cell Biochem Suppl* 2000; 34:80–83.
2. Lovato LC, Hill K, Hertert S, et al. Recruitment for controlled clinical trials: literature summary and annotated bibliography. *Control Clin Trials* 1997;18:328–352.
3. Rimer BK. Participant enrollment, participation, and compliance in chemoprevention trials. *Adv Exp Med Biol* 1992;320:111–117.
4. Prout TE. Patient recruitment techniques in clinical trials. *Control Clin Trials* 1981;1:313–318.
5. Ellis PM, Butow PN, Tattersol MHN, et al. Randomized clinical trials in oncology: understanding and attitudes predict willingness to participate. *J Clin Oncol* 2001;19: 3554–3561.
6. Tilley BC, Peterson EL, Kleerekoper M, et al. Designing clinical trials of treatment for osteoporosis: recruitment and follow-up. *Calcif Tissue Int* 1990;47:327–331.
7. Trauth JM, Musa D, Siminoff L, et al. Public attitudes regarding willingness to participate in medical research studies. *J Health Soc Policy* 2000;12:23–43.
8. Hudmon KS, Stoltzfus C, Chamberlain RM, et al. Participants' perceptions of a Phase I colon cancer chemoprevention trial. *Control Clin Trials* 1996;17:494–508.
9. Tangrea JA, Adrianza ME, Helsel WE. Patients' perceptions on participation in a cancer chemoprevention trial. *Cancer Epidemiol Biomarkers Prev* 1992;1:325–330.
10. Arnold A, Johnstone B, Stoskopf B, et al. Recruitment for an efficacy study in chemoprevention—the concerned smoker study. *Prev Med* 1989;18:700–710.
11. Tangrea JA. Patient participation and compliance in cancer chemoprevention trials: issues and concerns. *Proc Soc Exp Biol Med* 1997;216:260–265.
12. Britton A, McKee M, Black N, et al. Threats to applicability of randomised trials: exclusions and selective participation. *J Health Serv Res Policy* 1999;4:112–121.
13. King AC, Harris RB, Haskell WL. Effect of recruitment strategy on types of subjects entered into a primary prevention clinical trial. *Ann Epidemiol* 1994;4:312–320.
14. Rudick C, Anthonisen NR, Manfreda J. Recruiting healthy participants for a large clinical trial. *Control Clin Trials* 1993;14:68S–79S.
15. Boles M, Getchell WS, Feldman G, et al. Primary prevention studies and the healthy elderly: evaluating barriers to recruitment. *J Community Health* 2000;25:279–292.
16. Kaakko T, Murtomaa H, Milgrom P, et al. Recruiting phobic research subjects: effectiveness and cost. *Anesth Prog* 2001;48:3–8.
17. Kinney AY, Richards C, Vernon SW, Vogel VG. The effect of physician recommendation on enrollment in the breast cancer chemoprevention trial. *Prev Med* 1998;27:713–719.
18. Wadland WC, Hughes JR, Secker-Walker RH, et al. Recruitment in a primary care trial on smoking cessation. *Fam Med* 1990;22:201–204.
19. McBride PE, Massoth KM, Underbakke G, et al. Recruitment of private practices for primary care research: experience in a preventive services clinical trial. *J Fam Pract* 1996; 43:389–395.
20. Gerace TA, George VA, Arango IG. Response rates to six recruitment mailing formats and two messages about a nutrition program for women 50–79 years old. *Control Clin Trials* 1995;16:422–431.
21. Garrett SK, Thomas AP, Cicuttini F, et al. Community-based recruitment strategies for a longitudinal interventional study: the VECAT experience. *J Clin Epidemiol* 2000;53:541–548.
22. Daly M, Seay J, Balshem A, et al. Feasibility of a telephone survey to recruit health maintenance organization members into a tamoxifen chemoprevention trial. *Cancer Epidemiol Biomarkers Prev* 1992;1:413–416.
23. Silagy CA, Campion K, McNeil JJ, et al. Comparison of recruitment strategies for a large-scale clinical trial in the elderly. *J Clin Epidemiol* 1991;44:1105–1114.
24. Newcomb PA, Love RR, Phillips JL, Buckmaster BJ. Using a population-based cancer registry for recruitment in a pilot cancer control study. *Prev Med* 1990;19:61–65.
25. Sugarman J, Regan K, Parker B, et al. Ethical ramifications of alternative means of recruiting research participants from cancer registries. *Cancer* 1999;86:647–651.
26. Simpson NK, Johnson CC, Ogden SL, et al. Recruitment strategies in the prostate, lung, colorectal and ovarian (PLCO) cancer screening trial: the first six years. *Control Clin Trials* 2000;21:356S–378S.
27. Loescher LJ, Graham VE, Aickin M, et al. Development of a contingency recruitment plan for a Phase III chemopreven-

tion trial of cervical dysplasia. *Prog Clin Biol Res* 1990;339: 151–163.

28. Thornquist MD, Patrick DL, Omenn GS. Participation and adherence among older men and women recruited to the beta-carotene and retinol efficacy trial (CARET). *Gerontologist* 1991;31:593–597.

29. Paskett ED, DeGraffinreid C, Tatum CM, Margitic SE. The recruitment of African-Americans to cancer prevention and control studies. Prev Med 1996;25:547–553.

30. Roberson NL. Clinical trial participation. Viewpoints from racial/ethnic groups. *Cancer* 1994;74:2687–2691.

31. Mouton CP, Harris S, Rovi S, et al. Barriers to black women's participation in cancer clinical trials. *J Natl Med Assoc* 1997;89:721–727.

32. Zhu K, Hunter S, Bernard LJ, et al. Recruiting elderly African-American women in cancer prevention and control studies: a multifaceted approach and its effectiveness. *J Natl Med Assoc* 2000;92:169–175.

33. Fitzgibbon ML, Prewitt TE, Blackman LR, et al. Quantitative assessment of recruitment efforts for prevention trials in two diverse black populations. *Prev Med* 1998;27:838–845.

34. Lewis CE, George V, Fouad M, et al. Recruitment strategies in the women's health trial: feasibility study in minority populations. WHT:FSMP Investigators Group. *Control Clin Trials* 1998;19:461–476.

35. Stallings FL, Ford ME, Simpson NK, et al. Black participation in the prostate, lung, colorectal and ovarian (PLCO) cancer screening trial. *Control Clin Trials* 2000;21:379S–389S.

36. Outlaw FH, Bourjolly JN, Barg FK. A study on recruitment of black Americans into clinical trials through a cultural competence lens. *Cancer Nurs* 2000;23:444–451.

37. Moinpour CM, Lovato LC, Thompson IM Jr, et al. Profile of men randomized to the prostate cancer prevention trial: baseline health-related quality of life, urinary and sexual functioning, and health behaviors. *J Clin Oncol* 2000;18: 1942–1953.

38. Moinpour CM, Atkinson JO, Thomas SM, et al. Minority recruitment in the prostate cancer prevention trial. *Ann Epidemiol* 2000;10:S85–S91.

39. Holcombe RF, Jacobson J, Li A, Moinpour CM. Inclusion of black Americans in oncology clinical trials: the Louisiana State University Medical Center experience. *Am J Clin Oncol* 1998;22:18–21.

40. Brown DR, Fouad MN, Basen-Engquist K, Tortolero-Luna G. Recruitment and retention of minority women in cancer screening, prevention, and treatment trials. *Ann Epidemiol* 2000;10:S13–S21.

41. Lerman C, Rimer BK, Daly M, et al. Recruiting high risk women into a breast cancer health promotion trial. *Cancer Epidemiol Biomarkers Prev* 1994;3:271–276.

42. McCabe MS, Varricchio CG, Padberg RM. Efforts to recruit the economically disadvantaged to national clinical trials. *Semin Oncol Nurs* 1994;10:123–129.

43. Petchers MK, Milligan SE. Access to health care in a black urban elderly population. *Gerontologist* 1988;28:213–217.

44. Valanis B, Blank J, Glass A. Mailing strategies and costs of recruiting heavy smokers in CARET, a large chemoprevention trial. *Control Clin Trials* 1998;19:25–38.

45. Vogel VG, Parker LS. Ethical issues of chemoprevention clinical trials. *Cancer Control* 1997;4:142–149.

46. Weed DL. Ethics and chemoprevention research. *Semin Oncol* 1983;10:355–359.

47. Tambor ES, Bernhardt BA, Geller G, et al. Should women at increased risk for breast and ovarian cancer be randomized to prophylactic surgery? An ethical and empirical assessment. *J Womens Health Gend Based Med* 2000;9:223–233.

48. Parascandola M. Ethics and breast cancer risk assessment. *Ann Epidemiol* 2000;10:461.

49. Nyrén O. Chemoprevention trials in cancer research—ethical considerations. *Acta Oncol* 1998;37:235–239.

50. Guest S. Compensation for subjects of medical research: the moral rights of patients and the power of research ethics committees. *J Med Ethics* 1997;23:181–185.

51. Fitzmaurice JM. A new twist in US health care data standards development: adoption of electronic health care transactions standards for administrative simplification. *Int J Med Inform* 1998;48:19–28.

52. Gostin LO. National health information privacy: regulations under the health insurance portability and accountability act. *JAMA* 2001;285:3015–3021.

53. Melton LJ III. The threat to medical-records research. *N Engl J Med* 1997;337:1466–1470.

54. Korn D. Medical information privacy and the conduct of biomedical research. *Acad Med* 2000;75:963–968.

55. Loprinzi CL, Love RR, Therneau TM, Verma AK. Inhibition of human skin ornithine decarboxylase activity by alpha-difluoromethylornithine. *Cancer Ther Control* 1989;1: 75–80.

56. Love RR, Carbone PP, Verma AK, et al. Randomized Phase I chemoprevention dose-seeking study of alpha-difluoromethylornithine. *J Natl Cancer Inst* 1993;85:732–737.

57. Carbone PP, Douglas JA, Larson PO, et al. Phase I chemoprevention study of piroxicam and alpha-difluoromethylornithine. *Cancer Epidemiol Biomarkers Prev* 1998;7: 907–912.

58. Love RR, Jacoby R, Newton MA, et al. A randomized, placebo-controlled trial of low-dose alpha-difluoromethylornithine in individuals at risk for colorectal cancer. *Cancer Epidemiol Biomarkers Prev* 1998;7:989–992.

59. Messing EM, Love RR, Tutsch KD, et al. Low-dose difluoromethylornithine and polyamine levels in human prostate tissue. *J Natl Cancer Inst* 1999;91:1416–1417.

60. Carbone PP, Pirsch JD, Thomas JP, et al. Phase I chemoprevention study of difluoromethylornithine in subjects with organ transplants. *Cancer Epidemiol Biomarkers Prev* 2001;10:657–661.

61. Loprinzi CL, Messing EM, O'Fallon JR, et al. Toxicity evaluation of difluoromethylornithine: doses for chemoprevention trials. *Cancer Epidemiol Biomarkers Prev* 1996;5: 371–374.

62. Carbone PP. Chemoprevention of skin cancers with DFMO: a controlled, randomized clinical trial (NCI Contract no. U01-CA-77158) (personal communication), 2001.

63. Carbone PP. Phase III randomized, double-blind study of DFMO vs placebo in low-grade superficial bladder cancer (NCI Contract no. N01-CN-25434-01-Phase C) (personal communication), 2001.

64. Mansour EG. Barriers to clinical trials. Part III: knowledge and attitudes of health care providers. *Cancer* 1994;74: 2672–2675.

II   CANCER CHEMOPREVENTION AT MAJOR CANCER TARGET SITES

Prostate

15 Prostate Cancer Prevention

*William G. Nelson, MD, PhD, Angelo M. de Marzo, MD, PhD,
and Scott M. Lippman, MD*

CONTENTS

1. INTRODUCTION

Prostate cancer, one of the most significant health threats for aging men in the developed world, is the second most common cancer in United States (US) men, who have a 1 in 6 lifetime risk of a prostate cancer diagnosis and a 1 in 30 lifetime risk of prostate cancer death *(1)*. Over the past decade, increased use of serum prostate-specific antigen (PSA) testing for prostate cancer screening has increased the fraction of men diagnosed with localized prostate cancer; concomitantly, prostate cancer mortality rates have begun to fall *(1–3)*. Despite this progress, approx 189,000 prostate cancer diagnoses and 30,200 prostate cancer deaths were anticipated in the US in 2002 *(1)*. Prostate cancer incidence and mortality rates differ substantially among various ethnic groups, with African-American men having the highest rates in the world.

As these data suggest, the genetic, environmental, nutritional, and biologic variables of this disease are not well understood. Important psychosocial and quality-of-life consequences of the disease process and its treatment add to the burden of prostate cancer on public health.

Accumulating insights into the epidemiology, genetics, and molecular pathogenesis of prostate cancer all strongly suggest that it may be one of the most preventable of all human cancers. In this chapter, we review epidemiological evidence implicating such environment and lifestyle factors as diet and prostate inflammation in the etiology of prostate cancer; we present recent advances in efforts to identify and characterize prostate cancer susceptibility genes; and we examine emerging concepts in the molecular pathogenesis of prostate cancer, particularly the effect of prostate inflammation and loss of carcinogen

From: Cancer Chemoprevention, Volume 2: Strategies for Cancer Chemoprevention
Edited by: G. J. Kelloff, E. T. Hawk, and C. C. Sigman © Humana Press Inc., Totowa, NJ

detoxification capacity, to neoplastic transformation and malignant prostate cancer progression. After exploring the mechanisms underlying prostatic carcinogenesis, we consider opportunities for discovering, developing, and testing new prostate cancer prevention strategies.

2. DIET AND PROSTATE CANCER DEVELOPMENT

Geographic epidemiology data support a major role for environment and lifestyle in prostate cancer development. Prostate cancer risk varies greatly in different regions of the world, with high rates of incidence and mortality consistently reported for the US and Western Europe, and low rates of morbidity and mortality reported for most of Asia (4). Furthermore, men who immigrate from low prostate cancer risk regions to high-risk regions tend to adopt higher prostate cancer risks; for example, Asian immigrants to North America have substantially higher rates of prostate cancer morbidity and mortality than Asian residents (5,6). The stereotypical US diet, high in animal fats and meats and low in fruits and vegetables, has long been suspected to foster prostate cancer development, although some epidemiologic and intervention secondary analysis data (7) conflict with this view. Is the US diet also rich in prostate carcinogens and/or poor in prostate cancer-preventing micronutrients? Unfortunately, the mechanism(s) by which dietary components influence prostatic carcinogenesis have only begun to be studied intensely. Clearly, if dietary prostate carcinogens could be identified and characterized, risk reduction might be accomplished by carcinogen exposure avoidance. Also, discovery of dietary prostate cancer-preventing micronutrients could make prevention possible through supplementation.

Some tantalizing clues concerning dietary prostate carcinogens have begun to emerge. The Health Professionals Follow-up Study, the Physicians Health Study, and a large cohort study in Hawaii found that red meat consumption was consistently associated with increased prostate cancer risk (8–10). High-temperature cooking or charcoal broiling of red meat forms a number of heterocyclic aromatic amine (HAA) and polycyclic aromatic hydrocarbon (PAH) carcinogens (11–13). One of these carcinogens, 2-amino-1-methyl-6-phenylimidazo[4,5-b]pyridine (PhIP), has been reported to cause prostate cancer when fed to laboratory rats (14,15). Exposure to N-hydroxy-PhIP, a liver metabolite of PhIP, causes PhIP-DNA adducts in human

prostate tissues and prostate cancer cells (16). Thus far, an association between consumption of well-done red meats and prostate cancer risk has been difficult to demonstrate in epidemiology studies, in part because of a lack of reliable measures of exposure to HAA and PAH carcinogens. Hopefully, as new biomarkers of exposure to these compounds are discovered, more definitive tests of the prostate cancer risk associated with exposure can be undertaken. Of course, if one or more of the HAAs and/or PAHs appearing in well-done red meats is shown to act as a human prostatic carcinogen, then prostate cancer risk might be reduced by simply avoiding the practice of cooking or charbroiling red meat at very high temperatures but still preserving protection against microbial infection (17).

Specific dietary components may also protect against prostate cancer development (18). One vegetable component that may reduce prostate cancer risk is lycopene, an antioxidant carotenoid. The Physicians Health Study found that high lycopene blood levels, resulting from consumption of cooked tomatoes, were associated with reduced prostate cancer risk, including a reduced risk for aggressive prostate cancer (19). Also, in a proof-of-principle clinical trial, men who consumed tomato-sauce-based pasta dishes for 3 wk before radical prostatectomy were found to have increased lycopene levels in blood and prostate, decreased oxidative genome damage in leukocytes and prostate cells, and a reduced serum PSA (20). In another, similarly designed preprostatectomy trial, 26 patients were randomly assigned to either lycopene (30 mg/d) or control (no treatment). Positive results in the lycopene arm (vs the control arm) included significantly higher lycopene levels in prostate tissue and nonsignificant trends of reduced plasma PSA levels and increased connexin 43 expression in prostate tissue (21). The isothiocyanate sulforaphane may be another vegetable component that reduces prostate cancer risk. Sulforaphane, which is present at high levels in cruciferous vegetables, prevents cancers in several animal models by inducing the expression of carcinogen-detoxification enzymes, including glutathione (GSH)-S-transferases (GSTs) and quinone oxidoreductases, which protect against cell and genome damage inflicted by carcinogens (22,23). Consumption of cruciferous vegetables has been associated with reduced prostate cancer risk in a case-control study in King County, WA (24).

A reasonable hypothesis supported by epidemiological data is that diet may influence prostate cancer pathogenesis via effects on prostate cell and genome damage. Intake of dietary carcinogens, such as the

HAAs and/or PAHs present in well-done red meats, might cause cell and genome damage promoting development and progression of prostate cancer; intake of antioxidant and carcinogen-protective micronutrients, such as lycopene and sulforaphane, might lead to reduced cell and genome damage, attenuating the development and progression of prostate cancer. If this hypothesis proves correct, then prostate cancer prevention strategies focused on increasing protection against oxidant and electrophilic carcinogens might be a rational approach to reduce prostate cancer morbidity and mortality.

3. INHERITED PROSTATE CANCER SUSCEPTIBILITY GENES

A number of twin studies, comparing prostate cancer risks of monozygotic twins and dizygotic twins, have indicated a significant hereditary contribution to prostate cancer development (25–28). In 1990, Steinberg et al. reported that men with prostate cancer, when compared to their spouses, were more likely to have a brother or father with prostate cancer (29). Furthermore, prostate cancer risk for first-degree relatives was increased 2-, 5-, or 11-fold, depending on whether one, two, or three family members were affected (29). Similar findings have been reported in a number of additional studies (30–35). Clearly, men with a strong family history of prostate cancer might be good candidates for new prostate cancer prevention strategies. To ascertain whether familial clusters of prostate cancer might be the result of one or more inherited prostate cancer susceptibility genes, modes of prostate cancer risk inheritance were discriminated using several complex segregation analyses. In the first such analysis, prostate cancer inheritance in a collection of prostate cancer families was best explained by a rare autosomal dominant risk gene accounting for 9% of all prostate cancers, and as many as 43% of prostate cancers appearing at an early age (<55 yr) (36). Additional segregation analyses have confirmed this result, and have further suggested that an X-linked gene might be responsible for inherited prostate cancer susceptibility in some families (37–41).

To identify prostate cancer susceptibility genes, genetic linkage studies involving prostate cancer families were initiated at several centers. The first report from a genome-wide screen of polymorphic markers at approx 10 cM resolution (the human genome encompasses about 3300 cM) targeted 66 families with hereditary prostate cancer (HPC), defined as having three or more first-degree relatives diagnosed with prostate cancer, or having two or more brothers with prostate cancer diagnosed at age 55 or younger (42). The chromosomal region 1q24-25 exhibited the highest linkage to prostate cancer (a LOD score of 2.75) and was designated the locus of the HPC1 gene. Additional linkage screens involving other prostate cancer families have now also identified PCAP at 1q42–43 (43), CaPB at 1p36 (44), HPCX at Xq27–28 (45), HPC20 at 20q13 (46), HPC2 at 17p (47), and a gene at 8p22–23 (48), as candidate prostate cancer susceptibility genes.

Of the genetic loci thought to affect prostate cancer susceptibility, three genes have been tentatively identified. ELAC2 encodes a predicted 826 amino acid polypeptide of unknown function with sequence motifs shared by metallo-β-lactamases, DNA interstrand crosslink repair proteins, and mRNA cleavage and polyadenylation specificity factors; it has been proposed as a candidate for HPC2 (47). However, a number of studies of prostate cancer risks associated with variant ELAC2 alleles, including population-based case-control analyses, have yielded inconsistent and conflicting results, leading to uncertainty as to whether ELAC2 is a prostate cancer susceptibility gene (49–53). HPC1 appears likely to be RNASEL, encoding a widely expressed latent endoribonuclease L, a component of a 2′,5′-oligoadenylate-dependent RNA decay pathway induced by interferon that, on viral infection, is thought to degrade viral RNA (54–59). $RnaseL^{-/-}$ mice have not been reported to develop prostate cancer, though they have exhibited reduced interferon-α antiviral activity in comparison to $RnaseL^{+/+}$ mice (60). Furthermore, cells from $RnaseL^{-/-}$ mice appear resistant to apoptosis induction by a variety of different stimuli (60). MSR1, located at 8p22, has emerged as a candidate susceptibility gene for prostate cancer (61). It encodes class A macrophage scavenger receptor subunit polypeptides, capable of binding bacterial lipopoylsaccharide and lipoteichoic acid, and of binding oxidized high-density (HDL) and low-density (LDL) serum lipoproteins (62). Like $RnaseL^{-/-}$ mice, $Msr-A^{-/-}$ mice have not been found to develop prostate cancer, and most intriguingly, also exhibit defective responses to pathogenic organisms as do $RnaseL^{-/-}$ mice, showing increased sensitivity to serious infection with Listeria monocytogenes, Staphylococcus aureus, Escherichia coli, and Herpes simplex virus type 1 (62–65). In the prostate, MSR1 expression appears restricted to macrophages, particularly in areas of prostate inflammation. Although the precise function of MSR1 in the pathogenesis of prostate cancer has not been ascertained, available data implicate inefficient disposition of pathogenic organisms and/or altered oxidized serum lipoprotein metabolism in the prostate as possible etiologic factors. Furthermore, finding prostate cancer susceptibility associated with genes encoding defective macrophage receptors suggests that genetic variation in host cells as well as in cancer cells may play an important role in prostate cancer development.

In addition to the genes thought responsible for hereditary prostate cancer syndromes, polymorphic variants of three genes involved in androgen action, *AR, CYP17*, and *SRD5A2*, have been implicated in genetic epidemiology studies as increasing prostate cancer risk. For *AR*, encoding the androgen receptor (AR), both polymorphic polyglutamine (CAG) repeats, varying in lengths from 11 to 31 amino acids, and polymorphic polyglycine (GGC) repeats, varying in lengths from 10 to 22 amino acids, have been proposed to affect prostate cancer risk *(66–72)*. Shorter AR polyglutamine repeats, possibly associated with increased AR function, tend to be common in African-Americans, who have a high prostate cancer risk, and uncommon in Asians, who have a lower prostate cancer risk *(73–76)*. A polymorphic variant of the transcriptional promoter of *CYP17*, encoding the sex steroid biosynthesis enzyme cytochrome P450c17α, an enzyme that catalyzes key reactions in sex steroid biosynthesis, may also affect prostate cancer risk *(77–83)*. Polymorphic variants of *SRD5A2* encoding 5-α-reductase, an enzyme expressed in the prostate that converts testosterone to the more potent dihydrotestosterone, have been correlated with increased prostate cancer risk and poor prognosis *(84,85)*. Androgenic hormones are essential for normal prostate growth and development. The tendency for polymorphic variants of genes mediating androgen action to be associated with increased prostate cancer risk is consistent with the key role of androgenic hormones in prostate cancer development. Androgen signal pathways clearly constitute attractive targets for prostate cancer chemoprevention drugs.

4. SOMATIC *GSTP1* INACTIVATION AND LOSS OF CARCINOGEN-DETOXIFICATION CAPACITY DURING PROSTATIC CARCINOGENESIS

Small prostate cancers have been detected at autopsy in as many as 30% of men between the ages of 30 and 40 *(86)*. Because most prostate cancer diagnoses are made in men between the ages of 60 and 70, cancer cells present at the time of diagnosis might be expected to manifest the effects of as many as 30 or more years

of exposure to high-risk diet and lifestyle habits. Cancer cells present at the time of prostate cancer diagnosis typically contain myriad somatic genome alterations, including gene mutations, deletions, and amplifications; chromosomal rearrangements; and changes in DNA methylation. The most commonly reported chromosomal abnormalities in newly diagnosed prostate cancers appear to be gains at 7p, 7q, 8q, and Xq, and losses at 8p, 10q, 13q, and 16q *(87)*. Additional somatic genome alterations occur with prostate cancer progression, including gains at 8q, and losses of 7q, 8p, 13q and 16q *(88–92)*. Differences in the patterns of chromosome gains and losses in prostate cancers–from case to case, and from lesion to lesion, and primary tumor to metastatic tumor in an individual patient–suggest a marked heterogeneity in the molecular pathogenesis of the disease. The acquisition of such a wide variety of somatic genome lesions over 30 or more years, in a manner so sensitive to environment and lifestyle, may indicate that prostate cancers arise as a consequence of either chronic or recurrent exposure to genome-damaging stresses, defective protection against genome damage, or some combination of both processes.

Hypermethylation of a CpG island at *GSTP1*, encoding the π-class GST, is the most common somatic genome change associated with prostate cancer *(93–96)*. GSTP1 is normally expressed in prostate basal epithelial cells, and can be induced to high-level expression in columnar secretory epithelial cells. In more than 90% of cases, prostate cancer cells appear incapable of GSTP1 expression as a consequence of transcriptional silencing accompanying somatic *GSTP1* CpG island hypermethylation *(95)*. *GSTP1* CpG island hypermethylation has also been detected in prostatic intraepithelial neoplasia (PIN) lesions, candidate precursors to prostate cancer *(97)*.

Although *GSTP1* inactivation may offer some sort of selective growth or survival advantage at some point during pathogenesis of prostate cancer, *GSTP1* does not appear simply to act as a tumor-suppressor gene, because although π-class GSTs have been reported to modulate intracellular growth and stress signaling pathways in some cells, such as fibroblasts, forced GSTP1 expression in LNCaP prostate cancer cells has not been found to reduce growth in vitro or in vivo *(95,98–100)*. Rather than act as a tumor suppressor gene, *GSTP1* most likely serves as a "caretaker" gene *(101)*, defending prostate cells against genome damage mediated by carcinogens such as HAA and PhIP, which is known to cause prostate cancer in Copenhagen rats *(14,15)*. Forced GSTP1 expression in LNCaP prostate cancer cells has afforded substantial protection against DNA adducts inflicted by metabolically activated PhIP *(17)*. Lending further support to the general caretaker role for π-class GSTs, mice carrying disrupted *GSTP* genes displayed increased skin tumors compared with wild-type mice after treatment with the carcinogen 7,12 dimethyl-benz[*a*]anthracene (DMBA) *(102)*. Loss of π-class GST caretaker function also appears to provide a survival advantage in the face of injurious stresses, including oxidative stress. Mice carrying disrupted *GSTP* genes manifest less hepatocyte damage after high-dose acetaminophen administration than wild-type mice *(103)*. In addition, after prolonged exposure to oxidant stress, LNCaP prostate cancer cells carrying defective *GSTP1* genes display increased survival compared to those genetically modified to express GSTP1 (Dr. Theodore DeWeese and colleagues, Johns Hopkins, personal communication). The mechanisms by which π-class GSTs couple cell and genome damage to cell death have not been established.

5. CANDIDATE PROSTATE CANCER TUMOR-SUPPRESSOR GENES

The best candidate gatekeeper gene for prostate cancer development, analogous to *APC* in colorectal cancer development, may be *NKX3.1*, located at 8p21 *(101,104,105)*, which encodes a prostate-specific homeobox gene that is likely essential for normal prostate development *(104,105)*. Mice carrying one or two disrupted *Nkx3.1* alleles have been reported to manifest prostatic epithelial hyperplasia and dysplasia *(106,107)*. Loss of 8p21 genomic sequences carrying *NKX3.1* alleles has been detected in as many as 63% of PIN lesions and more than 90% of prostatic carcinomas *(108)*. Furthermore, loss of NKX3.1 expression has been reported for 20% of PIN lesions, 6% of low-stage prostate cancers, 22% of high stage prostate cancers, 34% of androgen-independent prostate cancers, and 78% of prostate cancer metastases *(109)*. Despite these findings, *NKX3.1* has not been established as the somatic gene target at 8p21 for inactivation during prostatic carcinogenesis because no somatic *NKX3.1* mutations accompanying allelic losses have been identified *(110–112)*.

Phosphatase and tensin homolog (PTEN) may be a critical target for somatic dysfunction during prostate cancer progression. Both protein and lipid phosphatase, PTEN appears to be present in normal prostatic epithelial cells and in most PIN lesion cells. PTEN has been proposed to act as a general tumor suppressor gene by

inhibiting the phosphatidylinositol 3′-kinase/protein kinase B (PI3K/Akt) signaling pathway needed for cell cycle proliferation and cell survival *(113–116)*. Mice carrying one disrupted *Pten* allele display prostatic hyperplasia and dysplasia, and both *Pten*$^{+/-}$*Nkx3.1*$^{+/-}$ mice and *Pten*$^{+/-}$*Nkx3.1*$^{-/-}$ mice develop intra-acinar and intraductal prostatic carcinomas *(117–119)*. In addition, TRAMP mice, which have an *SV40 T-antigen* transgene controlled by a prostate-specific transcriptional promoter and spontaneously develop prostate cancer, appear to have poorer prostate cancer survival when carrying a disrupted *Pten* allele than when carrying wild-type *Pten* genes *(120)*. In human prostate cancers, PTEN levels appear reduced, or heterogeneously expressed, particularly in cells present in high-grade or high-stage prostate cancers *(121,122)*. Furthermore, somatic PTEN alterations, including homozygous deletions, loss of heterozygosity, mutations, and probable CpG island hypermethylation, have been detected more commonly in prostate cancer metastases at autopsy than in newly diagnosed prostate cancers *(128–132)*.

p27, a cyclin-dependent kinase inhibitor encoded by *CDKN1B*, may also act as a tumor suppressor gene during prostatic carcinogenesis. Mice carrying disrupted *Cdkn1b* alleles develop prostatic hyperplasia, and *Pten*$^{+/-}$*Cdkn1b*$^{-/-}$ mice develop prostate cancers by 3 mo of age *(133,134)*. Abnormally low levels of p27 appear common in human prostate cancers, particularly in those with poor prognosis *(133,135–139)*. Somatic loss of DNA sequences at 12p12–13, encompassing *CDKN1B*, has been described in 23% of localized prostate cancers, 30% of prostate cancer regional lymph node metastases, and 47% of distant prostate cancer metastases *(140)*. In prostate cancers with low PTEN levels, the reduction in p27 levels may be partly the result of inappropriate activation of the PI3K/Akt signaling pathway, leading to a failure to repress Forkhead transcription factors needed to promote increases in *CDKN1B* mRNA and p27 protein half-life *(114,116,141–143)*.

6. SOMATIC ALTERATIONS IN ANDROGEN RECEPTOR ACCOMPANYING PROSTATE CANCER PROGRESSION TO ANDROGEN INDEPENDENCE

AR is expressed in most androgen-dependent and -independent prostate cancers *(144–146)*. Transgenic mice exhibiting high-level AR expression in prostatic epithelial cells develop PIN lesions *(147)*. Somatic AR alterations, particularly mutations and gene amplifications, have been reported for human prostate cancers, especially cancers that progress after prostate cancer treatment with androgen suppression and/or antiandrogens (148–161). Many reported AR mutations appear to lead to an altered specificity for agonist ligands, resulting in promiscuous AR activation by a variety of agents (162–165). AR amplification accompanied by overexpression is thought to increase prostate cancer cells' sensitivity to growth-promoting effects of low levels of circulating androgens (149).

7. PROSTATIC INFLAMMATION AND PROSTATIC CARCINOGENESIS

Chronic or recurrent inflammation promotes development of liver, esophagus, stomach, large intestine, and bladder cancers; prostatic inflammation has long been thought to somehow contribute to prostate cancer development (166). However, although prostatic inflammation and prostate cancer both commonly appear in prostates in US men, an association between prostatic inflammation and prostate cancer has been difficult to assess. One limitation for epidemiology studies is that prostatic inflammation may not always be symptomatic; when symptoms are present, their severity may not always reflect the intensity of inflammation. Symptomatic prostatitis has been reported in as many as 9% or more of men between the ages of 40 and 79; as many as 50% of these men suffer recurrent symptomatic episodes of prostatitis by age 80 (167). No infectious cause can be identified for many of these symptomatic episodes. Asymptomatic prostatitis is usually discovered during biopsy to detect prostate cancer or radical prostatectomy to treat it. Why some men suffer symptoms of prostatic inflammation while others do not has not been discerned. Also unknown is the prevalence of asymptomatic prostatitis, as there is no validated diagnostic biomarker for it (168,169). For these and other reasons, neither symptomatic nor asymptomatic prostatitis has yet been linked with prostate cancer in epidemiology studies.

There are several hints that inflammation may play some role in prostatic carcinogenesis. For example, two candidate prostate cancer susceptibility genes identified thus far, RNase L and MSR1, encode proteins with critical functions in host immune responses to infections (54,60–62). Epidemiology studies have suggested that infections such as those caused by sexually transmitted pathogens may increase prostate cancer risk (170,171). In response to infection, inflammatory cells produce activated oxygen and nitrogen, including superoxide, nitric oxide, peroxynitrite, etc., that might cause cell and genome damage in the prostate (172,173). Perhaps not surprisingly, intake of a variety of antioxidants or nonsteroidal antiinflammatory drugs (NSAIDs) may reduce prostate cancer risk (20,174–179).

Proliferative inflammatory atrophy (PIA) prostate lesions may provide a link between prostatic inflammation and cancer (166,180,181). These focal chronic inflammatory lesions containing proliferating epithelial cells that fail to fully differentiate into columnar secretory cells are usually found in the prostate periphery, where cancers more commonly arise, and are often directly adjacent to PIN lesions and/or prostate cancers (180,182–185). Epithelial cells found in PIA lesions often express high levels of GSTP1, GSTA1, and cyclooxygenase 2 (COX-2), perhaps as a manifestation of stress triggered by inflammatory oxidants and cytokines (180,186,187). Though the etiology of PIA has not been established, the lesions have been proposed to arise as either the consequence of prostatic inflammation, with regenerative proliferation of prostate epithelial cells in response to injury inflicted by inflammatory oxidants, or as the cause of prostatic inflammation, with epithelial regeneration and inflammation triggered by some other process that damages the prostate epithelium (180). In support of a causal role for prostatic inflammation in prostatic carcinogenesis, PIA may be a precursor to PIN or prostate cancer. Somatic genome abnormalities, similar to those appearing in PIN and prostate cancer cells, have been detected in PIA cells (185). Also, prostatic inflammation accompanied by focal epithelial atrophy has been described in association with prostate cancer development in rats (188,189). Of interest, PIA cells usually contain high GSTP1 levels, while PIN and prostate cancer cells are typically devoid of GSTP1. Loss of GSTP1 expression, as a consequence of de novo somatic GSTP1 CpG island hypermethylation, may demarcate the transition between PIA and PIN or prostate cancer.

8. ANTIOXIDANTS AND PROSTATE CANCER PREVENTION

Since it is likely that prostate cancers arise among cells with defenses crippled by reactive chemical species that must confront a barrage of inflammatory oxidants, it is not surprising that a variety of antioxidants and antiinflammatory drugs may protect against prostate cancer development. Epidemiological studies have suggested that increased consumption of antioxidants selenium and vitamin E decreases prostate cancer risk (19,190–192). The protective effects of these agents against prostate cancer development have been further supported by the secondary results of Phase III clinical prevention trials (174–176,193). One study randomly tested the ability of selenium (200 mcg/d) in brewer's yeast (vs placebo) to reduce skin cancer development in 1312 men and women with a history of nonmelanoma skin cancer (175). Remarkably, although selenium supplementation failed to prevent second skin cancers, men receiving the selenium supplements had a 67% reduced incidence of prostate cancer ($p = 0.002$). In another clinical study, α-tocopherol, β-carotene, the combination of α-tocopherol and β-carotene, or placebo was administered to 29,133 male Finnish smokers to prevent lung cancer (193). Again, although neither α-tocopherol nor β-carotene supplementation reduced lung cancer development in the trial, men receiving α-tocopherol had a 32% reduced incidence of prostate cancer and 41% reduced prostate cancer mortality (176). These preventive effects appeared within 2 yr of starting and disappeared within 2 yr of stopping the intervention. Since secondary findings indicated no protective effect against urinary tract (bladder, ureter, renal pelvis, and renal cell) cancers, the genitourinary effects of α-tocopherol appear to have been specific for prostate cancer (194). β-carotene, the other antioxidant in this trial, did not improve prostate cancer incidence or mortality (176,193).

Further support for vitamin E and selenium comes from secondary analyses of large Phase III cancer prevention trials testing antioxidant combinations that included one or both of these agents. One such complex trial of 29,584 people in Linxian, China, tested several combinations to prevent esophageal cancer. The primary outcome was not statistically significant, but one of the combinations (selenium, β-carotene, α-tocopherol) produced a significant 13% reduction in overall cancer mortality (195). A recently reported Phase III heart disease prevention study including approximately 15,500 men made a secondary finding of a nonsignificant 9% decrease in prostate cancer risk associated with taking vitamins E and C and β-carotene for 5 yr (196). Recent preclinical and clinical studies have provided biological plausibility for the epidemiologic and Phase III secondary findings on selenium and α-tocopherol effects in the prostate—these agents are potent inducers of apoptosis in prostate cancer cells (197). A recently completed randomized pharmacodynamic study of short-term (14–31 d) administration of selenium in the preprostatectomy model showed that selenium selec-

tively and significantly accumulates in the prostate vs plasma or seminal vesicles (198).

Formal hypothesis-testing trials of selenium and vitamin E for prostate cancer prevention are under way. Selenium is being studied in five clinical settings—prostate cancer in the preprostatectomy/pharmacodynamic model (selenium with and without vitamin E); increased PSA and negative biopsies; high-grade PIN; low-grade cancer and a life expectancy less than 10 yr (watchful waiting); and relatively good health and no signs or symptoms of prostate cancer (Selenium and Vitamin E Cancer Prevention Trial, SELECT) (199).

SELECT is a Phase III, placebo-controlled, intergroup (multicenter), 12-yr trial to determine whether selenium and/or vitamin E can prevent prostate cancer (200). Supported by NCI and coordinated by the Southwest Oncology Group, SELECT plans to enroll 32,400 men (55 yr or older, except African-American men, who may be 50 yr or older) from more than 500 sites in the US (including centers of four other major cooperative oncology groups and the Veterans Affairs Cooperative Studies Group), Puerto Rico, and Canada. SELECT is a 2×2 factorial design to allow prespecified primary-analysis comparisons of prostate cancer incidence, including vitamin E vs placebo, selenium vs placebo, combined vitamin E and selenium vs placebo, the combination vs vitamin E, and the combination vs selenium. The study is powered at 89% (0.05 α) to detect a 25% difference in prostate cancer incidence between the combination arm and either single-agent arm. This allows for even greater statistical power for any other pair-wise comparison, e.g., SELECT has a 96% power to detect a 25% difference between either single agent and placebo. SELECT's important prespecified secondary endpoints include prostate cancer-specific survival, lung and colon cancer incidence and survival, overall survival, overall cancer incidence and cancer survival, and cardiovascular deaths. Important SELECT ancillary-study endpoints include translational/molecular epidemiology endpoints reviewed elsewhere (200) and Alzheimer's disease.

9. ANTIINFLAMMATORY DRUGS AND PROSTATE CANCER PREVENTION

Epidemiologic and animal data suggest that inflammation and polyunsaturated fats in the diet can promote carcinogenesis, supporting strategies that target polyunsaturated fatty acid metabolic pathways with drugs such as NSAIDs for prostate cancer prevention. Targets of interest within these fatty acid pathways include COX-2 and 5-, 12-, and 15-lipoxygenase (LOX). Our understanding of the role of COX-2 as a target of NSAID activity in the prostate is complicated by conflicting data from in vitro, animal, and clinical studies of COX expression and NSAID activity. A number of NSAID studies in various animal prostate cancer models indicate that selective COX-2-inhibiting, nonselective COX-inhibiting, and non-COX-inhibiting NSAIDs are active in prostate cancer prevention (201). The data on COX-2 expression in human prostate cancer are conflicting (186,201,202). In a recent report, COX-2 expression in prostate cancer and PIN was low, comparable to that in adjacent normal prostate tissue in 144 human prostate cancer cases. This study also provocatively found that epithelial and inflammatory cells in PIA, the inflammatory prostate lesion that may be a precursor to PIN and/or prostate cancer, express high levels of COX-2 (186). Furthermore, intake of nonselective COX inhibitors has been associated with diminished prostate cancer risk in several epidemiology studies (177,178,201,203), including a recent cohort study in more than 90,000 men that found a significant 25% prostate cancer risk reduction associated with regular use of aspirin (203). Recently, new selective inhibitors of COX-2, celecoxib (Celebrex®; Pfizer Corporation) and rofecoxib (Vioxx®; Merck & Company), have become available. These drugs possess the antiinflammatory and analgesic properties of the nonselective COX inhibitors but elicit fewer side effects such as gastroduodenal irritation and ulceration. With this attractive safety profile, selective COX-2 inhibitors will eventually be tested for efficacy in attenuating human prostatic carcinogenesis. In addition to selective COX-2 inhibitors, R-flurbiprofen, an antiinflammatory agent that does not inhibit COX, appears to reduce prostate tumor formation in TRAMP mice (204). Exisulind (sulindac sulfone; OSI), a sulindac metabolite devoid of COX-inhibiting activity that may target cGMP phosphodiesterase, has demonstrated provocative preclinical activity against prostate cancer (201,205,206). The promising preclinical results led to a recently reported multicenter placebo-controlled double-blind Phase III trial of sulindac sulfone vs placebo in 96 patients with a rising PSA following radical prostatectomy (D_0 disease). Sulindac sulfone suppressed PSA levels (the primary study endpoint) compared with placebo ($p = 0.017$) (207).

Fatty acid metabolic enzymes 5-, 12- and 15-LOX also have been implicated in prostate carcinogenesis. 5- and 12-LOX are overexpressed in prostate cancer cells; inhibiting these enzymes induces apoptosis and inhibits

growth of prostate cancer cells (208–210). In contrast to 5- and 12-LOX, 15-LOX-2 expression is reduced in prostate cancer and high-grade PIN; its product 15-S-hydroxyeicosatetraenoic acid inhibits proliferation of prostate cancer cells in vitro (210). Inducible nitric oxide synthetase (iNOS), an enzyme expressed at high levels by inflammatory cells in the prostate, may offer a new target for new prostate cancer prevention drugs (211).

10. 5α-REDUCTASE INHIBITORS AND ANTI-ANDROGENS FOR PROSTATE CANCER PREVENTION

Androgen signaling pathways have been targeted by a number of drugs, including US Food and Drug Administration (FDA)-approved drugs for treating benign prostatic hyperplasia (BPH), advanced prostate cancer, and other conditions such as male pattern baldness. Finasteride (Merck & Company), which has been marketed as Proscar® for BPH and as Propecia® for alopecia, is a selective inhibitor of type II 5α-reductase, the enzyme responsible for converting testosterone to dihydrotestosterone in the prostate. Because finasteride has few worrisome side effects and may reduce the serum PSA in men with prostate cancer (212,213), it is being studied for prostate cancer chemoprevention as part of the Prostate Cancer Prevention Trial (PCPT) (214). The PCPT, which targeted ≥55-yr-old men in the general population, has completed accrual with the enrollment of 18,882 subjects. As part of the clinical trial design, after 7 yr of treatment with finasteride or placebo, all those in the trial are to undergo prostate biopsy. Results of the trial, expected by 2004, should reveal whether finasteride treatment reduces the period prevalence of prostate cancer. Other clinical trial data featuring finasteride treatment have not been very encouraging. In one prospective, randomized, placebo-controlled trial of finasteride for BPH ($n = 3040$), a secondary analysis revealed that 4.7% of men treated with finasteride and 5.1% of men treated with placebo were ultimately diagnosed with prostate cancer ($p = 0.7$) (215). In another randomized trial ($n = 52$), men with an elevated serum PSA but no cancer on prostate biopsies received finasteride or no treatment for 12 mo (216). Prostate biopsies obtained at study end were remarkable in detecting cancer in 30% of men treated with finasteride vs 4% of men left untreated ($p = 0.025$). A trial with men whose original biopsy revealed PIN found that finasteride treatment did not appear to affect the PIN lesions. Furthermore, prostate cancer was evident after 12 mo in six to eight men with PIN treated with finasteride vs none of five men with PIN who were left untreated *(216)*.

Anti-androgens such as bicalutamide (Casodex®; AstraZeneca International) and flutamide (Eulexin®; Schering-Plough Corporation), are in NCI prostate cancer prevention studies. Androgens are required for normal prostate development. Thus, antiandrogens and androgen-lowering drugs used at an early age or before puberty may prevent prostate cancer development as well. However, the drugs are associated with side effects upon prolonged use, including loss of bone and muscle mass, loss of libido, and breast pain/tenderness or gynecomastia, that will almost certainly limit their utility for prostate cancer prevention. A recent randomized placebo-controlled double-blind trial tested the ability of flutamide (250 mg/d) to decrease progression of high-grade PIN to prostate cancer. This randomized trial did not suggest any benefit of flutamide, in contrast to PIN reduction in a retrospective androgen-deprivation study. Although typical androgen deprivation toxicities increased in the flutamide arm of the randomized study, there were no changes in quality-of-life indicators (Dr. Charles L. Loprinzi and colleagues, unpublished observations).

11. CARCINOGEN-DETOXIFICATION ENZYME INDUCERS AND PROSTATE CANCER PREVENTION

Loss of GSTP1 caretaker activity during prostatic carcinogenesis emphasizes the critical role of carcinogen metabolism in protecting prostate cells against neoplastic transformation, and suggests that therapeutic compensation for inadequate GSTP1 caretaker function may help prevent prostate cancer. Augmentation of carcinogen-detoxification capacity, using a variety of chemoprotective compounds including isothiocyanates, 1,2-dithiole-3-thiones, terpenoids, etc., prevents a variety of cancers in different animal models by triggering expression of many different carcinogen-detoxification enzymes *(217,218)*. Oltipraz, an inducer of carcinogen-detoxification enzymes in liver tissues, has been shown to reduce aflatoxin B_1 damage when administered to a human clinical study cohort at high risk for aflatoxin exposure and liver cancer development in China *(219–221)*. Sulforaphane, an isothiocyanate present in large amounts in cruciferous vegetables, is also a potent inducer of carcinogen-detoxification enzymes *(22,23)*. Diets rich in carcinogen-detoxification enzyme inducers like sulforaphane have been associated with decreased cancer risks *(24)*. Such carcinogen-detoxification

enzyme inducers need to be developed and tested in prostate cancer prevention clinical trials.

12. CLINICAL DEVELOPMENT OF NEW AGENTS FOR PROSTATE CANCER PREVENTION

The four major clinical models (and their major endpoints) currently in use to test prostate cancer prevention agents include preprostatectomy (pharmacodynamic endpoints), high-grade PIN (prostate cancer and PIN), elevated PSA/negative biopsy (prostate cancer and PIN), and men in the general population with elevated risk based on age and race (prostate cancer, PIN, and PIA). The preprostatectomy model uses pharmacodynamic, -kinetic endpoints allowing generally smaller sample sizes, whereas the three other major models use more traditional efficacy endpoints of PIN and cancer requiring generally far higher sample sizes. Another clinical model for testing preventive agents—post-radical prostatectomy/rising PSA (D_0)—involves a setting that traditionally is used for cancer therapy. Table 1 summarizes the status of major completed and ongoing randomized clinical studies of potential prostate cancer preventive agents.

The preprostatectomy model involves patients scheduled for radical prostatectomy following a diagnosis of biopsy-proven prostate cancer. Generally, preprostatectomy studies are 2–4-wk interventions (between diagnosis and surgery) involving patients randomly assigned to a study agent(s) or no-treatment control arm (25–50 patients in each arm), who are assessed for prostate uptake of the agent(s), biologic agent effects in the prostate (e.g., on proliferation, apoptosis, or high-grade PIN), and relevant molecular agent mechanisms (e.g., effects of NSAIDs on polyunsaturated fatty acid metabolites). As shown in Table 1, this is an active model for testing preventive agents.

The model with the greatest potential public health impact is healthy men in the general population with elevated risk based on age and race. Very large-scale, randomized, placebo-controlled, double-blind clinical trials in this setting almost certainly will be required to test the efficacy and safety of prostate cancer prevention drugs. The primary goal of such trials will be to estimate differences in the rates of prostate cancer development between men treated with candidate prevention drugs vs placebos. A number of limitations encumber this straightforward approach. One problem is that prostate cancer has a very long natural history.

Table 1
Randomized Controlled Trials of Prostate Cancer Prevention Agents

Setting	Agent(s)	Primary Endpoint	Accrual[a]	Result(s) (vs Control)	Reference
Preprostatectomy	SeMet	Pharmacokinetic/ dynamic	66	Selective Se uptake in prostate	2002 (198)
Preprostatectomy	Lycopene	Pharmacokinetic/ dynamic	26	Increased lycopene in prostate	2001 (21)
Preprostatectomy	Sulindac sulfone, celecoxib, vitamin E, genistein, toremifene, bicalutamide/DFMO, vitamin D analog	Pharmacokinetic/ dynamic	Several trials in progress	Pending	—
Post-prostatectomy (D$_0$, elevated PSA)	Sulindac sulfone	PSA	96	Reduced PSA ($p=0.017$)	2001 (207)
Elevated PSA, negative biopsy	Selenium yeast	Prostate cancer	358/700	Pending	—
Elevated PSA, negative biopsy	Finasteride	Prostate cancer	52	Increased cancer, 30% vs 4% ($p=0.025$)	1998 (216)
High-grade PIN	Flutamide	Prostate cancer	57	14% vs 10% ($p=$NS)	2002 (Unpublished observations, see text)
High-grade PIN	SeMet	Prostate cancer	133/466	Pending	—
Healthy, high-risk	Finasteride	Prostate cancer	18,884[b]	Pending	—
Healthy, high-risk	Selenium, vitamin E	Prostate cancer	14,939/32, 400	Pending	—

[a]Accrual figures as of September 2002; single numbers indicate completed trials; two numbers (x/y) indicate present accrual/planned sample size.

[b]Accrual completed, but not treatment/follow-up.

Small prostate cancers appear to be present in as many as 30% of men between the ages of 30 and 40 yr even though most prostate cancer diagnoses are not made until men are between the ages of 60 and 70 yr (86). At what age should a prostate cancer prevention drug be started? A clinical trial that enrolls healthy men between the ages of 20 and 30 yr, provides 40–50 yr of candidate prostate cancer prevention treatment, and monitors men for prostate cancer development or death is not practical. Fortunately, early clinical studies hint that brief (5–7 yr) exposures for antioxidants like selenium and vitamin E, started at ages above 50 yr, might still be adequate to reduce or retard prostate cancer development (174,176). However, it is not known whether brief exposures of older men to other types of agents, such as 5α-reductase inhibitors, will similarly attenuate prostatic carcinogenesis.

Another problem for clinical trials testing prostate cancer prevention agent efficacy concerns the most appropriate subjects to be recruited for study. For trials involving men in the general population, the relatively low primary endpoint (prostate cancer development and/or prostate cancer mortality) rates require large populations and long follow-ups to achieve the necessary statistical power to discern significant differences in these rates between treatment and control arms. As examples, PCPT enrolled 18,882 men and SELECT has targeted 32,400 men (200,222). Clearly, new risk-stratification tools that can identify men at high risk for prostate cancer development, analogous to the Gail model used for identifying women at high risk for breast cancer development, will permit more efficient prostate cancer prevention trials (223). Also, without such risk-stratification tools incorporated into clinical trial designs, the results of pivotal clinical trials of prostate cancer prevention agents may be difficult to reduce to clinical practice. For example, if a drug with significant side effects appears to prevent prostate cancer development after 5–7 yr of treatment in otherwise unselected men above age 50, practicing physicians will be prone to recommend this drug to men with increased prostate cancer risks, and men with increased prostate cancer risks will be prone to request the drug. Such men may not enjoy the same benefits of the prevention drug as unselected men in the general population recruited to the clinical trial. One great hope is that new molecular biomarkers, discovered and developed with new genomics and proteomics technologies, might be useful as prostate cancer risk-stratification tools. For example, as inherited prostate cancer susceptibility genes, like *RNASEL* and *MSR*, are discovered and characterized, otherwise healthy men with high-risk genotypes may be definable as study subjects for prostate cancer prevention clinical trials. High-risk men may also be definable using serum markers, such as serum PSA levels, serum insulin-like growth factor-1 (IGF-1) levels, serum selenium levels, or perhaps even new serum "proteomics" profiles *(190,224–227)*.

The diagnosis and treatment of premalignant lesions is an active area of prevention research in many human cancers *(228)*. However, although evidence has accumulated to suggest that PIN, and perhaps PIA, are precursors to prostate cancer, specific treatment of PIN or PIA to prevent prostate cancer will prove difficult because the only method currently available to detect, diagnose, and monitor PIN or PIA is prostate biopsy. For PIN, it is not clear whether current prostate biopsy sampling strategies are sufficient to assess the extent of PIN or its progression to prostate cancer. Thus, clinical trials designed to ascertain whether a candidate prostate cancer prevention agent reduces the extent (or histological grade) of PIN on repeated prostate biopsies may not yield useful information. Of interest, a randomized clinical trial with repeat prostate biopsies found that the 5α-reductase inhibitor finasteride, currently being tested as a prostate cancer prevention drug in PCPT, appeared to have little effect on PIN *(216)*. Randomized, controlled clinical trials designed to ascertain whether a candidate prostate cancer prevention agent reduces the extent of PIN at the time of radical prostatectomy for prostate cancer, where the whole prostate gland can be assessed for the presence of PIN, may be more informative. In these trials, men are administered the candidate prostate cancer prevention agent(s) for several weeks before surgery for prostate cancer. In spite of limitations in serially assessing PIN by prostate biopsy, this method clearly identifies men at high risk for ultimately developing prostate cancer. For this reason, clinical trials targeting men whose biopsies reveal PIN but not prostate cancer may be best designed to test whether prostate cancer prevention drugs reduce prostate cancer development or death. New methods, such as noninvasive imaging techniques that can detect and monitor PIA, PIN, and prostate cancer lesions, are desperately needed.

With increasing molecular understanding of signal transduction pathways involving NKX3.1, PTEN, and p27 contributing to the malignant phenotype of prostate cancer cells, new drugs targeting these pathways potentially will be discovered and developed as treatments for established prostate cancer. Many of these drugs may be sufficiently safe and effective to serve as candidates for prostate cancer prevention, and Phase I clinical development of these drugs may serve both therapy and prevention objectives *(197)*. Our increasing molecular understanding of mechanisms underlying preinvasive prostatic carcinogenesis (such as the likely contribution of genome damage) mediated by dietary carcinogens and inflammatory oxidants in the face of compromised carcinogen defenses, will potentially lead to discovering new drugs targeting prostatic carcinogenesis itself. Examples include antioxidants, antiinflammatory drugs, and dietary carcinogen-detoxification enzyme inducers. To accommodate this growing pipeline of agents, the development and prioritization of drugs targeting prostatic carcinogenesis will require the use of new validated biomarkers of the disease process. One important approach is to give candidate drugs targeting prostatic carcinogenesis to men with established prostate cancer before radical prostatectomy to test proof-of-principle endpoints, such as levels of genome damage or carcinogen-detoxification enzymes *(20)*. This paradigm is analogous to the discovery and development of drugs that treat atherosclerosis to prevent heart attacks and strokes, in which serum cholesterol and blood pressure are used as disease biomarkers.

13. SUMMARY AND CONCLUSIONS

Prostate cancer ought to be preventable. Epidemiology data indicate that environment has a critical role in prostate cancer development. Emerging understanding of prostate cancer susceptibility genetics and of molecular pathogenesis of prostate cancer supports a hypothesis that relentless genome-damaging stresses arising from consumption of dietary carcinogens and from

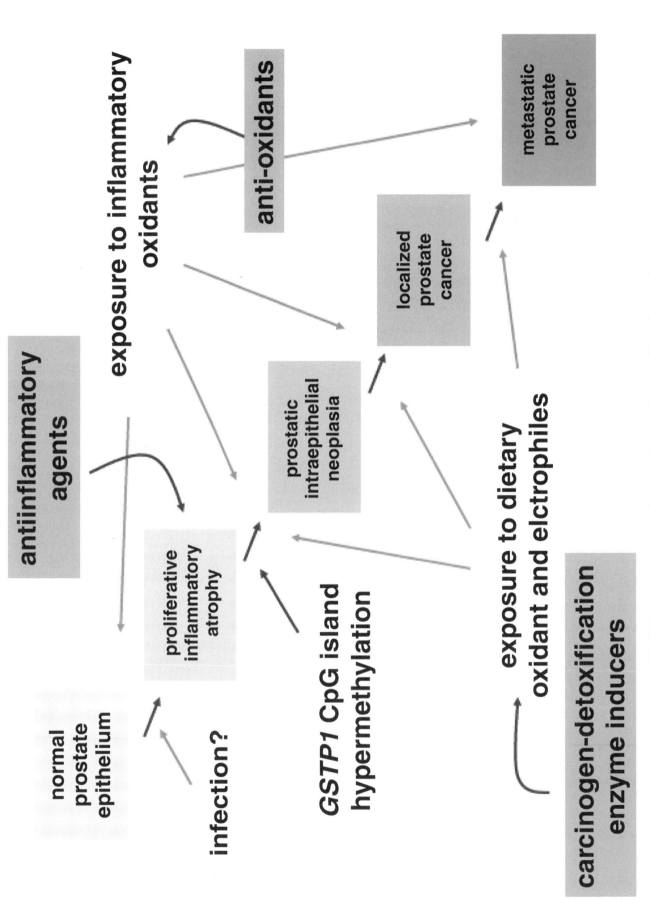

Fig. 1. Prostate cancer prevention strategies targeting prostatic carcinogenesis.

prostatic inflammation might promote prostatic carcinogenesis. If this hypothesis is correct, antioxidants, anti-inflammatory drugs, and carcinogen-detoxification enzyme inducers may act to attenuate prostatic carcinogenesis and prevent or delay prostate cancer development. SELECT, in which men will receive selenium, α-tocopherol, the combination of selenium and α-tocopherol, or a placebo, will provide one test of this hypothesis. The efficient discovery and development of drugs that target the prostatic carcinogenesis process will likely require new validated biomarkers to identify candidates for treatment and to use as treatment endpoints. Otherwise, prostate cancers, which may appear in men as early as age 30, display a marked sensitivity to androgenic hormones. For this reason, antiandrogens and androgen-lowering drugs, which can treat established advanced prostate cancers, may be useful in preventing the development of life-threatening prostate cancer, if strategies to minimize drug-associated side effects can be developed. PCPT, in which men will receive the 5α-reductase inhibitor finasteride, a drug with few side effects, or a placebo, will provide a test of this strategy. New drugs targeting abnormal signal transduction pathways in prostate cancer cells may also serve both to treat and to prevent prostate cancer, if side effects are tolerable *(197)*.

ADDENDUM IN PROOF

The PCPT was completed and reported after this chapter had been prepared for publication *(229,230)*. The prevalence of prostate cancer over the seven-year period of the trial was reduced by 24.8% in the finasteride arm (18.4% rate, or 803 of 4368 men) vs in the placebo arm (24.4% rate, or 1147 of 4692 men) ($p < 0.001$). Higher-grade tumors (Gleason grades 7, 8, 9, or 10), however, occurred in more men on finasteride (6.4%) than on placebo (5.1%) ($p = 0.005$). Finasteride-treated men had more sexual side effects; men on placebo had more urinary symptoms. Although finasteride prevented or delayed the appearance of prostate cancer, the investigators concluded that the benefits of finasteride must be considered along with the increases in sexual side effects and high-grade prostate cancer also seen with this agent.

REFERENCES

1. Jemal A, Thomas A, Murray T, Thun M. Cancer statistics, 2002. *CA Cancer J* Clin 2002;52:2–47.
2. Hankey BF, Feuer EJ, Clegg LX, et al. Cancer surveillance series: interpreting trends in prostate cancer—Part I: Evidence of the effects of screening in recent prostate cancer incidence, mortality, and survival rates. *J Natl Cancer Inst* 1999;91:1017–1024.
3. Bartsch G, Horninger W, Klocker H, et al. Prostate cancer mortality after introduction of prostate-specific antigen mass screening in the Federal State of Tyrol, Austria. *Urology* 2001;58:417–424.
4. Hsing AW, Tsao L, Devesa SS. International trends and patterns of prostate cancer incidence and mortality. *Int J Cancer* 2000;85:60–67.
5. Whittemore AS, Kolonel LN, Wu AH, et al. Prostate cancer in relation to diet, physical activity, and body size in blacks, whites, and Asians in the United States and Canada. *J Natl Cancer Inst* 1995;87:652–661.
6. Shimizu H, Ross RK, Bernstein L, et al. Cancers of the prostate and breast among Japanese and white immigrants in Los Angeles County. *Br J Cancer* 1991;63:963–966.
7. Shike M, Latkany L, Riedel E, et al. Lack of effect of a low-fat, high-fruit, -vegetable, and -fiber diet on serum prostate-specific antigen of men without prostate cancer: results from a randomized trial. *J Clin Oncol* 2002;20:3592–3598.
8. Giovannucci E, Rimm EB, Colditz GA, et al. A prospective study of dietary fat and risk of prostate cancer [see comments]. *J Natl Cancer Inst* 1993;85:1571–1579.
9. Gann PH, Hennekens CH, Sacks FM, et al. Prospective study of plasma fatty acids and risk of prostate cancer. *J Natl Cancer Inst* 1994;86:281–286.
10. Le Marchand L, Kolonel LN, Wilkens LR, et al. Animal fat consumption and prostate cancer: a prospective study in Hawaii. *Epidemiology* 1994;5:276–282.
11. Morgenthaler PM, Holzhauser D. Analysis of mutations induced by 2-amino-1-methyl-6-phenylimidazo[4,5- b]pyridine (PhIP) in human lymphoblastoid cells. *Carcinogenesis* 1995;16:713–718.
12. Knize MG, Salmon CP, Mehta SS, Felton JS. Analysis of cooked muscle meats for heterocyclic aromatic amine carcinogens. *Mutat Res* 1997;376:129–134.
13. Lijinsky W, Shubik P. Benzo(a)pyrene and other polynuclear hydrocarbons in charcoal-broiled meat. *Science* 1964;145:53–55.
14. Stuart GR, Holcroft J, de Boer JG, Glickman BW. Prostate mutations in rats induced by the suspected human carcinogen 2- amino-1-methyl-6-phenylimidazo[4,5-b]pyridine. *Cancer Res* 2000;60:266–268.
15. Shirai T, Sano M, Tamano S, et al. The prostate: a target for carcinogenicity of 2-amino-1-methyl-6- phenylimidazo[4,5-b]pyridine (PhIP) derived from cooked foods. *Cancer Res* 1997;57:195–198.
16. Nelson CP, Kidd LC, Sauvageot J, et al. Protection against 2-hydroxyamino-1-methyl-6-phenylimidazo[4,5-b]pyridine cytotoxicity and DNA adduct formation in human prostate by glutathione *S*-transferase P1. *Cancer Res* 2001;61:103–109.
17. Salmon CP, Knize MG, Panteleakos FN, et al. Minimization of heterocyclic amines and thermal inactivation of *Escherichia coli* in fried ground beef. *J Natl Cancer Inst* 2000;92:1773–1778.
18. Chan JM, Giovannucci EL. Vegetables, fruits, associated micronutrients, and risk of prostate cancer. *Epidemiol Rev* 2001;23:82–86.
19. Gann PH, Ma J, Giovannucci E, et al. Lower prostate cancer risk in men with elevated plasma lycopene levels: results of a prospective analysis. *Cancer Res* 1999;59:1225–1230.
20. Chen L, Stacewicz-Sapuntzakis M, Duncan C, et al. Oxidative DNA damage in prostate cancer patients consuming tomato

sauce-based entrees as a whole-food intervention. *J Natl Cancer Inst* 2001;93:1872–1879.

21. Kucuk O, Sarkar FH, Sakar W, et al. Phase II randomized clinical trial of lycopene supplementation before radical prostatectomy. *Cancer Epidemiol Biomarkers Prev* 2001; 10:861–868.

22. Zhang Y, Kensler TW, Cho CG, et al. Anticarcinogenic activities of sulforaphane and structurally related synthetic norbornl isothiocyanates. *Proc Natl Acad Sci USA* 1994;91: 3147–3150.

23. Zhang Y, Talalay P, Cho CG, Posner GH. A major inducer of anticarcinogenic protective enzymes from broccoli: isolation and elucidation of structure. *Proc Natl Acad Sci USA* 1992;89:2399–2403.

24. Cohen JH, Kristal AR, Stanford JL. Fruit and vegetable intakes and prostate cancer risk. *J Natl Cancer Inst* 2000;92:61–68.

25. Lichtenstein P, Holm NV, Verkasalo PK, et al. Environmental and heritable factors in the causation of cancer—analyses of cohorts of twins from Sweden, Denmark, and Finland. *N Engl J Med* 2000;343:78–85.

26. Page WF, Braun MM, Partin AW, et al. Heredity and prostate cancer: a study of World War II veteran twins. *Prostate* 1997;33:240–245.

27. Ahlbom A, Lichtenstein P, Malmstrom H, et al. Cancer in twins: genetic and nongenetic familial risk factors. *J Natl Cancer Inst* 1997;89:287–293.

28. Gronberg H, Damber L, Damber JE. Studies of genetic factors in prostate cancer in a twin population. *J Urol* 1994;52: 1484–1489.

29. Steinberg GD, Carter BS, Beaty TH, et al. Family history and the risk of prostate cancer. *Prostate* 1990;17:337–347.

30. Lesko SM, Rosenberg L, Shapiro S. Family history and prostate cancer risk. *Am J Epidemiol* 1996;144: 1041–1047.

31. Ghadirian P, Howe GR, Hislop TG, Maisonneuve P. Family history of prostate cancer: a multi-center case-control study in Canada. *Int J Cancer* 1997;70:679–681.

32. Glover FE, Jr., Coffey DS, Douglas LL, et al. Familial study of prostate cancer in Jamaica. *Urology* 1998;52:441–443.

33. Rodriguez C, Calle EE, Miracle-McMahill HL, et al. Family history and risk of fatal prostate cancer. *Epidemiology* 1997; 8:653–657.

34. Whittemore AS, Wu AH, Kolonel LN, et al. Family history and prostate cancer risk in black, white, and Asian men in the United States and Canada. *Am J Epidemiol* 1995;141: 732–740.

35. Spitz MR, Currier RD, Fueger JJ, et al. Familial patterns of prostate cancer: a case-control analysis. *J Urol* 1991;146: 1305–1307.

36. Carter BS, Beaty TH, Steinberg GD, et al. Mendelian inheritance of familial prostate cancer. *Proc Natl Acad Sci USA* 1992;89:3367–3371.

37. Cui J, Staples MP, Hopper JL, et al. Segregation analyses of 1,476 population-based Australian families affected by prostate cancer. *Am J Hum Genet* 2001;68:1207–1218.

38. Monroe KR, Yu MC, Kolonel LN, et al. Evidence of an X-linked or recessive genetic component to prostate cancer risk. *Nat Med* 1995;1:827–829.

39. Gronberg H, Damber L, Damber JE, Iselius L. Segregation analysis of prostate cancer in Sweden: support for dominant inheritance. *Am J Epidemiol* 1997;146:552–557.

40. Schaid DJ, McDonnell SK, Blute ML, Thibodeau SN. Evidence for autosomal dominant inheritance of prostate cancer. *Am J Hum Genet* 1998;62:1425–1438.

41. Verhage BA, Baffoe-Bonnie AB, Baglietto L, et al. Autosomal dominant inheritance of prostate cancer: a confirmatory study. *Urology* 2001;57:97–101.

42. Smith JR, Freije D, Carpten JD, et al. Major susceptibility locus for prostate cancer on chromosome 1 suggested by a genome-wide search. *Science* 1996;274:1371–1374.

43. Berthon P, Valeri A, Cohen-Akenine A, et al. Predisposing gene for early-onset prostate cancer, localized on chromosome 1q42.2-43. *Am J Hum Genet* 1998;62:1416–1424.

44. Gibbs M, Stanford JL, McIndoe RA, et al. Evidence for a rare prostate cancer-susceptibility locus at chromosome 1p36. *Am J Hum Genet* 1999;64:776–787.

45. Xu J, Meyers D, Freije D, et al. Evidence for a prostate cancer susceptibility locus on the X chromosome. *Nat Genet* 1998;20:175–179.

46. Berry R, Schroeder JJ, French AJ, et al. Evidence for a prostate cancer-susceptibility locus on chromosome 20. *Am J Hum Genet* 2000;67:82–91.

47. Tavtigian SV, Simard J, Teng DH, et al. A candidate prostate cancer susceptibility gene at chromosome 17p. *Nat Genet* 2001;27:172–180.

48. Xu J, Zheng SL, Hawkins GA, et al. Linkage and association studies of prostate cancer susceptibility: evidence for linkage at 8p22–23. *Am J Hum Genet* 2001;69:341–350.

49. Wang L, McDonnell SK, Elkins DA, et al. Role of HPC2/ELAC2 in hereditary prostate cancer. *Cancer Res* 2001;61:6494–6499.

50. Rokman A, Ikonen T, Mononen N, et al. ELAC2/HPC2 involvement in hereditary and sporadic prostate cancer. *Cancer Res* 2001;61:6038–6041.

51. Suarez BK, Gerhard DS, Lin J, et al. Polymorphisms in the prostate cancer susceptibility gene HPC2/ELAC2 in multiplex families and healthy controls. *Cancer Res* 2001;61: 4982–4984.

52. Xu J, Zheng SL, Carpten JD, et al. Evaluation of linkage and association of HPC2/ELAC2 in patients with familial or sporadic prostate cancer. *Am J Hum Genet* 2001;68: 901–911.

53. Rebbeck TR, Walker AH, Zeigler-Johnson C, et al. Association of HPC2/ELAC2 genotypes and prostate cancer. *Am J Hum Genet* 2000;67:1014–1019.

54. Carpten J, Nupponen N, Isaacs S, et al. Germline mutations in the ribonuclease L gene in families showing linkage with HPC1. *Nat Genet* 2002;30:181–184.

55. Silverman RH, Jung DD, Nolan-Sorden NL, et al. Purification and analysis of murine 2-5A-dependent RNase. *J Biol Chem* 1988;263:7336–7341.

56. Jacobsen H, Czarniecki CW, Krause D, et al. Interferon-induced synthesis of 2-5A-dependent RNase in mouse JLS-V9R cells. *Virology* 1983;125:496–501.

57. Floyd-Smith G, Slattery E, Lengyel P. Interferon action: RNA cleavage pattern of a (2'-5')oligoadenylate-dependent endonuclease. *Science* 1981;212:1030–1032.

58. Clemens MJ, Williams BR. Inhibition of cell-free protein synthesis by pppA2'p5'A2'p5'A: a novel oligonucleotide synthesized by interferon-treated L cell extracts. *Cell* 1978;13:565–572.

59. Zhou A, Hassel BA, Silverman RH. Expression cloning of 2-5A-dependent RNAase: a uniquely regulated mediator of interferon action. *Cell* 1993;72:753–765.

60. Zhou A, Paranjape J, Brown TL, et al. Interferon action and apoptosis are defective in mice devoid of 2',5'- oligoadenylate-dependent RNase L. *EMBO J* 1997;16: 6355–6363.

61. Xu J, Zheng SL, Komiya A, et al. Germline mutations of the macrophage scavenger receptor 1 gene are associated with prostate cancer risk. *Nat Genet* 2002;32:321–325.

62. Platt N, Gordon S. Is the class A macrophage scavenger receptor (SR-A) multifunctional? The mouse's tale. *J Clin Invest* 2001;108:649–654.

63. Suzuki H, Kurihara Y, Takeya M, et al. A role for macrophage scavenger receptors in atherosclerosis and susceptibility to infection. *Nature* 1997;386:292–296.

64. Peiser L, Gough PJ, Kodama T, Gordon S. Macrophage class A scavenger receptor-mediated phagocytosis of *Escherichia coli*: role of cell heterogeneity, microbial strain, and culture conditions in vitro. *Infect Immun* 2000;68: 1953–1963.

65. Thomas CA, Li Y, Kodama T, et al. Protection from lethal Gram-positive infection by macrophage scavenger receptor-dependent phagocytosis. *J Exp Med* 2000;191:147–156.

66. Edwards A, Hammond HA, Jin L, et al. Genetic variation at five trimeric and tetrameric tandem repeat loci in four human population groups. *Genomics* 1992;12:241–253.

67. Hsing AW, Gao YT, Wu G, et al. Polymorphic CAG and GGN repeat lengths in the androgen receptor gene and prostate cancer risk: a population-based case-control study in China. *Cancer Res* 2000;60:5111–5116.

68. Hakimi JM, Schoenberg MP, Rondinelli RH, et al. Androgen receptor variants with short glutamine or glycine repeats may identify unique subpopulations of men with prostate cancer. *Clin Cancer Res* 1997;3:1599–1608.

69. Giovannucci E, Stampfer MJ, Krithivas K, et al. The CAG repeat within the androgen receptor gene and its relationship to prostate cancer. *Proc Natl Acad Sci USA* 1997;94: 3320–3323.

70. Stanford JL, Just JJ, Gibbs M, et al. Polymorphic repeats in the androgen receptor gene: molecular markers of prostate cancer risk. *Cancer Res* 1997;57:1194–1198.

71. Irvine RA, Yu MC, Ross RK, Coetzee GA. The CAG and GGC microsatellites of the androgen receptor gene are in linkage disequilibrium in men with prostate cancer. *Cancer Res* 1995;55:1937–1940.

72. Platz EA, Giovannucci E, Dahl DM, et al. The androgen receptor gene GGN microsatellite and prostate cancer risk. *Cancer Epidemiol Biomarkers Prev* 1998;7:379–384.

73. Chamberlain NL, Driver ED, Miesfeld RL. The length and location of CAG trinucleotide repeats in the androgen receptor N-terminal domain affect transactivation function. *Nucleic Acids Res* 1994;22:3181–3186.

74. Kazemi-Esfarjani P, Trifiro MA, Pinsky L. Evidence for a repressive function of the long polyglutamine tract in the human androgen receptor: possible pathogenetic relevance for the (CAG)n-expanded neuronopathies. *Hum Mol Genet* 1995;4:523–527.

75. Irvine RA, Ma H, Yu MC, et al. Inhibition of p160-mediated coactivation with increasing androgen receptor polyglutamine length. *Hum Mol Genet* 2000;9:267–274.

76. Beilin J, Ball EM, Favaloro JM, Zajac JD. Effect of the androgen receptor CAG repeat polymorphism on transcriptional activity: specificity in prostate and non-prostate cell lines. *J Mol Endocrinol* 2000;25:85–96.

77. Stanford JL, Noonan EA, Iwasaki L, et al. A polymorphism in the CYP17 gene and risk of prostate cancer. *Cancer Epidemiol Biomarkers Prev* 2002;11:243–247.

78. Kittles RA, Panguluri RK, Chen W, et al. Cyp17 promoter variant associated with prostate cancer aggressiveness in

African Americans. *Cancer Epidemiol Biomarkers Prev* 2001;10:943–947.

79. Haiman CA, Stampfer MJ, Giovannucci E, et al. The relationship between a polymorphism in CYP17 with plasma hormone levels and prostate cancer. *Cancer Epidemiol Biomarkers Prev* 2001;10:743–748.

80. Habuchi T, Liqing Z, Suzuki T, et al. Increased risk of prostate cancer and benign prostatic hyperplasia associated with a CYP17 gene polymorphism with a gene dosage effect. *Cancer Res* 2000;60:5710–5713.

81. Gsur A, Bernhofer G, Hinteregger S, et al. A polymorphism in the CYP17 gene is associated with prostate cancer risk. *Int J Cancer* 2000;87:434–437.

82. Wadelius M, Andersson AO, Johansson JE, et al. Prostate cancer associated with CYP17 genotype. *Pharmacogenetics* 1999;9:635–639.

83. Lunn RM, Bell DA, Mohler JL, Taylor JA. Prostate cancer risk and polymorphism in 17 hydroxylase (CYP17) and steroid reductase (SRD5A2). *Carcinogenesis* 1999;20: 1727–1731.

84. Nam RK, Toi A, Vesprini D, et al. V89L polymorphism of type-2, 5-alpha reductase enzyme gene predicts prostate cancer presence and progression. *Urology* 2001;57: 199–204.

85. Makridakis NM, Ross RK, Pike MC, et al. Association of mis-sense substitution in SRD5A2 gene with prostate cancer in African-American and Hispanic men in Los Angeles, USA. *Lancet* 1999;354:975–978.

86. Sakr WA, Grignon DJ, Crissman JD, et al. High grade prostatic intraepithelial neoplasia (HGPIN) and prostatic adenocarcinoma between the ages of 20–69: an autopsy study of 249 cases. *In Vivo* 1994;8:439–443.

87. Elo JP, Visakorpi T. Molecular genetics of prostate cancer. *Ann Med* 2001;33:130–141.

88. Dong JT, Chen C, Stultz BG, et al. Deletion at 13q21 is associated with aggressive prostate cancers. *Cancer Res* 2000;60:3880–3883.

89. Elo JP, Harkonen P, Kyllonen AP, et al. Three independently deleted regions at chromosome arm 16q in human prostate cancer: allelic loss at 16q24.1–q24.2 is associated with aggressive behaviour of the disease, recurrent growth, poor differentiation of the tumour and poor prognosis for the patient. *Br J Cancer* 1999;79:156–160.

90. Takahashi S, Shan AL, Ritland SR, et al. Frequent loss of heterozygosity at 7q31.1 in primary prostate cancer is associated with tumor aggressiveness and progression. *Cancer Res* 1995;55:4114–4119.

91. Nupponen NN, Kakkola L, Koivisto P, Visakorpi T. Genetic alterations in hormone-refractory recurrent prostate carcinomas. *Am J Pathol* 1998;153:141–148.

92. Takahashi S, Qian J, Brown JA, et al. Potential markers of prostate cancer aggressiveness detected by fluorescence in situ hybridization in needle biopsies. *Cancer Res* 1994;54: 3574–3579.

93. Millar DS, Ow KK, Paul CL, et al. Detailed methylation analysis of the glutathione S-transferase pi (GSTP1) gene in prostate cancer. *Oncogene* 1999;18:1313–1324.

94. Lee WH, Morton RA, Epstein JI, et al. Cytidine methylation of regulatory sequences near the pi-class glutathione *S*-transferase gene accompanies human prostatic carcinogenesis. *Proc Natl Acad Sci USA* 1994;91:11733–11737.

95. Lin X, Tascilar M, Lee WH, et al. GSTP1 CpG island hypermethylation is responsible for the absence of GSTP1

expression in human prostate cancer cells. *Am J Pathol* 2001;159:1815–1826.

96. Nelson WG, De Marzo AM, DeWeese TL. The molecular pathogenesis of prostate cancer: Implications for prostate cancer prevention. *Urology* 2001;57:39–45.

97. Brooks JD, Weinstein M, Lin X, et al. CG island methylation changes near the GSTP1 gene in prostatic intraepithelial neoplasia. *Cancer Epidemiol Biomarkers Prev* 1998; 7:531–536.

98. Adler V, Yin Z, Fuchs SY, et al. Regulation of JNK signaling by GSTp. *EMBO J* 1999;18:1321–1334.

99. Ruscoe JE, Rosario LA, Wang T, et al. Pharmacologic or genetic manipulation of glutathione S-transferase P1-1 (GSTpi) influences cell proliferation pathways. *J Pharmacol Exp Ther* 2001;298:339–345.

100. Wang T, Arifoglu P, Ronai Z, Tew KD. Glutathione S-transferase P1-1 (GSTP1-1) inhibits c-Jun N-terminal kinase (JNK1) signaling through interaction with the C terminus. *J Biol Chem* 2001;276:20,999–21,003.

101. Kinzler KW, Vogelstein B. Cancer-susceptibility genes. Gatekeepers and caretakers [see comments]. *Nature* 1997;386:761, 763.

102. Henderson CJ, Smith AG, Ure J, et al. Increased skin tumorigenesis in mice lacking pi class glutathione S-transferases. *Proc Natl Acad Sci USA* 1998;95:5275–5280.

103. Henderson CJ, Wolf CR, Kitteringham N, et al. Increased resistance to acetaminophen hepatotoxicity in mice lacking glutathione S-transferase Pi. *Proc Natl Acad Sci USA* 2000;97:12,741–12,745.

104. Bieberich CJ, Fujita K, He WW, Jay G. Prostate-specific and androgen-dependent expression of a novel homeobox gene. *J Biol Chem* 1996;271:31,779–31,782.

105. Sciavolino PJ, Abrams EW, Yang L, et al. Tissue-specific expression of murine Nkx3.1 in the male urogenital system. *Dev Dyn* 1997;209:127–138.

106. Bhatia-Gaur R, Donjacour AA, Sciavolino PJ, et al. Roles for Nkx3.1 in prostate development and cancer. *Genes Dev* 1999;13:966–977.

107. Abdulkadir SA, Magee JA, Peters TJ, et al. Conditional loss of Nkx3.1 in adult mice induces prostatic intraepithelial neoplasia. *Mol Cell Biol* 2002;22:1495–1503.

108. Emmert-Buck MR, Vocke CD, Pozzatti RO, et al. Allelic loss on chromosome 8p12-21 in microdissected prostatic intraepithelial neoplasia. *Cancer Res* 1995;55:2959–2962.

109. Bowen C, Bubendorf L, Voeller HJ, et al. Loss of NKX3.1 expression in human prostate cancers correlates with tumor progression. *Cancer Res* 2000;60:6111–6115.

110. He WW, Sciavolino PJ, Wing J, et al. A novel human prostate-specific, androgen-regulated homeobox gene (NKX3.1) that maps to 8p21, a region frequently deleted in prostate cancer. *Genomics* 1997;43:69–77.

111. Ornstein DK, Cinquanta M, Weiler S, et al. Expression studies and mutational analysis of the androgen regulated homeobox gene NKX3.1 in benign and malignant prostate epithelium. *J Urol* 2001;165:1329–1334.

112. Voeller HJ, Augustus M, Madike V, et al. Coding region of NKX3.1, a prostate-specific homeobox gene on 8p21, is not mutated in human prostate cancers. *Cancer Res* 1997;57: 4455–4459.

113. Furnari FB, Huang HJ, Cavenee WK. The phosphoinositol phosphatase activity of PTEN mediates a serum- sensitive G1 growth arrest in glioma cells. *Cancer Res* 1998;58: 5002–5008.

114. Li DM, Sun H. PTEN/MMAC1/TEP1 suppresses the tumorigenicity and induces G1 cell cycle arrest in human glioblastoma cells. *Proc Natl Acad Sci USA* 1998;95: 15,406–15,411.

115. Ramaswamy S, Nakamura N, Vazquez F, et al. Regulation of G1 progression by the PTEN tumor suppressor protein is linked to inhibition of the phosphatidylinositol 3-kinase/Akt pathway. *Proc Natl Acad Sci USA* 1999;96:2110–2115.

116. Sun H, Lesche R, Li DM, et al. PTEN modulates cell cycle progression and cell survival by regulating phosphatidylinositol 3,4,5,-trisphosphate and Akt/protein kinase B signaling pathway. *Proc Natl Acad Sci USA* 1999;96:6199–6204.

117. Podsypanina K, Ellenson LH, Nemes A, et al. Mutation of Pten/Mmac1 in mice causes neoplasia in multiple organ systems. *Proc Natl Acad Sci USA* 1999;96:1563–1568.

118. Di Cristofano A, Pesce B, Cordon-Cardo C, Pandolfi PP. Pten is essential for embryonic development and tumour suppression. *Nat Genet* 1998;19:348–355.

119. Kim MJ, Cardiff RD, Desai N, et al. Cooperativity of Nkx3.1 and Pten loss of function in a mouse model of prostate carcinogenesis. *Proc Natl Acad Sci USA* 2002;99:2884–2889.

120. Kwabi-Addo B, Giri D, Schmidt K, et al. Haploinsufficiency of the Pten tumor suppressor gene promotes prostate cancer progression. *Proc Natl Acad Sci USA* 2001;98: 11,563–11,568.

121. McMenamin ME, Soung P, Perera S, et al. Loss of PTEN expression in paraffin-embedded primary prostate cancer correlates with high Gleason score and advanced stage. *Cancer Res* 1999;59:4291–4296.

122. Wu X, Senechal K, Neshat MS, et al. The PTEN/MMAC1 tumor suppressor phosphatase functions as a negative regulator of the phosphoinositide 3-kinase/Akt pathway. *Proc Natl Acad Sci USA* 1998;95:15,587–15,591.

123. Steck PA, Pershouse MA, Jasser SA, et al. Identification of a candidate tumour suppressor gene, MMAC1, at chromosome 10q23.3 that is mutated in multiple advanced cancers. *Nat Genet* 1997;15:356–362.

124. Teng DH, Hu R, Lin H, et al. MMAC1/PTEN mutations in primary tumor specimens and tumor cell lines. *Cancer Res* 1997;57:5221–5225.

125. Myers MP, Pass I, Batty IH, et al. The lipid phosphatase activity of PTEN is critical for its tumor supressor function. *Proc Natl Acad Sci USA* 1998;95:13,513–13,518.

126. Myers MP, Stolarov JP, Eng C, et al. P-TEN, the tumor suppressor from human chromosome 10q23, is a dual-specificity phosphatase. *Proc Natl Acad Sci USA* 1997;94: 9052–9057.

127. Maehama T, Dixon JE. The tumor suppressor, PTEN/MMAC1, dephosphorylates the lipid second messenger, phosphatidylinositol 3,4,5-trisphosphate. *J Biol Chem* 1998;273: 13,375–13,378.

128. Cairns P, Okami K, Halachmi S, et al. Frequent inactivation of PTEN/MMAC1 in primary prostate cancer. *Cancer Res* 1997;57:4997–5000.

129. Suzuki H, Freije D, Nusskern DR, et al. Interfocal heterogeneity of PTEN/MMAC1 gene alterations in multiple metastatic prostate cancer tissues. *Cancer Res* 1998;58: 204–209.

130. Wang SI, Parsons R, Ittmann M. Homozygous deletion of the PTEN tumor suppressor gene in a subset of prostate adenocarcinomas. *Clin Cancer Res* 1998;4:811–815.

131. Gray IC, Stewart LM, Phillips SM, et al. Mutation and expression analysis of the putative prostate tumour-suppressor gene PTEN. *Br J Cancer* 1998;78:1296–1300.

132. Whang YE, Wu X, Suzuki H, et al. Inactivation of the tumor suppressor PTEN/MMAC1 in advanced human prostate cancer through loss of expression. *Proc Natl Acad Sci USA* 1998;95:5246–5250.

133. Cordon-Cardo C, Koff A, Drobnjak M, et al. Distinct altered patterns of p27KIP1 gene expression in benign prostatic hyperplasia and prostatic carcinoma. *J Natl Cancer Inst* 1998;90:1284–1291.

134. Di Cristofano A, De Acetis M, Koff A, et al. Pten and p27KIP1 cooperate in prostate cancer tumor suppression in the mouse. *Nat Genet* 2001;27:222–224.

135. Yang RM, Naitoh J, Murphy M, et al. Low p27 expression predicts poor disease-free survival in patients with prostate cancer. *J Urol* 1998;159:941–945.

136. Cheville JC, Lloyd RV, Sebo TJ, et al. Expression of p27kip1 in prostatic adenocarcinoma. *Mod Pathol* 1998;11:324–328.

137. Cote RJ, Shi Y, Groshen S, et al. Association of p27Kip1 levels with recurrence and survival in patients with stage C prostate carcinoma. *J Natl Cancer Inst* 1998;90:916–920.

138. Guo Y, Sklar GN, Borkowski A, Kyprianou N. Loss of the cyclin-dependent kinase inhibitor p27(Kip1) protein in human prostate cancer correlates with tumor grade. *Clin Cancer Res* 1997;3:2269–2274.

139. De Marzo AM, Meeker AK, Epstein JI, Coffey DS. Prostate stem cell compartments: expression of the cell cycle inhibitor p27Kip1 in normal, hyperplastic, and neoplastic cells. *Am J Pathol* 1998;153:911–919.

140. Kibel AS, Faith DA, Bova GS, Isaacs WB. Loss of heterozygosity at 12P12-13 in primary and metastatic prostate adenocarcinoma. *J Urol* 2000;164:192–196.

141. Graff JR, Konicek BW, McNulty AM, et al. Increased AKT activity contributes to prostate cancer progression by dramatically accelerating prostate tumor growth and diminishing p27Kip1 expression. *J Biol Chem* 2000;275:24,500–24,505.

142. Gottschalk AR, Basila D, Wong M, et al. p27Kip1 is required for PTEN-induced G1 growth arrest. *Cancer Res* 2001;61: 2105–2111.

143. Nakamura N, Ramaswamy S, Vazquez F, et al. Forkhead transcription factors are critical effectors of cell death and cell cycle arrest downstream of PTEN. *Mol Cell Biol* 2000;20:8969–8982.

144. Amler LC, Agus DB, LeDuc C, et al. Dysregulated expression of androgen-responsive and nonresponsive genes in the androgen-independent prostate cancer xenograft model CWR22-R1. *Cancer Res* 2000;60:6134–6141.

145. Mousses S, Wagner U, Chen Y, et al. Failure of hormone therapy in prostate cancer involves systematic restoration of androgen responsive genes and activation of rapamycin sensitive signaling. *Oncogene* 2001;20:6718–6723.

146. van der Kwast TH, Schalken J, de Winter JAR, et al. Androgen receptors in endocrine-therapy-resistant human prostate cancer. *Int J Cancer* 1991;48:189–193.

147. Stanbrough M, Leav I, Kwan PW, et al. Prostatic intraepithelial neoplasia in mice expressing an androgen receptor transgene in prostate epithelium. *Proc Natl Acad Sci USA* 2001;98: 10,823–10,828.

148. Visakorpi T, Hyytinen E, Koivisto P, et al. In vivo amplification of the androgen receptor gene and progression of human prostate cancer. *Nat Genet* 1995;9:401–406.

149. Koivisto P, Kononen J, Palmberg C, et al. Androgen receptor gene amplification: a possible molecular mechanism for androgen deprivation therapy failure in prostate cancer. *Cancer Res* 1997;57:314–319.

150. Haapala K, Hyytinen ER, Roiha M, et al. Androgen receptor alterations in prostate cancer relapsed during a combined androgen blockade by orchiectomy and bicalutamide. *Lab Invest* 2001;81:1647–1651.

151. Marcelli M, Ittmann M, Mariani S, et al. Androgen receptor mutations in prostate cancer. *Cancer Res* 2000;60: 944–949.

152. Taplin ME, Bubley GJ, Shuster TD, et al. Mutation of the androgen-receptor gene in metastatic androgen-independent prostate cancer. *N Engl J Med* 1995;332:1393–1398.

153. Taplin ME, Bubley GJ, Ko YJ, et al. Selection for androgen receptor mutations in prostate cancers treated with androgen antagonist. *Cancer Res* 1999;59:2511–2515.

154. Tilley WD, Buchanan G, Hickey TE, Bentel JM. Mutations in the androgen receptor gene are associated with progression of human prostate cancer to androgen independence. *Clin Cancer Res* 1996;2:277–285.

155. Veldscholte J, Ris-Stalpers C, Kuiper GG, et al. A mutation in the ligand binding domain of the androgen receptor of human LNCaP cells affects steroid binding characteristics and response to anti-androgens. *Biochem Biophys Res Commun* 1990;173:534–540.

156. Schoenberg MP, Hakimi JM, Wang S, et al. Microsatellite mutation (CAG24→18) in the androgen receptor gene in human prostate cancer. *Biochem Biophys Res Commun* 1994;198:74–80.

157. Suzuki H, Akakura K, Komiya A, et al. Codon 877 mutation in the androgen receptor gene in advanced prostate cancer: relation to antiandrogen withdrawal syndrome. *Prostate* 1996;29:153–158.

158. Suzuki H, Sato N, Watabe Y, et al. Androgen receptor gene mutations in human prostate cancer. *J Steroid Biochem Mol Biol* 1993;46:759–765.

159. Newmark JR, Hardy DO, Tonb DC, et al. Androgen receptor gene mutations in human prostate cancer. *Proc Natl Acad Sci USA* 1992;89:6319–6323.

160. Gaddipati JP, McLeod DG, Heidenberg HB, et al. Frequent detection of codon 877 mutation in the androgen receptor gene in advanced prostate cancers. *Cancer Res* 1994;54: 2861–2864.

161. Evans BA, Harper ME, Daniells CE, et al. Low incidence of androgen receptor gene mutations in human prostatic tumors using single strand conformation polymorphism analysis. *Prostate* 1996;28:162–171.

162. Tan J, Sharief Y, Hamil KG, et al. Dehydroepiandrosterone activates mutant androgen receptors expressed in the androgen-dependent human prostate cancer xenograft CWR22 and LNCaP cells. *Mol Endocrinol* 1997;11: 450–459.

163. Veldscholte J, Voorhorst-Ogink MM, Bolt-de Vries J, et al. Unusual specificity of the androgen receptor in the human prostate tumor cell line LNCaP: high affinity for progestagenic and estrogenic steroids. *Biochim Biophys Acta* 1990;1052:187–194.

164. Culig Z, Hobisch A, Cronauer MV, et al. Mutant androgen receptor detected in an advanced-stage prostatic carcinoma is activated by adrenal androgens and progesterone. *Mol Endocrinol* 1993;7:1541–1550.

165. Shi XB, Ma AH, Xia L, et al. Functional analysis of 44 mutant androgen receptors from human prostate cancer. *Cancer Res* 2002;62:1496–1502.

166. Gardner WA, Bennett BD. The prostate overview: recent insights and speculations. In *Pathology and Pathobiology of the*

Urinary Bladder and Prostate. Weinstein RS, Gardner WA, eds. Williams and Wilkins, Baltimore; 1992: pp. 129–148.

167. Roberts RO, Lieber MM, Rhodes T, et al. Prevalence of a physician-assigned diagnosis of prostatitis: the Olmsted County Study of Urinary Symptoms and Health Status Among Men. *Urology* 1998;51:578–584.

168. Giovannucci E. Medical history and etiology of prostate cancer. *Epidemiol Rev* 2001;23:159–162.

169. Hoekx L, Jeuris W, Van Marck E, Wyndaele JJ. Elevated serum prostate specific antigen (PSA) related to asymptomatic prostatic inflammation. *Acta Urol Belg* 1998;66:1–2.

170. Hayes RB, Pottern LM, Strickler H, et al. Sexual behaviour, STDs and risks for prostate cancer. *Br J Cancer* 2000;82: 718–725.

171. Dennis LK, Dawson DV. Meta-analysis of measures of sexual activity and prostate cancer. *Epidemiology* 2002;13:72–79.

172. Xia Y, Zweier JL. Superoxide and peroxynitrite generation from inducible nitric oxide synthase in macrophages. *Proc Natl Acad Sci USA* 1997;94:6954–6958.

173. Eiserich JP, Hristova M, Cross CE, et al. Formation of nitric oxide-derived inflammatory oxidants by myeloperoxidase in neutrophils. *Nature* 1998;391:393–397.

174. Clark LC, Dalkin B, Krongrad A, et al. Decreased incidence of prostate cancer with selenium supplementation: results of a double-blind cancer prevention trial. *Br J Urol* 1998;81: 730–734.

175. Clark LC, Combs GF Jr, Turnbull BW, et al. Effects of selenium supplementation for cancer prevention in patients with carcinoma of the skin. A randomized controlled trial. Nutritional Prevention of Cancer Study Group [published erratum appears in *JAMA* 1997;277:1520]. *JAMA* 1996;276:1957–1963.

176. Heinonen OP, Albanes D, Virtamo J, et al. Prostate cancer and supplementation with alpha-tocopherol and beta-carotene: incidence and mortality in a controlled trial [see comments]. *J Natl Cancer Inst* 1998;90:440–446.

177. Roberts RO, Jacobson DJ, Girman CJ, et al. A population-based study of daily nonsteroidal anti-inflammatory drug use and prostate cancer. *Mayo Clin Proc* 2002;77:219–225.

178. Nelson JE, Harris RE. Inverse association of prostate cancer and non-steroidal anti- inflammatory drugs (NSAIDs): results of a case-control study. *Oncol Rep* 2000;7:169–170.

179. Norrish AE, Jackson RT, McRae CU. Non-steroidal anti-inflammatory drugs and prostate cancer progression. *Int J Cancer* 1998;77:511–515.

180. De Marzo AM, Marchi VL, Epstein JI, Nelson WG. Proliferative inflammatory atrophy of the prostate: implications for prostatic carcinogenesis. *Am J Pathol* 1999;155: 1985–1992.

181. Franks LM. Atrophy and hyperplasia in the prostate proper. *J Pathol Bacteriol* 1954;68:617–621.

182. Feneley MR, Young MP, Chinyama C, et al. Ki-67 expression in early prostate cancer and associated pathological lesions. *J Clin Pathol* 1996;49:741–748.

183. Ruska KM, Sauvageot J, Epstein JI. Histology and cellular kinetics of prostatic atrophy. *Am J Surg Pathol* 1998;22: 1073–1077.

184. Putzi MJ, De Marzo AM. Morphologic transitions between proliferative inflammatory atrophy and high-grade prostatic intraepithelial neoplasia. *Urology* 2000;56:828–832.

185. Shah R, Mucci NR, Amin A, et al. Postatrophic hyperplasia of the prostate gland: neoplastic precursor or innocent bystander? *Am J Pathol* 2001;158:1767–1773.

186. Zha S, Gage WR, Sauvageot J, et al. Cyclooxygenase-2 is up-regulated in proliferative inflammatory atrophy of the prostate, but not in prostate carcinoma. *Cancer Res* 2001;61:8617–8623.

187. Parsons JK, Nelson CP, Gage WR, et al. GSTA1 expression in normal, preneoplastic, and neoplastic human prostate tissue. *Prostate* 2001;49:30–37.

188. Wilson MJ, Ditmanson JV, Sinha AA, Estensen RD. Plasminogen activator activities in the ventral and dorsolateral prostatic lobes of aging Fischer 344 rats. *Prostate* 1990;16:147–161.

189. Reznik G, Hamlin MH 2nd, Ward JM, Stinson SF. Prostatic hyperplasia and neoplasia in aging F344 rats. *Prostate* 1981;2:261–268.

190. Brooks JD, Metter EJ, Chan DW, et al. Plasma selenium level before diagnosis and the risk of prostate cancer development. *J Urol* 2001;166:2034–2038.

191. Chan JM, Stampfer MJ, Ma J, et al. Supplemental vitamin E intake and prostate cancer risk in a large cohort of men in the United States. *Cancer Epidemiol Biomarkers Prev* 1999;8: 893–899.

192. Helzlsouer KJ, Huang HY, Alberg AJ, et al. Association between alpha-tocopherol, gamma-tocopherol, selenium, and subsequent prostate cancer. *J Natl Cancer Inst* 2000;92: 2018–2023.

193. The effect of vitamin E and beta carotene on the incidence of lung cancer and other cancers in male smokers. The Alpha-Tocopherol, Beta Carotene Cancer Prevention Study Group. *N Engl J Med* 1994;330:1029–1035.

194. Virtamo J, Edwards BK, Virtanen M, et al. Effects of supplemental alpha-tocopherol and beta-carotene on urinary tract cancer: incidence and mortality in a controlled trial (Finland). *Cancer Causes Control* 2000;11:933–939.

195. Blot WJ, Li Jy, Taylor PR, et al. Linxian nutrition intervention trials: supplementation with specific vitamin/mineral combinations, cancer incidence, and disease-specific mortality in the general population. *J Natl Cancer Inst* 1993;85: 1483–1492.

196. Heart Protection Study Collaborative Group. MRC/BHF heart protection study of antioxidant vitamin supplementation in 20 536 high-risk individuals: a randomised placebo-controlled trial. *Lancet* 2002;360:23–33.

197. Lippman SM, Hong WK. Cancer prevention science and practice. *Cancer Res* 2002;62:5119–5125.

198. Sabichi AL, Lee JJ, Taylor RJ, et al. Selenium accumulates in prostate tissue of prostate cancer patients after short-term administration of *l*-selenomethionine. *Proc Am Assoc Cancer Res* 2002;43:1007–1008.

199. Clark LC, Marshall JR. Randomized, controlled chemoprevention trials in populations at very high risk for prostate cancer: elevated prostate-specific antigen and high-grade prostatic intraepithelial neoplasia. *Urology* 2001;57: 185–187.

200. Hoque A, Albanes D, Lippman SM, et al. Molecular epidemiologic studies within the Selenium and Vitamin E Cancer Prevention Trial (SELECT). *Cancer Causes Control* 2001;12:627–633.

201. Sabichi AL, Lippman SM. COX-2 inhibitors and other NSAIDs in bladder prostate cancer. In *COX-2*. Dannenberg AJ, DuBois RN, eds. Karger, Basel, 2003; pp. 163–178.

202. Subbarayan V, Sabichi AL, Llansa N, et al. Differential expression of cyclooxygenase-2 and its regulation by tumor

necrosis factor-alpha in normal and malignant prostate cells. *Cancer Res* 2001;61:2720–2726.

203. Habel LA, Zhao W, Stanford JL. Daily aspirin use and prostate cancer risk in a large, multiracial cohort in the US. *Cancer Causes Control* 2002;13:427–434.

204. Wechter WJ, Leipold DD, Murray ED Jr, et al. E-7869 (R-flurbiprofen) inhibits progression of prostate cancer in the TRAMP mouse. *Cancer Res* 2000;60:2203–2208.

205. Goluboff ET, Shabsigh A, Saidi JA, et al. Exisulind (sulindac sulfone) suppresses growth of human prostate cancer in a nude mouse xenograft model by increasing apoptosis. *Urology* 1999;53:440–445.

206. Lim JT, Piazza GA, Han EK, et al. Sulindac derivatives inhibit growth and induce apoptosis in human prostate cancer cell lines. *Biochem Pharmacol* 1999; 58:1097–1107.

207. Goluboff ET, Prager D, Rukstalis D, et al. Safety and efficacy of exisulind for treatment of recurrent prostate cancer after radical prostatectomy. *J Urol* 2001;166:882–886.

208. Ghosh J, Myers CE. Inhibition of arachidonate 5-lipoxygenase triggers massive apoptosis in human prostate cancer cells. *Proc Natl Acad Sci USA* 1998;95:13182–13187.

209. Nie D, Che M, Grignon D, et al. Role of eicosanoids in prostate cancer progression. *Cancer Metastasis Rev* 2001;20:195–206.

210. Shureiqi I, Lippman SM. Lipoxygenase modulation to reverse carcinogenesis. *Cancer Res* 2001;61:6307–6312.

211. Aaltoma SH, Lipponen PK, Kosma VM. Inducible nitric oxide synthase (iNOS) expression and its prognostic value in prostate cancer. *Anticancer Res* 2001; 21:3101–3106.

212. Andriole G, Lieber M, Smith J, et al. Treatment with finasteride following radical prostatectomy for prostate cancer. *Urology* 1995;45:491–497.

213. Presti JC, Jr., Fair WR, Andriole G, et al. Multicenter, randomized, double-blind, placebo controlled study to investigate the effect of finasteride (MK-906) on stage D prostate cancer. *J Urol* 1992; 148:1201–1204.

214. Feigl P, Blumenstein B, Thompson I, et al. Design of the Prostate Cancer Prevention Trial (PCPT). *Control Clin Trials* 1995;16:150–163.

215. Andriole GL, Guess HA, Epstein JI, et al. Treatment with finasteride preserves usefulness of prostate-specific antigen in the detection of prostate cancer: results of a randomized, double-blind, placebo-controlled clinical trial. PLESS Study Group. Proscar Long-term Efficacy and Safety Study. *Urology* 1998;52:195–202.

216. Cote RJ, Skinner EC, Salem CE, et al. The effect of finasteride on the prostate gland in men with elevated serum prostate-specific antigen levels. *Br J Cancer* 1998;78:413–418.

217. Kensler TW. Chemoprevention by inducers of carcinogen detoxication enzymes. *Environ Health Perspect* 1997;105 Suppl 4:965–970.

218. Ramos-Gomez M, Kwak MK, Dolan PM, et al. From the Cover: sensitivity to carcinogenesis is increased and chemoprotective efficacy of enzyme inducers is lost in nrf2 transcription factor-deficient mice. *Proc Natl Acad Sci USA* 2001;98:3410–3415.

219. Jacobson LP, Zhang BC, Zhu YR, et al. Oltipraz chemoprevention trial in Qidong, People's Republic of China: study design and clinical outcomes. *Cancer Epidemiol Biomarkers Prev* 1997;6:257–265.

220. Kensler TW, He X, Otieno M, et al. Oltipraz chemoprevention trial in Qidong, People's Republic of China: modulation of serum aflatoxin albumin adduct biomarkers. *Cancer Epidemiol Biomarkers Prev* 1998;7:127–134.

221. Wang JS, Shen X, He X, et al. Protective alterations in phase 1 and 2 metabolism of aflatoxin B1 by oltipraz in residents of Qidong, People's Republic of China. *J Natl Cancer Inst* 1999;91:347–354.

222. Coltman CA Jr, Thompson IM Jr, Feigl P. Prostate Cancer Prevention Trial (PCPT) update. *Eur Urol* 1999;35:544–547.

223. Gail MH, Brinton LA, Byar DP, et al. Projecting individualized probabilities of developing breast cancer for white females who are being examined annually. *J Natl Cancer Inst* 1989;81:1879–1886.

224. Chan JM, Stampfer MJ, Giovannucci E, et al. Plasma insulin-like growth factor-I and prostate cancer risk: a prospective study. *Science* 1998;279:563–566.

225. Gann PH, Hennekens CH, Stampfer MJ. A prospective evaluation of plasma prostate-specific antigen for detection of prostatic cancer. *JAMA* 1995;273:289–294.

226. Ross KS, Carter HB, Pearson JD, Guess HA. Comparative efficiency of prostate-specific antigen screening strategies for prostate cancer detection. *JAMA* 2000;284:1399–405.

227. Petricoin EF, Ardekani AM, Hitt BA, et al. Use of proteomic patterns in serum to identify ovarian cancer. *Lancet* 2002;359:572–577.

228. O'Shaughnessy JA, Kelloff GJ, Gordon GB, et al. Treatment and prevention of intraepithelial neoplasia: an important target for accelerated new agent development. *Clin Cancer Res* 2002;8:314–346.

229. Thompson IM, Goodman PJ, Tangen CM, et al. The influence of finasteride on the development of prostate cancer. *N Engl J Med* 2003;349:215–224.

230. Scardino PT. The prevention of prostate cancer—The dilemma continues. *N Engl J Med* 2003;349:297–299.

16 Use of PSA to Evaluate Risk and Progression of Prostate Cancer

Bulent Akduman, MD, Abelardo Errejon, MD, and E. David Crawford, MD

1. INTRODUCTION

During the past two decades, a better understanding of tumor biology has led to increased interest in the concept of cancer prevention. Chemoprevention involves inhibiting carcinogenesis through application of noncytotoxic nutrients and pharmacologic compounds, thereby preventing the development and progression of malignant cells. Prostate cancer is one of the primary targets for chemopreventive studies. It has a long latency period, and autopsy series demonstrate that the probable precursors to prostate cancer are identifiable decades before presence of the disease. It was reported that prostatic epithelial neoplasia (PIN), a premalignant condition, can occur in men as young as 30 yr of age *(1)*. Because it takes a long time to go from the precursor lesion to cancer development, therapies do not reverse the premalignant condition, though the type of disease presentation affects ultimate survival. Along with interest in cancer chemoprevention have come a number of new challenges, including identification of high-risk groups as well as assessing response to intervention. Chemoprevention should benefit men

in the general population, especially those with high risk of developing cancer. Those with high-grade PIN in a prostate biopsy specimen, men with a family history of prostate cancer, and African-American men may gain additional benefits from chemopreventive measures.

Results of studies in the United States suggest that prostate cancer screening of men older than 50 yr of age decreases the incidence of advanced disease *(2)*. It has been proposed that annual prostate-specific antigen (PSA) measurement and digital rectal examination (DRE) have helped shift the majority of prostate cancer cases at diagnosis to being locally confined with potentially curative options *(3)*. Between 1990 and 1995, prostate cancer mortality declined 6.3% *(4)*. Labrie et al. found a 2.7-fold advantage in favor of screening and early treatment by examining the annual death rates of men in screened and unscreened groups *(5)*. Several other studies found that early detection increased the number of early-stage cancers diagnosed; the majority of these cancers involved potentially significant disease *(6–8)*. The value of early diagnosis of indolent prostate cancer varieties that otherwise might never be clinically detected is debatable. Moreover, critical questions still

From: Cancer Chemoprevention, Volume 2: Strategies for Cancer Chemoprevention
Edited by: G. J. Kelloff, E. T. Hawk, and C. C. Sigman © Humana Press Inc., Totowa, NJ

remain regarding treatment-associated morbidity, cost-effectiveness, and the psychosocial impact of screening. Because of these drawbacks to conventional therapy, chemoprevention of prostate cancer has become an attractive alternative.

Serum tumor markers are a most helpful tool in evaluating and managing patients with any type of neoplasm. No single biological marker has revolutionized cancer treatment to such an extent as PSA. It has established utility both as an immunohistochemical marker and as a method of monitoring patients with established malignancy. Use of PSA to diagnose and stage prostate cancer is currently undergoing detailed investigation.

2. PROSTATE-SPECIFIC ANTIGEN

PSA, a serine protease of the human kallikrein gene hKLK3, is a 34-kDa glycoprotein specific to prostatic epithelium. PSA manifests chymotrypsin-like proteolytic enzyme activity that is believed to be directed mainly against the major gel-forming proteins, semenogelin I and II and fibrinonectin, in freshly ejaculated semen (9). Proteolysis of these proteins induces liquefaction of semen, which results in the subsequent release of progressively motile spermatozoa (10). After it is synthesized in the ductal epithelium and acini of the prostate, most PSA remains in the lumen of the prostate gland, but a small portion can be detected in serum. Normal levels of serum PSA are <4 ng/mL, which is about 10^{-6} less than in seminal fluid. However, this tight compartmentalization of PSA in the normal prostate is altered in prostatic disease, allowing increased amounts of PSA to enter the serum. Elevations in serum PSA levels represent a spectrum of changes that include tumor size, grade, and inflammation as well as growth factors. These complexities may make the interpretation of results more difficult. It was reported that DRE was not associated with erroneous elevation of PSA (11,12). On the other hand, significant prostatic perturbations, such as prostate needle biopsy, urethral instrumentation, and transurethral resection of the prostate, cause significant elevation of serum PSA. Ellis and Brawer studied 127 men following ultrasound-guided transrectal prostate needle biopsies and noted a ≥20% elevation in serum PSA levels 28 d after the procedure, when compared with prebiopsy level (13). In contrast, ejaculation can lead to a significant decrease in serum PSA measured on the next day (14). Manipulation of the hormonal environment by treating benign prostatic hyperplasia (BPH) with finasteride, a

5α-reductase inhibitor, also lowers serum PSA levels by 50% after 12 mo of treatment (15). Patients treated with finasteride should have baseline PSA measured before initiation of treatment and should be followed with serial PSA measurement.

One problem with serum PSA assays is lack of an international standard. Numerous different assays are available to determine serum PSA, creating substantial problems in interpretation. Potential differences between different manufacturers' assays are caused by a number of factors, including assay calibration, incubation time, and nonequilibrium or different affinities of various PSA isoforms (16,17).

The natural history of changes in PSA might make it a useful surrogate endpoint for prostate cancer in the setting of chemoprevention trials. Since PSA is not exclusive for cancer, techniques to increase its sensitivity and specificity are desirable.

3. AGE-SPECIFIC PSA REFERENCE RANGES

One approach to enhance PSA's performance is age-specific PSA reference ranges. Serum PSA levels increase with age due to an increase in prostate size. In addition, other factors such as prostate infection, prostate infarction, microscopic prostate cancer, and leaking of the prostate epithelium need to be considered. Oesterling et al. studied a large cohort of men of all ages without prostate cancer to establish normal age-specific PSA reference ranges and suggested different cutoffs for different age groups: age 40–50 yr, 0–2.5 ng/mL; age 50–60, 0–3.5 ng/mL; age 60–70, 0–4.5 ng/mL; age 70–80, 0–6.5 ng/mL (18). It has been suggested that age-specific PSA reference ranges may lead to increased cancer detection in younger men more likely to benefit from treatment and minimize unnecessary evaluations in older men less likely to benefit from treatment. However, considerable disagreement exists over the benefit of using age-specific PSA reference ranges. Catalona et al. and Littrup et al. reported that this adjustment conferred no additional benefit over use of the adopted cutoff value of 4.0 ng/mL in detecting prostate cancer (19,20). However, for younger men, PSA levels below 4 ng/mL warrant greater scrutiny because the relative risk of cancer increases even at PSA levels between 2.0 and 4.0 ng/mL (21). These patients also have the most to gain from a diagnosis of prostate cancer (22).

Age-specific PSA reference ranges help establish baseline data for patients undergoing chemoprevention trials. As PSA variance increases with age, this is a more useful biomarker for prostate cancer chemoprevention in the 30–50-yr age range *(23)*. PSA was also compared by race in this study, and the greatest variability was found among African-Americans, which may complicate the usefulness of PSA in this subset of high-risk subjects.

4. PSA VELOCITY

PSA velocity (PSAV) is the change over time of several measurements of PSA. PSAV allows longitudinal measurements of serum PSA levels and therefore provides a more dynamic PSA interpretation than does a single measurement. This concept was first introduced by Carter et al. *(24)*, who found that a velocity of 0.75 ng/mL or more per year as measured with the Hybertech Tandem-R assay was highly suggestive of cancer. To obtain maximal benefit using PSAV, measurements should be obtained at least three times over a 2-yr period or spaced at least 12–18 mo apart. In addition, PSAV rises in a steeper fashion for advanced cases than for localized or regionally advanced cases of prostate cancer. A major limitation of PSAV is the significant degree of biological variation observed in serum PSA levels of normal men. These variations can be as high as 30% when the same assay is used on different days *(25)*. For PSAV to be useful in chemoprevention trials, the frequency of determinations and careful assay variability analysis is required.

5. PSA DENSITY AND TRANSITION ZONE PSA DENSITY

PSA density (PSAD) was introduced as a method by which the ratio of serum PSA and transrectal ultrasound-determined prostate volume could improve our ability to differentiate BPH from prostate cancer via noninvasive methods *(26)*. Although conceptually promising, PSAD alone showed no advantage in predicting prostate cancer *(27)*.

Since BPH is almost exclusively the result of hyperplasia of the transition zone, outer gland production of PSA is relatively constant as the gland enlarges due to BPH. PSA changes due to BPH are introduced by the effect on transition zone elements. Transition zone PSA density (TZPSAD) is defined as serum PSA divided by the volume of the transition zone determined by transrectal ultrasound. Although initial reports were encouraging, Lin et al. have been unable to reproduce these data in their series *(28–30)*.

Despite early enthusiasm for PSAD and TZPSAD, enhanced performances suggested by the initial investigators may not be reproducible. The usefulness of PSAD and TZPSAD in chemoprevention trials has similar limitations to PSA alone.

6. MOLECULAR FORMS OF PSA

PSA circulates in a variety of molecular forms. The majority of PSA does not occur in the free form found in the ejaculate, but rather is complexed to protease inhibitors including α_2-macroglobulin (A2M), α_1-antichymotrypsin (ACT), and α_1-antitrypsin. The majority of PSA in the systemic circulation is complexed to ACT. In PSA-ACT, two epitopes remain unmasked, and this complex can be detected with immunoassays. When PSA is complexed with A2M (PSA-A2M), all epitopes are sterically hindered, so that this moiety is undetectable by currently available assays. Studies have illustrated the potential benefits of using free-to-total PSA ratio to enhance the clinical utility of PSA in early prostate cancer detection *(31–33)*. Though these studies reported that free-to-total PSA ratio is lower in men with prostate cancer than in men with benign disease, there is considerable controversy as to how much lower. It is generally accepted that a ratio of <0.20 is associated with prostate cancer.

There is increasing interest in assays that measure the complex form of PSA. The Seattle group performed a study on archival serum in men who had undergone previous ultrasound-guided prostate needle biopsy using the Bayer complex PSA assay *(34)*. These results were compared with the Hybritech Tandem-R free and total PSA assays. At the 95% sensitivity level, total PSA specificity was 22%. The free-to-total PSA ratio required a 28% cutoff to afford the sensitivity and provided only a 15.6% specificity. In contrast, the complex PSA of 2.52 offered a 26.7% specificity. The value of molecular forms of PSA in the setting of chemoprevention trials is not known.

7. PSA REVERSE TRANSCRIPTION-POLYMERASE CHAIN REACTION ASSAY

When circulating prostate cancer cells are present in peripheral blood, these cells can be identified by reverse transcription of circulating PSA mRNA to complementary DNA and amplification of DNA coding for PSA by polymerase chain reaction (RT-PCR). PCR analysis for PSA has been negative in women and in men with no evidence of prostate cancer. A positive PCR-PSA assay appears to be specific for prostate cancer cells and correlates directly with the pathologic extent of the disease *(35)*. However, its use in prostate

Table 1
Risk Factors for Prostate Cancer

Age
Race, African-American
Genetics, family history
High-grade PIN
High PSA levels

Table 2
Advantages and Disadvantages of PSA
for Chemoprevention Trials

Advantages	Disadvantages
Noninvasive	Racial variability
Inexpensive	Age variability
Frequent monitoring	Affected by hormones
Reproducible	Affected by differentiation agents

cancer management is investigational. Because the role of RT-PCR in prostate cancer is not completely understood, it is difficult to apply this concept to chemoprevention studies. Further studies are indicated to evaluate the role of this technique.

8. IDENTIFYING HIGH-RISK COHORTS FOR CHEMOPREVENTION TRIALS

The launch of a chemoprevention trial on prostate cancer needs extra effort, as sample size and duration of follow-up are so extensive. Because healthy individuals are involved, refusal, loss to follow-up, and inadequate adherence may be substantial. Inclusion of high-risk patients serves to reduce the number of subjects required in trials to evaluate chemopreventive strategies. Age, race, family history, high-grade PIN, and high PSA levels are well-defined risk factors (Table 1). As an example, including men with familial prostate cancer where the risk approaches nearly 50%, a trial to demonstrate a 20–30% reduction in the incidence of prostate cancer would require only several hundred men. However, if the general population were studied, the required number would exceed 10,000 subjects in a randomized trial. Challenges face such a trial with high-risk patients—not only recruitment, but also possible failure in that the group may not represent the general population. Nevertheless strategies are being developed to study these cohorts. To find a 25% reduction in period prevalence between subjects taking the chemoprevention drug or placebo, 18,000 men are needed (36). If the estimated difference is smaller, a study population of 50,000 men or more would be necessary. These large sample sizes can be achieved only when chemoprevention studies are done on a multi-center basis.

Ideally, cancer incidence should be the endpoint for prostate cancer chemoprevention trials. However, 10 or more years of testing a chemoprevention drug might be necessary to reach this endpoint. To gain time, intermediate endpoints could be chosen. Unfortunately, it seems that no reliable biomarker has been validated for use to replace definitive endpoints. PSA appears to be a useful surrogate for following patients on chemoprevention trials. A rising level increases risk of progression and/or development of prostate cancer. Table 2 lists the advantages and disadvantages of utilizing initial serum PSA levels to define high-risk cohorts for chemoprevention trials. The major advantage is ability to utilize an inexpensive, noninvasive method of selection. The disadvantage is that this group does not represent the normal population.

The risk of prostate cancer is recognized to parallel PSA level. Men with an initial PSA of >10 ng/mL have nearly a 50% risk of disease (36). Using serum PSA levels to define high-risk groups has been considered; a study by Gann et al. found that patients with PSA between 2.0 and 4.0 ng/mL had a 12-fold increased risk of developing prostate cancer after 10 yr of follow-up, when compared with patients whose baseline PSA was <1.0 ng/mL (37). This group seems to represent an ideal cohort to include in chemoprevention trials.

REFERENCES

1. Sakr WA, Haas GP, Cassin BF, et al. The frequency of carcinoma and intraepithelial neoplasia of the prostate in young male patients. *J Urol* 1993;150:379–385.
2. Smart CR. The results of prostate carcinoma screening in the US as reflected in the surveillance, epidemiology, and end results program. *Cancer* 1997;80:1835–1844.
3. Eyre HJ. The American Cancer Society's prostate cancer position (Editorial). *CA Cancer J Clin* 1997;47:259–260.
4. Mettlin CJ, Murphy GP, Babaian RJ, et al. Observations on the early detection of prostate cancer from the American Cancer Society National Cancer Detection Project. *Cancer* 1997;80:1814–1817.
5. Labrie F, Dupont A, Candas B, et al. Decrease of prostate cancer death by screening. First data from the Quebec prospective and randomized study. *Proc Am Soc Clin Oncol* 1998;17:2A.
6. Smith DS, Humphry PA, Catalona WJ. The early detection of prostate carcinoma with prostate specific antigen. *Cancer* 1997;80:1852–1856.

7. Newcomer LM, Stanford LJ, Blumenstein BA, et al. Temporal trends in the rate of prostate cancer: declining incidence of advanced stage disease. *J Urol* 1997;158:1427–1430.

8. Reissigle A, Horninger W, Fink K, et al. Prostate carcinoma screening in the county of Tyrol, Austria: experience and results. *Cancer* 1997;80:1818–1829.

9. Lilja H. A kallikrein-like serine protease in prostatic fluid cleaves the predominant seminal vesicle protein. *J Clin Invest* 1985;76:1899–1903.

10. Lilja H, Laurell CB. Liquefaction of coagulated human semen. S*cand J Clin Lab Invest* 1984;44:447–452.

11. Brawer M, Schifman R, Ahmann F, et al. The effect of digital rectal examination on serum levels of prostate-specific antigen. *Arch Pathol Lab Med* 1988;112:1110–1112.

12. Crawford ED, Schutz M, Drago J, et al. The effect of digital rectal examination on PSA. *J Urol* 1991;145:398A.

13. Ellis WJ, Brawer MK. The role of tumor markers in the diagnosis and treatment of prostate cancer. In *Prostate Diseases*. 1st ed. Lepor H, ed. Saunders, Philadelphia, 1993, pp. 276–292.

14. Simak R, Madersbacher S, Zhang ZF, Maier U. The impact of ejaculation on serum prostate specific antigen. *J Urol* 1993;150:895–897.

15. Guess HA, Heyse JF, Gormley GJ, et al. Effect of finasteride on serum PSA concentration in men with benign prostatic hyperplasia: results from the North American Phase III Clinical Trial. *Urol Clin North Am* 1993;20:627–636.

16. Wener MH, Daum PR, Close B, Brawer MK. Method to method and lot to lot variation in assays for prostatic specific antigen. *Am J Clin Pathol* 1994;101:387–388.

17. Brawer MK, Daum P, Petteway JC, Wener MH. Assay variability in serum PSA determination. *Prostate* 1995;27:1–6.

18. Oesterling JE, Jacobsen SJ, Chute CG, et al. Serum PSA in a community-based population of healthy men: establishment of age-specific reference ranges. *JAMA* 1993;270:860–864.

19. Catalona WJ, Richie JP, Ahmann FR, et al. Comparison of digital rectal examination and serum prostate specific antigen in the early detection of prostate cancer: results of a multicenter clinical trial of 6630 men. *J Urol* 1994;151:1283–1290.

20. Littrup PJ, Kane RA, Mettlin CJ. Cost-effective prostate cancer detection. *Cancer* 1994;74:3146–3158.

21. Gann PH, Hennekens CH, Stumpfer MJ. A prospective evaluation of plasma prostate-specific antigen for detection of prostate cancer. *JAMA* 1995;273:289–294.

22. Gronberg H, Damber JE, Jonsson H, Lenner P. Patient age as a prognostic factor in prostate cancer. *J Urol* 1994;152:892–895.

23. De Antoni EP, Crawford ED, Stone NN, et al. Prostate cancer awareness week, summary of key findings. *Clin Invest Med* 1994;16:448–457.

24. Carter HB, Pearson JD, Metter EJ, et al. Longitudinal evaluation of prostate-specific antigen levels in men with and without prostate disease. *JAMA* 1992;267:2215–2220.

25. Stamey TA. Second Stanford Conference on international standardization of prostate-specific antigen immunoassays. *Urology* 1995;45:173–184.

26. Benson M, Whang I, Pantuck A, et al. Prostate specific antigen density: a means of distinguishing benign prostate hypertrophy and prostate cancer. *J Urol* 1992;147:815–816.

27. Brawer MK, Aramburu E, Chen G. The inability of prostate specific antigen index to enhance the predictive value of prostate specific antigen in the diagnosis of prostatic carcinoma. *J Urol* 1993;150:369–373.

28. Kalish J, Cooner WH, Graham SD Jr. Serum PSA adjusted for volume of transition zone (PSAT) is more accurate than PSA adjusted for total gland volume (PSAD) in detecting adenocarcinoma of the prostate. *Urology* 1994;43:601–606.

29. Djavan B, Zlotta AR, Byttebier G, et al. Prostate specific antigen density of the transition zone for early detection of prostate cancer. *J Urol* 1998;160:411–419.

30. Lin DW, Gold MH, Ransom S, et al. Transition zone PSA density. Lack of utility in prediction of prostatic carcinoma. *J Urol* 1998;160:77–82.

31. Stenman UH, Leinonen J, Afthan H, et al. A complex between prostate-specific antigen and alpha1-antichymotrypsin is the major form of prostate-specific antigen in the serum of patients with prostate cancer: assay of the complex improves clinical sensitivity for cancer. *Cancer Res* 1991;51:222–226.

32. Catalona WJ, Smith DS, Wolfert RL. Evaluation of percentage of serum prostate-specific antigen to improve specificity of prostate cancer screening. *JAMA* 1995;274:1214–1220.

33. Lilja H, Christensson A, Dahlen U. Prostate specific antigen in human serum occurs predominantly in complex with alpha1-antichymotrypsin. *Clin Chem* 1991;37:1618–1625.

34. Brawer MK, Meyer GE, Letran JE, et al. Measurement of complexed PSA improves specificity for early detection of prostate cancer. *Urology* 1998;52:372–378.

35. Smith MR, Biggar S, Hussain M. Prostate-specific antigen messenger RNA is expressed in non-prostate cells: implication for detection of micrometastasis. *Cancer Res* 1995;55:2640–2644.

36. Feigl P, Blumenstein B, Thompson I, et al. Design of the Prostate Cancer Prevention Trial (PCPT). *Control Clin Trials* 1995;16:150–163.

37. Gann PH, Hennekens CH, Stampfer MJ. A prospective evaluation of plasma prostate specific antigen for detection of prostatic cancer. *JAMA* 1995;273:1309–1315.

BREAST

17 Clinical Approaches to Discovering and Testing New Breast Cancer Prevention Drugs

Carol J. Fabian, MD, Bruce F. Kimler, PhD, Matthew S. Mayo, PhD, William E. Grizzle, MD, PhD, Shahla Masood, MD, and Giske Ursin, MD, PhD

CONTENTS

1. WHY NEW BREAST CANCER PREVENTION AGENTS AND MODELS TO TEST THEM ARE NEEDED

It was estimated that 211,000 women would be diagnosed with invasive breast cancer and 47,000 diagnosed with ductal carcinoma *in situ* (DCIS) in 2003 *(1)*. Furthermore, more than 39,000 women were expected to die from breast cancer in that year *(1)*. Approximately 70% of these cancers were anticipated to be estrogen receptor (ER)-positive *(2)*. If a proportion of those tumors could be prevented, morbidity resulting from surgery, radiation, and chemotherapy, as well as breast cancer-related mortality, could be reduced.

Tamoxifen, a selective estrogen receptor modulator (SERM), has been shown to reduce the incidence of breast cancer in some groups of high-risk women *(3)*. It is currently the only FDA-approved drug for breast cancer risk reduction in women ages 35–70 who have a minimum 5-yr estimated Gail risk of ≥1.66% and/or a history of lobular carcinoma *in situ* (LCIS) *(4)*. In the National Surgical Adjuvant Breast Project (NSABP) P-1 study, women randomized to receive 5 yr of tamoxifen were observed to have a 49% reduction in invasive

and a 50% reduction in noninvasive breast cancer relative to placebo at a median follow-up of 3.6 yr. Women with a prior biopsy indicating hyperplasia with atypia or LCIS enjoyed the greatest risk reduction at 86% and 56%, respectively *(3)*. King et al. *(5)* have also reported that BRCA-2 mutation carriers in this study had a 64% reduction in breast cancer incidence. Tamoxifen reduced the incidence of ER-positive breast cancer by 69% but did not reduce the incidence of ER-negative breast cancer *(3)*.

Only 26% of Caucasian women and 10% of African-American women with a Gail risk of ≥1.67% are predicted to benefit from tamoxifen *(6)*. Given the increased risk of uterine cancer and thromboembolism associated with tamoxifen in women over age 50, Gail et al. *(7)* have suggested that before considering the drug, women over 50 without a uterus should have a calculated 5-yr risk of approx 2.5%; for women with a uterus, it should be 5%. Women ages 35–50 would have a favorable risk:benefit ratio if their calculated 5-yr Gail risk is ≥1.66%. Using data from the Nurses Health Study, Rockhill et al. *(8)* observed that only a small minority of women developing breast cancer would have met these criteria and been eligible for tamoxifen

From: Cancer Chemoprevention, Volume 2: Strategies for Cancer Chemoprevention
Edited by: G. J. Kelloff, E. T. Hawk, and C. C. Sigman © Humana Press Inc., Totowa, NJ

risk reduction therapy 5 yr before their cancer occurred. This is because high Gail risk estimates are primarily driven by number of affected first-degree relatives and prior biopsies; the majority of women developing breast cancer for the first time have had neither of these prior to diagnosis (8). Thus, although the Gail risk model is validated at a population level, its discriminatory value at the individual level is modest (8,9).

Challenges for investigators working in the area of breast cancer prevention are to develop more sensitive and specific risk and response biomarkers; identify agents that have fewer side effects and/or a different side effect profile than tamoxifen; identify drugs/agents that will reduce the incidence of ER-negative as well as ER-positive cancers; and use biomarkers to develop more efficient clinical trial models that could then be used to test new agents.

A large number of potential prevention agents have been identified by the National Cancer Institute (NCI), industry, and individual investigators, but the majority will never be tested for efficacy unless more efficient clinical trial models are developed using biomarkers to help select cohorts and monitor response (10–12). At the present time, biomarker modulation is generally used as an indicator of response in Phase I and II trials, but breast cancer incidence is still the main endpoint in Phase III trials. It is hoped, however, that modulation of breast intraepithelial neoplasia (IEN), e.g., prevention or reversal of atypical hyperplasia, might be used as an indicator of response in Phase III trials in the future (13).

2. TYPES OF BIOMARKERS USED IN CLINICAL PREVENTION TRIALS

Several types of biomarkers are used in developing drugs for use as preventive agents. These include risk biomarkers to select subjects most appropriate for prevention drug therapy; surrogate endpoint biomarkers to monitor response to prevention agents; predictive biomarkers to select subcohorts of high-risk women likely to respond to a particular type of agent; and biochemical activity markers to provide an indication of systemic drug activity.

2.1. Risk Markers

Risk biomarkers vary considerably in latency and strength of linkage to invasive cancer. Biomarkers highly correlated with short-term risk are ideal for prevention trials and if reversible, can also be used as response indicators or surrogate endpoint biomarkers. Examples of risk biomarkers useful for cohort selection but not for

response endpoints would be germline mutations in BRCA1 or BRCA2 and/or prior treated DCIS or invasive cancer in a contralateral breast. Women with a deleterious BRCA1 or BRCA2 mutation have a risk of breast cancer of 2.5–3% per year between the ages of 30–60 (14,15), and women with prior contralateral cancer unselected for family history have a risk of approximately 0.7–0.8% per year for at least 10 yr after the original diagnosis (16–18). Risk biomarkers subject to modulation have the greatest potential for use in chemoprevention studies and include IEN, proliferation, mammographic breast density, nipple aspirate fluid (NAF) production with associated biomarkers (e.g., methylated genes, hormone levels), serum insulin-like growth factor (IGF)-1 and the ratio of IGF-1 to IGF binding protein-3 (IGFBP-3), and markers of estrogen exposure such as bone mineral density and serum bioavailable estradiol (for postmenopausal women) (19–30).

2.2. Surrogate Endpoint Biomarkers

Ideal properties of a surrogate endpoint biomarker (10,11,31) include biologic plausibility, differential expression in low- vs high-risk populations (or normal vs precancerous tissue), association with cancer in prospective studies, and expression in a reasonable proportion of the high-risk population to be studied, with expression minimally influenced by normal physiologic processes. An ideal biomarker should be quantifiable and easily and repetitively sampled, and its favorable modulation should be associated with lowered cancer risk.

Current risk markers that are strong candidates for use as surrogate endpoint biomarkers in Phase II breast cancer chemoprevention trials are IEN, tissue proliferation within foci of IEN, mammographic density, serum IGF-1:IGFBP-3 ratio (premenopausal women), serum bioavailable estradiol (postmenopausal women), and NAF hormone levels and other proteins (Table 1). IEN is the strongest candidate for surrogate endpoint biomarker status in Phase III trials.

2.2.1. INTRAEPITHELIAL NEOPLASIA

IEN spans a continuum from simple hyperplasia through *in situ* cancer (32,33) (Fig. 1). The majority of invasive cancers are thought to evolve from IEN over several decades. Increasing intraepithelial morphologic abnormality is associated with a progressive increase in relative risk and a decrease in latency (20,34–38).

Occult IEN, highly prevalent in autopsy series and reported in 55–84% of asymptomatic adult women (39–41), is found in 57% of women from hereditary breast cancer families (42). As sampled by random

Table 1
Feasibility of Commonly Used Response Markers

	IEN	Proliferation	Mammographic Density	Serum IGF-1: IGFBP-3	SerumE2	NAF
Biologically plausible	Y	Y	Y	Y	Y	Y
Strong statistical association with cancer	Y	Y	Y	+/–	+/–	+/–
Not affected by normal physiologic processes	Y	N	+/–	N	N	N
Present in majority of at risk population to be studied	Y	Y	Y	Y	Y	+/–
Modulated by known prevention agents	Y	Y	Y	Y	Y	Y
Quantified	+/–	Y	+/–	Y	Y	+/–
Easily sampled	N	N	Y	Y	Y	Y

periareolar fine-needle aspiration (FNA), occult IEN may be found in up to 70% of high-risk women *(25)* and appears to be more prevalent in high-risk women than in low-risk controls *(43)*.

Tamoxifen, an agent with proven efficacy in breast cancer risk reduction, has been reported to reduce the incidence of biopsy-proven hyperplasia with or without atypia by approximately one-third compared to placebo in the NSABP P-1 trial *(44)*. These reductions were seen at all time points, starting as early as 1 yr after initiating tamoxifen *(44)*. Since tamoxifen was also shown to reduce breast cancer incidence in the same trial by 49% *(3)*, this observation supplies important supportive evidence toward validating IEN as a surrogate endpoint biomarker for prevention studies.

There are drawbacks to using IEN as a surrogate endpoint biomarker. An invasive procedure is generally required to obtain tissue. IEN is not readily quantitated, although attempts have been made to do so with semi-quantitative indexes *(45,46)* and image morphometry *(47–49)*. Substantial intra- and interobserver variation exists among experts classifying cytologic and histologic breast IEN *(50–53)*. Little information is available regarding the time it might take for tissue to normalize following initiation of an effective agent, and/or how frequently IEN may resolve without an intervention. Heterogeneity in benign breast tissue results in sampling variance.

Perhaps the thorniest issue is how best to sample breast tissue for the presence of occult IEN in an asymptomatic population. Although random core needle biopsies would seem likely to provide the most material for analysis, substantial numbers of terminal-lobular duct units are not necessarily obtained unless the biopsy is directed toward a dense area of the breast visualized by mammogram or ultrasound *(54,55)*. To date, most trials in which benign tissue has been repeatedly sampled by core needle biopsy have not accrued at a rapid rate *(56)*, although small pilot trials have been completed using this technique *(55)*. NAF collection, random periareolar FNA, and ductal lavage are less invasive than core biopsies and are more likely to be acceptable to asymptomatic individuals as methods for repeated tissue sampling. Hyperplasia and hyperplasia with atypia have been observed in approximately 49% and 21% of high-risk women undergoing random periareolar FNA, respectively, with 94% of women producing sufficient ductal cells for cytologic analysis *(25)*. Furthermore, evidence of hyperplasia with atypia in random periareolar FNA has been associated with subsequent cancer development/detection in a prospective study *(25)*. Twenty-four percent (24%) of women successfully undergoing ductal lavage also were found to have atypia *(57)*, and a prospective trial correlating presence of lavage atypia with subsequent cancer development is ongoing. Repeatedly lavaging the same duct might be expected to reduce sampling variability. However, there is little information on how readily the same duct may be recannulated within a 6–12-mo interval between baseline and follow-up lavage, and still provide

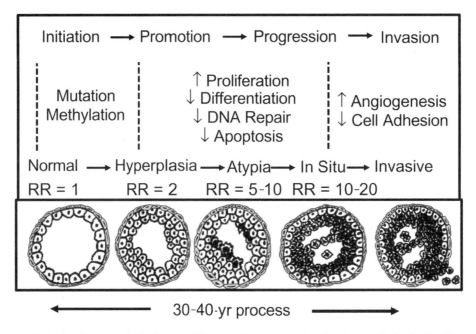

Fig. 1. Pathway for neoplasia development in the breast. The stepwise progression that is morphologically discernable is associated with processes of initiation, promotion, progression, and invasion. Increasing morphologic abnormality (shown schematically in the lower panel), increases relative risk of invasive breast cancer development. The various biological processes may occur over a 30–40 yr span before reaching the *in situ* stage and subsequently progressing to invasive breast cancer *(28)*.

adequate material for analysis. Furthermore, ductal lavage is easily performed only in women yielding NAF. NAF production has been reported in 39–66% of women without regard to risk *(29,58)* and up to 84% of high-risk women *(57)*. Up to 92% of subjects producing NAF are able to undergo duct cannulation for lavage, but 22% of those undergoing lavage do not yield sufficient material (≥10 ductal cells) for analysis *(57)*. Dooley et al. reported that 299 of 500 (60%) high-risk women in whom a NAF attempt was to be followed by lavage actually underwent both procedures and produced adequate material for cytologic characterization. Ductal lavage does appear to more frequently produce adequate cellular material for assessment than NAF. Seventy-two percent (72%) of NAF producers undergoing lavage had adequate material for cytologic characterization, but only 22% of NAF specimens in the same series had adequate cellular material for cytologic characterization *(57)*. The prevalence of atypical cells in NAF was approximately half of that observed in the ductal lavage samples *(57)*. Nonetheless, prospective studies by Wrensch et al. observed that women whose cell clusters exhibited hyperplasia or hyperplasia with atypia in their NAF had an increased risk of breast cancer compared with non-NAF producers or those with normal cytology *(29,59)*. Additional studies are needed to

determine the most sensitive and reproducible methods to sample breast tissue for presence of IEN and to assess morphologic change in short- and longer-term prevention studies.

2.2.2. Proliferation

IEN is associated with a progressive increase in the proportion of proliferating cells, decreasing apoptosis, or both *(60,61)*. The proportion of cells expressing the proliferation marker Ki-67/MIB-1 ranges from 0.8–2% in normal terminal lobular duct units in adult, nonpregnant, nonlactating breast, to 5–29% in carcinoma *in situ (30,62–64)*. Hyperplasia with or without atypia is associated with a modest increase in proliferation over that observed in normal breast tissue, averaging 2–5% in biopsy material utilizing the Ki-67/MIB-1 monoclonal antibody *(30,64)*. Proliferation in hyperplastic foci, but not normal lobules, was observed to be a risk factor for breast cancer in a case control study published by Shaaban et al. *(30)*. A median of 3.8% of cells expressed Ki-67/MIB-1 in hyperplastic foci from women subsequently developing breast cancer vs 0.8% of cells in hyperplastic foci from women not developing cancer *(30)*. Proliferation also may be measured by antibodies to proliferating cell nuclear antigen (PCNA), which has a longer half life and is generally associated with more diffuse tissue staining than Ki-67/MIB-1

(65). PCNA has been reported to be expressed in 3–27% of cells in biopsies exhibiting proliferative breast disease *(66,67)*. Duration of fixation substantially affects the intensity of PCNA staining. PCNA may also be expressed in response to injury in nonproliferating cells *(68)*. If only intensely stained cells (those with a nuclear replicon pattern) are counted, PCNA's correlation with other proliferation markers improves *(69)*. Ki-67/MIB-1 may be the preferred proliferation marker if sufficient cells (≥500) are present, as the observer does not need to make an assessment of stain intensity to score cells as positive *(70)*.

Affected by age and phase of the menstrual cycle, proliferation is highest in the midluteal phase (approx d 20) and lowest in the follicular phase *(71,72)*. Consequently, if proliferation is used as a response indicator in prevention trials, tissue must be sampled in the same portion of the menstrual cycle before and after the intervention. Reduction in proliferation has been correlated with later clinical response in neoadjuvant cancer treatment trials in response to a variety of chemotherapeutic and antihormonal agents *(73–75)*. Relative decreases of 20–46% in the proportion of cells staining for Ki-67/MIB-1 have been observed in breast cancer biopsy specimens following short-term tamoxifen administration *(73,76)*. Reduction in proliferation has yet to be studied in Phase III chemoprevention studies in relation to breast cancer incidence; thus at present, proliferation cannot be considered a validated surrogate endpoint for Phase III prevention trials. It is currently widely used in Phase I trials for dose range finding *(77)* as well as Phase II studies as an indicator of response *(55,78,79)*.

2.2.3. MAMMOGRAPHIC BREAST DENSITY

Mammographic breast density is a reflection of the ratio of stroma and epithelial tissue (which appear radiologically dense) to fat (which appears radiologically lucent) *(22,80)*. Mammographic density varies with proliferative activity and is thus higher in the luteal than in the follicular phase of the menstrual cycle *(81,82)*. Mammographic density generally decreases after menopause and with advancing age *(83)*, but postmenopausal decline may be delayed or prevented with hormone replacement therapy (HRT) *(84,85)*. Women with a very high area of mammographic density relative to total breast area (60–75%) have a four to six times greater relative risk of breast cancer than women with minimal (5–10%) breast density *(21,22,86)*. Approximately 30% of women who develop breast cancer will have had a prediagnostic mammogram exhibiting

≥50% area of increased breast density *(21,22)*. Boyd et al. have suggested that for every 1% increase in dense breast area there will be an associated 2% increase in relative risk of cancer *(22)*. High breast density area is positively correlated with other risk factors including proliferative breast disease *(87–89)*, HRT *(84,85,90,91)*, family history of breast cancer *(92,93)*, nulliparity *(94)*, and levels of serum IGF-1 and IGF-1:IGFBP-3 molar ratio in premenopausal women *(95)*.

Tamoxifen, an established agent for breast cancer risk reduction, is associated with a reduction in dense breast area in preliminary studies *(96–98)*. In a cohort of 69 women participating in the NSABP-P1 trial, those randomized to tamoxifen for an average of 3 yr had a mean reduction in estimated dense breast area of 9.4% compared to a mean reduction of 3.6% in the placebo group *(98)*.

Several operator-assisted computer image analysis software programs have been developed to estimate the proportion of the breast considered dense in mammographic images *(86,99,100)*. While these programs provide the opportunity for a systematic evaluation of mammographic density on a large scale, none of them quantify actual density or ratio of stroma-epithelium to fat in a given volume of tissue. This may be critical in assessing density changes in short-term Phase I and II prevention studies, as changes in intensity within the area of density may be more informative than simply the percent of area considered dense.

A number of pilot and Phase II prevention studies have been initiated with reduction in dense breast area as a primary endpoint *(99,101–103)*. Although breast density is a biologically plausible risk marker, further prospective studies with established prevention agents need to be performed linking reduction in dense breast area to reduced cancer incidence before breast density can be considered a validated response biomarker for Phase III chemoprevention trials. If breast density is used as a primary endpoint, the Phase II trial design should have several requirements: minimum breast density for trial participation; stratification by dense breast area that similarly distributes women with large areas of increased density between the control and experimental arms; adjustment for weight gain or loss; measurement of density during the same phase of the menstrual cycle; and for postmenopausal women, a restriction that HRT not be started or stopped for at least 6 mo prior to or during the trial period *(104)*. Uniformity of positioning, compression, and equipment would reduce measurement variation but are difficult to specify and enforce in a multi-institutional trial.

In order to accrue the appropriate number of participants prior to initiating a trial with breast density area as a response endpoint, the assay technique's variability in the study population to be assessed over the observation period of the trial should be known.

2.2.4. IGF-1 AS A POTENTIAL SURROGATE ENDPOINT BIOMARKER FOR PREMENOPAUSAL WOMEN

IGF-1 is a powerful breast epithelial cell mitogen when combined with its receptor IGF-1R (105,106). Ninety percent (90%) of circulating IGF-1 is bound to IGFBP-3, which in turn prevents binding with IGF-1R, since IGFBP-3 has a higher affinity for IGF-1 (107). The liver is the main source of circulating IGF-1 and IGFBP-3 (108). Regulation of IGF-1 and IGFBP-3 levels under similar conditions of estrogen exposure is complex, affected by a variety of genetic polymorphisms, age (growth hormone), alcohol intake, phase of menstrual cycle, and exogenous hormone use. Oral contraceptive use in premenopausal women and oral HRT in postmenopausal women decreases serum IGF-1 (109–111), whereas transdermal estradiol increases serum IGF-1 (108,112).

IGF-1 is produced in the breast by stromal elements, whereas IGF-1 receptor (IGF-1R) is expressed primarily in the epithelial cells (105). IGF-1 bioactivity in breast tissue is controlled by levels of IGF-1R, IGF binding proteins (especially IGFBP-3), local IGFBP-3 proteases, and estrogen (105,107). Estrogen induces expression of IGF-1R and decreases IGFBP-3 (105,107,113). There is considerable cross-talk between the ERα and IGF-1 signaling systems (114–116). Loss of ERα is associated with diminished IGF signal transduction (114). IGF-1 increases local breast estrogen levels by increasing estradiol 17 β-hydroxysteroid dehydrogenase (117). IGF-1 can also act synergistically with estrogen to enhance proliferation in ERα-positive breast cancer cells (117-119). Premenopausal women with serum IGF-1 levels and/or IGF-1:IGFBP-3 ratios in the upper tertile of the normal range (i.e., IGF-1 levels >207 ng/mL or >27 nM) have an increased risk of breast cancer relative to those in the lowest tertile (23). It is thus assumed for premenopausal women that the serum IGF-1:IGFBP-3 ratio is a surrogate for tissue IGF-1 bioactivity. However, serum IGF-1:IGFBP-3 ratios do not correlate with risk in postmenopausal women (106). The reasons for this lack of correlation of serum IGF-1 and IGF-1:IGFBP-3 ratio with postmenopausal breast cancer risk (23) are not clear, but local production of estrogen may increase local IGF-1 and IGF-1R bioactivity with-

out influencing systemic levels (105,107). Local estrogen production may be due to postmenopausal increases in breast aromatase and sulfatase activity (19,120–123). Tamoxifen has been reported to decrease serum IGF-1 levels by 21% compared to a <1% decrease in placebo-treated controls (124), and also increases serum IGFBP-3 largely because of its effects on hepatic synthesis of these proteins. Tamoxifen also causes reduction in IGF-1R expression at the tissue level (125–127).

Favorable modulation of serum IGF-1 level and/or IGF-1:IGFBP-3 ratio may be a potential response biomarker for SERMs and possibly other chemoprevention agents, at least for premenopausal women. However, to be validated as a surrogate marker for Phase III studies, reduction in IGF-1 level or IGF-1:IGFBP-3 ratio would need to correlate with reduced cancer incidence. A recent study reported by Decensi et al. (128) showed reduction in serum IGF-1 levels and cancer incidence with the retinoid fenretinide; however, there was no significant correlation between reduction in serum IGF-1 levels and reduction in cancer incidence.

2.2.5. SERUM HORMONE LEVEL AS A POTENTIAL SURROGATE BIOMARKER FOR POSTMENOPAUSAL WOMEN

Postmenopausal women with bioavailable (non-sex-hormone-binding globulin-bound) estradiol and free testosterone levels in the upper portion of the normal range are at increased risk relative to those with lower levels (24,129). Furthermore, breast cancer incidence in the placebo group in the Multiple Outcomes of Raloxifene Evaluation (MORE) trial in elderly average-risk osteoporotic women was directly related to serum estrogen levels. Those women with estradiol levels >2.7 pg/mL had an observed risk more than four times that of women with estradiol levels <2.7 pg/mL (130). Serum, tissue, and NAF estradiol levels are attractive potential surrogate endpoint biomarkers, especially for prevention trials of aromatase and sulfatase inhibitors and other types of agents whose mechanism of action includes reduction of estrogen levels.

2.2.6. NAF PRODUCTION

NAF production in adult nonpregnant nonlactating women has been associated with a modest increased risk for breast cancer (29,59). The ability to produce NAF is associated with many factors, including younger age, prior childbirth and lactation, ethnicity, cerumen type, and local concentrations of prolactin, estrogen, and other hormones and cytokines; not all of these factors are necessarily linked to an increased risk for breast cancer *(19,131)*. Increases in breast estrogen in postmenopausal women may be the result of increased breast sulfatase or aromatase activity *(122)*. NAF is produced in only 60–84% of high-risk women; though an unreliable source of epithelial cells, it is valuable for studying change in hormones, growth factors, and other proteins bathing the breast terminal lobule duct unit cells. These factors could be used in the future as indicators of risk, drug activity, or response to a prevention intervention *(29,132,133)*.

2.3. Predictive Biomarkers

One of the strongest arguments for sampling breast fluid or tissue is the potential to identify individual molecular abnormalities and target them with appropriate agents (i.e., using a SERM against overexpression of ER, a cyclooxygenase (COX)-2 inhibitor against COX-2 overexpression, etc.). This approach would allow appropriate selection of cohorts most likely to respond to a particular agent, presuming its mechanism of action is known.

Tamoxifen's efficacy in reducing breast cancer risk is largely a result of its ability to competitively bind ER and inhibit transcriptional activity through preferential binding of co-repressors *(134,135)*. Clinical response in women with breast cancer is predicted by the level of ER and progesterone receptor expression in pretreatment biopsies *(2,64,136)*. Although this is also likely to be the case in hyperplasia, correlation of reduction in cancer incidence after tamoxifen treatment has yet to be demonstrated with ER content in benign breast tissue.

Identification of subjects with potential tamoxifen resistance is important. Mechanisms of tamoxifen resistance in breast cancer include increased ligand-independent ERα activation resulting from growth factor and/or activated growth factor receptor-mediated activation of the PI3K/AKT and mitogen-activated protein (MAP) kinase pathways *(137,138)*; increased coactivator levels and/or binding induced by increased estrogen or growth factor levels *(75,137,139–141)*; increased proportion of cells expressing ERβ *(142,143)* or the hypersensitive ERα variant *(144,145)*; loss of ER expression through methylation of the gene promoter *(145)*; and reduction in co-repressors that repress transcription through recruitment of histone deacetylases to target promoters *(147)*.

New proteomics tools such as surface-enhanced laser desorption ionization combined with time-of-flight mass spectrometry (SELDI-TOF-MS) would potentially allow detection of activated MAP kinase and AKT pathways as well as many of the other molecular abnormalities which appear to be important in tamoxifen resistance *(148)*; such diagnoses may be carried out in snap-frozen or ethanol-fixed tissue *(149)*. Methylation-specific polymerase chain reaction (PCR) might also be used in conjunction with immunocytochemical or histochemical staining for ER to determine the reason for any prevalent loss of ER expression in precancerous tissue *(27)*.

While these exciting and promising new methodologies are being further developed and validated for use in cancer diagnosis and prevention, simple immunocytochemical tests for protein expression targeting a drug's mechanism of action may be helpful in selecting women most likely to respond to a particular agent, thus reducing the sample size needed to demonstrate an effect.

2.4. Biochemical Activity Markers

Markers of biochemical activity are fully quantitative measures of drug activity usually linked to one or more of the drug's mechanisms of action *(12,150)*. Biochemical activity markers should also vary with dose but may or may not be associated with modulation of the precancerous process at the breast tissue level. Biochemical activity markers are generally obtained from serum or urine and are helpful in establishing an appropriate dose range in Phase I trials as well as compliance monitoring in Phase II and III trials. Examples of biochemical activity markers would include urine polyamines for ornithine decarboxylase inhibitors and serum prostaglandins for COX-2 inhibitors. Some biochemical activity markers might also be risk biomarkers. For example, aromatase inhibitors given to postmenopausal women might reduce high serum estradiol levels, that have been associated with an increased risk of breast cancer development.

3. DEVELOPMENT OF NEW AGENTS TARGETING MOLECULAR ABNORMALITIES IN PRECANCEROUS BREAST TISSUE

Molecular abnormalities (*see* Fig. 2) that are attractive targets for prevention include increased histone deacetylation and methylation of gene promotors, resulting in diminished expression of several tumor suppression genes responsible for differentiation, apoptosis, and DNA repair *(146,151–156)*; increased activity of aromatase and other enzymes responsible

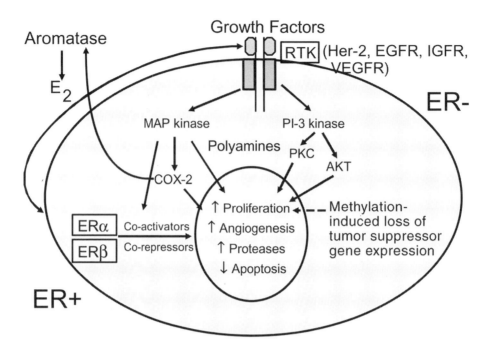

Fig. 2. Molecular abnormalities expressed in breast IEN *(28)*.

for *in situ* breast estrogen synthesis, as a result of increased in inflammatory cytokines *(117,157–165)*; increased proportion of cells that express ERα *(30,64,166)* and/or a hypersensitive ERα variant *(144)*; and increased proportion of cells expressing proliferation antigens as well as concomitant ERα and proliferation antigens *(30,167–169)*. Also good targets are concomitant expression of ERα and epidermal growth factor receptor (EGFR) by the same epithelial cells, resulting in dysfunctional signaling in both receptor pathways *(170,171)*; increased cytokines, growth factors, and growth factor receptors including interleukin (IL)-6, tumor necrosis factor (TNF)-α, transforming growth factor (TGF)α, COX-2, IGF-1, IGF-1R, EGF, and EGFR *(58,172–176)*; alterations of integrins and other cytoskeletal protein patterns *(177,178)*; and increased angiogenic and protease activity *(172,179–182)*.

3.1. Future Chemoprevention Agents

Given molecular abnormalities in breast IEN, several types of drugs offer potential chemoprevention approaches; they are listed in Table 2 in order of molecular abnormality. Agents such as second- and third-generation SERMs, aromatase and sulfatase inhibitors, luteinizing hormone releasing hormone agonists, and retinoids are currently in Phase II or III prevention trials for efficacy in precancerous tissue.

Raloxifene, a second-generation SERM developed primarily to prevent osteoporosis, exhibits estrogen antagonist effects in the breast and estrogen agonist effects on bone and lipids. It has less estrogen-like agonist activity in the uterus than tamoxifen *(183–187)*. No significant antitumor activity was demonstrated for raloxifene in metastatic breast cancer *(188,189)*, but the MORE trial associated 60–120 mg/d of raloxifene with a 74% reduction in breast cancer incidence relative to placebo in elderly osteoporotic women *(190,192)*. Reduced cancer incidence was observed only in women with estradiol levels >2.7 pg/mL at study entry *(130)*. Like tamoxifen, raloxifene is associated with increased incidence of hot flashes and thromboembolic phenomena without decreasing ER-negative breast cancers *(190–192)*. It is currently being compared to tamoxifen in the NSABP Study of Tamoxifen and Raloxifene (STAR) prevention trial in postmenopausal women *(193)*.

Third-generation SERMs such as arzoxifene, EM-652, and EM-800 are potent breast antiestrogens that block ER transcription in breast tissue and exhibit estrogen agonist effects on bone and lipids, but are estrogen antagonists or at least lack agonist activity in the uterus *(194)*. Arzoxifene, more potent than tamoxifen or raloxifene in animal tumor models *(195)*, has also shown efficacy in metastatic breast cancer trials *(196)*. However, like tamoxifen and raloxifene, third-generation

Table 2
Potential Prevention Agents Directed at Putative Targets/Molecular Abnormalities in Precancerous Breast Tissue

Drug Class	Abnormality/Putative Target
SERMs, ERDRs Aromatase inhibitors/inactivators	↑ ER, ER transcription
Aromatase inhibitors/inactivators (postmenopausal women)	↑ Tissue estrogen via ↑ aromatase activity
LHRH agonists (premenopausal women)	
Sulfatase inhibitors/tibilone	↑ Tissue estrogen via ↑ sulfatase activity
Retinoids, rexanoids +/– histone deacelytase inhibitors	Reduced retinoid receptor expression, differentiation, apoptosis
COX-2 inhibitors (Celecoxib)	Increased COX-2 activity
Polyamine synthesis inhibitors (DFMO)	Increased tissue polyamines
Soy or derivatives, receptor tyrosine kinase inhibitors	Increased growth factor and tyrosine kinase receptor activation
Histone deacetylase inhibitors and demethylating agents	Silenced tumor suppressor genes 2° methylation abnormalities

SERMs also are associated with hot flashes and procoagulant effects. Arzoxifene is reported to have some efficacy in tamoxifen-resistant animal models (197). Phase II prevention trials of arzoxifene utilizing modulation of biomarkers as endpoints are currently ongoing in the US (26).

ER downregulators (ERDRs) bind ER but block receptor dimerization. ER is then rapidly degraded, thus blocking ER-directed gene transcription (198,199). Fulvestrant, an ERDR, is active in tamoxifen-resistant metastatic disease (200–202), but lacks uterine agonist activity, and does not produce hot flashes as it does not cross the blood–brain barrier (199,203). However, its parenteral mode of administration makes it less attractive for prevention. Its generalized ERα antagonist activity also limits its usefulness in a healthy population.

Aromatase inhibitors decrease bioavailable estrogen and have been shown to have greater antitumor activity than tamoxifen in postmenopausal adjuvant and metastatic treatment trials (74,204–206). Aromatase inhibitor-induced decreases in bioavailable estrogen may reduce receptor tyrosine kinase activity and AP-1 activation, which in turn may be responsible for some forms of tamoxifen resistance (139,207,208). Nonsteroidal aromatase inhibitors lack procoagulant and uterine agonist activity but also lack estrogen agonist

activity in bone (209). The Arimidex, Tamoxifen Alone or Combination (ATAC) adjuvant trial reported a statistically significant increase in fractures with anastrazole compared to tamoxifen (206). However, the steroidal aromatase inactivator exemestane has been reported to exhibit agonist properties on bone and lipids in ovariectomized rats (210). Prevention studies with aromatase inhibitors/inactivators are likely to target high-risk postmenopausal women. Preclinical studies with letrozole in transgenic mice engineered to overexpress aromatase indicate potential risk reduction in a high estrogen environment, indicating potential use in premenopausal women or postmenopausal women receiving HRT (211,212).

Several trials with aromatase inhibitors/inactivators have recently been initiated, including a trial of exemestane vs placebo in postmenopausal BRCA1 and BRCA2 mutation carriers with cancer incidence as an endpoint (213). Also recently initiated are a randomized study of exemestane with reduction in breast density as an endpoint, and a pilot trial with letrozole in high-risk women having FNA evidence of atypical hyperplasia with reduction in proliferation as the main endpoint. Theoretically, SERMs and aromatase inhibitors/inactivators should make ideal prevention partners. However, preclinical studies fail to show superiority for tamoxifen combined with anastrazole or letrozole vs either aromatase inhibitor as a single agent *(214,215)*. Tamoxifen also was found to reduce blood levels of letrozole in postmenopausal women *(216)*.

Sulfatase inhibitors block conversion of estrone sulfate to estrone and thus decrease bioavailable estrogen *(217,218)*. Several SERMs and progestins decrease sulfatase activity *(219,220)*. Tibolone, a novel steroidal molecule with tissue-specific sulfatase inhibitory properties, inhibits breast sulfatase activity, increases apoptosis *(221,222)*, and prevents estradiol-induced increased proliferation *(223)*. It has inhibited tumor formation in the rat 7,12-dimethylbenz [*a*] anthracene mammary tumor model *(224)*. Clinical trials have suggested that tibolone is able to reduce hot flashes and vaginal dryness and prevent postmenopausal bone loss but has no stimulatory effects on the endometrium *(225)*.

Gonadotropin-releasing hormone agonists (GnRHA) reduce circulating sex hormone levels in premenopausal women. A Phase II clinical trial in premenopausal women of a GnRHA plus "add-back" low-dose HRT with a primary endpoint of mammographic breast density is currently ongoing following favorable pilot results *(226–228)*.

Retinoids and their derivatives have multiple chemoprevention properties, including reduction of proliferation and induction of differentiation and apoptosis *(229–231)*. They are likely to be most effective in breast epithelium expressing ER *(230)*. Preclinical studies indicate efficacy for some retinoid derivatives in ER-negative as well as ER-positive tamoxifen-resistant cell lines *(229,233,234)*. An Italian Phase III adjuvant trial was unable to demonstrate reduction in contralateral breast cancer incidence for women randomized to fenretinide vs placebo, although there was some suggestion of benefit in premenopausal women *(235)*. Side effects may limit the use of many retinoids and rexanoids for prevention *(231)*. A Phase II trial of targretin, an RXR-selective ligand *(234)*, is currently under way in high-risk women (Dr. Powel Brown, Randomized Chemoprevention Study of Bexarotene in Women at High Genetic Risk for Breast Cancer, Baylor College of Medicine, www.clinicaltrials.gov).

Several classes of agents are of particular interest in treating ER-negative or hormone-independent precancerous tissue, although they might show activity in ER-positive precancerous tissue as well. These agents inhibit polyamine synthesis, COX-2, lipoxygenase, receptor tyrosine kinase, histone deacetylase, and metalloproteinase activity *(237–253)*.

A biomarker modulation study of difluromethylornithine (DFMO), an inhibitor of polyamine synthesis, showed no evidence of modulation of breast cytology, mammographic density, or IGF-1 levels relative to placebo *(78,79)*.

Celecoxib, a selective COX-2 inhibitor, is currently in Phase I and II biomarker modulation chemoprevention trials. COX-2 expression has been observed in proliferative breast disease and breast cancer *(241,254,255)*; and celecoxib has been associated with reduction in mammary cancer in preclinical models *(256)*. Celecoxib also has a favorable toxicity profile *(257–259)* with minimal gastrointestinal toxicity at doses which reduced polyps in individuals with familial polyposis *(260)*.

Many anti-GFR antibodies as well as inhibitors of receptor tyrosine kinases, metalloproteases, and histone deacetylases may be too toxic for prevention trials in doses currently used for anticancer treatment *(245,249,261)*. However, for many of these agents, the optimal biologic dose for prevention is likely to be much lower than for treatment of established cancer. ZD1839 (Iressa), an oral anilinoquinazolone that selectively inhibits EGFR receptor tyrosine kinase activity, is of great interest in this regard. Pharmacodynamic effects on MAP kinase have been noted even at low doses (e.g., 150 mg/d) not generally associated with toxicity *(262)*. Iressa has been observed to have a profound effect on proliferation and activated MAP kinase activity in nude mouse xenografts of human ER-negative and ER-positive DCIS and adjacent normal tissue *(251)*. Soy protein produces few subjective side effects and contains genistein, a naturally occurring inhibitor of receptor tyrosine kinase activity *(263,264)* as well as lunasin, a histone deacetylase inhibitor. Soy is of particular interest as a prevention agent in premenopausal women; consumption of soy products containing >150 mg of isoflavones/d may reduce endogenous estrogen production and the midcycle surge of luteinizing hormone *(265–267)*.

Other agents of interest include sulindac sulfone, which induces apoptosis in preclinical prevention models *(268)*, as well as recombinant β-human chorionic gonadotropin, which induces differentiation in the terminal lobule duct unit *(269)*.

Combinations of agents with different mechanisms of action may be additive or synergistic. Combinations of synergistic agents may allow use of reduced doses of each with the potential of reducing side effects while maintaining efficacy. At the mechanistic level, SERMs are attractive partners for retinoids, aromatase inhibitors, vitamin D$_3$ analogs, and demethylating agents/histone deacetylase inhibitors *(195,270–274)*. COX-2 and

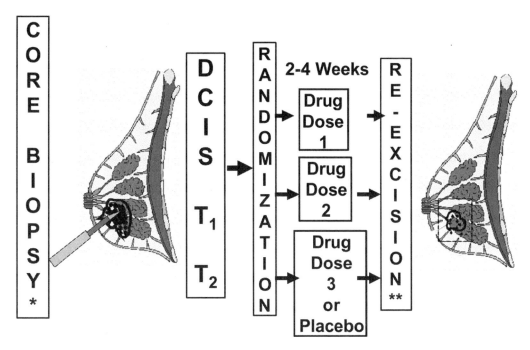

* Proliferation (Ki-67/PCNA) and biomarkers   ** Repeat Biomarkers
consistent with drug mechanism of action

Fig. 3. Schematic of the presurgical model of Phase I chemoprevention trials. Eligible subjects are randomized to one of several drug doses in the interval between tissue samplings. A nonrandomized but contemporaneous no-treatment control arm may be added (IA) or may be included in the randomization scheme (IB). The endpoints are modulation of proliferation and other biomarkers chosen based on the presumed mechanism of action of the agent under investigation *(54)*.

aromatase inhibitors deserve joint testing, as do retinoids and demethylating agents/histone deacetylaase inhibitors or retinoids and vitamin D_3 analogs *(275,276)*.

3.2. Clinical Models for Phase I and II Trials
3.2.1. PHASE I

For most Phase I prevention trials, the toxicity profile of the agent in question is known from other clinical settings. Since even minimal side effects are unacceptable when a prevention agent is to be administered to a healthy population over a protracted period of time, the major focus of Phase I trials is establishing the lowest dose at which the drug reliably modulates risk biomarkers *(10,11)*. Phase IA trials generally explore the effects of dose on biochemical activity and/or response biomarkers, and Phase IB trials confirm that a given dose of drug reliably modulates a response biomarker *(10,11)*.

To date, the so-called "presurgical" model is the most popular Phase IA clinical model. In this model, women with DCIS or a small invasive cancer who have undergone a core biopsy are randomized between one of several drug doses in the 2 to 4 wk between biopsy and re-excision. An optional, nonrandomized, no-treatment

control arm may be employed as well *(see* Fig. 3) *(56)*. The primary outcome measure for these trials is often modulation of biochemical activity markers and/or reduction in proliferation between baseline and re-excision sample. The optional nonrandomized control group is employed to ensure that tissue recovery from the core biopsy or other factors (such as stopping HRT) are not producing similar effects as the study drug on proliferation or other assessed biomarkers. The rationale behind use of the presurgical model to select a dose for prevention trials is that if the marker is modulated in cancer it is likely to be modulated in precancerous tissue. Generally 10–12 subjects are entered at each dose level. If 8 out of 10 or 9 out of 12 subjects exhibit modulation of a marker, there is 90% confidence of at least 50% probability of favorable modulation in this population. The dose selected from Phase IA may be used for a Phase II trial or further explored in a Phase IB trial.

Although the presurgical model Phase I design seems relatively straightforward, there are multiple practical problems. Many women are reluctant to take part in an experimental protocol at a highly emotional time when they are trying to make decisions regarding definitive treatment for their cancer. Also problematic are non-drug-related changes in proliferation between the initial biopsy and re-excision related to difference in menstrual cycle phase *(72,277)*, discontinuation of HRT between biopsy and re-excision *(278)*, tumor heterogeneity, minimal tumor at re-excision, fixation/processing differences between the core biopsy and re-excision sample *(279,280)*, and tissue reaction to injury *(281)*.

Fewer than 10% of women screened for Phase I trials utilizing the presurgical model are eligible and willing to participate, which makes this a difficult and labor-intensive endeavor for investigators and their research personnel *(282,283)*. In our experience, 10–20% of eligible women entering such a trial will not have sufficient tumor at re-excision to reassay the marker. Further, baseline tumor characteristics in the nonrandomized control group often differ from the treatment group *(77)*.

In the Phase IB design, the number of subjects is expanded at the dose level selected in IA. Biomarker modulation with the experimental drug may be compared in a blinded randomized fashion to placebo. Once again, the main study endpoint is often to demonstrate consistent reduction in proliferation (or modulation of other biomarkers of interest) with the study agent relative to placebo. A 2:1 (drug:placebo) randomization design may facilitate accrual. Restriction of entry to either non-high-grade or high-grade lesions may reduce the wide variation in baseline Ki-67 (MIB-1) values seen in breast cancer, irrespective of tumor grade, thus allowing the statistical objectives to be met with fewer subjects. Assuming 40 evaluable subjects in each group, a mean baseline Ki-67/MIB-1 value of 4% with a standard deviation of 9%, and a 6% standard deviation for the change in Ki-67/MIB-1 values for non-high-grade tumors, a 50% reduction in proliferation in the treatment group could be detected compared to no reduction in the placebo group, with 91% power and a type I error rate of 5%. With a 2:1 design of 40 subjects in the treatment group and 20 in the placebo group, we would have 76% power of detecting the same 50% reduction in proliferation. The preceding considerations presume fair homogeneity of the subject population with a reasonable chance of responding to the test agent. Given the necessity of entering subjects immediately after diagnosis, it is not possible to require centralized or even noncentralized biomarker assay prior to entry.

Although it is assumed that biomarkers modulated in breast cancer specimens are likely to be modulated to a similar degree in benign breast tissue, this may not always be the case. Furthermore, the prevalence of a biomarker in benign high-risk tissue is often much lower and more heterogeously distributed than in breast cancer. Phase I biomarker modulation models utilizing high-risk subjects need to be developed to allow determination of biomarker prevalence and variation in this population, as well as the magnitude of effect that might be anticipated from drug treatment. This in turn would allow better estimation of sample size requirements for Phase II and III trials. If proliferation is the main outcome marker in a Phase II study, statistical distribution of proliferation for benign tissue should be established in the study population, at baseline and over time, both for the study agent and a no-treatment group. Single-arm Phase I studies in high-risk populations may be very useful in this regard. For example, the drug dose may be known or anticipated, as is common with antihormonal agents, but the magnitude of its effect on proliferation in high-risk women with benign breast disease is unknown. Distribution of values (with the assay to be used in the Phase II trial) is then determined at baseline; the magnitude of effect is determined by the change and its standard deviation between baseline and end-of-study tissue sample. If the average baseline proliferation index in a benign tissue sample was 3%, an effect size of 0.5 standard deviation could be detected with 34 subjects, and an effect size of 0.33 standard deviation with 75 subjects. Assuming that the standard deviation for the change is 3%, an effect size of 0.5 standard deviation is equivalent to detecting a 50% reduction in proliferation with 34 subjects.

3.2.2. PHASE II TRIALS

Phase II studies are generally randomized, double-blind, placebo-controlled trials in which 100–200 high-risk subjects are enrolled, usually for an intervention period of 6–12 mo *(10,11)*. To date, biomarker response endpoints most often employed include modulation of tissue morphology in women with IEN, proliferation and apoptotic markers, mammographic breast density area, and serum IGF-1 level and IGF-1:IGFBP-3 ratio *(12,55,78,101–103,124,150)*. One or more serum or urine biochemical activity markers may also be used to ensure that sufficient drug is being received to modulate the biochemical pathway by which the drug is presumed to act. This may be very valuable in a situation where no effect is seen on response biomarkers.

Most Phase II trials initiated to date and either completed or accruing on schedule have used high-risk women with random periareolar FNA evidence of hyperplasia with or without atypia as the study cohort, with improvement in cytologic morphology as the main study endpoint and modulation of proliferation,

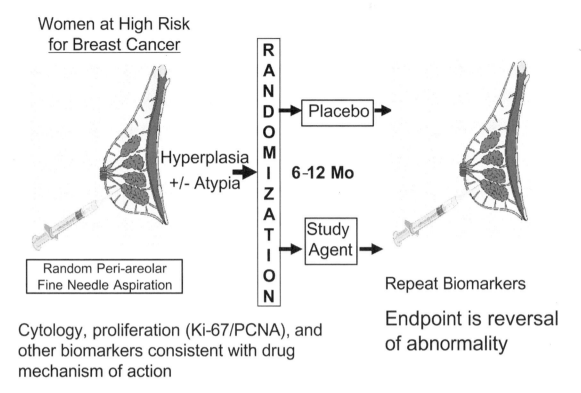

Fig. 4. Schematic of the FNA model for Phase II chemoprevention trials. Eligible subjects are randomized between a placebo group and the investigational agent (typically at a set dose) for six months between tissue samplings by random periareolar FNA. The endpoints are modulations of cytologic morphology, proliferation, and other biomarkers based on the presumed mechanism of action (e.g., ER/PR, EGFR, COX-2, Her-2) *(27)*.

mammographic breast density, and serum IGF-1:IGFBP-3 ratio as secondary endpoints (Fig. 4). The rationale for use of cytologic morphology sampled by random periareolar FNA as the main study endpoint is based on the prospective study of Fabian et al. *(25)* in which high-risk women with random FNA evidence of hyperplasia with atypia had a five times greater short-term risk of breast cancer development than women without random FNA evidence of atypia. In this study, 83% of women were willing to have the procedure repeated 6–12 mo later. This type of Phase II trial design requires stratification at the time of randomization on the basis of baseline cytologic morphology and other factors likely to affect response (i.e., menopausal status, hormone use, key predictive markers).

The number of subjects required for such a trial depends on variability in morphology inherent in the tissue sampling technique and cytopathology assessment, likelihood that the drug might favorably modulate morphology in a short interval (e.g., 6 mo), and number of subjects who actually complete the study with sufficient material evaluable for biomarkers. A Phase II study with DFMO randomized high-risk

women whose FNA revealed hyperplasia with or without atypia to 6 mo of DFMO or placebo with a defined primary endpoint of improvement in cytomorphology defined by a reduction in category (hyperplasia with atypia to simple hyperplasia or simple hyperplasia to nonproliferative) or a decrease in the semiquantitative Masood score *(45)* of three or more points. The Masood system assigns one to four points to each of six cytologic characteristics. Nonproliferative lesions generally score between 6 and 10, hyperplasia 11–14, hyperplasia with atypia 15–18, and cancer 19–24 *(45)*. Baseline FNA was allowed up to 9 mo prior to randomization. Approximately four women underwent aspiration for every woman placed on study. One hundred nineteen (119) women with a median age of 46 were accrued in 23 months in a single institution; half had initial FNA evidence of hyperplasia and half had hyperplasia with atypia. The median baseline Masood score index was 13.4. Ninety-six percent (96%) of participants completed the study and had a follow-up FNA 6 mo after randomization *(78,79)*. Overall, 28% of samples from subjects randomized to placebo were interpreted as showing improvement using traditional categories of nonproliferative, hyperplasia, or hyperplasia with atypia

(284), and 18% of placebo subjects were interpreted as showing improvement when improvement was defined as a decrease of three or more Masood score points *(79)*. Although this observed magnitude of variation in the placebo group is well within the range of interpretive discordance reported for benign breast disease specimens *(53)*, this amount of discordance would require an improvement in cytologic category in 60% of the treatment group in order to detect a significant difference in modulatory effect between placebo and treatment group given the modest sample size employed in this study, using an 80% power and 5% type I error rate. However, the placebo group had minimal variability in change in Masood score index (mean decrease of 0.46 points, standard deviation of 2.5 points). If change in mean Masood score is used as the primary endpoint, and if placebo is associated with a mean reduction of 0.5 points and standard deviation of 2.5 points, and if an active agent were to show a reduction of 2.0 points from an average baseline of 13.5 points, this degree of improvement relative to placebo could be detected with 90 evaluable subjects at 80% power and a type I error rate of 5%. Unfortunately, the semiquantitative Masood scoring system has yet to be evaluated as a risk biomarker in a prospective trial. If "improvement" in cytomorphology continues to be used as a response biomarker in Phase II studies, the number of subjects should increase to offset inherent variation and/or other methods of tissue sampling and morphologic assessment, and response definition should be developed in an effort to reduce variation in the control group.

Ductal lavage offers the potential to reduce sampling variance that theoretically exists with random periareolar FNA. However, studies have not yet been completed to determine how frequently the same NAF-producing duct may be recannulated, or even if atypia observed in lavage samples predicts later clinical development of cancer. Furthermore, since lavage is readily accomplished only in women producing NAF, it is unclear if this technique will be useful in chemoprevention studies if the agent to be tested reduces either prolactin levels (SERMs) or estrogen levels (aromatase inhibitors), which would be expected to reduce or curtail NAF production *(19,285)*. Finally, given that occult hyperplasia with or without atypia is generally multifocal and multicentric *(40,41)*, it is possible that modulation of a field effect as assessed by random tissue sampling may have as much or more implication for risk reduction as elimination of a specific focus of atypia in a single duct.

Use of modified consensus panel criteria for diagnostic FNA biopsies (quantity not sufficient [QNS], benign, indeterminate/atypia, and suspicious) *(286)* has been reported to have low interobserver discordance (11%) when applied to ductal lavage samples from high-risk women *(57)*. The consensus panel criteria essentially group most cases of nonproliferative cytology and hyperplasia without atypia into a single category of "benign" and may solve the problem of trying to differentiate cases of borderline hyperplasia versus hyperplasia with atypia by including both in the indeterminate/atypia category. However, grouping both proliferative cases without atypia and nonproliferative cases into a single category may not be optimal for prevention trials. Use of nuclear morphometry to quantitate subtle cytologic change via difference in Z scores is also a promising way to reduce variability in morphologic assessment *(287)* (Fig. 5).

Given the theoretical differences in what we wish to accomplish in cohorts with baseline hyperplasia without atypia (prevention of progression) and those with hyperplasia with atypia (reversal of atypia), prevention trials with modulation of morphology as an endpoint should separate rather than mix these two cohorts. Separation would facilitate sample size estimation and statistical analysis. For the prevention of progression model, women with benign (consensus panel criteria) or hyperplasia without atypia (traditional criteria) cytology would serve as the cohort. The primary endpoint would be reduction in the proportion of women found to have atypia in their later specimens. This model would require 335 subjects to detect a 50% reduction in incidence of women showing atypia at the 6-mo aspiration, assuming a 25% incidence in the placebo group and using a conservative estimate of variance observed with the DFMO trial and traditional cytologic criteria *(13)*.

Alternatively, a reversal of hyperplasia with atypia trial in which all subjects had atypia at entry would require as few as 130 subjects to detect a 50% reduction in FNA atypia relative to placebo, even with as much as a 50% decrease in random FNA atypia in the placebo arm; if detection of a 33% reduction in atypia is desired, 280 subjects would need to be entered *(13)*. More than twice as many subjects would need to be screened for a Phase II trial requiring FNA hyperplasia with atypia at entry vs hyperplasia without atypia at entry. Furthermore, it is currently unknown if atypical hyperplasia can be reversed in as little as 6 mo. This may not be likely unless pro-apoptotic agents are being utilized and/or growth factors such as estrogen are being withdrawn.

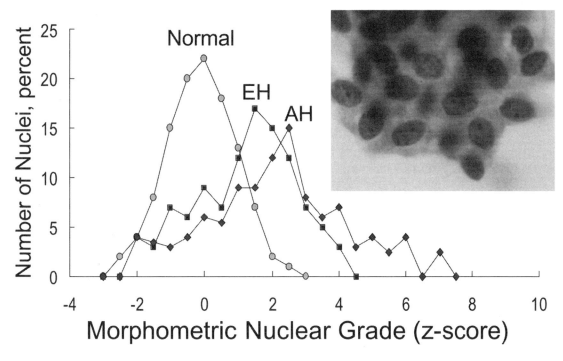

Fig. 5. Distribution of nuclei according to morphometric nuclear grade. Breast epithelial cells obtained by random FNA were classified as either normal (nonproliferative), epithelial hyperplasia without atypia, and epithelial hyperplasia with atypia (inset). The morphometric deviation from normal is characterized by a z-score. Courtesy of Dr. James Bacus of Bacus Laboratories, Inc., Elmhurst, IL.

Given the large number of subjects required for a meaningful modulation of morphology trial under either of the two scenarios, newly designed Phase II trials often employ modulation of proliferation as an endpoint since reduction in proliferation in weeks to months has been associated with later clinical response in neoadjuvant cancer trials *(73–75)*. It is unknown, however, if reduction in proliferation is associated with improved cytologic morphology or reduced cancer incidence in prevention studies. MIB-1 is an attractive proliferation marker because of its reproducibility *(288,289)*. However, because a low number of positive cells can be expected in women with hyperplasia with or without atypia (mean of 1–5%), a minimum of 500–1000 ductal epithelial cells are needed to reliably measure Ki-67/MIB-1 *(30,64)*. In a consecutive series of 100 high-risk subjects undergoing random periareolar FNA over 6 mo at the University of Kansas Medical Center, four ThinPrep™ slides (one for cytology, three for immunocytochemistry) with equal distribution of material were made from each aspirate, and cell number was prospectively categorized. Sixty-two percent (62%) of all aspirates had ≥1000 cells on the cytology slide. Women with hyperplasia had a median of 1000–5000 cells on the cytology slide, and those with hyperplasia

plus atypia a median of >5000 cells. Furthermore, women with >1000 ductal cells on their cytology slide generally had >500 cells on each of the other three slides; the vast majority had hyperplasia with or without atypia. Thus by limiting entry to women with >1000 cells on the cytology slide, sufficient cells should be present to assess proliferation as well as one or two other predictive biomarkers.

Our preliminary studies in 11 high-risk premenopausal women with ≥1000 cells on the corresponding cytology slide using a DAKO monoclonal antibody and antigen retrieval indicate a median Ki-67/MIB-1 value of 3.5% (range 2–12%) with a standard deviation of 3.6%. Assuming a similar standard deviation for the treated group, a 33% reduction in proliferation relative to placebo could be detected with 200 evaluable subjects with an 80% power and 5% type I error rate, whereas a 50% reduction would require approx 100 evaluable subjects.

Dooley et al. have published a ductal lavage series in which an estimated median of 13,500 cells were collected per duct with a median of 1.5 ducts per subject. Thirty-eight percent (38%) of lavages were performed under general anesthesia *(57)*. The cell processing technique used a millipore filter system that captured all cells in a filter paper that was subsequently dissolved on the slide. Dissolving the filter makes the cells so obtained unsuitable for immunochemistry, although the process very efficiently captures all cells present in the solution. Using Cytospin™ or ThinPrep™ techniques to process cells results in cell loss from the sample but produces a slide suitable for immunocytochemistry. It is likely that cell numbers obtained from ductal lavage and FNA are similar, but a head-to-head comparison utilizing the same cell processing techniques on the same study subjects has not been performed. As part of a recently initiated single-arm study of celecoxib sponsored by NCI, the relative suitability of FNA and ductal lavage will be compared for Phase II chemoprevention trials. High-risk premenopausal women first undergo NAF/ductal lavage followed by FNA the same day. Cells will be processed for cytology characterizations, plus ER, COX-2, and MIB-1 expression. Women with ≥1000 cells on the FNA cytology slide will be eligible for study. Baseline and follow-up specimens will be compared as to cell number category, morphology, and immunocytochemistry.

We observed only a mean 2% variation in area of mammographic density over a 6-mo study period in the placebo group in our Phase II DFMO study (79), using a computerized analysis program developed by Boyd et al. (86). Given the low variation in breast density in our trial and several other small preliminary studies (97,98), and the importance of high breast density (>60%) as a risk factor regardless of menopausal status, mammographic breast density area is a strong contender as a response biomarker in Phase II studies. If the mean baseline breast density is 46% with a standard deviation of 9% (as observed in our high-risk cohort in the DFMO trial), and if a 2% change is anticipated for the placebo group over 6 mo with a standard deviation of 3.5%, then one would need to enter 81 evaluable subjects in each arm (total of 162) to detect an absolute reduction in the treatment arm of 6% with 80% power and a type I error rate of 5%.

3.2.3. PHASE III TRIALS

Although cancer incidence will continue to be the gold standard for chemoprevention trials, given the substantial increased risk for women found to have occult (by random FNA) or clinical (by biopsy of abnormal palpable or mammographic lesions) evidence of atypical hyperplasia, Phase III trials with an endpoint of reversing atypical hyperplasia or preventing its appearance are attractive. The duration of such trials would depend on resources available and the study population.

In the failure-to-progress model, high-risk women without atypia in their baseline aspiration are randomized between control (or placebo) and experimental agent similarly to the schema depicted for Phase II studies. When the study is placebo-controlled, a trial of 6 mo duration is attractive to high-risk subjects if a period of open-label study drug is automatically built in at the conclusion of the study's randomized portion. Assuming a 25% detection of atypical hyperplasia in the follow-up aspirate in the placebo arm, entry of 336 evaluable subjects would allow detection of a 50% reduction in subsequent detection of atypia and 808 subjects would allow detection of a 33% reduction in subsequent detection of atypia with a 5% type I error rate and 80% power. A comparison with a drug known to be efficacious in reducing risk (i.e., tamoxifen) might be envisioned with a longer treatment period but would require substantially more subjects. For example, if 12 mo of tamoxifen were assumed to reduce the risk of subsequent detection of atypia by 30%, then 1242 subjects would be needed to reduce the subsequent detection of atypia by 33% relative to tamoxifen.

A reversal-of-atypia model similar to that depicted for Phase II trials could also be used for Phase III trials when the model is validated by demonstrating that it is possible to reliably reverse atypia after 6–12 mo of drug treatment with commonly used classes of chemopreventive agents and that failure to detect subsequent atypia by random tissue sampling is associated with reduced cancer incidence.

Other Phase III models could use contralateral breast cancer incidence as an endpoint in women previously treated for breast cancer, requiring fewer than the 16,000–22,000 subjects enrolled in the large NSABP primary prevention studies. For sample size calculations, assumptions would include 0.7% per year incidence of contralateral cancer and no treatment after surgery with or without radiation for a T1a or T1b invasive ER-negative cancer. Using these assumptions, a 50% reduction in contralateral breast cancer incidence could be detected with approx 3000 subjects randomized to placebo or experimental agent, assuming a 3-yr accrual period, a 5-yr follow-up, 10% loss to follow-up per year, 80% power, and a type 1 error rate of 5%. A reduction in contralateral breast cancer incidence trial for women with ER-positive tumors would require substantially more subjects, as antihormonal treatment is standard and would reduce the likelihood of contralateral cancer incidence by 50% or more, i.e., to an incidence of 0.35% per year (290). Thus the new agent would likely be compared to standard antihormonal therapy and approx 6000 subjects would be needed to show a 50% reduction from a 0.35% incidence to 0.175% incidence per year assuming a 10% subject dropout per year, 3 yr of accrual, 5-yr follow-up, 80% power and type I error rate of 5%.

4. SUMMARY

A large number of new agents targeting molecular abnormalities in precancerous breast tissue are available for clinical testing. Agents that lack antihormonal, uterine agonist, or procoagulant side effects are of particular interest, as are agents whose mechanism of action predicts activity in tamoxifen-resistant cells.

Clinical paradigms for new-agent evaluation need to shift from those used to evaluate traditional anticancer agents. Modulation of proliferation and other key biomarkers are used to define an optimal yet minimally toxic dose in Phase I trials. Modulation of proliferation or other key molecular markers in high-risk women with breast IEN in randomized, placebo-controlled trials is likely to be the main response endpoint in Phase II trials. Biomarkers predictive of response to the class of drug being tested should be used along with risk biomarkers to select cohorts for these studies. Sophisticated gene expression arrays and proteomic studies performed as part of these studies will help us to better understand a drug's mechanism of action, offering the potential to use specific gene and/or protein expression as future response biomarkers.

At present, reduction in cancer incidence continues to be the gold standard for Phase III trials. Two Phase III models using morphology (prevention of progression to or reversal of atypical hyperplasia) as the response endpoint are presented as alternatives to traditional cancer incidence trials. Central to the rationale behind these models is the observation that atypical hyperplasia obtained by a diagnostic biopsy or random tissue sampling dramatically increases a woman's short-term risk for breast cancer. Thus, preventing or treating early breast IEN will have the ultimate effect of reducing the incidence of breast cancer.

REFERENCES

1. *Cancer Facts & Figures 2003*. American Cancer Society, Atlanta, 2003.
2. Osborne CK, Yochmowitz MG, Knight WA 3rd, McGuire WL. The value of estrogen and progesterone receptors in the treatment of breast cancer. *Cancer* 1980;46(Suppl): 2884–2888.
3. Fisher B, Costantino JP, Wickerham DL, et al. Tamoxifen for prevention of breast cancer: Report of the National Surgical Adjuvant Breast and Bowel Project P-1 Study. *J Natl Cancer Inst* 1998;90:1371–1388.
4. Gail MH, Briton LA, Byar DP, et al. Projecting individualized probabilities of developing breast cancer for white females who are being examined annually. *J Natl Cancer Inst* 1989;81:1879–1886.
5. King M-C, Wieand S, Hale K, et al. Tamoxifen and breast cancer incidence among women with inherited mutations in BRCA1 and BRCA2. *JAMA* 2001;286:2251–2256.
6. Freedman AN, Graubard BI, Rao SR, et al. Estimates of the number of US women who could benefit from tamoxifen for breast cancer chemoprevention. *J Natl Cancer Inst* 2003;95:526–532.
7. Gail MH, Costantino JP, Bryant J, et al. Weighing the risks and benefits of tamoxifen treatment for preventing breast cancer. *J Natl Cancer Inst* 1999;91:1829–1846.
8. Rockhill B, Spiegelman D, Byrne C, et al. Validation of the Gail et al. model of breast cancer risk prediction and implications for chemoprevention. *J Natl Cancer Inst* 2001;93: 358–366.
9. Costantino JP, Gail MH, Pee D, et al. Validation studies for models projecting the risk of invasive and total breast cancer incidence. *J Natl Cancer Inst* 1999;91:1541–1548.
10. Kelloff GJ, Boone CW, Steele VE, et al. Mechanistic considerations in chemopreventive drug development. *J Cell Biochem Suppl* 1994;20:1–24.
11. Kelloff GJ, Boone CW, Steele VE, et al. Progress in cancer chemoprevention: perspectives on agent selection and short-term clinical intervention trials. *Cancer Res* 1994;54(Suppl): 2015S–2024S.
12. Kelloff GJ, Boone CW, Crowell JA, et al. Risk biomarkers and current strategies for cancer chemoprevention. *J Cell Biochem* 1996;25:1–14.
13. O'Shaughnessy JA, Kelloff GJ, Gordon GB, et al. Treatment and prevention of intraepithelial neoplasia: an important target for accelerated new agent development. *Clin Cancer Res* 2002;8:314–346.
14. Meijers-Heijboer H, van Geel B, van Putten WL, et al. Breast cancer after prophylactic bilateral mastectomy in women with a BRCA1 or BRCA2 mutation. *N Engl J Med* 2001;345:159–164.
15. Brekelmans CT, Seynaeve C, Bartels CC, et al. Effectiveness of breast cancer surveillance in BRCA1/2 gene mutation carriers and women with high familial risk. *J Clin Oncol* 2001;19:924–930.
16. Fisher ER, Fisher B, Sass R, Wickerham L. Pathologic findings from the National Surgical Adjuvant Breast Project (Protocol No. 4). XI. Bilateral breast cancer. *Cancer* 1984;54:3002–3011.
17. Broet P, de la Rochefordiere A, Scholl SM, et al. Contralateral breast cancer: annual incidence and risk parameters. J Clin Oncol 1995;13:1578–1583.
18. Obedian E, Fischer DB, Haffty BG. Second malignancies after treatment of early-stage breast cancer: lumpectomy and radiation therapy versus mastectomy. *J Clin Oncol* 2000;18:2406–2412.
19. Ernster VL, Wrensch MR, Petrakis NL, et al. Benign and malignant breast disease: initial study results of serum and breast fluid analyses of endogenous estrogens. *J Natl Cancer Inst* 1987;79:949–960.
20. Page DL, Dupont WD. Anatomic markers of human premalignancy and risk of breast cancer. *Cancer* 1990;66: 1326–1335.

21. Byrne C, Schairer C, Wolfe J, et al. Mammographic features and breast cancer risk: effects with time, age and menopause status. *Natl Cancer Inst* 1995;87:1622–1629.

22. Boyd NF, Lockwood GA, Bying JW, et al. Mammographic densities and breast cancer risk. *Cancer Epidemiol Biomarkers Prev* 1998;7:1133–1144.

23. Hankinson SE, Willett WC, Colditz GA, et al. Circulating concentrations of insulin-like growth factor-I and risk of breast cancer. *Lancet* 1998;351:1393–1396.

24. Cauley JA, Lucas FL, Kuller LH, et al. Elevated serum estradiol and testosterone concentrations are associated with a high risk for breast cancer. *Ann Intern Med* 1999;130:270–277.

25. Fabian CJ, Kimler BF, Zalles CM, et al. Short-term breast cancer prediction by random periareolar fine-needle aspiration cytology and the Gail risk model. *J Natl Cancer Inst* 2000;92:1217–1227.

26. Fabian CJ, Kimler BF. Beyond tamoxifen. New endpoints for breast cancer chemoprevention, new drugs for breast cancer prevention. *Ann NY Acad Sci* 2001;952:44–59.

27. Evron E, Dooley WC, Umbricht CB, et al. Detection of breast cancer cells in ductal lavage fluid by methylation-specific PCR. *Lancet* 2001;357:1335–1336.

28. Fabian CJ, Kimler BF. Breast cancer chemoprevention: current challenges and a look towards the future. *Clin Breast Cancer* 2002;3:120–131.

29. Wrensch MR, Petrakis NL, Miike R, et al. Breast cancer risk in women with abnormal cytology in nipple aspirates of breast fluid. *J Natl Cancer Inst* 2001;93:1791–1798.

30. Shaaban AM, Sloane JP, West CR, Foster CS. Breast cancer risk in usual ductal hyperplasia is defined by estrogen receptor-alpha and Ki-67 expression. *Am J Pathol* 2002;160: 597–604.

31. Boone CW, Kelloff GJ. Intraepithelial neoplasia, surrogate endpoint biomarkers, and cancer chemoprevention. *J Cell Biochem Suppl* 1993;17F:37–48.

32. Wellings SR, Jensen HM, Marcum RG. An atlas of subgross pathology of the human breast with special reference to possible precancerous lesions. *J Natl Cancer Inst* 1975;55: 231–273.

33. Boone CW, Bacus JW, Bacus JV, et al. Properties of intraepithelial neoplasia relevant to cancer chemoprevention and to the development of surrogate end points for clinical trials. *Proc Soc Exp Biol Med* 1997;216:151–165.

34. Page DL, Dupont WD, Rogers LW, Rados MS. Atypical hyperplastic lesions of the female breast. A long-term follow-up study. *Cancer* 1985;55:2698–2708.

35. Page DL, Kidd TE Jr, Dupont WD, et al. Lobular neoplasia of the breast: higher risk for subsequent invasive cancer by more extensive disease. *Hum Pathol* 1991;22:1232–1239.

36. Tavassoli FA, Norris HJ. A comparison of the results of long-term followup for atypical intraductal hyperplasia and intraductal hyperplasia of the breast. *Cancer* 1990;65: 518–529.

37. Ottesen GL, Graversen HP, Blichert-Toft M, et al. Lobular carcinoma in situ of the female breast. Short-term results of a prospective nationwide study. The Danish Breast Cancer Cooperative Group. *Am J Surg Pathol* 1993;17:14–21.

38. Modan B, Lubin F, Alfandary E, et al. Breast cancer following benign breast disease—a nationwide study. *Breast Cancer Res Treat* 1997;46:45.

39. Kramer WM, Rush BF. Mammary duct proliferation in the elderly. A histopathologic study. *Cancer* 1973;31:130–137.

40. Bhathal PS, Brown RW, Lesueur GC, Russell TS. Frequency of benign and malignant breast lesions in 207 consecutive autopsies in Australian women. *Br J Cancer* 1985;51: 271–278.

41. Nielsen M, Thomsen JL, Primdahl S, et al. Breast cancer and atypia among young and middle-aged women: a study of 110 medicolegal autopsies. *Br J Cancer* 1987;56:814–819.

42. Hoogerbrugge N, Bult P, deWidt-Levert LM, et al. High prevalence of premalignant lesions in prophylactically removed breasts from women at hereditary risk for breast cancer. *J Clin Oncol* 2003;21:41–45.

43. Fabian C, Zalles C, Kamel S, et al. Biomarker and cytologic abnormalities in women at high and low risk for breast cancer. *J Cell Biochem* 1993;17(Suppl G):153–160.

44. Tan-Chiu E, Costantino J, Wang J, et al. The effect of tamoxifen on benign breast disease. Findings from the National Surgical Adjuvant Breast and Bowel Project (NSABP) Breast Cancer Prevention Trial. *Breast Cancer Res Treat* 2001;69:210 (abstract).

45. Masood S, Frykberg ER, McLellan GL, et al. Prospective evaluation of radiologically directed fine-needle aspiration biopsy of nonpalpable breast lesions. *Cancer* 1990;66: 1480–1487.

46. Masood S. Cytomorphology of fibrocystic change, high risk, and premalignant breast lesions. *Breast J* 1995;1: 210–221.

47. King EB, Chew KL, Duarte LA, et al. Image cytometric classification of premalignant breast disease in fine needle aspirates. *Cancer* 1988;62:114–124.

48. Bacus JW, Bacus JV. A method of correcting DNA ploidy measurements in tissue sections. *Mod Pathol* 1994;7: 652–664.

49. Bacus JW, Bacus JV, Stoner GD, et al. Quantitation of preinvasive neoplastic progression in animal models of chemical carcinogenesis. *J Cell Biochem Suppl* 1997;28-29:21–38.

50. Page DL, Rogers LW. Combined histologic and cytologic criteria for the diagnosis of mammary atypical ductal hyperplasia. *Hum Pathol* 1992;23:1095–1097.

51. Schnitt J, Connolly L, Tavassoli FA, et al. Interobserver reproducibility in the diagnosis of ductal proliferative breast lesions using standardized criteria. *Am J Surg Pathol* 1992;16: 1133–1143.

52. Tavassoli FA. Mammary intraepithelial neoplasia: a translational classification system for the intraductal epithelial proliferations. *Breast J* 1997;3:48–58.

53. Sidawy MK, Stoler MH, Frable WJ, et al. Interobserver variability in the classification of proliferative breast lesions by fine-needle aspiration: results of the Papanicolaou Society of Cytopathology Study. *Diagn Cytopathol* 1998;18: 150–165.

54. Mansoor S, Ip C, Stomper PC. Yield of terminal ductal lobule units (TDLU) in normal breast stereotactic core biopsy specimens: implications of biomarker studies. *Breast J* 2000;6: 220–224.

55. Harper-Wynne C, Ross A, Sacks N, Dowsett M. A pilot prevention study of the aromatase inhibitor letrozole: effects on breast cell proliferation and bone/lipid indices in healthy postmenopausal women. *Breast Cancer Res Treat* 2001;69: 225 (abstract).

56. Fabian CJ, Kimler BF, Elledge RM, et al. Models for early chemoprevention trials in breast cancer. *Hematol Oncol Clin North Am* 1998;12:993–1017.

57. Dooley WC, Ljung BM, Veronesi U, et al. Ductal lavage for detection of cellular atypia in women at high risk for breast cancer. *J Natl Cancer Inst* 2001;93:1624–1632.

58. Rose DP. Hormones and growth factors in nipple aspirates from normal women and benign breast disease patients. *Cancer Detect Prev* 1992;16:43–51.

59. Wrensch M, Petrakis NL, King EB, et al. Breast cancer risk associated with abnormal cytology in nipple aspirates of breast fluid and prior history of breast biopsy. *Am J Epidemiol* 1993;137:829–833.

60. Allan DJ, Howell A, Roberts SA, et al. Reduction in apoptosis relative to mitosis in histologically normal epithelium accompanies fibrocytstic change and carcinoma of the premenopausal human breast. *J Pathol* 1992;167:25–32.

61. Mommers EC, van Diest PJ, Leonhart AM, et al. Balance of cell proliferation and apoptosis in breast carcinogenesis. *Breast Cancer Res Treat* 1999;58:163–169.

62. Pavelic ZP, Pavelic L, Lower EE, et al. c-myc, c-erbB-2, and Ki-67 expression in normal breast tissue and in invasive and noninvasive breast carcinoma. *Cancer Res* 1992;52: 2597–2602.

63. Siziopikou KP, Schnitt SJ. MIB-1 proliferation index in ductal carcinoma *in situ* of the breast: relationship to the expression of the apoptosis-regulating proteins bcl-2 and p53. *Breast J* 2000;6:400–406.

64. Allred DC, Mohsin SK, Fuqua SA. Histological and biological evolution of human premalignant breast disease. *Endocr Relat Cancer* 2001;8:47–61.

65. Tuccari G, Rizzo A, Muscara M, et al. PCNA/cyclin expressin in breast carcinomas: its relationships with Ki-67, ER, PgR immunostaining and clinico-pathologic aspects. *Pathologica* 1993;85(1095):47–55.

66. Dawson AE, Norton JA, Weinber DS. Comparative assessment of proliferation and DNA content in breast carcinoma by image analysis and flow cytometry. *Am J Pathol* 1990;136:1115–1124.

67. Shrestha P, Yamada K, Wada T, et al. Proliferating cell nuclear antigen in breast lesions: correlation of c-erbB-2 oncoprotein and EGF receptor and its clinicopathological significance in breast cancer. *Virchows Arch A Pathol Anat Histopathol* 1992;421:193–202.

68. Wolf HK, Dittrich KL. Detection of proliferating cell nuclear antigen in diagnostic histopathology. *J Histochem Cytochem* 1992;40:1269–1273.

69. Gee JM, Douglas-Jones A, Hepburn P, et al. A cautionary note regarding the application of Ki-67 antibodies to paraffin-embedded breast cancers. *J Pathol* 1995;177:285–293.

70. Yu CC, Dublin EA, Camplejohn RS, Levison DA. Optimization of immunohistochemical staining of proliferating cells in paraffin sections of breast carcinoma using antibodies to proliferating cell nuclear antigen and the Ki-67 antigen. *Anal Cell Pathol* 1995;9:45–52.

71. Meyer JS. Cell proliferation in normal human breast ducts, fibroadenomas, and other ductal hyperplasias measured by nuclear labeling with tritiated thymidine. Effects of menstrual phase, age, and oral contraceptive hormones. *Hum Pathol* 1977;8:67–81.

72. Potten CS, Watson RJ, Williams GT, et al. The effect of age and menstrual cycle upon proliferative activity of the normal human breast. *Br J Cancer* 1988;58:163–170.

73. Chang J, Powles TJ, Allred DC, et al. Prediction of clinical outcome from primary tamoxifen by expression of biologic markers in breast cancer patients. *Clin Cancer Res* 2000;6:616–621.

74. Ellis MJ, Coop A, Singh B, et al. Letrozole is more effective neoadjuvant endocrine therapy than tamoxifen for ErbB-1-and/or ErbB-2-positive, estrogen receptor-positive primary breast cancer: evidence from a Phase III randomized trial. *J Clin Oncol* 2001;19:3808–3816.

75. Dowsett M, Bundred NJ, Decensi A, et al. Effect of raloxifene on breast cancer cell Ki67 and apoptosis: a double-blind, placebo-controlled, randomized clinical trial in postmenopausal patients. *Cancer Epidemiol Biomarkers Prev* 2001;10:961–966.

76. Clarke RB, Laidlaw IJ, Jones LJ, et al. Effect of tamoxifen on Ki-67 labelling index in human breast tumours and its relationship to oestrogen and progesterone receptor status. *Br J Cancer* 1993;67:606–611.

77. Fabian CJ, Kimler BF, Anderson J, et al. Phase I biomarker and toxicity evaluation of LY353381 (a 3rd generation selective estrogen receptor modulator, SERM) in breast cancer. *Proc Am Soc Clin Oncol* 2000;19:75a.

78. Kimler BF, Zalles CM, Masood S, et al. Phase II chemoprevention trial of α-difluoromethylornithine (DFMO) in women at high risk for breast cancer: surrogate endpoint biomarkers. *Proc Am Assoc Cancer Res* 2001;42:826:abstr. no. 4437.

79. Fabian CJ, Kimler BF, Brady DA, et al. A Phase II breast cancer chemoprevention trial of oral α-difluoromethylornithine: breast tissue, imaging, and serum and urine biomarkers. *Clin Cancer Res* 2002;8:3105–3117.

80. Oza AM, Boyd NF. Mammographic parenchymal patterns: a marker of breast cancer risk. *Epidemiol Rev* 1993;15: 196–208.

81. White E, Velentgas P, Mandelson MT, et al. Variation in mammographic breast density by time in menstrual cycle among women aged 40-49 years. *J Natl Cancer Inst* 1998;90:906–910.

82. Ursin G, Parisky YR, Pike MC, Spicer DV. Mammographic density changes during the menstrual cycle. *Cancer Epidemiol Biomarkers Prev* 2001;10:141–142.

83. Gertig DM, Stillman IE, Byrne C, et al. Association of age and reproductive factors with benign breast tissue composition. *Cancer Epidemiol Biomarkers Prev* 1999;8:873–879.

84. Persson I, Thurfjell E, Holmberg L. Effect of estrogen and estrogen-progestin replacement regimens on mammographic breast parenchymal density. *J Clin Oncol* 1997;15: 3201–3207.

85. Sterns EE, Zee B. Mammographic density changes in perimenopausal and postmenopausal women: is effect of hormone replacement therapy predictable? *Breast Cancer Res Treat* 2000;59:125–132.

86. Boyd NF, Byng JW, Jong RA, et al. Quantitative classification of mammographic densities and breast cancer risk: results from the Canadian National Breast Screening Study. *J Natl Cancer Inst* 1995;87:670–675.

87. Bland KI, Kuhns JG, Buchanan JB, et al. A clinicopathologic correlation of mammographic parenchymal patterns and associated risk factors for human mammary carcinoma. *Ann Surg* 1982;195:582–594.

88. Boyd NF, Jensen HM, Cooke G, Han HL. Relationship between mammographic and histological risk factors for breast cancer. *J Natl Cancer Inst* 1992;84:1170–1179.

89. Lee MM, Petrakis NL, Wrensch MR, et al. Association of abnormal nipple aspirate cytology and mammographic pattern and density. *Cancer Epidemiol Biomarkers Prev* 1994;3: 33–36.

90. Laya MB, Gallagher JC, Schreiman JS, et al. Effect of postmenopausal hormonal replacement therapy on mammographic density and parenchymal pattern. *Radiology* 1995;196:433–437.

91. Greendale GA, Reboussin BA, Sie A, et al. Effects of estrogen and estrogen-progestin on mammographic parenchymal density. Postmenopausal Estrogen/Progestin Interventions (PEPI) Investigators. *Ann Intern Med* 1999;130: 262–269.

92. Hainline S, Myers L, McLelland R, et al. Mammographic patterns and risk of breast cancer. *AJR Am J Roentgenol* 1978;130:1157–1158.

93. Pankow JS, Vachon CM, Kuni CC, et al. Genetic analysis of mammographic breast density in adult women: evidence of a gene effect. *J Natl Cancer Inst* 1997;89:549–556.

94. Kelsey JL, Gammon MD, John EM. Reproductive factors and breast cancer. *Epidemiol Rev* 1993;15:36–47.

95. Byrne C, Colditz GA, Willet WC, et al. Plasma insulin-like growth factor (IGF) I, IGF-binding protein 3, and mammographic density. *Cancer Res* 2000;60:3744–3748.

96. Ursin G, Pike MC, Spicer DV, et al. Can mammographic densities predict effects of tamoxifen on the breast? *J Natl Cancer Inst* 1996;88:128–129.

97. Atkinson C, Warren R, Bingham SA, Day NE. Mammographic patterns as a predictive biomarker of breast cancer risk: effect of tamoxifen. *Cancer Epidemiol Biomarkers Prev* 1999;8:863–866.

98. Brisson J, Brisson B, Cote G, et al. Tamoxifen and mammographic breast densities. *Cancer Epidemiol Biomarkers Prev* 2000;9:911–915.

99. Ursin G, Astrahan MA, Salane M, et al. The detection of changes in mammographic densities. *Cancer Epidemiol Biomarkers Prev* 1998;7:43–47.

100. Zhou C, Chan HP, Petrick N, et al. Computerized image analysis: estimation of breast density on mammograms. *Med Phys* 2001;28:1056–1069.

101. Cassano E, Coopmans de Yoldi G, et al. Mammographic patterns in breast cancer chemoprevention with fenretinide (4-HPR). *Eur J Cancer* 1993;29A:2161–2163.

102. Boyd NF, Greenberg C, Lockwood G, et al. Effects at two years of a low-fat, high-carbohydrate diet on radiologic features of the breast: results from a randomized trial. *J Natl Cancer Inst* 1997;89:488–496.

103. Spicer DV, Ursin G, Parisky YR, et al. Changes in mammographic densities induced by a hormonal contraceptive designed to reduce breast cancer risk. *J Natl Cancer Inst* 1994;86:431–436.

104. Harvey JA, Pinkerton JV, Herman CR. Short-term cessation of hormone replacement therapy and improvement of mammographic specificity. *J Natl Cancer Inst* 1997;89: 1623–1625.

105. Gamroudi F, Cullen KJ. Insulin-like growth factors in breast cancer. *J Womens Cancer* 2000;2:41–52.

106. Pollak M. Insulin-like growth factor physiology and cancer risk. *Eur J Cancer* 2000;36:1224–1228.

107. Yu H, Rohan T. Role of the insulin-like growth factor family in cancer development and progression. *J Natl Cancer Inst* 2000;92:1472–1489.

108. Jernstrom H, Deal C, Wilkin F, et al. Genetic and nongenetic factors associated with variation of plasma levels of insulin-like growth factor-I and insulin-like growth factor-binding protein-3 in healthy premenopausal women. *Cancer Epidemiol Biomarkers Prev* 2001;10:377–384.

109. White E, Malone K, Weiss N, Daling J. Breast cancer among young U.S. women in relation to oral contraception use. *J Natl Cancer Inst* 1994;86:505–514.

110. Wang HS, Lee JD, Soong YK. Serum levels of insulin-like growth factor-binding protein-1 and -3 in women with regular menstrual cycles. *Fertil Steril* 1995;63:1204–1209.

111. Thierry van Dessel HJ, Chandrasekher Y, Yap OW, et al. Serum and follicular fluid levels of insulin-like growth factor I (IGF-I), IGF-II, and IGF-binding protein-1 and -3 during the normal menstrual cycle. *J Clin Endocrinol Metab* 1996;81:1224–1231.

112. Janssen YJ, Helmerhorst F, Frolich M, Roelfsema F. A switch from oral (2 mg/day) to transdermal (50 microg/day) 17beta-estradiol therapy increases serum insulin-like growth factor-I levels in recombinant human growth hormone (GH)-substituted women with GH deficiency. *J Clin Endocrinol Metab* 2000;85:464–467.

113. van den Berg HW, Claffie D, Boylan M, et al. Expression of receptors for epidermal growth factor and insulin-like growth factor I by ZR-75-1 human breast cancer cell variants is inversely related: the effect of steroid hormones on insulin-like growth factor I receptor expression. *Br J Cancer* 1996;73:477–481.

114. Lee AV, Jackson JG, Gooch JL, et al. Enhancement of insulin-like growth factor signaling in human breast cancer: estrogen regulation of insulin receptor substrate-1 expression in vitro and in vivo. *Mol Endocrinol* 1999;13:787–796.

115. Yee D, Lee AV. Crosstalk between the insulin-like growth factors and estrogens in breast cancer. *J Mammary Gland Biol Neoplasia* 2000;5:107–115.

116. Oesterreich S, Zhang P, Guler RL, et al. Re-expression of estrogen receptor alpha in estrogen receptor alpha-negative MCF-7 cells restores both estrogen and insulin-like growth factor-mediated signaling and growth. *Cancer Res* 2001;61: 5771–5777.

117. Singh A, Blench I, Morris HR, et al. Synergistic interaction of growth factors and albumin in regulating estradiol synthesis in breast cancer cells. *Mol Cell Endocrinol* 1992;85:165–173.

118. Stewart AJ, Johnson MD, May FE, Westley BR. Role of insulin-like growth factors and the type I insulin-like growth factor receptor in the estrogen-stimulated proliferation of human breast cancer cells. *J Biol Chem* 1990;265: 21,172–21,178.

119. Stewart AJ, Westley BR, May FE. Modulation of the proliferative response of breast cancer cells to growth factors by oestrogen. *Br J Cancer* 1992;66:640–648.

120. van Landeghem AA, Poortman J, Nabuurs M, Thijssen JH. Endogenous concentration and subcellular distribution of estrogens in normal and malignant human breast tissue. *Cancer Res* 1985;45:2900–2906.

121. Yue W, Wang JP, Hamilton CJ, et al. *In situ* aromatization enhances breast tumor estradiol levels and celular proliferation. *Cancer Res* 1998;58:927–932.

122. Santen RJ, Martel J, Hoagland M, et al. Demonstration of aromatase activity and its regulation in breast tumor and benign breast fibroblasts. *Breast Cancer Res Treat* 1998;49(Suppl 1):S93–S99.

123. Brodie A, Long B, Lu Q. Aromatase expression in the human breast. *Breast Cancer Res Treat* 1998; 49:S85–S91.

124. Bonanni B, Johansson H, Gandini S, et al. Effect of low dose tamoxifen on the insulin-like growth factor system in healthy women. *Breast Cancer Res* Treat 2001;69:21–27.

125. Daughaday WH, Rotwein P. Insulin-like growth factors I and II. Peptide, messenger ribonucleic acid and gene structures, serum, and tissue concentrations. *Endocr Rev* 1989;10:68–91.

126. Guvakova MA, Surmacz E. Tamoxifen interferes with the insulin-like growth factor I receptor (IGF-IR) signaling pathway in breast cancer cells. *Cancer Res* 1997;57:2606–2610.

127. Resnik JL, Reichart DB, Huey K, et al. Elevated insulin-like growth factor I receptor autophosphorylation and kinase activity in human breast cancer. *Cancer Res* 1998;58:1159–1164.

128. Decensi A, Mariani L, Johansson H, et al. Role of plasma IGF-1 as a surrogate biomarker of second breast cancer in a prevention trial of fenretinide. *Proc Am Assoc Cancer Res* 2002;43:821:abstr. no. 4078.

129. The Endogenous Hormones and Breast Cancer Collaborative Group. Endogenous sex hormones and breast cancer in postmenopausal women: reanalysis of nine prospective studies. *J Natl Cancer Inst* 2002; 94:606–616.

130. Cummings SR, Duong T, Kenyon E, et al. Serum estradiol level and risk of breast cancer during treatment with raloxifene. *JAMA* 2002;287:216–220.

131. Gann P, Chatterton R, Vogelsong K, et al. Mitogenic growth factors in breast fluid obtained from healthy women: evaluation of biological and extraneous sources of variability. *Cancer Epidemiol Biomarkers Prev* 1997;6:421–428.

132. Paweletz CP, Trock B, Pennanen M, et al. Proteomic patterns of nipple aspirate fluids obtained by SELDI-TOF for new biomarkers to aid in diagnosis of breast cancer. *Dis Markers* 2001;17:301–307.

133. Elia M, Handpour S, Terranova P, et al. Marked variation in nipple aspirate fluid (NAF) estrogen concentration and NAF/serum ratios between ducts in high risk women. *Proc Am Assoc Cancer Res* 2002;43:820:abstr. no. 4072.

134. Shiau AK, Barstad D, Loria PM, et al. The structural basis of estrogen receptor/coactivator recognition and the antagonism of this interaction by tamoxifen. *Cell* 1998;95:927–937.

135. Starcevic SL, Elferink C, Novak RF. Progressive resistance to apoptosis in a cell lineage model of human proliferative breast disease. *J Natl Cancer Inst* 2001;93:776–782.

136. Harvey JM, Clark GM, Osborne CK, Allred DC. Estrogen receptor status by immunohistochemistry is superior to the ligand-binding assay for predicting response to adjuvant endocrine therapy in breast cancer. *J Clin Oncol* 1999;17:1474–1481.

137. Newby JC, Johnston SR, Smith IE, Dowsett M. Expression of epidermal growth factor receptor and c-erbB2 during the development of tamoxifen resistance in human breast cancer. *Clin Cancer Res* 1997;3:1643–1651.

138. Sun M, Paciga JE, Feldman RI, et al. Phosphatidylinositol-3-OH kinase (PI3K)/AKT2, activated in breast cancer, regulates and is induced by estrogen receptor alpha (ERalpha) via interaction between ERalpha and PI3K. *Cancer Res* 2001;61:5985–5991.

139. Tonetti DA, Jordan VC. Possible mechanisms in the emergence of tamoxifen-resistant breast cancer. *Anticancer Drugs* 1995;6:498–507.

140. Brzozowski AM, Pike AC, Dauter Z, et al. Molecular basis of agonism and antagonism in the oestrogen receptor. *Nature* 1997;389:753–758.

141. Takimoto GS, Graham JD, Jackson TA, et al. Tamoxifen resistant breast cancer: coregulators determine the direction of transcription by antagonist-occupied steroid receptors. *J Steroid Biochem Mol Biol* 1999;69:45–50.

142. Leygue E, Dotzlaw H, Watson PH, Murphy LC. Altered estrogen receptor alpha and beta messenger RNA expression during human breast tumorigenesis. *Cancer Res* 1998;58: 3197–3201.

143. Speirs V, Malone C, Walton DS, et al. Increased expression of estrogen receptor beta mRNA in tamoxifen-resistant breast cancer patients. *Cancer Res* 1999;59:5421–5424.

144. Fuqua SA, Wiltschke C, Zhang QX, et al. A hypersensitive estrogen receptor-α mutation in premalignant breast lesions. *Cancer Res* 2000;60:4026–4029.

145. Hopp TA, Hilsenbeck S, Mohsin S, et al. A hypersensitive estrogen receptor α protein in premalignant breast lesions. *Breast Cancer Res Treat* 2000;64:33:abstr.

146. Nass SJ, Herman JG, Gabrielson E, et al. Aberrant methylation of the estrogen receptor and E-cadherin 5' CpG islands increases with malignant progression in human breast cancer. *Cancer Res* 2000;60:4346–4348.

147. Lavinsky RM, Jepsen K, Heinzel T, et al. Diverse signaling pathways modulate nuclear receptor recruitment of N-CoR and SMRT complexes. *Proc Natl Acad Sci USA* 1998;95:2920–2925.

148. Petricoin EF, Ardekani AM, Hitt BA, et al. Use of proteomic patterns in serum to identify ovarian cancer. *Lancet* 2002;359:572–577.

149. Gillespie JW, Best CJ, Bichsel VE, et al. Evaluation of nonformalin tissue fixation for molecular profiling studies. *Am J Pathol* 2002;160:449–457.

150. Kelloff GJ, Boone CW, Steele VE, et al. Development of breast cancer chemopreventive drugs. *J Cell Biochem Suppl* 1993;17G:2–13.

151. Xu XC, Sneige N, Liu X, et al. Progressive decrease in nuclear retinoic acid receptor beta messenger RNA level during breast carcinogenesis. *Cancer Res* 1997;15:4992–4996.

152. Widschwendter M, Berger J, Daxenbichler G, et al. Loss of retinoic acid receptor B expression in breast cancer and normal adjacent tissue but not in normal tissue distinct from the cancer. *Cancer Res* 1997;57:4158–4161.

153. Huschtscha LI, Noble JR, Neumann AA, et al. Loss of p16INK4 expression of methylation is associated with lifespan extension of human mammary epithelial cells. *Cancer Res* 1998;58:3508–3512.

154. Gobbi H, DuPont WD, Simpson JF, et al. Transforming growth factor-B and breast cancer risk in women with mammary epithelial hyperplasia. *J Natl Cancer Inst* 1999;91:2096–2101.

155. Gross JM, Yee D. How does the estrogen receptor work? *Breast Cancer Res* 2002;4:62–64.

156. Gasco M, Shami S, Crook T. The p53 pathway in breast cancer. *Breast Cancer Res* 2002;4:70–76.

157. Miller WR, O'Neill J. The importance of local synthesis of estrogen within the breast. *Steroids* 1987;50:537–548.

158. Miller WR. Biology of aromatase inhibitors: pharmacology/endocrinology within the breast. *Endocr Relat Cancer* 1999;6:187–195.

159. Reed MJ, Coldham NG, Patel SR, et al. Interleukin-1 and interleukin-6 in breast cyst fluid: their role in regulating aromatase activity in breast cancer cells. *J Endocrinol* 1992; 132:R5–R8.

160. Singh A, Purohit A, Ghilchik MW, Reed MJ. The regulation of aromatase activity in breast fibroblasts: the role of interleukin-6 and prostaglandin E2. *Endocr Relat Cancer* 1999;6:139–147.

161. Wei J, Xu H, Davies JL, Hemmings GP. Increase of plasma IL-6 concentration with age in healthy subjects. *Life Sci* 1992;51:1953–1956.

162. Zhao Y, Nichols JE, Bulun SE, et al. Aromatase P450 gene expression in human adipose tissue. Role of a Jak/STAT path-

way in regulation of the adipose-specific promoter. *J Biol Chem* 1995;270:16,449–16,457.

163. Zhao Y, Agarwal V, Mendelson C, Simpson ER. Estrogen synthesis proximal to a breast tumor is stimulated by PGE2 via cyclic AMP; leading to activation of promoter II CYP 19 (aromatase) gene. *Endocrinology* 1996;137:5739–5742.

164. Rubin GL, Zhao Y, Kalus AM, Simpson ER. Peroxisome proliferator-activated receptor gamma ligands inhibit estrogen biosynthesis in human breast adipose tissue: possible implications for breast cancer therapy. *Cancer Res* 2000;60: 1604–1608.

165. Purohit A, Newman SP, Reed MJ. The role of cytokines in regulating estrogen synthesis: implications for the etiology of breast cancer. *Breast Cancer Res* 2002;4:65–69.

166. Khan SA, Rogers MA, Khurana KK, et al. Estrogen receptor expression in benign breast epithelium and breast cancer risk. *J Natl Cancer Inst* 1998;90:37–42.

167. Clarke RB, Howell A, Potten CS, Anderson E. Dissociation between steroid receptor expression and cell proliferation in the human breast. *Cancer Res* 1997;57:4987–4991.

168. Russo J, Ao X, Grill C, Russo IH. Pattern of distribution of cells positive for estrogen receptor alpha and progesterone receptor in relation to proliferating cells in the mammary gland. *Breast Cancer Res Treat* 1999;53:217–227.

169. Shoker BS, Jarvis C, Clarke RB, et al. Estrogen receptor-positive proliferating cells in the normal and precancerous breast. *Am J Pathol* 1999;155:1811–1815.

170. Stoica A, Saceda M, Doraiswamy VL, et al. Regulation of estrogen receptor-alpha gene expression by epidermal growth factor. *J Endocrinol* 2000;165:371–378.

171. Oh AS, Lorant LA, Holloway JN, et al. Hyperactivation of MAPK induces loss of ERalpha expression in breast cancer cells. *Mol Endocrinol* 2001;15:1344–1359.

172. Scambia G, Benedetti Panici P, Ferrandina G, et al. Cathepsin D and epidermal growth factor in human breast cyst fluid. *Br J Cancer* 1991;64:965–967.

173. Parham DM, Jankowski J. Transforming growth factor alpha in epithelial proliferative diseases of the breast. *Clin Pathol* 1992;45:513–516.

174. Walker RA, Dearing SJ. Expression of epidermal growth factor receptor mRNA and protein in primary breast cancers. *Breast Cancer Res Treat* 1999; 53:167–176.

175. Stark A, Hulka BS, Joens S, et al. Her-2/neu amplification in benign breast disease and the risk of subsequent breast cancer. *J Clin Oncol* 2000;8:267–274.

176. Stoica A, Saceda M, Fakhro A, et al. Role of insulin-like growth factor-I in regulating estrogen receptor-alpha gene expression. *J Cell Biochem* 2000;76:605–614.

177. Koukoulis GK, Vertanen I, Korhonen M, et al. Immunohistochemical localization of integrins in the normal, hyperlastic and neoplastic breast: correlations with their functions as receptors and cell adhesion molecules. *Am J Pathol* 1991;139:787–799.

178. Simpson JF, Page DL. Altered expression of a structural protein (fodrin) within epithelial proliferation disease of the breast. *Am J Pathol* 1992;141:285–289.

179. Fregene TA, Kellogg CM, Pienta KJ. Microvessel quantification as a measure of angiogenic activity in benign breast tissue lesions: a marker for precancerous disease? *Int J Oncol* 1994;4:1999–2002.

180. Shekhar MPV, Werdell J, Tait L. Interaction with endothelial cells is a prerequisite for branching ductal-alveola morphogenesis and hyperplasia of preneoplastic human breast

epithelial cells: regulation by estrogen. *Cancer Res* 2000;60: 439–449.

181. Roger P, Daures JP, Maudelonde T, et al. Dissociated overexpression of cathepsin D and estrogen receptor alpha in preinvasive mammary tumors. *Hum Pathol* 2000;31: 593–600.

182. Monteagudo C, Merino MJ, San-Juan J, et al. Immunohistochemical distribution of type IV collagenase in normal, benign, and malignant breast tissue. *Am J Pathol* 1990;136: 585–592.

183. Clemens JA, Bennett DR, Black LJ, Jones CD. Effects of a new antiestrogen, keoxifene (LY156758), on growth of carcinogen-induced mammary tumors and on LH and prolactin levels. *Life Sci* 1983;32:2869–2875.

184. Draper MW, Flowers DE, Huster WJ, et al. A controlled trial of raloxifene HCl:impact on bone turnover and serum lipid profile in healthy postmenopausal women. *J Bone Mineral Res* 1996;11:835–842.

185. Walsh BW, Kuller LH, Wild RA, et al. Effects of raloxifene on serum lipids and coagulation factors in healthy postmenopausal women. *JAMA* 1998;279:145–151.

186. Khovidhunkit W, Shoback DM. Clinical effects of raloxifene hydrochloride in women. *Ann Intern Med* 1999;130:431–439.

187. Cano A, Hermenegildo C. Endometrial effects of SERMs. *Hum Reprod Update* 2000;6:244–254.

188. Buzdar AU, Marcus C, Holmes F, et al. Phase II evaluation of LY156758 in metastatic breast cancer. *Oncology* 1988;45: 344–345.

189. Gradishar W, Glusman J, Lu Y, et al. Effects of high dose raloxifene in selected patients with advanced breast carcinoma. *Cancer* 2000;88:2047–2053.

190. Cummings SR, Eckert S, Krueger KA, et al. The effect of raloxifene on risk of breast cancer in postmenopausal women: results from the MORE Randomized Trial. Multiple outcomes of raloxifene evaluation. *JAMA* 1999;281:2189–2197.

191. Cauley JA, Norton L, Lippman ME, et al. Continued breast cancer risk reduction in postmenopausal women treated with raloxifene: 4-year results from the MORE trial. Multiple outcomes of raloxifene evaluation. *Breast Cancer Res Treat* 2001;65:125–134.

192. Davies GC, Huster WJ, Lu Y, et al. Adverse events reported by postmenopausal women in controlled trials with raloxifene. *Obstet Gynecol* 1999;93:558–565.

193. Dunn BK, Ford LG. From adjuvant therapy to breast cancer prevention: BCPT and STAR. *Breast J* 2001;7:144-157.

194. Sato M, Turner CH, Wang TY, et al. LY353381.HCl: a novel raloxifene analog with improved SERM potency and efficacy in vivo. *J Pharmacol Exp Ther* 1998;287:1–7.

195. Suh N, Glasebrook AL, Palkowitz AD, et al. Arzoxifene, a new selective estrogen receptor modulator for chemoprevention of experimental breast cancer. *Cancer Res* 2001;61: 8412–8415.

196. Munster PN, Buzdar A, Dhingra K, et al. Phase I study of a third-generation selective estrogen receptor modulator, LY353381.HCL, in metastatic breast cancer. *J Clin Oncol* 2001;19:2002–2009.

197. Schafer JM, Lee ES, Dardes RC, et al. Analysis of crossresistance of the selective estrogen receptor modulators arzoxifene (LY353381) and LY117018 in tamoxifen-stimulated breast cancer xenografts. *Clin Cancer Res* 2001;7: 2505–2512.

198. Wakeling AE, Bowler J. Steroidal pure antiestrogens. *J Endocrinol* 1987;112:R7–R10.

199. Osborne CK, Zhao H, Fuqua SA. Selective estrogen receptor modulators: structure, function, and clinical use. *J Clin Oncol* 2000;18:3172–3186.

200. Osborne CK, Coronado-Heinsohn EB, Hilsenbeck SG, et al. Comparison of the effects of a pure steroidal antiestrogen with those of tamoxifen in a model of human breast cancer. *J Natl Cancer Inst* 1995;87:746–750.

201. Howell A, DeFriend D, Robertson J, et al. Response to a specific antioestrogen (ICI 182780) in tamoxifen-resistant breast cancer. *Lancet* 1995;345:29–30.

202. Howell A, DeFriend DJ, Robertson JF, et al. Pharmacokinetics, pharmacological and anti-tumour effects of the specific anti-oestrogen ICI 182780 in women with advanced breast cancer. *Br J Cancer* 1996;74:300–308.

203. Wade GN, Blaustein JD, Gray JM, Meredith JM. ICI 182,780: a pure antiestrogen that affects behaviors and energy balance in rats without acting in the brain. *Am J Physiol* 1993;265:R1392–R1398.

204. Nabholtz JM, Buzdar A, Pollak M, et al. Anastrozole is superior to tamoxifen as first-line therapy for advanced breast cancer in postmenopausal women: results of a North American multicenter randomized trial. *J Clin Oncol* 2000;18:3758–3767.

205. Mouridsen H, Gershanovich M, Sun Y, et al. Superior efficacy of letrozole versus tamoxifen as first-line therapy for post-menopausal women with advanced breast cancer: results of a Phase III study of the International Letrozole Breast Cancer Group. *J Clin Oncol* 2001;19:2596–3606.

206. The ATAC Trialists' Group. Anastrozole alone or in combination with tamoxifen versus tamoxifen alone for adjuvant treatment of postmenopausal women with early breast cancer: first results of the ATAC randomised trial. *Lancet* 2002;359:2131–2139.

207. Tzukerman MT, Esty A, Santiso-Mere D, et al. Human estrogen receptor transactivational capacity is determined by both cellular and promoter context and mediated by two functionally distinct intramolecular regions. *Mol Endocrinol* 1994;8:21–30.

208. Tsai EM, Wang SC, Lee JN, Hung MC. Akt activation by estrogen in estrogen receptor-negative breast cancer cells. *Cancer Res* 2001;61:8390–8392.

209. Bonneterre J, Thurlimann B, Robertson JF, et al. Anastrozole versus tamoxifen as first-line therapy for advanced breast cancer in 668 postmenopausal women: results of the tamoxifen or arimidex randomized group efficacy and tolerability study. *J Clin Oncol* 2000;18:3748–3757.

210. Goss P, Grynpas M, Qi S, Hu H. The effects of exemestane on bone and lipids in the ovariectomized rat. *Breast Cancer Res Treat* 2001;69:224:abstr. no. 132.

211. Kirma N, Mandava UK, Tekmal RR. Use of letrozole as a chemopreventive agent in the aromatase overexpression transgenic mouse model. *Breast Cancer Res Treat* 2001;69:289: abstr.

212. Kirma NB, Gill K, Mandava U, Tekmal RR. The overexpression of colony-stimulating factor 1 and/or its receptor c-fms leads to mammary hyperplasia in transgenic mice. *Proc Am Assoc Cancer Res* 2002;43:187:abstr. no. 940.

213. Bevilacqua G, Silingardi V, Marchetti P. Exemestane for the prevention of breast cancer in postmenopausal unaffected carriers of BRCA1/2 mutations—aromasin prevention study (ApreS). *Breast Cancer Res Treat* 2001;69:226 abstr.

214. Brodie A, Lu Q, Liu Y, et al. Preclinical studies using the intratumoral aromatase model for postmenopausal breast cancer. *Oncology (Huntingt)* 1998;12(3 Suppl 5):36–40.

215. Long BJ, Jelovac D, Thiantanawat A, Brodie AM. The effect of alternating letrozole and tamoxifen in comparison to sequential treatment with each drug alone or in combination. *Breast Cancer Res Treat* 2001;69:287:abstr. no. 444.

216. Ingle JN, Suman VJ, Johnson PA, et al. Evaluation of tamoxifen plus letrozole with assessment of pharmacokinetic interaction in postmenopausal women with metastatic breast cancer. *Clin Cancer Res* 1999;5:1642–1649.

217. Purohit A, Hejaz HA, Woo LW, et al. Recent advances in the development of steroid sulphatase inhibitors. *J Steroid Biochem Mol Biol* 1999;69:227–238.

218. Pasqualini JR. Recent developments of the biological role of progestins in human breast cancer. *J Woman's Cancer* 2000;2:135–143.

219. Prost-Avallet O, Oursin J, Adessi GL. In vitro effect of synthetic progestogens on estrone sulfatase activity in human breast carcinoma. *J Steroid Biochem Mol Biol* 1991;39:967–973.

220. Santner SJ, Santen RJ. Inhibition of estrone sulfatase and 17 beta-hydroxysteroid dehydrogenase by antiestrogens. *J Steroid Biochem Mol Biol* 1993;45:383–390.

221. Gompel A, Kandouz M, Siromachkova M, et al. The effect of tibolone on proliferation, differentiation and apoptosis in normal breast cells. *Gynecol Endocrinol* 1999;1:77–79.

222. Gompel A, Siromachkova M, Lombet A, et al. Tibolone actions on normal and breast cancer cells. *Eur J Cancer* 2000;36: S76–S77.

223. Dobson R, Chan K, Knox WR, et al. Tibolone does not stimulate epithelial proliferation in the breast. *Breast Cancer Res Treat* 2001;69:292:abstr. no. 461.

224. Deckers GH, Verheul HAM, van Aalst GBT, et al. Tibolone and 5alpha-dihydrotestosterone alone or in combination with an antiandrogen in a rat breast tumour model. *Eur J Cancer* 2002;38: 443-448.

225. Kloosterboer HJ. Tibolone: a steroid with a tissue-specific mode of action. *J Steroid Biochem Mol Biol* 2001;76:231–238.

226. Spicer DV, Pike MC. Future possibilities in the prevention of breast cancer. Luteinizing hormone-releasing hormone agonists. *Breast Cancer Res* 2000;2:264–267.

227. Weitzel JN, Pike MC, Daniels, AM, et al. Safety of a gonadotropin-releasing hormone agonist (GnRHA)-based hormonal chemoprevention regimen for young women at high genetic risk for breast cancer. *Breast Cancer Res Treat* 2000;64:48: abstr. no. 150.

228. Gram IT, Ursin G, Spicer DV, Pike MC. Reversal of gonadotropin-releasing hormone agonist induced reductions in mammographic densities on stopping treatment. *Cancer Epidemiol Biomarkers Prev* 2001;10:1117–1120.

229. Bischoff ED, Heyman RA, Lamph WW. Effect of retinoid X receptor-selective ligand LGD1069 on mammary carcinoma after tamoxifen failure. *J Natl Cancer Inst* 1999;91:2118–2123.

230. Mehta RG, Williamson E, Patel MK, Koeffler HP. A ligand of peroxisome proliferator-activated receptor γ, retinoids and prevention of preneoplastic mammary lesions. *J Natl Cancer Inst* 2000;92:418–423.

231. Brown PH, Lippman SM. Chemoprevention of breast cancer. *Breast Cancer Res Treat* 2000;62:1–17.

232. van der Leede BJ, Folkers GE, van den Brink CE, et al. Retinoic acid receptor alpha 1 isoform is induced by estradiol and confers retinoic acid sensitivity in human breast cancer cells. *Mol Cell Endocrinol* 1995;109:77–86.

233. Wu K, Kim HT, Rodriquez JL, et al. 9-*cis*-Retinoic acid suppresses mammary tumorigenesis in C3(1)-simian virus 40 T antigen-transgenic mice. *Clin Cancer Res* 2000;6: 3696–3704.

234. Wu K, Kim HT, Rodriquez JL, et al. Suppression of mammary tumorigenesis in transgenic mice by the RXR-selective retinoid, LGD1069. *Cancer Epidemiol Biomarkers Prev* 2002;11:467–474.

235. Veronesi U, DePalo G, Marubini E, et al. Randomized trial of fenretinide to prevent second breast malignancy in women with early breast cancer. *J Natl Cancer Inst* 1999;91:1847–1856.

236. Gottardis MM, Bischoff ED, Shirley MA, et al. Chemoprevention of mammary carcinoma by LGD1069 (Targretin): an RXR-selective ligand. *Cancer Res* 1996;56:5566–5570.

237. Manni A, Grove R, Kunselman S, Aldaz M. Involvement of the polyamine pathway in breast cancer progression. *Cancer Lett* 1995;92:49–57.

238. Klohs WD, Fry DW, Kraker AJ. Inhibitors of tyrosine kinase. *Curr Opin Oncol* 1997;9:562–568.

239. Meyskens FL, Gerner EW. Development of difluoromethylornithine (DFMO) as a chemoprevention agent. *Clin Cancer Res* 1999;5:945–951.

240. Steele VE, Holmes CA, Hawk ET, et al. Lipoxygenase inhibitors as potential cancer chemopreventives. *Cancer Epidemiol Biomarkers Prev* 1999;8:467–483.

241. Koki AT, Leahy KM, Masferrer JL. Potential utility of COX-2 inhibitors in chemoprevention and chemotherapy. *Expert Opin Invest Drugs* 1999;8:1623–1638.

242. Leveque J, Foucher F, Havouis R, et al. Benefits of complete polyamine deprivation in hormone responsive and hormone resistant MCF-7 human breast adenocarcinoma in vivo. *Anticancer Res* 2000;20:97–101.

243. Marks PA, Richon JM, Rifkind RA. Histone deacetylase inhibitors: inducers of differentiation or apoptosis of transformed cells. *J Natl Cancer Inst* 2000;92:1210–1216.

244. Nelson AR, Fingleton B, Rothenberg ML, Matrisian LM. Matrix metalloproteinases: biologic activity and clinical implications. *J Clin Oncol* 2000;18:1135–1149.

245. Cherrington JM, Strawn LM, Shawver LK. New paradigms for the treatment of cancer: the role of anti-angiogenesis agents. *Adv Cancer Res* 2000;79:1–38.

246. Harris RE, Alshafie GA, Hussen AI, Seibert K. Chemoprevention of breast cancer in rats by celecoxib, a cyclooxygenase 2 inhibitor. *Cancer Res* 2000;60:2101–2103.

247. Davis T, Kennedy C, Chiew YE, et al. Histone deacetylase inhibitors decrease proliferation and modulate cell cycle gene expression in normal mammary epithelial cells. *Clin Cancer Res* 2000;6:4334–4342.

248. Duffy MJ, Maguire TM, Hill A, et al. Metalloproteinases: role in breast carcinogenesis, invasion and metastasis. *Breast Cancer Res* 2000;2:252–257.

249. Baselga J. Targeting the epidermal growth factor receptor: a clinical reality. *J Clin Oncol* 2001;19:41S–44S.

250. Chan KC, Knox WF, Gandhi A, et al. Blockade of growth factor receptors in ductal carcinoma *in situ* inhibits epithelial proliferation. *Br J Surg* 2001;88:412–418.

251. Chan KC, Knox WF, Gee JM, et al. Effect of epidermal growth factor receptor tyrosine kinase inhibition on epithelial proliferation in normal and premalignant breast. *Cancer Res* 2002;62:122–128.

252. Munster PN, Troso-Sandoval T, Rosen N, et al. The histone deacetylase inhibitor suberoylanilide hydroxamic acid induces differentiation of human breast cancer cells. *Cancer Res* 2001;61:8492–8497.

253. Paridaens R, Uges DR, Barbet N, et al. A Phase I study of a new polyamine biosynthesis inhibitor, SAM486A, in cancer patients with solid tumours. *Br J Cancer* 2000;83: 594–601.

254. Soslow RA, Dannenberg AJ, Rush D, et al. COX-2 is expressed in human pulmonary, colonic and mammary tumors. *Cancer* 2000;89:2637–2645.

255. Ristimaki A, Sivula A, Lundin J, et al. Prognostic significance of elevated cyclooxygenase-2 expression in breast cancer. *Cancer Res* 2002;62:632–635.

256. Hwang D, Scollard D, Byrne J, Levine E. Expression of cyclo-oxygenase-1 and cyclo-oxygenase-2 in human breast cancer. *J Natl Cancer Inst* 1998;90:455–460.

257. Simon LS, Lanza FL, Lipsky PE, et al. Preliminary study of the safety and efficacy of SC 58635, a novel cycloogenase 2 inhibitor. *Arthritis Rheum* 1998;41:1591–1602.

258. Silverstein FE, Faich G, Goldstein JL, et al. Gastrointestinal toxicity with celecoxib vs nonsteroidal anti-inflammatory drugs for osteoarthritis and rheumatoid arthritis: the CLASS study: a randomized controlled trial. *JAMA* 2000;284: 1247–1255.

259. Feldman M, McMahon AT. Do cyclooxygenase-2 inhibitors provide benefits similar to those of traditional nonsteroidal anti-inflammatory drugs, with less gastrointestinal toxicity? *Ann Intern Med* 2000;132:134–143.

260. Steinbach G, Lynch PM, Phillips RK, et al. The effect of celecoxib, a cyclooxygenase-2 inhibitor, in familial adenomatous polyposis. *N Engl J Med* 2000;342:1946–1952.

261. Shalinsky DR, Shetty B, Pithavola Y, et al. A potent and selective matrix metalloproteinase inhibitor—preclinical and clinical development for oncology. In *Cancer Drug Discovery and Development: Matrix Metalloproteinases in Cancer Therapy*. Clendenin NJ, Appelt K, eds. Humana Press Inc., Totowa, NJ, 2000; pp.143–173.

262. Albanell J, Rojo F, Averbuch S, et al. Pharmacodynamic studies of the epidermal growth factor receptor inhibitor ZD1839 in skin from cancer patients: histopathologic and molecular consequences of receptor inhibition. *J Clin Oncol* 2001;20:110–124.

263. Akiyama T, Ishida J, Nakagawa S, et al. Genistein, a specific inhibitor of tyrosine-specific protein kinases. *J Biol Chem* 1987;262:5592–5595.

264. Fotsis T, Pepper M, Adlercreutz H, et al. Genistein, a dietary-derived inhibitor of in vitro angiogenesis. *Proc Natl Acad Sci USA* 1993;90:2690–2694.

265. Duncan AM, Merz BE, Xu X, et al. Soy isoflavones exert modest hormonal effects in premenopausal women. *J Clin Endocrinol Metab* 1999;84:192–197.

266. Lu LJ, Anderson KE, Grady JJ, et al. Decreased ovarian hormones during a soya diet: implications for breast cancer prevention. *Cancer Res* 2000;60:4112–4121.

267. Galvez AF, Chen N, Macasieb J, de Lumen BO. Chemopreventive property of a soybean peptide (lunasin) that binds to deacetylated histones and inhibits acetylation. *Cancer Res* 2001;61:7473–7478.

268. Thompson HJ, Jiang C, Lu J, et al. Sulfone metabolite of sulindac inhibits mammary carcinogenesis. *Cancer Res* 1997;57:267–271.

269. Russo IH, Russo J. Hormonal approach to breast cancer prevention. *J Cell Biochem* 2000;77(S34):1–6.

270. Ferguson AT, Lapidus RG, Baylin SB, Davidson NE. Demethylation of the estrogen receptor gene in estrogen receptor-negative breast cancer cells can reactivate estro-

gen receptor gene expression. *Cancer Res* 1995;55: 2279–2283.

271. Anzano MA, Peer CW, Smith JM, et al. Chemoprevention of mammary carcinogenesis in the rat: combined use of raloxifene and 9-CIS-retinoic acid. *J Natl Cancer Inst* 1996;88:123–125.

272. Love-Schimenti CD, Gibson DF, Ratnam AV, Bikle DD. Antiestrogen potentiation of antiproliferative effects of vitamin D_3 analogues in breast cancer cells. *Cancer Res* 1996;56:2789–2794.

273. Conley B, O'Shaughnessy J, Prindiville S, et al. Pilot trial of the safety, tolerability, and retinoid levels of *N*-(4-hydroxyphenyl) retinamide in combination with tamoxifen in patients at high risk for developing invasive breast cancer. *J Clin Oncol* 2000;18:275–283.

274. Wang Q, Lee D, Sysounthone V, et al. 1,25-Dihydroxyvitamin D_3 and retinoic acid analogues induce differentiation in breast cancer cells with function- and cell-specific additive effects. *Breast Cancer Res Treat* 2001;67:157–168.

275. Brueggemeier RW, Quinn AL, Parrett ML, et al. Correlation of aromatase and cyclooxygenase gene expression in human breast cancer specimens. *Cancer Lett* 1999;140:27–35.

276. Sporn MB. Retinoids and demethylating agents—looking for partners. *J Natl Cancer Inst* 2000;92:780–781.

277. Pike MC, Spicer DV, Dahmoush L, Press MF. Estrogens, progestins, normal breast cell proliferation, and breast cancer risk. *Epidemiol Rev* 1993;15:17–35.

278. Boland GP, McKeown A, Chan KC, et al. Oestrogen withdrawal reduces cell proliferation in oestrogen receptor (ER) positive ductal carcinoma *in situ* (DCIS). *Breast Cancer Res Treat* 2001;69:251: abstr. no. 257.

279. Grizzle WE, Meyers RB, Oelschlager DK. Prognostic biomarkers in breast cancer: factors affecting immunohistochemical evaluation. *Breast* J 1995;1:243–250.

280. Grizzle WE, Myers RB, Manne U, et al. Factors affecting immunohistochemical evaluation of biomarker expression in neoplasia. In *John Walker's Methods in Molecular Medicine— Tumor Marker Protocols.* Hanausek M, Walaszek Z, eds. Humana Press, Inc., Totowa, NJ; 1998; pp.161–179.

281. Urban D, Myers R, Manne U, et al. Evaluation of biomarker modulation by fenretinide in prostate cancer patients. *Eur J Urol* 1999;35:429–438.

282. Singletary E, Lieberman R, Atkinson N, et al. Novel translational model for breast cancer chemoprevention study: accrual to a presurgical intervention with tamoxifen and *N*-(4-hydroxyphenyl) retinamide. *Cancer Epidemiol Biomarkers Prev* 2000;9:1087–1090.

283. Singletary SE, Atkinson EN, Hoque A, et al. Phase II clinical trial of *N*-(4-hydroxyphenyl)retinamide and tamoxifen administration before definitive surgery for breast neoplasia. *Clin Cancer Res* 2002;8:2835–2842.

284. Zalles C, Kimler BF, Kamel S, et al. Cytologic patterns in random aspirates from women at high and low risk for breast cancer. *Breast J* 1995;1:343–349.

285. Pasqualini JR, Cortes-Prieto J, Chetrite G, et al. Concentrations of estrone, estradiol and their sulfates, and evaluation of sulfatase and aromatase activities in patients with breast fibroadenoma. *Int J Cancer* 1997;70:639–643.

286. Final Version: the uniform approach to breast fine-needle aspiration biopsy. *Breast J* 1997;3:149–168.

287. Bacus JW, Boone CW, Bacus JV, et al. Image morphometric nuclear grading of intraepithelial neoplastic lesions with applications to cancer chemoprevention trials. *Cancer Epidemiol Biomarkers Prev* 1999;8:1087–1094.

288. Keshgegian AA, Cnaan A. Proliferation markers in breast carcinoma. Mitotic figure count, S-phase fraction, proliferating cell nuclear antigen, Ki-67 and MIB-1. *Am J Clin Pathol* 1995;104:42–49.

289. Biesterfeld S, Kluppel D, Koch R. Rapid and prognostically valid quantification of immunohistochemical reactions by immunohistometry of the most positive tumour focus. A prospective follow-up study on breast cancer using antibodies against MIB-1, PCNA, ER, and PR. *J Pathol* 1998;185: 25–31.

290. Fisher B, Dignam J, Wolmark N, et al. Tamoxifen in treatment of intraductal breast cancer: National Surgical Adjuvant Breast and Bowel Project B-24 randomised controlled trial. *Lancet* 1999;353:1993–2000.

18 Ductal Lavage

Its Role in Breast Cancer Risk Assessment and Risk Reduction

Joyce O'Shaughnessy, MD and Andrea Decensi, MD

CONTENTS

1. BREAST INTRAEPITHELIAL NEOPLASIA

One of the best established risk factors of developing invasive breast cancer is the presence of biopsy-proven atypical ductal or lobular hyperplasia. Atypical hyperplasia is a form of breast intraepithelial neoplasia (IEN) that, with invasive breast cancer, features overexpression of the estrogen receptor (ER) and coexpression of ER with receptor tyrosine kinase overexpression, e.g., epidermal growth factor receptor (EGFR) and insulin-like growth factor receptor (IGFR), as well as loss of heterozygosity in multiple chromosomal locations *(1–3)*. Within atypical hyperplasia lesions, the balance of proliferation and apoptosis is disrupted; atypical cells ranging from mildly atypical to frankly dysplastic in their appearance accumulate within the terminal duct lobular unit.

Autopsy studies have suggested that atypical hyperplasia may be an obligate precursor of invasive breast cancer. In one study of 110 women ages 20 to 54 who died of nonbreast-cancer-related causes in Denmark, 7% of the women had evidence of breast atypical hyperplasia, 18% *in situ*, noninvasive breast cancer, and 2% frank invasive breast cancer *(4)*. Ninety-five percent (95%) of women whose breasts contained *in situ* or invasive carcinoma had synchronous atypical hyperplasia, compared with only 9% of women who did not have *in situ* or invasive carcinoma (Fig. 1).

Based on the age-related peak of clinical breast cancer incidence in Denmark, it was hypothesized that IEN precedes invasive breast cancer incidence by 15–20 yr.

Several long-term prospective studies have demonstrated a fivefold increased relative risk of developing invasive breast cancer in women with biopsy-proven atypical hyperplasia *(5)*. This risk increases to 11-fold if the woman with atypical hyperplasia also has a first-degree relative with breast cancer. Biopsy-proven atypical hyperplasia is associated with a 0.5 to 1% risk per yr of developing invasive breast cancer *(6)*. In addition, a finding of atypical hyperplasia on breast biopsy approximately doubles a woman's 5-yr and lifetime Gail risk for developing invasive breast cancer.

Atypical ductal and lobular hyperplasia are generally clinically silent lesions. Only approx 10–12% of atypical hyperplasia lesions are detectable as mammographic or palpable abnormalities. In the United States, (US) approx 60,000 breast biopsies per year contain atypical hyperplasia, generally found incidentally, while 360,000 biopsies reveal epithelial hyperplasia without atypia *(7)*.

Two large studies have prospectively evaluated the predictive value of cytologically identified atypical breast epithelial cells. Fabian et al. have demonstrated a 21% incidence of occult hyperplasia with atypia on random periareolar breast fine-needle aspiration (FNA) in high-risk women *(8)*. Women with a 5-yr Gail

From: Cancer Chemoprevention, Volume 2: Strategies for Cancer Chemoprevention
Edited by: G. J. Kelloff, E. T. Hawk, and C. C. Sigman © Humana Press Inc., Totowa, NJ

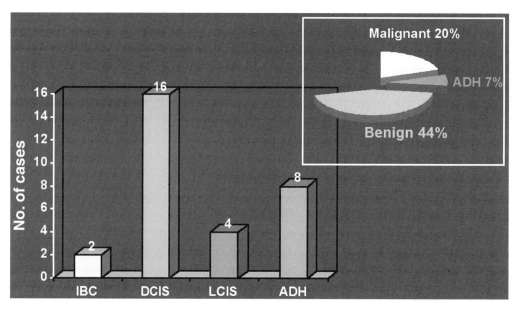

Fig. 1. Prevalence of intraepithelial neoplasia in an autopsy series of 110 asymptomatic women aged 20–54 (median 30 yr) *(4)*.

risk >2% had an approx 3% per yr risk of developing breast cancer over the 4-yr following FNA-detected hyperplasia with atypia. This prospective study in high-risk women demonstrated that finding cytologically atypical breast epithelial cells was an important risk marker for breast cancer that was independent of a woman's 5-yr Gail risk in a multivariate analysis.

A second longitudinal prospective study by Wrensch et al. has also shown that women with epithelial cell atypia in their nipple aspirate fluid (NAF) have a fivefold elevated risk of developing breast cancer compared to women without evidence of cellular atypia *(9,10)*. Both the Fabian and Wrensch studies showed that cytologically defined atypia elevates invasive breast cancer risk to the same extent as that demonstrated by Dupont and Page in their studies of pathologically defined atypical hyperplasia. Table 1 summarizes the risk ratio of developing breast cancer in women with cellular atypia as detected by random FNA or NAF in prospective studies compared with biopsy-proven atypical ductal hyperplasia.

2. BREAST IEN: A NOVEL TREATMENT ENDPOINT

Atypical hyperplasia incidence in high-risk women is an attractive endpoint for breast cancer risk reduction clinical trials that aim to test the effectiveness of new treatment agents. This is because atypical hyperplasia appears to be a near-obligate precursor of invasive breast cancer, has a defined relationship with elevated breast cancer risk, and clearly identifies a subgroup of women

who benefit from treatment with antiestrogen therapy. The National Surgical Adjuvant Breast Project (NSABP) P1 Breast Cancer Prevention Trial demonstrated an 86% reduction in invasive breast cancer risk in women with biopsy-proven atypical hyperplasia treated with 5-yr of tamoxifen. Treatment reduced the incidence of biopsy-proven atypical hyperplasia by about 25%, and reduced the overall need for breast biopsies by 22% compared with placebo in high-risk women in this study *(11)*. These data are the first to show that 5-yr of tamoxifen treatment can reduce atypical hyperplasia incidence in high-risk women. It is especially important that this reduction in atypical hyperplasia incidence occurred in conjunction with the documented 49% reduction in invasive breast cancer incidence with tamoxifen treatment *(6)*. The different magnitude of risk reduction might be explained by the lag time to elicit a true preventive effect by tamoxifen as opposed to the therapeutic effect on occult invasive cancer that was observed as early as after 1-yr of intervention with the P1 trial *(6)*.

As atypical hyperplasia doubles a woman's 5-yr and lifetime risk of developing invasive breast cancer, and this risk can be decreased substantially with tamoxifen treatment, it is of high clinical interest to identify women who have occult atypical ductal or lobular hyperplasia in order to define a group for whom the benefits of 5-yr of tamoxifen treatment likely outweigh the risks.

Successful eradication of atypical hyperplasia by an effective breast IEN treatment agent would be expected to confer clinical benefit because atypical hyperplasia is

Table 1
Atypical Cells on Cytology Confer Similar Increase
in Risk to ADH on Biopsy

Wrensch *(9,10)*	4.9 RR with atypia on NAF
Fabian *(8)*	5.0 RR with atypia on FNA
Dupont, Page *(5)*	3–5.3 RR with ADH on biopsy

RR; relative risk; NAF; nipple aspirate fluid; FNA; fine-needle aspiration. ADH; atypical ductal hypzerplasia.

an established risk marker that has a well-defined relationship to invasive breast cancer. A Phase II clinical trial that enrolled approximately 300 women with documented cytological atypia on FNA or ductal lavage would have sufficient statistical power to detect a 50% reduction in incidence of hyperplasia with atypia after administration of an effective treatment agent. Such a clinical trial design, if successful, could considerably accelerate the development of new agents to treat breast precancer, because it would involve hundreds and not thousands of high-risk women and could be conducted over 2 to 3 yr. This clinical trial design is currently being utilized to test the effectiveness of 6 to 12 mo of arzoxifene, a novel selective ER modulator (SERM), in reducing incidence of hyperplasia with atypia compared to placebo in high-risk women who have random, peri-areolar FNA-detected epithelial hyperplasia with or without atypia. It is not yet known whether 6 to 12 mo of treatment with an effective SERM or any other breast precancer treatment agent can eradicate breast atypical hyperplasia in a proportion of high-risk women. The use of placebo as a control arm in such a trial would also provide essential information on the reproducibility and variability of atypia within subjects over time.

3. CLINICAL DEVELOPMENT OF DUCTAL LAVAGE

The feasibility of reliably identifying high-risk women who have occult atypical hyperplasia has not been established using noninvasive means. Although the volume of dense breast tissue on mammography correlates with increased breast cancer risk, it has not been established that dense breast tissue represents proliferative breast disease, either epithelial hyperplasia or atypical hyperplasia. The ability to use atypical hyperplasia incidence as a definitive endpoint in breast precancer treatment trials has been significantly hampered by our current inability to measure the extent of atypical hyperplasia in the breast and to follow it reliably and longitudinally. To date, no published data

demonstrate the feasibility of reproducibly detecting atypical hyperplasia on serial breast biopsies, FNAs, or NAFs.

Ductal lavage is a new diagnostic procedure that holds promise as a method of collecting breast ductal epithelial cells for cytologic analysis in a reproducible fashion. Breast ductal lavage involves using a handheld suction device to perform nipple suction aspiration, followed by cannulation of fluid-yielding ducts with a microcatheter to lavage the ducts with normal saline. The effluent from the duct is collected with breast massage, which returns the saline back into the microcatheter, where it is collected for cytologic analysis. Figure 2 illustrates the main phases of the clinical procedure.

Dooley and colleagues recently summarized their study, which was conducted in 507 high-risk women and compared the utility of ductal lavage and NAF in detecting abnormal breast epithelial cells *(12)*. Results of this study are summarized in Table 2. Fifty-seven percent (57%) of high-risk women had a personal history of breast cancer and were not on tamoxifen, and 39% had a 5-yr Gail risk for breast cancer of 1.7% or above. In this study, 84% of the high-risk women yielded NAF and more than 90% of women with NAF successfully underwent ductal lavage. Both NAF and ductal lavage samples were successfully collected from 383 women. Adequate samples for diagnosis (at least 10 breast epithelial cells collected) were obtained from 27% of women with NAF and from 78% of women with ductal lavage. The ductal lavage samples were much more cellular, having a median of 13,500 epithelial cells per duct compared with 120 epithelial cells per breast with NAF. An example of the cytological appearance of the two methods is illustrated in Fig. 3. Notably, 23% of the women were found to have atypical breast epithelial cells with ductal lavage compared with 9% with NAF. This study showed that ductal lavage collected adequate epithelial cells for cytologic analysis from substantially more women than was possible with NAF and that ductal lavage was 3.2 times more likely to identify women who had atypical cells compared with NAF.

The tolerability of the procedure was excellent with the use of a topical anesthetic cream. The women reported their level of discomfort with these procedures using a 100-mm visual analog scale with 0 representing "no pain" and 100 mm representing "most severe pain." The median pain score with nipple aspiration was 8 mm and with ductal lavage was 24 mm. Twenty-nine percent (29%) of women reported that ductal lavage was more comfortable than mammography, 20% said it was as comfortable, and 51% said it was less comfortable.

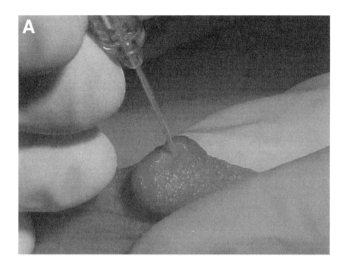

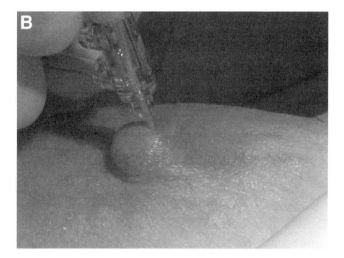

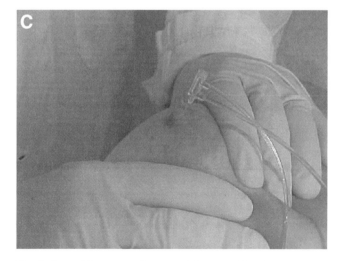

Fig. 2. Ductal lavage, main steps. **(A)** The guidewire catheter is introduced into the desired duct. **(B)** After gradual advancement, the catheter is completely seated in the duct. **(C)** After gentle saline infusion of 1–2 cc, the breast is massaged toward the nipple for 30 s to ensure maximum cell recovery.

Table 2
Cytological Findings Comparing Nipple Aspirate Fluid and Ductal Lavage *(12)*

Cytologic Diagnosis	NAF	Ductal Lavage
Number of women	417	383
ICMD[a]	306 (73%)	84 (22%)
Benign	70 (17%)	207 (54%)
Atypical (mild)	27 (6%)	66 (17%)
Atypical (marked)	12 (3%)	24 (6%)
Malignant	2 (<1%)	2 (<1%)
Median number epithelial cells	120/breast	13,500/duct

[a]ICMD: Insufficient cellular material for diagnosis, defined as fewer than 10 epithelial cells.

Subsequent unpublished data collected at the European Institute of Oncology among 220 at-risk women have confirmed the incidence of atypical cell specimens at 28%. A total of 5% of the procedures was unsuccessful and another 14% was inadequate for a cytological diagnosis. Atypical specimens tend to exhibit a higher expression of Ki67 compared with normal samples, indicating that additional biomarkers of proliferation can be measured to further refine risk and assess the activity of preventive intervention. A total of 13 adverse events occurred, all of mild grade, including hematoma and ecchymosis. These results underscore the feasibility and safety of the procedure, which can successfully be implemented in a clinical center after appropriate training. It is well established that the presence of atypical epithelial cells defined on histology or cytology significantly elevates a woman's risk for developing breast cancer. However, only a subset of women with atypical epithelial cells, approx 20–30% depending as well on family history, will develop breast cancer *(5,8,10,17)*.

Ductal lavage specimens are prepared for cytologic interpretation in a similar fashion to that for breast FNAs and NAF. While millipore filtration or the cytospin technique may be utilized, Thin Prep™ is the method most commonly used at present, along with Papanicolaou staining. A web-based tutorial has been prepared with representative cell images from each of the cytology diagnostic categories to facilitate the training of pathologists in interpreting ductal lavage specimens. The criteria used for cytologic interpretation of ductal lavage specimens are based on the 1997 National Cancer Institute (NCI) Consensus Criteria for FNA Cytology *(13)*. To date, more than 250 pathologists have taken the web-based certification study program.

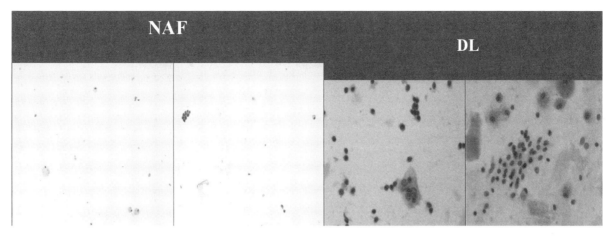

Fig. 3. An example of cytological smears comparing nipple aspirate fluid (**NAF**) with ductal lavage (**DL**) from the same subjects.

Certification as a ductal lavage cytologist requires central cytology review of a specified number of ductal lavage samples at the University of California, San Francisco in order to assure consistency and quality in cytologic interpretations. To date, an 81% level of concordance in interpretation between the central reference and local pathology laboratories has been found *(14)*.

One of the potential advantages of ductal lavage is the ability to map the lavaged duct on a grid and to photograph the position of the duct orifice to enable repeated sampling. Studies have been initiated to assess the reproducibility of cytology findings with serial lavage of the same duct, and are important to the clinical development of this diagnostic tool. In the comparative study of ductal lavage and NAF, only ducts that yielded NAF were cannulated for ductal lavage. Fluid-yielding ducts were targeted because of ease in locating these ducts for cannulation, and because the prospective study by Wrensch et al. had demonstrated that women who produced NAF were at higher risk for developing breast cancer than those who did not. The current working hypothesis is that breast ducts that contain proliferating abnormal ductal epithelial cells produce more fluid than ducts with normal ductal epithelium. Studies are underway to perform ductal lavage on non-fluid-yielding ducts to assess their incidence of atypia.

4. INCORPORATING DUCTAL LAVAGE INTO CLINICAL MANAGEMENT OF HIGH-RISK WOMEN

Figure 4 illustrates the way in which ductal lavage findings can be used for clinical applications. These management pathways represent the majority opinion of a group of breast cancer risk assessment experts who used ductal lavage in clinical trials and in the clinical

management of high-risk women *(15)*. Of note is the recommendation that high-risk women in whom ductal lavage reveals atypical cells should more strongly consider undergoing 5 yr of tamoxifen treatment or participation in the Study of Tamoxifen and Raloxifene (STAR) trial. At present, the greatest clinical utility of ductal lavage is to identify a subset of women at very high risk for developing breast cancer who are most likely to benefit from antiestrogen treatment. Although the Gail risk model has been validated and proven accurate in estimating a woman's high risk of developing breast cancer, this tool has been shown to have modest discriminatory utility for any particular woman *(16)*. In addition, the Gail risk model can underestimate breast cancer risk in women with a personal history of breast cancer, lobular carcinoma *in situ*, or ductal carcinoma *in situ*, and may underestimate risk in women with multiple second-degree relatives, or a family history of ovarian cancer or early-onset breast cancer. Therefore, additional risk assessment tools are needed to provide individualized risk stratification information.

In spite of the proven effectiveness of tamoxifen in substantially reducing invasive breast cancer in high-risk women, the vast majority of high-risk women decline tamoxifen therapy due to concerns about side effects. From a clinical risk management standpoint, the promise of ductal lavage stems from its potential to provide individual information to high-risk women about the presence or absence of breast epithelial cell atypia to aid them in making a decision about undergoing 5 yr of antiestrogen therapy. For example, a 55-yr-old woman with a 2.0% 5-yr and 13% lifetime Gail risk of developing invasive breast cancer would see that risk approximately double after a finding of atypical

Ductal Lavage Algorithm

Benign	➡	Repeat ductal lavage in 1–3 yr
Mildly Atypical	➡	Strongly consider tamoxifen or prevention trial unless contraindicated Repeat ductal lavage in 6–12 mo to confirm findings
Markedly Atypical	➡	Repeat ductal lavage to confirm findings Additional imaging (ductogram, MRI, ductoscopy) Biopsy if abnormality found Strongly consider tamoxifen or prevention trial unless contraindicated.
Malignant	➡	Repeat ductal lavage to confirm findings Additional imaging (ductogram, MRI, ductoscopy) Surgical excision or exploration if warranted Strongly consider tamoxifen or prevention unless contraindicated
ICMD	➡	Repeat lavage at next opportunity. If again ICMD and good fluid exchange observed, f/u in 1–3 yr

Fig. 4. Management pathway for incorporating ductal lavage into clinical care of high-risk women.

hyperplasia *(17)*. The increased relative risk for breast cancer, defined on the basis of cytologic atypia on FNA and NAF as well as a histologic diagnosis of atypical hyperplasia, strongly suggests that a finding of cytologic atypia on ductal lavage has the same clinical implications as a breast biopsy showing atypical hyperplasia. Such a finding places this woman into a higher-risk category and may influence her decision about risk reduction therapy. These assumptions are being explored in a large ongoing prospective Ductal Lavage Outcomes Tracking Study. Current information suggests that ductal lavage may substantially enable clinicians to better refine breast cancer risk management in an individual subject.

The sensitivity of ductal lavage in identifying cytologically atypical epithelial cells in high-risk women is not known. It is of interest that the 23% incidence of atypical hyperplasia in the ductal lavage study by Dooley et al. is very similar to the 21% incidence of FNA-detected cytologic atypia described by Fabian and colleagues in their cohort of high-risk women. A case control study is taking place to address the issue of whether atypia incidence is indeed higher in at-risk women as compared to average-risk women. Women at increased risk of breast cancer based on BRCA1/2 mutation, or >10% probability of mutation, or because of a Gail probability >1.7% in 5-yr, are being compared

with age-matched population-based women with no known risk factors for breast cancer. We assumed a 25% incidence of atypia in the case group and 5% in the control group. With 70 case subjects and 30 control subjects, the study has sufficient statistical power to detect such a difference as significant. If proven, such a difference would provide further rationale for using atypia as a risk marker and a potential surrogate biomarker for chemoprevention interventions.

At present, no prospective data yet indicate that a cytologic finding of only benign cells on ductal lavage decreases breast cancer risk in a woman with elevated risk based on her Gail risk or other factors. Two other prospective studies evaluating breast cytology by FNA and NAF did demonstrate that absence of cytologically atypical cells placed women into a substantially lower-risk category for developing breast cancer than did the presence of cytologically atypical cells *(8,9)*. The ongoing prospective Ductal Lavage Outcomes Tracking Study will provide insight into the currently unanswered question of whether a woman at elevated risk who has only benign cells found on ductal lavage can safely forgo antiestrogen risk reduction therapy.

Ductal lavage should be offered to women as a risk stratification tool only if their risk of developing breast cancer is elevated. This includes women who have a 5-yr Gail risk >1.7%, those with an elevated-risk Claus model that incorporates both first- and second- degree relatives and their ages at diagnosis *(18)*, a personal history of invasive breast cancer or ductal carcinoma *in situ* for whom tamoxifen risk reduction therapy would be appropriate, women with elevated mammographic density (i.e., >75%), and women who have been on combined estrogen and progesterone hormonal replacement therapy for 10 yr or more. Aside from controlled clinical trials, ductal lavage should be offered only to women for whom a finding of cytologically atypical cells will alter their clinical management. These alterations could include initiation of antiestrogen therapy, discontinuing hormone replacement therapy, and increased breast cancer surveillance with more frequent clinical breast examinations, and breast imaging modalities such as digital mammography, ultrasound, or magnetic resonance imaging.

The sensitivity and specificity of ductal lavage for detecting occult malignancy are not known. Given the small area covered by a breast duct, however, ductal lavage is not a screening tool for breast cancer and neither substitutes for nor complements mammography. In addition, an association between a cytologic finding of marked atypia on ductal lavage and a histologic finding of malignancy on a subsequent breast biopsy has not been established. For this reason, considerable caution should be exercised in utilizing ductal lavage as a diagnostic tool to clarify the appropriateness of prophylactic mastectomy. Ductal lavage and breast cancer risk reduction investigators have concluded that there are inadequate data regarding the correlation between malignant lavage cytology and a histologic diagnosis of malignancy to recommend either surgical exploration of the affected duct or prophylactic mastectomy in women with malignant cells in their lavage fluid *(14,15)*. High-risk women with markedly atypical or malignant cytology on ductal lavage are recommended to repeat lavage of the same duct to confirm the finding, followed by ductography to determine whether a filling defect is apparent in the duct to guide biopsy, as well as breast imaging with MRI, ultrasound, and/or digital mammography. A biopsy of any abnormality found on breast imaging is indicated. For women not found to have an abnormality on ductography and breast imaging studies, treatment with tamoxifen as well as enhanced surveillance with breast examinations and imaging procedures is recommended. A 6- to 12-mo surveillance with repeated ductal lavage is reasonable in the absence of other abnormal signs.

Because the ductal system is highly complex, with multiple branching segments extending from the nipple areolar complex to the chest wall, the location of the duct orifice does not provide guidance regarding the anatomic location of the ductal system containing the abnormality. For this reason, blind duct exploration is not recommended as a surgical method for evaluating a highly atypical or malignant lavage finding *(14)*.

The clinical utility of ductal lavage in the clinical management of women with a known BRCA1 or BRCA-2 germline mutation is unknown. A finding of cytologic atypia on ductal lavage could aid a woman who is a mutation carrier in making a decision about prophylactic mastectomy, although it is not known whether cytologic atypia further increases risk in BRCA1/2 mutation carriers. Conversely, it is not known whether the absence of cytologic atypia on ductal lavage lowers the short- or long-term breast cancer risk in a BRCA1/2 mutation carrier. Women opting for prophylactic mastectomy because of their mutation status would be an ideal cohort to assess the relationship between results of ductal lavage and subsequent histological examination of the whole gland.

While the 5-yr Gail risk is the only breast cancer risk assessment tool that has been prospectively validated, several other promising risk markers are under intensive study, including serum insulin-like growth factor-1 (IGF-1) levels in premenopausal women, serum estradiol levels in postmenopausal women, quantitative breast density on mammography, and bone density *(19–23)*. It is likely that some of these risk markers will be incorporated into standard breast cancer risk assessment formulas once they are prospectively validated. Several studies have prospectively confirmed that a cytologic finding of atypia increases breast cancer risk to the same extent as a pathologic finding of atypical hyperplasia *(8,9)*. In addition, cytologic atypia provides risk assessment information that is independent of a woman's 5-yr Gail risk. It is not yet known whether a cytologic finding of atypia on ductal lavage will provide risk information that is independent of other important risk markers such as serum estradiol and IGF-1 levels, and quantitative breast density on mammography.

A potential strength of ductal lavage as a risk assessment tool is its ability to provide adequate cellular material for cytologic diagnosis, as well as sufficient cellular material for molecular analysis in a high proportion of high-risk women. It is likely that the predictive value of cytologic atypia can be further refined in the future on the basis of biomarkers of increased proliferation (Ki67) or reduced apoptosis, altered biochemical expression (e.g., ER, HER-2, etc.), and altered cytometric and nuclear morphometric parameters, as well as important molecular analyses such as loss of heterogygosity and gene expression profile *(24)*. Availability of abnormal breast epithelial cells will facilitate the further stratification of atypical cells into those with a high likelihood of progression to breast cancer vs those with a lower risk. In addition, molecular characterization of the atypical cells may help guide therapy selection in the future. Overexpression of ER, EGFR, IGFR, cyclooxygenase (COX)-2, and HER-2 have all been demonstrated on atypical breast epithelial cells (Dr. Carol Fabian, personal communication) *(1–3,25–27)*. Inhibitors of these constitutive proliferative and survival pathways are undergoing clinical development in patients with breast cancer and in high-risk women with breast IEN. Ductal lavage holds promise as an attractive tool for risk stratification in women at elevated risk who are weighing the risks and benefits of tamoxifen treatment, beginning or stopping hormone replacement therapy, or the need for more intensive breast imaging surveillance. A recent study has documented women's reluctance to take tamoxifen risk reduction therapy due to concern about side effects, even if they are at substantially elevated risk *(28)*. Ductal lavage is another risk assessment option for the approximate 30 million women in the US who are at elevated risk on the basis of their 5-yr Gail risk score.

5. DUCTAL LAVAGE AS A RISK ASSESSMENT AND INTERVENTION RESEARCH TOOL

Several ongoing and planned clinical trials will incorporate ductal lavage into intervention studies that test the effectiveness of new precancer treatment agents. In one study, postmenopausal women at elevated breast cancer risk will undergo ductal lavage and will then be treated with the aromatase inhibitor letrozole vs placebo for 12 mo. The primary endpoint of this study is the incidence of cytologic atypia in women who undergo letrozole treatment for 12 mo. An approximate 20% incidence of cytologic atypia is expected after 12 mo of placebo treatment in these high-risk women. A similar study is planned with the steroidal aromatase inhibitor exemestane.

In another trial, the ability of the COX-2 inhibitor celecoxib to decrease incidence of cytologic epithelial hyperplasia with and without atypia will be evaluated by both bilateral breast random periareolar FNA and bilateral breast ductal lavage. This study will evaluate the effectiveness of celecoxib in reversing the cytologic

findings of breast IEN, and will also compare the usefulness of breast FNA and ductal lavage within the context of a therapeutic intervention trial. Ductal lavage may also facilitate the study of novel preventive agents in women at increased risk for developing ER-negative breast cancer, such as those carrying a BRCA1 mutation or those with prior ER-negative DCIS, where the effect of tamoxifen and other hormonal agents is likely to be null if not detrimental.

In a cancer detection pilot study, ductal lavage fluid from breast cancer patients frequently contained methylated alleles of cyclin D2, RAR-β, and Twist genes *(29)*. Among 56 samples of ductal lavage fluid obtained from high-risk women with normal mammograms and breast examinations, methylation-specific PCR detected four of six samples that were found to contain cytologically atypical or malignant cells. Two of the women with abnormal cytology findings and methylated cyclin D2 and/or RAR-β genes on PCR were subsequently diagnosed with breast cancer. This study suggested that methylation-specific PCR of ductal lavage fluid might provide further risk stratification information and may be worthy of study as an early detection tool for breast cancer in very high-risk women.

REFERENCES

1. Stark A, Hulka BS, Joens S, et al. Her-2/neu amplification in benign breast disease and the risk of subsequent breast cancer. *J Clin Oncol* 2000;8:267–274.
2. van Agthoven T, Timmermans M, Foekens JA, et al. Differential expression of estrogen, progesterone and epidermal growth factor receptor in normal, benign, and malignant human breast tissues using dual staining immunohistochemistry. *Am J Pathol* 1994;144:1238–1246.
3. O'Connell P, Pekkel V, Fuqua SA, et al. Analysis of loss of heterozygosity in 399 premalignant breast lesions at 15 genetic loci. *J Natl Cancer Inst* 1998;90:697–703.
4. Nielsen M, Thomsen JL, Primdahl S, et al. Breast cancer and atypia among young and middle-aged women: a study of 110 medicological autopsies. *Br J Cancer* 1987;56:814–819.
5. Dupont WD, Parl FF, Hartmann WH, et al. Breast cancer risk associated with proliferative breast disease and atypical hyperplasia. *Cancer* 1993;71:1258–1265.
6. Fisher B, Costantino JP, Wickerham DL, et al. Tamoxifen for prevention of breast cancer: report of the National Surgical Adjuvant Breast and Bowel Project P-1 Study. *J Natl Cancer Inst* 1998:90:1371–1388.
7. Boerner S, Fornage BD, Singletary E, Sneige N. Ultrasound-guided fine-needle aspiration (FNA) of nonpalpable breast lesions: a review of 1885 FNA cases using the National Cancer Institute-supported recommendations on the uniform approach to breast FNA. *Cancer* 1999; 87:19–24.
8. Fabian CJ, Kimler BF, Zalles CM, et al. Short-term breast cancer prediction by random periareolar fine-needle aspiration cytology and the Gail risk model. *J Natl Cancer Inst* 2000;92:1217–1227.

9. Wrensch MR, Petrakis NJ, King EB, et al. Breast cancer incidence in women with abnormal cytology in nipple aspirates of breast fluid. *Am J Epidemiol* 1992;135:130–134.

10. Wrensch MR, Petrakis NJ, King EB, et al. Breast cancer risk in women with abnormal cytology in nipple aspirates of breast fluid. *J Natl Cancer Inst* 2001;93:1791–1798.

11. Tan-Chiu E, Costantino J, Wang J, et al. The effect of tamoxifen on benign breast disease. Findings from the National Surgical Adjuvant Breast and Bowel Project (NSABP) Breast Cancer Prevention Trial (BCPT). *Breast Cancer Res Treat* 2001;69:210. (abstr. no. 7).

12. Dooley WC, Ljung BM, Veronesi U, et al. Ductal lavage for detection of cellular atypia in women at high risk for breast cancer. *J Natl Cancer Inst* 2001;93:1624–1632.

13. National Cancer Institute. The uniform approach to breast fine-needle aspiration biopsy. NIH Consensus Development Conference. *Am J Surg* 1997;174:371–385.

14. Morrow M, Vogel V, Ljung BM, O'Shaughnessy JA. Evaluation and management of the woman with abnormal ductal lavage. *J Am Coll Surg* 2002;194:648–656.

15. O'Shaughnessy JA, Ljung BM, Dooley WC, et al. Ductal lavage and the clinical management of women at high risk for breast carcinoma. A Commentary. *Cancer* 2002;94:2:292–298.

16. Costantino JP, Gail MH, Pee D, et al. Validation studies for models projecting the risk of invasive and total breast cancer incidence. *J Natl Cancer Inst* 1999;91:1541–1548.

17. Gail MH, Brinton LA, Byar DP, et al. Projecting individualized probabilities of developing breast cancer for white females who are being examined annually. *J Natl Cancer Inst* 1989;81:1879–1886.

18. Claus EB, Schildkraut JM, Thompson WD, Risch NJ. The genetic attributable risk of breast and ovarian cancer. *Cancer* 1996:77:2318–2324.

19. Hankinson SE, Willett WC, Golditz GA, et al. Circulatory concentrations of insulin-like growth factor-1 and risk of breast cancer. *Lancet* 1998;9:1393–1396.

20. Cauley JA, Lucas FL, Kuller LH, et al. Elevated serum estradiol and testosterone concentrations are associated with a high risk for breast cancer. *Ann Intern Med* 1999;130:270–277.

21. Boyd NF, Lockwood GA, Martin LJ, et al. Mammographic densities and risk of breast cancer among subjects with a family history of this disease. *J Natl Cancer Inst* 1999;191:1404–1408.

22. Cauley JA, Lucas FL, Kuller LH, et al. Bone mineral density and risk of breast cancer in older women; the study of osteoporotic fractures. *JAMA* 1996;276:1404–1408.

23. Zhang Y, Kiel DP, Kreger BE, et al. Bone mass and the risk of breast cancer among postmenopausal women. *N Engl J Med* 1997;336:611–617.

24. Gherardi G, Marveggio C. Cytologic score and DNA-image analysis in the classification of borderline breast lesions: a prospective study on 47 fine-needle aspirates. *Diagn Cytopathol* 1999;20A:212–218.

25. Khan SA, Rogers MA, Obando JA, Tamsen A. Estrogen receptor expression of benign breast epithelium and its association with breast cancer. *Cancer Res* 1994;54:993-997.

26. Athanassiadou PP, Veneti SZ, Kyrkou KA, et al. Presence of epidermal growth factor receptor in breast smears of cyst fluids: relationship to electrolyte ratios and pH concentration. *Cancer Detect Prev* 1992;16:113–118.

27. Monaghan P, Perusinghe NP, Nicholson RI, et al. Growth factor stimulation of proliferating cell nuclear antigen (PCNA) in human breast epithelium organ culture. *Cell Biol Int Rep* 1991;15:561–570.

28. Port ER, Montgomery LL, Heerdt AS, Borgen PL. Patient reluctance toward tamoxifen use for breast cancer primary prevention. *Ann Surg Oncol* 2001;8:580–584.

29. Sabo AB, Hung DT, Ljung BM, et al. Detection of breast cancer cells in ductal lavage fluid by methylation-specific PCR. *Lancet* 2001;357:1335–1336.

19 Counteracting Estrogen as Breast Cancer Prevention

Kathrin Strasser-Weippl, MD
and Paul E. Goss, MD, PhD, FRCPC, FRCP (UK)

CONTENTS

ESTROGEN AND THE RISK OF BREAST CANCER
AGENTS
COMPLETED AND ONGOING CHEMOPREVENTION TRIALS
NEW BIOMARKERS AND COHORTS
CONSIDERATIONS FOR THE FUTURE
REFERENCES

1. ESTROGEN AND THE RISK OF BREAST CANCER

The association between estrogen and breast cancer growth has been appreciated for more than 100 yr, since George Beatson produced remission of advanced breast cancer by performing bilateral oophorectomy in premenopausal patients *(1)*. Since that time, a body of evidence has accumulated supporting the hypothesis that estrogen and its metabolites are related in a complex fashion to both the initiation and promotion of breast cancer.

1.1. Epidemiological Evidence

Epidemiological studies point to an important role for estrogens in breast cancer development and growth. The almost 150-fold greater incidence of breast cancer in women compared to men reflects the relationship between female sex steroids and breast cancer. A number of clinical markers of excessive cumulative lifetime exposure to estrogens are linked to an individual's breast cancer risk. These include early menarche and late menopause *(2)*, high bone density *(3)*, and obesity in menopause *(4)*, which are all surrogates for exposure to estrogens. In addition, elevated levels of plasma estrogens are themselves directly associated with a raised risk of breast cancer *(5–7)* and it may well be that, in postmenopausal women, plasma estrogen levels are the most

reliable intermediate biomarker of breast cancer risk. This is discussed in more detail below. In support of this finding, a correlation has been shown between high levels of urinary estrogens *(8)* and breast cancer risk.

The relationship between exogenous estrogens and breast cancer risk has also been investigated in several large epidemiological studies. Three cohort studies and four case-control studies have shown that using hormone replacement therapy (HRT) in menopause increases breast cancer risk by one-third *(9–16)*. Recently published data from the Women's Health Initiative (WHI), a prospective study in which 16,608 postmenopausal women were randomized to HRT vs placebo, confirmed this excess breast cancer risk (HR 1.29 after a median follow-up of 5.2 yr) *(17)*. In one of the epidemiologic studies discussed above, the increased risk was higher in women with a lower body mass index, which could mean that lower body fat, and thus lower levels of endogenous estrogens, might lead to higher sensitivity to increased breast cancer risk caused by exogenous estrogens. It was also reported that increased risk in women using estrogen/progestin therapy is higher than in those using estrogen therapy alone *(10)*. Hysterectomized postmenopausal women on the WHI study receiving estrogen-only therapy (ERT) vs placebo continue on study; this arm of the trial will report in 2005. Elevated breast cancer risk in women who have stopped taking HRT normalizes 5 yr after

From: Cancer Chemoprevention, Volume 2: Strategies for Cancer Chemoprevention
Edited by: G. J. Kelloff, E. T. Hawk, and C. C. Sigman © Humana Press Inc., Totowa, NJ

249

cessation of therapy *(18)*. Longer follow-up of the WHI study will provide more information in this regard.

The relationship between oral contraceptive use and breast cancer is less clear, because studies addressing this issue have produced varying results. Several studies suggested a very slight increase in breast cancer risk with oral contraceptive use, irrespective of duration *(12,13,19)*. However, in a recently published population-based study including more than 9000 women *(20)*, breast cancer risk was not elevated in current or previous users of oral contraceptives. These findings did not differ according to duration of use, estrogen dose, race, or family history of breast cancer. A summary of available information on hormonally mediated indicators of elevated breast cancer risk is shown in Table 1.

In addition to exogenous factors increasing breast cancer risk, epidemiological studies have also identified certain dietary agents that decrease breast cancer risk. These primarily include flaxseed and soy, for which a high intake has been noted in geographic regions with a low breast cancer risk. Available data on the chemopreventive properties of these dietary supplements will be included in this review.

Epidemiologic studies have also indicated that certain genetic polymorphisms of enzymes involved in estrogen synthesis and metabolism may increase breast cancer risk. For example, results of two case-control studies indicated that carriers of the A1 variant of the aromatase gene face an elevated risk of developing breast cancer *(21,22)*. Numerous other studies demonstrated correlations between certain polymorphisms of estrogen-catabolizing enzymes and breast cancer risk *(23–27)*. However, an equal number of studies were unable to confirm these associations. It will take larger cohorts and the consideration of post-transcriptional influences on enzyme activity in order to clarify this important issue.

1.2. Evidence From Animal Studies

Apart from epidemiological studies, another line of evidence linking estrogen to breast cancer comes from animal studies. Estrogen and its metabolites induce breast cancer in several animal models. For example, tumors of the mammary gland in female ACI rats develop rapidly on exposure to estrogen *(28)*. In several other animal models of tumor carcinogenesis, tumor development or growth is enhanced by estrogen *(29)*. In the kidney of the male Syrian golden hamster, estrogen (E_2), estrone (E_1) and 2-hydroxy-catechol estrogen (2-OHCE, an estrogen metabolite) are carcinogenic

Table 1
Hormonally Mediated Risk Factors for Breast Cancer

Factor	Approximate Relative Risk Estimate
Premenopausal obesity	1.2
Postmenopausal obesity	1.2
Use of oral contraceptives	1.0
Hormone replacement therapy	1.1–1.4
Oophorectomy prior to age 40	0.5
Young age at menarche	Risk ↑ 4–5%/year
Old age at menopause	Risk ↑ 4–5%/year
Age at first birth <20	1.0
>20 and Multiparous	1.6
Nulliparous ≥35	1.9
Bone mass	2–3.5
Breast density	~5
Postmenopausal levels of estradiol	~3

(30–32). When 2-OH- and 4-OH-CEs were compared, the 4-OH-metabolites were significantly more carcinogenic *(29,31,33)*, indicating that the specific pathway of estrogen metabolism might be important with respect to breast cancer risk. Interestingly, tumor formation decreased in hamsters treated with estrogen plus inhibitors of its metabolism, compared with hamsters exposed to estrogen alone *(34–36)*. This observation demonstrates a role for estrogen metabolites in carcinogenesis. In early 2003, the US National Institutes of Health (NIH) National Toxicology Program's 10th Report on Carcinogens placed conjugated estrogens, estradiol, estrone, ethinylestradiol, and mestranol on the list of probable cancer-causing substances because they met the criteria for registration as human carcinogens *(37)*.

1.3. Molecular Evidence

Important data on molecular mechanisms of estrogen-induced carcinogenesis have been generated in the past few years. The classical paradigm was that estrogens manifest their effect on breast cancer via the estrogen receptor (ER). In this model, breast cells' exposure to estrogen leads to DNA synthesis and cell proliferation. Proliferating cells are susceptible to DNA damage; with a high rate of proliferation, DNA repair diminishes. Ultimately, accumulating uncorrected genetic errors lead to a malignant phenotype *(38)*. In recent years, data have indicated two important new points. First, receptor-mediated signal transduction is not the most important pathway of estrogen carcinogenesis. Secondly, estrogen metabolites are at least as carcinogenic as their parent compounds.

The first clue to receptor-independent pathways of estrogen carcinogenesis came from studies showing that ER-positive cells in the normal mammary gland are not the ones that proliferate in response to estrogen as measured by Ki67-positivity (39,40). Furthermore, estrogen-induced mammary tumors in ER-knockout mice develop independently of the ER (41).

The role of estrogen metabolites in carcinogenesis has been extensively studied in the male Syrian hamster kidney and in the uterus of CD-1 mice (29–33). In these models, the 2-OH and 4-OH CEs, signaling molecules working through the ER, are able to induce malignant tumors. The fact that 4-OH catechols are much more potent carcinogens than 2-OH catechols is important when discussing individual differences in estrogen metabolism and implications for breast cancer risk. The CEs themselves give rise to genotoxic quinones, which can subsequently generate reactive oxygen species, causing oxidative damage (42,43). Numerous studies have shown that both estrogen and its catechol metabolites cause multiple direct genotoxic effects, such as aneuploidy (44,45), structural chromosomal aberrations (44–47), gene amplification (48), and microsatellite instability (49). Apart from nonspecific genetic damage, certain specific mutations triggered by estrogens have also now been confirmed (50). Genetic damage caused by estrogen metabolites might be an important step in the development of breast cancer, as genetic lesions are known to cause cancer in humans (51). Tumors may be initiated by estrogen metabolites and proliferate in response to ER-mediated stimuli.

Apart from circulating endogenous and exogenous estrogens, other tissue-related estrogenic factors have been implicated in the initiation of hormone-dependent breast cancer. The level of tissue expression of the aromatase enzyme, which is responsible for the synthesis of estrogens from androgens, might be important in this regard. It has been shown that aromatase expression and activity are higher in breast tumors than in peritumoral fat, and that peritumoral aromatase levels are higher in the quadrant where the tumor is located than in other quadrants of the breast (52–56). In addition, increasing evidence indicates that this local estrogen production may play a major role in tumor proliferation (57–60). The exact mechanisms involved in estrogen production within the breast are still not well understood. Tissue-specific promoters of the aromatase gene are regulated by transcription factors, some of which have been demonstrated to be tumor-related (61). It has been hypothesized that the aromatase gene may be constitutively activated in the breast in certain women, causing an exaggerated estrogen stimulus on the breast and thereby acting as an oncogene to induce cancer.

2. AGENTS

Since it is clear that antagonizing estrogen is an anti-breast cancer strategy, several agents have been evaluated to treat hormone-sensitive breast cancer. In clinical development, these agents have classically been tested as second-line and then first-line therapy for advanced disease, and thereafter evaluated as adjuvant and neoadjuvant (preoperative) treatment. Tamoxifen, the first hormonal agent approved for the adjuvant treatment of ER-positive breast cancer, was also among the first hormonal agents to be tested in chemoprevention in the mid-1990s. In the interim, numerous antiestrogens have been developed, many of them promising a superior therapeutic index. Because of the mixed agonist/antagonist effects of these agents on different organs of the body, they are being tested either primarily as breast cancer preventives, or for their effects on other hormone-dependent organs important to women's health. In addition to these new selective estrogen receptor modulators (SERMs), the aromatase inhibitors, already established hormonal agents in breast cancer treatment, are also beginning to be tested in chemoprevention.

Several agents with prospects as breast cancer preventives will be discussed in this section, with a focus on the data suggesting their efficacy in chemoprevention, and subsequently their therapeutic index with respect to actions on other end-organs.

2.1. Chemopreventive Efficacy of Agents

Tamoxifen citrate is the lead compound in the SERM class of agents, which binds to the ER and exerts either estrogenic or antiestrogenic effects depending on the specific organ. Having been first approved by the FDA for use in advanced breast cancer in 1978, tamoxifen is now the most widely studied antiestrogenic treatment in breast cancer. The National Surgical Adjuvant Breast Project (NSABP) B-14 study, one of the initial large trials examining tamoxifen's benefits as adjuvant therapy, randomized 2818 pre- and postmenopausal patients with primary, ER-positive, node-negative breast cancer to 5 yr of tamoxifen or placebo (62). A significant difference in disease-free survival in favor of patients receiving tamoxifen was detected (a 26% reduction in treatment failure at 4 yr, *p* > 0.00001). This significant beneficial effect of adjuvant tamoxifen was confirmed in the Scottish trial of 1987 and in a large meta-analysis including more than 30,000 patients *(63,64)*. Importantly, in addition to a reduction in local and distant treatment failure, tumor incidence in the contralateral breast also decreased in these studies.

These findings generated the hypothesis that tamoxifen might serve as a breast tumor-preventive agent. Results of four prospective placebo-controlled trials evaluating tamoxifen's chemopreventive potential in breast cancer have now been published *(65–68)*. In the two larger trials, NSABP P-1 *(65)* and the International Breast Intervention Study 1 (IBIS-1) *(66)*, tamoxifen was able to reduce the incidence of ER-positive breast cancer by about one-third to one-half in women at an elevated risk of developing the disease. While initial results from the two smaller trials did not confirm these findings, a recent update has confirmed a reduction from tamoxifen in all four trials (unpublished data). The completed prevention studies will be discussed in more detail in Section 3.

Additional evidence of tamoxifen's chemopreventive effects has been obtained from trials in women with ductal carcinoma *in situ* (DCIS), in particular in the NSABP B-24 study *(69)*. Women with DCIS were not eligible for prevention trials, but their 5-yr 3.4% risk of contralateral breast cancer falls into the inclusion criteria of the largest of the studies, NSABP P-1. Among 1804 patients with DCIS treated with lumpectomy and radiation in B-24, tamoxifen significantly reduced subsequent invasive breast cancers by 47% *(65,69)*.

2.1.1. RALOXIFENE

Raloxifene, a SERM differing slightly from tamoxifen in its estrogenic and antiestrogenic properties, was originally developed for osteoporosis prevention because of its proestrogenic effect on bone.

In the Multiple Outcomes of Raloxifene Evaluation (MORE) study, 7705 postmenopausal women with osteoporosis and no history of breast or endometrial cancer were randomized to receive either raloxifene (60 or 120 mg) or placebo daily for 3 yr. The MORE trial was designed primarily to test the bone-preserving effects of raloxifene; breast cancer occurrence was a secondary endpoint. After a median follow-up of 40 mo, women receiving raloxifene had substantially fewer invasive cancers (risk ratio [RR] = 0.24; 95% CI 0.13–0.44; *p* < 0.001) than those taking placebo. This

Table 2
Results of the MORE trial *(70)*

Type of Event	Placebo N = 2576	Raloxifene N = 5129	Risk Ratio
Invasive breast cancer	27	13	0.24
Invasive endometrial cancer	4	6	0.8
New vertebral fracture	10.1%	5.4/6.6%[a]	0.7/0.51[a]
Deep-vein thrombosis and pulmonary embolism	8	55	3.1

aFor groups receiving raloxifene 60 mg/d and 120 mg/d respectively.

difference was entirely attributable to a 90% reduction in ER-positive invasive breast cancers (RR = 0.1; 95% CI 0.04–0.24) by raloxifene with no difference in the occurrence of ER negative tumors *(70)*. Results of the MORE trial are presented in Table 2.

Data from the MORE trial have to be taken cautiously, as breast cancer prevention was only a secondary endpoint. However, a partially overlapping analysis reviewing data from nine raloxifene trials (including MORE) has confirmed a significant reduction in newly diagnosed breast cancers in women on raloxifene, validating MORE data *(71)*. Interestingly, a recent update of the MORE trial found that only those women with elevated levels of plasma estrogen at baseline benefited from the breast cancer risk reduction of raloxifene *(72)*.

Based on these data, which suggest that raloxifene and tamoxifen have similar efficacy in reducing receptor-positive breast tumor incidence, a confirmatory study comparing raloxifene to tamoxifen is under way (see below).

2.1.2. FASLODEX

Faslodex (ICI 182,780) is a steroidal estrogen antagonist belonging to the newly defined group of selective estrogen receptor downregulators (SERDs), which, in contrast to SERMs, are devoid of estrogen agonist activity. Their mode of action is to bind to the ER, inhibit its dimerization, and increase its degradation *(73–75)*. Preclinical studies have shown that cell lines resistant to or stimulated by tamoxifen remain sensitive to faslodex *(76,77)*. Two studies in postmenopausal women with tamoxifen-resistant breast cancer have shown that faslodex is at least as good as the third-generation aromatase inhibitor anastrozole in this setting *(78–80)*. Based on these data, faslodex was recently approved in the US to treat postmenopausal, hormone-sensitive breast cancer following an antiestrogen. Results of trials of faslodex vs tamoxifen as first-line therapy in advanced disease are awaited with interest. To date there are no data testing the chemopreventive efficacy of faslodex.

2.1.3. EM-652

EM-652 (SCH57068) is a very promising SERM in clinical development. In a preclinical study that also tested tamoxifen, toremifene, raloxifene, droloxifene, idoxifene, and GW-5638, SCH57068 was the only compound that decreased the tumor size of ZR-75-1 human breast cancer xenografts in ovariectomized nude mice. Over a treatment period of 23 wk, the six other SERMs tested were able only to decrease the progression rate of the tumors stimulated by estrone *(81)*. EM-800, the parent compound of EM-652, has shown clinical benefit in patients with tamoxifen-resistant breast cancer *(82,83)*.

2.1.4. LASOFOXIFENE

Lasofoxifene is a SERM being developed to treat postmenopausal osteoporosis. Only preclinical data are available regarding its efficacy in breast cancer treatment and prevention. In the *N*-methyl-*N*-nitrosourea (MNU)-induced rat mammary tumor model, lasofoxifene was able to delay tumor incidence and reduce tumor multiplicity to a similar extent as tamoxifen. When existing tumors were treated with lasofoxifene in this model, 50% of the tumors regressed, compared to none of the untreated tumors *(84)*.

2.1.5. ARZOXIFENE

Arzoxifene (formerly known as SERM III) is a third-generation SERM that exerts greater tumor inhibitory effects in the MNU-induced rat mammary tumor model than does raloxifene *(85)*. The ability of arzoxifene to reverse ductal hyperplasia in high risk women who have fine-needle aspiration cytologic evidence of ductal hyperplasia is currently being evaluated in a Phase II clinical study.

2.1.6. MIPROXIFENE

Miproxifene phosphate, or TAT-59, is a SERM developed in Japan. In preclinical studies, TAT-59 was able to inhibit the proliferation of estrogen-dependent MCF-7 tumor xenografts in ovariectomized nude mice to a greater extent than tamoxifen. Moreover, R-27 and FST-1 tumors, which are resistant to tamoxifen, responded strongly to TAT-59 *(86)*. The drug was also evaluated in comparison with tamoxifen in patients with advanced ER-positive or ER-unknown breast cancer.

TAT-59's response rate was similar to that of tamoxifen in a Phase II study of 195 patients (30.1% vs 26.5% in the TAT-59 and TAM group, respectively; n.s.) *(87)*.

2.1.7. OTHER SERMS AND SERDS

Aside from the compounds discussed above, a number of other SERMs have been developed in the hope of improving the efficacy and therapeutic index of ER modulators. After the introduction of tamoxifen, several other first-generation SERMs were developed, including droloxifene *(88)*, levormeloxifene, and idoxifene. These agents could not demonstrate superiority in treating advanced breast cancer, and plans to develop them for such treatment have been discontinued. Several of the more promising second and third-generation compounds have been discussed above. Others include bazedoxifene (formerly TSE-424), an agent being developed in combination with Premarin® as a non-uterine-stimulating HRT; SERM 3339; ERA 923; LY 326,315; and SR 16234, which combines antiangiogenic and SERM properties. Published data are very limited for all of these agents.

2.1.8. ANTIESTROGENIC DIETARY SUPPLEMENTS

Flaxseed is a source of plant lignans, estrogenic compounds in plants called phytoestrogens. Secoisolariciresinol diglucoside (SDG), the most important lignan contained in flaxseed, is chemically similar to tamoxifen and exerts antiestrogenic effects in part by binding to the ER and inhibiting estrogen synthesis *(89)*.

Numerous preclinical studies have shown that flaxseed has chemopreventive effects on mammary tumor development *(90–92)*. In humans, flaxseed increases total urinary estrogen excretion and lengthens the luteal phase of the menstrual cycle *(93,94)*.

Postmenopausal women consuming 5 g or 10 g of ground flaxseed/day for 7 wk showed significant reductions in blood concentrations of estradiol *(95)*. Preliminary results in a more recent study of 116 premenopausal women showed that those taking 25 g/d of ground flaxseed for 1 yr had longer menstrual cycles, but no reduction in estradiol levels or breast density was seen *(96)*. In a similar protocol, premenopausal women with cyclical mastalgia experienced a significant reduction in pain after 4 mo of flaxseed consumption *(97)*. Women with breast cancer who ate flaxseed-containing muffins preoperatively showed notable reductions in breast cancer cell proliferation and increased apoptosis in another study *(98)*. Therefore, flaxseed ingestion is a potential way of reducing breast cancer risk, at least in part through its hormonal effects. Larger studies will be needed to determine the true effect of regular flaxseed intake on parameters of breast cancer risk.

Soy, which contains the phytoestrogens genistein and daidzein, was initially reported to have cytostatic activity in mammary cancer cell lines and to inhibit growth and progression of mammary tumors in rodents *(99–101)*. However, a breast cancer-stimulating effect of genistein and daidzein was observed in other preclinical studies *(102–105)*. In two studies, genistein antagonized the tumor-inhibitory effects of tamoxifen on breast cancer cells *(106,107)*, but in one of these studies, genistein was—at higher doses—tumor inhibitory itself *(106)*. In a study using the 7,12-dimethyl-benz[*a*]anthracene (DMBA)-induced rat mammary tumor model, chemoprevention was demonstrated after prepubertal and combined prepubertal and adult genistein treatments but not after prenatal- or adult-only treatments, indicating that the timing of exposure to genistein might be important for breast cancer chemoprevention. In this study, genistein's cellular mechanism of action was found to be mammary gland and cell differentiation *(108)*.

In clinical studies, soy milk supplements have been shown to reduce serum estradiol levels in premenopausal women *(109)*. Also, several population-based case-control studies in Asian women showed a significant correlation between high intake of soy during adolescence and reduced breast cancer risk *(110,111)*. This correlation could not be confirmed in a Caucasian population *(112)*.

Altogether, it seems that phytoestrogens contained in soy may have chemopreventive properties if consumed at high doses. In women with a history of breast cancer, however, soy products may have a detrimental effect due to the proestrogenic effects they exert on breast cancer cells in preclinical models.

2.1.9. AROMATASE INHIBITORS

In principle, the use of estrogen synthetase (aromatase) inhibitors in breast cancer is based on the same rationale as the use of ER antagonists. However, in addition to preventing estradiol from stimulating its receptor, aromatase inhibitors also reduce formation of estrogen's genotoxic metabolites. This ability to target two different mechanisms of estrogen-induced carcinogenesis might indicate that aromatase inhibitors are more effective chemopreventives than SERMs. Currently, anastrozole and letrozole, nonsteroidal aromatase inhibitors, and exemestane, a steroidal aromatase inactivator, are in clinical use for the treatment of metastatic breast cancer.

As all of them have been shown to be superior in terms of toxicity or efficacy to traditional second-line hormonal therapy *(113)*, they are widely used after tamoxifen in hormone-sensitive breast cancer. Recently, aromatase inhibitors were also found to be superior to tamoxifen as first-line treatment of metastatic breast cancer *(114–117)*.

Exemestane may, as a steroidal agent, have advantages over the nonsteroidal aromatase inhibitors as it does not compete with endogenous aromatase and it irreversibly inhibits the enzyme. It has been shown that intratumoral aromatase is upregulated in the presence of nonsteroidal aromatase inhibitors *(118)*, implicating a possible mechanism of tumor resistance circumvented by exemestane. In addition, being an androgenic steroid may make exemestane superior to the other inhibitors in terms of side effects caused by estrogen depletion of other target tissues.

At least eight ongoing adjuvant trials are testing aromatase inhibitors in early-stage postmenopausal receptor-positive breast cancer. To date, only the Arimidex, Tamoxifen Alone or in Combination (ATAC) trial, in which anastrozole was compared to tamoxifen in 9366 patients, has published data available *(119)*. After a median follow-up of 33 mo, anastrozole significantly lengthened disease-free survival ($p = 0.013$). Importantly, the incidence of contralateral new primary breast cancer was significantly lower with anastrozole than with tamoxifen (OR 0.42, $p = 0.0068$). All the data showing that aromatase inhibitors are superior to tamoxifen in treating breast cancer imply that they might also be superior in the chemopreventive setting. The reduction in contralateral breast cancer incidence in the ATAC trial is especially promising in this regard. In addition to clinical studies, a significant body of data on the chemopreventive properties of aromatase inhibitors comes from preclinical studies. In the MNU- and DMBA-carcinogen-induced mammary tumor models, inhibition of both the appearance of new tumors and their multiplicity has been shown with the aromatase inhibitors letrozole, aminoglutethimide, fadrozole, and vorozole; the last three are no longer widely used in breast cancer therapy *(120–126)*.

2.2. Therapeutic Index of New Agents

To assess the overall value of a breast cancer prevention agent, it is necessary to consider not only its efficacy against tumor development, but also positive and negative effects on other organ systems and general toxicities. In the case of endocrine agents, desirable endocrinologic effects such as preventing osteoporosis and lowering cardiovascular risk are particularly important. It has long been known that tamoxifen exerts estrogenic and antiestrogenic effects on organs other than the breast. These effects are of limited clinical importance in treating advanced breast cancer. However, when treating healthy women in the chemopreventive setting, any agent needs to be evaluated carefully to ensure not just reduction in cancer but also a net health benefit. Therefore, newly developed endocrine agents are carefully tested with regard to potentially harmful antiestrogenic effects on hormone-sensitive tissues. Available information on the therapeutic index of the aforementioned agents is presented in the following section. Beneficial and detrimental endocrinological effects as well as nonendocrinological side effects are discussed.

2.2.1. ENDOCRINOLOGICAL EFFECTS OTHER THAN THOSE ON THE BREAST

The most comprehensive antiestrogen data on the therapeutic index is available on tamoxifen. In the P-1 study, tamoxifen's effects on uterus, bone, lipid metabolism, thromboembolic risk, cataract incidence, and quality of life were carefully evaluated (65). Participants in P-1 who received tamoxifen had a 2.53 times greater risk of developing invasive endometrial cancer (95% CI 1.35–4.97) than those receiving placebo; this effect was more pronounced in women >50 yr of age than in younger women (RR 4.01 vs 1.21). All invasive endometrial cancers were International Federation of Gynecology and Obstetrics (FIGO) stage I; none resulted in a death. Data from the other three prevention trials (66–68) and the overview of adjuvant breast cancer trials by the Early Breast Cancer Trialists' Collaborative Group (EBCTCG) (127) confirm this excess of endometrial cancer risk (OR 2.41).

In the P-1 tamoxifen group, pulmonary embolism (PE) was three times as common (RR = 3.01, 95% CI 1.15–9.27) and strokes nearly twice as frequent among women >50 yr of age (RR 1.75; 95% CI 0.98–3.20). In addition, more women receiving tamoxifen developed deep-vein thrombosis (DVT, RR 1.6; 95% CI 0.91–2.86). Overall, the increase in vascular events in those receiving tamoxifen was comparable to that seen with HRT (65,128). The International Breast Cancer Intervention Study (IBIS-1) trial confirmed this higher endometrial and thromboembolic risk (66).

While retrospective analyses of three randomized tamoxifen trials found a reduction in coronary heart disease (CHD), no benefit was demonstrated in P-1 (65,129–132). In the EBCTCG overview of 1998,

mortality rates for causes "not attributed to breast or endometrial cancer" were nearly identical in patients receiving tamoxifen or placebo in the adjuvant setting (127). In view of recently published data from the WHI study (17), it is uncertain whether tamoxifen's favorable influence on lipid metabolism will translate into a true reduction in CHD.

Tamoxifen has been shown to preserve bone mineral density (BMD) in postmenopausal breast cancer patients (133–135). P-1 is the only prospective trial that evaluated the effect of tamoxifen on bone fractures vs placebo and showed a reduction in the risk of long bone and symptomatic vertebral fractures of borderline statistical significance (RR = 0.81, 95% CI 0.63–1.05) (65). To date, tamoxifen has not been evaluated in a prospective trial in women with osteoporosis.

Many data on raloxifene's side effects were collected in the MORE trial. As anticipated from preclinical testing, raloxifene did not increase the risk of endometrial cancer (RR = 0.8; 95% CI 0.2–2.7) during the first 3 yr of the MORE trial, but the total number of cases was small (70). Several smaller clinical studies have confirmed that raloxifene has a negligible or no stimulatory effect on the endometrium of postmenopausal women (136–138). It has not yet been established, however, whether animal models and clinical endometrial proliferation are reliable predictors of endometrial cancer, especially in view of limited follow-up.

In the MORE trial, relative risk of a thromboembolic event (including PE and DVT) for women on raloxifene was 3.1 (95% CI 1.5–6.2) (70). The Study of Tamoxifen and Raloxifene (STAR, see below) trial will provide a direct comparison between tamoxifen and raloxifene on vascular events. Available data indicate a similar increase in these serious side effects from the two drugs.

Raloxifene is approved for preventing osteoporosis in postmenopausal women, because the MORE trial showed women on raloxifene had a significant increase in bone mineral density of the lumbar spine and decrease in clinical vertebral fractures (70). Like tamoxifen, raloxifene has been shown to have a favorable influence on serum lipid levels (137,139,140). In the prospective, placebo-controlled Raloxifene Use for The Heart (RUTH) trial, raloxifene is being tested for its effects on CHD in high-risk postmenopausal women (141). This trial will report in approx 4 yr.

A pooled analysis from several clinical trials demonstrated that raloxifene had a tamoxifen-like effect on symptoms of menopause in postmenopausal women (142). As the greatest increase in hot flashes in the tamoxifen group of P-1 was seen in premenopausal women *(65)*, a similar effect of raloxifene can be expected in this setting.

Very little data is available on the effects of faslodex on organs other than breast. Based on preclinical data showing the purely antiestrogenic nature of faslodex, similar antiestrogenic effects can be expected on bone, endometrial tissue, and serum lipids.

SCH57068 does not have agonistic effects on endometrial tissue as measured by endometrial epithelial thickness *(81)*. When administered to ovariectomized mice, EM-652 prevents bone loss, lowers cholesterol and triglyceride levels *(82)*, decreases insulin resistance and prevents ovariectomy-induced obesity *(143)*. Because of its pure estrogen-antagonistic effects on breast and uterine tissue and beneficial effects on bone and potentially on cardiovascular risk, EM-652 might be an ideal candidate for prevention of breast and uterine cancers.

Lasofoxifene was found to be more effective than raloxifene in improving spinal bone density and reducing vertebral fractures in Phase II clinical studies. In addition, lasofoxifene leads to a significantly greater decrease in low-density lipoprotein (LDL) cholesterol compared to raloxifene, and has similar endometrial effects. Lasofoxifene is now undergoing Phase III evaluation in the treatment of osteoporosis.

Very limited data are available on the clinical side effect profile of arzoxifene. Reports about arzoxifene's effects on uterine tissue are inconclusive *(85,144)* and there are no data regarding other endocrinological side effects.

Miproxifene's short-term side effect profile was similar to that of tamoxifen in a Phase II study *(87)*. Its effects on uterus and bone have not been investigated in clinical studies, but preclinical data indicate that its estrogenic activity in these organs is comparable to that of tamoxifen.

The recently discovered nonsteroidal third-generation SERM CHF 4056 has profound antiestrogenic effects on uterine tissue while lowering cholesterol levels and protecting bone. No data are available on CHF 4056 regarding breast tissue *(145)*.

ERA-239, also briefly mentioned above as one of the new SERMs, has no uterotrophic effects in immature rats and ovariectomized mice *(146)*. No data are available on other endocrinologic side effects.

Although aromatase inhibitors are often discussed together, their side effect profiles may contain important differences, particularly between steroidal and nonsteroidal inhibitors.

Anastrozole was the first agent for which results in the adjuvant setting were presented. Toxicity data in comparison to tamoxifen, which were collected in the ATAC trial *(119)*, are particularly important, as these postmenopausal women were disease-free and healthy. Women receiving anastrozole had a significantly lower risk of developing endometrial cancer than those taking tamoxifen ($p = 0.02$). The nonstimulatory effect of anastrozole on the endometrium was also reflected by a significantly decreased rate of vaginal bleeding during the trial (4.5% vs 8.2%, $p < 0.0001$). In addition, both ischemic cerebrovascular and venous thromboembolic events (including DVT) were significantly rarer in the anastrozole group (1.0% vs 2.1% and 2.1% vs 3.5% respectively, both $p = 0.00006$). However, women taking anastrozole were significantly more likely to suffer from musculoskeletal disorders (27.8% vs 21.3%, $p < 0.000001$), in particular fractures (5.9% vs 3.7%, $p < 0.0001$). The ATAC trial has not reported any influences of either anastrozole or tamoxifen on the serum lipid profile. Another study found no influence of anastrozole on the lipid profile *(147)*.

The effects of letrozole and exemestane on organs other than breast have not been studied as comprehensively. Similarly to anastrozole, letrozole has been shown to significantly increase parameters of bone resorption in several studies *(148,149)*. When letrozole was given to healthy women for 3 mo, no influence was seen on their lipid profiles *(150)*. However, in another study including 20 women with breast cancer, letrozole significantly increased total and LDL cholesterol levels, as well as the atherogenic risk ratios of total/high-density lipoprotein (HDL) and LDL/HDL cholesterol *(151)*. Effects of letrozole on bone metabolism and parameters of cardiovascular risk are being extensively studied in the ongoing adjuvant placebo-controlled National Cancer Institute-Canada (NCIC)-MAP.17 trial cited under Subheading 3.2.

Exemestane's effect on excretion of pyridinoline, a marker of bone metabolism, was studied in a preclinical trial. In ovariectomized rats, exemestane was able to prevent increased pyridinoline excretion compared to non-ovariectomized rats by 96% ($p < 0.0001$ vs OVX control) *(152)*. Likewise, exemestane seems to have opposite effects of other aromatase inhibitors in terms of lipid metabolism. An EORTC companion study compared exemestane to tamoxifen in breast cancer patients. After a treatment period of 24 wk, exemestane had beneficial effects on triglycerides and a stabilizing effect on HDL and total cholesterol levels *(153)*. Overall, as an androgenic steroid, exemestane may be superior to other inhibitors in terms of side effects caused by estrogen depletion of other target tissues.

2.2.2. OTHER SIDE EFFECTS

Aside from their effects on hormone-sensitive tissues, hormonal agents have a number of nonendocrinologic side effects. These include toxicities such as skin rashes, gastrointestinal toxicity, and musculoskeletal disorders.

For example, a slightly increased risk of cataracts (RR 1.14, 95% CI 1.01–1.29) for women on tamoxifen was identified in the P-1 trial (65). Tamoxifen also significantly increased bothersome hot flashes and vaginal discharge, but this did not affect overall physical and emotional well being (154). The reported effects of tamoxifen on cognition are variable and depend on the parameters measured. Several ongoing studies are addressing this point.

In the MORE trial, raloxifene use was associated with a significantly higher rate of diabetes (0.5 vs 1.2%, $p =$ 0.009); levels of hemoglobin A_{1C} and the proportion of participants who began using insulin or oral hypoglycemic agents were the same in the two groups (70).

Clinical studies of other SERMs and SERDs have so far focused on parameters of efficacy; their tolerability cannot be assessed from published data.

Although a large body of data is available on aromatase inhibitors, their side-effect profiles reported from metastatic studies may not be applicable in the preventive setting. As yet, data from the adjuvant setting are available primarily on anastrozole (119). In the ATAC trial, investigators reported that anastrozole caused significantly fewer vasomotor symptoms than tamoxifen, although a parallel quality of life study by Fallowfield et al. did not confirm this (155). Incidences of cataracts, nausea/vomiting, fatigue, and mood disturbances were the same in both groups. For exemestane and letrozole, only data from studies in advanced breast cancer are available at present to ascertain their tolerability. In a first-line setting of a metastatic breast cancer study, exemestane induced fewer hot flashes and peripheral edema than tamoxifen. In terms of nausea and sweating, exemestane was also better tolerated than tamoxifen (156). When letrozole was compared to tamoxifen in advanced breast cancer, the two agents had similar tolerability with respect to nausea and hot flashes (116).

3. COMPLETED AND ONGOING CHEMOPREVENTION TRIALS

3.1. Completed Trials

In 1992, NSABP initiated the P-1 trial, in which women at increased risk for breast cancer were ran-

Table 3
Results of the NSABP P-1 Trial (65)

Type of Event	Placebo	Tamoxifen	Risk Ratio
Invasive breast cancer	175	89	0.51
Non-invasive breast cancer	69	35	0.50
Invasive endometrial cancer	15	36	2.53
Fractures	137	111	0.81
Stroke	24	38	1.59
Transient ischemic attack	25	19	0.76
Pulmonary embolism	6	18	3.01
Deep-vein thrombosis	22	35	1.60

domized to receive either tamoxifen (20 mg daily) or placebo for 5 yr (65). The average 5-yr risk of developing breast cancer in P-1 was 3.2%. When the P-1 trial was terminated in 1997, tamoxifen was found to have reduced the overall risk of invasive breast cancer by 49% ($p < 0.00001$). Cumulative breast cancer incidence rates in the two groups through 69 mo of follow-up were 43.4 vs 22.0 per 1000 women in the placebo and tamoxifen groups, respectively. The reduction in breast cancer incidence was confined to ER-positive tumors (69% less in the tamoxifen group), whereas noninvasive breast cancers (DCIS and lobular carcinoma in situ, LCIS) were reduced to the same extent as invasive cancers. The results of the P-1 trial are shown in Table 3 (65). Based on the data of P-1, on October 29, 1998, the FDA approved tamoxifen for reducing the incidence of breast cancer in women at high risk for the disease.

Two additional European trials have evaluated tamoxifen in breast cancer chemoprevention (67,68). Both failed to show any effect on breast cancer incidence. Tamoxifen's lack of effect on breast cancer incidence in the Italian trial (67) can be explained by the relatively small size compared to P-1 ($n = 5408$ vs 13,888), low-risk population (48.3% had had a bilateral oophorectomy and no specific risk factors were required) and limited compliance, with only 149 participants completing 5 yr of treatment. Interestingly, a subset analysis in this study showed a definite trend toward chemoprevention of breast cancer by tamoxifen in women taking concurrent HRT. In the UK trial (68), 2494 women received tamoxifen (20 mg orally) or placebo for up to 8 yr. Inclusion in this trial was based on a strong family history of breast cancer, a possible reason for differing results from the P-1 study.

Recently, preliminary results of the IBIS-1 trial were published *(66)*. In this study, more than 7000 women aged 35–65 yr with increased breast cancer risk or with specific changes seen on biopsy, such as LCIS, were randomized to tamoxifen or placebo. On average, women taking part in IBIS-1 had a fourfold increased risk of breast cancer, mostly because of a family history. After a median follow-up of 50 mo, incidence of newly diagnosed breast cancer was reduced by 33% ($p = 0.01$) in the tamoxifen arm. As in P-1, this reduction was confined to ER-positive tumors. The results were similar if age, nodal status, tumor size, and grading were taken into consideration. Importantly, a significant effect was also seen in women taking HRT during the trial (OR 0.73).

Data from all the prevention trials indicate that tamoxifen is able to reduce breast cancer incidence by approximately one-third to one-half in women at increased risk for the disease and that this effect is independent of age and HRT. Before the IBIS data were available, discrepancies between P-1 and the European trials were attributed to differences in inclusion criteria, particularly breast cancer risk at study entry and concomitant use of HRT. The results of IBIS-1, however, indicate that the difference in results most probably lies in the low number of person-years of follow-up and the low number of events in the European studies. The P-1 and IBIS trials are in line with the preclinical data and the Oxford overview, all indicating a chemopreventive effect of tamoxifen in breast cancer. It should be noted, however, that the effect of tamoxifen on overall or breast cancer-specific survival has not been ascertained by any of these trials.

3.2. Planned and Ongoing Trials

The encouraging results of the P-1 trial and data on breast cancer prevention by raloxifene from the MORE trial led NSABP to design and launch the STAR trial to directly compare the efficacy of the two agents in preventing breast cancer. A minimum age of 35 and postmenopausal status are required for study entry. Furthermore, participants must have a 5-yr risk of developing breast cancer of at least 1.67%, or a history of LCIS. The trial is designed to randomize a total of 22,000 women to either 20 mg of tamoxifen or 60 mg of raloxifene daily. The primary endpoint is breast cancer incidence; secondary endpoints include cardiovascular events and bone fractures. In addition, ancillary studies will look at cognitive function.

In the RUTH study, which has completed accrual of 10,011 postmenopausal women, breast cancer incidence

was added to cardiac disease as a second primary study end point. This trial is scheduled to report in 2005.

Positive preliminary results of the ATAC trial have triggered the IBIS-II study, in which anastrozole will be compared to placebo for prevention of breast cancer in women with increased risk. In the subgroup of women with a history of DCIS, anastrozole will be compared to tamoxifen. IBIS-II will prospectively evaluate risk factors for developing breast cancer, such as elevated serum estrogen levels, mammographic density, and presence of breast cancer susceptibility genes; ancillary studies will collect data on various categories of putative side effects.

The Clinical Trials Group of the National Cancer Institute of Canada (NCIC-CTG) is currently conducting a double-blind, multicenter proof-of-principle prevention trial (MAP.1) in which letrozole is compared to placebo in 120 women. This 1-yr study will include both healthy women and those with a past history of ER-positive breast cancer, and will evaluate letrozole's ability to reduce mammographic density in women with increased breast density (grade 4–6). The similarly designed MAP.2, launched in North America, compares exemestane to placebo in healthy postmenopausal women with moderate or high breast density. Ongoing pilot trials in women with breast cancer risk factors include a study of letrozole in women with preinvasive breast lesions and a study combining raloxifene with exemestane.

4. NEW BIOMARKERS AND COHORTS

The definition of "elevated breast cancer risk" for inclusion in the large breast cancer prevention trials of the 1990s was quite diverse among the studies. In the P-1 trial, inclusion was based on a 5-yr risk of breast cancer of at least 1.66% as calculated by the model of Gail et al. *(157)* (Fig. 1), age greater than 60 yr, or a history of LCIS *(65)*. Inclusion in the UK trial was based on a strong family history of breast cancer. No special risk factors were required for the Italian trial *(67,68)*. Differences in results of these trials were partly attributed to differing inclusion criteria, and it was concluded that the benefit of a SERM might vary according to individual risk factors. For example, several risk/benefit models of tamoxifen use have suggested that premenopausal women without a uterus and those with a higher risk of breast cancer benefit most from tamoxifen. Therefore, in a formal review by the American Society of Clinical Oncology (ASCO) Technology Assessment Group, tamoxifen use was not generally

- Age
- Age at menarche
- Number of first-degree relatives with breast cancer
- Nulliparity or age at first live birth
- Number of breast biopsies
- Pathologic diagnosis of atypical hyperplasia

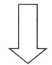

Five-Year Risk of Breast Cancer

Fig. 1. The breast cancer risk assessment tool of Gail et al. *(157)*.

recommended *(158)*. Our challenge is to identify women for chemopreventive therapies who will benefit most from that intervention. Future trials of novel SERMs would appropriately exclude women who did not experience a net health benefit in prior tamoxifen trials. In the IBIS II trial involving anastrozole, inclusion will not only be based on risk factors similar to those in the Gail model but also on mammographic density. Theoretically, all the factors known to be associated with elevated breast cancer risk can be used as surrogate markers for risk in prevention trials, both for inclusion criteria and as study end points. These clinical markers may also include a history of breast biopsies, prior radiation therapy to healthy breasts at a young age (for example, mantle field radiation for Hodgkin's disease) *(159)* and possibly all women taking prolonged HRT *(17)*. In addition, information gained from ductal lavage, fine-needle aspiration, or breast biopsy specimens can be used. Thus, any benign breast disease, loss of tumor suppressor genes, and activation of oncogenes as determined by DNA microarrays or increased expression of aromatase might be considered risk factors. Genetic risk factors that can be determined by blood analysis include not only the presence of BRCA1 or BRCA2 breast cancer susceptibility genes, but also certain genetic polymorphisms of estrogen metabolism. Measuring the genotype of estrogen metabolism might in fact be a more accurate method of determining exposure to endogenous estrogens.

5. CONSIDERATIONS FOR THE FUTURE

The proof of principle that breast cancer can be reduced by chemoprevention has been established by the demonstrated effects of tamoxifen. Both large tamoxifen trials and the recently reported WHI HRT study, however, have emphasized the need to determine the net health benefit and not just cancer prevention in therapeutic interventions in healthy individuals. From an efficacy standpoint, there is a need to improve on the achievements of tamoxifen as we enter the second generation of trials. In view of the apparent superiority of aromatase inhibitors over tamoxifen in ER-positive breast cancer treatment, this new class of agents may well be more effective than tamoxifen in reducing the occurrence of ER-positive breast cancer. Achieving a reduction in ER-negative tumors, however, is an important future goal as these tumors disproportionately account for breast cancer mortality. Combining antiestrogen agents with other potential cancer preventives may achieve these goals. For example, the cyclooxygenase (COX)-2 inhibitor celecoxib, recently approved for prevention of familial polyposis coli, has been shown to have antiproliferative effects on ER-negative breast cancer cells in vitro *(160)* and to act synergistically with the aromatase inhibitor exemestane in treatment and prevention of DMBA hormone-dependent tumors in vivo *(161)*. This combination will be tested as adjuvant therapy in early-stage breast cancer and holds promise as a chemopreventive combination. Other combinations with retinoids or retinomimetics, or other biologic pathway inhibitors, may likewise show synergism and reduction in ER-negative cancer.

Achieving a net health benefit must be the objective of cancer prevention. By virtue of their effects on estrogen-dependent tissues, hormonal agents have pleiotropic actions that need to be carefully balanced against cancer reduction. Prevention trials with tamoxifen have shown us that subsets of women are more vulnerable to benefits and toxicities, so more careful selection of women and agents with better therapeutic profiles are needed. Aromatase inhibitors are promising in this regard. They are likely to reduce all estrogen-dependent diseases, e.g., breast and endometrial cancer, and, lacking an estrogen agonist effect, are unlikely to cause uterine cancer or thromboembolism. Their drawback may be from effects of estrogen depletion on bone and lipid metabolism, cognitive function, and other end-organ functions. The nonsteroidal inhibitors are now being tested in early-stage breast cancer with bone-preserving agents in an attempt to overcome this problem. Exemestane may have inherent properties to protect against these effects, making it potentially the most promising novel agent in this regard.

Increasingly, markers of cumulative estrogen exposure, such as dense bones in postmenopausal women, are being recognized as predictors of breast cancer risk and general organ health. Most importantly, elevated levels of postmenopausal serum estrogen are predictive of breast cancer risk and of reduction of incidence by raloxifene, and low levels of estrogen have been associated with osteoporosis. There may be an ideal individual normal or "eu-estrogenic" state of health; titration of estrogen into an optimal therapeutic range in menopause may be the best strategy for women. Estrogen replacement therapy has been available for some time; the advent of aromatase agents makes the ability to reduce estrogen available. It is also known that the breast itself produces estrogen in an autocrine manner, creating a high breast-to-plasma ratio of estrogen. It has therefore been suggested that complete blockade of endogenous estrogen production, both peripherally and in the breast, followed by physiologic replacement of estrogen would be a way of affording normal estrogen delivery to most organs but reducing breast-specific estrogen and thereby breast cancer risk. These and other endocrine strategies will be the subject of a new generation of research studies attempting to reduce breast cancer risk and optimize women's health.

REFERENCES

1. Beatson G. On the treatment of inoperable cases of the mamma: suggestions for a new method of treatment with illustrative cases. *Lancet* 1896;2:104–107,162–165.
2. Pfaffenberger RS Jr, Kampert JB, Chang HG. Characteristics that predict risk of breast cancer before and after the menopause. *Am J Epidemiol* 1980;112:258–268.
3. Zhang Y, Kiel DP, Kreger BE, et al. Bone mass and the risk of breast cancer among postmenopausal women. *New Engl J Med* 1997;336:611–617.
4. Magnusson C, Baron J, Persson I, et al. Body size in different periods of life and breast cancer risk in post-menopausal women. *Int J Cancer* 1998;76:29–34.
5. Toniolo PG, Levitz M, Zeleniuch-Jacquotte A, et al. A prospective study of endogenous estrogens and breast cancer in postmenopausal women. *J Natl Cancer Inst* 1995;87:190–197.
6. Thomas HV, Key TJ, Allen DS, et al. A prospective study of endogenous serum hormone concentrations and breast cancer risk in post-menopausal women on the island of Guernsey. *Br J Cancer* 1997;76:401–405.
7. The Endogenous Hormones and Breast Cancer Collaborative Group. Endogenous sex hormones and breast cancer in postmenopausal women: reanalysis of nine prospective studies. *J Natl Cancer Inst* 2002;94(8):606–616.
8. Adlercreutz H, Gorbach SL, Goldin BR, et al. Estrogen metabolism and excretion in Oriental and Caucasian women. *J Natl Cancer Inst* 1994;86:1076–1082.
9. Schairer C, Lubin J, Troisi R, et al. Menopausal estrogen and estrogen-progestin replacement therapy and breast cancer risk. *JAMA* 2000;283:485–491.
10. Persson I, Weiderpass E, Bergkvist L, et al. Risks of breast and endometrial cancer after estrogen and estrogen-progestin replacement. *Cancer Causes Control* 1999;10:253–260.
11. Gapstur SM, Morrow M, Sellers TA. Hormone replacement therapy and risk of breast cancer with a favorable histology: results of the Iowa Women's Health Study. *JAMA* 1999;281:2091–2097.
12. Brinton LA, Brogan DR, Coates RJ, et al. Breast cancer risk among women under 55 years of age by joint effects of usage of oral contraceptives and hormone replacement therapy. *Menopause* 1998;5:145–151.
13. Titus-Ernstoff L, Longnecker MP, Newcomb PA, et al. Menstrual factors in relation to breast cancer risk. *Cancer Epidemiol Biomarkers Prev* 1998;7:783–789.
14. Henrich JB, Kornguth PJ, Viscoli CM, Horwitz RI. Postmenopausal estrogen use and invasive versus *in situ* breast cancer risk. *J Clin Epidemiol* 1998;51:1277–1283.
15. Magnusson C, Baron JA, Correia N, et al. Breast-cancer risk following long-term oestrogen- and oestrogen-progestin-replacement therapy. *Int J Cancer* 1999;81:339–344.
16. IARC Monographs on the Evaluation of Carcinogenic Risks to Humans. 1999: Hormonal Contraception and Postmenopausal Hormone Therapy 1999;72:474–530.
17. Writing Group for the Women's Health Initiative Investigators. Risks and benefits of estrogen plus progestin in healthy postmenopausal women: principal results from the Women's Health Initiative randomized controlled trial. *JAMA* 2002;288: 321–333.
18. Colditz GA. Relationship between estrogen levels, use of hormone replacement therapy, and breast cancer. *J Natl Cancer Inst* 1998;90:814–823.
19. Rohan TE, Miller AB. A cohort study of oral contraceptive use and risk of benign breast disease. *Int J Cancer* 1999;82: 191–196.
20. Marchbanks PA, McDonald JA, Wilson HG, et al. Oral contraceptives and the risk of breast cancer. *N Engl J Med* 2002; 346:2025–2032.
21. Kristensen VN, Andersen TI, Lindblom A, et al. A rare CYP19 (aromatase) variant may increase the risk of breast cancer. *Pharmacogenetics* 1998;8:43–48.
22. Siegelmann-Danieli N, Buetow KH. Constitutional genetic variation at the human aromatase gene (Cyp19) and breast cancer risk. *Br J Cancer* 1999;79:456–463.
23. Taioli E, Trachman J, Chen X, et al. A CYP1A1 restriction fragment length polymorphism is associated with breast cancer in African-American women. *Cancer Res* 1995;55: 3757–3758.
24. Ishibe N, Hankinson SE, Colditz GA, et al. Cigarette smoking, cytochrome P450 1A1 polymorphisms, and breast cancer risk in the Nurses' Health Study. *Cancer Res* 1998;58: 667–671.
25. Feigelson HS, Coetzee GA, Kolonel LN, et al. A polymorphism in the CYP17 gene increases the risk of breast cancer. *Cancer Res* 1997;57:1063–1065.
26. Lavigne JA, Helzlsouer KJ, Huang HY, et al. An association between the allele coding for a low activity variant of catechol-O-methyltransferase and the risk for breast cancer. *Cancer Res* 1997;57:5493–5497.
27. Thompson PA, Shields PG, Freudenheim JL, et al. Genetic polymorphisms in catechol-O-methyltransferase, menopausal status, and breast cancer risk. *Cancer Res* 1998;58:2107–2110.
28. Harvell DM, Strecker TE, Tochacek M, et al. Rat strain-specific actions of 17beta-estradiol in the mammary gland:

correlation between estrogen-induced lobuloalveolar hyperplasia and susceptibility to estrogen-induced mammary cancers. *Proc Natl Acad Sci USA* 2000;97:2779–2784.

29. Liehr JG, Fang WF, Sirbasku DA, Ari-Ulubelen A. Carcinogenicity of catechol estrogens in Syrian hamsters. *J Steroid Biochem* 1986;24:353–356.

30. Kirkman H. Hormone-related tumors in Syrian hamsters. *Prog Exp Tumor Res* 1972;16:201–240.

31. Li JJ, Li SA. Estrogen carcinogenesis in hamster tissues: role of metabolism. *Fed Proc* 1987;46:1858–1863.

32. Kirkman H. Estrogen-induced tumors of the kidney. III. Growth characteristics in the Syrian hamster. *Natl Cancer Inst Monogr* 1959;1:1–57.

33. Newbold RR, Liehr JG. Induction of uterine adenocarcinoma in CD-1 mice by catechol estrogens. *Cancer Res* 2000;60: 235–237.

34. Newbold RR, Bullock BC, McLachlan JA. Uterine adenocarcinoma in mice following developmental treatment with estrogens: a model for hormonal carcinogenesis. *Cancer Res* 1990;50:7677–7681.

35. Liehr JG, Gladek A, Macatee T, et al. DNA adduct formation in liver and kidney of male Syrian hamsters treated with estrogen and/or α-naphthoflavone. *Carcinogenesis* 1991;21: 385–389.

36. Liehr JG, Wheeler WJ. Inhibition of estrogen-induced renal carcinoma in Syrian hamsters by vitamin C. *Cancer Res* 1983;43:4638–4642.

37. National Institutes of Environmental Health Toxicology Program. Tenth Report on Carcinogens. Dept. of Health and Human Services, Washington DC, 2002.

38. Feigelson HS, Henderson BE. Estrogens and breast cancer. *Carcinogenesis* 1996;17:2279–2284.

39. Clarke RB, Howell A, Potten CS, Anderson E. Dissociation between steroid receptor expression and cell proliferation in the human breast. *Cancer Res* 1997;57(22):4987–4991.

40. Russo J, Ao X, Grill C, Russo IH. Pattern of distribution of cells positive for estrogen receptor alpha and progesterone receptor in relation to proliferating cells in the mammary gland. *Breast Cancer Res Treat* 1999;53:217–227.

41. Bocchinfuso WP, Hively WP, Couse JF, et al. A mouse mammary tumor virus-Wnt-1 transgene induces mammary gland hyperplasia and tumorigenesis in mice lacking estrogen receptor-alpha. *Cancer Res* 1999;59:1869–1876.

42. Cavalieri EL, Stack DE, Devanesan PD, et al. Molecular origin of cancer: catechol estrogen-3,4-quinones as endogenous tumor initiators. *Proc Natl Acad Sci USA* 1997;94: 10,937–10,942.

43. Wang MY, Liehr JG. Induction by estrogens of lipid peroxidation and lipid peroxide-derived malonaldehyde-DNA adducts in male Syrian hamsters: role of lipid peroxidation in estrogen-induced kidney carcinogenesis. *Carcinogenesis* 1995;16:1941–1945.

44. Banerjee SK, Banerjee S, Li SA, Li JJ. Induction of chromosome aberrations in Syrian hamster renal cortical cells by various estrogens. *Mutat Res* 1994;311:191–197.

45. Li JJ, Gonzalez A, Banerjee S, et al. Estrogen carcinogenesis in the hamster kidney: role of cytotoxicity and cell proliferation. *Environ Health Perspect* 1993;101(suppl 5):259–264.

46. Tsutsui T, Barret JC. Neoplastic transformation of cultured mammalian cells by estrogens and estrogenlike chemicals. *Environ Health Perspect* 1997;105:619–624.

47. Tsutsui T, Tamura Y, Hagiwara M, et al. Induction of mammalian cell transformation and genotoxicity by 2-

methoxyestradiol, an endogenous metabolite of estrogen. *Carcinogenesis* 2000;21:735–740.

48. Li JJ, Hou X, Banerjee SK, et al. Overexpression and amplification of c-myc in the Syrian hamster kidney during estrogen carcinogenesis: a probable critical role in neoplastic transformation. *Cancer Res* 1999;59:2340–2346.

49. Russo J, Lareef MH, Tahin Q, et al. 17-β-estradiol is carcinogenic in human breast epithelial cells. *J Steroid Biochem Mol Biol* 2002;1656:1–17.

50. Kong LY, Szaniszlo P, Albrecht T, Liehr JG. Frequency and molecular analysis of hprt mutations induced by estradiol in Chinese hamster V79 cells. *Int J Oncol* 2000;17:1141–1149.

51. Lengauer C, Kinzler KW, Vogelstein B. Genetic instabilities in human cancers. *Nature* 1998;396:643–649.

52. Bulun SE, Price TM, Mahendroo MS, et al. A link between breast cancer and local estrogen biosynthesis suggested by quantification of breast adipose tissue aromatase cytochrome P450 transcripts using competitive polymerase chain reaction after reverse transcription. *J Clin Endocrinol Metab* 1993;77:1622–1628.

53. Harada N. Aberrant expression of aromatase in breast cancer tissues. *J Steroid Biochem Mol Biol* 1997;61:175–184.

54. James VHT, McNeill JM, Lai LC, et al. Aromatase activity in normal breast and breast tumor tissues: in vivo and in vitro studies. *Steroids* 1987;50:269–279.

55. Miller WR, O'Neill J. The importance of local synthesis of estrogen within the breast. *Steroids* 1987;50:537–548.

56. Miller WR, Mullen P, Sourdaine P, et al. Regulation of aromatase activity within the breast. *J Steroid Biochem Mol Biol* 1997;61:193–202.

57. Brodie A, Lu Q, Liu Y, Long B. Aromatase inhibitors and their antitumor effects in model systems. *Endocr Relat Cancer* 1999;6:205–210.

58. Tekmal RR, Ramachandra N, Gubba S, et al. Overexpression of *int-5/aromatase* in mammary glands of transgenic mice results in the induction of hyperplasia and nuclear abnormalities. *Cancer Res* 1996;56:3180–3185.

59. Tekmal RR, Kirma N, Gill K, et al. Aromatase overexpression and breast hyperplasia, an in vivo model–continued overexpression of aromatase is sufficient to maintain hyperplasia without circulating estrogens, and aromatase inhibitors abrogate these preneoplastic changes in mammary glands. *Endocr Relat Cancer* 1999;6:307–314.

60. Santner SJ, Pauley RJ, Tait L, et al. Aromatase activity and expression in breast cancer and benign breast tissue stromal cells. *J Clin Endocrinol Metab* 1997;82:200–208.

61. Jin T, Zhang X, Li H, Goss PE. Characterization of a novel silencer element in the human aromatase gene PII promoter. *Breast Cancer Res Treat* 2000;62:151–159.

62. Fisher B, Costantino J, Redmond C, et al. A randomized clinical trial evaluating tamoxifen in the treatment of patients with node-negative breast cancer who have estrogen-receptor-positive tumors. *N Engl J Med* 1989;320: 479–484.

63. Breast Cancer Trials Committee, Scottish Cancer Trials Office (MRC), Edinburgh. Adjuvant tamoxifen in the management of operable breast cancer: The Scottish Trial. *Lancet* 1987;2:171–175.

64. Early Breast Cancer Trialists' Collaborative Group. Systemic treatment of early breast cancer by hormonal, cytotoxic, or immune therapy: 133 randomised trials involving 31000 recurrences and 24000 deaths among 75000 women. *Lancet* 1992;339:1–15, 71–78.

65. Fisher B, Costantino J, Wickerham L, et al. Tamoxifen for prevention of breast cancer: report of the National Surgical Adjuvant Breast and Bowel Project P-1. *J Natl Cancer Inst* 1998;90:1371–1388.

66. Cuzick J. The prevention of breast cancer. Program and abstracts of the 3rd European Breast Cancer Conference, March 19–23, 2002; Barcelona, Spain.

67. Veronesi U, Maisonneuve P, Costa A, et al. Prevention of breast cancer with tamoxifen: preliminary findings from the Italian randomised trial among hysterectomised women. Italian Tamoxifen Prevention Study. *Lancet* 1998;352:93–97.

68. Powles T, Eeles R, Ashley S, et al. Interim analysis of the incidence of breast cancer in the Royal Marsden Hospital tamoxifen randomised chemoprevention trial. *Lancet* 1998;352:98–101.

69. Fisher B, Dignam J, Wolmark N, et al. Tamoxifen in treatment of intraductal breast cancer: National Surgical Adjuvant Breast and Bowel Project B-24 randomised controlled trial. *Lancet* 1999;353:1993–2000.

70. Cummings R, Eckert S, Krueger K, et al. The effect of raloxifene on risk of breast cancer in postmenopausal women. Results from the MORE randomized trial. *JAMA* 1999;281:2189–2197.

71. Jordan VC, Glusman, JE, Eckert S, et al. Raloxifene reduces incident primary breast cancer: integrated data from multicenter, double-blind, placebo-controlled, randomized trials in postmenopausal women. *Breast Cancer Res Treat* 1998;50:227 (abstr 2).

72. Cummings SR, Duong T, Kenyon E, et al. Serum estradiol level and risk of breast cancer during treatment with raloxifene. The Multiple Outcomes of Raloxifene Evaluation (MORE) Trial. *JAMA* 2002;287:1528.

73. Pink JJ, Jordan VC. Models of estrogen receptor regulation by estrogen and antiestrogens in breast cancer cell lines. *Cancer Res* 1996;56:2321–2330.

74. Parker MG. Action of "pure" antiestrogens in inhibiting estrogen receptor action. *Breast Cancer Res Treat* 1993;26:131–137.

75. Dauvois S, White R, Parker MG. The antiestrogens ICI 182,780 disrupts estrogen receptor nucleocytoplasmic shuttling. *J Cell Sci* 1993;106:1377–1388.

76. Coopman P, Garcia M, Brunner N, et al. Anti-proliferative and anti-estrogenic effects of ICI 164,384 and ICI 182,780 in 4-OH-tamoxifen resistant human breast cancer cells. *Int J Cancer* 1994;56:295–300.

77. Hu XF, Veroni M, de Luise M, et al. Circumvention of tamoxifen resistance by the pure anti-estrogen ICI 182,780. *Int J Cancer* 1993;55:873–876.

78. Osborne CK, Pippen J, Jones SE, et al. Double-blind, randomized trial comparing the efficacy and tolerability of fulvestrant versus anastrozole in postmenopausal women with advanced breast cancer progressing on prior endocrine therapy: results of a North American trial. *J Clin Oncol* 2002;20:3386–3395.

79. Howell A, Robertson JF, Quaresma Albano J, et al. Fulvestrant, formerly ICI 182,780, is as effective as anastrozole in postmenopausal women with advanced breast cancer progressing after prior endocrine treatment. *J Clin Oncol* 2002;20:3396–3403.

80. Howell A, Robertson JFR, Albano JQ, et al. Comparison of efficacy and tolerability of Faslodex (ICI 182,780) with Arimidex (anastrozole) in postmenopausal women with

advanced breast cancer—preliminary results. *Breast Cancer Res Treat* 2000;64:27 (abstr 6).

81. Gutman M, Couillard S, Roy J, et al. Comparison of the effects of EM-652 (SCH57068), tamoxifen, toremifene, droloxifene, idoxifene, GW-5638 and raloxifene on the growth of human ZR-75-1 breast tumors in nude mice. *Int J Cancer* 2002;99:273–278.

82. Martel C, Picard S, Richard V, et al. Prevention of bone loss by EM-800 and raloxifene in the ovariectomized rat. *J Steroid Biochem Mol Biol* 2000;74:45–56.

83. Labrie F, Labrie C, Belanger A, et al. EM-652 (SCH57068), a pure SERM having complete antiestrogenic activity in the mammary gland and endometrium. *Steroid Biochem Mol Biol* 2001;79:213–225.

84. Cohen LA, Pittman B, Wang, CX, et al. LAS, a novel selective estrogen receptor modulator with chemopreventive and therapeutic activity in the *N*-nitroso-*N*-methylurea-induced rat mammary tumor model. *Cancer Res* 2001;61:8683–8688.

85. Suh N, Glasebrook AL, Palkowitz AD, et al. Arzoxifene, a new selective estrogen receptor modulator for chemoprevention of experimental breast cancer. *Cancer Res* 2001;61:8412–8415.

86. Shibata J, Toko T, Saito H, et al. Estrogen agonistic/antagonistic effects of miproxifene phosphate (TAT-59). *Cancer Chemother Pharmacol* 2000;45:133–141.

87. Noguchi S, Koyama H, Nomura Y, et al. Late Phase II study of TAT-59 (new antiestrogen) in advanced or recurrent breast cancer patient: a double-blind comparative study with tamoxifen citrate. *Breast Cancer Res Treat* 1998;50:307 (abstr 446).

88. Buzdar A, Hyes D, El-Khoudary A, et al. Phase III randomized trial of droloxifene and tamoxifen as first-line endocrine treatment of ER/PgR-positive advanced beast cancer. *Breast Cancer Res Treat* 2002;73:161–175.

89. Brzezinski A, Debi A. Phytoestrogens: the "natural" selective estrogen receptor modulators? *Eur J Obstet Gynecol Reprod Biol* 1999;85:47–51.

90. Serraino M, Thompson LU. The effect of flaxseed supplementation on the initiation and promotional stages of mammary tumorigenesis. *Nutr Cancer* 1992;17:153–159.

91. Hirano T, Fukuoka K, Oka K, et al. Antiproliferative activity of mammalian lignan derivatives against the human breast carcinoma cell line, ZR-75-1. *Cancer Invest* 1990;8:595–602.

92. Thompson LU, Rickard SE, Orcheson LJ, Seidl MM. Flaxseed and its lignan and oil components reduce mammary tumor growth at a late stage of carcinogenesis. *Carcinogenesis* 1996;17:1373–1376.

93. Haggans CJ, Hutchins AM, Olson BA, et al. Effect of flaxseed consumption on urinary estrogen metabolites in postmenopausal women. *Nutr Cancer* 1999;33:188–195.

94. Phipps WR, Martini MC, Lampe JW, et al. Effect of flax seed ingestion on the menstrual cycle. *J Clin Endocrinol Metab* 1993;77:1215–1219.

95. Hutchins AM, Martini MC, Olson BA, et al. Flaxseed consumption influences endogenous hormone concentrations in post-menopausal women. *Nutr Cancer* 2001;39:58–65.

96. Goss PE, Li T, Theriault M, et al. Effects of dietary flaxseed in women with cyclical mastalgia. *Breast Cancer Res Treat* 2000;64:49 (abstr 153).

97. Goss PE, Thompson LU. The effects of dietary flaxseed on mammographic density. *Breast Cancer Res Treat* 2001;69:223 (abstr 125).

98. Thompson L, Li T, Chen J, Goss PE. Biological effects of dietary flaxseed in patients with breast cancer. *Breast Cancer Res Treat* 2000;64:50 (abstr 157).

99. Lamartiniere CA, Moore JB, Brown NM, et al. Genistein suppresses mammary cancer in rats. *Carcinogenesis* 1995; 16:2833–2840.

100. Hawrylewicz EJ, Zapata JJ, Blair WH. Soy and experimental cancer: animal studies. *J Nutr* 1995;125(Suppl 3): 698–708.

101. Gallo D, Giacomelli S, Cantelmo F, et al. Chemoprevention of DMBA-induced mammary cancer in rats by dietary soy. *Breast Cancer Res Treat* 2001;69:153–164.

102. Ju YH, Allred CD, Allred KF, et al. Physiological concentrations of dietary genistein dose-dependently stimulate growth of estrogen-dependent human breast cancer (MCF-7) tumors implanted in athymic nude mice. *J Nutr* 2001;131:2957–2962.

103. Allred CD, Ju YH, Allred KF, et al. Dietary genistein stimulates growth of estrogen-dependent breast cancer tumors similar to that observed with genistein. *Carcinogenesis* 2001;22:1667–1673.

104. Allred CD, Allred KF, Ju YH, et al. Soy diets containing varying amounts of genistein stimulate growth of estrogen-dependent (MCF-7) tumors in a dose-dependent manner. *Cancer Res* 2001;61:5045–5050.

105. de Lemos ML. Effects of soy phytoestrogens genistein and daidzein on breast cancer growth. *Ann Pharmacother* 2001;35:1118–1121.

106. Jones JL, Daley BJ, Enderson BL, et al. Genistein inhibits tamoxifen effects on cell proliferation and cell cycle arrest in T47D breast cancer cells. *Am Surg* 2002;68:575–577.

107. Ju YH, Doerge DR, Allred KF, et al. Dietary genistein negates the inhibitory effect of tamoxifen on growth of estrogen-dependent human breast cancer (MCF-7) cells implanted in athymic mice. *Cancer Res* 2002;62:2474–2477.

108. Lamartiniere CA, Cotroneo MS, Fritz WA, et al. Genistein chemoprevention: timing and mechanisms of action in murine mammary and prostate. *J Nutr* 2002;132: 552S–558S.

109. Kumar NB, Cantor A, Allen K, et al. The specific role of isoflavones on estrogen metabolism in premenopausal women. *Cancer* 2002;94:1166–1174.

110. Shu XO, Jin F, Dai Q. Soyfood intake during adolescence and subsequent risk of breast cancer among Chinese women. *Cancer Epidemiol Biomarkers Prev* 2001;10:483-488.

111. Shanghai Dai Q, Shu XO, Jin F. Population-based case-control study of soyfood intake and breast cancer risk. *Br J Cancer* 2001;85:372–378.

112. Horn-Ross PL, John EM, Lee M. Phytoestrogen consumption and breast cancer risk in a multiethnic population: the Bay Area Breast Cancer Study. *Am J Epidemiol* 2001; 154: 434–441.

113. Goss PE, Strasser K. Aromatase inhibitors in the treatment and prevention of breast cancer. *J Clin Oncol* 2001;19: 881–894.

114. Nabholtz JM, Buzdar A, Pollak M. Anastrozole is superior to tamoxifen as first-line therapy for advanced breast cancer in postmenopausal women: results of a North American multi-center randomized trial. Arimidex Study Group. *J Clin Oncol* 2000;18:3758–3767.

115. Bonneterre J, Buzdar A, Nabholtz JM, et al. Arimidex Writing Committee. Anastrozole is superior to tamoxifen as first-line therapy in hormone receptor positive advanced breast carcinoma. Investigators Committee Members. *Cancer* 2001;92:2247–2258.

116. Mouridsen H, Gershanovich M, Sun Y, et al. Superior efficacy of letrozole versus tamoxifen as first-line therapy for postmenopausal women with advanced breast cancer: results of a Phase III study of the International Letrozole Breast Cancer Group. *J Clin Oncol* 2001;19:2596–2606.

117. Dirix L, Piccart MJ, Lohrisch C, et al. Efficacy of and tolerance to exemestane (E) versus tamoxifen (T) in 1st line hormone therapy (HT) of postmenopausal metastatic breast cancer (MBC) patients (pts): a European Organisation for the Research and Treatment of Cancer (EORTC Breast Group) Phase II trial with Pharmacia and Upjohn. *Proc Am Soc Clin Oncol* 2001;20:29a (abstr 114).

118. Miller WR, Dixon JM. Local endocrine effects of aromatase inhibitors within the breast. *J Steroid Biochem Mol Biol* 2001;79:93–102.

119. The ATAC Trialists' Group. Arimidex, tamoxifen alone or in combination. Anastrozole alone or in combination with tamoxifen versus tamoxifen alone for adjuvant treatment of postmenopausal women with early breast cancer: first results of the ATAC randomised trial. *Lancet* 2002;359:2131–2139.

120. Gunson DE, Steele RE, Chau RY. Prevention of spontaneous tumours in female rats by fadrozole hydrochloride, an aromatase inhibitor. *Br J Cancer* 1995;72:72–75.

121. Moon RC, Steele VE, Kelloff GJ, et al. Chemoprevention of MNU-induced mammary tumorigenesis by hormone response modifiers: toremifene, RU 16117, tamoxifen, aminoglutethimide and progesterone. *Anticancer Res* 1994;14:889–894.

122. De Coster R, Van Ginckerl RF, Callens MJ, et al. Antitumoral and endocrine effects of (+)-vorozole in rats bearing dimethylbenzanthracene-induced mammary tumors. *Cancer Res* 1992;52:1240–1244.

123. Lubet RA, Steele VE, Casebolt TL, et al. Chemopreventive effects of the aromatase inhibitors vorozole (R-83842) and 4-hydroxyandrostenedione in the methylnitrosourea (MNU)-induced mammary tumor model in Sprague-Dawley rats. *Carcinogenesis* 1994;15:2775–2780.

124. Schieweck K, Bhatnagar AS, Matter A. CGS 16949A, a new nonsteroidal aromatase inhibitor: effects on hormone-dependent and -independent tumors in vivo. *Cancer Res* 1988;48:834–838.

125. Schieweck K, Bhatnagar AS, Batzl C, et al. Anti-tumor and endocrine effects of non-steroidal aromatase inhibitors on estrogen-dependent rat mammary tumors. *J Steroid Biochem Mol Biol* 1993;44:633–636.

126. Bhatnagar AS, Hausler A, Schieweck K, et al. Highly selective inhibition of estrogen biosynthesis by CGS 20267, a new non-steroidal aromatase inhibitor. *J Steroid Biochem Mol Biol* 1990;31:1021–1027.

127. Early Breast Cancer Trialists' Collaborative Group. Tamoxifen for early breast cancer: an overview of the randomised trials. *Lancet* 1998;351:1451–1467.

128. Chlebowski RT, Collyar DE, Somerfield MR, et al. American Society of Clinical Oncology technology assessment on breast cancer risk reduction strategies: tamoxifen and raloxifene. *J Clin Oncol* 1999;17:1939–1955.

129. McDonald CC, Alexander FE, Whyte BW, et al. Cardiac and vascular morbidity in women receiving adjuvant tamoxifen for breast cancer in a randomised trial: the Scottish Cancer Trials Breast Group. *Br Med J* 1995;311:977–980.

130. McDonald CC, Stewart HJ. Fatal myocardial infarction in the Scottish adjuvant tamoxifen trial: The Scottish Breast Cancer Committee. *Br Med J* 1991;303:435–437.

131. Costantino JP, Kuller LH, Ives DG, et al. Coronary heart disease mortality and adjuvant tamoxifen therapy. *J Natl Cancer Inst* 1997;89:776–782.

132. Ruqvist LE, Matteson A. Cardiac and thromboembolic morbidity among postmenopausal women with early-stage breast cancer in a randomized trial of adjuvant tamoxifen: The Stockholm Breast Cancer Study Group. *J Natl Cancer Inst* 1993;85:1398–1406.

133. Love RR, Barden HS, Mazess RB, et al. Effect of tamoxifen on lumbar spine bone mineral density in postmenopausal women after 5 years. *Arch Intern Med* 1994;154:2585–2588.

134. Love RR, Mazess RB, Barden HS, et al. Effects of tamoxifen on bone mineral density in postmenopausal women with breast cancer. *N Engl J Med* 1992;326:852–856.

135. Love RR, Mazess RB, Torney DC, et al. Bone mineral density in women with breast cancer treated with adjuvant tamoxifen for at least two years. *Breast Cancer Res Treat* 1998;12:297–302.

136. Chittacharoen A, Theppisai U, Manonai J. Transvaginal color Doppler sonographic evaluation of the uterus in postmenopausal women on daily raloxifene therapy. *Climacteric* 2002;5:156–159.

137. Delmas PD, Bjarnasan NG, Mitlak BH, et al. Effects of raloxifene on bone mineral density, serum cholesterol concentrations, and uterine endometrium in postmenopausal women. *N Engl J Med* 1997;337:1641–1647.

138. Boss SM, Huster WJ, Neild JA, et al. Effects of raloxifene hydrochloride on the endometrium of postmenopausal women. *Am J Obstet Gynecol* 1997;177:1458–1464.

139. Draper MW, Flowers DE, Huster WJ, et al. A controlled trial of raloxifene (LY13948I) HCl: impact on bone turnover and serum lipid profile in healthy postmenopausal women. *J Bone Mineral Res* 1996;11:835–842.

140. Walsh BW, Kuller LH, Wild RA, et al. Effects of raloxifene on serum lipids and coagulation factors in healthy postmenopausal women. *JAMA* 1998;279:1445–1485.

141. Mosca L. Rationale and overview of the Raloxifene Use for the Heart (RUTH) trial. *Ann NY Acad Sci* 2001;949:181–185.

142. Glusman JE, Huster WJ, Paul S. Raloxifene effects on vasomotor and other climacteric symptoms in postmenopausal women. *Prim Care Update Ob Gyns* 1998;5:166.

143. Picard F, Deshaies Y, Lalonde J, et al. Effects of the estrogen antagonist EM-652.HCl on energy balance and lipid metabolism in ovariectomized rats. *Int J Obes Relat Metab Disord* 2000;24:830–840.

144. Dardes RC, Bentrem D, O'Regan RM, et al. Effects of the new selective estrogen receptor modulator LY353381.HCl (Arzoxifene) on human endometrial cancer growth in athymic mice. *Clin Cancer Res* 2001;7:4149–4155.

145. Galbiati E, Caruso PL, Amari G, et al. Effects of 3-phenyl-4-[[4-[2-(1-piperidinyl)ethoy]phenyl]methyl]-2H-1-benzopyran-7-ol (CHF4056), a novel nonsteroidal estrogen agonist/antagonist, on reproductive and nonreproductive tissue. *J Pharmacol Exp Ther* 2002;300:802–809.

146. Greenberger LM, Annable T, Collins I, et al. A new antiestrogen, 2-(4-hydroxy-phenyl)-3-methyl-1-[4-(2-piperidin-1-yl-ethoxy)-benzyl]-1H-indol-5-ol hydrochloride (ERA-923), inhibits the growth of tamoxifen-sensitive and-resistant tumors and is devoid of uterotrophic effects in mice and rats. *Clin Cancer Res* 2001;7:3166–3177.

147. Dewar J, Nabholtz J-MA, Monneterre J, et al. The effect of anastrozole (Arimidex™) on serum lipids—data from a randomized comparison of anastrozole (AN) vs tamoxifen (TAM) in postmenopausal (PM) women with advanced breast cancer (ABC). *Breast Cancer Res Treat* 2000;64:51 (abstr 164).

148. Heshmati HM, Khosla S, Robins SP, et al. Endogenous residual estrogen levels determine bone resorption even in late postmenopausal women. *J Bone Mineral Res* 1997;12:S121 (abstr 76).

149. Harper-Wynne C, Ross G, Sacks N, Dowsett M. A pilot prevention study of the aromatase inhibitor letrozole: effects on breast cell proliferation and bone/lipid indices in healthy postmenopausal women. *Breast Cancer Res Treat* 2001;69:225 (abstr 136).

150. Harper-Wynne C, Ross G, Sacks N, et al. Effects of the aromatase inhibitor letrozole on normal breast epithelial cell proliferation and metabolic indices in postmenopausal women: a pilot study for breast cancer prevention. *Cancer Epidemiol Biomarkers Prev* 2002;11:614–621.

151. Elisaf MS, Bairaktari ET, Nicolaides C, et al. Effect of letrozole on the lipid profile in postmenopausal women with breast cancer. *Eur J Cancer* 2001;37:1510–1513.

152. Goss PE, Grynpas M, Qi S, Hu H. The effects of exemestane on bone and lipids in the ovariectomized rat. *Breast Cancer Res Treat*, 2001;69:224 (abstr 132).

153. Lohrisch C, Paridaens R, Dirix LY. No adverse impact on serum lipids of the irreversible aromatase inactivator Aromasin® (exemestane [E]) in 1st line treatment of metastatic breast cancer (MBC): companion study to a European Organization of Research and Treatment of Cancer (Breast Group) Trial with Pharmacias' Upjohn. *Proc Am Soc Clin Oncol* 2001;20:43a (abstr 167).

154. Day R, Ganz PA, Costatino JP, et al. Health-related quality of life and tamoxifen in breast cancer prevention: a report from the National Surgical Adjuvant Breast and Bowel Project P-1 Study. *J Clin Oncol* 1999;17:2659–2669.

155. Fallowfield L and ATAC Trialists' Group. Assessing the quality of life (QOL) of postmenopausal (PM) women randomized into the ATAC ("Arimidex", tamoxifen, alone or in combination) adjuvant breast cancer (BC) trial. *Proc Am Soc Clin Oncol* 2002;21:40a (abstr 159).

156. Paridaens R, Dirix L, Beex L, et al. Promising results with exemestane in the first-line treatment of metastatic breast cancer: a randomized phase II EORTC trial with a tamoxifen control. *Clin Breast Cancer* 2000;1(Suppl 1):S19–S21.

157. Gail MH, Brinton LA, Byar DP, et al. Projecting individualized probabilities of developing breast cancer for white females who are being examined annually. *J Natl Cancer Inst* 1989;81:1879–1886.

158. Chlebowski RT, Col N, Winer EP. American Society of Clinical Oncology technology assessment of pharmacologic interventions for breast cancer risk reduction including tamoxifen, raloxifene, and aromatase inhibitors. *J Clin Oncol* 2002;20:3328–3343.

159. Goss PE, Sierra S. Current perspectives on radiation-induced breast cancer. *J Clin Oncol* 1998;16:338–347.

160. Arun B, Zhang H, Mirza NQ, et al. Growth inhibition of breast cancer cells by celecoxib. *Breast Cancer Res Treat* 2001;69:234 (abstr 171).

161. Pesenti E, Masferrer JL, di Salle E. Effect of exemestane and celecoxib alone or in combination on DMBA-induced mammary carcinoma in rats. *Breast Cancer Res Treat* 2001;69:288 (abstr 445).

COLORECTAL

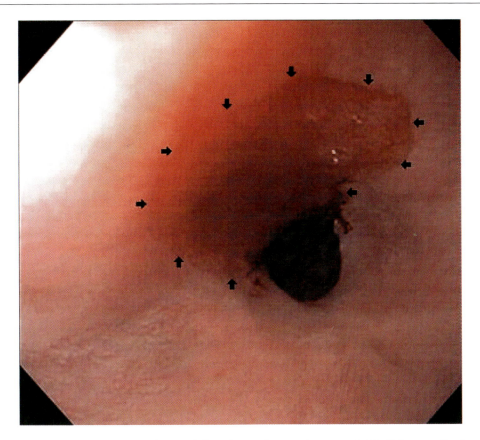

Color Plate 5, Fig. 1. (*see* discussion in Ch. 26 on p. 343 and complete caption on p. 344). Columnar-lined mucosa in Barrett's esophagus.

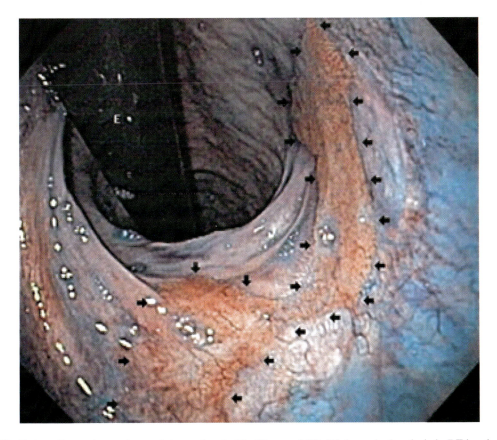

Color Plate 5, Fig. 3. (*see* discussion and complete caption in Ch. 26 on p. 347). High-grade dysplasia in BE by chromoendoscopy.

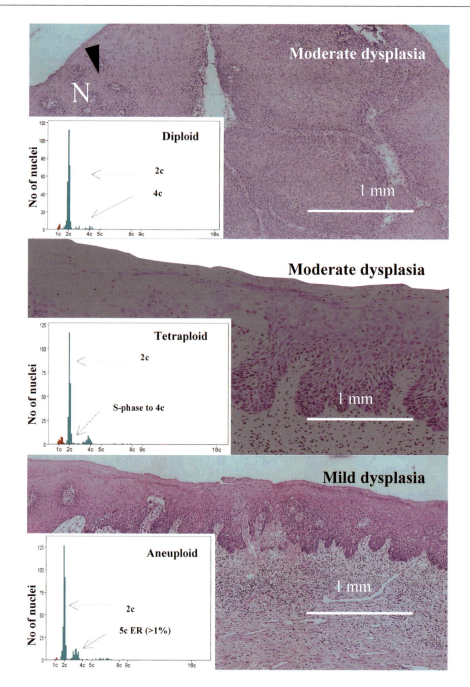

Color Plate 6, Fig. 4. (*see* discussion in Ch. 29 on p. 388 and complete caption on p. 389). Moderate (**top, middle**) and mild (**lower**) dysplasia: DNA ploidy and histological findings. With permission.

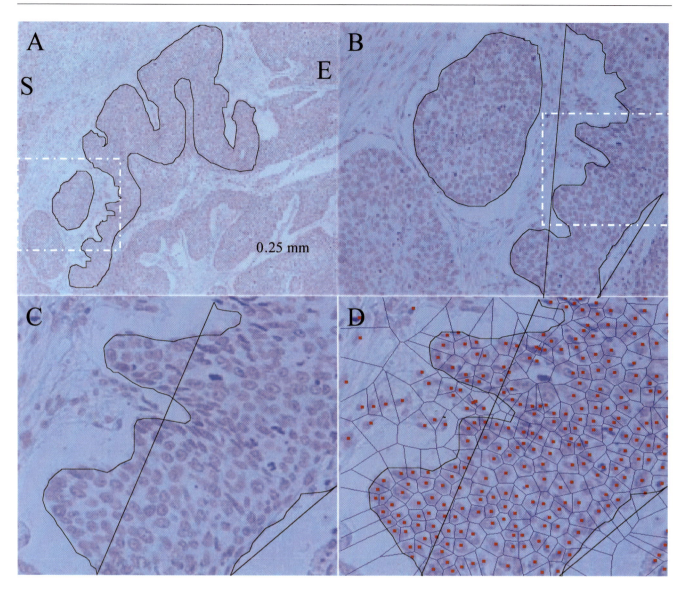

Color Plate 7, Fig. 6. (*see* discussion in Ch. 29 on pp. 391–392 and full caption on p. 392). Voronoi diagrams used to quantify cellular interactions in tissues.

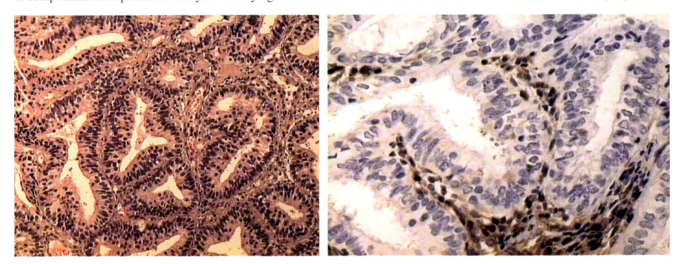

| Specimen Number: | 99-4312 |
| Patient name: | Smith-Jensen |

Input parameters:

Volume % Stroma: 43
S.D. short nuclear axis: 1.3
Outer surface density: 14 mm_ per mm_

D-Score: - 0.6

Progression risk   HIGH   UNCERTAIN   LOW

D-score :   -2.00   0.00   1.00   4.00

Present Case

Results:

Conclusion: Risk on progression to cancer is high

Color Plate 8, Fig. 1. (*see* full caption and discussion in Ch. 34 on p. 465). Routine laboratory presentation to requesting clinician of computerized morphometric analysis identifying a multivariate combination of architectural and nuclear features (DS).

Color Plate 8, Fig. 2. (*see* discussion in Ch. 34 on pp. 465–466 and full caption on p. 466). Endometrial epithelial neoplasia reported by DS as high risk.

20 Chemoprevention of Colorectal Cancer

Clinical Strategies

Monica M. Bertagnolli, MD and Stanley R. Hamilton, MD

CONTENTS

1. THE MAGNITUDE OF THE PROBLEM

It is a disturbing reality that one of the most preventable cancers is also one of the most common and deadly. Worldwide, approx 950,000 people are diagnosed with colorectal cancer (CRC) each year, and deaths from CRC number almost 500,000 per year *(1)*. The prevalence of this disease is disproportionately highest in more-developed countries, which account for 20% of the world's population but 64% of CRC cases and 60% of deaths due to the disease *(2)*. Because CRC produces few, if any, symptoms until the disease is advanced, 35% of newly diagnosed cases already exhibit regional lymph node metastases, and 20% of new cases are stage IV, representing incurable disease *(3)*. Data from migratory populations suggest that adaptation to a lifestyle characteristic of developed Western nations is associated with increased CRC incidence. For example, colon cancer incidence in Japanese men and women who have been lifetime residents of the United States now exceeds that of the US white population *(3)*. In addition, the incidence of CRC in Japan has increased over the past 25 yr in concert with Westernization and is presently equivalent to that of Western Europe *(3)*. These observations support a strong environmental role in CRC development and suggest that the problem is likely to increase as Western cultural and dietary influences expand.

Despite these grim figures, it may be possible to achieve great improvements in CRC incidence and outcome with tools presently at our disposal. Substantial data support the hypothesis that CRC develops by progression of an initiated cell through a visible adenoma stage *(4)*. Most importantly, strong data indicate that removal of these precursor lesions by endoscopic polypectomy decreases cancer risk *(5)*. From early tumor initiation to emergence of an invasive phenotype is typically a long interval, estimated at 15–25 yr in an individual with intact DNA repair capability. It is increasingly clear that administration of chemopreventive agents to individuals at risk for adenoma formation can prevent these tumors, and theoretically also reduce cancer incidence in this population. Finally, improved awareness and understanding of heritable contributions to CRC will allow specific interventions to target at-risk populations.

Improvement in CRC mortality will require intervention at all stages of tumor formation. Primary prevention of CRC is defined as an intervention that reduces the risk of incident CRC *(6)*. Secondary prevention involves discovering cancers at an early, readily curable stage. Tertiary prevention generally involves interventions

From: Cancer Chemoprevention, Volume 2: Strategies for Cancer Chemoprevention
Edited by: G. J. Kelloff, E. T. Hawk, and C. C. Sigman © Humana Press Inc., Totowa, NJ

Table 1
Genetic Changes Associated With CRC Development

Genetic change	Effect on associated protein	Effect on cell behavior
APC mutation	Loss of APC-facilitated degradation of β-catenin	Increased expression of oncoproteins such as c-myc, cyclin D1, PPARs, MMP7
K-*ras* mutation	Constitutive activation of MAP kinase pathway	Increased cell proliferation
TP53 mutation	Loss of p53 protein or increased expression of abnormal p53	Increased cell survival and genetic instability
SMAD-4 loss	Inability to initiate gene transcription in response to TGF-β	Loss of response to growth control by TGF-β
h*MSH2*, h*MLH1* mutation	Loss of mismatch repair protein expression	Inability to repair DNA mismatches contributing to loss of function of genes such as TGFβR-II (growth suppressor) or BAX (apoptosis inducer)
Promoter hypermethylation with transcriptional silencing	Loss of protein expression	Loss of important growth regulators such as APC, p16, IGF2, MyoD, or estrogen receptor; or creation of mismatch repair deficiency due to loss of hMLH1

that reduce cancer morbidity and/or increase lifespan for individuals with more advanced disease. The focus of this review is primary prevention of CRC. Specifically, this chapter will address anticancer strategies that use dietary or pharmacologic agents to prevent or reverse premalignant colorectal lesions.

2. CRC BIOLOGY: CHARACTERISTICS OF EARLY NEOPLASIA

Colorectal carcinogenesis is the process during which epithelial cells in the large bowel acquire the characteristics of malignant behavior, which are defined, at a minimum, by the ability to invade the underlying basement membrane. This multifactoral process involves the accumulation of alterations in DNA structure that contribute to loss of normal controls over cell proliferation and migratory capacity (Table 1).

Studies of persons at risk for colorectal neoplasia suggest that early tumor-associated phenotypic changes in colorectal cells include increased colonocyte proliferation (7,8), reduced colonocyte apoptosis (9,10), and altered expression of mucosal differentiation markers (11,12). These changes are found in persons with genetic predisposition for CRC and in those who have dietary risk factors such as high fat and low calcium intake (12–15). The specificity of these tissue characteristics for colorectal tumorigenesis is

unknown, and similar features are often observed in other disease states, such as inflammatory bowel disease (16,17). The earliest morphologically visible evidence of colonocyte clonal expansion is the presence of aberrant crypt foci (ACF), clusters of enlarged, irregularly shaped colonic crypts. When examined by magnification endoscopy, crypts characteristic of ACF have oval or slit-like lumen and are elongated above the level of the surrounding colorectal mucosa (Fig. 1). Incidence and multiplicity of ACF may be increased in persons at high risk for colorectal adenomas and carcinoma. Some ACF are composed of cells with histopathologic features of intraepithelial neoplasia/dysplasia, and they can also harbor cancer-associated gene mutations, such as loss of wild-type *APC* and K-*ras* mutations (18–20). Despite this, progression of an ACF to an adenoma is thought to be a rare event. For individuals reaching 65 yr of age living in the US, ACF incidence may be as much as 66% (21), whereas adenoma incidence is 30–50% (22,23), and carcinoma is 3–5% (24).

Recent studies using microarray technology have compared gene expression patterns for nonneoplastic colonic mucosa to those found in colorectal adenomas and cancers (25). These studies suggest that most biochemical changes in carcinogenesis occur during the transition from normal mucosa to adenoma. These changes may reflect metabolic and structural requirements of actively proliferating adenoma cells

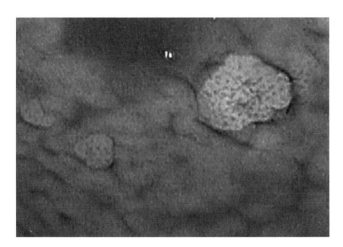

Fig. 1. View of aberrant crypt foci obtained using magnification chromoendoscopy (location = distal rectum; dye = indigo carmine; field magnified approx ×50).

compared to normal mucosa, largely a terminally differentiated mixed cell population. Differences in gene expression between adenomas and carcinomas are more limited, and may involve more specific changes in membrane function required for invasion of the basement membrane or initiation of angiogenesis. Studies of gene expression differences in the colorectal mucosa of high- and low-risk individuals remain to be reported.

Despite our present understanding of colorectal carcinogenesis, we have not yet identified the optimal times or methods for preventive intervention. Endoscopic polypectomy is an effective way to prevent the adenoma-carcinoma transition at a relatively late stage in the carcinogenic process, after a premalignant neoplasm has already developed (5,26). The most effective chemopreventive regimen is likely to be one that can target both the early initiating factors leading to intraepithelial neoplasia, as well as those events responsible for the adenoma-carcinoma transition. The multifactoral nature of carcinogenesis suggests that effective CRC prevention will involve a combination of strategies. Fortunately, studies of colorectal tumor biology using animal tumor models, human observational studies, and human therapeutic trials show that a wide variety of interventions can alter the course of premalignant disease.

3. MARKERS FOR EFFICACY OF CHEMOPREVENTIVE AGENTS

The ultimate endpoint of CRC chemoprevention is a reduction in the risk of incident CRC in a treated population. Because of strong evidence suggesting that

adenomatous polyps can progress to invasive cancer, adenomas are considered a validated surrogate endpoint for the development of CRC (reviewed in ref. 27). The use of adenoma development as a predictive biomarker for CRC permits a 3-yr period of treatment and follow-up for human trials of agent efficacy in sporadic disease (28). Although this is a substantial improvement over the 10–15 yr required of studies with a cancer endpoint, these trials are still lengthy, logistically complicated, and expensive. As a consequence, few potential chemopreventive regimens have been evaluated in prospective, randomized clinical trials. In addition, these studies target suppression of recurrent adenomas that are known to have a relatively low malignant potential, rather than high-risk precursor lesions.

Studies of persons at increased risk of CRC development are also important to chemopreventive agent development. Examples of these populations include persons with germline mutation of either the *APC* tumor suppressor gene, which results in familial adenomatous polyposis (FAP), or nucleotide mismatch repair genes responsible for hereditary nonpolyposis colorectal cancer (HNPCC) syndrome, or those with chronic inflammatory bowel disease (ulcerative colitis or Crohn's disease). Because these populations carry an increased risk of colorectal neoplasia, conclusions concerning the efficacy of a chemopreventive regimen may be reached through trials of shorter duration and smaller sample size than are required of trials in sporadic disease. More important, these cohorts provide an opportunity to examine the effect of chemopreventive agents in the setting of specific cancer-associated mutations or disease states that promote tumorigenesis. As our understanding of heritable or disease-associated causes of cancer increases, so will our ability to identify gene-specific or disease-specific treatments to inhibit tumorigenesis.

Improved understanding of earlier stages of CRC may lead to the identification of surrogate endpoint biomarkers that will permit more rapid evaluation of chemopreventive agents (Table 2). Biomarkers currently under investigation in human studies include measures of colonocyte proliferation (e.g., Ki-67 expression, apoptosis assessment), differentiation (e.g., expression of sialyl mucins), or oncogenic protein expression (e.g., cyclooxygenase [COX]-2, vascular endothelial growth factor [VEGF], phospho-Akt). Identification of these potential biomarkers proceeds in concert with mechanism-directed therapy, as in the example of COX-2 expression in ACF from subjects treated with a selective COX-2 inhibitor.

Table 2
Markers of Chemopreventive Agent Efficacy In Vivo

IEN Description	Present use
Adenomatous polyp	These lesions carry a spectrum of CRC risk depending on their degree of dysplasia, histologic subtype, size, multiplicity, and the genetic background of the individual in which they arise. Adenomatous polyps are currently used as validated endpoints in CRC prevention trials.
Aberrant crypt foci	Investigation of these lesions as indicators of CRC risk are ongoing. A relationship between number and persistence of these lesions and increased adenoma and CRC risk is suggested, but ACF are heterogeneous and have not yet been tested as an indicator of CRC or adenoma treatment outcome.
Cell growth and differentiation markers	Although studies of enterocyte proliferation, apoptosis, and differentiation antigen expression suggest a correlation between these markers and cancer or adenoma risk, these markers have not been validated as indicators of CRC or adenoma treatment outcome.
Cancer-associated mutations and other forms of DNA modification	Tumors typically accumulate particular mutations, such as those in APC, K-*ras*, and *p53*, or DNA modifications, such as specific promoter hypermethylation. Unfortunately, there are little or no data concerning the prevalence of these mutations in subpopulations of epithelial cells in non-neoplastic mucosa, or for the mutations in isolation. Studies addressing these issues are central to development of prevention strategies.
Tumor-associated protein expression	Tumor-associated changes in oncoprotein expression may provide insight into optimal chemopreventive approaches, and can be used as target-specific biomarkers of treatment response. Examples include increased serum expression of enterocyte growth factors such as insulin-like growth factor-1 (IGF-1), or upregulation in adenomas or ACF of growth factor receptors such as EGFR, mitogenic proteins such as COX-2 and β-catenin, and angiogenesis promoters such as VEGF.

4. CLUES FROM EPIDEMIOLOGY

Much of the hypothesis generation concerning dietary or drug modulation of colorectal neoplasia stems from human observational studies. One of the first major insights was the report by Armstrong and Doll in 1975 indicating that differences in dietary constituents varied geographically in a pattern similar to that observed for CRC incidence (29). These and other studies of cancer epidemiology suggested that residents of industrialized nations with a high incidence of CRC have diets high in animal fats and red meat, whereas societies whose diet lacks these factors have a lower CRC incidence (30,31). This association is supported by corresponding changes in diet that occur when individuals migrate from low-risk to high-risk regions of the world (32). Despite these compelling data, determining the relationship between diet and cancer is difficult because of the long interval required for carcinogenesis, as well as the existence of multiple confounding interactions between dietary constituents. As a result, findings in studies of the relationship between single dietary

constituents and CRC are inconsistent. For a few key dietary components, however, strong cumulative data from both human epidemiology and animal studies link consumption levels to CRC risk. These components include high consumption of saturated fats and red meat, and low consumption of fruits and vegetables (33,34). In addition, several micronutrients, such as selenium, calcium, folate, and vitamin D, may be important (33–40). Human cancer epidemiology also identifies some potential nondietary means of modulating colorectal neoplasia. These include associations between CRC and lifestyle factors, such as physical activity, and alcohol or medication use (34,41). One of the most consistent observations is the inverse association between use of nonsteroidal antiinflammatory drugs (NSAIDs) and CRC incidence (reviewed in 42) (Table 3).

5. IDENTIFICATION OF SPECIFIC CHEMOPREVENTIVE AGENTS

Primary prevention therapies must meet a stringent set of requirements in order to be both safe and effective

Table 3
Major Prospective Observational Studies of CRC Risk

Study	Cohort description	CRC results					
		Dietary fat intake	Fruit & vegetable intake	Dietary fiber intake	Folate/methionine intake	Antioxidants	NSAIDs
Nurses' Health Study, 121,700 subjects, initiated 1976 (43–58)	Female nurses—United States	2-fold ↑ CRC risk for highest vs lowest 20% of dietary fat intake	No association between dietary fruit or vegetable consumption and CRC risk	No association between dietary fiber intake and CRC or adenoma risk	↓ adenoma risk highest vs lowest 25% intake; 85%↓ CRC with ≥ 15yr use folate supplements		↓ CRC risk following 10–20 yr ASA use, greatest ↓ with 4–6 tablets/wk
Cancer Prevention Study II, 1,185,124 initiated subjects, 1982 (59–65)	Males and females—United States	No association between fat intake and risk of CRC mortality	↓risk of CRC mortality for lowest vs highest 20% of vegetable consumption	↓ risk of CRC mortality with ↑ consumption of high fiber grains			↑ risk of CRC at mortality with ASA use of ≥16/mo for least 1 yr
Health Follow-up Study, Professionals 51,529 subjects, initiated 1986 (44,56,66–71)	Male health care professionals—United States	↑ adenoma but not CRC risk with high fat intake	↓ adenoma but not CRC risk for those with highest consumption of folate-rich vegetables	↓ adenoma risk with highest consumption of total fiber	↓ adenoma highest vs lowest risk 25% intake	No decrease in CRC for vitamins C,D,E	↓ CRC incidence and mortality with ≥2/wk ASA use
Iowa Women's Health Study, 41,837 subjects, initiated 1986 (72–77)	Women recruited from Iowa Department of Transportation driver's license registration		No association between dietary fruit or vegetable consumption and CRC risk			↓ CRC highest vs lowest third of vitamin E intake	
Netherlands Cohort Study, 120,852 subjects, initiated 1986 (78–85)	Males and females recruited from 204 municipal registries—Netherlands		No association between consumption of Allium genus vegetables and CRC risk			No association between toenail selenium levels and CRC risk	

271

(43–65). These regimens may require administration to otherwise healthy individuals over long periods of time, and must therefore be extremely well tolerated in a patient population with a broad range of general health and comorbid diseases. Because agents are likely to be used in an older population, possible interactions with common medications such as antihypertensives, cholesterol-lowering drugs, exogenous hormones, and cardioprotective aspirin must be considered. Chemopreventives must also be cost effective for prolonged administration and, to foster long-term compliance, these regimens must provide minimal impact on lifestyle.

Dietary interventions appear to be a relatively straightforward approach to CRC prevention, and one likely to have other significant health benefits such as reduction in diabetes and cardiovascular disease. In almost all respects, dietary intervention is the ideal chemoprevention strategy, as it is safe, cost-effective, and readily available. Many different dietary strategies have been examined in a variety of case-control, cohort, and interventional studies of CRC or adenoma reduction. Unfortunately, these studies have not conclusively identified optimal dietary guidelines for CRC risk reduction, and compliance with dietary changes is problematical. At least a partial explanation is the complex nature of diet, a component of human behavior that is refractory to long-term change. The identification of specific dietary antitumor components in animal tumor models has led to several dietary supplementation trials in humans. Although studies with individual agents have yielded neither consistent nor dramatic reductions in adenoma recurrence, some of these strategies may be beneficial in particular risk populations, either alone or in combination with chemopreventive drugs. Dietary intervention may exert effects early in the process of tumorigenesis by lessening initiation of preneoplastic events in colorectal mucosa despite absence of efficacy against adenoma emergence *(66–85)*.

Chemopreventive drugs, chosen to target specific biological changes in the carcinogenesis process, may be used in addition to dietary counseling, particularly for high-risk populations. The agents currently under investigation target a range of cell functions, including epithelial cell proliferation and apoptosis, DNA modification, induction of detoxifying enzyme synthesis, and reduction of oxidative injury *(86–103)*. Further study of these agents promises to decrease CRC mortality and also increase our understanding of the relative contribution of these processes to colorectal carcinogenesis.

5.1. Dietary Agents

5.1.1. FIBER

One of the striking differences between the diets of countries with a low incidence of CRC and that of the Western world is the amount of dietary fiber. This observation led to the hypothesis that high fiber protects against CRC, possibly by binding to or diluting carcinogenic luminal contents, reducing intestinal transit time, or stabilizing postprandial serum insulin levels *(104–106)*. Case-control and cohort studies have yielded conflicting results concerning the relationship between dietary fiber intake and risk of colorectal neoplasia (Table 4, p.274). Although several case-control studies found that high intake of dietary fiber is associated with decreased CRC incidence, this result failed to be confirmed in several prospective dietary intervention trials. In the largest study, the Polyp Prevention Trial, 2079 patients with a history of colorectal adenomas were randomized following endoscopic polypectomy to receive counseling to achieve a low fat, high-fiber, high-vegetable intake diet, or to receive no intervention other than an informational brochure. Colonoscopy after 1 and 4 yr showed no difference in adenoma recurrence between the two study arms *(88)*. A randomized study by the Phoenix Colon Cancer Prevention Physicians Network directly addressed fiber intake by randomizing adenoma patients postpolypectomy to receive either 2.0 g or 13.5 g of supplemental fiber daily *(90)*. Follow-up colonoscopy performed after 3 yr of treatment showed no difference in recurrent adenoma formation between the low- and high-fiber groups.

5.1.2. FRUITS AND VEGETABLES

Fruits and vegetables contain a wide variety of compounds with potential to reduce epithelial neoplasia. These constituents include antioxidant vitamins, anthocyanins, flavonoids, glucosinolates, and allyl sulfides. Compounds from each of these classes demonstrate antitumor activity in a variety of CRC models *(107)*. In observational studies, vegetable consumption has been one of the most consistent dietary predictors of decreased CRC risk *(34,108)*. Results from prospective cohort studies *(57,61,71,75)* have been mixed, however, and no conclusive data have emerged from studies of specific vegetable types such as *Allium* genus (e.g., garlic, onions) *(32,67,75,81,109–115)* or *Brassica* genus (e.g., broccoli, cabbage, cauliflower) *(116)*. The potential role of a vegetable-rich diet was addressed in the Polyp Prevention Trial *(88)*. After 4 yr on intervention, during which participants in the intervention arm achieved a substantial dietary change, the incidence of recurrent colorectal adenomas was no different from that of the control arm *(88)*.

5.1.3. CALCIUM AND VITAMIN D

Data from human epidemiology and animal intestinal tumor models suggest that diets deficient in calcium and vitamin D increase spontaneous intestinal tumor formation *(117,118)*. In addition, case-control and cohort studies show risk reductions ranging from 25–50% for individuals with the highest quintile of calcium intake *(75,76,119–121)*. The benefit of calcium in chemoprevention may occur through its ability to counteract the genotoxic effects of intestinal bile acids. Secondary bile acids increase cell proliferation in human CRC cell lines and in carcinogen-induced spontaneous rodent intestinal tumor models *(117)*. The microflora of the large intestine convert luminal secondary bile acids to diacylglycerol (DAG), an activator of protein kinase C (PKC), a key inducer of mitogen-activated protein (MAP) kinase signal transduction and an important promoter of cell proliferation and tumor formation *(118,122,123)*. Bile acids are mucosal irritants and may also contribute to tumor initiation by inhibiting the activity of xenobiotic metabolizing enzymes such as glutathione-*S*-transferase (GST) and UDP-glucuronyltransferase (UGT) *(124)*. Secondary bile acid production is increased by high dietary fat intake, and is therefore a possible mechanism of carcinogenesis associated with the diet of Western nations. A clinical trial of ursodeoxycholic acid to alter fecal bile acid profiles in humans is currently in progress.

Calcium binds fatty acids and bile acids to form insoluble soaps *(33)*, thereby neutralizing their effect on the intestinal mucosa. In humans with sporadic colorectal adenomas, calcium may significantly decrease fecal bile acids *(125)*, and ingestion of approx 1 g of elemental calcium daily decreases colonic epithelial cell proliferation and normalizes the distribution of proliferating cells in the lower colonic crypt *(126)*. Calcium may also have intracellular effects. These potentially protective effects were supported by the results of a recent randomized trial, in which patients with a history of colorectal adenomas who received 1200 mg of elemental calcium daily achieved a modest but significant decrease in adenoma recurrence *(30)*.

Vitamin D is an important regulator of intestinal cell differentiation that may decrease tumor formation by regulating PKC activity *(127,128)*. Administered alone, vitamin D protects against tumors in carcinogen-induced rodent intestinal tumor models *(128,129)*. With

calcium, vitamin D suppresses the activity of ornithine decarboxylase (ODC), an enzyme that mediates cell proliferation induced in response to mitogenic stimuli, oncogenic viruses, and chemical carcinogens *(117)*. At present, clinical trials are under way to evaluate the combination of calcium and vitamin D for prevention of colorectal carcinogenesis.

5.1.4. ANTIOXIDANTS AND OTHER MICRONUTRIENTS

Normal cellular metabolism requires a careful balance of intra- and extracellular oxidation and reduction. Loss of this balance produces DNA-damaging reactive oxygen species that promote tumor formation *(130)*. Oxidative balance in healthy cells is maintained by a protective system of enzymes, such as GST, that guard the cell against significant oxidative damage. Certain states of "oxidative stress," however, can overcome the cell's ability to neutralize genotoxic metabolites. One such situation arises with the presence of polymorphisms in genes encoding proteins such as GST. These polymorphisms can produce gene products with sub-normal activity and therefore disrupt cellular metabolism and alter the cell's ability to process carcinogenic substances without sustaining harm *(131)*.

Antioxidant compounds enhance the resistance of cultured cells to oxidative stress. These compounds include such antioxidant vitamins as A, C, and E, and micronutrients such as the trace metal selenium and a variety of plant-derived compounds. Examples of naturally occurring antioxidants include compounds present in curry (phenolics such as curcumin), onions and garlic (sulfides such as allyl sulfide), and tea (catechins). Most of these substances are also anti-inflammatory, as they exert varying degrees of COX and lipoxygenase (LOX) inhibition *(132)*. Data from human cancer cell lines, animal cancer models, and some human observational studies suggest that nutrients with antioxidant properties prevent tumors *(133–135)*. Case-control and prospective studies of antioxidants and other micronutrients have reported conflicting findings for endpoints of prevalent or recurrent adenomas and CRC *(38,75,76,134–137)*. Similarly, data from large human intervention trials with adenoma or CRC endpoints have shown no benefit to dietary supplementation with β-carotene *(87,96,97,138,139)*, and minor or no effect from administration of vitamin A, C, or E, or combinations of these with other micronutrients *(87,94,134,140,141)*. Selenium, in the form of selenocysteine, is required for the activity of the antioxidant enzyme glutathione peroxidase *(142)*. Several observational studies *(143,144)* and one prospective randomized

Table 4
Randomized Trials of Adenoma Modulation

Study	Intervention	Cohort	Endpoint	Result
McKeown-Eyssen (86)	"Typical" Western diet vs low fat (50 g/d), high fiber (>50 g/d)	Prior history of adenomas/201 subjects randomized	Adenoma recurrence	No difference between treatment arms
Australian Polyp Prevention Trial (87)	Low fat (<25% total calories) vs fiber supplement (20 g/d) vs β-carotene supplement	Prior history of adenomas/424 subjects randomized	Adenoma recurrence	No differences among treatment arms
Polyp Prevention Trial (88)	Western diet vs low fat (≤20% total calories), high fiber (18g/1000 kcal), high fruit & vegetable intake (5–8 servings/d)	Prior history of adenomas/2,079 subjects randomized	Adenoma recurrence	No difference between treatment arms
DeCosse (89)	Small amount fiber (2.2 g/d) vs small amount fiber (2.2 g/d) + vitamins C (4 g/d) and E (400 mg/d) vs high fiber (22.5 g/d) + vitamins C (4 g/d) and E (400 mg/d)	Familial adenomatous polyposis/58 subjects randomized	Adenoma regression	Trend toward ↓ in adenoma burden for high fiber + anti-oxidant vitamin arm
Alberts (90)	2 g/d fiber vs 13.5 g/d fiber	Prior history of adenomas/1429 subjects randomized	Adenoma recurrence	No difference between intervention arms
European Cancer Prevention Organization (91,92)	Placebo vs fiber supplement (3.8 g/d) vs calcium supplement (2 g/d)	Prior history of adenomas/655 subjects randomized	Adenoma recurrence	Slight nonsignificant 34% ↓ in adenomas for calcium arm, significant 67% ↑ in adenomas for fiber arm
Thomas (93)	Calcium 1.5 g/d vs placebo	Familial adenomatous polyposis/25 subjects randomized	Adenoma regression	No difference between intervention and control arms after 6 mo treatment

274

Study	Intervention	Population/subjects randomized	Outcome	Results
Baron (37)	Calcium 3 g/d vs placebo	Prior history of adenomas/930 subjects randomized	Adenoma recurrence	19% reduction in adenoma recurrence in treatment arm
Hofstad (94,95)	Calcium 1.6g/d + β-carotene 15 mg/d + vitamin C 150 mg/d + vitamin E 75 mg/d + selenium 100 mcg/d	Retained adenomas <1 cm in size/116 subjects randomized	Adenoma regression	No difference in growth of small adenomas in intervention arm
Hennekens (96)	β-carotene 50 mg/qod	Male physicians/ 22,071 subjects randomized	Cancer incidence	No effect on cancer incidence after 60 mo
Women's Health Study (97,98)	β-carotene 50 mg/qod	Female health professionals ≥45 years old/39,876 subjects randomized	Cancer incidence	No effect on cancer incidence after median 24 mo follow-up
Labayle (99)	Sulindac 100 mg/tid × 4 mo	Familial adenomatous polyposis/9 subjects randomized	Adenoma regression	Reduced adenoma number and size
Giardiello (100,101)	Sulindac 150 mg/bid × 9 mo	Familial adenomatous polyposis/22 subjects randomized	Adenoma regression	Reduced adenoma number and size
Nugent (102)	Sulindac 200 mg/bid × 6 mo	Familial adenomatous polyposis/14 subjects randomized	Adenoma regression	Reduced adenoma number and size
Steinbach (103)	Celecoxib 100 mg/bid vs celecoxib 400 mg/bid vs placebo × 6 mo	Familial adenomatous polyposis/77 subjects randomized	Adenoma regression	Reduced adenoma number and size in 400 mg/bid arm

trial, the Nutritional Prevention of Cancer (NPC) Trial *(145,146)*, suggest that adequate amounts of dietary selenium are important for CRC prevention. Despite these favorable results, caution must be exercised in interpreting selenium studies as evidence for recommending selenium supplementation as a chemopreventive therapy. Background dietary selenium levels vary considerably, based upon local soil concentrations in areas of food production. The NPC Trial, for instance, was conducted in a region of low selenium soil concentration, possibly contributing to the positive result.

5.1.5. FOLATE AND METHIONINE

Folate or folic acid is a micronutrient present in fruits and vegetables, and is particularly abundant in leafy green vegetables such as spinach. Methionine is present in high concentrations in red meat, chicken, and fish. Folate and methionine are methyl donors that contribute to nucleotide synthesis and proper methylation of DNA. Diets deficient in folate have the potential to produce methylation defects such as hypomethylation of CCGG sites *(147)*. Methionine deficiency is characterized by changes in deoxynucleotide availability *(148)*; these changes may alter DNA function or repair capability, or even inhibit efficient DNA transcription enough to foster the acquisition of tumor-associated mutations.

Evidence from human epidemiology strongly supports a role for dietary folate in CRC prevention. In the Nurses' Health Study, individuals taking folate supplements demonstrated a significant reduction of CRC risk (RR = 0.25) after 15 yr of supplement use *(38)*. The chemopreventive benefits of folate supplementation may be most important for patients carrying increased genetic risk for CRC because of inefficient DNA repair. The importance of folate metabolism to CRC risk is illustrated by the presence of a particular polymorphism of methylenetetrahydrofolate reductase (MTHFR). In certain individuals, MTHFR facilitates the conversion of 5,10-methylenetetrahydrofolate to 5-methyltetrahydrofolate, which then serves as a methyl donor for methionine synthase, allowing conversion of homocysteine to methionine. Patients homozygous for particular polymorphisms of MTHFR or of the enzyme methionine synthase have an approximately 50% decreased risk of CRC *(149–151)*. The association of these polymorphisms with altered folate synthesis is further supported by the observation that this genotype-specific benefit is lost for individuals with inadequate folate intake *(152)*. Interventional trials of folate supplementation for the prevention of colorectal adenoma recurrence are currently under way *(153)*.

5.2. Pharmacologic Agents
5.2.1. NONSTEROIDAL ANTIINFLAMMATORY DRUGS

At the present time, NSAIDs are the most promising class of agents for CRC prevention. Consistent results showing NSAID-associated reductions in CRC incidence and precursor adenoma formation in the range of 30–60% are evident in a wide variety of case-control and cohort studies (reviewed in *42*). Most striking is the finding of decreased CRC mortality among NSAID users, a result reported in at least three separate studies *(58,60,68)*.

NSAIDs are widely available and frequently used treatments for relief of musculoskeletal pain and prevention of thrombosis of coronary and cerebral vessels. Their broad clinical use both facilitates and hinders studies of NSAID efficacy for chemoprevention. On one hand, NSAIDs have a well-known toxicity profile, making it relatively easy to weigh the risks and benefits of their use in a particular study cohort. On the other hand, the widespread use of NSAIDs makes it difficult to maintain compliance in a placebo-control arm, particularly as prospective randomized trials of adenoma prevention typically require a 3-yr intervention interval.

The first direct evidence of NSAID-associated modulation of colorectal tumors came from studies of patients with FAP. As a result of germline *APC* mutation, these individuals develop hundreds to thousands of colorectal adenomas, with progression to CRC in the absence of intervention. FAP patients were first given the NSAID sulindac for treatment of desmoid tumors, an APC-related neoplasm characterized by extensive tissue fibrosis suggesting inflammation as a pathogenetic factor *(154)*. Although sulindac only modestly attenuates the natural history of desmoids, FAP patients taking sulindac at antiinflammatory doses showed regression of coexisting rectal polyps, a result that was later confirmed by randomized trials *(99,100)*. Similar results were recently reported following treatment of FAP patients with celecoxib, a selective COX-2 inhibitor *(103)*. The overall level of adenoma reduction in these studies was 25–35%, with some patients achieving complete resolution of visible polyps while others showed no response or even disease progression. These studies are important for several reasons. First, they show that therapeutic modulation of the adenoma–carcinoma sequence can occur relatively late, as these patients showed significant regression of existing premalignant lesions. Second, because *APC* loss also occurs in the majority of sporadic CRCs, results achieved in FAP patients may be relevant to prevention of sporadic disease. Finally, these studies show that some adenomas are not responsive to NSAID use. In fact, although the overall effect of these agents in FAP patients is reduction of number and size of adenomas, the benign neoplasms persist in most patients and the progression to invasive carcinoma during therapy has been reported *(101,155,156)*. Clinical trials are under way to determine whether NSAIDs such as aspirin or selective COX-2 inhibitors prevent the development of sporadic colorectal adenomas.

The exact mechanism of NSAID-associated cancer prevention is unknown. NSAIDs exert many effects on the pathways governing cell proliferation, differentiation, and mobility that may be related to tumor development. One important activity of NSAIDs is suppression of prostaglandin synthesis. Certain prostaglandins, such as PGE_2 and $PGF_{2\alpha}$, are associated with epithelial tumorigenesis, possibly by inducing cell proliferation, suppressing apoptosis, or reducing tumor immune surveillance *(157–161)*. The tumor-preventing activity of NSAIDs may result from inhibition of COX-2, one of the key enzymes of arachidonic acid metabolism. In contrast to COX-1, which is a constitutively expressed enzyme responsible for gastric mucosal protection and platelet function, COX-2 is the product of an intermediate-early response gene that is induced in response to inflammation or mitogenic stimuli *(162)*. COX-2 expression is increased during the course of tumor development in a variety of epithelial tissues (reviewed in *163*), and colorectal tumors overexpress COX-2 as well as PGE_2 *(164)*. COX-2 may be responsible for apoptosis suppression in enterocytes *(10)*, an effect counteracted by NSAIDs such as sulindac *(165)*. A critical link between COX-2 activity and intestinal tumor prevention was provided by a study of COX-2 expression in *Apc*-deficient mice *(166)*. In this study, animals homozygous for a germline mutation in murine *Apc* developed multiple intestinal tumors, each exhibiting loss of wild-type *Apc*. When these animals were crossed with a mouse altered by genetic knockout of COX-2, intestinal tumor incidence was dramatically decreased. A similar magnitude of tumor reduction was also observed for *Apc*-deficient mice treated with selective inhibitors of COX-2 *(167)*.

Other antitumor effects by NSAIDs may be independent of prostaglandin activity. Several NSAIDs, including aspirin, indomethacin, and selective COX-2 inhibitors, block the carcinogen-induced activation of AP-1, a transcription factor regulating growth-associated genes *(168,169)*. Aspirin and sodium salicylate alter cell proliferation by inhibiting the activity of the NFκB activating enzyme, IκB kinase β, in a prostaglandin-independent fashion *(170)*. In addition, sulindac sulfone/exisulind, a metabolite of sulindac that does not alter prostaglandin synthesis, protects against carcinogen-induced tumors in rodents *(171)*. This agent may inhibit tumors by inactivating cyclic GMP phosphodiesterase and activating PKG *(171)*. In a recent Phase II trial, sulindac sulfone also reduced adenoma burden in FAP patients *(172)*.

5.2.2. EXOGENOUS ESTROGENS

The mortality from CRC among women living in developed countries has declined substantially in recent years *(34,173)*. Although NSAID use is more prevalent in women than in men, this trend has also been attributed to the use of menopausal hormone replacement therapy (HRT), a practice that began in the 1970s *(174)*. In support of this hypothesis, numerous observational studies of CRC incidence show a protective effect of menopausal HRT. A recent meta-analysis of studies published up to December 1996 suggests that HRT reduces CRC risk by as much as 25%, with a summary relative risk (RR) of 0.85 (95% CI 0.73;0.99) *(175)*. Studies identifying the duration of HRT use also suggest a dose response, with a RR of 0.69 (95% C.I. 0.52;0.91) among current or recent HRT users compared to 0.88 (95% CI 0.64;1.21) for short-term users *(175,176)*.

The mechanism responsible for HRT-associated reduction in CRC incidence is unknown. One possibility is that estrogens influence intestinal carcinogenesis by an indirect mechanism. Estrogens are metabolized to a variety of compounds that have different half-lives and receptor affinities, and produce tissue-specific effects upon cell proliferation. Studies of cancer cell lines and animal tumor models suggest that some of these metabolites may have tumor-promoting activity, while others may be chemopreventive *(177–179)*. Estrogenic compounds also decrease bile acid levels *(180)*, potentially lowering the concentration of these tumorigenic compounds in the colorectum. In addition, estrogens may serve as differentiation factors for intestinal cells *(181)* or induce reduction of serum insulin-like growth factors that may stimulate enterocyte proliferation *(182)*. More definitive conclusions concerning the role of HRT in CRC prevention may come from the Women's Health Initiative, a trial involving approximately 45,000 postmenopausal women randomized to receive either calcium and vitamin D or placebo for a mean of 9 yr. This ongoing trial will gather data on concomitant HRT use and will evaluate the incidence of several diseases common to this cohort, including osteoporosis, breast cancer, and CRC *(183)*.

5.2.3. DIFLUOROMETHYLORNITHINE

Difluoromethylornithine (DFMO) is an irreversible inhibitor of ODC that has potent antitumor activity against cancer cell lines and in animal cancer models *(184–186)*. ODC is essential for the synthesis of polyamines, which in turn are required for the proliferation and function of epithelial cells. Agents that block polyamine synthesis produce an inhibition of cell proliferation that can be restored by addition of exogenous polyamines. Inhibition of polyamine synthesis also alters epidermal growth factor signaling activity, disrupts the epithelial cell cytoskeleton, and suppresses matrilysin expression *(187,188)*. Low-dose DFMO has been studied in combination with other chemopreventive agents, resulting in synergistic antitumor activity with NSAIDs such as piroxicam, aspirin, or selenium *(189–193)*. Phase II trials of DFMO in patients with a history of colorectal adenomas confirmed decreased polyamine levels in the rectal mucosa of treated subjects *(194)*. Unfortunately, 12.5% of participants receiving DFMO (0.5 g/m^2/d) developed reversible hearing loss. Two NCI-sponsored clinical trials are currently testing low-dose DFMO combined with NSAIDs for prevention of sporadic colorectal adenomas and regression of adenomas in persons with FAP.

5.2.4. URSODEOXYCHOLIC ACID

Evidence from animal tumor models and cancer cell line studies suggests that bile acids influence intestinal tumor formation. Unconjugated bile acids, such as deoxycholic acid, are mutagenic and cytotoxic when applied to intestinal epithelium *(195–197)*. Ursodeoxycholic acid is a 7β-epimer of chenodeoxycholic acid commonly used to manage biliary stasis due to primary biliary sclerosis. Unlike other bile acids, ursodeoxycholic acid may inhibit intestinal tumorigenesis; the exact mechanism of this activity is unknown. Ursodeoxycholic acid suppressed intestinal tumor formation in rodents treated with carcinogens *(198,199)*. When the effect of this agent on intestinal mucosa was examined, reductions in mucosal PGE$_2$, iNOS, phospholipase A$_2$, and activated isoforms of PKC were observed *(200–206)*. A recent study of patients with ulcerative colitis and sclerosing cholangitis suggested that ursodeoxycholic acid reduced colonic dysplasia *(207)*. This therapy is presently under evaluation in two ongoing Phase III trials for prevention of postpolypectomy adenoma recurrence *(208)*.

5.2.5. OTHER POSSIBILITIES

A variety of additional agents are of interest in CRC prevention due to mechanistic support for their antitumor activity in intestinal tissues. Some of the most promising include HMG-CoA reductase inhibitors, perillyl alcohol, and matrix metalloproteinase (MMP) inhibitors. HMG-CoA reductase inhibitors, currently used as cholesterol-lowering agents, suppress tumor growth in several neoplasia models, including carcinogen-induced murine tumors *(209–213)*. Perillyl alcohol, a hydroxylated derivative of *d*-limonene, selectively inhibits post-translational isoprenylation of small guanine nucleotide binding proteins, including the *ras* oncogene product *(214,215)*. In intestinal tumor models, both perillyl alcohol and *d*-limonene inhibit tumor cell proliferation, induce apoptosis, and induce carcinogen-metabolizing enzymes *(216,217)*. Protease inhibitors, such as the Bowman-Birk inhibitor (BBI), inhibit both carcinogen- and APC-associated intestinal tumorigenesis in mice *(218–220)*. This well-tolerated agent may inhibit tumorigenesis through the activity of a trypsin inhibitory domain *(219)*. Finally, MMPs are endogenous enzymes capable of disrupting basement membrane structures and may be associated with the development of invasive tumor behavior. MMPs have recently been implicated in early as well as late stages of tumorigenesis *(221)*. For example, expression of the MMP family member matrilysin was localized by immunohistochemistry to the luminal surface of dysplastic enterocytes, but was absent from this location in normal epithelium *(222)*. Batimistat, a synthetic MMP inhibitor, suppresses intestinal tumor multiplicity in a spontaneous murine intestinal tumor model, suggesting that these agents may prove useful in CRC chemoprevention *(223,224)*.

6. OPTIMIZING CHEMOPREVENTION STRATEGIES

Progress in chemoprevention occurs in concert with new insights into the multifactoral process of tumorigenesis and the resulting identification of rational targets for intervention. The study of persons with inherited cancer predisposition syndromes such as FAP continues to help define molecular elements of tumor progression and to aid in identifying promising new treatments for prevention of sporadic as well as hereditary disease. For example, the relationship between folate intake and the MTHFR polymorphism illustrates that important new but subtle risk factors can be expected from the continued identification of new genetic-susceptibility loci. In addition, the development of biologic response modifiers with specificity for cancer-associated changes will benefit both primary prevention and treatment of established cancers. Potential new chemoprevention therapies include antitumor vaccines, as well as selective inhibitors of angiogenesis, COX-2 activity *(166,225)*, β-catenin/Tcf transcriptional activation *(226,227)*, farnesyltransferase *(228,229)*, epidermal growth factor receptor signaling *(230–232)*, insulin-like growth factor activity *(233,234)*, and telomerase *(235,236)*.

Although recent contributions to CRC chemoprevention are very promising, many challenges remain, and it is important to keep these issues in mind as the achievements of the past are reviewed. Will the reduction in incidence of adenomas achieved by chemopreventive agents produce a decrease in cancer incidence equal to or better than that of endoscopic polypectomy? Which agent or (more likely) combination of agents best balances the risks, costs, and benefits of chemoprevention? At what age should chemopreventive agents be administered, and for how long? Is there an identifiable subpopulation of individuals most likely to benefit from a particular chemopreventive regimen because of the specific characteristics of their process of tumorigenesis? At what phase in tumorigenesis (preneoplastic mucosa, ACF, adenoma) will various agents demonstrate efficacy? Finally, what is the role of endoscopic surveillance for individuals treated with chemopreventive agents? The field of chemoprevention has advanced to the point where it is clear that substantial improvements in CRC incidence and mortality are a possibility. Realization of these goals will require completion of the difficult task of answering these and other questions in human clinical trials.

REFERENCES

1. Ferlay J, Bary F, Pisani P, et al. GLOBOCAN 2000: Cancer incidence, mortality and prevalence worldwide, version 1.0; IARC CancerBase No. 5. IARC Press, Lyon, 2001.
2. McDevitt TM. US Bureau of the Census, Report WP/98. World Population Profile: 1998. US Government Printing Office, Washington, DC, 1999.
3. Greenlee RT, Bolden S, Wingo PA. Cancer statistics. *CA Cancer J Clin* 2000;50:7–33.
4. Kelloff GJ. Perspectives on cancer chemoprevention research and drug development. *Adv Cancer Res* 2000;78:199–334.
5. Winawer SJ, Zauber AG, O'Brien MJ, et al. Prevention of colorectal cancer by colonoscopic polypectomy. The National Polyp Study Workgroup. *N Engl J Med* 1993;329: 1977–1981.
6. US Preventive Services Task Force. Methodology. Guide to Clinical Preventive Services: Report of the US Preventive Services Task Force. Williams & Wilkins, Baltimore, 1996;xl–xli.
7. Alberts DS, Einspahr J, Ritenbaugh C, et al. The effect of wheat bran fiber and calcium supplementation on rectal

8. Karagas MR, Tosteson TD, Greenberg ER, et al. Effects of milk and milk products on rectal mucosal cell proliferation in humans. *Cancer Epidemiol Biomarkers Prev* 1998;7: 757–766.
9. Liu LU, Holt PR, Krivosheyev V, Moss SF. Human right and left colon differ in epithelial cell apoptosis and in expression of Bak, a pro-apoptotic Bcl-2 homologue. *Gut* 1999;45: 45–50.
10. Bedi A, Pasricha A, Akhtar AJ, et al. Inhibition of apoptosis during development of colorectal cancer. *Cancer Res* 1995;55:1811–1816.
11. Holt PR, Atillasoy EO, Gilman J, et al. Modulation of abnormal colonic epithelial cell proliferation and differentiation by low-fat dairy foods: a randomized controlled trial. *JAMA* 1998;280:1074–1079.
12. Baldus SE, Hanisch FG, Putz C, et al. Immunoreactivity of Lewis blood group and mucin peptide core antigens: correlations with grade of dysplasia and malignant transformation in the colorectal adenoma-carcinoma sequence. *Histol Histopathol* 2002;17:191–198.
13. Alberts DS, Einspahr J, Rees-McGee S, et al. Effects of dietary wheat bran fiber on rectal epithelial cell proliferation in patients with resection for colorectal cancers. *J Natl Cancer Inst* 1990;82:1280–1285.
14. Lipkin M, Newmark H. Effect of added dietary calcium on colonic epithelial-cell proliferation in subjects at high risk for familial colonic cancer. *N Engl J Med* 1985;313:1381–1384.
15. Thomas MG, Thomson JP, Williamson RC. Oral calcium inhibits rectal epithelial proliferation in familial adenomatous polyposis. *Br J Surg* 1993;80:499–501.
16. Fogt F, Poremba C, Shibao K, et al. Expression of survivin, YB-1, and KI-67 in sporadic adenomas and dysplasia-associated lesions or masses in ulcerative colitis. *Appl Immunohistochem Mol Morphol* 2001;9:143–149.
17. Ierardi E, Principi M, Francavilla R, et al. Epithelial proliferation and ras p21 oncoprotein expression in rectal mucosa of patients with ulcerative colitis. *Dig Dis Sci* 2001;46: 1083–1087.
18. Nucci MR, Robinson CR, Longo P, et al. Phenotypic and genotypic characteristics of aberrant crypt foci in human colorectal mucosa. *Hum Pathol* 1997;28:1396–1407.
19. Hao XP, Pretlow TG, Rao JS, Pretlow TP. Beta-catenin expression is altered in human colonic aberrant crypt foci. *Cancer Res* 2001;61:8085–8088.
20. Shpitz B, Bomstein Y, Shalev M, et al. Oncoprotein coexpression in human aberrant crypt foci and minute polypoid lesions of the large bowel. *Anticancer Res* 1999;19: 3361–3366.
21. Takayama T, Katsuki S, Takahashi Y, et al. Aberrant crypt foci of the colon as precursors of adenoma and cancer. *N Engl J Med* 1998;339:1277–1284.
22. Blatt LJ. Polyps of the colon and rectum: incidence and distribution. *Dis Colon Rectum* 1961;4:277–282.
23. Bernstein MA, Feczko PJ, Halpert RD, et al. Distribution of colonic polyps: increased incidence of proximal lesions in older patients. *Radiology* 1985;155:35–38.
24. Colon and rectum cancer. In *Cancer Facts & Figures, 1999*. American Cancer Society, Atlanta, 1999; pp. 18–23.
25. Notterman DA, Alon U, Sierk AJ, Levine AJ. Transcriptional gene expression profiles of colorectal adenoma, adenocarci-

noma, and normal tissue examined by oligonucleotide arrays. *Cancer Res* 2001;61:124–3130.

26. Bond JH. Polyp guidelines: diagnosis, treatment, and surveillance for patients with colorectal polyps. Practice Parameters Committee of the American College of Gastroenterology. *Am J Gastroenterol* 2000;95:3053–3063.

27. O'Shaughnessy JA, Kelloff GJ, Gordon GB, et al. Treatment and prevention of intraepithelial neoplasia: an important target for accelerated new agent development. Recommendations of the American Association for Cancer Research Task Force on the Treatment and Prevention of Intraepithelial Neoplasia. *Clin Cancer Res* 2002;8:314–346.

28. Winawer SJ, Zauber AG, O'Brien MJ, et al. Randomized comparison of surveillance intervals after colonoscopic removal of newly diagnosed adenomatous polyps. *N Engl J Med* 1993;328:901–906.

29. Armstrong B, Doll R. Environmental factors and cancer incidence and mortality in different countries, with special reference to dietary practices. *Int J Cancer* 1975;15: 617–631.

30. Haenszel W, Correa P. Cancer of the large intestine: epidemiologic findings. *Dis Colon Rectum* 1973;16:371–377.

31. Willett W. The search for the causes of breast and colon cancer. *Nature* 1989;338:389–394.

32. Haenszel W, Berg JW, Segi M, et al. Large-bowel cancer in Hawaiian Japanese. *J Natl Cancer Inst* 1973;51:1765–1779.

33. Newmark HL, Wargovich MJ, Bruce WE. Colon cancer and dietary fat, phosphate, and calcium: a hypothesis. *J Natl Cancer Inst* 1984;72:1323–1325.

34. Potter JD, Slattery ML, Bostick RM, Gapstur SM. Colon cancer: a review of the epidemiology. *Epidemiol Rev* 1993;15:499–545.

35. Richter F, Newmark HL, Richter A, et al. Inhibition of Western-diet induced proliferation and hyperplasia in mouse colon by two sources of calcium. *Carcinogenesis* 1995;16: 2685–2689.

36. Shabahang M, Buras RR, Davoodi F, et al. 1,25-Dihydroxyvitamin D_3 receptor as a marker of human colon carcinoma cell line differentiation and growth inhibition. *Cancer Res* 1993;53:3712–3718.

37. Baron JA, Beach M, Mandel JS, et al. Calcium supplements for the prevention of colorectal adenomas. Calcium Polyp Prevention Study Group. *N Engl J Med* 1999;340:101–107.

38. Giovannucci E, Stampfer ME, Colditz GA, et al. Multivitamin use, folate, and colon cancer in women in the Nurses' Health Study. *Ann Intern Med* 1998;129:517–524.

39. Nomura A, Heilbrun LK, Morris S, Stemmerman GN. Serum selenium and the risk of cancer, by specific sites: case-control analysis of prospective data. *J Natl Cancer Inst* 1987;79:103–108.

40. Giovannucci E, Willett WC. Dietary factors and risk of colon cancer. *Ann Med* 1994;26:443–452.

41. Slattery ML, Edwards SL. Boucher KM, et al. Lifestyle and colon cancer: an assessment of factors associated with risk. *Am J Epidemiol* 1999;150:869–877.

42. Baron JA, Sandler RS. Nonsteroidal anti-inflammatory drugs and cancer prevention. *Annu Rev Med* 2000;51:511–523.

43. Colditz GA, Manson JE, Hankinson SE. The Nurses' Health Study: 20-year contribution to the understanding of health among women. *J Woman's Health* 1997;6:49–62.

44. Giovannucci E, Stampfer MJ, Colditz GA, et al. Folate, methionine, and alcohol intake and risk of colorectal adenoma. *J Natl Cancer Inst* 1993;85:875–884.

45. Giovannucci E, Martinez ME. Tobacco, colorectal cancer, and adenomas: a review of the evidence. *J Natl Cancer Inst* 1996;88:1717–1730.

46. Giovannucci E, Colditz GA, Stampfer MJ, et al. A prospective study of cigarette smoking and risk of colorectal adenoma and colorectal cancer in U.S. women. *J Natl Cancer Inst* 1994;86:192–199.

47. Giovannucci E, Colditz GA, Stampfer MJ, Willett WC. Physical activity, obesity, and risk of colorectal adenoma in women (United States). *Cancer Causes Control* 1996;7: 253–263.

48. Platz EA, Martinez ME, Grodstein F, et al. Parity and other reproductive factors and risk of adenomatous polyps of the distal colorectum (United States). *Cancer Causes Control* 1997;8:894–903.

49. Grodstein F, Martinez ME, Platz EA, et al. Postmenopausal hormone use and risk for colorectal cancer and adenoma. *Ann Intern Med* 1998;128:705–712.

50. Fuchs CS, Giovannucci EL, Colditz GA, et al. Dietary fiber and the risk of colorectal cancer and adenoma in women. *N Engl J Med* 1999;340:169–176.

51. Platz EA, Hankinson SE, Rifai N, et al. Glycosylated hemoglobin and risk of colorectal cancer and adenoma (United States). *Cancer Causes Control* 1999;10:379–386.

52. Giovannucci E, Pollak MN, Platz EA, et al. A prospective study of plasma insulin-like growth factor-1 and binding protein-3 and risk of colorectal neoplasia in women. *Cancer Epidemiol Biomarkers Prev* 2000;9:345–349.

53. Martinez ME, Giovannucci E, Spiegelman D, et al. Leisure-time physical activity, body size, and colon cancer in women. Nurses' Health Study Research Group. *J Natl Cancer Inst* 1997;89:948–955.

54. Hu FB, Manson JE, Liu S, et al. Prospective study of adult onset diabetes mellitus (type 2) and risk of colorectal cancer in women. *J Natl Cancer Inst* 1999;91:542–547.

55. Willett WC, Stampfer MJ, Colditz GA, et al. Relation of meat, fat, and fiber intake to the risk of colon cancer in a prospective study among women. *N Engl J Med* 1990;323: 1664–1672.

56. Fuchs CS, Giovannucci EL, Colditz GA, et al. A prospective study of family history and the risk of colorectal cancer. *N Engl J Med* 1994;331:1669–1674.

57. Michels KB, Giovannucci E, Joshipura KJ, et al. Prospective study of fruit and vegetable consumption and incidence of colon and rectal cancers. *J Natl Cancer Inst* 2000;92: 1706–1707.

58. Giovannucci E, Egan KM, Hunter DJ, et al. Aspirin and the risk of colorectal cancer in women. *N Engl J Med* 1995;333: 609–614.

59. Cancer Prevention Study II. The American Cancer Society Prospective Study. *Stat Bull Metrop Insur Co* 1992;73:21–29.

60. Thun MJ, Namboodiri MM, Heath CWJ. Aspirin use and reduced risk of fatal colon cancer. *N Engl J Med* 1991;325:1593–1596.

61. Thun MJ, Calle EE, Namboodiri MM, et al. Risk factors for fatal colon cancer in a large prospective study. *J Natl Cancer Inst* 1992;84:1491–1500.

62. Calle EE, Miracle-McMahill HL, Thun MJ, Heath CWJ. Estrogen replacement therapy and risk of fatal colon cancer in a prospective cohort of postmenopausal women. *J Natl Cancer Inst* 1995;87:517–523.

63. Stellman SD, Demers PA, Colin D, Boffetta P. Cancer mortality and wood dust exposure among participants in the

American Cancer Society Cancer Prevention Study-II (CPS-II). *Am J Ind Med* 1998;34:229–237.

64. Kahn HS, Tatham LM, Thun MJ, Heath CWJ. Risk factors for self-reported colon polyps. *J Gen Intern Med* 1998;13: 303–310.

65. Thun MJ, Namboodiri MM, Calle EE, et al. Aspirin use and risk of fatal cancer. *Cancer Res* 1993;53:1322–1327.

66. Giovannucci E, Rimm EB, Stampfer MJ, et al. A prospective study of cigarette smoking and risk of colorectal adenoma and colorectal cancer in U.S. men. *J Natl Cancer Inst* 1994;86:183–191.

67. Giovannucci E, Rimm EB, Stampfer MJ, et al. Intake of fat, meat, and fiber in relation to risk of colon cancer in men. *Cancer Res* 1994;54:2390–2397.

68. Giovannucci E, Rimm EB, Stampfer MJ, et al. Aspirin use and the risk for colorectal cancer and adenoma in male health professionals. *Ann Intern Med* 1994;121:241–246.

69. Giovannucci E, Ascherio A, Rimm EB, et al. Physical activity, obesity, and risk for colon cancer and adenoma in men. *Ann Intern Med* 1995;122:327–334.

70. Giovannucci E, Rimm EB, Ascherio A, et al. Alcohol, low-methionine, low-folate diets, and risk of colon cancer in men. *J Natl Cancer Inst* 1995;87:265–273.

71. Platz EA, Giovannucci E, Rimm EB, et al. Dietary fiber and distal colorectal adenoma in men. *Cancer Epidemiol Biomarkers Prev* 1997;6:661–670.

72. Bostick RM, Potter JD, Kushi LH, et al. Sugar, meat, and fat intake, and non-dietary risk factors for colon cancer incidence in Iowa women (United States). *Cancer Causes Control* 1994;5:38–52.

73. Steinmetz KA, Kushi LH, Bostick RM, et al. Vegetables, fruit, and colon cancer in the Iowa Women's Health Study. *Am J Epidemiol* 1994;139:1–15.

74. Doyle TJ, Zheng W, Cerhan JR, et al. The association of drinking water source and chlorination by-products with cancer incidence among postmenopausal women in Iowa: a prospective cohort study. *Am J Public Health* 1997;87: 1168–1176.

75. Sellers TA, Bazyk AE, Bostick RM, et al. Diet and risk of colon cancer in a large prospective study of older women: an analysis stratified on family history (Iowa, United States). *Cancer Causes Control* 1998;9:357–367.

76. Zheng W, Anderson KE, Kushi LH, et al. A prospective cohort study of intake of calcium, vitamin D, and other micronutrients in relation to incidence of rectal cancer among postmenopausal women. *Cancer Epidemiol Biomarkers Prev* 1998;7:221–225.

77. Gapstur SM, Potter JD, Folsom AR. Alcohol consumption and colon and rectal cancer in postmenopausal women. *Int J Epidemiol* 1994;23:50–57.

78. van den Brandt PA, Goldbohm RA, van 't Veer P, et al. A large-scale prospective cohort study on diet and cancer in the Netherlands. *J Clin Epidemiol* 1990;43:285–295.

79. van den Brandt PA, Goldbohm RA, van 't Veer P, et al. A prospective cohort study on toenail selenium levels and risk of gastrointestinal cancer. *J Natl Cancer Inst* 1993;85: 224–229.

80. Kampman E, Goldbohm RA, van den Brandt PA, van 't Veer P. Fermented dairy products, calcium, and colorectal cancer in The Netherlands Cohort Study. *Cancer Res* 1994;54: 3186–3190.

81. Dorant E, van den Brandt PA, Goldbohm RA. A prospective cohort study on the relationship between onion and leek consumption, garlic supplement use and the risk of colorectal carcinoma in the Netherlands. *Carcinogenesis* 1996;17: 477–484.

82. Goldbohm RA, van den Brandt PA, van 't Veer P, et al. Cholecystectomy and colorectal cancer: evidence from a cohort study on diet and cancer. *Int J Cancer* 1993;53: 735–739.

83. Goldbohm RA, van den Brandt PA, van 't Veer P, et al. A prospective cohort study on the relation between meat consumption and the risk of colon cancer. *Cancer Res* 1994;54:718–723.

84. Goldbohm RA, Hertog MG, Brants HA, et al. Consumption of black tea and cancer risk: a prospective cohort study. *J Natl Cancer Inst* 1996;88:93–100.

85. Goldbohm RA, van den Brandt PA, van 't Veer P, et al. Prospective study on alcohol consumption and the risk of cancer of the colon and rectum in the Netherlands. *Cancer Causes Control* 1994;5:95–104.

86. McKeown-Eyssen GE, Bright-See E, Bruce WR, et al. A randomized trial of a low fat high fibre diet in the recurrence of colorectal polyps. Toronto Polyp Prevention Group [published erratum appears in J Clin Epidemiol 1995 Feb;48(2):i]. *J Clin Epidemiol* 1994;47:525–536.

87. MacLennan R, Macrae F, Bain C, et al. Randomized trial of intake of fat, fiber, and beta carotene to prevent colorectal adenomas. The Australian Polyp Prevention Project. *J Natl Cancer Inst* 1995;87:1760–1766.

88. Schatzkin A, Lanza E, Corle D, et al. Lack of effect of a low-fat, high-fiber diet on the recurrence of colorectal adenomas. Polyp Prevention Trial Study Group. *N Engl J Med* 2000;342:1149–1155.

89. DeCosse JJ, Miller HH, Lesser ML. Effect of wheat fiber and vitamins C and E on rectal polyps in patients with familial adenomatous polyposis. *J Natl Cancer Inst* 1989;81:1290–1297.

90. Alberts DS, Martinez ME, Roe DJ, et al. Lack of effect of a high-fiber cereal supplement on the recurrence of colorectal adenomas. Phoenix Colon Cancer Prevention Physicians' Network. *N Engl J Med* 2000;342:1156–1162.

91. Faivre J, Couillault C, Kronborg O, et al. Chemoprevention of metachronous adenomas of the large bowel: design and interim results of a randomized trial of calcium and fibre. ECP Colon Group. *Eur J Cancer Prev* 1997;6:132–138.

92. Bonithon-Kopp C, Kronborg O, Giacosa A, et al. Calcium and fibre supplementation in prevention of colorectal adenoma recurrence: a randomised intervention trial. European Cancer Prevention Organisation Study Group. *Lancet* 2000;356: 1300–1306.

93. Thomas MG, Thomson JP, Williamson RC. Oral calcium inhibits rectal epithelial proliferation in familial adenomatous polyposis. *Br J Surg* 1993;80:499–501.

94. Hofstad B, Almendingen K, Vatn M, et al. Growth and recurrence of colorectal polyps: a double-blind 3-year intervention with calcium and antioxidants. *Digestion* 1998;59: 148–156.

95. Hofstad B, Vatn MH, Andersen SN, et al. The relationship between faecal bile acid profile with or without supplementation with calcium and antioxidants on recurrence and growth of colorectal polyps. *Eur J Cancer Prev* 1998;7: 287–294.

96. Hennekens CH, Buring JE, Manson JE, et al. Lack of effect of long-term supplementation with beta carotene on the incidence of malignant neoplasms and cardiovascular disease. *N Engl J Med* 1996;334:1145–1149.

97. Lee IM, Cook NR, Manson JE, et al. Beta-carotene supplementation and incidence of cancer and cardiovascular disease: the Women's Health Study. *J Natl Cancer Inst* 1999;91: 2102–2106.

98. Rexrode KM, Lee IM, Cook NR, et al. Baseline characteristics of participants in the Women's Health Study. *J Womens Health Gend Based Med* 2000;9:19–27.

99. Labayle D, Fischer D, Vielh P, et al. Sulindac causes regression of rectal polyps in familial adenomatous polyposis. *Gastroenterology* 1991;101:635–639.

100. Giardiello FM, Hamilton SR, Krush AJ, et al. Treatment of colonic and rectal adenomas with sulindac in familial adenomatous polyposis. *N Engl J Med* 1993;328:1313–1316.

101. Giardiello FM, Spannhake EW, DuBois RN, et al. Prostaglandin levels in human colorectal mucosa: effects of sulindac in patients with familial adenomatous polyposis. *Dig Dis Sci* 1998;43:311–316.

102. Nugent KP, Farmer KC, Spigelman AD, et al. Randomized controlled trial of the effect of sulindac on duodenal and rectal polyposis and cell proliferation in patients with familial adenomatous polyposis. *Br J Surg* 1993;80:1618–1619.

103. Steinbach G, Lynch PM, Phillips RK, et al. The effect of celecoxib, a cyclooxygenase-2 inhibitor, in familial adenomatous polyposis. *N Engl J Med* 2000;342:1946–1952.

104. Kritchevsky D. Dietary fibre and cancer. *Eur J Cancer Prev* 1997;6:435–441.

105. Chaplin MF. Bile acids, fibre and colon cancer: the story unfolds. *J R Soc Health* 1998;118:53–61.

106. Giovannucci E. Insulin and colon cancer. *Cancer Causes Control* 1995;6:164–179.

107. Heber D, Bowerman S. Applying science to changing dietary patterns. *J Nutr* 2001;131:3078S–3081S.

108. Potter JD. Colorectal cancer: molecules and populations. *J Natl Cancer Inst* 1999;91:916–932.

109. Steinmetz KA, Potter JD. Food-group consumption and colon cancer in the Adelaide Case-Control Study. I. Vegetables and fruit. *Int J Cancer* 1993;53:711–719.

110. Graham S, Dayal H, Swanson M, et al. Diet in the epidemiology of cancer of the colon and rectum. *J Natl Cancer Inst* 1978;61:709–714.

111. Tuyns AJ, Kaaks R, Haelterman M. Colorectal cancer and the consumption of foods: a case-control study in Belgium. *Nutr Cancer* 1988;11:189–204.

112. Manousos O, Day NE, Trichopoulos D, et al. Diet and colorectal cancer: a case-control study in Greece. *Int J Cancer* 1983;32:1–5.

113. Tajima K, Tominaga S. Dietary habits and gastro-intestinal cancers: a comparative case-control study of stomach and large intestinal cancers in Nagoya, Japan. *Jpn J Cancer Res* 1985;76:705–716.

114. Hu JF, Liu YY, Yu YK, et al. Diet and cancer of the colon and rectum: a case-control study in China. *Int J Epidemiol* 1991;20:362–367.

115. Le Marchand L, Wilkens LR, Kolonel LN, et al. Associations of sedentary lifestyle, obesity, smoking, alcohol use, and diabetes with the risk of colorectal cancer. *Cancer Res* 1997;57:4787–4794.

116. Lin HJ, Probst-Hensch NM, Louie AD, et al. Glutathione transferase null genotype, broccoli, and lower prevalence of colorectal adenomas. *Cancer Epidemiol Biomarkers Prev* 1998;7:647–652.

117. Pence BC. Role of calcium in colon cancer prevention: experimental and clinical studies. *Mutat Res* 1993;290:87–95.

118. Lipkin M, Yang K, Edelmann W, et al. Preclinical mouse models for cancer chemoprevention studies. *Ann NY Acad Sci* 1999;889:14–19.

119. Kato I, Akhmedkhanov A, Koenig K, et al. Prospective study of diet and female colorectal cancer: the New York University Women's Health Study. *Nutr Cancer* 1997;28: 276–281.

120. Pietinen P, Malila N, Virtanen M, et al. Diet and risk of colorectal cancer in a cohort of Finnish men. *Cancer Causes Control* 1999;10:387–396.

121. Hyman J, Baron JA, Dain BJ, et al. Dietary and supplemental calcium and the recurrence of colorectal adenomas. *Cancer Epidemiol Biomarkers Prev* 1998;7:291–295.

122. Ochsenkuhn T, Bayerdorffer E, Maining A, et al. Colonic mucosal proliferation is related to serum deoxycholic acid levels. *Cancer* 1999;85:1664–1669.

123. Martinez JD, Stratagoules ED, LaRue JM, et al. Different bile acids exhibit distinct biological effects: the tumor promoter deoxycholic acid induces apoptosis and the chemopreventive agent ursodeoxycholic acid inhibits cell proliferation. *Nutr Cancer* 1998;31:111–118.

124. Baijal PK, Fitzpatrick DW, Bird RP. Modulation of colonic xenobiotic metabolizing enzymes by feeding bile acids: comparative effects of cholic, deoxycholic, lithocholic, and ursodeoxycholic acids. *Food Chem Toxicol* 1998;36: 601–607.

125. Alberts DS, Ritenbaugh C, Story JA, et al. Randomized, double-blinded, placebo-controlled study of effect of wheat bran fiber and calcium on fecal bile acids in patients with resected adenomatous colon polyps. *J Natl Cancer Inst* 1996;88:81–92.

126. Bostick R, Potter J, Fosdick L, et al. Calcium and colorectal epithelial cell proliferation: a preliminary randomized, double-blinded, placebo-controlled clinical trial. *J Natl Cancer Inst* 1993;85:132–141.

127. Slater SJ, Kelly MB, Taddeo FJ, et al. Direct activation of protein kinase C by 1,25-dihydroxy Vitamin D_3. *J Biol Chem* 1995;270:6639–6643.

128. Sitrin MD, Halline AG, Abrahams C, Brasitus TA. Dietary calcium and vitamin D modulate 1,2 dimethylhydrazine-induced colonic carcinogenesis in the rat. *Cancer Res* 1991;51:5608–5613.

129. Belleli A, Shany S, Levy J, et al. A protective role of 1,25 dihydroxy vitamin D3 in chemically induced rat colon carcinogenesis. *Carcinogenesis* 1992;13:2293–2298.

130. Aw TY. Molecular and cellular responses to oxidative stress and changes in oxidation-reduction imbalance in the intestine. *Am J Clin Nutr* 1999;70:557–565.

131. Hengstler JG, Arand M, Herrero ME, Oesch F. Polymorphisms of *N*-acteyltransferases, glutathione *S*-transferases, microsomal epoxide hydrolase and sulfotransferases: influence on cancer susceptibility. *Recent Results Cancer Res* 1998;154: 47–85.

132. Bravo L. Polyphenols: chemistry, dietary sources, metabolism, and nutritional significance. *Nutr Rev* 1998;56:317–333.

133. Tanaka T. Effect of diet on human carcinogenesis. *Crit Rev Oncol Hematol* 1997;25:73–95.

134. Enger SM, Longnecker MP, Chen MJ, et al. Dietary intake of specific carotenoids and vitamins A, C, and E, and the prevalence of colorectal adenomas. *Cancer Epidemiol Biomarkers Prev* 1996;5:147–153.

135. Lupulescu A. The role of hormones, growth factors, and vitamins in carcinogenesis. *Crit Rev Oncol Hematol* 1996;23: 95–130.

136. Tseng M, Murray SC, Kupper LL, Sandler RS. Micronutrients and the risk of colorectal adenomas [published erratum appears in *Am J Epidemiol* 1997;146:788]. *Am J Epidemiol* 1996;144:1005–1014.

137. Greenberg ER, Baron JA, Tosteson TD, et al. A clinical trial of antioxidant vitamins to prevent colorectal adenoma. Polyp Prevention Study Group. *N Engl J Med* 1994;331:141–147.

138. Malila N, Virtamo J, Virtanen M, et al. The effect of alpha-tocopherol and beta-carotene supplementation on colorectal adenomas in middle-aged male smokers. *Cancer Epidemiol Biomarkers Prev* 1999;8:489–493.

139. Albanes D, Malila N, Taylor PR, et al. Effects of supplemental alpha-tocopherol and beta-carotene on colorectal cancer: results from a controlled trial (Finland). *Cancer Causes Control* 2000;11:197–205.

140. McKeown-Eyssen G, Holloway C, Jazmaji V, et al. A randomized trial of vitamins C and E in the prevention of recurrence of colorectal polyps. *Cancer Res* 1988;48:4701–4705.

141. Roncucci L, Di Donato P, Carati L, et al. Antioxidant vitamins or lactulose for the prevention of the recurrence of colorectal adenomas. Colorectal Cancer Study Group of the University of Modena and the Health Care District 16. *Dis Colon Rectum* 1993;36:227–234.

142. Combs GF Jr. Chemopreventive agents: selenium. *Pharmacol Ther* 1998;79:179–192.

143. Nomura A, Heilbrun LK, Morris S, Stemmerman GN. Serum selenium and the risk of cancer, by specific sites: case-control analysis of prospective data. *J Natl Cancer Inst* 1987;79:103–108.

144. Ghadirian P, Masionneuve P, Perret C, et al. A case-control study of toenail selenium and cancer of the breast, colon, and prostate. *Cancer Detect Prev* 2000;24:305–313.

145. Clark LC, Combs GF, Turnbull BW, et al. Effects of selenium supplementation for cancer prevention in patients with carcinoma of the skin. *JAMA* 1996;276:1957–1963.

146. Clark LC, Dalkin B, Krongrad A, et al. Decreased incidence of prostate cancer with selenium supplementation: results of a double-blind cancer prevention trial. *Br J Urol* 1998;81:730–734.

147. Christman JK, Sheikhnejad G, Diznik M, et al. Reversibility of changes in nucleic acid methylation and gene expression induced in rat liver by severe dietary methyl deficiency. *Carcinogenesis* 1993;14:551–557.

148. Song J, Sohn KJ, Medline A, et al. Chemopreventive effects of dietary folate on intestinal polyps in Apc+/–Msh2–/– mice. *Cancer Res* 2000;60:3191 3199.

149. Ma J, Stampfer MJ, Giovannucci E, et al. Methylenetetrahydrofolate reductase polymorphism, dietary interactions, and risk of colorectal cancer. *Cancer Res* 1997;57:1098–1102.

150. Ma J, Stampfer MJ, Christensen B, et al. A polymorphism of the methionine synthase gene: association with plasma folate, vitamin B12, homocyst(e)ine, and colorectal cancer risk. *Cancer Epidemiol Biomarkers Prev* 1999;8:825–829.

151. Slattery ML, Potter JD, Samowitz W, et al. Methylenetetrahydrofolate reductase, diet, and risk of colon cancer. *Cancer Epidemiol Biomarkers Prev* 1999;8:513–518.

152. Chen J, Giovannucci E, Hankinson SE, et al. A prospective study of methylenetetrahydrofolate reductase and methionine synthase gene polymorphisms, and risk of colorectal adenoma. *Carcinogenesis* 1998;19:2129–2132.

153. Kelloff GJ, Boone CW, Sigman CC, Greenwald P. Chemoprevention of colorectal cancer. In Young GP, Rozen P, Levin B, eds. *Prevention and Early Detection of Colorectal Cancer* W.B. Saunders Company Ltd., London, 1996;115–139.

154. Waddell WR, Loughry RW. Sulindac for polyposis of the colon. *J Surg Oncol* 1983;24:83–87.

155. Tonelli F, Valanzano R, Messerini L, Ficari F. Long-term treatment with sulindac in familial adenomatous polyposis: is there an actual efficacy in prevention of rectal cancer? *J Surg Oncol* 2000;74:15–20.

156. Lynch HT, Thorson AG, Smyrk T. Rectal cancer after prolonged sulindac chemoprevention. A case report. *Cancer* 1995;75:936–938.

157. Furstenberger G, Gross M, Marks F. Eicosanoids and multistage carcinogenesis in NMRI mouse skin: role of prostaglandins E and F in conversion (first stage of tumor promotion) and promotion (second stage of tumor promotion). *Carcinogenesis* 1989;10:91–96.

158. Sheng H, Shao J, Morrow JD, et al. Modulation of apoptosis and Bcl-2 expression by prostaglandin E2 in human colon cancer cells. *Cancer Res* 1998;58:362–366.

159. Botti C, Seregni E, Ferreri L, et al. Immunosuppressive factors: role in cancer development and progression. *Int J Biol Markers* 1998;13:51–69.

160. Yang VW, Shields JM, Hamilton SR, et al. Size-dependent increase in prostanoid levels in adenomas of patients with familial adenomatous polyposis. *Cancer Res* 1998;58:1750–1753.

161. Yang VW, Geiman DE, Hubbard WC, et al. Tissue prostanoids as biomarkers for chemoprevention of colorectal neoplasia: correlation between prostanoid synthesis and clinical response in familial adenomatous polyposis. *Prostaglandins Other Lipid Mediat* 2000; 60:83–96.

162. Kujubu DA, Fletcher BS, Varnum BC, et al. TIS 10, a phorbol ester tumor promoter-inducible mRNA from Swiss 3T3 cells, encodes a novel prostaglandin synthase/cyclooxygenase homologue. *J Biol Chem* 1991;266:12,866–12,872.

163. Marks F, Furstenberger G. Cancer chemoprevention through interruption of multistage carcinogenesis: the lessons learnt by comparing mouse skin carcinogenesis and human large bowel cancer. *Eur J Cancer* 2000;36:314–329.

164. Sheng H, Shao J, Morrow JD, et al. Modulation of apoptosis and Bcl-2 expression by prostaglandin E2 in human colon cancer cells. *Cancer Res* 1998;58:362–366.

165. Pasricha PJ, Bedi A, O'Connor K, et al. The effects of sulindac on colorectal proliferation and apoptosis in familial adenomatous polyposis. *Gastroenterology* 1995;109:994–998.

166. Oshima M, Dinchuk JE, Kargman SL, et al. Suppression of intestinal polyposis in APC$^{\Delta 716}$ knockout mice by inhibition of cyclooxygenase-2 (COX-2). *Cell* 1995;83:493–501.

167. Jacoby RF, Seibert K, Cole CE, et al. The cyclooxygenase-2 inhibitor celecoxib is a potent preventive and therapeutic agent in the min mouse model of adenomatous polyposis. *Cancer Res* 2000;60:5040–5044.

168. Huang C, Ma WY, Hahnenberger D, et al. Inhibition of untraviolet B-induced activator protein-1 (AP-1) activity by aspirin in AP-1-luciferase transgenic mice. *J Biol Chem* 1997;272: 26,325–26,331.

169. Xie W, Herschman HR. Transcriptional regulation of prostaglandin-2 gene expression by platelet-derived growth factor and serum. *J Biol Chem* 1996;271: 31,742–31,748.

170. Kipp E, Gosh S. Inhibition of NF-kappa B by sodium salicylate and aspirin. *Science* 1994;265:956–959.

171. Piazza GA, Alberts DS, Hixson LJ, et al. Sulindac sulfone inhibits azoxymethane-induced colon carcinogenesis in rats

without reducing prostaglandin levels. *Cancer Res* 1997;57:2909–2915.

172. Stoner GD, Budd GT, Ganapathi R, et al. Sulindac sulfone induced regression of rectal polyps in patients with familial adenomatous polyposis. *Adv Exp Med Biol* 1999;470:47–53.

173. Potter JD. Hormones and colon cancer. *J Natl Cancer Inst* 1995;87:1039–1040.

174. McMichael AJ, Potter JD. Reproduction, endogenous and exogenous sex hormones, and colon cancer: a review and hypothesis. *J Natl Cancer Inst* 1980;65:1201–1207.

175. Grodstein F, Newcomb PA, Stampfer, MJ. Postmenopausal hormone therapy and the risk of colorectal cancer: a review and meta-analysis. *Am J Med* 1999;106:574–582.

176. Hebert-Croteau N. A meta-analysis of hormone replacement therapy and colon cancer in women. *Cancer Epidemiol Biomarkers Prev* 1998;7:653–659.

177. Zhu BT, Conney AH. Is 2-methoxyestradiol an endogenous estrogen metabolite that inhibits mammary carcinogenesis? *Cancer Res* 1998;58:2269–2277.

178. Telang NT, Suto A, Wong GY, et al. Induction by estrogen metabolite 16α-hydroxyestrone of genotoxic damage and aberrant proliferation in mouse mammary epithelial cells. *J Natl Cancer Inst* 1992;84:634–638.

179. Klauber N, Paragni S, Flynn E, et al. Inhibition of angiogenesis and breast cancer in mice by the microtubule inhibitors 2-methoxyestradiol and taxol. *Cancer Res* 1997;57:81–86.

180. Okolicsanyi L, Lirussi F, Strazzabosco M, et al. The effect of drugs on bile flow and composition. An overview. *Drugs* 1986;31:430–448.

181. Issa JP, Ottaviano YL, Celano P, et al. Methylation of the oestrogen receptor CpG island links ageing and neoplasia in human colon. *Nat Genet* 1994;7:536–540.

182. Campagnoli C, Biglia N, Cantamessa C, et al. Effect of progestins on IGF-I serum level in estrogen-treated postmenopausal women. *Zentralbl Gynakol* 1997;119:7–11.

183. Design of the Women's Health Initiative clinical trial and observational study. The Women's Health Initiative Study Group. *Control Clin Trials* 1998;19:61–109.

184. Kelloff GJ, Boone CW, Steele VE, et al. Mechanistic considerations in chemopreventive drug development. *J Cell Biochem Suppl* 1994;20:1–24.

185. Thompson H, Ronan A. Effect of D,L-2-difluoromethylornithine and endocrine manipulation on the induction of mammary carcinogenesis by 1-methyl-1-nitrosourea. *Carcinogenesis* 1986;7:2003–2006.

186. Reddy B, Nayini J, Tokumo K, et al. Chemoprevention of colon carcinogenesis by concurrent administration of piroxicam, a nonsteroidal antiinflammatory drug with D,l-a-difluoromethylornithine, an ornithine decarboxylase inhibitor, in diet. *Cancer Res* 1990;50:2562–2568.

187. McCormack SA, Blanner PM, Zimmerman BJ, et al. Polyamine deficiency alters EGF receptor distribution and signaling effectiveness in IEC-6 cells. *Am J Physiol* 1998;274:C192–205.

188. Wallon UM, Shassetz LR, Cress AE, et al. Polyamine-dependent expression of the matrix metalloproteinase matrilysin in a human colon cancer-derived cell line. *Mol Carcinog* 1994;11:138–144.

189. Nigro ND, Bull AW, Boyd ME. Inhibition of intestinal carcinogenesis in rats: effect of difluoromethylornithine with piroxicam or fish oil. *J Natl Cancer Inst* 1986;77:1309–1313.

190. Rao CV, Tokumo K, Rigotty J, et al. Chemoprevention of colon carcinogenesis by dietary administration of piroxicam, alpha-difluoromethylornithine, 16 alpha-fluoro-5-androsten-17-one, and ellagic acid individually and in combination. *Cancer Res* 1991;51:4528–4534.

191. Li H, Schut HA, Conran P, et al. Prevention by aspirin and its combination with alpha- difluoromethylornithine of azoxymethane-induced tumors, aberrant crypt foci and prostaglandin E2 levels in rat colon. *Carcinogenesis* 1999;20:425–430.

192. Jacoby RF, Cole CE, Tutsch K, et al. Chemopreventive efficacy of combined piroxicam and difluoromethylornithine treatment of Apc mutant Min mouse adenomas, and selective toxicity against Apc mutant embryos. *Cancer Res* 2000;60:1864–1870.

193. McGarrity TJ, Peiffer LP. Selenium and difluoromethylornithine additively inhibit DMH-induced distal colon tumor formation in rats fed a fiber-free diet. *Carcinogenesis* 1993;14:2335–2340.

194. Love RR, Jacoby R, Newton MA, et al. A randomized, placebo-controlled trial of low-dose alpha-difluoromethylornithine in individuals at risk for colorectal cancer. *Cancer Epidemiol Biomarkers Prev* 1998;7:989–992.

195. Watabe J, Bernstein H. The mutagenicity of bile acids using a fluctuation test. *Mutat Res* 1985;158:45–51.

196. Martinez JD, Stratagoules ED, LaRue JM, et al. Different bile acids exhibit distinct biological effects: the tumor promoter deoxycholic acid induces apoptosis and the chemopreventive agent ursodeoxycholic acid inhibits cell proliferation. *Nutr Cancer* 1998;31:111–118.

197. Ochsenkuhn T, Bayerdorffer E, Meining A, et al. Colonic mucosal proliferation is related to serum deoxycholic acid levels. *Cancer* 1999;85:1664–1669.

198. Earnest DL, Holubec H, Wali RK, et al. Chemoprevention of azoxymethane-induced colonic carcinogenesis by supplemental dietary ursodeoxycholic acid. *Cancer Res* 1994;54:5071–5074.

199. Narisawa T, Fukaura Y, Terada K, Sekiguchi H. Inhibitory effects of ursodeoxycholic acid on N-methylnitrosourea-induced colon carcinogenesis and colonic mucosal telomerase activity in F344 rats. *J Exp Clin Cancer Res* 1999;18:259–266.

200. Guldutuna S, Zimmer G, Imhof M, et al. Molecular aspects of membrane stabilization by ursodeoxycholate. *Gastroenterology* 1993;104:1736–1744.

201. Leuschner U, Fischer H, Kurtz W, et al. Ursodeoxycholic acid in primary biliary cirrhosis: results of a controlled double-blind trial. *Gastroenterology* 1989;97:1268–1274.

202. Rigas B, Tsioulias GJ, Allan C, et al. The effect of bile acids and piroxicam on MHC antigen expression in rat colonocytes during colon cancer development. *Immunology* 1994;83:319–323.

203. Brasitus TA. Primary chemoprevention strategies for colorectal cancer: ursodeoxycholic acid and other agents. *Gastroenterology* 1995;109:2036–2038.

204. Wali RK, Frawley BPJ, Hartmann S, et al. Mechanism of action of chemoprotective ursodeoxycholate in the azoxymethane model of rat colonic carcinogenesis: potential roles of protein kinase C-alpha, -beta II, and -zeta. *Cancer Res* 1995;55:5257–5264.

205. Ikegami T, Matsuzaki Y, Shoda J, et al. The chemopreventive role of ursodeoxycholic acid in azoxymethane- treated rats: suppressive effects on enhanced group II phospholipase A2 expression in colonic tissue. *Cancer Lett* 1998;134:129–139.

206. Invernizzi P, Salzman AL, Szabo C, et al. Ursodeoxycholate inhibits induction of NOS in human intestinal epithelial cells and in vivo. *Am J Physiol* 1997;273: G131–G138.

207. Tung BY, Emond MJ, Haggitt RC, et al. Ursodiol use is associated with lower prevalence of colonic neoplasia in patients with ulcerative colitis and primary sclerosing cholangitis. *Ann Intern Med* 2001;134:89–95.

208. Hawk ET, Viner JL. Chemoprevention in ulcerative colitis: narrowing the gap between clinical practice and research. *Ann Intern Med* 2001;134:158–160.

209. Kikuchi T, Nagata Y, Abe T. In vitro and in vivo antiproliferative effects of simvastatin, an HMG- CoA reductase inhibitor, on human glioma cells. *J Neurooncol* 1997;34: 233–239.

210. Newman A, Clutterbuck RD, Powles RL, et al. A comparison of the effect of the 3-hydroxy-3-methylglutaryl coenzyme A (HMG-CoA) reductase inhibitors simvastatin, lovastatin and pravastatin on leukaemic and normal bone marrow progenitors. *Leuk Lymphoma* 1997;24:533–537.

211. Rubins JB, Greatens T, Kratzke RA, et al. Lovastatin induces apoptosis in malignant mesothelioma cells. *Am J Respir Crit Care Med* 1998;157:1616–1622.

212. Narisawa T, Fukaura Y, Terada K, et al. Prevention of 1,2-dimethylhydrazine-induced colon tumorigenesis by HMG-CoA reductase inhibitors, pravastatin and simvastatin, in ICR mice. *Carcinogenesis* 1994;15:2045–2048.

213. Narisawa T, Fukaura Y, Tanida N, et al. Chemopreventive efficacy of low dose of pravastatin, an HMG-CoA reductase inhibitor, on 1,2-dimethylhydrazine-induced colon carcinogenesis in ICR mice. *Tohoku J Exp Med* 1996;180:131–138.

214. Gould MN. Cancer chemoprevention and therapy by monoterpenes. *Environ Health Perspect* 105 Suppl 1997;4: 977–979.

215. Crowell PL. Prevention and therapy of cancer by dietary monoterpenes. *J Nutr* 1999;129:775S–778S.

216. Kawamori T, Tanaka T, Hirose Y, et al. Inhibitory effects of d-limonene on the development of colonic aberrant crypt foci induced by azoxymethane in F344 rats. *Carcinogenesis* 1996;17:369–372.

217. Reddy BS, Wang CX, Samaha H, et al. Chemoprevention of colon carcinogenesis by dietary perillyl alcohol. *Cancer Res* 1997;57:420–425.

218. Weed HG, McGandy RB, Kennedy AR. Protection against dimethylhydrazine-induced adenomatous tumors of the mouse colon by the dietary addition of an extract of soybeans containing the Bowman-Birk protease inhibitor. *Carcinogenesis* 1985;6:1239–1241.

219. St. Clair WH, Billings PC, Carew JA, et al. Suppression of dimethylhydrazine-induced carcinogenesis in mice by dietary addition of the Bowman-Birk protease inhibitor. *Cancer Res* 1990;50:580–586.

220. Kennedy AR, Beazer-Barclay Y, Kinzler KW, Newberne PM. Suppression of carcinogenesis in the intestines of min mice by the soybean-derived Bowman-Birk inhibitor. *Cancer Res* 1996;56:679–682.

221. Newell KJ, Witty JP, Rodgers WH, Matrisian LM. Expression and localization of matrix-degrading metalloproteinases during colorectal tumorigenesis. *Mol Carcinog* 1994;10:199–206.

222. Wilson CL, Heppner KJ, Labosky PA, et al. Intestinal tumorigenesis is suppressed in mice lacking the metalloproteinase matrilysin. *Proc Natl Acad Sci USA* 1997;94: 1402–1407.

223. Goss KJ, Brown PD, Matrisian LM. Differing effects of endogenous and synthetic inhibitors of metalloproteinases on intestinal tumorigenesis. *Int J Cancer* 1998;8:629–635.

224. Fingleton BM, Heppner Goss KJ, Crawford HC, Matrisian LM. Matrilysin in early stage intestinal tumorigenesis. *APMIS* 1999;107:102–110.

225. Dannenberg AJ, Zakim D. Chemoprevention of colorectal cancer through inhibition of cyclooxygenase-2. *Semin Oncol* 1999;26:499–504.

226. Green DW, Roh H, Pippin JA, Drebin JA. Beta-catenin antisense treatment decreases beta-catenin expression and tumor growth rate in colon carcinoma xenografts. *J Surg Res* 2001;101:16–20.

227. Roh H, Green DW, Boswell CB, et al. Suppression of beta-catenin inhibits the neoplastic growth of APC-mutant colon cancer cells. *Cancer Res* 2001;61:6563–6568.

228. Bos JL. ras Oncogenes in human cancer: a review [published erratum appears in *Cancer Res* 1990;50:1352]. *Cancer Res* 1989;49:4682–4689.

229. Rowinsky EK, Windle JJ, Von Hoff DD. Ras protein farnesyltransferase: a strategic target for anticancer therapeutic development. *J Clin Oncol* 1999;17:3631–3652.

230. Kelloff GJ, Fay JR, Steele VE, et al. Epidermal growth factor receptor tyrosine kinase inhibitors as potential cancer chemopreventives. *Cancer Epidemiol Biomarkers Prev* 1996;5: 657–666.

231. Huang SM, Harari PM. Epidermal growth factor receptor inhibition in cancer therapy: biology, rationale and preliminary clinical results. *Invest New Drugs* 1999;17:259–269.

232. Torrance CJ, Jackson PE, Montgomery E, et al. Combinatorial chemoprevention of intestinal neoplasia. *Nat Med* 2000;6: 1024–1028.

233. Pollak M. Insulin-like growth factor physiology and cancer risk. *Eur J Cancer* 2000;36:1224–1228.

234. Kath R, Hoffken K. The significance of somatostatin analogues in the antiproliferative treatment of carcinomas. *Recent Results Cancer Res* 2000;153:23–43.

235. Tang R, Cheng AJ, Wang JY, Wang TC. Close correlation between telomerase expression and adenomatous polyp progression in multistep colorectal carcinogenesis. *Cancer Res* 1998;58:4052–4054.

236. Hahn WC, Stewart SA, Brooks MW, et al. Inhibition of telomerase limits the growth of human cancer cells. *Nat Med* 1999;5:1164–1170.

21 Screening in Risk Evaluation and Prevention of Colorectal Cancer

Bernard Levin, MD

CONTENTS

INTRODUCTION
SECONDARY PREVENTION
IMPLEMENTATION OF SCREENING
EMERGING TECHNOLOGIES
CONCLUSION
REFERENCES

1. INTRODUCTION

Colorectal cancer (CRC) is the second leading cause of cancer death in the United States *(1)*. In 2002, 148,000 new cases and 57,000 deaths were estimated to occur from this disease. CRC incidence and mortality rates increase with age, markedly so after age 60. Overall CRC death rates decreased by 1.8% per year from 1992 to 1998 *(2)*; however, the death rates for CRC remain higher for African-Americans than for other ethnic groups.

Many new cases and deaths of CRC could be averted by more timely use of screening tests *(3)*, lifestyle modifications, and potentially by chemoprevention *(4)*. Currently only 37% of CRC are discovered in the earliest stage (Fig. 1).

The lifetime probability (magnitude of absolute risk) of US men and women for developing CRC is about 6% *(3)*. Risk factors for CRC development are listed in Table 1.

2. SECONDARY PREVENTION

Screening and early detection (secondary prevention) are of importance in influencing the outcome of patients with CRC. A screening test is intended to distinguish the most likely population to have a neoplastic lesion. Those with abnormal tests are recommended to undergo diagnostic tests to confirm the presence or absence of cancer. The screening process is detailed in Table 2.

Several existing screening methods have demonstrated effectiveness in reducing mortality from CRC. Detection and removal of adenomatous polyps before they become invasive is an extremely important strategy. Detection and surgical resection of CRC when still highly curable also has a major impact on the outcome. Symptomatic malignancies are often locally advanced or have spread to distant sites.

Among the four screening tests currently in routine use, the strongest evidence exists for fecal occult blood testing. Intermediate-level evidence is available for flexible sigmoidoscopy; only indirect evidence supports the use of colonoscopy and double-contrast barium enema (Table 3).

2.1. Fecal Occult Blood Test (FOBT)

Because large adenomas and most cancers bleed intermittently, screening is based on the presence of blood in the stool. Small adenomas rarely bleed. The major features of different types of FOBTs are outlined in Table 4; usage issues related to the two major types of FOBT are indicated in Table 5.

Guaiac-based tests for peroxidase activity have been the most commonly used in population screening. These results have been obtained using the traditional three-card test performed at home. In major randomized controlled trials, FOBT has been shown to reduce CRC mortality *(5–7)*. The results of these trials are presented in Table 6. A recent update to the Danish Fecal

From: Cancer Chemoprevention, Volume 2: Strategies for Cancer Chemoprevention
Edited by: G. J. Kelloff, E. T. Hawk, and C. C. Sigman © Humana Press Inc., Totowa, NJ

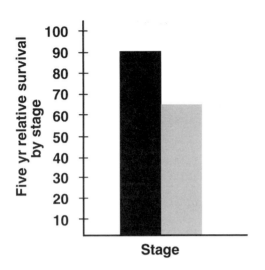

Fig. 1. Colorectal cancer survival. Only 37% of colorectal cancers are discovered in the earliest stage.

Occult Blood Trial indicated that the relative risk for death from CRC in participants who adhered to all seven screening rounds was reduced by 30% compared with controls. The reduction in mortality for CRC proximal to the sigmoid colon was 28%; it was only 8% for cancers of the rectum and sigmoid. In this trial, the cumulative risk for a positive test was 5.1% after seven rounds; 4.8% of patients underwent at least one colonoscopy *(8)*.

Annual testing is recommended because randomized trials have demonstrated that testing every 2 yr is less

Table 1
Risk Factors for Colorectal Cancer

Average Risk	≥50 years of age
Decreased Risk	High vegetable consumption
	Oral contraceptive use
	Estrogen replacement
	Multivitamins containing folic acid
	Long-term use of NSAIDs
Increased Risk	Family History
	– Colorectal cancer
	– Colorectal adenomas
	Personal History
	– Colorectal adenomas
	– Ovarian, uterine cancers
	Familial adenomatous polyposis
	Peutz-Jeghers syndrome
	Juvenile polyposis
	Inflammatory bowel disease
	Physical inactivity (<3 hours per week)
	Obesity
	Smoking
	Alcohol (>1 drink/day)

Table 2
The Screening Process

Target those at risk for colorectal cancer

Invite participation in screening program

Ensure that special circumstances such as symptoms or family history are identified early in the process

Perform the screening test, which is safe, effective, acceptable and affordable

Use the result to identify those who should undertake the diagnostic process

Ensure compliance with the appropriate diagnostic follow-up

Ensure adequate subsequent treatment

Offer rescreening at appropriate intervals

Monitor the outcomes of the program

Data from *3*.

effective. Annual testing may allow detection of disease that, though undetected on prior occasions, has not reached an incurable stage. Meta-analysis of mortality results from the randomized controlled trials shows that those allocated to screening had a decrease in CRC

Table 3
Evidence Supporting Effectiveness of Colorectal Cancer Screening Tests[a]

Test	Quality of Evidence[b]	Benefit/ Comments
FOBT	I	33% reduction in CRC mortality with annual rehydrated FOBT
	I	15%–18% reduction in CRC mortality with biennial, unrehydrated FOBT
Sigmoidoscopy	I	80% reduction in CRC incidence with flexible sigmoidoscopy
	II	60–95% reduction in mortality for cases of distal CRC
Colonoscopy	III	Sensitivity 27%–47% greater than that of 60 cm flexible sigmoidoscopy for advanced adenomas
DCBE	III	Sensitivity for adenomatous polyps lower than that of colonoscopy but much higher than that of FOBT

[a]DCBE = double-contrast barium enema; FOBT = fecal occult blood test.

[b]I = randomized, controlled trial, II = controlled observational study (case-control or corhort); III = descriptive study.

Data from *36*.

Table 4
Main Features of Different Types of Fecal Occult Blood Tests (FOBTs)

Type of FOBT	Basis	Stool-Sampling Method	Endpoint
Chemical	Guaiac; detects peroxidase	Wooden spatula and fecal smear for most	Blue blush of color on paper card
Immunochemical	Antihemoglobin antibody	Wooden spatula, probe, spoon, or brush	Latex or red cell agglutination
			Solid-phase immuno-chromatography
			Enzyme-linked immuno-sorsorbent sorbent assay (ELISA)

Data from *3*.

mortality of 16% (RR = 0.84, CI = 0.77–0.93). When adjusted for screening attendance in the individual studies, the mortality reduction is 23% (RR = 0.77, CI = 0.57–0.89) *(9)*.

Estimates of the sensitivity of FOBT have ranged from 25% to over 90%. Studies that show higher sensitivity usually refer to "program sensitivity" or the effectiveness of repeated FOBT over several years. One concern of tests with low sensitivity is that those who have a false negative test may be falsely reassured. Another concern has been lack of specificity associated with a high false positive rate, which means that many with no colorectal neoplasia will undergo screening colonoscopy with associated risks and disruption to lifestyle. It is estimated that if 10,000 people were offered inclusion in a biennial Hemoccult Screening Program and two thirds attended

for at least one Hemoccult test, 8.5 deaths (CI = 3.6–13.5) from CRC would be prevented over 10 yr. Data from the Minnesota trial shows that such screening would also result in 2800 participants having at least one colonoscopy, which would generate 3.4 colonoscopy complications (perforation or hemorrhage) *(9)*. Compared with endoscopic tests, FOBT detects relatively few adenomas; the principal benefit of an FOBT program is to increase detection of early-stage cancers.

Newer FOBTs use enhanced guaiac reagents that improve sensitivity without much negative impact on specificity if recommended dietary measures are followed. The sensitivity of immunochemical FOBTs is better than that of Hemoccult without an unacceptable decline in specificity *(3)*. Newer immunochemical FOBTs can be read by automated techniques.

Table 5
Usage Issues of Different Types of FOBTs

Type of FOBT	Diet Restrictions	Drug Interference	Site of Bleeding Detectable	Endpoint for Test Result
Chemical	Must avoid red meats; possibly avoid certain raw plant foods[a]	Vitamin C; possibly NSAIDs[b]	Rectum > colon > stomach (in decreasing order of sensitivity)	Subjective and transient[c]
Immunochemical	None required	None required	Colon and rectum	Agglutination tests[c]— can be difficult to read Immunochromatography—easy to read ELISA—machine-read

[a]Delaying development for 72 h minimizes interference from plant foods and avoids the need for their restriction.

[b]NSAIDs: low-dose aspirin is not a problem, but therapeutic doses for rheumatic disorders may be so.

[c]The tests generally provide a qualitative result, but newer immunochromatographic tests may be quantifiable.

Data from *3*.

Table 6
Summary of Three Randomized Trials (refs. 5–7) of FOBT

	Minnesota: Mandel et al. 1975–1992 (5)	United Kingdom: Hardcastle et al. 1981–1995 (6)	Denmark: Kronborg et al. 1985–1995 (7)
Participants (n)	46,551	152,850	137,000
Type of Test	Hemoccult II	Hemoccult	Hemoccult II
Positivity Rate	2–10%	2%	0.8–5.1%
Colonoscopy Rate	28–38%	4%	5%
Sensitivity	81–92%	67%	51%
PPV[a] for CRC	2–6%	10–15%	8–18%
Decrease In:			
• Mortality Rate			
Annual	33%	—	—
Biennial	21%	15%	15%
• Incidence	17–20%	—	—

[a]PPV = positive predictive value.

2.2. Endoscopic Screening Tests

Examination of the large bowel by flexible sigmoidoscopy or colonoscopy permits direct visualization of the mucosa as well as photodocumentation, biopsy of suspicious lesions, and endoscopic polypectomy.

2.2.1. FLEXIBLE SIGMOIDOSCOPY

Case-control studies have demonstrated an association between sigmoidoscopic examination of the rectum or rectosigmoid and a reduction in the chance of dying from CRC that occurs within reach of the instrument. A case-control study from the Kaiser Permanente program demonstrated a 70% risk reduction for cancers within reach of the sigmoidoscope, and data suggested that the benefit may last as long as 10 yr (10). A prospective study from the US Health Professionals Study showed that screening (primarily with flexible sigmoidoscopy) was associated with a 60% reduction in distal CRC incidence (11). In a prospective randomized trial in Norway, CRC incidence was reduced 80% compared to unscreened controls in 400 patients who had flexible sigmoidoscopy screening followed by colonoscopy when polyps were detected (12).

Two large-scale prospectively randomized controlled studies are examining the efficacy of flexible sigmoidoscopy. In the US, the Prostate, Lung, Colorectal, Ovary (PLCO) trial has enrolled 154,000 individuals aged 55 to 74 yr. Final results will not be available for several years (13). Baseline findings of a multicenter trial in the United Kingdom (UK) were recently reported. Distal adenomas were detected in 12% and distal cancers in 0.3% of approx 40,000 individuals screened. Proximal adenomas were detected in 19% of those undergoing colonoscopy and proximal cancer in 0.4%; 62% of cancers were early (Dukes' Stage A). There was one perforation after flexible sigmoidoscopy and four after colonoscopy (14).

Sigmoidoscopy detects 70–85% of advanced lesions throughout the colon (15). Individuals with an advanced distal adenoma have a 6–10% chance of having an advanced proximal adenoma. When a nonadvanced adenoma is found during sigmoidoscopy, the chance of a proximal advanced lesion is lower, viz. 4.7%. Screening colonoscopy studies have suggested that individuals with an apparently normal sigmoidoscopy have a 1–2% risk of having an advanced proximal lesion (16). In contrast, among patients with advanced distal polyps, the prevalence of advanced proximal neoplasia was 11.5%.

Obstacles to more widespread use of flexible sigmoidoscopy include lack of training and relatively low reimbursement rates. Training of nonphysician personnel to perform flexible sigmoidoscopy, especially in high-volume centers, may facilitate more widespread use of this technique.

The impact of combining fecal occult blood testing with flexible sigmoidoscopy is advocated (Table 7), but the impact on mortality has not been critically examined.

2.2.2. COLONOSCOPY

The effectiveness of colonoscopy has been demonstrated by several observational studies. In the National Polyp Study (NPS), 1418 patients were prospectively

Table 7
American Cancer Society Recommendations for Early Cancer Detection in Average-Risk, Asymptomatic People

Cancer Site	Population	Test or Procedure	Frequency
Colorectal	Men and women	FOBT and flexible sigmoidoscopy[a]	Annual FOBT and flexible sigmoidoscopy every 5 yr, starting at age 50
		-or-	
		Flexible sigmoidoscopy	Every 5 yr, starting at age 50
		-or-	
		FOBT	Annual, starting at age 50
		-or-	
		Colonoscopy	Colonoscopy every 10 yr, starting at age 50,
		-or-	
		Double contrast barium enema (DCBE)	DCBE every 5 yr, starting at age 50

[a]Flexible sigmoidoscopy together with FOBT is preferred over FOBT or flexible sigmoidoscopy alone.

Data from *24*.

followed after a colonoscopic polypectomy during which one or more adenomas were removed. The observed incidence of CRC in the NPS cohort was compared with the expected rates based on three noconcurrent reference groups. A reduction in incidence of 76–90% was observed *(17)*. A Veterans Administration (VA) case-control study described a reduction in CRC incidence of 50% *(18)*. Two recent colonoscopy studies from Italy and Denmark have reported reduction in CRC incidence after polypectomy *(19,20)*.

Three nonrandomized studies have reported baseline results of screening colonoscopy. In a study of 3212 US veterans (almost all male) with a mean age of 63 yr, Lieberman et al. reported an adenoma incidence rate of 37% *(15)*. Advanced adenoma incidence (diameter at least 10 mm, villous features, high-grade dysplasia or cancer) was 10.5%. A Navy study of 1,322 women reported an adenoma incidence rate of 21% and an advanced adenoma incidence of 3% *(21)*. In a 1994 study of pharmaceutical industry workers (mean age 60 yr, about 60% men), Imperiale et al. reported an adenoma incidence of 17% and advanced adenoma incidence of 5.6% *(16)*.

A randomized controlled trial of screening colonoscopy to examine efficacy has not been performed, although a pilot study is in progress in three centers *(22)*.

2.2.3. DOUBLE-CONTRAST BARIUM ENEMA (DCBE)

There has not been a formal trial of barium enema as a population screen. A comparison was performed of colonoscopy and DCBE for surveillance after polypectomy *(23)*. The proportion of examinations in which

adenomatous polyps were detected by barium enema and colonoscopy was significantly related to the size of the adenomas. The rate was 53% for those in which the largest adenomas detected were 0.6 to 1.0 cm and 48% for those in which the largest adenomas exceeded 1.0 cm. Although listed as an option for screening, lack of junior radiologists trained in this technique is likely to further limit its use in the future.

3. IMPLEMENTATION OF SCREENING

The options discussed above for CRC screening, including FOBT, endoscopic visualization by flexible sigmoidoscopy and colonoscopy, and DCBE, differ in sensitivity, specificity, cost, and complexity. They also have different limitations and potential harms (*see* Table 8). However, much data supports the efficacy and cost effectiveness of screening for CRC. Several organizations have published CRC screening recommendations *(24–26)* (Table 7). All endorse regular screening for average-risk adults 50 years of age and older. The most recent endorsement of CRC screening has come from the US Preventive Services Task Force (USPSTF) *(26)*.

Despite the acknowledged benefits, the majority of Americans are not being screened for CRC. Data from the 1999 Behavioral Risk Factor Surveillance System Survey indicated that only 21% of respondents had undergone a FOBT within the prior year and approximately 34% had undergone sigmoidoscopy or colonoscopy within the prior 5 yr (Table 9) *(27)*. There remains a significant challenge to enhance screening

Table 8
Comparison of Characteristics of Screening Options

Screening Test	Effectiveness	Strength of Evidence	Risk of Complication	Complexity[a]	Cost
FOBT	Moderate	High	Low	Low	Low
Flexible sigmoidoscopy					
FOBT & flexible sigmoidoscopy	↓	↑	↓	↓	↓
DCBE					
Colonoscopy	High	Moderate	High	High	High

[a]Complexity involves patient discomfort, preparation, and inconvenience, as well as facilities and equipment needed.

Adapted from materials created by the Massachusetts Colorectal Cancer Working Group.

Table 9
Prevalence (%) of Cancer Screening among US Adults, Behavioral Risk Factor Surveillance System (BRFSS), 1999 and 2000

Colorectal Cancer	Age	Males Median	(Range)	Females Median	(Range)	Total Median	(Range)
Either a flexible sigmoidoscopy or colonoscopy[a]	50+	34.2	(25.7–49.0)	30.3	21.1–37.0	32.3	(22.6–46.2)
FOBT (homekit)[b]	50++	17.1	(9.8–35.6)	2.3	(13.1–37.2)	19.0	(11.6–35.8)

[a]Recent sigmoidoscopy or colonoscopy test within the preceding five years. Source: BRFSS, 1999.

[b]Recent fecal occult blood test using a home-kit test performed within the preceding year. Source: BRFSS, 1999.

Data from (24).

rates for average-risk individuals in the US. Guidelines on screening and surveillance for those at increased risk are indicated in Table 10.

3.1. Cost-Effectiveness of CRC Screening

Cost analyses of CRC screening programs have been carried out to provide a basis from which legislation can be influenced and health benefit plans can be constructed. The cost-effectiveness of CRC screening is estimated to be approx $20,000–$40,000 per year of life gained. This compares favorably with the cost of other usually accepted preventive services such as end-stage renal dialysis or mammography (28).

4. EMERGING TECHNOLOGIES

4.1. Molecular Detection Methods

Detecting gene mutations in the stool has been possible for over a decade (29). Recent studies have indicated the technical feasibility of detecting adenomatous polyposis coli (APC) and p53 mutations in addition to K-ras mutations (29–31). In addition, right-sided lesions can be detected by identifying BAT 26 mutations (32). Systematic large-scale population-based studies are in progress to compare DNA mutation techniques with colonoscopy. The cost of such techniques is high at present, but it is possible that their effectiveness may offset these costs.

4.2. Virtual Colonoscopy—Computed Tomography (CT) Colonography

CT colonography relies on sophisticated graphics software to assemble an endoluminal image from a fast CT scan, including surface and volume characteristics (33,34). Recent data suggest a sensitivity of 90% for lesions larger than 1 cm. Maintenance of a high specificity (more than 90%) will be of great importance in reducing the need for follow-up colonoscopic examination.

5. CONCLUSION

According to the 2000 US Census, approx 77 million Americans are age 50 and older. By the year 2030, the total US population is predicted to increase by about 40%, with about a 200% increase in those over 65 yr of age. Clearly, wider use of currently available screening technologies, as well as development and

Table 10
American Cancer Society Guidelines on Screening and Surveillance for Early Detection of Colorectal Adenomas
and Cancer—Women and Men at Increased or High Risk

Risk Category	Age to Begin	Recommendation	Comment
Increased Risk			
People with a single, small (<1 cm) adenoma	3–6 yr after initial polypectomy	Colonoscopy[a]	Patients with normal exams can thereafter be screened using average-risk guidelines
People with a large (1 cm+) adenoma, multiple adenomas, with high-grade dysplasia or villous change	Within 3 yr after initial polypectomy	Colonoscopy[a]	Repeat normal exam in 3 yr; if normal then, patient can thereafter be screened using average-risk guidelines
Personal history of curative -intent resection of CRC resection of CRC	Within 1 yr after cancer resection	Colonoscopy[a]	Repeat normal exam in 3 yr; if normal then, repeat every 5 yr
Either CRC or adenomatous polyps in any first-degree relative before age 60 or in two or more first-degree relatives at any age (if not a hereditary syndrome)	Age 40, or 10 yr before the youngest case in immediate family	Colonoscopy[a]	Every 5–10 yr. Colorectal cancer in relatives more distant than first-degree does not increase risk substantially above the average-risk group.
High Risk			
Family history of familial adenomatous polyposis (FAP)	Puberty	Early surveillance with endoscopy, and counseling to consider genetic testing	If genetic test is positive, colectomy is indicated. These patients are best referred to a center with experience in FAP management
Family history of hereditary nonpolyposis colon cancer (HNPCC)	Age 21	Colonoscopy and counseling to consider genetic testing	If genetic test is positive or if patient has not had genetic testing every 1–2 yr until age 40, then annually. These patients are best referred to a center with experience in HNPCC management
Inflammatory bowel disease Chronic ulcerative colitis Crohn's disease	Cancer risk becomes significant 8 yr after pancolitis onset, or 12–15 yr after left-sided colitis onset	Colonoscopy with biopsies for dysplasia	Every 1–2 yr. These patients are best referred to a center with experience in surveillance and management of inflammatory bowel disease

[a]If colonoscopy is unavailable, not feasible, or not desired by the patient, DCBE alone, or combined flexible sigmoidoscopy and DCBE, are acceptable alternatives. Adding flexible sigmoidoscopy to DCBE may provide a more comprehensive diagnostic evaluation than DCBE alone in finding significant lesions. Supplementary DCBE may be needed if a colonoscopic exam fails to reach the cecum, and supplementary colonoscopy may be needed if DCBE identifies a possible lesion, or does not adequately visualize the entire colorectum.

Data from (24).

application of even more sensitive and specific tests, will help to reduce the very significant impact of CRC on the population.

The US National Cancer Institute estimates that CRC can shorten an affected individual's life by approx 13 yr. In 2002, the USPSTF strongly recommended that clinicians screen men and women aged 50 and older for CRC (26). If these recommendations are widely imple-

mented, it is likely that morbidity and mortality will be reduced (35).

The impact of novel screening methods such as gene mutation detection and CT colonography will emerge over the next 5 yr. It is likely that these techniques may serve to enhance the effectiveness of colonoscopy by targeting those most likely to benefit from an invasive procedure.

REFERENCES

1. Colon and rectum cancer. In *Facts and Figures 2002*. American Cancer Society, Atlanta, 2002:26–29.

2. Howe H, Wingo P, Thun M, et al. Annual report to the nation on the status of cancer (1973–1998), featuring cancers with recent increasing trends. *J Natl Cancer Inst* 2001;93: 824–842.

3. Young GP, Rozen P, Levin B. How should we screen for early colorectal neoplasia? In *Colorectal Cancer in Clinical Practice: Prevention, Early Detection and Management* Rozen P, Young G, Levin B, Spann S, eds. Martin Dunitz, Ltd, London, 2002; pp. 77–99.

4. Gatof D, Ahnen D. Primary prevention of colorectal cancer: diet and drugs. *Gastroenterol Clin North Am* 2002;31: 587–623.

5. Mandel JS, Bond JH, Church TR, et al. Reducing mortality from colorectal cancer by screening for fecal occult blood. *N Engl J Med* 1993;278:1365–1372.

6. Hardcastle JD, Chamberlain JD, Robinson NHI, et al. Randomized controlled trial of faecal occult blood screening for colorectal cancer. *Lancet* 1996;348:1472–1477.

7. Kronborg O, Fenger C, Olsen J, et al. Randomized study of screening for colorectal cancer with fecal-occult blood test. *Lancet* 1996;348:1467–1471.

8. Jorgensen OD, Kronborg O, Fenger C, et al. A randomized study of screening for colorectal cancer using faecal occult blood testing. Results after 13 years and 7 biennial screening rounds. *Gut* 2002; 50:29–32.

9. Towler BP, Irwig L, Glasziou P, et al. Screening for colorectal cancer using the faecal occult blood test, hemoccult. *Cochrane Database Syst Rev* 2002;2:CD001216.

10. Selby JV, Fredman GD, Quesenbery CP Jr, et al. A case control study of screening sigmoidoscopy and mortality from colorectal cancer. *N Engl J Med* 1992;326:653–657.

11. Kavanagh AM, Giovannucci E, Fuchs CS, Colditz GA. Screening endoscopy and risk of colorectal cancer in United States men. *Cancer Causes Control* 1998;9: 455–461.

12. Thiis-Evenson E, Hoff GS, Sauar J, et al. Population-based surveillance by colonoscopy: Effect on the incidence of colorectal cancer. Telemark Polyp Study I. *Scand J Gastroenterol* 1999;34:414–420.

13. Prorok PC, Andriole GL, Bresalier RS, et al. Design of the prostate, lung, colorectal and ovarian (PLCO) cancer screening trial. *Control Clin Trials* 2000;21:2735–3095.

14. UK Flexible Sigmoidoscopy Screening Trial Investigators. Single flexible sigmoidoscopy screening to prevent colorectal cancer: baseline findings of a UK multicenter randomized trial. *Lancet* 2002;359:1291–1300.

15. Lieberman DA, Weiss DG, Bond JH, et al. Use of colonoscopy to screen asymptomatic adults for colorectal cancer. VA Cooperative Study Group 380. *N Engl J Med* 2000;343:162–168.

16. Imperiale TF, Wagner DR, Lin CY, et al. Risk of advanced proximal neoplasms in asymptomatic adults according to the distal colorectal findings. *N Engl J Med* 2000; 334: 169–174.

17. Winawer SJ, Zauber AG, Ho MN, et al. Prevention of colorectal cancer by colonoscopic polypectomy. *N Engl J Med* 1993; 329:1997–1981.

18. Muller AD, Sonnenberg A. Prevention of colorectal cancer by flexible endoscopy and polypectomy. *Ann Intern Med* 1995; 23:904–910.

19. Citarda F, Tomaselli G, Capocaccia R, et al. Efficacy in standard clinical practice of colonoscopic polypectomy in reducing colorectal cancer incidence. *Gut* 2001;48: 812–815.

20. Jorgensen OD, Kronborg O, Fenger C. The Funen adenoma follow-up study: incidence and death from colorectal carcinoma in an adenoma surveillance program. *Scand J Gastroenterol* 1993;28:869–871.

21. Cash B, Schoenfeld PS, Dobhan R, et al. Colorectal neoplasia screening with colonoscopy in asymptomatic women at regional naval medical centers. *Gastroenterology* 2001; 120:A509.

22. Winawer SJ, Zauber AG, Church TR, et al. National Colonoscopy Study (NCS) Preliminary Results: a randomized controlled trial of general population screening colonoscopy. *Gastroenterology* 2002;122:T–1560.

23. Winawer SJ, Stewart ET, Zauber AG, et al. A comparison of colonoscopy and double-contrast barium enema for surveillance after polypectomy. *N Engl J Med* 2000;342: 1766–1772.

24. Smith RA, Cokkinides V, Von Eschenbach AC, et al. American Cancer Society Guidelines for the Early Detection of Cancer. *CA Cancer J Clin* 2002;52:8–22.

25. Winawer SJ, Fletcher RH, Miller L, et al. Colorectal cancer screening: guidelines and rationale. *Gastroenterology* 1997;112:594–642.

26. Screening for colorectal cancer: rcommendation and rationale. US Preventive Services Task Force. *Ann Intern Med* 2002; 129–131.

27. Trends in screening for colorectal cancer—United States 1997 and 1999. *JAMA* 2001;295:1570–1571.

28. Spann S, Rozen P, Levin B, Young G. The pros and cons of population-based colorectal cancer preventative strategies. In *Colorectal Cancer in Clinical Practice: Prevention, Early Detection and Management* Rozen P, Young G, Levin B, Spann S, eds. Martin Dunitz Ltd, London, 2002;10: pp. 115–129.

29. Sidransky D, Tokino T, Hamilton SR, et al. Identification of *ras* oncogene mutations in the stool of patients with curable colorectal tumors. *Science* 1992;256:102–105.

30. Ahlquist DA, Shuber AP. Stool screening for colorectal cancer: evolution from occult blood to molecular markers. *Clin Chim Acta* 2002;315:157–168.

31. Traverso G, Shuber A, Levin B, et al. Detection of APC mutations in fecal DNA of patients with colorectal tumors. *N Engl J Med* 2002;346:311–320.

32. Traverso G, Shuber A, Olsson L, et al. Detection of proximal colorectal cancer through the analysis of faecal DNA. *Lancet* 2002;359:403–404.

33. Fletcher JG, Johnson CD, Welch TJ, et al. Optimization of CT colonography technique: prospective trial in 180 patients. *Radiology* 2000;216:704–711.

34. Gluecker T, Dorta G, Keller W, et al. Performance of multidetection computed tomography colonography compared with conventional colonoscopy. *Gut* 2002;51:207–211.

35. Levin B, Smith RA, Feldman GE, et al. Promoting early detection tests for colorectal cancer and adenomatous polyps: a framework for action—the strategic plan of the National Colorectal Cancer Roundtable. *Cancer* 2002;95: 1618–1628.

36. Selby JV. Colorectal cancer screening: keeping the options open. *Eff Clin Pract* 2001;4:39–41.

LUNG

22 Strategies in Lung Cancer Chemoprevention

Edward S. Kim, MD, Faye M. Johnson, MD, PhD,
Waun Ki Hong, MD, and Fadlo R. Khuri, MD

CONTENTS

1. INTRODUCTION

Lung cancer is the leading cause of cancer deaths worldwide. It has overtaken breast cancer as the leading cause of cancer death in women, due largely to increased incidence of smoking among women, as well as adolescents of both sexes. Though the relationship between lung cancer and tobacco is well described, smoking cessation efforts have had limited success. Lung cancer incidence for 2002 was estimated to be 174,300; the projected number of deaths was 157,700 (1). Early detection methods have also been largely unsuccessful—no benefit of screening with chest radiographs or CT scans has been demonstrated, although studies are ongoing. Over the past 40 yr, the overall survival rate has improved only slightly as surgery, radiation therapy, and chemotherapy remain the mainstays of current treatment. Therapies with novel targeted agents are currently under active investigation in all settings of treatment. Primary lung cancer prevention efforts focus on educating people not to begin smoking; secondary prevention involves cessation efforts; and chemoprevention targets reversal of premalignant lesions and prevention of second primary tumors (SPTs) in patients with a prior history of cancer.

Chemoprevention uses natural or synthetic agents to interrupt the process of carcinogenesis and to prevent or delay tumor occurrence. Researchers in basic science and clinical settings collaborate to study lung cancer biology with the goal of uncovering the mechanisms of carcinogenesis and formulating new strategies for prevention and treatment. This chapter will review the biology of carcinogenesis, review completed clinical trials, and explore future strategies in lung cancer prevention.

2. BIOLOGICAL BASIS FOR LUNG CANCER

In 1912, researchers first proposed a potential role of tobacco in bronchogenic carcinoma (2), and observed that cessation of smoking could prevent lung carcinoma. In the 1930s, Ochsner and DeBakey hypothesized that increased cigarette sales might be related to the rising incidence of lung cancer (3). The carcinogenic link between smoking and lung cancer development is explained in terms of two concepts: field cancerization and the model of multistep carcinogenesis.

2.1. Field Cancerization

In the 1950s, Auerbach and others introduced the concept of field cancerization, which applies to cancers of the aerodigestive tract and states that carcinogen exposure results in diffuse injury to the epithelium throughout the aerodigestive tract (4). Genetic changes and premalignant and malignant lesions in one region of the field increase risk of cancer development in the entire field. Areas of carcinoma *in situ* and metaplasia occurring in the bronchial epithelium after prolonged exposure to

From: Cancer Chemoprevention, Volume 2: Strategies for Cancer Chemoprevention
Edited by: G. J. Kelloff, E. T. Hawk, and C. C. Sigman © Humana Press Inc., Totowa, NJ

inhaled carcinogens, specifically cigarette smoke, are causally related to lung cancer development (5,6).

2.2. Multistep Carcinogenesis

The multistep model of carcinogenesis holds that cancer development is a multistep process in which exposure to a carcinogen (in lung cancer, for example, any of the carcinogens identified in cigarette smoke) results in repeated damage and repair until the accumulated exposure triggers a transformation from normal to premalignant cells (i.e., from normal cells to metaplasia and dysplasia) and eventually to frank carcinoma. An example of multistep carcinogenesis on the molecular level has best been described in colon cancer by Vogelstein and colleagues.

3. STRATEGIES IN LUNG CANCER CHEMOPREVENTION

The rationale for preventing lung cancer is similar to that of head and neck cancer. In both diseases, chronic exposure to tobacco is the major risk factor, and dysplastic epithelial lesions are thought to represent a premalignant stage. Preclinical data indicate that retinoids reverse dysplastic bronchial epithelial lesions. Despite these data, placebo-controlled, randomized trials in smokers have revealed that retinoid treatment adds no significant clinical benefit to smoking cessation, nor does it reverse bronchial metaplasia. In light of results demonstrating that retinoids reduce SPTs in patients with resected lung cancer, bronchial metaplasia may not accurately reflect the chemopreventive effects of retinoids on bronchial epithelium. Research is under way to identify intermediate markers that may predict retinoid chemopreventive effects on bronchial epithelial cells.

3.1. Reversal of Premalignant Lesions

Early detection of lung cancer by chest X-ray has not significantly changed the outcome for patients with lung cancer. However, premalignant markers detectable by sputum cytology studies or found in bronchial metaplasia have been investigated as early predictors of lung cancer. Reversal of these premalignant lesions through treatment modalities may prevent progression to lung cancer. Studies have included various agents to treat sputum atypia (4–7) or bronchial squamous metaplasia (8–11). One study even showed improvement of bronchial epithelium metaplasia in smokers taking folate and vitamin B12 (12). However, because of problems with consistency of the endpoints, positive results must be viewed with caution. Larger trials of biologic endpoints are needed to confirm treatment efficacy. Reversal of premalignant head and neck lesions using retinoids has met with some success. It may be that lessons learned from studies in the upper aerodigestive tract can be transplanted into the arena of lung cancer (13).

Studies showing that low-dose 13-cis-retinoic acid (13-cRA) decreased oral premalignancy when employed as a maintenance regimen (14) have led to translational lung cancer trials based on the biological activity of 13-cRA in the aerodigestive tract. Trials targeting intermediate biologic markers, including molecular indicators of genetic damage, may well be the most promising element in control of lung cancer.

In 2003, Kurie et al. reported the results of a large trial in former smokers who received 9-cis-retinoic acid (9-cRA) or 13-cRA with α-tocopherol. The endpoint of the trial was upregulation of retinoic acid receptor (RAR)-β, loss of which in the bronchial epithelium is considered a biomarker of preneoplasia. Of 177 evaluable patients, those treated with 9-cRA were found to have restored RAR-β expression ($p = 0.03$) and reduced metaplasia ($p = 0.01$) (15). Based on these results, further investigations with 9-cRA are warranted in former smokers.

The β-Carotene and Retinol Efficacy Trial (CARET) and the α-Tocopherol β-Carotene Trial (ATBC) produced similar results for β-carotene. CARET, a randomized, double-blind, placebo-controlled trial, tested the combination of β-carotene (30 mg) and retinyl palmitate (25,000 IU) against placebo in 18,314 men and women aged 50–69 yr at high risk for lung cancer (16). A majority of participants had a smoking history of at least 20 pack-years and were either current or recent ex-smokers. Extensive occupational exposure to asbestos was noted in 4060 men (17). This trial was stopped 21 mo earlier than planned due to evidence of no benefit or possible harm. Lung cancer incidence, the primary endpoint, increased 28% in the active intervention group. The overall mortality rate also increased 17% in this group. Given these results and those of the ATBC trial described below, high-dose β-carotene is not recommended for patients at high risk who continue to smoke.

The ATBC cancer prevention study was a randomized, double-blind, placebo-controlled, primary-prevention trial in which 29,133 Finnish male smokers received either α-tocopherol (50 mg/d) alone, β-carotene (20 mg/d) alone, both α-tocopherol and β-carotene, or a placebo (18). Male participants were 50–69 years of age, and all smoked five or more cigarettes a day. Patients received follow-up observations for 5 to 8 yr. Lung cancer incidence, the primary endpoint, did not change with the addition of α-tocopherol alone, nor did the overall mortality rate. However, both groups who received β-carotene supplementation (alone or with α-tocopherol) had an 18% increase in lung cancer incidence. β-Carotene appeared to have a stronger adverse effect in men who smoked more than 20 cigarettes a day. This trial raised the serious issue that pharmacologic doses of β-carotene could potentially be harmful in active smokers.

The Physicians' Health Study, a randomized, double-blind, placebo-controlled trial, studied 22,071 healthy male physicians. Half of participants (11,036) received β-carotene (50 mg) on alternate days and the other half (11,035) received placebos. The use of supplemental β-carotene showed virtually no adverse or beneficial effects on cancer incidence or overall mortality during a 12-yr follow-up period *(19)*.

Subgroup analysis of the above-mentioned studies, especially ATBC and CARET, has provided few explanations for increased lung cancer incidence. It seems β-carotene has a harmful effect only in high-risk heavy smokers or those with previous exposure to asbestos. Current recommendations are for these people to avoid supplemental β-carotene in large doses *(16)*. Including the results of EUROSCAN mentioned below, much work is needed before chemoprevention agents can be instituted in lung cancer. Currently, an Eastern Cooperative Group (ECOG) trial is studying the effect of daily selenium supplementation in patients with stage I lung cancer.

Chemoprevention and treatment trials of the aerodigestive tract will continue as these cancers continue to be a challenge. Use of natural and synthetic agents may indeed reduce cancer risk in high-risk individuals, though the optimal dosage and maintenance schedules need further clarification. Through this approach we hope to identify accurate biomarkers and establish effective treatment regimens for aerodigestive tract carcinogenesis.

3.2. Second Primary Tumors

Patients with aerodigestive tract cancers (lung and head and neck) who have undergone successful treatment remain at a significantly elevated risk for developing additional tumors in the same area *(20–26)*. The concept of multistep field cancerization explains the development of multiple independent tumor sites within the aerodigestive tract. In fact, despite occurring in all

treatment stages of head and neck cancer, SPTs have the greatest impact on patients treated for early-stage disease (stage I or II), which is usually curative *(25,26)*. Initially described by Warren and Gates in the 1930s, SPT occurrence helps to explain high rates of multiple oral cancers (both synchronous and metachronous) *(27)*. An SPT is either a new cancer of a different histological type, or a cancer, regardless of site, that occurs more than 3 yr after the primary cancer. In head and neck cancer, an SPT lesion is separated from the initial primary tumor by more than 2 cm of clinically normal epithelium. In lung, an SPT must be of squamous cell histological type, develop within 3 yr, and present as a solitary mass. The patient must be free of local or regional disease, and changes consistent with dysplasia or carcinoma *in situ* must be found within the bronchial epithelium. Using these criteria, the risk of local recurrence seems to decline over time, whereas the risk of SPT is constant for the first 8 yr following initial head and neck cancer *(28)*.

The lifetime risk of developing an SPT in head and neck squamous cell cancer (HNSCC) is 20% and the annual rate is 4–6%. One oral cancer study reported rates of 3.6% per year *(29)*. SPTs are the major cause of death after curative surgery in head and neck cancer and are the leading cause of death in early-stage disease, more so than recurrence *(25,26,28–31)*. Retinoids have proven active in oral premalignancy. These facts provided the basis for chemoprevention trials in head and neck cancer evaluating SPTs and the impact of smoking. In resected non-small-cell lung cancer (NSCLC) patients, SPTs occur at the rate of 2–4% per year. Similar to its effects in head and neck cancer patients, retinoid treatment reduces the incidence of SPTs in lung cancer patients who have undergone resection.

Because of morbidity associated with development of SPTs in head and neck cancer, the first Phase III adjuvant chemoprevention trial was performed by Hong et al. in 1990 *(32)*. This randomized, placebo-controlled, double-blind study followed 103 patients with stage I through IV (M0) head and neck cancer randomized to receive high-dose 13-cRA (100 mg per m² per day) or placebo for 1 yr after definitive local therapy. 13-cRA dosage was reduced to 50 mg per m² per day after 13 of the first 44 patients experienced intolerable side effects. Primary endpoints were primary recurrence and SPT development. No difference in local recurrence development or distant metastases was found in the two treatment arms. However, patients treated with 13-cRA had a dramatically lower incidence of SPTs. Of 103 patients followed

Table 1
Selected Major Chemoprevention Trials

Trial	Endpoint	Compounds	End Result
Intergroup Study (40)	Prevention of second primary tumors	13-cRA	Harmful?
EUROSCAN (39)	Prevention of second primary tumors	Retinyl palmitate N-acetylcysteine	Negative
Hong 1990 (32)	Second primary tumors	13-cRA	Positive
Pastorino 1993 (44)	Second primary tumors	Retinyl palmitate	Positive
Bolla 1994 (45)	Second primary tumors	Etretinate	Negative
ATBC (19)	Lung cancer	β-carotene α-tocopherol	Negative
CARET (16)	Lung cancer	β-carotene Vitamin A	Negative
Physicians' Health (18)	Epithelial cancer	β-carotene	Negative
Arnold (7)	Sputum atypia	Etretinate	Negative
Kurie (42)	Metaplasia	4-HPR	Negative
McLarty (43)	Sputum atypia	β-carotene Retinol	Negative

for a median of 42 mo, 6% (3 of 49) developed SPTs in the 13-cRA arm, whereas 28% (14 of 51) developed SPTs in the placebo arm. Consistent with field carcinogenesis, most SPTs in the placebo group (14 of 17) developed in the upper aerodigestive tract (UADT), esophagus, and lung, and were histologically squamous cell type. Additionally, none of the patients receiving 13-cRA developed an SPT during the year of active treatment. Despite only 47% of patients in the 13-cRA treatment arm completing therapy as prescribed, reduction in SPT development was still significant.

A randomized chemoprevention trial in HNSCC, based on the important findings of the previous study and designed to prevent SPT development, was instituted through the University of Texas M. D. Anderson Cancer Center and its affiliated Community Clinical Oncology Program (CCOP) and the Radiation Therapy Oncology Group (RTOG) (33,34). This randomized, double-blind trial was launched in 1991 and studied the effect of low-dose 13-cRA to prevent SPTs in patients who had been definitively treated for stage I or II HNSCC within 3 yr before participation (T1N0M0 or T2N0M0). Patients received 13-cRA (30 mg/d) or placebo for 3 yr and were followed for an additional 4 yr. This study recently completed accrual with 1190 randomized and 1384 registered patients. The annual primary tumor recurrence rate was 2.8%, and the SPT occurrence rate was 5.1% annually. Stage II HNSCC had a higher rate of SPT development than did stage I. Additionally, active smokers had a significantly higher recurrence rate than former and never smokers (4.3% vs 3.3% vs 1.9%).

This prospective study demonstrated for the first time the impact of active smoking status and SPT development. The SPT rate was significantly higher in smokers vs former smokers ($p = 0.018$) and was marginally significant between former and never-smokers ($p = 0.11$). The site of SPT also differed by the primary index tumor. Patients with primary laryngeal cancers were most likely to develop an SPT in either lung or larynx, whereas patients with oral cavity primaries were most likely to develop second primaries in either the oral cavity or lung. Finally, patients with an index primary tumor of the pharynx developed SPTs in lung, oral cavity, pharynx, or esophagus. Compared to previous trials, SPTs occurred more frequently than expected at the index primary sites of the oral UADT. The lower 13-cRA dose was also well tolerated with few grade 3 toxicities. This trial was scheduled to be unblinded in 2002 (35–38).

Other reported major Phase III studies include EUROSCAN and the US-Intergroup NCI 91-0001 trial. EUROSCAN, a randomized adjuvant chemoprevention study of the European Organization for Research and Treatment of Cancer (EORTC) Head/Neck and Lung Cancer Groups, studied the effects of vitamin A (retinyl palmitate) and N-acetylcysteine (NAC) in patients with early-stage head and neck and lung cancer (39). In the trials, 2592 patients with cancers of the larynx (Tis-T3, N0-N1), oral cavity (Tis-T2, N0-N1), and NSCLC (T1-T2, N0-N1) received retinyl palmitate (300,000 IU/d in year 1; 150,000 IU/d in yr 2), NAC (600 mg/d for 2 yr), both drugs, or placebo. No endpoint differences were detected between the three active treatment arms and the placebo group in terms of lung cancer incidence, occurrence of second primary cancer, and survival. A statistically significant difference was found in time to development of SPTs within the carcinogen-exposed field ($p = 0.045$) in favor of the retinoid-treated group. The majority (93%) of patients was considered regular smokers; at least half had greater than 43 pack-years of tobacco exposure. Problems with the study included differences in medication adherence across the three treatment groups and the testing of NAC, a drug with little established efficacy in chemoprevention, in 1300 patients at risk.

US-Intergroup NCI 91-0001, a randomized, double-blind study using low-dose 13-cRA after complete resection of stage I NSCLC, completed accrual in April 1997 with 1486 participants *(40)*. Study objectives were to evaluate 13-cRA efficacy in reducing SPT incidence after complete resection of stage I NSCLC, to examine qualitative and quantitative toxicity of daily low-dose 13-cRA (30 mg/d), and to compare overall survival rates of patients receiving 13-cRA with those receiving a placebo. Randomization of 1304 patients was completed in June 1997. Patients were required to have complete resection of primary stage I NSCLC (postoperative T1 or T2, N0) 6 wk to 3 yr prior to registering. Eleven hundred sixty-six patients with pathologic stage I NSCLC (6 wk to 3 yr from definitive resection with no prior radiotherapy or chemotherapy) were evaluated. Patients took the study drug for 3 yr and were stratified at randomization by tumor stage, histology, and smoking status. No statistically significant differences between placebo and isotretinoin arms were found after a median follow-up of 3.5 yr with respect to time to SPTs, recurrences, or mortality. Multivariate analyses showed that the rate of SPTs was unaffected by any stratification factor. Recurrence rate was affected by tumor stage (HR for T2 vs T1 = 1.77 [95% CI = 1.35–2.31]) and a treatment-by-smoking interaction (HR for treatment-by-current vs never-smoking status = 3.11 [95% CI = 1.00–9.71]). Mortality was affected by tumor stage, histology, and a treatment-by smoking interaction. The authors concluded that isotretinoin did not improve overall survival rates of SPTs, recurrences, or mortality in stage I NSCLC; subset analyses showed it was possibly harmful in current smokers and beneficial in never-smokers.

In a randomized, double-blind, placebo-controlled trial, researchers at Yale University studied the efficacy of β-carotene (50 mg/d) in reducing local recurrence and SPTs in head and neck cancer *(41)*. Two hundred sixty-four patients (some recruited from the state tumor registry) with curatively treated early-stage squamous cell carcinoma of the oral cavity, pharynx, or larynx were randomized to receive β-carotene (50 mg/d) or placebo and followed for 90 mo for development of SPTs and local recurrences. After a median follow-up of 51 mo, there was no difference between the two groups in time to failure (SPTs and local recurrences). In site-specific analyses, supplemental β-carotene had no significant effect on second head and neck cancer or lung cancer. Total mortality was not significantly affected by the drug intervention. Based on the point estimates, the authors concluded that a statistically non-significant decrease in risk of second head and neck cancer as well as a possible increase in lung cancer risk was suggested.

Other retinoid studies have been described by Kurie et al., McLarty et al., Pastorino et al., and Bolla et al. (reviewed in refs. *42–45*).

4. FUTURE STRATEGIES IN LUNG CANCER CHEMOPREVENTION

Development of chemopreventive strategies is essential in order to increase survival rates in lung cancer, an increasingly difficult disease to treat with conventional therapies. Molecular or targeted therapies are the next step in therapy and prevention. Epidermal growth factor receptor (EGFR) has been identified as an attractive target for lung cancer and is also present in early bronchial neoplasia, including metaplastic bronchial epithelium, in moderate to early premalignant lesions *(46)*. *Ras* oncogene mutations, the most frequently described mutations in cancer, have been demonstrated in lung adenocarcinomas. Based on this biology, members of the Lung Cancer Biomarkers Chemoprevention Consortium (LCBCC), an intra-SPORE (Specialized Programs of Research Excellence) National Cancer Institute (NCI)-funded program, elected to develop two compounds, ZD1839 (Iressa), an EGFR-tyrosine kinase inhibitor, and R115777 (Zarnestra), a farnesyl transferase inhibitor, in the setting of lung cancer chemoprevention. Two randomized, double-blinded, placebo-controlled multi-institutional Phase IIB trials are planned to investigate reversal of premalignant lesions. The primary endpoint is improvement in bronchial histology, with the secondary endpoint being assessment of Ki-67, an indicator of proliferation. Patients must have a prior definitively treated tobacco-related cancer (lung, head and neck, bladder, esophagus), a 30 pack-year smoking history, and presence of sputum atypia. Patients will be treated for 6–12 mo on study with serial bronchoscopies. These trials were planned to open by late 2002.

Cyclooxygenase (COX) inhibitors are also being studied. An increasing body of evidence indicates that nonsteroidal antiinflammatory drugs (NSAIDs) can prevent cancer in humans (47). Most epidemiological studies examining NSAIDs as chemopreventive agents have examined the roles of these agents in colorectal cancer. Both retrospective and prospective studies have shown that aspirin, sulindac, and celecoxib can prevent colon cancer and colorectal polyps in humans (48–51). In addition, a prospective study of 12,668 subjects showed that lung, breast, and colon cancer incidence was lower in those who reported aspirin use (52). The exact mechanism of action of NSAIDs in cancer prevention is unclear, although it is likely that inhibition of COX-2 is at least partly responsible for their chemopreventive effects.

Most NSAIDs have pleiotropic biological effects, including inhibition of the COX-1 and COX-2 enzymes. Most tissues express COX-1 constitutively. COX-2 is inducible; increased levels are seen with inflammation and in many types of cancer, including NSCLC. Due to the NSAID side effect of bleeding, attributed to COX-1 inhibition in platelets, selective COX-2 inhibitors have been developed (e.g., celecoxib and rofecoxib). A variety of preclinical studies have examined the effect of COX-2 inhibition on several tumor types, including NSCLC.

Examination of human NSCLC tumor tissue by immunohistochemistry, in situ hybridization for mRNA, or RT-PCR by several independent investigators, has shown that COX-2 is frequently expressed in NSCLC and in premalignant lesions (53–56). COX-2 expression correlates with a worse prognosis, at least in those with early-stage disease (57–59). In contrast, adjacent histologically normal epithelium, as well as histologically normal epithelium from smokers without known cancer, shows negligible COX-2 expression (60,61).

Inhibition of COX-2 by genetic and pharmacological methods has led to decreased growth, invasion, and angiogenesis, increased tumor lymphocyte infiltration, and increased apoptosis of NSCLC cancer cells in vitro and in vivo in human tumor xenografts in mice (62–69). Interestingly, significant data suggest that the effects of NSAIDs and even selective COX-2 inhibitors may be independent of COX-2 inhibition (70–72). However, despite this controversy about mech-anism, the biological effects of NSAIDs have been clearly seen in preclinical models of NSCLC by many independent investigators.

Based on clinical and preclinical data outlined above, chemopreventive trials for NSCLC using selective COX-2 inhibitors are well supported. These agents are well tolerated for sustained use with relatively few side effects and may have the added benefit of preventing multiple types of cancer (50,52). An ongoing trial at M. D. Anderson Cancer Center is examining the bronchial histology of current and former smokers before, during, and after treatment with celecoxib.

Molecularly targeted agents will also be used in settings other than chemoprevention, including maintenance therapy and adjuvant treatment, to reduce incidence of recurrence as well as SPTs. It is hoped that these strategies will make a meaningful impact in our knowledge of cancer biology and ultimately in cancer survival.

5. CONCLUSIONS

Reducing lung cancer mortality is the major goal. This will require a combination of smoking cessation, early detection, chemoprevention, and improved treatment of established disease.

Lung cancer treatment is an ever-challenging issue; progress in stemming overall mortality has been disappointing. As this is a major public health problem in the United States, prevention methods such as smoking cessation campaigns for current smokers and preventing nonsmokers from starting may have a profound impact on lung cancer incidence. Exposure to tobacco and the tobacco-related illnesses that follow contributes to lung cancer's excessive morbidity and mortality. Patients with early-stage cancers can still be "cured"; however, these patients are at high risk for recurrence and SPTs. Cost-effective and efficacious screening strategies have yet to be developed.

Chemoprevention has demonstrated some efficacy in preventing lung cancer SPTs, which, underscoring the principle of field cancerization, have emerged as an increasingly important problem, despite curative local therapy. Chemopreventive agents such as antioxidants and retinoic acid have been studied, but their role in preventing SPTs needs further definition. Small-molecule compounds that target specific receptors or mutations may play a significant role in treatment, as their side effect profiles are tolerable. Development of a risk model is important to help guide and tailor therapy for patients with various risk profiles, thus allowing stratification based on risk factors. A multidisciplinary approach from clinicians and basic researchers is needed to study the biology of lung cancer before chemoprevention can be incorporated into a societal standard of care.

REFERENCES

1. Jemal A, Thomas A, Murray T, et al. Cancer statistics, 2002. *CA Cancer J Clin* 2002;52:23–47.

2. Adler I. *Primary Malignant Growths of the Lung and Bronchi*. Longmans, Green and Co., New York, 1912.

3. Ochsner A, DeBakey M. Carcinoma of the lung. *Arch Surgery* 1940:209–258.

4. Auerbach O, Gere JB, Forman JB, et al. Changes in the bronchial epithelium in relation to smoking and cancer of the lung. *N Engl J Med* 1957;256:98–104.

5. Auerbach O, Hammond EC, Garfinkel L. Changes in bronchial epithelium in relation to cigarette smoking, 1955–1960 vs 1970–1977. *N Engl J Med* 1979;300:381–386.

6. Auerbach O, Stout AP, Hammond EC, et al. Changes in bronchial epithelium in relation to cigarette smoking and in relation to lung cancer. *N Engl J Med* 1961;265:253–267.

7. Arnold AM, Browman GP, Levine MN, et al. The effect of the synthetic retinoid etretinate on sputum cytology: results from a randomised trial. *Br J Cancer* 1992;65:737–743.

8. Gouveia J, Hercend T, Lemaigre G, et al. Degree of bronchial metaplasia in heavy smokers and its regression after treatment with a retinoid. *Lancet* 1982;1:710–712.

9. Lee JS, Lippman SM, Benner SE, et al. A randomized placebo-controlled trial of isotretinoin in chemoprevention of bronchial squamous metaplasia. *J Clin Oncol* 1994;12:937–945.

10. Mathe G, Gouveia J, Hercend R, et al. Correlation between precancerous bronchial metaplasia and cigarette consumption, and preliminary results of retinoid treatment. *Cancer Detect Prev* 1982;5:461–466.

11. Misset JL, Santelli G, Homasson JP, et al. Regression of bronchial epidermoid metaplasia in heavy smokers with etretinate treatment. *Cancer Detect Prev* 1986;9:167–170.

12. Heimberger DC, Alexander CB, Birch R, et al. Improvement in bronchial squamous metaplasia in smokers treated with folate and vitamin B12: report of a preliminary randomized double-blind intervention trial. *JAMA* 1988; 259:1525–1530.

13. Hong WK, Endicott J, Itri LM, et al. 13-*cis*-Retinoic acid in the treatment of oral leukoplakia. *N Engl J Med* 1986; 315:1501–1505.

14. Lippman SM, Batsakis JG, Toth BB, et al. Comparison of low-dose isotretinoin with beta carotene to prevent oral carcinogenesis. *N Engl J Med* 1993;328:15–20.

15. Kurie JM, Lotan R, Lee JJ, et al. Treatment of former smokers with 9-*cis*-retinoic acid reverses loss of retinoic acid receptor-beta expression in the bronchial epithelium: results from a randomized placebo-controlled trial. *J Natl Cancer Inst* 2003;95:178–179.

16. Omenn GS, Goodman GE, Thornquist MD, et al. Effects of a combination of beta carotene and vitamin A on lung cancer and cardiovascular disease. *N Engl J Med* 1996;334:1150–1155.

17. Goodman M, Morgan RW, Ray R, et al. Cancer in asbestos-exposed occupational cohorts: a meta-analysis. *Cancer Causes Control* 1999;10:453–465.

18. The Alpha-Tocopherol, Beta-Carotene Cancer Prevention Study Group. The effect of Vitamin E and beta carotene on the incidence of lung cancer and other cancers in male smokers. *N Engl J Med* 1994;330:1029–1035.

19. Hennekans CH, Buring JE, Manson JE, et al. Lack of long-term supplementation with beta-carotene on the incidence of malignant neoplasms and cardiovascular disease. *N Engl J Med* 1996;334:1145–1149.

20. Decker J, Goldstein JC. Risk factors in head and neck cancer. *N Engl J Med* 1982;306:1151–1155.

21. Wynder EL, Stellman SD. Impact of long-term filter cigarette usage on lung and larynx cancer risk. A case-control study. *J Natl Cancer Inst* 1979;62:471–477.

22. Boice JD, Fraumeni JF. Second cancer following cancer of the respiratory system in Connecticut, 1935–1982. *Natl Cancer Inst Monogr* 1985;68:83–98.

23. Gluckman JL, Crissman JD. Survival rates in 548 patients with multiple neoplasms of the upper aerodigestive tract. *Laryngoscope* 1983;93:71–74.

24. De Vries N, Snow GB. Multiple primary tumours in laryngeal cancer. *J Laryngol Otol* 1986;100:915–918.

25. Yellin A, Hill LR, Benfield JR. Bronchogenic carcinoma associated with upper aerodigestive cancers. *J Thorac Cardiovasc Surg* 1986;91:674–683.

26. Vokes EE, Weichselbaum RR, Lippman SM, Hong WK. Head and neck cancer. *N Engl J Med* 1993;328:184–193.

27. Warren S, Gates O. Multiple primary malignant tumors: a survey of the literature and statistical study. *Am J Cancer* 1932;16:1358–1403.

28. Vikram B: Changing patterns of failure in advanced head and neck cancer. *Arch Otolaryngol Head Neck Surg* 1984; 110:564–565.

29. Lippman SM, Hong WK. Not yet standard: retinoids versus second primary tumors. *J Clin Oncol* 1993;11:1204–1207.

30. Lippman SM, Hong WK. Second malignant tumors in head and neck squamous cell carcinoma: the overshadowing threat for patients with early stage disease. *Int J Radiat Oncol Biol Phys* 1989;17:691–694.

31. Larson JT, Adams GL, Fattah HA. Survival statistics for multiple primaries in head and neck cancer. *Otolaryngol Head Neck Surg* 1990;103:14–24.

32. Hong WK, Lippman SM, Itri LM, et al. Prevention of second primary tumors with isotretinoin in squamous-cell carcinoma of the head and neck. *N Engl J Med* 1990;323:795–801.

33. Benner SE, Lippman SM, Hong WK. Current status of chemoprevention of head and neck cancer. *Oncology* 1992;6:61–66.

34. Benner SE, Pajak TF, Stetz J, et al. Toxicity of isotretinoin in a chemoprevention trial to prevent second primary tumors following head and neck cancer. *J Natl Cancer Inst* 1994; 86:1799–1801.

35. Khuri FR, Lee JJ, Winn RJ, et al. Interim analysis of randomized chemoprevention trial of HNSCC. *Proc Annu Meet Am Soc Clin Oncol* 1999;abstr 1503.

36. Kim ES, Khuri FR, Lee JJ, et al. Second primary tumor incidence related to primary index tumor and smoking status in a randomized chemoprevention study of head and neck squamous cell cancer. *Proc Ann Meet Am Soc Clin Oncol* 2000;19:abstr 1642.

37. de Vries N, van Zandwijk N, Pastorino U. Chemoprevention of head and neck and lung (pre)cancer. *Recent Results Cancer Res* 1999;151:13–25.

38. Khuri FR, Kim ES, Lee JJ, et al. The impact of smoking status, disease stage, and index tumor site on second primary tumor incidence and tumor recurrence in the head and neck retinoid chemoprevention trial. *Cancer Epidemiol Biomarkers Prev* 2001;10:823–829.

39. van Zandwijk N, Dalesio O, Pastorino U, et al. EUROSCAN, a randomized trial of vitamin A and *N*-acetylcysteine in patients with head and neck cancer or lung cancer. For the European Organization for Research and Treatment of Cancer

Head and Neck and Lung Cancer Cooperative Groups. *J Natl Cancer Inst* 2000;92:977–986.

40. Lippman SM, Lee JJ, Karp DD, et al. Randomized phase III intergroup trial of isotretinoin to prevent second primary tumors in stage I non-small cell lung cancer. *J Natl Cancer Inst* 2001;93:605–618.

41. Mayne ST, Cartmel B, Baum M, et al. Randomized trial of supplemental beta-carotene to prevent second head and neck cancer. *Cancer Res* 2001;61:1457–1463.

42. Kurie JM, Lee JS, Khuri FR, et al. N-(4-hydroxyphenyl) retinamide in the chemoprevention of squamous metaplasia and dysplasia of the bronchial epithelium. *Clin Cancer Res* 2000;6:2973–2979.

43. McLarty JW, Holiday DB, Girard WM, et al. Beta-carotene, vitamin A, and lung cancer chemoprevention: results of an intermediate endpoint study. *Am J Clin Nutr* 1995;62: 1431S–1438S.

44. Pastorino U, Infante M, Maioli M, et al. Adjuvant treatment of stage I lung cancer with high dose vitamin A. *J Clin Oncol* 1993;11:1216–1222.

45. Bolla M, Lefur R, Ton Van J, et al. Prevention of second primary tumours with etretinate in squamous cell carcinoma of the oral cavity and oropharynx. Results of a multicentric double-blind randomized study. *Eur J Cancer* 1994;30A: 767–772.

46. Kurie JM, Shin HJ, Lee JS, et al. Increased epidermal growth factor receptor expression in metaplastic bronchial epithelium. *Clin Cancer Res* 1996;2:1787–1793.

47. Vainio H. Chemoprevention of cancer: a controversial and instructive story. *Br Med Bull* 1999;55:593–599.

48. Giardiello FM, Hamilton SR, Krush AJ, et al. Treatment of colonic and rectal adenomas with sulindac in familial adenomatous polyposis. *N Engl J Med* 1993;328:1313–1316.

49. Giovannucci E, Egan KM, Hunter DJ, et al. Aspirin and the risk of colorectal cancer in women. *N Engl J Med* 1995; 333:609–614.

50. Steinbach G, Lynch PM, Phillips RK, et al. The effect of celecoxib, a cyclooxygenase-2 inhibitor, in familial adenomatous polyposis. *N Engl J Med* 2000;342:1946–1952.

51. Thun MJ, Namboodiri MM, Heath CW Jr. Aspirin use and reduced risk of fatal colon cancer. *N Engl J Med* 1991;325: 1593–1596.

52. Schreinemachers DM, Everson RB. Aspirin use and lung, colon, and breast cancer incidence in a prospective study. *Epidemiology* 1994;5:138–146.

53. Hida T, Yatabe Y, Achiwa H, et al. Increased expression of cyclooxygenase 2 occurs frequently in human lung cancers, specifically in adenocarcinomas. *Cancer Res* 1998;58: 3761–3764.

54. Hosomi Y, Yokose T, Hirose Y, et al. Increased cyclooxygenase 2 (COX-2) expression occurs frequently in precursor lesions of human adenocarcinoma of the lung. *Lung Cancer* 2000; 30:73–81.

55. Watkins DN, Lenzo JC, Segal A, et al. Expression and localization of cyclo-oxygenase isoforms in non-small cell lung cancer. *Eur Respir J* 1999;14:412–418.

56. Wolff H, Saukkonen K, Anttila S, et al. Expression of cyclooxygenase-2 in human lung carcinoma. *Cancer Res* 1998;58:4997–5001.

57. Achiwa H, Yatabe Y, Hida T, et al. Prognostic significance of elevated cyclooxygenase 2 expression in primary, resected lung adenocarcinomas. *Clin Cancer Res* 1999;5:1001–1005.

58. Brabender J, Park J, Metzger R, et al. Prognostic significance of cyclooxygenase 2 mRNA expression in non-small cell lung cancer. *Ann Surg* 2002;235:440–443.

59. Khuri FR, Wu H, Lee JJ, et al. Cyclooxygenase-2 overexpression is a marker of poor prognosis in stage I non-small cell lung cancer. *Clin Cancer Res* 2001;7:861–867.

60. Hasturk S, Kemp B, Kalapurakal SK, et al. Expression of cyclooxygenase-1 and cyclooxygenase-2 in bronchial epithelium and nonsmall cell lung carcinoma. *Cancer* 2000;94: 1023–1031.

61. Soslow RA, Dannenberg AJ, Rush D, et al. COX-2 is expressed in human pulmonary, colonic, and mammary tumors. *Cancer* 2000;89:2637–2645.

62. Berman KS, Verma UN, Harburg G, et al. Sulindac enhances tumor necrosis factor-alpha-mediated apoptosis of lung cancer cell lines by inhibition of nuclear factor-kappaB. *Clin Cancer Res* 2002;8:354–360.

63. Eli Y, Przedecki F, Levin G, et al. Comparative effects of indomethacin on cell proliferation and cell cycle progression in tumor cells grown in vitro and in vivo. *Biochem Pharmacol* 2001;61:565–571.

64. Williams CS, Tsujii M, Reese J, et al. Host cyclooxygenase-2 modulates carcinoma growth. *J Clin Invest* 2000;105: 1589–1594.

65. Tsubouchi Y, Mukai S, Kawahito Y, et al. Meloxicam inhibits the growth of non-small cell lung cancer. *Anticancer Res* 2000;20:2867–2872.

66. Hida T, Kozaki K, Muramatsu H, et al. Cyclooxygenase-2 inhibitor induces apoptosis and enhances cytotoxicity of various anticancer agents in non-small cell lung cancer cell lines. *Clin Cancer Res* 2000;6:2006–2011.

67. Stolina M, Sharma S, Lin Y, et al. Specific inhibition of cyclooxygenase 2 restores antitumor reactivity by altering the balance of IL-10 and IL-12 synthesis. *J Immunol* 2000; 164:361–370.

68. Dohadwala M, Luo J, Zhu L, et al. Non-small cell lung cancer cyclooxygenase-2-dependent invasion is mediated by CD44. *J Biol Chem* 2001;276:20,809–20,812.

69. El-Bayoumy K, Rose DP, Papanikolaou N, et al. Cyclooxygenase-2 expression influences the growth of human large and small cell lung carcinoma lines in athymic mice: impact of an organoselenium compound on growth regulation. *Int J Oncol* 2002;20:557–561.

70. Grosch S, Tegeder I, Niederberger E, et al. COX-2 independent induction of cell cycle arrest and apoptosis in colon cancer cells by the selective COX-2 inhibitor celecoxib. *Faseb J* 2001;15:2742–2744.

71. Song X, Lin HP, Johnson AJ, et al. Cyclooxygenase-2, player or spectator in cyclooxygenase-2 inhibitor-induced apoptosis in prostate cancer cells. *J Natl Cancer Inst* 2002; 94:585–591.

72. Waskewich C, Blumenthal RD, Li H, et al. Celecoxib exhibits the greatest potency amongst cyclooxygenase (COX) inhibitors for growth inhibition of COX-2-negative hematopoietic and epithelial cell lines. *Cancer Res* 2002;62:2029–2033.

23 Lung Cancer Chemoprevention

An Opportunity for Direct Drug Delivery

James L. Mulshine, MD and Luigi M. De Luca, PhD

CONTENTS

1. INTRODUCTION

Lung cancer is the leading cause of cancer death in the world and accounts for more than 150,000 deaths annually in the United States *(1)*. Global progress in improving lung cancer outcomes has been exceedingly difficult *(2,3)*. Progress in the specific area of chemoprevention research has also been challenging. Despite a vast at-risk population of current or past users of tobacco products (or perhaps because this population is so vast), it is difficult to assemble an appropriate-sized cohort of at-risk individuals to efficiently conduct a definitive chemoprevention trial *(4,5)*. In breast cancer, the key dynamic in launching initial chemoprevention research was the utility of tamoxifen in reducing second breast cancers *(6,7)*. Since lung cancer is more frequently lethal than breast cancer, there is no large pool of initial survivors at risk for a second lung cancer. This difficulty in conducting lung cancer chemoprevention trials, though a major detriment to developing more effective lung cancer chemoprevention, is only one of a number of reasons for the lack of significant pharmaceutical industry efforts to develop a lung cancer chemoprevention drug *(8)*.

In this chapter, we will consider chemoprevention issues ranging from conceptual to pragmatic. Progress in improving lung cancer outcomes with chemoprevention has thus far not been encouraging.

Though results from major lung cancer chemoprevention trials have been negative, some approaches were excluded; some logical and compelling options remain to be evaluated *(9,10)*. However, the real engine for positive change in early lung cancer management may turn out to be improved technical capability to routinely detect lung cancer at an earlier stage *(10–14)*. The use of spiral computerized tomography (CT) to detect early lung cancer has had a profound effect on disease management. While developments in lung cancer screening have evoked considerable concern *(15,16)*, from a translational research perspective, enhanced detection of early cancers along with development of objective measurement tools *(17)* has rekindled investigative possibilities in this major public health challenge. As a byproduct of renewed interest in lung cancer screening research, identifying large cohorts with extraordinary risk for lung cancer has become more routine. The availability of large numbers of potential candidates for chemoprevention trials could greatly accelerate research opportunities.

From: Cancer Chemoprevention, Volume 2: Strategies for Cancer Chemoprevention
Edited by: G. J. Kelloff, E. T. Hawk, and C. C. Sigman © Humana Press Inc., Totowa, NJ

2. IMPACT OF SPIRAL CT DETECTION OF SMALLER PRIMARY LUNG CANCERS

The first positive pilot reports for improved lung imaging came from New York and Tokyo, where investigators explored the enhanced imaging sensitivity of spiral CT *(10–14)*. In both of these preliminary experiences, investigators demonstrated that spiral CT could screen high-risk populations and consistently find early-stage lung cancer. In Japan and New York, the frequency of stage I lung cancer detected was in excess of 80%. Based on historical experience, finding early-stage cancers is associated with increased long-term survival. If individuals can be diagnosed by annual screening, the size of detected primary lung cancers may even be smaller than the prevalent cases *(6,7,11)*. Major screening trials to validate spiral CT and determine its actual benefit are being launched. Given the time needed to complete such trials, it is important to conduct this type of research in parallel to make effective lung cancer chemoprevention approaches available if these screening measures prove beneficial. The National Cancer Institute (NCI) has convened a series of workshops to consider these emerging issues; summaries of key meetings are available on its Web site (http://prg.nci.nih.gov/lung/finalreport.html and http://www.webtie.org/sots/Meetings/Lung/June%2019%202001/Default.htm). Review of these documents links the pace and direction of lung cancer chemoprevention research to innovations in lung cancer imaging for the foreseeable future.

3. IMPLICATIONS OF FIELD CARCINOGENESIS ON CHEMOPREVENTION RESEARCH

Field carcinogenesis implies that long after a primary resection, the cancer patient has a greater chance of manifesting a subsequent primary lung cancer; these cancers can arise in multiple locations throughout the airway *(18,19)*. Published accounts have found that risk of subsequent lung cancer is cumulative and likely to be on the order of 1–3% per year *(20)*. As more people have small primary lung cancers excised, more tissue from other foci of early lung cancer will be available for pathological and molecular analysis, as discussed at the recent NCI State-of-the-Science workshop on new management for screen-detected small-volume lung cancer (http://www.webtie.org/sots/Meetings/Lung/June%2019%202001/Default.htm). This situation will result in the availability of previously unstudied early cancer tissue. Given the robust development of in vitro diagnostics,

considerable new biological information will enable the research community to develop diagnostic and therapeutic targets for evolving lung cancer. Currently, we do not know which events activate early lung cancer, so the selection of chemoprevention targets has been empiric. Driven by renewed interest in lung cancer screening, more frequent evaluation of early lung cancer patients is an important opportunity and a profound challenge for new chemoprevention research.

Since there are no validated lung cancer chemoprevention agents, we will look at new strategies for addressing the challenges of arresting early lung cancer progression based on a critical evaluation of unsuccessful past efforts.

4. CONVENTIONAL APPROACHES TO LUNG CANCER CHEMOPREVENTION

For many years, retinoids have been lead candidates for lung cancer chemoprevention *(21–23)*; much of the clinical work evaluating this approach has been conducted at M. D. Anderson Cancer Center *(5,10,20, 24–30)*. In a large and rigorous body of work, the M. D. Anderson group has made important contributions in terms of chemoprevention study design and refinement of biomarker-based intermediate endpoint analysis. Hong and coworkers have tested various retinoids in several sites in the upper aerodigestive tract *(5,25–30)*. Despite a number of studies, promising initial results have not been confirmed *(10)*. An important problem in these efforts has been frequent occurrence of significant clinical toxicity with all of the evaluated retinoids *(9,10,28,30,31)*.

The consistent occurrence of drug side effects is a particular problem for chemoprevention agents. Candidates for chemoprevention approaches are otherwise fit and fully functional people unwilling to tolerate unpleasant side effects from chronic drug administration. The original trial of 100 mg/m^2 13-*cis*-retinoic acid (13-cRA) in a group of curatively treated head and neck cancer patients with significant risk of developing a second lung cancer lowered the retinoid dosage to 50 mg/m^2 as a result of unacceptable toxicity *(30)*. This trial did show a statistically significant reduction in the frequency of second primary aerodigestive cancers in the retinoid trial arm. However, side effects included headache, sores around the mouth, severe itching, and elevated serum lipids. To avoid these complications in the follow-up trial (US-Intergroup NCI 91-0001), 13-cRA was further reduced to 30 mg as a total daily dose *(10)*. In this randomized trial of 1304 curatively resected stage I non-small-cell lung cancer (NSCLC) patients, there was no significant reduction in frequency of second aerodigestive cancers in the retinoid arm compared with the placebo arm. Even the lower retinoid dose used in this follow-up multicenter validation trial still caused unpleasant side effects *(10)*.

Reducing a dosing schedule by over 50% in a cancer therapeutics trial raises ongoing concerns about losing the therapeutic effect and failing to establish the requisite dose of the relevant drug needed to achieve a successful chemopreventive effect. This is not a unique situation for retinoids. Unfortunately, the rationale for chemoprevention trial drug dosing in general has not been rigorously determined, so the least effective dose for any chemopreventive drug is not evident.

An important question in the wake of this effort is whether chemoprevention with retinoids just does not work, or whether retinoids do work but only at a dose that causes unacceptable side effects with oral administration. Some years ago, we reported that the effective dose to mediate growth inhibition in vitro for a number of lung cancer cell lines was much lower if retinoid exposure to the cancer cells was done in serum-free rather than serum-containing media *(32)*, an effect due to albumin binding of the retinoid. This interaction of retinoid with albumin was well known, but it was not well understood that retinoid binding to albumin decreased the potency of the retinoid in mediating antiproliferative effects within cancer cells *(33)*. This observation that retinoids can still mediate significant growth inhibitory effects in fully transformed lung cancer cells has been reported by others *(34)*, and the effect of albumin binding on retinoid potency has also been confirmed, but clinical implications have still not been fully assessed *(32,33)*. Issues with cancer therapy and vitamin A availability have been well reported in treating acute promelocytic anemia *(35,36)*. In this disease, vitamin A delivered orally as all-*trans*-retinoic acid (ATRA) has been associated with a significant complete response rate, which in many instances is of brief duration. The serum presence of this vitamin A derivative is short, and further shortened by accelerated induction of the cytochrome P450 system, making it impossible to maintain a critical concentration of this retinoid on a chronic basis *(36–38)*. The pharmacological nature of this resistance is confirmed by in vivo experiments with promyelocytic cells harvested from patients who no longer respond clinically to ATRA, but whose cells still exhibit sensitivity to ATRA exposure in vitro *(39,40)*. Strategies that increase ATRA exposure to malignant cell populations have met with some clinical success.

In recognition of the pharmacological challenges that retinoids present, the M. D. Anderson group is using more potent retinoids in an effort to achieve a more favorable clinical response *(24,28,29)*. For example, Kurie and coworkers evaluated 4-hydroxyphenylretinamide (4-HPR) in treating bronchial dysplasia *(28)*. Initial reports of 4-HPR indicated that it was a particularly potent inducer of apoptosis in lung cancer cells *(25,41)*. In the M. D. Anderson trials, the chemopreventive dose of 4-HPR was based on a previously reported breast cancer prevention trial and calibrated to minimize clinical side effects *(28,31)*, the most disturbing of which is lack of dark adaptation, more commonly known as night blindness. From the laboratory work, a dose of about 1 μM was thought to be required for maximal apoptotic effect; an oral dose of 200 mg per d was expected to easily achieve this serum level. However, observed drug levels from the trial were on the order of 104.5 ± 64.0 ng/mL (mean ± SD) *(28)*. It is important to note that these drug measurements are from the bloodstream, whereas critical drug exposure occurs in tissues. In practice, we have little information about the dynamics of drug penetration into tissue, but it is reasonable to expect that serum drug levels represent a "best case" relative to tissue levels.

5. MODELING EFFORTS WITH EXPERIMENTAL PHARMACOLOGY

In the early days of serotherapy with monoclonal antibodies, an important effort was made to better understand the kinetics of drug delivery into target tissues. This work was enabled by the fact that the antibodies could be directly labeled and then followed through time. Weinstein, Dedrick, Jain, and colleagues found that drug penetration into target tissue was surprisingly inefficient *(42–46)*. While systemic drug administration may improve this situation *(45)*, such research strongly suggests theoretical benefits with regional delivery as well. Weinstein's work demonstrated that delivery efficiency varied within different body compartments. The final problem was percolation of the agent from blood vessels into nodules of the tumor *(42,43,47)*. Reviewing these issues in the setting of early cancer, Weinstein suggests that the challenge in chemopreventive drug delivery is much more favorable in regard to intractable percolation *(48)*. Given the localized distribution of most early epithelial cancers, the efficiency of drug delivery could also be modified as a function of the route of administration. For example, efficiencies of drug delivery could be consistently enhanced by at least two orders of magnitude if antibodies were delivered regionally instead of systemically *(43,49,50)*. Dedrick and coworkers proposed that a route of drug delivery that restricts the drug initially to a smaller compartment has theoretical advantages *(51,52)*.

6. PHARMACOLOGICAL ADVANTAGE OF REGIONAL DRUG DELIVERY

Clinical work with ovarian cancer therapeutics provided an opportunity to demonstrate the relevance of pharmacological models in evaluating the benefit of changing route of administration for regional drug delivery *(52)*. Specifically, regional chemotherapy delivery for either intra-arterial or intracavitary administration as proposed by Dedrick initially concentrated the drug dose in the compartment of interest before it distributed throughout the rest of the body.

6.1. Equations Showing Pharmacokinetic Advantage of Regional Drug Administration:

$$R_d = 1 + CL_{TB}/K(1 - E)* \qquad (1)$$

R_d = pharmacokinetic advantage (defined as the ratio of tissue exposure to systemic exposure following regional drug delivery divided by the same ratio following systemic delivery)

CL_{TB} = total body clearance following intravenous drug administration

K = intercompartment transport parameter

E = irreversible extraction of drug by the target region.

*Exposure may be measured by AUC of plasma that would be in equilibrium with the tissue.

If there is no extraction by the region ($E = 0$), Equation (1) becomes simply

$$R_d = 1 + CL_{TB}/K \qquad (2)$$

This equation assumes the derivation of the basic equation for pharmacokinetic advantage. These include: (1) constant CL_{TB} and K; (2) linearity of the underlying biological processes such as metabolism, binding, and transport; and (3) a uniform concentration of drug in the target region.

The analytical basis of Dedrick's observation is outlined in the above equations. The second equation shows that the pharmacokinetic advantage depends on the ratio of clearance (CL_{TB}) to transport (K). If K were the same for two drugs, then the agent with larger clearance from the body would be kinetically preferred. Therefore, the advantage of regional delivery from a first-pass drug effect through a compartment containing the

target epithelial cell population relates directly to therapeutic index. (For this discussion, the definition of therapeutic index is the ratio of a drug favorably affecting a target relative to the drug's side-effect profile.) In Dedrick's analysis, the absorbed drug acts as a systemic dose. From this perspective, larger clearance of the absorbed drug will lead to lower equilibrium concentration in the serum, making it less likely that the drug will cause systemic toxicity. Current clinical management tools have not been optimized to exploit this predicted advantage.

While the advantage of regional drug delivery can be evaluated in many potential situations, we tested whether aerosol delivery technology for early lung cancer was an appropriate model to determine benefit from the pharmacological advantage predicted by Dedrick. Our research question is whether progression of clonal lung cancer growing in the bronchial epithelium can be arrested by using aerosolized or nebulized drug delivery strategies as a specific example of regional drug delivery *(53)*. The target of this drug delivery strategy would be the "field" of cancer injury, which includes the extent of airway tissue in the direct path of tobacco-combustion products chronically deposited on the respiratory epithelium *(18,19,53)*.

The rationale for aerosol drug delivery is conveyed in Fig. 1. Lung cancer due to tobacco exposure is an aerosolized carcinogen-induced disease. The drop zone for tobacco combustion-derived carcinogens and aerosol drug delivery can be designed to overlap. This target volume is vastly smaller than the corresponding volume for distribution of orally administered drug. Aerosolized delivery could provide a significant first-pass pharmacological advantage by virtue of asymmetric volumes of relevant compartments; for saturation with oral drug delivery, these are either the intravascular compartment or some fraction of the total body compartment, depending on agent chemistry. These compartments vastly exceed the respiratory epithelium's volume of interstitial fluid, about 15 mL. This interstitial fluid, which bathes all the cells at risk of emerging as lung cancer, is the exclusive location for much of the natural history of lung carcinogenesis. Aerosol delivery, as suggested by Dedrick, involves a much more favorable situation because the drug sees the small volume of the respiratory epithelium first and then drops off across the rest of the body. Side effects would be minimized, as the respiratory epithelium would receive an enormous drug concentration while eventual serum drug levels would be modest. The research challenge is to formulate the drug for aerosol

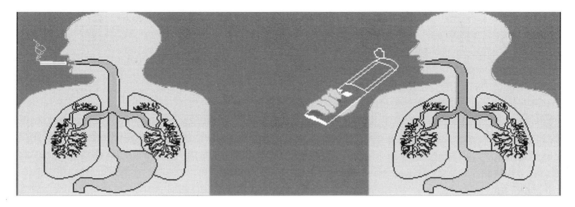

Fig. 1. Rationale for aerosol drug delivery.

delivery to ensure a favorable drug respiratory epithelial cell area-under-the-curve (AUC) exposure *(54–56)*.

However, this is a new area, and actual clinical data on these issues for cancer applications are generally not available. For example, total body retinoid clearance in human subjects has generally not been measured, since intravenous formulations are not available; but, as we reported in a previous review, approximate estimates can be derived from oral data *(38,57)*. Kinetic studies of absorption of drugs and other chemicals from the lung of several species are available following both intratracheal and aerosolized delivery *(58)*. As we reported, these suggest the effect of molecular size and lipid solubility, but the rate is expressed as a first-order rate constant (min^{-1}) *(53)*. To determine the transport parameter, K (mL/min) requires that the effective volume is known. The rate of absorption of retinoids from the lung is not known for either normal lung or in a smoker's chronically damaged respiratory epithelium. Previous rodent studies for a variety of retinoids found that gross measurements of plasma and lung concentrations track closely, but the fine detail of actual retinoid uptake in the epithelial cells is not known *(37,59–61)*. A further limitation of these experimental data is that the precise disposition of the retinoid and what fraction is bound to interstitial albumin or intracellular binding proteins is not known. Application of the model is confounded by the spatially distributed nature of drug distribution within the airways, existence of high-affinity binding proteins, and concentration gradients that exist during drug absorption from the airway surfaces. In principle, one would like to know the (free) drug concentration at epithelial sites of action and its variation with time. In light of these factors and the molecular pharmacology of retinoid effect, definition of the pharmacokinetic advantage in terms of AUC drug exposure may not adequately address the biological

effect of retinoids. Furthermore, how these data in healthy animals relate to retinoid dynamics in the airway of a heavy smoker is speculative.

Despite this complexity, our analysis suggests that a critical feature of direct epithelial delivery will be the first-pass concentration of the drug. From this perspective, features such as drug half-life or distribution profile in lipid may convey an advantage for particular analogs, but actual experimental data are necessary to sort out the clinically dominant feature in drug suitability for aerosolized delivery. Aerosolized antibiotic delivery has been used with great success in managing the pulmonary infections of cystic fibrosis, where chronic parenteral administration of antibiotics resulted in severe side effects *(55,56,62–66)*. By preferentially targeting the cancer field through use of aerosolized delivery technologies and other local delivery approaches, higher drug levels can be administered with minimal systemic toxicity. Preclinical work in corticosteroid delivery in rodent carcinogenesis models has also been associated with a favorable chemopreventive effect *(67)*.

7. RESPIRATORY ISSUES WITH AEROSOLIZED DRUG DELIVERY

The ability of pulmonary delivery technology to mirror the location of carcinogenic injury from tobacco smoke is the intuitively appealing aspect of achieving dose deposition where incipient cancers are likely to arise. Under a National Institutes of Health (NIH) cooperative research and development agreement, we have been working with Battelle Pulmonary Therapeutics (BPT) to develop an electrohydrodynamic delivery system. Understanding the details of direct drug delivery via the airway is the goal of this collaboration; to this end, we used relevant animal models to determine if candidate drugs have a favorable effect while preserving a favorable therapeutic index. The first work of this collaboration involved pulmonary delivery of retinoids with carcinogen-induced bronchial tumor models. Using AJ mice with lung cancer induced by tobacco-related carcinogens 4-(methylnitrosamino)-1-(3-pyridyl)-1-butanone (NNK) and benzo(*a*)pyrene (B*a*P), we showed that nebulized 13-cRA significantly reduced the number of lung tumor nodules in the majority of mice compared to aerosolized vehicle control *(68)*. In other findings from this collaboration, we reported that airway-delivered retinoid had a reproducible effect on activating nuclear retinoic acid receptors of the lung; this pattern of activation was markedly different from nuclear retinoid activation seen with oral retinoid administration *(69)* As this favorable anticancer response has not been seen with orally administered retinoids in rodents, further clinical validation of this approach is warranted. A recent report by Kohlhaulf and co-workers using retinyl palmitate over a three-month period showed reversal of bronchoscopy-detected sites of bronchial metaplasia and dysplasia in airways of 11 smokers *(70)*. While this was a single-arm pilot trial studying only 11 cases, no appreciable drug side effects were noted.

The evolving picture of histological distribution in lung cancer cases may have some important implications. Filtered smoke containing smaller mean particle size may deliver carcinogens to more distal aspects of the airways, resulting in more adenocarcinomas of the lung *(71)*. This represents a challenge for standard pulmonary delivery technology, such as metered dose inhalers (MDIs), as they deliver most of their dose in the oropharynx and central airways *(55,63,72)*. For this reason, we have been interested in pulmonary delivery technology with a greater capability of distal respiratory tract delivery. Our collaborators at BPT have developed such a device. Using a process similar to electrospray, which differs from propellant-driven MDIs, the BPT device generates small, neutrally charged drug particles and delivers them into the lung under isokinetic conditions, mirroring the characteristics of tobacco smoke, which also delivers small particles under isokinetic conditions. In contrast to the MDI device, which deposits a high percentage of delivered drug in the back of the throat with only a small fraction reaching the deep lung, the BPT device efficiently delivers most of the drug to the distal epithelium. The electrospray-like device can be configured as a standard benchtop respiratory delivery-type instrument or as a small handheld device for ambulatory use. For chemoprevention applications, the handheld device is attractive not only for convenience and efficiency but also for cost. Ease of

operation is comparable to that for an MDI. Design features of this device make it practical for use in broad public health applications.

8. CONCLUSION

The field of lung cancer chemoprevention merits a serious and rapid reconsideration in light of recent advances in pulmonary drug delivery capability, global pharmacological considerations, preliminary results from retinoid exposures in the mouse adenoma model, and results from oral and aerosolized retinoid chemoprevention. Orally administered retinoid failed to achieve high enough concentrations in the respiratory epithelium to arrest the progression of field carcinogenesis, and had unacceptable clinical toxicity as well. In contrast, direct pulmonary drug delivery is associated with a more favorable chemoprevention effect in pilot studies with mice and in the clinic *(68,69,72)*. Parallel in vivo work with aerosolized steroids has also achieved favorable chemopreventive results *(67)*.

Lists of candidate targets for lung cancer chemoprevention have been compiled at a number of recent expert meetings (http://prg.nci.nih.gov/lung/finalreport.html and http://www.webtie.org/sots/Meetings/Lung/June%2019%202001/Default.htm). The therapeutic index advantages of pulmonary delivery compared to systemic delivery are generic for direct drug delivery for early lung cancer. There is a strong rationale to give first preference to direct drug delivery in aerosol form for candidate drugs proposed for early lung cancer chemoprevention. This statement is made with full understanding that a host of research questions remain. A number of parameters such as molecular size and lipid solubility will affect the efficiency of drug delivery, but these issues can be assessed experimentally. New opportunities have arisen to alter drug formulation, maximizing drug partitioning to achieve more favorable drug residence times in the critical epithelial cell interface. This was shown by using topical skin delivery to increase drug access to basal cell populations, as basal cells comprise the microenvironment driving field carcinogenesis in the skin *(73–75)*. Many of these questions can be answered only through human trials; the actual condition of a smoker's respiratory epithelium cannot be easily emulated with current in vivo models. Despite these questions, candidate constructs exist today that could begin the clinical investigation for this approach.

In terms of lung cancer screening, a recent survey from the American Cancer Society determined that close to 15% of current or former smokers have had spiral CT recommended by their personal physicians, and the vast majority of those 15% are getting those scans. We have no systematic information from the clinical care of all but the smallest fraction of these individuals. If only a small fraction from that large cohort of early cancer patients entered chemoprevention trials of aerosolized agents, we could quickly find out if aerosolized drug delivery is as exciting in practice as the theory suggests.

REFERENCES

1. Jemal A, Thomas A, Murray T, Thun M. Cancer statistics, 2002. *CA Cancer J Clin* 2002;52:23–47.
2. Chute JP, Chen T, Feigal E, et al. Twenty years of Phase III trials for patients with extensive-stage small-cell lung cancer: perceptible progress. *J Clin Oncol* 1999;17:1794–1801.
3. Carney DN. Lung cancer—time to move on from chemotherapy. *N Engl J Med* 2002;346:126–128.
4. Peto R, Chen ZM, Boreham J. Tobacco—the growing epidemic. *Nature Med* 1999;5:15–17.
5. Hong WK. Chemoprevention of lung cancer. *Asian Am Pac Isl J Health* 1998; 6:322–326.
6. Jordan C. Historical perspective on hormonal therapy of advanced breast cancer. *Clin Ther* 2002;24 (Suppl A): A3–A16.
7. Fisher B, Redmond C. New perspective on cancer of the contralateral breast: a marker for assessing tamoxifen as a preventive agent. *J Natl Cancer Inst* 1991;83:1278–1280.
8. Mulshine JL. Fostering chemoprevention agent development: how to proceed? *J Cell Biochem* 1995;22:254–259.
9. van Zandwijk N, Dalesio O, Pastorino U, et al. EUROSCAN, a randomized trial of vitamin A and N-acetylcysteine in patients with head and neck cancer or lung cancer. For the European Organization for Research and Treatment of Cancer Head and Neck and Lung Cancer Cooperative Groups. *J Natl Cancer Inst* 2000;92:977–986.
10. Lippman SM, Lee JJ, Karp DD, et al. Randomized Phase III intergroup trial of isotretinoin to prevent second primary tumors in stage I non-small-cell lung cancer. *J Natl Cancer Inst* 2001;93:605–618.
11. Henschke CI, McCauley DI, Yankelevitz DF, et al. Early Lung Cancer Action Project: overall design and findings from baseline screening. *Lancet* 1999;354:99–105.
12. Henschke CI, Naidich DP, Yankelevitz DF, et al. Early lung cancer action project. *Cancer* 2001;92:153–159.
13. Kaneko M, Kusumoto M, Kobayashi T, et al. Computed tomography screening for lung carcinoma in Japan. *Cancer* 2000;89(Suppl 11):2485–2488.
14. Okamoto N, Suzuki T, Hasegawa T, et al. Evaluation of a clinic-based screening program for lung cancer with a case-control design in Kanagawa, Japan. *Lung Cancer* 1999;25: 77–85.
15. Woloshin W, Schwartz LM, Welch HG. Tobacco money: up in smoke. *Lancet* 2002;359:2108–2111.
16. Lee TH, Brennan TA. Direct-to-consumer marketing of high-technology screening tests. *N Engl J Med* 2002;346: 529–531.
17. Yankelevitz DF, Reeves AP, Kostis WJ, et al. Small pulmonary nodules: volumetrically determined growth rates based on CT evaluation. *Radiology* 2000;217:251–256.
18. Slaughter DP, Southwick HW, Smejkal W. "Field cancerization" in oral stratified squamous epithelium. *Cancer* 1953;6: 963–968.
19. Auerbach O, Gere JB, Forman JB, et al. Changes in the bronchial epithelium in relation to smoking and cancer of the lung. *N Engl J Med* 1957;256:97–104.
20. Tockman MS, Mulshine JL, Piantadosi S, et al. Prospective detection of preclinical lung cancer: results from two studies of heterogeneous nuclear ribonucleoprotein A2/B1 overexpression. *Clin Cancer Res* 1997;3:2237–2246.
21. DeLuca LM. Retinoids and their receptors in differentiation, embryogenesis and neoplasia. *FASEB J* 1991;5:2924–2933.
22. McDowell E, Coleman B, Chang S, et al. Effects of retinoid acid on the growth and morphology of hamster tracheal epithelia cells in primary culture. *Virchows Arch B* 1987;54:38–51.
23. Moon RC, McCormick DL, Mehta RG. Inhibition of carcinogenesis by retinoids. *Cancer Res* 1983, 43:24,696–24755.
24. Oridate N, Suzuki S, Higuchi M, et al. Involvement of reactive oxygen species in *N*-(4-hydroxyphenyl)retinamide-induced apoptosis in cervical carcinoma cells. *J Natl Cancer Inst* 1997;89:1191–1198.
25. Oridate N, Lotan D, Xu XC, et al. Differential induction of apoptosis by all-trans-retinoic acid and N-(4-hydroxyphenyl)retinamide in human head and neck squamous cell carcinoma cell lines. *Clin Cancer Res* 1996;2:855–863.
26. Lee JJ, Liu D, Lee JS, et al. Long-term impact of smoking on lung epithelial proliferation in current and former smokers. *J Natl Cancer Inst* 2001;93;1081–1088.
27. Lee HY, Dawson MI, Walsh GL, et al. Retinoic acid receptor- and retinoid X receptor-selective retinoids activate signaling pathways that converge on AP-1 and inhibit squamous differentiation in human bronchial epithelial cells. *Cell Growth Differ* 1996;7:997–1004.
28. Kurie JM, Lee JS, Khuri FR, et al. N-(4-hydroxyphenyl)retinamide in the chemoprevention of squamous metaplasia and dysplasia of the bronchial epithelium. *Clin Cancer Res* 2000;6:2973–2979.
29. Kurie JM, Lee JS, Griffin T, et al. Phase I trial of 9-cis retinoic acid in adults with solid tumors. *Clin Cancer Res* 1996;2: 287–293.
30. Hong WK, Lippman SM, Itri LM, et al. Prevention of second primary tumors with isotretinoin in squamous-cell carcinoma of the head and neck. *N Engl J Med* 1990;323:795–801.
31. Veronesi U, De Palo G, Marubini E, et al. Randomized trial of fenretinide to prevent second breast malignancy in women with early breast cancer. *J Natl Cancer Inst* 1999;91:1847–1856.
32. Avis I, Mathias A, Unsworth EJ, et al. Analysis of small cell lung cancer cell growth inhibition by 13-cis-retinoic acid: importance of bioavailability. *Cell Growth Differ* 1995;6:485–492.
33. Okamato K, Andreola F, Chiantore MV, et al. Differences in uptake and metabolism of retinoid acid between estrogen-positive and estrogen-negative human breast cancer cells. *Cancer Chemother Pharmacol* 2000;46:128–134.
34. Geradts J, Chen J-Y, Russell E, et al. Human lung cancer cell lines exhibit resistance to retinoic acid treatment. *Cell Growth Differ* 1993;4:799–809.
35. Warrell RP Jr, Maslak P, Eardley A, et al. Treatment of acute promyelocytic leukemia with all-*trans*-retinoic acid: an update of the New York experience. *Leukemia* 1994;8 Suppl 2:S33–S37.
36. Hansen LA, Sigman CC, Andreola F, et al. Retinoids in chemoprevention and differentiation therapy. *Carcinogenesis* 2000;21:1271–1279.
37. Kalin JR, Starling ME, Hill DL. Disposition of all-trans-retinoic acid in mice following oral doses. *Drug Metab Dispos* 1981;9:196–201.

38. Muindi JRF, Frankel SR, Huselton C, et al. Clinical pharmacology of oral all-*trans* retinoic acid in patients with acute promyelocytic leukemia. *Cancer Res* 1992;52:2138–2142.

39. Cornic M, Delva L, Castaigne S, et al. In vitro all-*trans* retinoic acid (ATRA) sensitivity and cellular retinoic acid binding protein (CRABP) levels in relapse leukemic cells after remission induction by ATRA in acute promyelocytic leukemia. *Leukemia* 1994;8 Suppl 2:S16–S19.

40. Ozpolat B, Lopez-Berestein G, Mehta K. ATRA(ouble) in the treatment of acute promyelocytic leukemia. *J Biol Regul Homeost Agents* 2001;15:107–122.

41. Zou CP, Kurie JM, Lotan D, et al. Higher potency of *N*-(4-hydroxyphenyl)retinamide than all-trans-retinoic acid in induction of apoptosis in non-small cell lung cancer cell lines. *Clin Cancer Res* 1998;4:1345–1355.

42. van Osdol WW, Sung C, Dedrick RL, Weinstein JN. A distributed pharmacokinetic model of two-step imaging and treatment protocols: application to streptavidin-conjugated monoclonal antibodies and radiolabeled biotin. *J Nucl Med* 1993;34:1552–1564.

43. Weinstein JN, Eger RR, Covell DG, et al. The pharmacology of monoclonal antibodies. *Ann N Y Acad Sci* 1987;507:199–210.

44. Dedrick RL, Flessner MF. Pharmacokinetic considerations on monoclonal antibodies. *Prog Clin Biol Res* 1989;288:429–438.

45. Netti PA, Hamberg LM, Babich JW, et al. Enhancement of fluid filtration across tumor vessels: implication for delivery of macromolecules. *Proc Natl Acad Sci USA* 1999;96:3137–3142.

46. Banerjee RK, van Osdol WW, Bungay PM, et al. Finite element model of antibody penetration in a prevascular tumor nodule embedded in normal tissue. *J Control Release* 2001;74:193–202.

47. Juweid M, Neumann R, Paik C, et al. Micropharmacology of monoclonal antibodies in solid tumors: direct experimental evidence for a binding site barrier. *Cancer Res* 1992;52:5144–5153.

48. Weinstein JN, van Osdol W. Early intervention in cancer using monoclonal antibodies and other biological ligands: micropharmacology and the "binding site barrier." *Cancer Res* 1992;52:2747–2751.

49. Keenan AM, Weinstein JN, Mulshine JL, et al. Immunolymphoscintigraphy in patients with lymphoma after subcutaneous injection of indium-111-labeled T101 monoclonal antibody. *J Nucl Med* 1987;28:42–46.

50. Mulshine JL, Carrasquillo JA, Weinstein JN, et al. Direct intralymphatic injection of radiolabeled 111In-T101 in patients with cutaneous T-cell lymphoma. *Cancer Res* 1991;51:688–695.

51. Dedrick RL, Myers CE, Bungay PM, DeVita VT Jr. Pharmacokinetic rationale for peritoneal drug administration in the treatment of ovarian cancer. *Cancer Treat Rep* 1978;62:1–11.

52. Alberts DS, Liu PY, Hannigan EV, et al. Intraperitoneal cisplatin plus intravenous cyclophosphamide versus intravenous cisplatin plus intravenous cyclophosphamide for stage III ovarian cancer. *N Engl J Med* 1996;335:1950–1955.

53. Mulshine JL, De Luca LM, Dedrick RL. Regional delivery of retinoids: a new approach to early lung cancer intervention. *Clin Biol Basis Lung Cancer Prev* 1998;24:273–283

54. Newman SP. *Delivery of Drugs to the Respiratory Tract.* Marcel Dekker, New York, 1996.

55. Adjei AL, Qiu Y, Gupta PK. *Bioavailability and Pharmacokinetics of Inhaled Drugs.* Marcel Dekker, New York, 1996.

56. O'Riordan TG. Inhaled antimicrobial therapy: from cystic fibrosis to the flu. *Respir Care* 2000;45:836–845.

57. Colburn WA, Vane FM, Bugge CJL, et al. Pharmacokinetics of 14C-isotretinoin in healthy volunteers and volunteers with biliary T-tube drainage. *Drug Metab Dispos* 1985;13:327–332.

58. Peng YM, Dalton WS, Alberts DS, et al. Pharmacokinetics of N-4-hydroxyphenylretinamide and the effects of its oral administration on plasma retinol concentration in cancer patients. *Int J Cancer* 1989;43:22–26.

59. Schanker LS, Mitchell EW, Brown RA. Species comparison of drug absorption from the lung after aerosol inhalation or intratracheal injection. *Drug Metab Dispos* 1986;14:79–88.

60. Tzimas G, Collins MD, Nau H. Developmental stage-associated differences in the transplacental distribution of 13-*cis*- and all-*trans*-retinoic acid as well as their glucuronides in rats and mice. *Toxicol Appl Pharmacol* 1995;133::91–101.

61. Swanson BN, Zaharevitz DW, Sporn MB. Pharmacokinetics of *N*-(4-hydroxyphenyl)-all-*trans*-retinamide in rats. *Drug Metab Dispos* 1980;8:168–172.

62. Geller DE, Pitlick WH, Nardella PA, et al. Pharmacokinetics and bioavailability of aerosolized tobramycin in cystic fibrosis. *Chest* 2002;122:219–26.

63. Kuhn RJ: Pharmaceutical considerations in aerosol drug delivery. *Pharmacotherapy* 2002;22:80S–85S.

64. Flume P, Klepser ME. The rationale for aerosolized antibiotics. *Pharmacotherapy* 2002;22:71S–79S.

65. Todisco T, Eslami A, Baglioni S, et al. Basis for nebulized antibiotics: droplet characterization and in vitro antimicrobial activity versus *Staphylococcus aureus, Escherichia coli,* and *Pseudomonas aeruginosa. J Aerosol Med* 2000;13:11–16.

66. Patton JS. Pulmonary delivery of drugs for bone disorders. *Adv Drug Deliv Rev* 2000;42:239–248.

67. Wattenberg LW, Wiedmann TS, Estensen RD, et al. Chemoprevention of pulmonary carcinogenesis by brief exposures to aerosolized budesonide or beclomethasone dipropionate and by the combination of aerosolized budesonide and dietary myo-inositol. *Carcinogenesis* 2000;21:179–182.

68. Dahl AR, Grossi IM, Houchens DP, et al. Inhaled isotretinoin (13-*cis* retinoic acid) is an effective lung cancer chemopreventive agent in A/J mice at low doses: a pilot study. *Clin Cancer Res* 2000;6:3015–6324.

69. Wang DL, Marko M, Dahl AR, et al. Topical delivery of 13-*cis*-retinoic acid by inhalation up-regulates expression of rodent lung but not liver retinoic acid receptors. *Clin Cancer Res* 2000;6:3636–3645.

70. Kohlhaulf M, Haussinger K, Stanzek F, et al. Inhalation of aerosolized vitamin A: reversibility of metaplasia and dysplasia of human respiratory epithelia—a prospective pilot study. *Eur J Med Res* 2002;7:72–78.

71. Stellman SD, Muscat JE, Hoffmann D, Wynder EL. Impact of filter cigarette smoking on lung cancer histology. *Prev Med* 1997;26:451–456.

72. Altiere RJ, Thompson DC. Physiology and Pharmacology of the Airways. In *Inhalation Aerosols.* Hickey AJ, ed. Marcel Dekker, New York, 1996:85–138.

73. McEwan LE, Smith JG. Topical diclofenac/hyaluronic acid gel in the treatment of solar keratoses. *Australas J Dermatol* 1997;38:187–189.

74. Brown MB, Marriott C, Martin GP. The effect of hyaluronan on the in vitro deposition of diclofenac within the skin. *Int J Tissue React* 1995;17:133–140.

75. Sakai S, Yasuda R, Sayo T, et al. Hyaluronan exists in the normal stratum corneum. *J Invest Dermatol* 2000;114:1184–1187.

BLADDER

24 Bladder Cancer

Clinical Strategies for Cancer Chemoprevention

H. Barton Grossman, MD, Anita L. Sabichi, MD, and Yu Shen, PhD

CONTENTS

NATURAL HISTORY
PRIMARY PREVENTION
SECONDARY PREVENTION
CONCLUSIONS
REFERENCES

1. NATURAL HISTORY

Bladder cancer is the fourth most common noncutaneous malignancy in men and the ninth most common in women in the United States *(1)*. The incidence in men is three to four times that seen in women. There is considerable evidence that bladder cancer is carcinogen-induced. However, the interval between carcinogen exposure and development of clinically evident bladder cancer can be 20 yr or more *(2)*. The major risk factor for bladder cancer is cigarette smoking. Epidemiologic studies have estimated that almost half of all bladder cancers are a result of tobacco use *(3)*.

Diagnosis of bladder cancer is usually by cystoscopy and biopsy. While cystoscopy is very effective at detecting the presence of cancer, it can miss some cancers, particularly carcinoma *in situ*. Urine cytology can be particularly helpful in the detection of high-grade disease (carcinoma *in situ*) *(4)*. New methods of cystoscopy using fluorescence to enhance the detection of superficial bladder cancer and carcinoma *in situ* are being explored and appear promising *(5)*.

Bladder cancers, particularly the relatively common noninvasive, papillary transitional cell carcinomas (Ta), are associated with a high rate of recurrence but a relatively low incidence of progression to muscle-invasive disease *(6)*. Accessibility of the bladder to diagnostic evaluation, strong association with carcinogen exposure, and the high rate of superficial recurrence provide unique opportunities for intervention with chemopreventive agents. Furthermore, recent evidence suggests that polyclonality of bladder cancer is common *(7,8)*. Preventing recurrent disease by relatively nontoxic therapy (chemoprevention) is appealing.

2. PRIMARY PREVENTION

2.1. Risk

Bladder cancer is strongly associated with environmental carcinogens, the most important being tobacco smoke. Approximately half of all bladder cancers have been attributed to tobacco use *(3)*. Although cigarette smoke has been the primary source implicated in bladder carcinogenesis, other forms of inhaled smoke (pipe and cigar) also apparently contribute to the development of this disease *(9)*. Importantly, this risk is not distributed evenly throughout the population. Susceptibility is related not only to the extent of smoking but also to individual genetic susceptibility. Smokers who have an *N*-acetyltransferase 2 polymorphism are slow acetylators and appear to be at increased risk due to decreased ability to detoxify carcinogenic aromatic amines in cigarette smoke *(10)*. GSTM1 deficiency is also associated with an increased risk of developing bladder cancer *(11)*. Women may be more susceptible to developing bladder cancer when controlling for the amount of

From: Cancer Chemoprevention, Volume 2: Strategies for Cancer Chemoprevention
Edited by: G. J. Kelloff, E. T. Hawk, and C. C. Sigman © Humana Press Inc., Totowa, NJ

tobacco exposure *(12)*. Smoking cessation is associated with a decreased incidence and lower recurrence rate of superficial bladder cancer *(13,14)*.

Occupational exposure to carcinogens is also associated with bladder cancer. High-risk industries include aromatic amine and dyestuff production, rubber, painting, leather and aluminum industries, and truck driving *(15)*. Latency between exposure and development of bladder cancer can be 20 yr or more *(2)*. The role of total fluid intake in modulating the risk of bladder cancer is controversial *(16,17)*.

2.2. Study Design/Endpoints

The obvious endpoint for primary prevention is the incidence of bladder cancer. An effective approach would decrease incidence of this disease. In the past, cystoscopy has proved to be more sensitive than cytology for detecting bladder cancers, especially those that are low-grade *(18)*. The low frequency of bladder cancer in the general population and the long latency between exposure and clinically apparent disease onset make population-based strategies an inefficient approach to development of new forms of chemoprevention. Targe-ting individuals at high risk (people exposed to carcinogens through occupational exposure or through tobacco use) provides a focused population that can be selected based on extent of exposure to a putative bladder carcinogen. However, routine cystoscopy is an invasive diagnostic approach that may be unacceptable as a screening test even in this high-risk population. Alternative approaches to early diagnosis have therefore been considered.

One approach has been to evaluate molecular biomarkers in exfoliated urothelial cells shed in the urine. A case-control study evaluated urine from a high-risk group of workers in China with occupational exposure to benzidine, using modulation of biomarkers as a measure to assess their risk of bladder cancer *(19)*. The study population, consisting of 1788 workers who had been exposed to benzidine and 373 without exposure, was evaluated over a period of 7 yr. The exposed cohort had been exposed to the carcinogen for at least 1 yr and was studied approx 20 yr after initial exposure. The exposed workers were classified as being at high (153), moderate (312), or low (1065) risk depending on their biomarker profile. Incidences of bladder cancer in the benzidine-exposed and control workers were 263 and 87 per 100,000 person-years, respectively, during the study time frame. In this study, 28 cancers were detected in exposed workers compared with two in nonexposed workers.

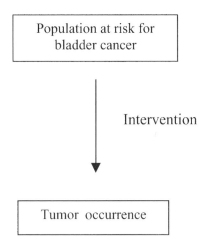

Fig. 1. Primary prevention: clinical endpoint.

Figure 1 depicts a classic design to assess the effect of a chemoprevention strategy on occurrence of bladder cancer. Study power is related to the number of events. Targeting a high-risk population will provide more statistical power than screening a similar-size cohort from the general population, because there will be more events due to the higher incidence of bladder cancer. Smokers and individuals exposed to putative carcinogens comprise such a cohort.

2.2.1. DESIGN AND ANALYSIS OF PRIMARY PREVENTION TRIALS OF BLADDER CANCER

The target cohort for primary prevention trials includes healthy individuals at high risk of developing bladder cancer. Many case-control studies suggest that smoking is the main risk factor for bladder cancer.

A primary clinical chemoprevention trial can be designed to allow randomized controlled evaluation of one or more interventions: the chemoprevention agent under study vs placebo (or other active therapy). In general, such prevention trials require a large sample size due to a low incidence of disease in the study cohort. Without sufficient sample size and duration of follow-up, the study will not have the statistical power to demonstrate a reasonable reduction in disease incidence. Participants in this type of clinical trial are generally followed through regularly scheduled examinations to monitor disease occurrence and possible adverse effects of the intervention.

Sample size is calculated based on a comparison of proportions of bladder cancer occurrence in two study groups using data from all participants *(20)*. We use such a setting for a conservative sample size calculation, but we do not recommend such a test of proportions for data analysis at end of trial.

Some assumptions are necessary in calculating power and sample size. Power is based on a two-sided 5% level test of significance with an average 10-yr follow-up. Based on the Surveillance, Epidemiology and End Results (SEER) Program registry, the age-adjusted bladder cancer incidence for men from 1973–1998 was approx 30 per 100,000 per year. In addition, the literature shows that 25% of men older than 17 yr of age are current smokers, and about 50% of men with bladder cancer are current smokers. Using these assumptions, we may roughly estimate the yearly incidence of bladder cancer among male smokers to be about 60 per 100,000. To detect a 50% reduction of incidence from an intervention, we need a total of 15,600 male smokers equally randomized to placebo and intervention with 80% power based on an average follow-up period of 10 yr, as shown in Table 1. From the SEER database, we note that incidence of bladder cancer increases with age. Thus, if we restrict our study population to smoking men ages 50 yr and older, the annual incidence will be higher than 60 per 100,000. Assuming an incidence of 80 per 100,000 per year for this cohort, the corresponding sample size and power calculation can be found in Table 1 as well. Table 1 also lists sample size requirements for an incidence reduction of 30%.

Gail *(20)* noted that binomial sample size calculations are generally larger than the size required for use with time to disease occurrence outcome (using the log-rank test). If a very high noncompliance rate is predicted, sample sizes calculated by the two methods are close to each other. In primary chemoprevention trials with relatively infrequent events and short intervention duration compared with mean event time, Gail showed that binomial sample size calculations suffice for use with the log-rank test statistic. Moreover, because the effectiveness of chemoprevention agents may require time to be manifest, the commonly used log-rank test may not be sensitive enough to detect the expected difference in time to tumor occurrence. Thus, a more conservative calculation of binomial sample size is appropriate.

There are some other important issues related to the design of this type of trial: duration of treatment, duration of follow-up, screening methods to detect the disease of interest during follow-up, frequency of screening, and compliance. Although the primary study endpoint may be to assess reduction of bladder

Table 1
Sample Size for Primary Prevention Trial With Two-Sided
Type I Error Rate of 0.05 and Average of 10 yr Follow-Up

Bladder cancer incidence/100,000		Power	
Placebo	Intervention	80%	90%
60	30	15,620	20,910
60	40	39,041	52,264
80	40	11,695	15,657
80	56	36,805	49,271

cancer incidence, considerable additional information can be gained by monitoring incidence of other diseases. Other considerations include loss to follow-up and competing risks (death from other causes) during the trials.

2.2.2. ANALYSIS PLAN

To compare the effect of chemoprevention regimens on bladder cancer incidence in the context of a randomized trial, the usual analysis methods for typical cancer clinical trials may not be the most efficient choices. Primary prevention trials typically involve tens of thousands of participants followed for up to 10 yr or more. As with secondary prevention trials (carried out in patients with a previous diagnosis of cancer), there is likely a delay from the start of the intervention and the time that any effects on cancer incidence are expected to be observed.

A basic test statistic to compare an intervention group to a corresponding control group will be a weighted log-rank statistic by stratification on year of follow-up. The weighting is intended to enhance test power. Some adaptive weighted log-rank tests *(21)* or maximum of the weighted Kaplan Meier test may be applicable for this purpose. Moreover, listed analysis methods in the following section on secondary prevention trials can be applied as well.

Biomarkers should be an integral component of most chemoprevention studies. Because no currently validated biomarkers exist for bladder cancer chemoprevention, potentially informative biomarkers must be validated by prospectively assessing their correlation with a clinical endpoint (bladder cancer occurrence). Once validated, biomarkers may expedite chemoprevention studies by providing a surrogate endpoint that can be reached faster than a clinical one. Such a design is shown in Fig. 2.

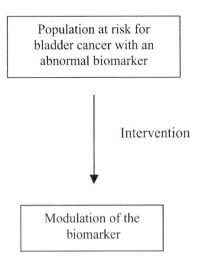

Fig. 2. Primary prevention: biomarker endpoint.

3. SECONDARY PREVENTION

3.1. Tumor Characteristics

Superficial bladder cancers (those that do not invade the muscularis propria) are associated with a high rate of recurrence related to characteristics of the primary tumor, e.g., multiplicity, size, grade, and invasion of the lamina propria *(22)*. Patients presenting with a solitary tumor have a risk of tumor recurrence approaching 50% at 4 yr *(23)*. Individuals with multiple adverse tumor characteristics have a 70% risk of tumor recurrence at 1 yr *(22)*. A large body of evidence suggests that many of these recurrences stem from a monoclonal origin *(24,25)*. However, recent evidence suggests that polyclonality of bladder cancer is common *(7,8)*. In routine patient care, distinction is not made between bladder cancer recurrences from a monoclonal origin and second primaries. They are all designated recurrent tumors.

Risk of recurrence is distinct from risk of progression *(6)*. Factors associated with increased risk of progression to muscle invasive disease are invasion of the lamina propria and alteration in expression of p53 and retinoblastoma proteins *(26,27)*. Intravesical Bacillus Calmette-Guerin (BCG) has been effective in decreasing the rate of bladder cancer recurrence *(28,29)*. BCG is commonly administered weekly for 6 wk. Although there is no consistent approach to maintenance BCG therapy, current results demonstrate that this approach is more effective than treatment with an induction course alone *(30)*. The effectiveness of BCG in decreasing incidence of progression to muscle invasive disease remains controversial *(31,32)*.

3.2. Study Design/Endpoints

Because patients with a diagnosis of bladder cancer have a high rate of recurrence but a low rate of progression to muscle-invasive disease, this population has been used for chemoprevention studies using a variety of designs. The control population has many events but is at relatively low risk for tumor progression if no therapy (placebo) is administered. The population is usually selected on clinical evidence of being free of disease by conventional assessment, i.e., negative cystoscopy. Conventional cystoscopy is, however, a flawed standard that will fail to identify some carcinoma *in situ* lesions and other areas of microscopic disease. Urine cytology will assist in this assessment by detecting many occult high-grade tumors. However, it has low sensitivity for low-grade lesions *(4)*. Several new modalities such as fluorescence cystoscopy *(5)* and urine assessment using fluorescence *in situ* hybridization *(33)* or microsatellite analysis *(34)* suggest that more sensitive and specific methods to detect bladder cancer are possible.

Two general strategies have been employed to study potential chemopreventive agents in this population. For patients at relatively low risk for recurrence, all gross disease is resected and subjects are then randomly assigned to chemoprevention or control groups. Patients with a high risk for recurrence have all gross disease resected followed by adjuvant intravesical therapy to maximize a disease-free state. They are then randomly assigned to the chemoprevention or control groups. Since risk of recurrence cannot be reliably determined on an individual basis, these two strategies are not mutually exclusive.

Lamm and associates *(35)* used a 2×2 design to evaluate BCG (intravesical vs intravesical and intradermal administration) and vitamins (megadose vs conventional dose). In this study, patients underwent tumor resection and were randomly assigned to treatment with BCG or to vitamin dose. In this small study of 65 patients, analysis of the vitamin dose group showed a significantly longer interval to recurrence in patients receiving megavitamins ($p = 0.0014$). The rate of recurrence in these two arms did not diverge until 9 mo after the study began, suggesting that vitamins were not effective in treating preexisting microscopic tumors but were effective in delaying or inhibiting progression of normal urothelium or early lesions to clinical cancer.

Studer and associates *(36)* employed a different strategy for preventing bladder cancer recurrence. After superficial tumors were resected, patients were ran-

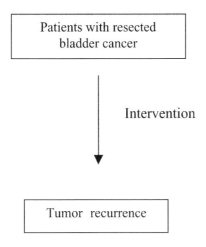

Fig. 3. Secondary prevention: clinical endpoint.

Table 2
Two-Sided Test With Type I Error Rate of 0.05
and Power of 80%

Accrual duration		Accrual rate	
		50/yr	80/yr
2 yr	Sample size	100	160
	Total trial duration	11 yr	4.3 yr
3 yr	Sample size	150	240
	Total trial duration	5.2 yr	3.4 yr

3.2.1. DESIGN AND ANALYSIS FOR SECONDARY PREVENTION

This section addresses study design and data analysis issues related to secondary prevention with the endpoint of time to tumor recurrence or death (Fig. 3). For patients with resected bladder cancer, the recurrence-free survival rate at 2.5 yr after surgery is about 40%. If we assume that a secondary preventive therapy will increase the recurrence-free survival rate to 60% at 2.5 yr after surgery and desire a power of 80% and two-sided type I error rate of 0.05, the relationship between sample size, accrual rate, and total study duration of a trial can be calculated (Table 2). In this situation, there is a clear tradeoff in sample size and study duration. Study duration is based on achieving an adequate number of events. For example, with an accrual rate of 50 patients per year and accrual duration of 2 yr, we need an additional 9 yr of follow-up after accrual to reach a power of 80%. On the other hand, if we can speed up accrual (with 80 patients per year) for 2 yr, total study duration is reduced to 4.3 yr.

3.2.2. ANALYSIS PLAN

As prior data suggested *(35,36)*, changes in the rate of tumor recurrence with secondary prevention may not be instantaneous but may require a phase-in period to show a treatment effect. Therefore, the commonly used log-rank test and Cox regression model with proportional hazards assumption are not the most efficient methods to do inference. Some non-rank-based test statistics, such as weighted Kaplan-Meier test statistics by Pepe and Fleming *(39)* and its extension when covariates are incorporated in the inference *(40)*, can be more sensitive to nonproportional hazard alternatives.

Just as in primary chemoprevention studies, biomarkers can facilitate studies of secondary chemoprevention. A general example is shown in Fig. 4. Biomarker data can be either binary or continuous. Biomarkers with continuous data offer the additional advantage of evaluating quantitative changes in the biomarker over time.

domly assigned to receive etretinate or placebo for 2 yr. Patients with recurrent bladder cancer had their tumors resected and continued on treatment unless their physicians elected to remove them from the study. Nine patients in the placebo arm (21%) and one in the etretinate arm (3%) were removed from the study during the first year of therapy. Mean time to first recurrence was similar in the two groups. However, mean time to second recurrence was significantly longer in the etretinate group. This delayed response to chemoprevention is similar to the finding in the Lamm study *(35)*. Furthermore, it suggests that there may be benefit in maintaining therapy even in the face of initial tumor recurrence.

Most studies have used tumor recurrence as the endpoint. The use of biomarkers as surrogate endpoints offers a quantitative measure that could, in theory, predict response much earlier than can clinical disease recurrence. While this concept is attractive, there are as yet no validated markers for this purpose. A Phase II study suggested that modulation of DNA content by flow cytometry could be used to monitor the efficacy of fenretinide *(37)*. However, a subsequent randomized trial did not confirm the efficacy of fenretinide or the utility of DNA flow cytometry as an intermediate endpoint *(38)*.

Figure. 3 shows the commonly employed strategy for studying an agent to prevent bladder cancer recurrence. Patients with resected bladder cancer tumors are enrolled. Depending on the risk of recurrence, additional interventions such as intravesical BCG can be added. The chemoprevention agent or agents are tested in comparison with a randomized control group. The endpoint is clinical tumor recurrence.

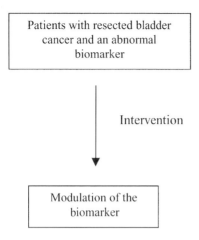

Fig. 4. Secondary prevention: biomarker endpoint.

The strategy of continuing patients on a chemoprevention trial after an initial recurrence is depicted in Fig. 5. This strategy assumes that initial recurrences are largely due to occult microscopic disease and that continued chemoprevention can delay or prevent subsequent occurrences. These second recurrences are likely to be second primaries that may be more susceptible to chemoprevention. In this type of study design, patients are continued on the study for a fixed period of time. Provided that patients have disease recurrence with noninvasive tumors that are resected, they are at low risk of progression in tumor stage and can be maintained on the study.

3.2.2.1. Statistical Design Issues for Time-to-Multiple Bladder Cancer Recurrences. When clinical trials involve times to multiple recurrences, methods of statistical analysis developed for time to a single event may not be the best choice. In particular, data may be analyzed in one of three ways: comparing frequencies of events that occurred; comparing time to the first event taking censoring into consideration; or comparing time to multiple recurrence events with potential of censoring and taking into account correlation between various times obtained from the same patient. Variable lengths of follow-up complicate comparison of the frequencies of events. It has been also recognized that using only time to the first event will generally result in loss of information. Therefore, we will focus on the third method in the following discussion.

Wei et al. *(41)* proposed to model the marginal distribution of times for each recurrence; time to each recurrence is measured from the same time origin. Hughes has discussed power and sample size estimation *(42)*; the analyses methods and interpretation for

treatment effect in the Cox model are well developed *(41)*, and software is widely available *(43)*.

3.2.2.2. Some Hypothetical Examples for Design Consideration Using Multivariate Time-to-Event Data. This example approximates the power of a clinical trial that aims to use multiple recurrent event data for comparing two treatments. We assume that each patient can potentially experience two recurrences. When analyzing such data, we will model data by marginal distributions of multivariate failure times with the Cox proportional hazards models while leaving the nature of dependence among related failure times unspecified *(42)*. The method is used in randomized clinical trials where the comparability of treatment groups is established at the time of randomization in assessing all events of interest, rather than using time to the first recurrence only.

Two types of hypothesis tests will be considered: a global test across all types of events, and a pooled test based on assessing an average treatment effect across events. For the global test, we test $H_0: \beta = 0$, where $\beta = (\beta_1, \beta_2)$, and β_1, β_2 denote the treatment effect for time to first recurrence and second recurrence, respectively. For the pooled test, assuming $\beta_1 = \beta_2 = \beta^*$, we test $H_0: \beta^* = 0$. If a global test is used, then it is important to consider what interpretation will be drawn from a significant finding. A valid conclusion is that there is some difference between the two treatments

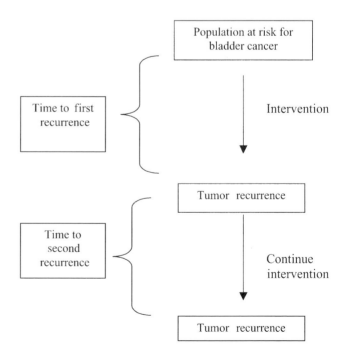

Fig. 5. Prevention with fixed duration of treatment.

Table 3
Hazard Ratio for First Event, $exp(\beta_1) = 1.5$, and No
Censorship, With Total Sample Size of 200

$exp(\beta_2)$	ρ	Power of global test	Power for pooled test	Power by using time to 1st event
1	0.33	0.781	0.393	0.800
1	0.63	0.915	0.291	0.800
1.25	0.33	0.737	0.772	0.800
1.25	0.63	0.725	0.689	0.800
1.50	0.33	0.901	0.944	0.800
1.50	0.63	0.816	0.881	0.800
1.75	0.33	0.956	0.969	0.800
1.75	0.63	0.960	0.965	0.800

being compared when rejecting the null hypothesis. For example, the effect of one treatment compared with another is detrimental for time to first recurrence but beneficial for time to second recurrence. The pooled test is particularly appropriate if the treatment differences are expected to be the same for all events being considered.

On the basis of the tables in Hughes (42), we found that the gain of power can be substantial for both global and pooled tests when the hazard ratio for the second event is equal to or greater than the hazard ratio for the first event when there is no censorship. However, it may lead to slight losses in power when the rank correlation between the first and second event is very strong (i.e., $\rho > 0.8$). In Table 3, we illustrate how, with some hypothetical parameters, power may be changed when multiple time-to-events data are used compared with the scenario when only time to first recurrence is used. Here, ρ is a rank correlation for time to first and second recurrence.

The results presented in Table 3 show that a total of 200 patients were randomly assigned to one of the two treatments. These patients were followed until each of the first and second recurrence times were obtained, and the hazard ratio for the first event, $exp(\beta_1)$, was set to 1.5. Choices of sample size mean that the power to detect the treatment effect ($\beta_1 = 0$) using just the first event is about 80%. For the hazard ratio of the second event, $exp(\beta_2)$, values of 1, 1.25, 1.5, and 1.75 were used. When there is no censorship and the treatment effect for the second recurrence is equal or greater than the treatment effect for the first recurrence, the power is generally greater when using time to multiple events

than using time to first recurrence only with the same sample size. However, a smaller treatment effect for the second recurrence may lead to a loss in power, especially for pooled tests.

4. CONCLUSIONS

Primary prevention of bladder cancer requires significant resources because of the long period of development and low incidence in the population. While the strategy of primary prevention is most desirable, progress in this area is unlikely until sufficient data justify evaluation of specific agents. These data will likely be developed in the strategy of secondary prevention (treating patients with a history of bladder cancer). Limited data suggest that effective chemoprevention in this setting results in a delayed response. The most efficient way of dealing with this phenomenon is to develop studies using methods that evaluate multiple recurrent events.

REFERENCES

1. Jemal A, Thomas A, Murray T, Thun M. Cancer statistics, 2002. *CA Cancer J Clin* 2002;52:23–47.
2. Miyakawa M, Tachibana M, Miyakawa A, et al. Re-evaluation of the latent period of bladder cancer in dyestuff-plant workers in Japan. *Int J Urol* 2001;8:423–430.
3. Marcus PM, Vineis P, Rothman N. NAT2 slow acetylation and bladder cancer risk: a meta-analysis of 22 case-control studies conducted in the general population. *Pharmacogenetics* 2000;10:115–122.
4. Bastacky S, Ibrahim S, Wilczynski SP, Murphy WM. The accuracy of urinary cytology in daily practice. *Cancer* 1999; 87:118–128.
5. Zaak D, Frimberger D, Stepp H, et al. Quantification of 5-aminolevulinic acid induced fluorescence improves the specificity of bladder cancer detection. *J Urol* 2001;166: 1665–1668.
6. Grossman HB. Superficial bladder cancer: decreasing the risk of recurrence. *Oncology* 1996;10:1617–1624.
7. Cheng L, Gu J, Ulbright TM, et al. Precise microdissection of human bladder carcinomas reveals divergent tumor subclones in the same tumor. *Cancer* 2002;94:104–110.
8. Paiss T, Wohr G, Hautmann RE, et al. Some tumors of the bladder are polyclonal in origin. *J Urol* 2002;167:718–723.
9. Pitard A, Brennan P, Clavel J, et al. Cigar, pipe, and cigarette smoking and bladder cancer risk in European men. *Cancer Causes Control* 2001;12:551–556.
10. Marcus PM, Hayes RB, Vineis P, et al. Cigarette smoking, N-acetyltransferase 2 acetylation status, and bladder cancer risk: a case-series meta-analysis of a gene-environment interaction. *Cancer Epidemiol Biomarkers Prev* 2000;9: 461–467.
11. Brockmoller J, Cascorbi I, Kerb R, Roots I. Combined analysis of inherited polymorphisms in arylamine N-acetyltransferase 2, glutathione S-transferases M1 and T1, microsomal epoxide hydrolase, and cytochrome P450 enzymes as modulators of bladder cancer risk. *Cancer Res* 1996;56: 3915–3925.

12. Castelao JE, Yuan JM, Skipper PL, et al. Gender- and smoking-related bladder cancer risk. *J Natl Cancer Inst* 2001; 93:538–545.

13. Brennan P, Bogillot O, Cordier S, et al. Cigarette smoking and bladder cancer in men: a pooled analysis of 11 case-control studies. *Int J Cancer* 2000;86:289–294.

14. Fleshner N, Garland J, Moadel A, et al. Influence of smoking status on the disease-related outcomes of patients with tobacco-associated superficial transitional cell carcinoma of the bladder. *Cancer* 1999;86:2337–2345.

15. Negri E, La Vecchia C. Epidemiology and prevention of bladder cancer. *Eur J Cancer Prev* 2001;10:7–14.

16. Michaud DS, Spiegelman D, Clinton SK, et al. Fluid intake and the risk of bladder cancer in men. *N Engl J Med* 1999; 340:1390–1397.

17. Geoffroy-Perez B, Cordier S. Fluid consumption and the risk of bladder cancer: results of a multicenter case-control study. *Int J Cancer* 2001;93:880–887.

18. Ward E, Halperin W, Thun M, et al. Screening workers exposed to 4,4′-methylenebis(2-chloroaniline) for bladder cancer by cystoscopy. *J Occup Med* 1990;32:865–868.

19. Hemstreet GP, Yin SN, Ma ZZ, et al. Biomarker risk assessment and bladder cancer detection in a cohort exposed to benzidine. *J Natl Cancer Inst* 2001;93:427–436.

20. Gail MH. Applicability of sample size calculations based on a comparison of proportions for use with the logrank test. *Control Clin Trials* 1985;6:112–119.

21. Self SG. An adaptive weighted log-rank test with application to cancer prevention and screening trials. *Biometrics* 1991; 47:975–986.

22. Allard P, Bernard P, Fradet Y, Tetu B. The early clinical course of primary Ta and T1 bladder cancer: a proposed prognostic index. *Br J Urol* 1998;81:692–698.

23. Morgan JD, Bowsher W, Griffiths DF, Matthews PN. Rationalisation of follow-up in patients with non-invasive bladder tumours. A preliminary report. *Br J Urol* 1991;67: 158–161.

24. Sidransky D, Frost P, Von Eschenbach A, et al. Clonal origin bladder cancer. *N Engl J Med* 1992;326:737–740.

25. Simon R, Eltze E, Schafer KL, et al. Cytogenetic analysis of multifocal bladder cancer supports a monoclonal origin and intraepithelial spread of tumor cells. *Cancer Res* 2001;61: 355–362.

26. Heney NM, Ahmed S, Flanagan MJ, et al. Superficial bladder cancer: progression and recurrence. *J Urol* 1983;130: 1083–1086.

27. Grossman HB, Liebert M, Antelo M, et al. p53 and RB expression predict progression in T1 bladder cancer. *Clin Cancer Res* 1998;4:829–834.

28. Lamm DL, Blumenstein BA, Crawford ED, et al. A randomized trial of intravesical doxorubicin and immunotherapy with bacille Calmette-Guerin for transitional-cell carcinoma of the bladder. *N Engl J Med* 1991;325:1205–1209.

29. Lamm DL, Blumenstein BA, Crawford ED, et al. Randomized intergroup comparison of bacillus Calmette-Guerin immunotherapy and mitomycin C chemotherapy prophylaxis in superficial transitional cell carcinoma of the bladder. A Southwest Oncology Group study. *Urol Oncol* 1995;1: 119–126.

30. Lamm DL, Blumenstein BA, Crissman JD, et al. Maintenance bacillus Calmette-Guerin immunotherapy for recurrent Ta, T1 and carcinoma in situ transitional cell carcinoma of the bladder: a randomized Southwest Oncology Group study. *J Urol* 2000;163:1124–1129.

31. Herr HW, Schwalb DM, Zhang ZF, et al. Intravesical bacillus Calmette-Guerin therapy prevents tumor progression and death from superficial bladder cancer: ten-year follow-up of a prospective randomized trial. *J Clin Oncol* 1995;13: 1404–1408.

32. Shelley MD, Kynaston H, Court J, et al. A systematic review of intravesical bacillus Calmette-Guerin plus transurethral resection vs transurethral resection alone in Ta and T1 bladder cancer. *BJU Int* 2001;88:209–216.

33. Bubendorf L, Grilli B, Sauter G, et al. Multiprobe FISH for enhanced detection of bladder cancer in voided urine specimens and bladder washings. *Am J Clin Pathol* 2001;116: 79–86.

34. Schneider A, Borgnat S, Lang H, et al. Evaluation of microsatellite analysis in urine sediment for diagnosis of bladder cancer. *Cancer Res* 2000;60:4617–4622.

35. Lamm DL, Riggs DR, Shriver JS, et al. Megadose vitamins in bladder cancer: a double-blind clinical trial. *J Urol* 1994; 151:21–26.

36. Studer UE, Jenzer S, Biedermann C, et al. Adjuvant treatment with a vitamin A analogue (etretinate) after transurethral resection of superficial bladder tumors. Final analysis of a prospective, randomized multicenter trial in Switzerland. *Eur Urol* 1995;28:284–290.

37. Decensi A, Bruno S, Costantini M, et al. Phase IIa study of fenretinide in superficial bladder cancer, using DNA flow cytometry as an intermediate end point. *J Natl Cancer Inst* 1994;86:138–140.

38. Decensi A, Torrisi R, Bruno S, et al. Randomized trial of fenretinide in superficial bladder cancer using DNA flow cytometry as an intermediate end point. *Cancer Epidemiol Biomarkers Prev* 2000;9:1071–1078.

39. Pepe MS, Fleming TR. Weighted Kaplan-Meier statistics: a class of distance tests for censored survival data. *Biometrics* 1989;45:497–507.

40. Shen Y, Fleming TR. Weighted mean survival test statistics: a class of distance tests for censored survival data. *J R Stat Soc* [Ser B] 1997;59:269–280.

41. Wei LJ, Lin DY, Weissfeld L. Regression analysis of multivariate incomplete failure time data by modeling marginal distributions. *J Am Stat Assoc* 1989;84:1065–1073.

42. Hughes MD. Power considerations for clinical trials using multivariate time-to-event data. *Stat Med* 1997;16: 865–882.

43. Therneau TM, Hamilton SA. rhDNase as an example of recurrent event analysis. *Stat Med* 1997;16:2029–2047.

ESOPHAGUS

25 Barrett's Esophagus

Strategies for Cancer Prevention

Brian J. Reid, MD, PhD

CONTENTS

1. INTRODUCTION

Barrett's esophagus (BE) is a condition in which the normal stratified squamous epithelium of the esophagus is replaced by a metaplastic columnar mucosa as a complication of chronic gastroesophageal reflux disease (GERD) (1,2). BE is the only known precursor to esophageal adenocarcinoma, which has greater than 90% mortality unless detected early (2–4).

During the past 50 yr, numerous observations have linked GERD to BE and esophageal adenocarcinoma. This evidence has been the basis for the postulated model of histological progression in BE (Fig. 1).

Under this construct, GERD is the inciting injury that leads to erosive esophagitis, BE, dysplasia, and esophageal adenocarcinoma. Only a subset of patients progress from each stage to the next, and factors modulating such progression are not well characterized. Several steps appear to be reversible, either spontaneously or as a result of events that are as yet incompletely understood. As will be discussed below, the vast majority of patients with GERD or BE do not progress to cancer during their lifetimes. A better understanding of environmental risk and protective factors as well as

the stages at which they act might be used to develop cost-efficient cancer prevention trials using surrogate endpoints. Improved knowledge of the molecular mechanisms of progression might also yield new targets for chemoprevention that could become the basis for tailored management of the cancer risk.

Cancer appears to arise in BE as a result of genomic instability and evolution of neoplastic cell lineages with accumulated somatic genetic lesions. Some neoplastic clones expand within the Barrett's segment and evolve progeny clones with additional genomic abnormalities, culminating in cancer, whereas other clones are either delayed in progression or represent evolutionary dead ends (5). Somatic genetic abnormalities predisposing to cancer in BE include lesions in the p16 and p53 tumor suppressor genes as well as DNA content abnormalities (aneuploidy, increased 4N fractions), among others (6–21). Another strategy for cancer prevention would be to develop interventions that modulate clonal evolution, favoring proliferation of more benign clones.

In this chapter we review a body of evidence suggesting strategies for preventing esophageal adenocarcinoma, with special attention to the concept that clinical management of BE may eventually be tailored to the

From: Cancer Chemoprevention, Volume 2: Strategies for Cancer Chemoprevention
Edited by: G. J. Kelloff, E. T. Hawk, and C. C. Sigman © Humana Press Inc., Totowa, NJ

Esophageal squamous epithelium

—

GERD

—

Squamous esophagitis

—

Barrett's esophagus

—

High-grade dysplasia

—

Esophageal adenocarcinoma

Fig. 1. Postulated model of histologic progression of GERD and Barrett's esophagus to esophageal adenocarcinoma.

risk status of individual patients. First, we examine the sudden and still largely unexplained emergence of GERD, BE, and esophageal adenocarcinoma in the latter half of the 20th century. We also review known or suspected risk and protective factors for esophageal adenocarcinoma. We discuss current clinical management of BE. We review advances in understanding the molecular genesis of BE and esophageal adenocarcinoma, including biomarkers that have recently been evaluated as predictors of progression to cancer. We then examine challenges and opportunities for cancer prevention in BE. Finally, we discuss multidisciplinary and interinstitutional collaborations that might be employed to more efficiently achieve the goal of tailored management of cancer risk in these patients.

2. DISEASES OF THE 20TH CENTURY

GERD, BE, and esophageal adenocarcinomas are diseases of the 20th century. Winklestein first described the clinical entity of GERD in 1935 *(22)*. In 1950, Barrett described the first four cases of the syndrome that was to bear his name *(23)*. Naef et al. provided the first large series linking GERD to BE and esophageal adenocarcinoma in 1975 *(24)*. By 1991, the incidence of esophageal adenocarcinoma was increasing more rapidly than that of any other cancer in the United

States (US) *(25)*. A review of cancer registries in 2001 found similar rapid increases in esophageal adenocarcinoma in many regions of the Western world *(26)*.

2.1. GERD

The high prevalence of heartburn in the US has been confirmed by scientific studies and public opinion polls. A 1988 Gallup poll reported that 44% of Americans have regular heartburn at least once a month *(27)*. Weekly heartburn has been reported in as many as 19% of the adult population *(28)*.

2.2. BE

"This paper concerns a condition whose existence is denied by some, misunderstood by others, and ignored by the majority of surgeons. It has been called a variety of names which have confused the story because they have suggested incorrect etiologic explanations...."
—N. R. Barrett, 1957 *(29)*

2.2.1. DEFINITIONS OF BE

Any evaluation of the natural history of GERD over the 65 and 50 yr, respectively, since reflux esophagitis and BE were initially described faces a challenge because the definition of BE has changed several times. BE was initially defined as an arbitrary length (usually 2–3 cm) of columnar lining in the esophagus without histologic specification of the nature of the columnar epithelium *(30,31)*. In the 1980s, it was proposed to limit the diagnosis of BE to patients in whom biopsies of the columnar lining showed intestinal metaplasia *(32)*. In the 1990s, several studies showed a high prevalence of intestinal metaplasia at the gastroesophageal junction, and the definition of BE was revised to include only those patients in whom biopsies of the esophagus showed intestinal metaplasia *(33)*. In this revision, BE was divided into short-segment (<3 cm) and long-segment (≥3 cm) cases.

2.2.2. PREVALENCE OF BE

By 1990, at least 15 studies, largely using the older definition of BE, had reported that the prevalence of BE in patients undergoing upper endoscopy for symptoms of GERD ranged from 2.5% to 23.8% *(24,34–45)*. Recently, Hirota et al. reported that the prevalence of long- and short-segment BE was 1.6% and 6%, respectively, of all patients undergoing diagnostic upper endoscopy *(46)*. Referral for endoscopy is a confounding factor for all of these estimates. However, Robinson et al. studied a population who were frequent users of over-the-counter antacids and reported that 6% had BE *(47)*. Two patients had dysplastic BE and esophageal adenocarcinoma, respectively.

Two relatively recent studies, both reported in abstract form only, have attempted to estimate the prevalence of BE in persons undergoing colorectal cancer screening *(48,49)*. In one study, patients undergoing flexible sigmoidoscopic screening were offered upper endoscopy *(48)*. Participants could not have reflux symptoms more than once monthly, take antisecretory medications, or have had a prior upper endoscopy. BE, defined as intestinal metaplasia from an endoscopically visible columnar segment in the esophagus, was found in 28 (25%) of the 109 participants, eight with long-segment BE (7%) and 20 with short-segment BE (18%). In the second study, patients undergoing screening colonoscopy were offered upper endoscopy *(49)*. Forty-nine of 500 patients (9.8%) had BE, including seven with long-segment BE (1.4%) and 42 with short-segment BE (8.4%). Reasons for the striking differences in prevalence of BE in these two studies are not readily apparent from the abstracts.

In 1992, Cameron and Lomboy examined the prevalence of BE, defined by columnar lining ≥3 cm in the esophagus, in 51,311 patients undergoing endoscopy at the Mayo Clinic between 1976 and 1989 *(50)*. Three hundred seventy-seven patients met the criteria for BE. The prevalence of BE increased with age in both sexes

to reach a plateau by the seventh decade. Estimated median age of BE onset was 40 yr *(50)*. Comparison of clinical and autopsy series suggests that a large reservoir of persons in the general population with clinically undetected BE live out their lives, dying of unrelated causes *(51)*.

In summary, the prevalence of BE appears to be approx 5–10% in patients with GERD and those undergoing diagnostic upper endoscopy. The median age of onset has been estimated at 40 yr and the prevalence increases with age, reaching a plateau by the seventh decade. There appears to be a large reservoir of undetected patients in the population, some of whom may be asymptomatic.

2.2.3. INCIDENCE OF BE

Data on the natural history of untreated patients with symptomatic GERD are sparse. Naef's classic series in 1975 and a few well-documented case reports in the 1960s and 1970s described patients with striking upward migrations of columnar lining within the esophagus over periods of 18 mo to 7 yr *(24,52–55)*. However, this phenomenon does not appear to have been well-documented in the peer-reviewed literature since 1975. In Cameron and Lomboy's study, the mean length of the Barrett's segment was similar in all age groups, and it did not change in follow-up even in the presence of esophagitis *(50)*.

Three studies have attempted to determine BE incidence in the population over successive time intervals. Increased use of endoscopy over the same time period has been a confounding factor for each of the studies, which reached different conclusions. Conio et al. evaluated the incidence of BE, defined as ≥3 cm of columnar lining in the esophagus, from 1965 to 1998 in Olmsted County, Minnesota *(56)*. The incidence of clinically diagnosed BE increased 28-fold from 0.37/100,000 person-years in 1965–1969 to 10.5/100,000 in 1995–1997. This paralleled the 22-fold increase in endoscopy during the same period; the authors concluded that the evidence suggested a detection phenomenon rather than a true increase in BE incidence. Caygill et al. used the United Kingdom (UK) BE Registry to investigate the prevalence of histologically proven BE during a 20-yr period (January 1977–December 1996) in a single center *(57)*. BE frequency increased steadily from 0.2% to 1.6% of all endoscopies per 5-yr band; the authors concluded that either incidence or recognition of BE was increasing. Prach et al. evaluated BE incidence in 53,433 upper GI endoscopies performed in a population of 384,000 in Tayside, Scotland from 1980 to 1993

(58). They reported a substantial increase in BE incidence, rising from 1/100,000 per year (1.4 per 1000 endoscopies) in 1980–1981 to 48/100,000 per year (42.7 per 1000 endoscopies) in 1992–1993. The authors concluded that the incidence of BE in Tayside did increase during this period, although education concerning endoscopic recognition of BE, enthusiasm over local interest in BE, changing referral patterns, and absence of consistent histologic confirmation might be confounding factors.

2.3. Esophageal Adenocarcinoma

2.3.1. INCIDENCE OF ESOPHAGEAL ADENOCARCINOMA IN THE POPULATION

Prior to the 1980s, esophageal adenocarcinoma was considered a rare illness, constituting fewer than 8% of all esophageal cancers; esophageal adenocarcinomas now comprise more than three of every five new esophageal cancers *(59–61)*. However, beginning in 1988, a series of studies reported an alarming increase in esophageal adenocarcinoma incidence in the US and other regions of the Western world *(26,62–72)*. By 1998, esophageal adenocarcinoma incidence among white males in the US had increased more than 350% since the mid-1970s *(61)*. The increase among white women was 300%, but the absolute magnitude of risk was lower than in white males. Incidence rates increased in black males, rising from 0.4 to 0.6, but based on only 7 and 16 cases, respectively.

2.3.2. INCIDENCE OF ESOPHAGEAL ADENOCARCINOMA IN PATIENTS WITH BE

Although BE is the only known precursor to esophageal adenocarcinoma, most persons with BE will not develop cancer during their lifetimes *(51,56,73)*. The annual incidence of esophageal adenocarcinoma in persons with BE ranged from 0.2% to 2.9% in 24 different studies *(74)*. A recent study reported possible publication bias in estimating esophageal adenocarcinoma incidence in BE patients because of selective reporting of series that have positive or extreme results *(75)*. Although the results of this study did not permit accurate determination of the true incidence, the authors suggested that an annual incidence of 0.5% might be reasonable. Four studies in the US have produced estimates on this order *(56,76–78)*. The possible contribution of regional variation has not been well studied, but one report suggests that the annual incidence of cancer in BE may be higher in the UK than in the US (1% vs 0.5%, respectively) *(79)*.

3. ETIOLOGY

3.1. Risk Factors

3.1.1. SYMPTOMATIC GERD

A strong relationship between gastroesophageal reflux and risk of esophageal adenocarcinoma has long been noted clinically, but has only recently been quantified in the general population. In a Swedish population-based study, frequency, duration, and severity of heartburn were all risk factors for developing esophageal adenocarcinoma *(80)*. Compared with persons with no weekly heartburn episodes, those with more than three episodes of heartburn had an odds ratio (OR) of 16.7 for developing esophageal adenocarcinoma (95% CI = 8.7, 28.3). Similarly, patients who had more than 20 yr of heartburn had a 16.4 OR for developing esophageal adenocarcinoma (95% CI = 8.3, 28.4) compared with those with no heartburn, and those who had the most severe heartburn had an OR of 20 (95% CI = 11.6, 34.6). Among persons with long-standing and severe reflux symptoms, the OR for developing esophageal adenocarcinoma was 43.5 (95% CI = 18.3, 103.5). Interestingly, however, 40% of persons with esophageal adenocarcinoma reported no history of reflux symptoms.

Similar trends were seen in the US Esophageal and Gastric Adenocarcinoma (EGA) study *(81)*. Both frequency and duration of heartburn were risk factors for esophageal adenocarcinoma, although the ORs were more modest than in the Swedish study. Persons who had reflux symptoms 105–364 d per year and 365+ d per year had ORs of 3.4 (95% CI = 1.9, 6.1) and 5.5 (95% CI = 3.2, 9.3), respectively. Similarly, patients with 20 or more years of heartburn had an OR of 2.7 (95% CI = 1.4, 5.0) for esophageal adenocarcinoma.

3.1.2. DUODENOGASTROESOPHAGEAL REFLUX (DGER)

A growing body of evidence implicates DGER in the pathogenesis and progression of BE *(82–84)*. Recent studies using 24-h spectrophotometric ("Bilitec") measurement of bilirubin (a surrogate for bile acids), hepatobiliary scanning techniques, and bile acid measurement indicate that persons whose refluxate contains bile may be at increased risk of BE and esophageal adenocarcinoma *(85–93)*. In the largest study, mean esophageal bile exposure increased progressively from GERD without mucosal injury ($N = 19$ patients) to erosive esophagitis ($N = 45$) to BE ($N = 33$), with the highest levels found in early esophageal adenocarcinoma ($N = 14$) ($p < 0.01$) *(93)*. At least three studies have

Table 1
NSAIDs and Risk of Esophageal Cancer

Study	NSAID	Type of cancer	Relative risk	(95% CI)
Langman[a]	All	SCC, Adeno	0.6	(0.4–1.0)
ACS Cohort[b]	Aspirin	SCC, Adeno	0.6	(0.3–1.0
NHANES 1 Cohort[c]	Aspirin	SCC, Adeno	0.1	(0.0–0.8)
EGA[c]	Aspirin	Adeno	0.4	(0.2–0.6)
EGA[d]	Other	Adeno	0.6	(0.3–1.0)

[a]Langman et al. *(105)*.

[b]Thun et al. *(106)*.

[c]Funkhouser et al. *(104)*.

[d]Farrow et al. *(103)*.

shown that treatment with proton pump inhibitors decreases DGER as well as acid reflux, probably by a volume effect *(87,94,95)*.

3.1.3. BODY MASS INDEX

Besides reflux, the strongest and most consistently identified risk factor for esophageal adenocarcinoma is increased body mass index (BMI). Both Swedish and US EGA studies found a strong dose-dependent relationship between increasing BMI and risk of esophageal adenocarcinoma *(96,97)*. In the US study, an OR of 2.9 (95% CI = 1.8–4.7) was observed comparing extreme quartiles of BMI (97). The association was even stronger in the Swedish study with an OR of 7.6 (95% CI = 3.8, 15.2) among persons with the highest BMI quartile compared to those in the lowest *(96)*. Others have noted similar results *(98,99)*.

3.1.4. TOBACCO

The potential role of cigarette smoking has been studied because it is a strong risk factor for esophageal squamous cell carcinoma. Studies in the US have consistently demonstrated a modest, approximately twofold increase in risk among current smokers *(98,100,101)*. Interestingly, it appears that the carcinogenic effect of smoking persists for 20–30 yr after cessation. In Sweden, the association between tobacco use and esophageal adenocarcinoma was weaker *(102)*.

3.2. Protective Factors

3.2.1. NONSTEROIDAL ANTIINFLAMMATORY DRUGS

Several epidemiology studies suggest that nonsteroidal antiinflammarory drugs (NSAIDS) may reduce the risk of esophageal cancer, including adenocarcinoma and squamous cell carcinoma (SCC) (Table 1) *(103–106)*.

3.2.2. DIET HIGH IN FRUITS AND VEGETABLES

Several studies suggest that a diet high in fat and low in fruits and vegetables increases the risk of esophageal adenocarcinoma *(107–111)*. In the US EGA study, higher intake of nutrients found primarily in plant-based foods was associated with decreased risk *(112)*. The association with esophageal adenocarcinoma was particularly strong for fiber, for which a 72% reduction in risk was observed comparing the 75th to the 25th percentile of intake. In contrast, a diet high in fat was found to be a risk factor for esophageal adenocarcinoma (OR 2.18; 95% CI = 1.27, 3.76) *(112)*.

3.3. Summary

Epidemiological data suggest that NSAIDs and a diet high in fruits and vegetables may be protective against esophageal adenocarcinoma, whereas GERD, increased BMI, a diet high in fat, and tobacco use are risk factors. All are potential targets for intervention to prevent esophageal adenocarcinoma, but there is a critical lack of data concerning the stages of neoplastic progression at which the different exposures act. As discussed below, such critical information could be obtained by interinstitutional, multidisciplinary collaborative cohort studies between gastroenterologists and epidemiologists to determine the stages of progression at which risk and protective factors appear to act in patients undergoing endoscopic biopsy surveillance.

4. CLINICAL MANAGEMENT

4.1. Endoscopic Surveillance

If BE is detected at endoscopy, lifetime endoscopic surveillance is recommended for early detection of cancer *(113)*. Because the median age of BE onset has been estimated at 40 yr *(50)*, lifetime surveillance can represent a substantial commitment of medical resources. Though several studies have shown that surveillance can detect esophageal adenocarcinomas at an early stage when the patients can be cured by esophagectomy *(114–116)*, the lifespan of most BE patients cannot be increased by endoscopic surveillance because they will die of other causes *(51,56,73)*. Further, several recent studies have challenged the efficacy of endoscopic surveillance for patients with BE *(73,117)*. Regardless, clinical practice surveys have shown that approximately 90% of BE patients are followed with endoscopy annually or biennially *(118)*, even though the results of decision analyses indicate that 5-yr surveillance would be more cost-effective *(119)*.

Clinical practice guidelines recommend endoscopic surveillance of BE based on a five-tiered classification of dysplasia—negative, indefinite, low-grade dysplasia (LGD), high-grade dysplasia (HGD), and cancer *(113)*. However, this five-tiered histologic classification appears to be poorly reproducible, especially for diagnoses less than HGD *(120–126)*. For example, we found only 48% interobserver agreement for the five-tiered classification system in a blinded study *(120)*. This increased to 86% when negative, indefinite, and LGD were combined and was greatest for the diagnosis of intramucosal cancer (95%). A study conducted more than a decade later reached similar conclusions *(126)*.

HGD is the only dysplasia grade shown by prospective studies to be a risk factor for progression to cancer, but the magnitude of risk varies substantially in different series. In our study, 5-yr cumulative incidences of cancer were 59% (95% CI = 44, 74) and 31% (95% CI = 14, 60) for patients with HGD detected at baseline endoscopy or during follow-up, respectively *(127)*. However, Schnell et al. reported that the 5-yr cumulative incidence of cancer was only 9% in a study of 79 patients with HGD seen over a 20-yr period *(128)*. Buttar et al. reported 3-yr cumulative cancer incidences of 56% and 14% for patients with diffuse and focal (affecting five or fewer crypts) HGD, respectively *(129)*. Weston et al. reported that 27% of 15 patients with unifocal HGD progressed to cancer and 47% regressed to less than HGD *(130)*. In general, rates of progression appear higher in centers with large referral populations *(127,129)* than in those where HGD is detected by screening a large primary population of BE patients *(128)*. Thus, although HGD appears to be a risk factor for esophageal adenocarcinoma, the magnitude of risk varies in different studies. The reasons for different magnitudes of risk are not completely clear. The

apparently higher rate of progression in centers with large referral populations suggests the possibility of referral bias in some studies *(128,129,131)*. Methodological variations may also play a role; for example, Schnell et al. excluded cancers arising in the first year as coexisting, whereas other studies included all cancers that were detected after the baseline endoscopy. Further, the studies used different pathologists, and somewhat different results are to be expected, given limitations in reproducibility of dysplasia diagnoses. Nevertheless, it appears clear that 40% to 90% of patients do not progress to cancer during follow-up, and some appear to regress.

The risk of patients whose biopsies do not have HGD progressing to cancer appears to be low, but not zero *(127,128,132)*. In one large study of more than 700 patients who had LGD diagnosed at any time during surveillance, only about 3% developed cancer *(128)*. In our study in Seattle, the 5-yr cumulative incidence of cancer in BE patients whose biopsies were negative, indefinite, or LGD was 3.8% (95% CI=1.6, 9), with no significant differences among the dysplasia grades *(120)*. Regression of LGD appears to occur more than 10 times as frequently as progression to frank cancer *(132)*. Nevertheless, 70% of gastroenterologists perform endoscopy every 3–6 mo for patients with LGD *(118)*. Transient diagnoses of dysplasia are a significant factor in increasing the cost of medical care because they trigger more frequent endoscopies *(133,134)*. In one study that modeled the care of 95 patients over a decade, 61% of all surveillance endoscopies were a result of transient dysplasia diagnoses *(133)*. The discounted incremental cost of more frequent surveillance for transient dysplasia diagnoses in this cohort of 95 patients over 10 yr was more than a half million dollars *(133)*. This estimate did not consider other costs, including increased absence from work and heightened patient anxiety.

4.2. Therapies for BE

Medical therapy for BE is directed toward reducing gastroesophageal reflux, usually by proton pump inhibitors, but existing medical therapies have not been shown to prevent progression to cancer, although they may decrease proliferation in the BE segment *(135)*. Recently, there has been enthusiasm for endoscopic therapies, including photodynamic therapy, argon plasma coagulation, multipolar electrocoagulation, and endoscopic mucosal resection *(136–142)*. Although some cases of apparently complete regression have been reported, it is common for residual BE metaplasia to be concealed beneath neosquamous epithelium, where it is difficult to detect by endoscopic biopsies *(136,137,143,144)*. Unfortunately, such concealed BE metaplasia has been reported to progress to HGD and cancer in some cases *(137,141,143,144)*. Though relatively little is known concerning the biology of either the residual BE or neosquamous epithelia, biomarker studies have suggested that there may be some abnormalities. Redevelopment of HGD after ablation has been reported to be associated with residual *p16*, p53, and ploidy abnormalities in BE epithelium *(145)*. Endoscopic therapies have been associated with a range of adverse events, including strictures, photosensitivity, GI bleeding, perforations, and rare deaths *(136,137,141,146)*. Esophagectomy is the only therapy proven to completely eliminate metaplastic epithelium, and several studies have shown that endoscopic surveillance combined with esophageal resection for either HGD or esophageal adenocarcinoma results in 5-yr disease-free survival rates that are markedly improved relative to patients whose cancers arise outside of surveillance *(114–116)*. However, esophagectomy has substantial morbidity and mortality, and mortality varies with the surgical volume of the institution. High-volume hospitals have surgical mortalities of 3%–5%, whereas low-volume institutions are in the 16%–20% range *(147–149)*. Unfortunately, more than 80% of esophagectomies appear to be performed in low-volume institutions *(149)*.

4.3. SUMMARY

Endoscopic biopsy surveillance is the mainstay of management for BE. However, our understanding of neoplastic progression in BE has been limited by excessive reliance on dysplasia, leading to paradoxes not easily resolved. Intraobserver agreement is typically greater than interobserver agreement in observer variation studies *(120,126)*. Further, it has been reported that the only way to achieve near-perfect agreement is to eliminate interobserver variation, leaving only the smaller effects of intraobserver variation while using a cut-off between low- and high-grade dysplasia *(126)*. Studies such as these appear to lead to paradoxical conclusions that are not easily resolved in practice. Thus, an individual study appears to be better off using a single experienced BE pathologist to increase diagnostic consistency by eliminating interobserver variation. This approach may be especially useful for studies managing large numbers of high-risk patients. Both BE teams (Seattle and Hines, VA) with more than a decade of experience in nonsurgical management of high-grade

dysplasia have used a single BE pathologist, who becomes part of the study team and participates in team conferences, because this approach increases diagnostic consistency and patient safety *(128,150)*. However, such results are not easily generalized to other institutions because of interobserver variation in pathologic interpretations.

Objective, reproducible biomarkers appear to be needed as adjuncts to histologic diagnosis to resolve this paradox. Validation and implementation of such prognostic biomarkers for clinical medicine would be greatly facilitated by interinstitutional, multidisciplinary collaborations between clinicians supervising large-scale endoscopic surveillance studies and molecular geneticists with the high-throughput capacity to characterize biomarkers in thousands of biopsies from hundreds of patients followed longitudinally.

5. MOLECULAR GENESIS

5.1. Genomic Instability and Clonal Evolution in BE

The conceptual framework for understanding the somatic genetic basis of human neoplastic progression was provided by Nowell, who hypothesized that cancer develops as a result of an acquired genetic instability that predisposes to the evolution of clones with accumulated genetic errors *(151)*. Some clones gain selective advantages and eventually a subclone evolves that becomes an early cancer.

There is now a substantial body of evidence that most human cancers, including esophageal adenocarcinoma, arise by a process of clonal evolution similar to that postulated by Nowell *(151)*. This process of genetic instability, clonal expansion, and clonal evolution leads to genome-wide abnormalities that accumulate with the evolution of new clones *(5)*.

A clone with lesions in both *p16* and p53 is usually the progenitor from which progeny clones with additional genetic abnormalities evolve. Some clones have selective advantages, whereas others are either delayed in progression or represent evolutionary dead ends. Incomplete ablation may result in residual BE containing any one or combination of these clones, which may be concealed beneath neosquamous epithelium. Better understanding of the differences in molecular phenotypes between clones that progress to cancer and those that remain stable or regress might identify molecular targets that could become the basis for tailored interventions to prevent progression to cancer. Microarray studies, including those in breast cancer and diffuse, large B-cell lymphoma, have identified gene expression profiles that predict subsequent progression, and such studies could also be performed in BE *(152,153)*.

It is likely that this genome-wide process of instability and clonal evolution is responsible for the more than 60 biomarkers that have been proposed for BE *(154,155)*. However, it is essential to distinguish random or background abnormalities that develop as a consequence of instability from those that are involved in the pathogenesis or progression of BE. As an example, tumor-suppressor genes are typically inactivated by a two-hit mechanism that involves mutation or methylation of one allele and loss of heterozygosity (LOH) of the other *(156)*. However, LOH can occur throughout the genome; in some cases it appears to be selected, whereas in others it appears to represent background or random LOH arising as a result of generalized instability *(156)*. Three studies of genome-wide LOH ("allelotypes") in esophageal adenocarcinoma *(157–159)* found that LOH involving chromosomes 9p, 17p, and 18q appeared to be selected, and two of the three also reported high-frequency loss involving 5q and 13q. Therefore, these chromosome arms are presumed to harbor loci involved in the pathogenesis or progression of BE. Other LOH events may be background in the sense that they occur randomly or were detected in a single study.

5.2. Proliferation

The intestinal metaplasia of BE has been shown to be hyperproliferative by a number of assays, including tritiated thymidine incorporation, PCNA immunostaining, DNA content flow cytometry (S phase), Ki67 immuno staining (G_1, S phase, G_2, mitosis), and Ki67/DNA content multiparameter flow cytometry (G_0, G_1, S phase, G_2, mitosis) *(160–164)*. One study reported that normalization of intraesophageal pH with proton pump inhibitor therapy decreased the proportion of BE epithelial cells in S phase *(135)*. This observation raises the possibility that proton pump inhibitor therapy may be a useful adjunct in chemoprevention, but its significance is not yet clear because S phase does not appear to be an independent predictor of progression to esophageal adenocarcinoma *(165)*.

5.3. p16 (*p16/CDKN2a/INK4a*)

This tumor suppressor negatively regulates progression from G_1 to S phase in the cell cycle by binding and inhibiting cyclin-dependent kinases 4 and 6 *(166)*. *p16* also appears to be involved in cellular senescence

(167–170). Its levels are increased in senescent cells and are low or undetectable in immortalized cells, and loss of *p16* function permits cells to escape early stages of senescence in vitro.

p16 is one of the most commonly inactivated tumor suppressor genes in human cancers; in esophageal adenocarcinomas, *p16* lesions are second in frequency only to those involving p53 *(157–159)*. *p16* lesions in BE include 9p21 LOH, *p16* mutation, and *p16* promoter (CpG island) methylation *(5,7,9,10,171,172)*. Although at least three candidate tumor suppressor genes on 9p21 (*p16, p15,* and *p14^ARF*) could be targeted by 9p21 LOH, promoter methylation and mutation occur frequently at *p16* and rarely at *p15* or *p14^ARF*, indicating that *p16* is the likely 9p21 target for inactivation *(171–174)*.

We investigated 107 patients with BE for 9p (*p16*) LOH, *p16* mutations, and *p16* methylation *(174)*. More than 85% of all BE segments at all histologic grades of dysplasia had *p16* lesions, making them the earliest known genetic/epigenetic lesions in BE. We found evidence for successive waves of clonal expansion in which *p16*+/− progenitor clones underwent expansion and evolved *p16*−/− progeny clones that also underwent expansion, typically throughout the BE segment. The *p16* genotype was also highly correlated with median BE segment length, increasing from 1.5 to 6.0 to 8.0 cm in *p16*+/+, *p16*+/−, and *p16*−/− clones, respectively, also suggesting that *p16* lesions confer a selective advantage. The expansion phenotype was observed in all clones with *p16* alterations, regardless of whether they were due to mutation, methylation, or LOH. These data suggest that *p16* lesions may be critical intermediates that allow "selective sweeps" to spread rapidly throughout the BE segment, possibly to reestablish mucosa denuded by chronic GERD.

5.4. Cyclin D1 Overexpression

Cyclin D1 promotes the transition from G_1 to S phase *(175,176)*. Cyclin D1 overexpression can be detected immunohistochemically in a subset of patients with BE and esophageal adenocarcinoma *(177,178)*. One recent small case-control study reported that patients with cyclin D overexpression were at increased risk for developing esophageal adenocarcinoma during follow-up (OR 6.85 [95% CI = 1.57–29.91], $p = 0.01$) *(179)*. Cyclin D1 overexpression may be a surrogate marker for *p16* null (*p16*−/−) clones because *p16* and cyclin D1 compete with each other for binding to a complex that promotes cell division *(176,180)*. When *p16* is present in the complex, it appears that cyclin D1 can be displaced and degraded leading to cell cycle arrest, but in the absence of *p16*, cyclin D1 is stabilized in the complex, where it promotes cell division.

5.5. p53

Like *p16*, p53 also causes G_1 arrest. In response to DNA breaks, p53 causes cells to arrest in the G_1 interval of the cell cycle, leading to terminal cell cycle arrest or apoptosis, both of which prevent transmission of genetic damage to daughter cells *(181)*. Loss of p53 function predisposes to genomic instability and the evolution of additional somatic genetic abnormalities *(5,181)*. Tobacco-related field carcinogenesis in the upper aerodigestive tract has been shown to be associated with development of p53 mutant clones in histologically normal epithelium *(182)*. In addition, endogenous telomere shortening, which can be accelerated by hyperproliferation and/or oxidative damage *(183,184)*, can lead to chromosome breaks that activate the p53-dependent cell cycle checkpoint, providing strong selective pressure in favor of abrogation of p53 function as well as a mechanism for generating the DNA breaks that lead to 17p LOH *(185–189)*. These observations suggest possible interventions to prevent cancer in BE by preventing the development of p53 lesions.

p53 mutations and 17p LOH are the most common genetic lesions in esophageal adenocarcinomas, occurring in approx 90% of cases *(5,6,13,14,157–159)*. Both p53 alleles are typically inactivated (mutation and 17p LOH) in advanced histologic lesions (HGD or cancer) *(5,6,12–14,190,191)*. Unlike *p16* lesions, the prevalence of 17p (p53) LOH increases with advancing histologic grade, increasing from 6% in metaplasia negative or indefinite for dysplasia to 20% in LGD and 57% in HGD *(192)*. Further, we have also shown by prospective studies that 17p (p53) LOH is a strong and significant predictor of progression to esophageal adenocarcinoma in BE (RR = 16; 95% CI = 6.2–39; $p < 0.001$) *(192)*. It is also a predictor of progression to increased 4N fractions and aneuploidy. In addition, p53 lesions appear to predispose to the evolution of other somatic genetic abnormalities in the BE segment, including 5q LOH, 13q LOH and 18q LOH *(5,11,12,15,190,193)*. These results are consistent with p53's known checkpoint functions and suggest that exposure to DNA breaks may lead to selection of clones lacking p53 function, which are then permissive for the evolution of new somatic genetic lesions that culminate in cancer *(5,11,12,192)*.

Three small studies have reported that patients with p53 protein overexpression (used as a surrogate for p53 mutations) tend to have an increased risk of progressing to HGD or cancer *(132,179,194)*. However, only two of the three reached statistical significance, possibly because of the high false-negative and false-positive rates for p53 protein overexpression in detecting p53 mutations in esophageal neoplasia *(13,195,196)*. The high false-negative and false-positive rates for p53 mutations make p53 immunostaining undesirable as a biomarker in BE *(197)*.

5.6. Aneuploidy and/or Increased 4N

Several studies have suggested that DNA content flow cytometry may be a useful adjunct to histology in assessing risk in BE *(16–18,163,198)*. Flow-cytometric abnormalities have also been shown to predict progression to intermediate endpoints in small studies, further suggesting that flow cytometry may be an objective aid in identifying patients at increased risk *(199,200)*. One study of 30 dysplasia-free patients followed for up to 13 yr reported that no patient whose biopsies remained diploid progressed to dysplasia or cancer, whereas 6 of 13 patients (46%) with aneuploidy progressed to dysplasia or cancer *(200)*. Increased 4N was a predictor of progression to aneuploidy in another study of 90 patients followed for a mean of 51.4 mo. Eleven of 15 patients who had or developed increased 4N during prospective surveillance progressed to aneuploidy, compared with eight of 75 whose 4N fractions remained normal ($p < 0.0001$) *(11)*. Recently, we extended these results by showing that increased 4N and aneuploidy, especially ploidies >2.7N, are strong and significant predictors of progression to cancer in BE *(127,165)*. Among patients whose biopsies were negative, indefinite, or LGD, those with increased 4N fractions and/or aneuploidy >2.7N had a relative risk of developing cancer of 25 (95% CI = 6.5–98) compared with patients whose biopsies were diploid and had normal 4N fractions *(165)*. Flow-cytometric analysis appears to be especially useful in patients without HGD; those without aneuploidy or increased 4N fractions had a 5-yr cumulative incidence of cancer of 0 (95% CI = 0–4.7), whereas those with aneuploidy and/or increased 4N had a 28% 5-yr cumulative incidence of cancer (95% CI = 12–55) *(127)*.

5.7. APC

LOH involving chromosome 5q has been shown to be selected during neoplastic progression in BE by several teams of investigators *(5,157,158,193,201,202)*. Recently, methylation of the *APC* gene on chromosome 5q has been reported in BE and esophageal adenocarcinoma *(203,204)*.

APC methylated DNA can be detected in the sera of some patients with esophageal adenocarcinoma and appears to be associated with a poor prognosis *(203)*.

5.8. Summary

Increased 4N fractions, aneuploidy, 17p (p53) LOH, and cyclin D1 overexpression have been reported to be predictors of progression to cancer in BE. *p16* lesions (methylation, mutation, 9p[p16]LOH) are the earliest known genetic/epigenetic abnormalities in BE, occurring in at least 85% of all BE segments regardless of grade of dysplasia. *p16* lesions appear to predispose to clonal expansion throughout the BE segment as well as to longer segments. p53 lesions (mutation, 17p[p53]LOH) are typically detected after *p16* lesions and appear to predispose to the evolution of new clones with other abnormalities, including 5q LOH, 13q LOH, 18q LOH, increased 4N fractions, and aneuploidy. This process of clonal expansion and evolution can result in a mosaic of clones within the BE segment, some of which progress to cancer, whereas others are either delayed in progression or represent evolutionary dead ends. Clonal evolution not only drives neoplastic progression, but it can also breed resistance to therapeutic interventions to prevent or cure cancer. It is unlikely that effective cancer prevention strategies can be implemented without a better appreciation of mechanisms of clonal evolution. For example, as discussed above, ablation studies suggest that residual clones can progress to HGD or cancer even in the absence of detectable high grade at the time of ablation *(143,145)*. Unfortunately, there is a paucity of knowledge concerning the factors that influence clonal evolution and whether or not it can be modulated to favor selection of benign clones in mosaics containing multiple clones.

A better understanding of the interactions between risk and protective factors and clonal selection might be obtained by interinstitution, multidisciplinary collaborations among epidemiologists, clinicians, and molecular geneticists in large-scale studies of BE cohorts in endoscopic surveillance. Such collaborations could elucidate the effects of environmental risk and protective factors on clonal selection in large numbers of patients followed longitudinally.

6. STRATEGIES FOR CANCER PREVENTION IN BE

6.1. Overview

In many ways, BE is an ideal condition in which to conduct efficient observation and prevention studies using surrogate biomarkers as endpoints. During the past decade, much has been learned from epidemiology studies of risk and protective factors for esophageal adenocarcinoma. Many of these risk and protective factors offer innovative new interventions, including NSAIDs, which can be evaluated in cancer prevention trials. Similarly, new medical therapies, including proton pump inhibitors and cyclooxygenase-2 inhibitors, offer exciting chemoprevention opportunities in BE, and there is reason to anticipate more candidate chemopreventive agents from targeted therapies developed in the biotechnology industry, possibly identified by microarray studies of different stages of neoplastic progression. Advances in genomics and the biotechnology revolution have also led to startling new discoveries of the molecular genesis of BE and esophageal adenocarcinoma. Since 1998, at least four candidate biomarkers—aneuploidy, increased 4N fractions, 17p (p53) LOH, and cyclin D1 overexpression—have been reported as predictors of progression to cancer in persons with BE. Such biomarkers may well serve as inclusion/exclusion criteria and surrogate endpoints in targeted prevention trials, as well as for risk stratification for endoscopic surveillance.

6.2. Challenges

In the 1970s and 1980s, BE and esophageal adenocarcinoma, considered rare diseases, were studied by relatively few investigators. With recognition of the large susceptible population (GERD) and the rapid increase in esophageal adenocarcinoma incidence, there have been significant advances in our understanding of the etiology, clinical management, and molecular genesis of these conditions. Funding for research on GERD, BE, and esophageal adenocarcinoma is still limited, although there are attempts to improve the situation. Also of concern in developing tailored management of cancer risk in BE are barriers to multidisciplinary and interinstitutional collaborations that could make design and execution of prevention trials more efficient and effective.

For example, we have increased knowledge of risk and protective factors, but little understanding of the stages at which they act in neoplastic progression, an essential element in designing targeted prevention trials. In addition, although several biomarkers have been evaluated in large-scale prospective or smaller case-control studies, many more have been proposed but not evaluated. At least two impediments to wider implementation of objective, reproducible biomarkers

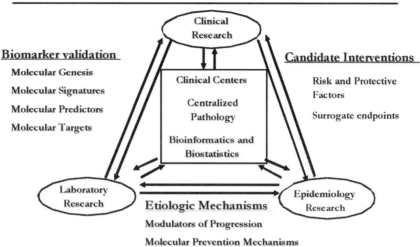

Fig. 2. Collaborative interinstitutional multidisciplinary centers of excellence in Barrett's esophagus. Interinstitutional, multidisciplinary collaborations between clinical, laboratory, epidemiology and cancer prevention researchers could facilitate development of tailored management of the cancer risk in Barrett's esophagus in several ways. Collaborations between clinical researchers taking care of large numbers of patients in endoscopic surveillance and molecular geneticists who have high-throughput capability to evaluate thousands of biopsies from hundreds of patients could validate molecular predictors of progression to cancer for tailored risk stratification. Similarly, collaborations between clinical researchers and biotechnology researchers using microarrays could improve our understanding of the molecular genesis of neoplastic progression by identifying molecular signatures of different stages of progression as well as potential targets for intervention to prevent cancer. Collaborations between epidemiologists and laboratory investigators could elucidate molecular mechanisms by which risk and protective factors modulate progression to cancer. Knowledge gained from these combined clinical, laboratory and epidemiologic investigations could then be used to develop cost-efficient prevention trials using surrogate endpoints with the goal of tailored interventions to prevent progression to cancer.

in BE exist. First, many biomarkers appear to have been developed by investigators at centers without cohorts of BE patients that can be investigated to determine the stage(s) at which biomarkers develop relative to other validated predictors of progression. Second, many centers do not have high-throughput capabilities to enable validation of biomarkers in large-scale studies involving hundreds of participants and thousands of biopsies. Finally, BE patients are typically cared for by gastroenterologists, but gastroenterologists have not been well represented in cancer control and prevention efforts previously. It seems likely that new platforms will be needed to engage gastroenterologists in front-line prevention research on BE and possibly other premalignant conditions of the gastrointestinal tract.

6.3. Opportunities

The vast majority of known BE patients have periodic endoscopic biopsy surveillance; many academic medical centers have specialized programs for these patients, headed by experts. To some extent, these programs are voluntarily self-aggregating into interinstitutional collaborative studies, although the degree to which this is possible is limited by lack of funding. Collaborative interinstitutional, multidisciplinary Centers of Excellence for BE with large numbers of endoscopic surveillance patients could be an enormous driving force for research on this condition (Fig. 2). Multidisciplinary collaborations between molecular geneticists with high-throughput capacity and clinical investigators who follow large numbers of patients by longitudinal endoscopic surveillance would permit new biomarkers to be rapidly evaluated for their utility in risk stratification and as surrogate endpoints, as well as developing new molecular targets for cancer prevention (Fig. 2; clinical-laboratory research collaborations). Other multidisciplinary collaborations between epidemiologists and molecular geneticists could facilitate elucidation of molecular mechanisms by which risk and protective factors act to modulate progression to cancer in vivo in human cohorts followed longitudinally (Fig. 2; epidemiology-laboratory research collaborations). This knowledge would be invaluable in designing efficient cancer prevention trials using surrogate endpoints (Fig. 2; clinical-epidemiology-laboratory collaborations). Finally, multidisciplinary, interinstitutional collaborations between cancer prevention researchers, clinical researchers, and laboratory researchers could greatly facilitate the conduct of cancer prevention trials themselves by bringing together large numbers of patients, candidate interventions, and surrogate endpoints for prevention trials. Centralized pathology, bioinformatics, and biostatistics could be essential elements of such a research platform (Fig. 2).

7. TAILORED MANAGEMENT FOR PATIENTS WITH BE

Conducting prevention studies in BE using cancer as an endpoint is difficult, as low cancer incidence would require large numbers of patients to be followed for prolonged periods of time. Trials with a cancer endpoint may be especially inefficient if the goal is tailored management of individual BE patients based on careful assessment of the risk of developing cancer relative to adverse effects of intervention. If tailored therapy is the goal, then smaller, efficient prevention studies using validated surrogate endpoints may be preferable initially. Such small, efficient, hypothesis-driven prevention trials using surrogate endpoints also provide a safeguard against an incorrect hypothesis or intervention that accelerates progression to cancer, as was observed in the β-carotene lung cancer prevention trials *(205–208)*.

The rapid increase in our understanding of the molecular genesis of BE and esophageal adenocarcinoma has given a glimpse into the exciting future of tailored management of cancer risk for patients with this condition. Tailored management depending on careful risk-benefit assessment might be extended to screening, surveillance, and counseling as well as medical, endoscopic, and surgical interventions. Thus, patients at low risk of cancer may be counseled and reassured of their low risk to reduce anxiety, placed in less frequent endoscopic surveillance, and treated with interventions that have excellent safety profiles. Patients at intermediate risk may undergo more frequent surveillance and be treated appropriately. More aggressive interventions may be warranted in patients at highest risk of cancer.

ACKNOWLEDGMENT

Dr. Reid is supported by NIH Grant R01 CA61202, "Predictors of Progression in Barrett's Esophagus."

REFERENCES

1. Phillips RW, Wong RK. Barrett's esophagus. Natural history, incidence, etiology, and complications. *Gastroenterol Clin North Am* 1991;20:791–816.
2. Morales TG, Sampliner RE. Barrett's esophagus: update on screening, surveillance, and treatment. *Arch Intern Med* 1999;159:1411–1416.
3. Farrow DC, Vaughan TL. Determinants of survival following the diagnosis of esophageal adenocarcinoma (United States). *Cancer Causes Control* 1996;7:322–327.
4. Reid BJ. Barrett's esophagus and esophageal adenocarcinoma. In *Gastroenterology Clinics of North America: Mucosal Diseases of the Esophagus.* Roy KHW, ed. WB Saunders Co., Philadelphia, 1991; pp. 817–834.
5. Barrett MT, Sanchez CA, Prevo LJ, et al. Evolution of neoplastic cell lineages in Barrett oesophagus. *Nat Genet* 1999;22:106–109.
6. Gleeson CM, Sloan JM, McGuigan JA, et al. Base transitions at CpG dinucleotides in the p53 gene are common in esophageal adenocarcinoma. *Cancer Res* 1995;55:3406–3411.
7. Klump B, Hsieh CJ, Holzmann K, et al. Hypermethylation of the CDKN2/p16 promoter during neoplastic progression in Barrett's esophagus. *Gastroenterology* 1998;115:1381–1386.
8. Muzeau F, Flejou JF, Potet F, et al. Profile of p53 mutations and abnormal expression of P53 protein in 2 forms of esophageal cancer. *Gastroenterol Clin Biol* 1996;20:430–437.
9. Muzeau F, Flejou JF, Thomas G, Hamelin R. Loss of heterozygosity on chromosome 9 and p16 (MTS1, CDKN2) gene mutations in esophageal cancers. *Int J Cancer* 1997;72:27–30.
10. Tarmin L, Yin J, Zhou X, et al. Frequent loss of heterozygosity on chromosome 9 in adenocarcinoma and squamous cell carcinoma of the esophagus. *Cancer Res* 1994;54:6094–6096.
11. Galipeau PC, Cowan DS, Sanchez CA, et al. 17p (p53) allelic losses, 4N (G2/tetraploid) populations, and progression to aneuploidy in Barrett's esophagus. *Proc Natl Acad Sci USA* 1996;93:7081–7084.
12. Galipeau PC, Prevo LJ, Sanchez CA, et al. Clonal expansion and loss of heterozygosity at chromosomes 9p and 17p in premalignant esophageal (Barrett's) tissue. *J Natl Cancer Inst* 1999;91:2087–2095.
13. Hamelin R, Flejou JF, Muzeau F, et al. TP53 gene mutations and p53 protein immunoreactivity in malignant and premalignant Barrett's esophagus. *Gastroenterology* 1994;107:1012–1018.
14. Neshat K, Sanchez CA, Galipeau PC, et al. p53 mutations in Barrett's adenocarcinoma and high-grade dysplasia. *Gastroenterology* 1994;106:1589–1595.
15. Prevo LJ, Sanchez CA, Galipeau PC, Reid BJ. p53 Mutant clones and field effects in Barrett's esophagus. *Cancer Res* 1999;59:4784–4787.
16. Menke-Pluymers MB, Mulder AH, Hop WC, et al. Dysplasia and aneuploidy as markers of malignant degeneration in

Barrett's oesophagus. The Rotterdam Oesophageal Tumour Study Group. *Gut* 1994;35:1348–1351.

17. Fennerty MB, Sampliner RE, Way D, et al. Discordance between flow cytometric abnormalities and dysplasia in Barrett's esophagus. *Gastroenterology* 1989;97:815–820.

18. Gimenez A, Minguela A, Parrilla P, et al. Flow cytometric DNA analysis and p53 protein expression show a good correlation with histologic findings in patients with Barrett's esophagus. *Cancer* 1998;83:641–651.

19. McKinley MJ, Budman DR, Grueneberg D, et al. DNA content in Barrett's esophagus and esophageal malignancy. *Am J Gastroenterol* 1987;82:1012–1015.

20. Rabinovitch PS, Reid BJ, Haggitt RC, et al. Progression to cancer in Barrett's esophagus is associated with genomic instability. *Lab Invest* 1989;60:65–71.

21. Robaszkiewicz M, Hardy E, Volant A. Analyse du contenu cellulaire en ADN par cytometrie en flux dans les endobrachyoesophages. *Gastroenterol Clin Biol* 1991;15:703–710.

22. Winkelstein A. Peptic esophagitis: a new clinic entity. *JAMA* 1935;104:906–909.

23. Barrett NR. Chronic peptic ulcer of the oesophagus and 'oesophagitis'. *Br J Surg* 1950–1951;38:175–182.

24. Naef AP, Savary M, Ozzello L. Columnar-lined lower esophagus: an acquired lesion with malignant predisposition. Report on 140 cases of Barrett's esophagus with 12 adenocarcinomas. *J Thorac Cardiovasc Surg* 1975;70:826–835.

25. Blot WJ, Devesa SS, Kneller RW, Fraumeni JF Jr. Rising incidence of adenocarcinoma of the esophagus and gastric cardia. JAMA 1991;265:1287–1289.

26. Bollschweiler E, Wolfgarten E, Gutschow C, Holscher AH. Demographic variations in the rising incidence of esophageal adenocarcinoma in white males. *Cancer* 2001;92: 549–555.

27. Gallup. A Gallup Organization national survey: heartburn across America. The Gallup Organization, Princeton, 1988.

28. Locke GR 3rd, Talley NJ, Fett SL, et al. Prevalence and clinical spectrum of gastroesophageal reflux: a population-based study in Olmsted County, Minnesota. *Gastroenterology* 1997;112:1448–1456.

29. Barrett NR. The lower esophagus lined by columnar epithelium. *Surgery* 1957;41:881–894.

30. Schmidt HG, Riddell RH, Walther B, et al. Dysplasia in Barrett's esophagus. *J Cancer Res Clin Oncol* 1985;110: 145–152.

31. McClave SA, Boyce HW Jr, Gottfried MR. Early diagnosis of columnar-lined esophagus: a new endoscopic diagnostic criterion. *Gastrointest Endosc* 1987;33:413–416.

32. Gottfried MR, McClave SA, Boyce HW. Incomplete intestinal metaplasia in the diagnosis of columnar lined esophagus (Barrett's esophagus). *Am J Clin Pathol* 1989;92:741–746.

33. Sharma P, Morales TG, Sampliner RE. Short segment Barrett's esophagus—the need for standardization of the definition and of endoscopic criteria. *Am J Gastroenterol,* 1998;93:1033–1036.

34. Burbige EJ, Radigan JJ. Characteristics of the columnar-cell lined (Barrett's) esophagus. *Gastrointest Endosc* 1979;25: 133–136.

35. Rothery GA, Patterson JE, Stoddard CJ, Day DW. Histological and histochemical changes in the columnar lined (Barrett's) oesophagus. *Gut* 1986;27:1062–1068.

36. Cooper BT, Barbezat GO. Barrett's oesophagus: a clinical study of 52 patients. *Q J Med* 1987;62:97–108.

37. Ovaska J, Miettinen M, Kivilaakso E. Adenocarcinoma arising in Barrett's esophagus. *Dig Dis Sci* 1989;34:1336–1339.

38. Herlihy KJ, Orlando RC, Bryson JC, et al. Barrett's esophagus: clinical, endoscopic, histologic, manometric, and electrical potential difference characteristics. *Gastroenterology* 1984;86:436–443.

39. Snyder JD, Goldman H. Barrett's esophagus in children and young adults. Frequent association with mental retardation. *Dig Dis Sci* 1990;35:1185–1189.

40. Starnes VA, Adkins RB, Ballinger JF, Sawyers JL. Barrett's esophagus. A surgical entity. *Arch Surg* 1984;119:563–567.

41. Sarr MG, Hamilton SR, Marrone GC, Cameron JL. Barrett's esophagus: its prevalence and association with adenocarcinoma in patients with symptoms of gastroesophageal reflux. *Am J Surg* 1985;149:187–193.

42. Gilchrist AM, Levine MS, Carr RF, et al. Barrett's esophagus: diagnosis by double-contrast esophagography. *Am J Roentgenol* 1988;150:97–102.

43. Winters C Jr, Spurling TJ, Chobanian SJ, et al. Barrett's esophagus. A prevalent, occult complication of gastroesophageal reflux disease. *Gastroenterology* 1987;92:118–124.

44. Mann NS, Tsai MF, Nair PK. Barrett's esophagus in patients with symptomatic reflux esophagitis. *Am J Gastroenterol* 1989;84:1494–1496.

45. Dahms BB, Greco MA, Strandjord SE, Rothstein FC. Barrett's esophagus in three children after antileukemia chemotherapy. *Cancer* 1987;60:2896–2900.

46. Hirota WK, Loughney TM, Lazas DJ, et al. Specialized intestinal metaplasia, dysplasia, and cancer of the esophagus and esophagogastric junction: prevalence and clinical data. *Gastroenterology* 1999;116:277–285.

47. Robinson M, Earnest D, Rodriguez-Stanley S, et al. Heartburn requiring frequent antacid use may indicate significant illness. *Arch Intern Med* 1998;158:2373–2376.

48. Gerson LB, Shelter K, Triadafilopoulos G. Screening for Barrett's esophagus in asymptomatic adults undergoing routine flexible sigmoidoscopy for colorectal cancer screening. *Gastrointest Endosc* 2001;53:AB61.

49. Ghorai S, Rex D, Cummings O, Rahmani E. Screening for Barrett's (B) in colonoscopy (CS) patients with and without heartburn (HB). *Gastrointest Endosc* 2001;53:AB61.

50. Cameron AJ, Lomboy CT. Barrett's esophagus: age, prevalence, and extent of columnar epithelium. *Gastroenterology* 1992;103:1241–1245.

51. Cameron AJ, Zinsmeister AR, Ballard DJ, Carney JA. Prevalence of columnar-lined (Barrett's) esophagus. Comparison of population-based clinical and autopsy findings. *Gastroenterology* 1990;99:918–922.

52. Endo M. A case of Barrett epithelization followed up for five years. *Endoscopy* 1974;6:48–51.

53. Goldman M. Barrett syndrome. *Case Reports* 1960;39: 104–110.

54. Mossberg SM. The columnar-lined esophagus (Barrett syndrome)—an acquired condition? *Gastroenterology* 1966;50: 671–676.

55. Halvorsen JF, Semb BK. The Barrett syndrome (the columnar-lined lower oesophagus): an acquired condition secondary to reflux oesophagitis. A case report with discussion of pathogenesis. *Acta Chir Scand* 1975;141:683–687.

56. Conio M, Cameron AJ, Romero Y, et al. Secular trends in the epidemiology and outcome of Barrett's oesophagus in Olmsted County, Minnesota. *Gut* 2001;48:304–309.

57. Caygill CP, Reed PI, Johnston BJ, et al. A single centre's 20 years' experience of columnar-lined (Barrett's) oesophagus diagnosis. *Eur J Gastroenterol Hepatol* 1999;11: 1355–1358.

58. Prach AT, MacDonald TA, Hopwood DA, Johnston DA. Increasing incidence of Barrett's oesophagus: education, enthusiasm, or epidemiology? *Lancet* 1997;350:933.

59. Bosch A, Frias Z, Caldwell WL. Adenocarcinoma of the esophagus. *Cancer* 1979;43:1557–1561.

60. Faintuch J, Shepard KV, Levin B. Adenocarcinoma and other unusual variants of esophageal cancer. *Semin Oncol* 1984;11:196–202.

61. Devesa SS, Blot WJ, Fraumeni JF Jr. Changing patterns in the incidence of esophageal and gastric carcinoma in the United States. *Cancer* 1998;83:2049–2053.

62. Yang PC, Davis S. Incidence of cancer of the esophagus in the US by histologic type. *Cancer* 1988;61:612–617.

63. Blot WJ, Devesa SS, Fraumeni JF Jr. Continuing climb in rates of esophageal adenocarcinoma: an update. *JAMA* 1993;270:1320.

64. McKinney A, Sharp L, Macfarlane GJ, Muir CS. Oesophageal and gastric cancer in Scotland 1960–1990. *Br J Cancer* 1995;71:411–415.

65. Moller H. Incidence of cancer of oesophagus, cardia and stomach in Denmark. *Eur J Cancer Prev* 1992;1:159–164.

66. Hansen S, Wiig JN, Giercksky KE, Tretli S. Esophageal and gastric carcinoma in Norway 1958-1992: incidence time trend variability according to morphological subtypes and organ subsites. *Int J Cancer* 1997;71:340–344.

67. Levi F, Randimbison L, La Vecchia C. Esophageal and gastric carcinoma in Vaud, Switzerland, 1976–1994. *Int J Cancer* 1998;75:160–161.

68. Thomas RJ, Lade S, Giles GG, Thursfield V. Incidence trends in oesophageal and proximal gastric carcinoma in Victoria. *Aust NZ J Surg* 1996;66:271–275.

69. Armstrong RW, Borman B. Trends in incidence rates of adenocarcinoma of the oesophagus and gastric cardia in New Zealand, 1978–1992. *Int J Epidemiol* 1996;25:941–947.

70. Bytzer P, Christensen PB, Damkier P, et al. Adenocarcinoma of the esophagus and Barrett's esophagus: a population-based study. *Am J Gastroenterol* 1999;94:86–91.

71. Powell J, McConkey CC. The rising trend in oesophageal adenocarcinoma and gastric cardia. *Eur J Cancer Prev* 1992;1:265–269.

72. Rios-Castellanos E, Sitas F, Shepherd NA, Jewell DP. Changing pattern of gastric cancer in Oxfordshire. *Gut* 1992;33:1312–1317.

73. van der Burgh A, Dees J, Hop WC, van Blankenstein M. Oesophageal cancer is an uncommon cause of death in patients with Barrett's oesophagus. *Gut* 1996;39:5–8.

74. Spechler SJ. Barrett's esophagus: an overrated cancer risk factor. *Gastroenterology* 2000;119:587–589.

75. Shaheen NJ, Crosby MA, Bozymski EM, Sandler RS. Is there publication bias in the reporting of cancer risk in Barrett's esophagus? *Gastroenterology* 2000;119:333–338.

76. Drewitz DJ, Sampliner RE, Garewal HS. The incidence of adenocarcinoma in Barrett's esophagus: a prospective study of 170 patients followed 4.8 years. *Am J Gastroenterol* 1997;92:212–215.

77. O'Connor JB, Falk GW, Richter JE. The incidence of adenocarcinoma and dysplasia in Barrett's esophagus: report on the Cleveland Clinic Barrett's Esophagus Registry. *Am J Gastroenterol* 1999;94:2037–2042.

78. Spechler SJ, Lee E, Ahnen D, et al. Long-term outcome of medical and surgical therapies for gastroesophageal reflux disease: follow-up of a randomized controlled trial. *JAMA* 2001;285:2331–2338.

79. Jankowski JA, Provenzale D, Moayyedi P. Esophageal adenocarcinoma arising from Barrett's metaplasia has regional variations in the west. *Gastroenterology* 2002;10:588–590.

80. Lagergren J, Bergstrom R, Lindgren A, Nyren O. Symptomatic gastroesophageal reflux as a risk factor for esophageal adenocarcinoma. *N Eng J Med* 1999;340: 825–831.

81. Farrow DC, Vaughan TL, Sweeney C, et al. Gastroesophageal reflux disease, use of H2 receptor antagonists, and risk of esophageal and gastric cancer. *Cancer Causes Control* 2000;11:231–238.

82. Vaezi, MF, Richter JE. Bile reflux in columnar-lined esophagus. *Gastroenterol Clin North Am* 1997;26:565–582.

83. Marshall RE, Anggiansah A, Owen WJ. Bile in the oesophagus: clinical relevance and ambulatory detection. *Br J Surg* 1997;84:21–28.

84. DeMeester SR. Management of Barrett's esophagus free of dysplasia. *Semin Thorac Cardiovasc Surg* 1997;9: 279–284.

85. Vaezi MF, Richter JE. Role of acid and duodenogastroesophageal reflux in gastroesophageal reflux disease. *Gastroenterology* 1996;111:1192–1199.

86. Vaezi MF, Singh S, Richter JE. Role of acid and duodenogastric reflux in esophageal mucosal injury: a review of animal and human studies. *Gastroenterology* 1995;108: 1897–1907.

87. Champion G, Richter JE, Vaezi MF, et al. Duodenogastroesophageal reflux: relationship to pH and importance in Barrett's esophagus. *Gastroenterology* 1994;107:747–754.

88. Caldwell MT, Lawlor P, Byrne PJ, et al. Ambulatory oesophageal bile reflux monitoring in Barrett's oesophagus. *Br J Surg* 1995;82:657–660.

89. Kauer WK, Peters JH, DeMeester TR, et al. Mixed reflux of gastric and duodenal juices is more harmful to the esophagus than gastric juice alone. The need for surgical therapy re-emphasized. *Ann Surg* 1995;222:525–531.

90. Kauer WK, Burdiles P, Ireland AP, et al. Does duodenal juice reflux into the esophagus of patients with complicated GERD? Evaluation of a fiberoptic sensor for bilirubin. *Am J Surg* 1995;169:98–104.

91. Muller-Lissner SA. Bile reflux is increased in cigarette smokers. *Gastroenterology* 1986;90:1205–1209.

92. Nehra D, Howell P, Williams CP, et al. Toxic bile acids in gastro-oesophageal reflux disease: influence of gastric acidity. *Gut* 1999;44:598–602.

93. Stein HJ, Kauer WKH, Feussner H, Siewert JR. Bile reflux in benign and malignant Barrett's esophagus: effect of medical acid suppression and nissen fundoplication. *J Gastrointest Surg* 1998;2:333–341.

94. Marshall RE, Anggiansah A, Manifold DK, et al. Effect of omeprazole 20 mg twice daily on duodenogastric and gastro-oesophageal bile reflux in Barrett's oesophagus. *Gut* 1998;43:603–606.

95. Menges M, Muller M, Zeitz M. Increased acid and bile reflux in Barrett's esophagus compared to reflux esophagitis, and

effect of proton pump inhibitor therapy. *Am J Gastroenterol* 2001;96:331–337.

96. Lagergren J, Bergstrom R, Nyren O. Association between body mass and adenocarcinoma of the esophagus and gastric cardia. *Ann Intern Med* 1999;130:883–890.
97. Chow WH, Blot WJ, Vaughan TL, et al. Body mass index and risk of adenocarcinomas of the esophagus and gastric cardia. *J Natl Cancer Inst* 1998;90:150–155.
98. Vaughan TL, Davis S, Kristal A, Thomas DB. Obesity, alcohol, and tobacco as risk factors for cancers of the esophagus and gastric cardia: adenocarcinoma versus squamous cell carcinoma. *Cancer Epidemiol Biomarkers Prev* 1995;4:85–92.
99. Brown LM, Swanson CA, Gridley G, et al. Adenocarcinoma of the esophagus: role of obesity and diet. *J Natl Cancer Inst* 1995;87:104–109.
100. Brown LM, Silverman DT, Pottern LM, et al. Adenocarcinoma of the esophagus and esophagogastric junction in white men in the United States: alcohol, tobacco, and socioeconomic factors. *Cancer Causes Control* 1994;5:333–340.
101. Gammon MD, Schoenberg JB, Ahsan H, et al. Tobacco, alcohol, and socioeconomic status and adenocarcinomas of the esophagus and gastric cardia. *J Natl Cancer Inst* 1997;89:1277–1284.
102. Lagergren J, Bergstrom R, Lindgren A, Nyren O. The role of tobacco, snuff and alcohol use in the aetiology of cancer of the oesophagus and gastric cardia. *Int J Cancer* 2000;85: 340–346.
103. Farrow DC, Vaughan TL, Hansten PD, et al. Use of aspirin and other nonsteroidal anti-inflammatory drugs and risk of esophageal and gastric cancer. *Cancer Epidemiol Biomarkers Prev* 1998;7:97–102.
104. Funkhouser EM, Sharp GB. Aspirin and reduced risk of esophageal carcinoma. *Cancer* 1995;76:1116–1119.
105. Langman MJ, Cheng KK, Gilman EA, Lancashire RJ. Effect of anti-inflammatory drugs on overall risk of common cancer: case-control study in general practice research database. *Br Med* J 2000;320:1642–1646.
106. Thun MJ, Namboodiri MM, Calle EE, et al. Aspirin use and risk of fatal cancer. *Cancer Res* 1993;53:1322–1327.
107. Brown JM, Lemmon MJ. Potentiation by the hypoxic cytotoxin SR 4233 of cell killing produced by fractionated irradiation of mouse tumors. *Cancer Res* 1990;50:7745–7749.
108. Mayne ST, Risch H, Dubrow R, et al. Nutrient intake and risk of adenocarcinomas of the esophagus and gastric cardia. *FASEB J* 1999;13:A1021.
109. Kabat GC, Ng SK, Wynder EL. Tobacco, alcohol intake, and diet in relation to adenocarcinoma of the esophagus and gastric cardia. *Cancer Causes Control* 1993;4:123–132.
110. Zhang ZF, Kurtz RC, Yu GP, et al. Adenocarcinomas of the esophagus and gastric cardia: the role of diet. *Nutr Cancer* 1997;27:298–309.
111. Tzonou A, Lipworth L, Garidou A, et al. Diet and risk of esophageal cancer by histologic type in a low-risk population. *Int J Cancer* 1996;68:300–304.
112. Mayne ST, Risch HA, Dubrow R, et al. Nutrient intake and risk of subtypes of esophageal and gastric cancer. *Cancer Epidemiol Biomarkers Prev* 2001;10:1055–1062.
113. Sampliner RE. Practice guidelines on the diagnosis, surveillance, and therapy of Barrett's esophagus. The Practice Parameters Committee of the American College of Gastroenterology. *Am J Gastroenterol* 1998;93: 1028–1032.
114. Corley DA, Levin TR, Habel LA, et al. Surveillance and survival in Barrett's adenocarcinomas: a population-based study. *Gastroenerology* 2002;122:633–640.
115. Peters JH, Clark GW, Ireland AP, et al. Outcome of adenocarcinoma arising in Barrett's esophagus in endoscopically surveyed and nonsurveyed patients. *J Thorac Cardiovasc Surg* 1994;108:813–822.
116. van Sandick JW, van Lanschot JJ, Kuiken BW, et al. Impact of endoscopic biopsy surveillance of Barrett's oesophagus on pathological stage and clinical outcome of Barrett's carcinoma. *Gut* 1998;43:216–222.
117. Macdonald CE, Wicks AC, Playford RJ. Final results from 10 year cohort of patients undergoing surveillance for Barrett's oesophagus: observational study. *Br Med J* 2000;321:1252–1255.
118. Falk GW, Ours TM, Richter JE. Practice patterns for surveillance of Barrett's esophagus in the United States. *Gastrointest Endosc* 2000;52:197–203.
119. Provenzale D, Schmitt C, Wong JB. Barrett's esophagus: a new look at surveillance based on emerging estimates of cancer risk. *Am J Gastroenterol* 1999;94:2043–2053.
120. Reid BJ, Haggitt RC, Rubin CE, et al. Observer variation in the diagnosis of dysplasia in Barrett's esophagus. *Hum Pathol* 1988;19:166–178.
121. Sagan C, Flejou JF, Diebold MD, et al. Observer variation in the diagnosis of dysplasia in Barrett's mucosa. *Gastroenterol Clin Biol* 1994;18:D31–D34.
122. Polkowski W., van Lanschot JJ, Ten Kate FJ, et al. The value of p53 and Ki67 as markers for tumour progression in the Barrett's dysplasia-carcinoma sequence. *Surg Oncol* 1995;4:163–171.
123. Polkowski W, Baak JP, van Lanschot JJ, et al. Clinical decision making in Barrett's oesophagus can be supported by computerized immunoquantitation and morphometry of features associated with proliferation and differentiation. *J Pathol* 1998;184:161–168.
124. Alikhan M, Rex D, Khan A, et al. Variable pathologic interpretation of columnar lined esophagus by general pathologists in community practice. *Gastrointest Endosc* 1999;50:23–26.
125. van Sandick JW, Baak JP, van Lanschot JJ, et al Computerized quantitative pathology for the grading of dysplasia in surveillance biopsies of Barrett's oesophagus. *J Pathol* 2000;190: 177–183.
126. Montgomery E, Bronner MP, Goldblum JR, et al. Reproducibility of the diagnosis of dysplasia in Barrett esophagus: a reaffirmation. *Hum Pathol* 2001;32: 368–378.
127. Reid BJ, Levine DS, Longton G, et al. Predictors of progression to cancer in Barrett's esophagus: baseline histology and flow cytometry identify low- and high-risk patient subsets. *Am J Gastroenterol* 2000;95:1669–1676.
128. Schnell TG, Sontag SJ, Chejfec G, et al. Long-term nonsurgical management of Barrett's esophagus with high-grade dysplasia. *Gastroenterology* 2001;120:1607–1619.
129. Buttar NS, Wang KK, Sebo TJ, et al. Extent of high-grade dysplasia in Barrett's esophagus correlates with risk of adenocarcinoma. *Gastroenterology* 2001;120:1630–1639.
130. Weston AP, Sharma P, Topalovski M, et al. Long-term follow-up of Barrett's high-grade dysplasia. *Am J Gastroenterol* 2000;95:1888–1893.

131. Reid BJ, Blount PL, Feng Z, Levine DS. Optimizing endoscopic biopsy detection of early cancers in Barrett's high-grade dysplasia. *Am J Gastroenterol* 2000;95:3089–3096.

132. Weston AP, Banerjee SK, Sharma P, et al. p53 protein overexpression in low grade dysplasia (LGD) in Barrett's esophagus: immunohistochemical marker predictive of progression. *Am J Gastroenterol* 2001;96:1355–1362.

133. Ofman JJ, Lewin K, Ramers C, et al. The economic impact of the diagnosis of dysplasia in Barrett's esophagus. *Am J Gastroenterol* 2000;95:2946–2952.

134. Eloubeidi MA, Homan RK, Martz MD, et al. A cost analysis of outpatient care for patients with Barrett's esophagus in a managed care setting. *Am J Gastroenterol* 1999;94:2033–2036.

135. Ouatu-Lascar R, Fitzgerald RC, Triadafilopoulos G. Differentiation and proliferation in Barrett's esophagus and the effects of acid suppression. *Gastroenterology* 1999;117: 327–335.

136. Sampliner RE, Faigel D, Fennerty B, et al. Effective and safe endoscopic reversal of nondysplastic Barrett's esophagus with thermal electrocoagulation combined with high dose acid inhibition: a multicenter study. *Gastrointest Endosc* 2001;53:554–558.

137. Overholt BF, Panjehpour M, Haydek JM. Photodynamic therapy for Barrett's esophagus: follow-up in 100 patients. *Gastrointest Endosc* 1999;49:1–7.

138. Gossner L, May A, Stolte M, et al. KTP laser destruction of dysplasia and early cancer in columnar-lined Barrett's esophagus. *Gastrointest Endosc* 1999;49:8–12.

139. Gossner L, Stolte M, Sroka R, et al. Photodynamic ablation of high-grade dysplasia and early cancer in Barrett's esophagus by means of 5-aminolevulinic acid. *Gastroenterology* 1998;114: 448–455.

140. Nijhawan PK, Wang KK. Endoscopic mucosal resection for lesions with endoscopic features suggestive of malignancy and high-grade dysplasia within Barrett's esophagus. *Gastrointest Endosc* 2000;52:328–332.

141. Ell C, May A, Gossner L, et al. Endoscopic mucosal resection of early cancer and high-grade dysplasia in Barrett's esophagus. *Gastroenterology* 2000;118:670–677.

142. Buttar NS, Wang KK, Lutzke LS, et al. Combined endoscopic mucosal resection and photodynamic therapy for esophageal neoplasia within Barrett's esophagus. *Gastrointest Endosc* 2001;54:682–688.

143. Van Laethem JL, Peny MO, Salmon I, et al. Intramucosal adenocarcinoma arising under squamous re-epithelialisation of Barrett's oesophagus. *Gut* 2000;46:574–577.

144. Ertan A, Zimmerman M, Younes M. Esophageal adenocarcinoma associated with Barrett's esophagus: long-term management with laser ablation. *Am J Gastroenterol* 1995;90:2201–2203.

145. Krishnadath KK, Wang KK, Taniguchi K, et al. Persistent genetic abnormalities in Barrett's esophagus after photodynamic therapy. *Gastroenterology* 2000;119:624–630.

146. Byrne JP, Armstrong GR, Attwood SE. Restoration of the normal squamous lining in Barrett's esophagus by argon beam plasma coagulation. *Am J Gastroenterol* 1998;93: 1810–1815.

147. Dimick JB, Cattaneo SM, Lipsett PA, et al. Hospital volume is related to clinical and economic outcomes of esophageal resection in Maryland. *Ann Thorac Surg* 2001;72: 334–341.

148. Begg CB, Cramer LD, Hoskins WJ, Brennan MF. Impact of hospital volume on operative mortality for major cancer surgery. *JAMA* 1998;280:1747–1751.

149. Patti MG, Corvera CU, Glasgow RE, Way LW. A hospital's annual rate of esophagectomy influences the operative mortality rate. *J Gastrointest Surg* 1998;2:186–192.

150. Rusch VW, Levine DS, Haggitt R, Reid BJ. The management of high grade dysplasia and early cancer in Barrett's esophagus. A multidisciplinary problem. *Cancer* 1994;74: 1225–1229.

151. Nowell PC. The clonal evolution of tumor cell populations. *Science* 1976;194:23–28.

152. van 't Veer LJ, Dai H, van de Vijver MJ, et al. Gene expression profiling predicts clinical outcome of breast cancer. *Nature* 2002;415:530–535.

153. Shipp MA, Ross KN, Tamayo P, et al. Diffuse large B-cell lymphoma outcome prediction by gene-expression profiling and supervised machine learning. *Nat Med* 2002;8:68–74.

154. van Lieshout EM, Jansen JB, Peters WH. Biomarkers in Barrett's esophagus (review). *Int J Oncol* 1998;13: 855–864.

155. Krishnadath K, Reid B, Wang K. Biomarkers in Barrett esophagus. *Mayo Clin Proc* 2001;76:438–446.

156. Deville P, Cleton-Jansen A-M, Cornelisse CJ. Ever since Knudson. *Trends Genet* 2001;17:569–573.

157. Barrett MT, Galipeau PC, Sanchez CA, et al. Determination of the frequency of loss of heterozygosity in esophageal adenocarcinoma by cell sorting, whole genome amplification and microsatellite polymorphisms. *Oncogene* 1996;12: 1873–1878.

158. Dolan K, Garde J, Gosney J, et al. Allelotype analysis of oesophageal adenocarcinoma: loss of heterozygosity occurs at multiple sites. *Br J Cancer* 1998;78:950–957.

159. Hammoud ZT, Kaleem Z, Cooper JD, et al. Allelotype analysis of esophageal adenocarcinomas: evidence for the involvement of sequences on the long arm of chromosome 4. *Cancer Res* 1996;56:4499–4502.

160. Herbst JJ, Berenson MM, McCloskey DW, Wiser WC. Cell proliferation in esophageal columnar epithelium (Barrett's esophagus). *Gastroenterology* 1978;75:683–687.

161. Gray MR, Hall PA, Nash J, et al. Epithelial proliferation in Barrett's esophagus by proliferating cell nuclear antigen immunolocalization. *Gastroenterology* 1992;103: 1769–1776.

162. Reid BJ, Sanchez CA, Blount PL, Levine DS. Barrett's esophagus: cell cycle abnormalities in advancing stages of neoplastic progression. *Gastroenterology* 1993;105: 119–129.

163. Reid BJ, Haggitt RC, Rubin CE, Rabinovitch PS. Barrett's esophagus. Correlation between flow cytometry and histology in detection of patients at risk for adenocarcinoma. *Gastroenterology* 1987;93:1–11.

164. Hong MK, Laskin WB, Herman BE, et al. Expansion of the Ki-67 proliferative compartment correlates with degree of dysplasia in Barrett's esophagus. *Cancer* 1995;75:423–429.

165. Rabinovitch PS, Longton G, Blount PL, et al. Cytometric predictors of Barrett's progression. *Am J Gatroenterol* 2001;96:3071–3083.

166. Serrano M, Hannon GJ, Beach D. A new regulatory motif in cell-cycle control causing specific inhibition of cyclin D/CDK4. *Nature* 1993;366:704–707.

167. Alcorta DA, Xiong Y, Phelps D, et al. Involvement of the cyclin-dependent kinase inhibitor p16 (INK4a) in replicative

senescence of normal human fibroblasts. *Proc Natl Acad Sci USA* 1996;93:13742–13747.

168. Foster SA, Wong DJ, Barrett MT, Galloway DA. Inactivation of p16 in human mammary epithelial cells by CpG island methylation. *Mol Cell Biol* 1998;18:1793–1801.

169. Reznikoff CA, Yeager TR, Belair CD, et al. Elevated p16 at senescence and loss of p16 at immortalization in human papillomavirus 16 E6, but not E7, transformed human uroepithelial cells. *Cancer Res* 1996;56:2886–2890.

170. Wong DJ, Foster SA, Galloway DA, Reid BJ. Progressive region-specific de novo methylation of the p16 CpG island in primary human mammary epithelial cell strains during escape from M(0) growth arrest. *Mol Cell Biol* 1999;19: 5642–5651.

171. Barrett MT, Sanchez CA, Galipeau PC, et al. Allelic loss of 9p21 and mutation of the CDKN2/p16 gene develop as early lesions during neoplastic progression in Barrett's esophagus. *Oncogene* 1996;13:1867–1873.

172. Wong DJ, Barrett MT, Stoger R, et al. p16INK4a Promoter is hypermethylated at a high frequency in esophageal adenocarcinomas. *Cancer Res* 1997;57:2619–2622.

173. Zhou X, Tarmin L, Yin J, et al. The MTS1 gene is frequently mutated in primary human esophageal tumors. *Oncogene* 1994;9:3737–3741.

174. Wong DJ, Paulson TG, Prevo LJ, et al. p16 INK4a lesions are common, early abnormalities that undergo clonal expansion in Barrett's metaplastic epithelium. *Cancer Res* 2001;61:8284–8289.

175. Sherr CJ. Cancer cell cycles. Science 1996;274:1672–1677.

176. Sherr CJ, Roberts JM. CDK inhibitors: positive and negative regulators of G1-phase progression. *Genes Dev* 1999;13: 1501–1512.

177. Morgan RJ, Newcomb PV, Hardwick RH, Alderson D. Amplification of cyclin D1 and MDM-2 in oesophageal carcinoma. *Eur J Surg Oncol* 1999;25:364–367.

178. Arber N, Lightdale C, Rotterdam H, et al. Increased expression of the cyclin D1 gene in Barrett's esophagus. *Cancer Epidemiol Biomarkers Prev* 1996;5:457–459.

179. Bani-Hani K, Martin IG, Hardie LJ, et al. Prospective study of cyclin D1 overexpression in Barrett's esophagus: association with increased risk of adenocarcinoma. *J Natl Cancer Inst* 2000;92:1316–1321.

180. Kitahara K, Yasui W, Yokozaki H, et al. Expression of cyclin D1, CDK4 and p27KIP1 is associated with the p16MTS1 gene status in human esophageal carcinoma cell lines. *J Exp Ther Oncol* 1996;1:7–12.

181. Ko LJ, Prives C. p53: puzzle and paradigm. *Genes Dev* 1996;10:1054–1072.

182. Waridel F, Estreicher A, Bron L, et al. Field cancerisation and polyclonal p53 mutation in the upper aero- digestive tract. *Oncogene* 1997;14:163–169.

183. Furumoto K, Inoue E, Nagao N, et al. Age-dependent telomere shortening is slowed down by enrichment of intracellular vitamin C via suppression of oxidative stress. *Life Sci* 1998;63:935–948.

184. von Zglinicki T, Saretzki G, Docke W, Lotze C. Mild hyperoxia shortens telomeres and inhibits proliferation of fibroblasts: a model for senescence? *Exp Cell Res* 1995;220:186–193.

185. Ducray C, Pommier JP, Martins L, et al. Telomere dynamics, end-to-end fusions and telomerase activation during the human fibroblast immortalization process. *Oncogene* 1999;18:4211–4223.

186. de Lange T, Jacks T. For better or worse? Telomerase inhibition and cancer. *Cell* 1999;98:273–275.

187. Chin L, Artandi SE, Shen Q, et al. p53 deficiency rescues the adverse effects of telomere loss and cooperates with telomere dysfunction to accelerate carcinogenesis. *Cell* 1999;97:527–538.

188. Blasco MA, Lee HW, Hande MP, et al. Telomere shortening and tumor formation by mouse cells lacking telomerase RNA. *Cell* 1997;91:25–34.

189. Martens UM, Zijlmans JM, Poon SS, et al. Short telomeres on human chromosome 17p. *Nat Genet* 1998;18:76–80.

190. Blount PL, Galipeau PC, Sanchez CA, et al. 17p allelic losses in diploid cells of patients with Barrett's esophagus who develop aneuploidy. *Cancer Res* 1994;54:2292–2295.

191. Prevo LJ, Sanchez CA, Galipeau PC, Reid BJ. p53-Mutant clones and field effects in Barrett's esophagus. *Cancer Res* 1999;59:4784–4787.

192. Reid BJ, Prevo LJ, Galipeau PC, et al. Predictors of progression in Barrett's esophagus II: Baseline 17p (p53) loss of heterozygosity identifies a patient subset at increased risk for neoplastic progression. *Am J Gastroenterol* 2001;96:2839–2848.

193. Blount PL, Meltzer SJ, Yin J, et al. Clonal ordering of 17p and 5q allelic losses in Barrett dysplasia and adenocarcinoma. *Proc Natl Acad Sci USA* 1993;90:3221–3225.

194. Younes M, Ertan A, Lechago LV, et al. p53 protein accumulation is a specific marker of malignant potential in Barrett's metaplasia. *Dig Dis Sci* 1997;42:697–701.

195. Coggi G, Bosari S, Roncalli M, et al. p53 protein accumulation and p53 gene mutation in esophageal carcinoma. A molecular and immunohistochemical study with clinicopathologic correlations. *Cancer* 1997;79:425–432.

196. Moore JH, Lesser EJ, Erdody DH, et al. Intestinal differentiation and p53 gene alterations in Barrett's esophagus and esophageal adenocarcinoma. *Int J Cancer* 1994;56:487–493.

197. Reid BJ. p53 and neoplastic progression in Barrett's esophagus. *Am J Gastroenterol* 2001;96:1321-1323.

198. Robaszkiewicz M, Hardy E, Volant A, et al. Flow cytometric analysis of cellular DNA content in Barret's esophagus. A study of 66 cases. *Gastroenterol Clin Biol* 1991;15:703–710.

199. Reid BJ, Blount PL, Rubin CE, et al. Flow-cytometric and histological progression to malignancy in Barrett's esophagus: prospective endoscopic surveillance of a cohort. *Gastroenterology* 1992;102:1212–1219.

200. Teodori L, Gohde W, Persiani M, et al. DNA/protein flow cytometry as a predictive marker of malignancy in dysplasia-free Barrett's esophagus: thirteen-year follow-up study on a cohort of patients. *Cytometry* 1998;34:257–263.

201. Boynton RF, Blount PL, Yin J, et al. Loss of heterozygosity involving the APC and MCC genetic loci occurs in the majority of human esophageal cancers. *Proc Natl Acad Sci USA* 1992;89:3385–3388.

202. Zhuang Z, Vortmeyer AO, Mark EJ, et al. Barrett's esophagus: metaplastic cells with loss of heterozygosity at the APC gene locus are clonal precursors to invasive adenocarcinoma. *Cancer Res* 1996;56:1961–1964.

203. Kawakami K, Brabender J, Lord RV, et al. Hypermethylated APC DNA in plasma and prognosis of patients with

esophageal adenocarcinoma. *J Natl Cancer Inst* 2000;92: 1805–1811.

204. Eads CA, Lord RV, Kurumboor SK, et al. Fields of aberrant CpG island hypermethylation in Barrett's esophagus and associated adenocarcinoma. *Cancer Res* 2000;60: 5021–5026.

205. The Alpha Tocopherol BC Cancer Prevention Study Group. The effect of vitamin E and beta carotene on the incidence of lung cancer and other cancers in male smokers. *N Engl J Med* 1994;330:1029–1035.

206. Omenn GS, Goodman GE, Thornquist MD, et al. Effects of a combination of beta carotene and vitamin A on lung can-cer and cardiovascular disease. *N Eng J Med* 1996;330: 1029–1035.

207. Albanes D, Heinonen OP, Taylor PR, et al. Alpha-tocopherol and beta-carotene supplements and lung cancer incidence in the Alpha-Tocopherol, Beta-Carotene Cancer Prevention study: effects of base-line characteristics and study compli-ance. *J Natl Cancer Inst* 1996;88:1513–1515.

208. Omenn GS, Goodman GE, Thornquist MD, et al. Risk fac-tors for lung cancer and for intervention effects in CARET, the Beta-Carotene and Retinol Efficacy Trial. *J Natl Cancer Inst* 1996;88:1550–1559.

26 Endoscopic Detection of Esophageal Neoplasia

Brian C. Jacobson, MD, MPH and Jacques Van Dam, MD, PhD

CONTENTS

1. INTRODUCTION

Endoscopic visualization of the esophagus has been practiced since the 19th century; the first illuminated views were obtained by Mikulicz in 1880 *(1)*. Esophagogastroduodenoscopy (EGD) or "upper endoscopy" is one of the most frequently performed semi-invasive procedures, currently accounting for approx 25% of all endoscopies conducted annually. Use of endoscopy to detect esophageal dysplasia in the United States is primarily limited to evaluation of Barrett's esophagus (BE), an eponym describing metaplastic replacement of normal squamous mucosa of the esophagus with a columnar epithelium resembling that found in the small intestine (Fig. 1) *(2)*. BE is the major predisposing condition for esophageal adenocarcinoma, one of the few cancers whose incidence has been increasing over the past few years *(3)*. BE carries a 30- to 40-fold higher risk of progression to adenocarcinoma than baseline, with an incidence of 0.5% per year *(4,5)*. The prevalence of BE among patients undergoing upper endoscopy for symptoms of gastroesophageal reflux is 3–6% *(6,7)* and is 0.3% among the general population *(8)*. Surveillance biopsies of Barrett's mucosa can identify foci of dysplasia and differentiate patients with dysplasia from those with adenocarcinoma *(9,10)*, providing indispensable information for patient management. Current guidelines therefore recommend upper endoscopy BE screening for all patients with long-standing reflux symptoms, particularly those over

50 yr of age *(11)*. Furthermore, patients with established BE undergo regular surveillance endoscopy with multiple biopsies at an interval based on presence and grade of dysplasia *(11)*.

Early squamous cell carcinoma of the esophagus can also be identified endoscopically, but there are currently no formal screening recommendations aside from patients with a personal history of tylosis *(12)*. Endoscopic screening may be useful for other high-risk individuals, such as those with a significant history of alcohol and cigarette use in addition to frequent consumption of maté (an extremely hot herbal infusion enjoyed in South America) *(13)*. In addition, patients with concurrent or prior nonesophageal squamous cell carcinomas may also benefit from screening *(14)*.

Endoscopic methods for viewing the esophagus have evolved greatly over the past few decades and today include much more than simple white-light endoscopy (WLE) imaging of the luminal surface of the gastrointestinal tract. High-resolution imaging and magnification endoscopy are two modern methods for improving detection of subtle mucosal abnormalities. The endoscopist's ability to visualize pathology can be augmented by spraying the mucosa with dyes or acetic acid in an attempt to distinguish normal from abnormal tissue. Endoscopic ultrasound, performed with dedicated echoendoscopes or miniature ultrasound probes, can reveal pathology below the mucosal surface and provide information about the submucosa and muscularis propria of the gastrointestinal tract. Finally, evolving

From: Cancer Chemoprevention, Volume 2: Strategies for Cancer Chemoprevention
Edited by: G. J. Kelloff, E. T. Hawk, and C. C. Sigman © Humana Press Inc., Totowa, NJ

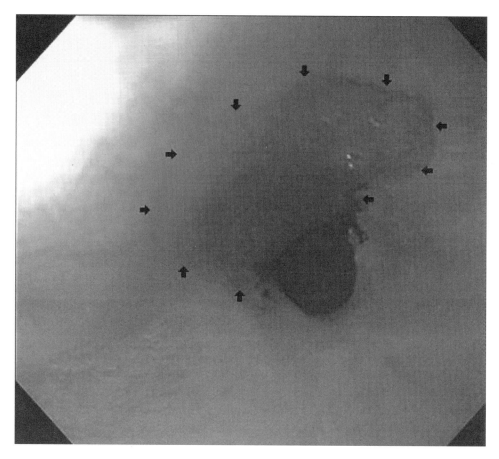

Fig. 1. Short-segment BE. An endoscopic view of the distal esophagus demonstrating a patch of columnar-lined mucosa (arrows), which appears red compared with the normal pink squamous epithelium. Biopsy of this region revealed specialized intestinal metaplasia consistent with BE.

endoscopic techniques such as optical coherence tomography and spectroscopy are being used to demonstrate findings at the microscopic and molecular levels. This chapter will review each of these entities, discussing how and when they are utilized (Table 1).

2. WLE AND TISSUE SAMPLING

WLE can be performed with a diagnostic endoscope (outer diameter 9 mm), a therapeutic endoscope (outer diameter 13 mm), or an ultrathin endoscope (outer diameter 6 mm) (Fig. 2). The ultrathin endoscope can be passed through either the mouth or the nose in a procedure typically performed without sedation. Endoscopic images considered within the context of a specific clinical picture may provide all the information necessary for a formal diagnosis *(15)*. More commonly, the endoscopist must sample tissue or remove a lesion in order to arrive at a diagnosis. Even normal-appearing mucosa may be shown to harbor pathology when a biopsy is analyzed microscopically, such as in mild celiac sprue. Pinch biopsies performed with biopsy forceps are the most frequently used form of endoscopic

tissue sampling *(15)*. Such biopsies are extremely safe; no biopsy-associated complications occurred in a study that included more than 50,000 consecutive biopsies *(16)*.

Pinch biopsies can be small or large (often referred to as "jumbo") depending on biopsy forceps size. All biopsy forceps have a similar design. The sampling portion has a paired set of teeth or cups that are in apposition when closed. They are passed through the accessory channel of an endoscope and can be directed toward the mucosa under direct vision. Endoscopic biopsy should yield a sample deep enough to contain muscularis mucosa except where the mucosal folds may be very thick (such as the gastric body) *(17)*. Submucosa may be sampled occasionally, but not consistently *(18)*. Standard biopsies are generally 4 to 8 mm in length depending on where they are obtained *(19,20)*. Jumbo biopsies are not necessarily deeper than standard biopsies but tend to include more mucosa for analysis. They are particularly useful during surveillance endoscopies for Barrett's dysplasia and appear to be a safe method for sampling esophageal mucosa *(16)*.

Table 1
Imaging Techniques to Detect Esophageal Neoplasia

Imaging Technique	Resolution	Advantages	Drawbacks
White-light endoscopy	Macroscopic lesions	Widely available	Dysplasia often microscopic or minuscule
Magnification endoscopy	Macroscopic lesions, but allows visualization of minuscule findings	Can be incorporated into standard endoscopes	Must have suspicion about a region to choose to visualize it magnified; dysplasia may be microscopic
Chromoendoscopy	Macroscopic lesions, but can detect microscopic qualities such as pit structure within a mucosa	Easy to employ; uses standard endoscopic equipment	May be difficult to learn; variation in results among users; dysplasia may be invisible to it
Optical coherence tomography	10 microns	Provides images similar to histologic sections	Not widely available; resolution may still miss early dysplasia
Spectroscopy	Biochemical content and sub-cellular structures can be analyzed	Provides information about the earliest stages of dysplasia	Not widely available; doesn't provide real-time information

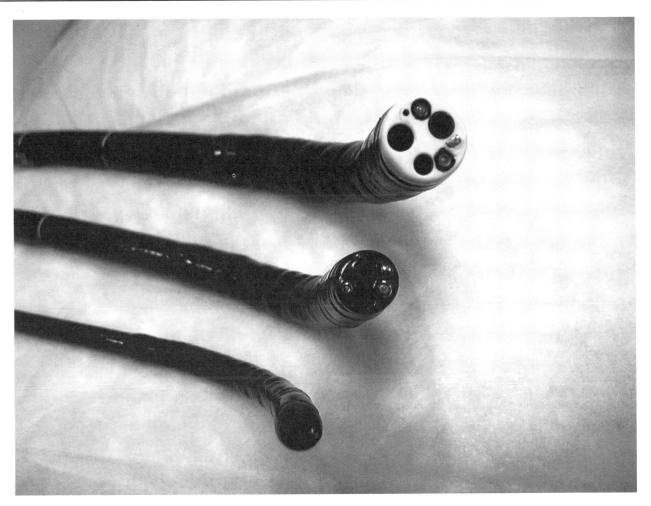

Fig. 2. Various endoscopes. Various endoscopes used for upper endoscopy are shown. The uppermost endoscope has an outer diameter of 13 mm and a large accessory channel for accommodating large ("jumbo") biopsy forceps. The middle endoscope has an outer diameter of 9 mm and is used for routine endoscopy. The lowest endoscope is a "thin caliber" endoscope with an outer diameter of 6 mm. This is used for unsedated and occasionally transnasal endoscopy.

However, jumbo biopsy forceps are larger than standard forceps and therefore require use of a diagnostic endoscope containing a larger accessory channel.

Endoscopic mucosal resection (EMR) is a newer technique for sampling tissue and removing small malignant and premalignant lesions confined to the mucosa or submucosa (21). In EMR, saline is injected into the submucosa beneath a lesion, thereby elevating it on a cushion of fluid and minimizing transmural cautery damage. EMR allows the endoscopist to attempt an en-bloc resection of small, early malignancies. This technique has been successful in removing lesions throughout the gastrointestinal tract, including the esophagus (22). When deep resection margins are still positive for dysplasia, surgical resection of the affected region is advocated (23). EMR can also provide a large specimen for pathologic analysis even in the absence of a complete resection.

3. ENHANCED ENDOSCOPY

While standard endoscopes are capable of detecting even tiny abnormalities within the gastrointestinal mucosa, dysplastic and early neoplastic lesions are commonly indistinguishable from their normal surroundings. Development of high-resolution and magnification endoscopes, along with use of special mucosal stains (chromoendoscopy), has proven useful for making these lesions visible endoscopically. These enhancements allow an endoscopist to target biopsies, thereby making screening or surveillance procedures more efficient.

3.1. High-Resolution Endoscopy

The resolution of an endoscopic image is defined as the ability to distinguish optically two closely approximated objects or points (24). Resolution is a function of the number of pixels used to portray a video image—higher density of pixels provides higher image resolution. High-resolution endoscopes use high-density charged-coupled devices (or video chips) to provide more detailed images of the gastrointestinal lumen. While standard endoscopes employ 100,000 to 200,000 pixels, high-resolution endoscopes have video chips with more than 400,000 pixels (25). Special tissue stains or chromoendoscopy (see Subheading 3.3.) used in conjunction with high-resolution endoscopy provides valuable information about subtle mucosal surface patterns that enable the endoscopist to predict histopathology more accurately (26). As is true for most technology, yesterday's breakthrough becomes today's standard. Most new endoscopes currently available use high-resolution video chips, while even higher image definition looms on the horizon. How this will translate into improved endoscopic surveillance remains to be seen.

3.2. Magnification Endoscopy

Magnification endoscopy is not necessarily high-resolution. Magnifying endoscopes use varying lenses to enlarge the video image. By using special dials or knobs on the endoscope, the endoscopist can zoom in on an image, magnifying it 1.5 to 105 times the original size (24). This feature may be used with chromoendoscopy to characterize Barrett's epithelium (27,28), small-bowel atrophy in patients with suspected malabsorption (29), and colonic polyps and aberrant crypt foci (25,30).

3.2.1. ENHANCED MAGNIFICATION ENDOSCOPY

Topical application of acetic acid is a standard adjunct during colposcopy to enhance contrast between normal and abnormal mucosa around a squamocolumnar junction. In a similar manner, acetic acid sprayed onto esophageal mucosa can detect small, ill-defined remnant islands of columnar epithelium after endoscopic ablation of BE (31). Acetic acid combined with magnification endoscopy can also highlight specific esophageal mucosal surface patterns, possibly permitting identification of BE within a columnar-lined esophagus (32). Whether this will have broader application in detecting dysplasia or neoplasia amid BE remains to be established.

3.3. Chromoendoscopy

Chromoendoscopy is the use of special dyes during endoscopy to highlight histologic entities within the gastrointestinal mucosa. A specific dye is applied to the mucosa using a spray catheter passed through the accessory channel of an endoscope. After dye application, endoscopic inspection is best carried out with a high-resolution or magnification endoscope. Based on the particular pathology sought, the choice of dye reflects different cell types and cell components to be stained.

3.3.1. METHYLENE BLUE

Methylene blue (MB) stains the mucus present in intestinal-type cells of the gastrointestinal tract. MB is taken up by goblet cells among the specialized columnar mucosa of BE, but not by normal esophageal squamous epithelium. Therefore, MB staining highlights the Barrett's epithelium amid unstained normal esophagus. For optimal staining, the mucosa is initially washed

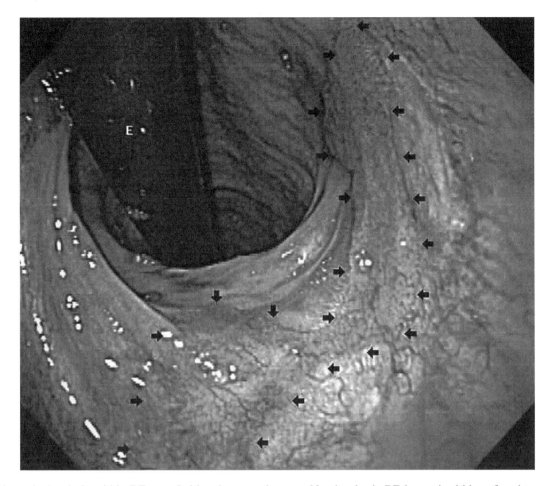

Fig. 3. High-grade dysplasia within BE revealed by chromoendoscopy. Nondysplastic BE has stained blue after the application of methylene blue. A region within the Barrett's epithelium failed to absorb the dye and appears quite different from its surroundings (arrows). Biopsies within this unstained patch revealed specialized columnar epithelium with high grade dysplasia. The endoscope (e) is retroflexed in the stomach to obtain this view of the gastroesophageal junction. Courtesy of David L. Carr-Locke, Brigham and Women's Hospital, Boston, MA.

free of overlying mucus using an agent such as 10% *N*-acetylcysteine. A 0.5–1% solution of MB is then sprayed onto the mucosa using a specially designed spray catheter. After 1–2 min, the dye is washed off with water or saline. Washing continues until the squamous mucosa appears free of dye and the staining pattern within columnar-lined mucosa is stable.

Using MB to improve detection of BE was first reported in 1996 *(33)*; subsequent studies have demonstrated that MB staining enables the endoscopist to diagnose BE with fewer biopsies than a random biopsy protocol *(28,34,35)*. MB staining may also be helpful in detecting intestinal metaplasia within short segments of columnar-lined esophagus *(36)*, although this indication has not yet been validated *(37)*.

As Barrett's epithelium becomes dysplastic, the nucleus-to-cytoplasm ratio increases and number of goblet cells decreases. This change results in decreased absorption of MB among dysplastic or neoplastic cells. MB chromoendoscopy may therefore be undertaken not only to detect BE, but also to highlight regions of dysplasia or neoplasia within Barrett's mucosa (see Fig. 3). Patches of dysplastic or neoplastic Barrett's mucosa may stain less darkly and more heterogeneously than nondysplastic Barrett's mucosa *(34,35)*. This finding may provide improved sensitivity in detecting dysplasia or neoplasia during BE surveillance endoscopy.

3.3.2. IODINE

Iodine staining is based on a chemical reaction between iodine and glycogen *(38)*. The glycogen-rich prickle-cell layer of stratified squamous esophageal epithelium stains brown after application of a 1.5–3% potassium iodide solution or Lugol's iodine. Dysplastic epithelium lacks the glycogen-rich granules in the prickle-cell layer and therefore fails to stain. The brown staining of normal squamous cells may not be complete, but the endoscopist can take biopsies targeted from the least-stained regions. Iodine chromoendoscopy can detect early squamous cell carcinoma in the esophagus that might otherwise go undetected by conventional endoscopy *(13,14,38)*. Iodine chromoendoscopy can also be helpful in defining the extent of an esophageal squamous cell carcinoma or in better defining the gastroesophageal junction. Patients may experience heartburn, tingling, or nausea; the technique should be avoided in those with an allergy to iodine.

3.3.3. COMBINATIONS OF DYES

Investigators occasionally use two different stains sequentially to create a double contrast effect. For instance, indigo carmine has been used in conjunction with Lugol's iodine to better define the fine mucosal pattern of Barrett's epithelium *(27)*. Crystal violet (0.05%) and methylene blue have also been applied together to the esophageal lumen to define the mucosal glandular pattern of neoplastic lesions *(39)*. The clinical efficacy of double staining remains to be established.

4. ENDOSCOPIC ULTRASOUND

Endoscopic ultrasound (EUS) is currently one of the most accurate methods for T- and N-staging of esophageal malignancies *(40)*. However, it also has a role in evaluating high-grade dysplasia or intramucosal carcinoma. Unsuspected submucosal invasion or lymph node involvement may be present in up to 23% of these patients *(41)*. EUS should therefore be performed for patients prior to undergoing nonsurgical management of high-grade dysplasia or intramucosal carcinoma. Particularly useful in this setting are small ultrasound probes, 2–3 mm in diameter, passed through the accessory channel of an endoscope. These probes obtain sonographic images at 12–30 MHz, revealing the particular depth of involvement of a lesion within the esophageal wall. Any involvement of the submucosa should preclude endoscopic ablation or EMR *(42,43)*. Lower ultrasound frequencies such as 7.5 MHz are required to visualize paraesophageal and celiac axis lymph nodes.

5. EMERGING TECHNIQUES

Currently, identification of dysplastic or neoplastic epithelium depends on histologic interpretation of a biopsy specimen by a pathologist. Unfortunately, since normal-appearing epithelium may still harbor dysplasia,

"blind" biopsy protocols are still the most common method of tissue sampling during surveillance endoscopies. Yet even the widely advocated systematic use of jumbo biopsy forceps can miss adenocarcinoma in the setting of BE *(44)*. Furthermore, significant interobserver variation exists among pathologists classifying degrees of dysplasia within histologic BE specimens *(45–47)*. This has led investigators to search for new methods to identify dysplasia and neoplasia that are independent of tissue processing and histologic interpretation. Optical coherence tomography (OCT), spectroscopy, and confocal microscopy are three such techniques providing information about tissue using optical techniques without the need of a biopsy.

5.1. OCT

Similar in imaging to ultrasound, OCT uses infrared light waves instead of sound waves to focus into the tissue. A principle known as interferometry measures the time delay between light leaving the imaging source and light returning from the tissue. This is accomplished by having a beam of incident light split into two. Half the beam travels to the target tissue while the other half travels to a moving reference mirror. The light reflecting back from both tissue and mirror is then analyzed. When light reflecting from within the tissue returns to a detector at the same time as light from the mirror, interference is generated. This interference represents the presence of a reflective structure within the tissue; knowing the mirror position, the depth of this structure can be determined and mapped. An optical beam scans across the tissue surface and as light reflects back, a two-dimensional image of the tissue architecture with approximately 10 µm resolution is obtained *(48)*.

OCT has been used to demonstrate tissue architecture within the gastrointestinal tract and can be performed with special probes passed through the accessory channel of a standard endoscope (Fig. 4) *(49–54)*. OCT can distinguish layers of the gastrointestinal wall in a similar manner to high-frequency ultrasound, with a resolution of 10 µm. Current OCT systems can accurately detect specialized intestinal metaplasia seen in BE *(50,55)*, and newer systems with 1µm resolution are being evaluated *(56)*.

5.2. Spectroscopy

Spectroscopy is the study of interactions between light and matter. Several forms of spectroscopy exist and represent the analysis of various fates of photons of light. When a photon strikes the surface of the gastrointestinal

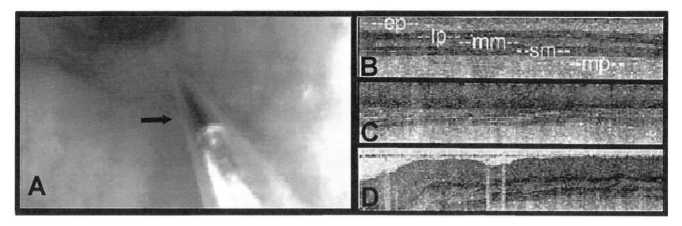

Fig. 4. OCT. **A.** An OCT probe (arrow) is shown protruding from the accessory channel of an endoscope during upper endoscopy. **B–D.** OCT images of normal esophageal mucosa. With a resolution of 10 microns, the various histologic layers of the esophageal wall are visualized. ep = epithelial surface; lp = lamina propria; mm = muscularis mucosa; sm = submucosa; mp = muscularis propria.

lumen, it can be absorbed or reflected by the tissue. Some of the light undergoes scattering within the tissue prior to being reflected. The degree of scattering depends on the density and size of space-occupying structures such as nuclei, connective tissue fibers, and mitochondria in the epithelium being illuminated. Scattering occurs when photons of light bounce off and pass through these structures. Studying bulk scattering components of reflected light provides information about the presence of large objects like collagen within the lamina propria or submucosa. This bulk scattering information combined with observed absorbance of specific wavelengths is the basis for reflectance spectroscopy and provides insight into the structural and biochemical composition of a particular tissue. For instance, reflectance spectroscopy can distinguish dysplastic from nondysplastic Barrett's epithelium *(57)*. Analysis of minute scattering events, representing measures of nuclear crowding and size, can be done after subtracting out bulk scattering followed by mathematical modeling *(58)*. This is the basis of light-scattering spectroscopy, a technique that has also been applied in the setting of BE *(57,59)*.

Finally, some photons of light excite tissue fluorophores, biochemical structures that emit longer wavelengths of light when excited by specific incident wavelengths of light. This is the basis of fluorescence spectroscopy.

5.2.1. FLUORESCENCE SPECTROSCOPY

Laser-induced fluorescence (LIF) spectroscopy occurs when laser light is used to excite tissue fluorophores. Laser light of one or various frequencies can

be directed onto a tissue surface; the resulting fluorescence can be analyzed as it is emitted from the tissue. Dysplastic epithelium fluoresces with a different intensity than nondysplastic epithelium, thereby providing a method for distinguishing these two entities (Fig. 5). Fluorophores that have proven particularly useful for distinguishing dysplastic and nondysplastic epithelium include collagen and NADH *(60,61)*. LIF can be conducted with the use of a specialized light-delivery probe that can pass through the accessory channel of a standard endoscope *(62)*. This form of LIF has been used to distinguish dysplastic from nondysplastic Barrett's mucosa *(57,63)* and esophageal carcinoma from normal esophagus *(64)*.

LIF methods require a "point-by-point" sampling of the mucosa with a fiber probe and to date have not provided real-time results. Another technique, laser-induced fluorescence endoscopy (LIFE), represents a true imaging method that allows the endoscopist to see tissue fluorescence during endoscopy. In LIFE, excitation and emission wavelengths travel through the light bundle of an endoscope instead of through a small fiber probe. The endoscopist can therefore shine specific wavelengths of light on a large region of tissue and visualize the fluorescence from the mucosa. Focal areas of dysplasia fluoresce differently than their surroundings and therefore appear visible *(65–67)*. LIFE has been used in the gastrointestinal tract to detect foci of high-grade dysplasia in BE, gastric adenocarcinoma, and flat colonic adenomas *(67)*. Various investigators have also administered exogenous fluorophores such as 5-aminolevulinic acid to enhance tissue fluorescence *(67–71)*.

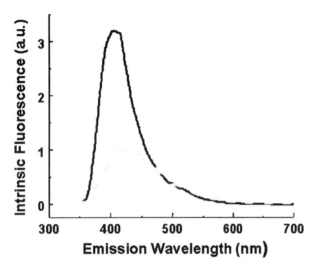

Fig. 5. Laser-induced fluorescence spectroscopy. The fluorescence intensities of various emission wavelengths resulting from the excitation of tissue during upper endoscopy with 337 nm light. The fluorescence of nondysplastic BE epithelium seen at 420 nm (—) is three times greater than that observed for Barrett's epithelium with high-grade dysplasia (- - -). Courtesy of Irene Georgakoudi, Massachusetts Institute of Technology, Cambridge, MA.

5.3. Confocal Endoscopy

Laser-scanning confocal microscopy (LCM) is an emerging technique using an argon beam directed at tissue sections *ex vivo (72)*. Light reflected from the tissue is used to create an image similar to that seen with standard histologic methods. LCM therefore provides a virtual histologic picture. The depth of laser light into the tissue is approximately 200–500 μm; resolution is similar to that seen in a × 500 light-microscopic image. LCM is currently being miniaturized for use with probes that can pass through the accessory channel of an endoscope. Ultimately this will allow an endoscopist to obtain a virtual biopsy without the need for tissue disruption.

REFERENCES

1. Modlin IM. *A Brief History of Endoscopy.* MultiMed, Milan; 2000.
2. Spechler SJ, Goyal RK. Barrett's esophagus. *N Engl J Med* 1986;315:362–371.
3. Blot WJ, Devesa SS, Kneller RW, Fraumeni JF Jr. Rising incidence of adenocarcinoma of the esophagus and gastric cardia. *JAMA* 1991;265:1287–1289.
4. Cameron A, Ott B, Payne W. The incidence of adenocarcinoma in columnar-lined (Barrett's) esophagus. *N Engl J Med* 1985; 313:857–859.
5. Shaheen N, Crosby M, Bozymski E, Sandler R. Is there publication bias in the reporting of cancer risk in Barrett's esophagus? *Gastroenterology* 2000;119:333–338.
6. Winters C, Spurling TJ, Cohbanian SJ, et al. Barrett's esophagus: a prevalent, occult complication of gastroesophageal reflux disease. *Gastroenterology* 1987;92:118–124.
7. Cameron A. Epidemiology of columnar-lined esophagus and adenocarcinoma. *Gastroenterol Clin North Am* 1997;26: 487–494.
8. Cameron AJ, Zinsmeister AR, Ballard DJ, Carney JA. Prevalence of columnar-lined (Barrett's) esophagus: comparison of population-based and autopsy findings. *Gastroenterology* 1990;99:918–922.
9. Reid BJ, Weinstein WM, Lewin KJ, et al. Endoscopic biopsy can detect high-grade dysplasia or early adenocarcinoma in Barrett's esophagus without grossly recognizable neoplastic lesions. *Gastroenterology* 1988;94:81–90.
10. Levine DS, Haggitt RC, Blount PL, et al. An endoscopic biopsy protocol can differentiate high-grade dysplasia from early adenocarcinoma in Barrett's esophagus. *Gastroenterology* 1993;105:40–50.
11. Sampliner RE and The Practice Parameters Committee of the American College of Gastroenterology. Practice guidelines on the diagnosis, surveillance, and therapy of Barrett's esophagus. *Am J Gastroenterol* 1998;93: 1028–1032.
12. Riddell RH. Early detection of neoplasia of the esophagus and gastroesophageal junction. *Am J Gastroenterol* 1996;91: 853–863.
13. Fagundes RB, de Barros SG, Putten AC, et al. Occult dysplasia is disclosed by Lugol chromoendoscopy in alcoholics at high risk for squamous cell carcinoma of the esophagus. *Endoscopy* 1999;31:281–285.
14. Shimizu Y, Tukagoshi H, Fujita M, et al. Endoscopic screening for early esophageal cancer by iodine staining in patients with other current or prior primary cancers. *Gastrointest Endosc* 2001;53:1–5.
15. Faigel DO, Eisen GM, Baron TH, et al. Tissue sampling and analysis. *Gastrointest Endosc* 2003;57:811–816.
16. Levine D, Blount P, Rudolf R, Reid B. Safety of a systemic endoscopic biopsy protocol in patients with Barrett's esophagus. *Am J Gastroenterol* 2000;95:1152–1157.
17. Weinstein W. Mucosal biopsy techniques and interaction with the pathologist. *Gastrointest Endosc Clin N Am* 2000;10:555–572.
18. Bernstein D, Barkin J, Reiner D, et al. Standard biopsy forceps vs large-capacity forceps with and without needle. *Gastrointest Endosc* 1995;41:573–576.
19. Woods K, Anand B, Cole R, et al. Influence of endoscopic biopsy forceps characteristics on tissue specimens: results of a prospective randomized study. *Gastrointest Endosc* 1999;49:177–183.
20. Ladas S, Tsamouri M, Kouvidou C, Raptis S. Effect of forceps size and mode of orientation on endoscopic small bowel biopsy evaluation. *Gastrointest Endosc* 1994;40: 51–55.
21. Soetikno R, Inoue H, Chang K. Endoscopic mucosal resection: current concepts. *Gastrointest Endosc Clin N Am* 2000;10:595–617.
22. Inoue H, Takeshita K, Hori H, et al. Endoscopic mucosal resection with a cap-fitted panendoscope for esophagus, stomach, and colon mucosal lesions. *Gastrointest Endosc* 1993;39:58–62.
23. Kojima T, Parra-Blanco A, Takahashi H, Fujita R. Outcome of endoscopic mucosal resection for early gastric cancer: review of the Japanese literature. *Gastrointest Endosc* 1998;48:550–554.

24. Nelson DB, Block KP, Bosco JJ, et al. Technology status evaluation report. High resolution and high-magnification endoscopy. *Gastrointest Endosc* 2000;52: 864–866.

25. Fleischer DE. Chromoendoscopy and magnification endoscopy in the colon. *Gastrointest Endosc* 1999;49: S45–S49.

26. Axelrad AM, Fleischer DE, Geller AJ, et al. High-resolution chromoendoscopy for the diagnosis of diminutive colon polyps: implications for colon cancer screening. *Gastroenterology* 1996;110:1253–1258.

27. Stevens PD, Lightdale CJ, Green PH, et al. Combined magnification endoscopy with chromoendoscopy for the evaluation of Barrett's esophagus. *Gastrointest Endosc* 1994;40:747–749.

28. Kiesslich R, Hahn M, Herrmann G, Jung M. Screening for specialized columnar epithelium with methylene blue: chromoendoscopy in patients with Barrett's esophagus and a normal control group. *Gastrointest Endosc* 2001;53: 47–52.

29. Siegel LM, Stevens PD, Lightdale CJ, et al. Combined magnification endoscopy with chromoendoscopy in the evaluation of patients with suspected malabsorption. *Gastrointest Endosc* 1997;46:226–230.

30. Takayama T, Katsuki S, Takahashi Y, et al. Aberrant crypt foci of the colon as precursors of adenoma and cancer. *N Engl J Med* 1998;339:1277–1284.

31. Guelrud M, Herrera I. Acetic acid improves identification of remnant islands of Barrett's epithelium after endoscopic therapy. *Gastrointest Endosc* 1998;47:512–515.

32. Guelrud M, Herrera I, Essenfeld H, Castro J. Enhanced magnification endoscopy: a new technique to identify specialized intestinal metaplasia in Barrett's esophagus. *Gastrointest Endosc* 2001;53:559–565.

33. Canto MI, Setrakian S, Petras R, et al. Methylene blue selectively stains intestinal metaplasia in Barrett's esophagus. *Gastrointest Endosc* 1996;44:1–7.

34. Canto MI, Setrakian S, Willis J, et al. Methylene blue-directed biopsies improve detection of intestinal metaplasia and dysplasia in Barrett's esophagus. *Gastrointest Endosc* 2000;51:560–568.

35. Canto MI, Setrakian S, Willis JE, et al. Methylene blue staining of dysplastic and nondysplastic Barrett's esophagus: an in vivo and ex vivo study. *Endoscopy* 2001;33:391–400.

36. Sharma P, Topalovski M, Mayo MS, Weston AP. Methylene blue chromoendoscopy for detection of short-segment Barrett's esophagus. *Gastrointest Endosc* 2001;54:289–293.

37. Wo JM, Ray MB, Mayfield-Stokes S, et al. Comparison of methylene blue-directed biopsies and conventional biopsies in the detection of intestinal metaplasia and dysplasia in Barrett's esophagus: a preliminary study. *Gastrointest Endosc* 2001;54:294–301.

38. Inoue H, Rey JF, Lightdale C. Lugol chromoendoscopy for esophageal squamous cell cancer. *Endoscopy* 2001;33:75–79.

39. Tabuchi M, Sueoka N, Fujimori T. Videoendoscopy with vital double dye staining (crystal violet and methylene blue) for detection of a minute focus of early stage adenocarcinoma in Barrett's esophagus: a case report. *Gastrointest Endosc* 2001;54:385–388.

40. Van Dam J, Brugge W. Endoscopy of the upper gastrointestinal tract. *N Engl J Med* 1999;341:1738–1747.

41. Scotiniotis I, Kochman M, Lewis J, et al. Accuracy of EUS in the evaluation of Barrett's esophagus and high-grade dysplasia or intramucosal carcinoma. *Gastrointest Endosc* 2001;54:689–696.

42. Murata Y, Suzuki S, Ohta M, et al. Small ultrasonic probes for determination of the depth of superficial esophageal cancer. *Gastrointest Endosc* 1996;44:23–28.

43. Waxman I, Saitoh Y. Clinical outcome of endoscopic mucosal resection for superficial GI lesions and the role of high-frequency US probe sonography in an American population. *Gastrointest Endosc* 2000;52:322–327.

44. Falk G, Rice T, Goldblum J, Richter J. Jumbo biopsy forceps protocol still misses unsuspected cancer in Barrett's esophagus with high-grade dysplasia. *Gastrointest Endosc* 1999;49:170–176.

45. Alikhan M, Rex D, Khan A, et al. Variable pathologic interpretation of columnar lined esophagus by general pathologists in community practice. *Gastrointest Endosc* 1999;50: 23–26.

46. Montgomery E, Bronner M, Goldblum J, et al. Reproducibility of the diagnosis of dysplasia in Barrett's esophagus: a reaffirmation. *Hum Pathol* 2001;32:368–378.

47. Reid B, Haggitt R, Rubin C, et al. Observer variation in the diagnosis of dysplasia in Barrett's esophagus. *Hum Pathol* 1988;9:166–178.

48. Jacobson BC, Van Dam J. Enhanced endoscopy in inflammatory bowel disease. *Gastrointest Endosc Clin N Am* 2002;12:573–578.

49. Bouma BE, Tearney GJ, Compton CC, Nishioka NS. High-resolution imaging of the human esophagus and stomach in vivo using optical coherence tomography. *Gastrointest Endosc* 2000;51:467–474.

50. Jäckle S, Gladkova N, Feldchtein F, et al. In vivo endoscopic optical coherence tomography of esophagitis, Barrett's esophagus, and adenocarcinoma of the esophagus. *Endoscopy* 2000;32:750–755.

51. Sivak MV Jr, Kobayashi K, Izatt JA, et al. High-resolution endoscopic imaging of the GI tract using optical coherence tomography. *Gastrointest Endosc* 2000;51:474–479.

52. Tearney G, Brezinski M, Bouma B, et al. In vivo endoscopic optical biopsy with optical coherence tomography. *Science* 1997;276:2037–2039.

53. Tearney GJ, Brezinski ME, Southern JF, et al. Optical biopsy in human gastrointestinal tissue using optical coherence tomography. *Am J Gastroenterol* 1997;92:1800–1804.

54. Zuccaro G, Gladkova N, Vargo J, et al. Optical coherence tomography of the esophagus and proximal stomach in health and disease. *Am J Gastroenterol* 2001;96: 2633–2639.

55. Poneros J, Brand S, Bouma B, et al. Diagnosis of specialized intestinal metaplasia by optical coherence tomography. *Gastroenterology* 2001;120:7–12.

56. Li X, Boppart S, Van Dam J, et al. Optical coherence tomography: advanced technology for the endoscopic imaging of Barrett's esophagus. *Endoscopy* 2000;32:921–930.

57. Georgakoudi I, Jacobson BC, Van Dam J, et al. Fluorescence, reflectance, and light-scattering spectroscopy for evaluating dysplasia in patients with Barrett's esophagus. *Gastroenterology* 2001;120:1620–1629.

58. Backman V, Wallace M, Perelman L, et al. Detection of preinvasive cancer cells: early warning changes in precancerous epithelial cells can now be spotted *in situ. Nature* 2000;406:35–36.

59. Wallace M, Perelman L, Backman V, et al. Endoscopic detection of dysplasia in patients with Barrett's esophagus using light-scattering spectroscopy. *Gastroenterology* 2000; 119:677–682.

60. Georgakoudi I, Jacobson B, Muller M, et al. NAD(P)H and collagen as in vivo quantitative fluorescent biomarkers of epithelial precancerous changes. *Cancer Res* 2002;62: 682–687.

61. Römer T, Fitzmaurice M, Cothren R, et al. Laser-induced fluorescence microscopy of normal colon and dysplasia in colonic adenomas: implications for spectroscopic diagnosis. *Am J Gastroenterol* 1995;90:81–87.

62. Cothren R, Richards-Kortum R, Sivak M, et al. Gastro-intestinal tissue diagnosis by laser-induced fluorescence spectroscopy at endoscopy. *Gastrointest Endosc* 1990;36: 105–111.

63. Panjehpour M, Overholt B, Vo-Dinh T, et al. Endoscopic fluorescence detection of high-grade dysplasia in Barrett's esophagus. *Gastroenterology* 1996;111:93–101.

64. Panjehpour M, Overholt B, Schmidhammer J, et al. Spectroscopic diagnosis of esophageal cancer: new classification model, improved measurement system. *Gastrointest Endosc* 1995;41:577–581.

65. Zeng H, Weiss A, Cline R, MacAulay C. Real-time endoscopic fluorescence imaging for early cancer detection in the gastrointestinal tract. *Bioimaging* 1998;6:151–165.

66. Wang T, Crawford J, Feld M, et al. In vivo identification of colonic dysplasia using fluorescence endoscopic imaging. *Gastrointest Endosc* 1999;49:447–455.

67. Haringsma J, Tytgat G, Yano H, et al. Autofluorescence endoscopy: feasibility of detection of GI neoplasms unapparent to white light endoscopy with an evolving technology. *Gastrointest Endosc* 2001;53:642–650.

68. Messmann H, Knüchel R, Bäumler W, et al. Endoscopic fluorescence detection of dysplasia in patients with Barrett's esophagus, ulcerative colitis, or adenomatous polyps after 5-aminolevulinic acid-induced protoporphyrin IX sensitization. *Gastrointest Endosc* 1999;49:97–101.

69. Messmann H, Kullmann F, Wild T, et al. Detection of dysplastic lesions by fluorescence in a model of colitis in rats after previous photosensitization with 5-aminolaevulinic acid. *Endoscopy* 1998;30:333–338.

70. Staël von Holstein C, Nilsson A, Andersson-Engels S, et al. Detection of adenocarcinoma in Barrett's oesophagus by means of laser induced fluorescence. *Gut* 1996;39: 711–716.

71. Tajiri H, Yokoyama K, Boku N, et al. Fluorescent diagnosis of experimental gastric cancer using a tumor-localizing photosensitizer. *Cancer Lett* 1997;111:215–220.

72. Inoue H, Igari T, Nishikage T, et al. A novel method of virtual histopathology using laser-scanning confocal microscopy in-vitro with untreated fresh specimens from the gastrointestinal mucosa. *Endoscopy* 2000;32:439–443.

27 Chemoprevention Strategies for Esophageal Squamous Cell Carcinoma

Paul J. Limburg, MD, MPH, Philip R. Taylor, MD, ScD, and Sanford M. Dawsey, MD

CONTENTS

1. INTRODUCTION

Esophageal cancer is the eighth most common form of malignant disease in the world, and squamous cell carcinoma is the predominant histologic subtype *(1–3)*. Esophageal squamous cell carcinoma (ESC) typically remains asymptomatic until the tumor reaches an advanced stage. Thus, patients often present with incurable disease, which is reflected by the ESC 5-yr survival rate of approximately 10%. Early detection programs have been implemented in select high-risk populations. However, such initiatives have been only modestly successful, primarily because an effective, affordable, and acceptable screening technique is not currently available. Existing data from a variety of sources suggest that chemoprevention may represent a viable approach to ESC prevention. In this chapter, current concepts regarding the key aspects of ESC chemoprevention are reviewed. Risk stratification and biomarker selection are discussed initially, followed by a more comprehensive overview of promising candidate agents for future ESC chemoprevention trials.

2. RISK STRATIFICATION

ESC incidence rates differ by more than 100-fold across global regions. High-risk areas include north central China, northeastern Iran, northeastern India, southern Brazil, and southeastern South Africa, where annual incidence rates can exceed 100 cases per 100,000 population *(4–8)*. Typically, ESC incidence rates are higher among men than among women, although minimal gender differences have been observed in some high-risk populations. In the United States, overall age-adjusted incidence rates are 2.2 and 0.9 cases per 100,000 population for men and women, respectively *(2)*; however, rates vary up to four- to fivefold by race/ethnicity. African Americans experience higher incidence rates, as well as lower 5-yr survival rates, than other racial/ethnic subgroups; these rates may relate to culturally mediated differences in environmental exposures *(9)*. Lower socioeconomic status has also been linked to increased ESC risk in both developed and underdeveloped societies *(9–11)*. In aggregate, these observations suggest that exogenous agents likely play a prominent role in esophageal squamous carcinogenesis. In addition, a limited number of host conditions have been associated with increased ESC risk. However, the utility of applying these risk factors to cohort selection for ESC chemoprevention trials remains to be determined.

2.1. Environmental Exposures

2.1.1. ALCOHOL AND TOBACCO

Cigarette smoking and alcohol consumption are the most consistent and important environmental risk factors

From: Cancer Chemoprevention, Volume 2: Strategies for Cancer Chemoprevention
Edited by: G. J. Kelloff, E. T. Hawk, and C. C. Sigman © Humana Press Inc., Totowa, NJ

for ESC in Western countries. Many epidemiological studies in Europe and the Americas have shown significant associations and strong dose-response relationships between these two exposures and the risk of ESC (12–16). Studies evaluating both factors have shown that the risks associated with tobacco and alcohol are independent and multiplicative (12–14,16) and, for men, attributable risks for one or both of these habits are estimated to be >90% (9,14). Studies of effects of different kinds of tobacco (dark or blond) or alcohol (spirits, wine, or beer) suggest greater risks for consumption of dark tobacco and distilled spirits (14,16). Several studies have shown that stopping tobacco and alcohol use significantly reduces ESC risk, with risks approaching those of nonusers after 10 or more years (16–18).

Most epidemiological studies in high-risk rural populations in China and central Asia have not shown strong associations between tobacco or alcohol consumption and ESC risk (4,19–21), possibly because many of these populations use or consume relatively little tobacco and alcohol. Indeed, though women in these societies are essentially not exposed to these agents, their ESC rates are similar to those of men. However, residents of these regions may be exposed to some of the major carcinogens in tobacco and alcohol (such as polycyclic aromatic hydrocarbons, or PAHs, and nitrosamines) in other ways, including eating pyrolysis residues from opium or tobacco pipes (22) and consuming foods with high levels of PAHs (23) and food and water with high levels of nitrosamines and nitrates (24). In contrast, studies in lower-risk urban China (where tobacco and alcohol consumption is higher) have found statistically significant associations between these lifestyle habits and ESC risk (25,26). Thus, in developed or "Westernized" populations, cigarette smoking and alcohol consumption represent important ESC risk factors and may form useful stratification criteria for chemoprevention trials.

2.1.2. Diet and Nutrition

A number of dietary components have been associated with ESC risk, at least in select populations. Early studies from China reported positive associations between ESC risk and consumption of pickled vegetables or moldy foods. These popular food items were subsequently found to contain high levels of nitrosamines and/or fungal contamination (27,28). Local public health education programs effectively reduced the ingestion of pickled vegetables and moldy foods in some areas. Accordingly, more recent studies have

observed less striking risk associations in these geographic regions (4,21). Residents of southern Brazil and neighboring countries often consume maté, an infusion of the herb *Ilex paraguayensis*, in large quantity (about 1 L/d). In a combined analysis of five case-control studies coordinated by the International Agency for Research on Cancer (IARC), ESC risks reportedly increased with the amount and temperature of ingested maté. Moreover, these risk associations were independent and multiplicative (8). Ecologic studies in South Africa and China have suggested that consumption of fumonisin-contaminated corn may be associated with esophageal squamous carcinogenesis (29). Fumonisins are toxins produced by *Fusarium verticillioides* (formerly *Fusarium moniliforme*), a fungus that commonly grows on corn. These fungal toxins disrupt sphingolipid metabolism, and they have been shown to cause several diseases in animals, including liver cancer in rats (30). Only one human study has evaluated the relationship of individual exposure to fumonisins and development of ESC. This prospective nested case-control study in a high-risk Chinese population found no association between serum sphingolipid levels (as biomarkers of fumonisins) and ESC risk (31).

Nitrosamines are potentially important esophageal carcinogens in both low- and high-risk populations. Among low-risk populations, the probable major route of exposure is cigarette smoke, which contains preformed nitrosamines. Among high-risk populations (wherein smoking is less common), a variety of possible sources may be important, including pickled vegetables, moldy foods, and contaminated drinking water (27). Poor oral health, which can alter the usual bacterial flora, may also increase upper gastrointestinal nitrosamine exposure (32). As mentioned above (*see* Section 2.1.1.), PAHs can be found in both tobacco smoke and alcohol. In Linxian, China, cooking methods (burning smoky coal in unvented stoves) also likely contribute to PAH exposure, as evidenced by the high PAH levels found in food samples from this high-risk region (23).

Physical irritants have been linked to increased ESC risk as well, although the available data are somewhat controversial. Hot liquids (regardless of beverage type) have been positively associated with ESC in a number of studies from high-risk regions (8,25,33–35), but no significant association was observed in a recent case-control study from Sweden (36). Silica fragments have been found in staple foods from select areas of China, Iran, and South Africa. Such fragments could increase ESC risk by causing repeated trauma or by stimulating excess proliferation in the esophageal mucosa *(37)*.

Limited exposure to potentially anticarcinogenic compounds has also been hypothesized as a modulator of ESC risk. For example, low fruit and vegetable intakes have been consistently associated with increased ESC risk *(8,19,25,26,36,38–40)*. However, the precise micronutrient(s) involved in this process remain incompletely defined. Dietary factors that may afford ESC chemopreventive benefits are discussed separately (see Section 4).

2.1.3. INFECTIOUS AGENTS

To date, the only infectious agent that has been rigorously evaluated in the context of ESC risk is human papillomavirus (HPV). A possible association between HPV and ESC was first proposed by Syrjanen in 1982, based on his observation of koilocytosis in the esophageal epithelia of patients with ESC that was morphologically similar to that seen in HPV-infected cervical epithelia *(41)*. This association has since been evaluated in both high- and low-risk populations using several different techniques. Three serologic studies found an increased risk for ESC in HPV16 seropositive individuals *(42–44)*. However, a fourth study (which included the largest sample size and most extensive consideration of potential confounders) reported no appreciable association *(45)*. Studies examining ESC tumor tissue for HPV (either by immunohistochemistry, *in situ* hybridization, or PCR) have also yielded conflicting results. Among high-risk populations, most recent PCR-based investigations have found evidence of HPV in a minority of tumor specimens (usually around 20%; occasional reports up to 60%) *(46–48)*, while similar studies from low-risk populations have found essentially no evidence of HPV involvement (0–4%) *(49–51)*. Only a few of these reports included evaluations of esophageal mucosa from non-cases, and none correlated serologic and tissue findings within the same individual. Nonetheless, Syrjanen recently proposed that existing data favor a possible etiologic role for HPV in esophageal squamous carcinogenesis *(52)*. Potential associations between ESC and Epstein-Barr virus (EBV), *Helicobacter pylori*, cytomegalovirus, and herpes simplex virus have not been fully explored, although scattered reports exist *(48,53,54)*.

2.1.4. OCCUPATIONAL EXPOSURES

Potential carcinogens in the workplace environment may come into direct contact with the esophageal mucosa through unintentional ingestion, deep inhalation, or a combination of both. Chemical compounds (such as organic solvents) and physical irritants (such as silica dust) have each been associated with increased esophageal cancer risk, although most early studies did not discriminate by histologic subtype. More recently, relatively high ESC mortality rates were observed among brick masons and stone masons, concrete and terrazzo finishers, roofers, and construction laborers. Higher-than-expected ESC mortality was further noted among janitors and cleaners, but to a lesser degree *(55)*. Specific agents, including sulfuric acid, carbon black, and PAHs, have been associated with increased ESC risks in recent case-control studies as well *(56,57)*. Although not definitive, these data support a possible causative link between occupational exposures and ESC. Further investigation is warranted to clarify the distribution and magnitude of job-related ESC risks.

2.1.5. OTHER FACTORS

Breast cancer radiotherapy and caustic substance ingestions have been associated with increased ESC risk after a decade or more from the time of initial exposure *(58–60)*. However, the fraction of ESC cases attributable to either of these exposures appears to be quite small. Thus, it seems unlikely that patients whose risk for ESC is defined solely by these risk factors would contribute meaningfully to the design of future chemoprevention trials.

2.2. Host Conditions

2.2.1. ACHALASIA

Achalasia is a motor disorder that affects smooth muscle fibers within the esophagus. Although epidemiological data are relatively limited, the global annual incidence rate is approximately 0.5 cases per 100,000 population *(61)*. ESC relative risk estimates range from 7 to 14.5 in the setting of longstanding achalasia (>15 yr), as compared to variably defined disease-free controls *(62,63)*. Mechanistically, achalasia is thought to induce carcinogenesis by causing prolonged intraluminal stasis, thereby allowing ingested toxicants to have greater contact time with the esophageal mucosa. Regular endoscopic surveillance to detect early signs of dysplasia has been recommended for achalasia patients *(63)*, which may afford the opportunity to conduct chemopreventive interventions in this high-risk population, at least at select referral centers.

2.2.2. CELIAC SPRUE

Also known as gluten-sensitive enteropathy, celiac sprue is a chronic inflammatory condition that affects small-bowel absorption in up to 1 in 250 persons in the

United States *(64)*. Symptoms may either present during childhood or later on in life. Among adults, typical manifestations of disease include diarrhea, weight loss, and iron-deficiency anemia. Patients with celiac sprue are known to be at markedly increased risk for small-bowel cancers (lymphoma and adenocarcinoma). Higher-than-expected ESC incidence rates have also been described *(65)*, but the relative rarity of these cancers makes celiac sprue an unlikely inclusion criterion for chemoprevention trials.

2.2.3. OTHER FACTORS

Focal nonepidermolytic palmoplantar keratoderma, otherwise know as tylosis, is associated with a 95% incidence of ESC by age 65 yr *(66)*. Although this condition has only been reported from three extended kindreds *(67)*, characterization of the "tylosis oesophageal cancer" *(TOC)* gene may provide novel insights regarding the molecular pathways involved in sporadic esophageal squamous carcinogenesis. Recent analyses suggest that the *TOC* gene is located on chromosome 17q25 *(68)*. Interestingly, loss of heterozygosity at microsatellite markers in close proximity to the proposed *TOC* locus has also been demonstrated in sporadic ESC *(69,70)*. Plummer-Vinson (or Patterson-Kelly) syndrome is characterized by dysphagia, glossitis, iron-deficiency anemia, and upper esophageal webs *(71)*. Approximately 10% of all patients with this syndrome develop upper aerodigestive tract malignancies, including ESC of the cervical esophagus *(72)*. For unknown reasons, incident cases of Plummer-Vinson syndrome seem to be on the decline *(73)*. A small number of case reports have described ESCs arising from esophageal diverticula, but a convincing risk association has yet to be demonstrated. Based on these data, tylosis, Plummer-Vinson syndrome, and esophageal diverticula appear to be of limited value for defining future ESC chemoprevention trial cohorts.

3. BIOMARKER SELECTION

3.1. Genetic Pathways

Although environmental factors appear to play the predominant role in the etiology of ESC, association *(74,75)*, familial aggregation *(76,77)*, cytogenetic *(78)*, and segregation analysis *(79)* studies all support a role for a Mendelian-transmitted gene in this malignancy. Identification of a major esophageal cancer susceptibility gene (or genes) may allow screening of populations in order to identify persons at particularly high risk who could then be targeted for chemoprevention trials or other

cancer prevention strategies. Similarly, an understanding of the molecular progression of esophageal cancer should permit targeting individuals with early molecular changes for chemoprevention. Regression (or lack of progression) of validated molecular markers following intervention could serve as a surrogate endpoint for establishing preliminary efficacy of candidate agents in short-term chemoprevention trials.

Loss of heterozygosity (LOH) indicates a region of genetic loss and may help to define potential loci for tumor suppressor genes *(80)*. Studies of allelic loss in ESC have shown generalized genetic instability with very high LOH throughout the genome, but with particularly high areas identified on chromosomes 13q, 9q, 9p, 5q, and 3p, as well as 17p *(81)*. Candidate tumor suppressor genes have been evaluated on most of these chromosomal arms. On 13q, for example, mutations have been found in *BRCA2* (9% of cases) *(82)*, *RNF6* (13% of cases) *(83)*, and *DICE1* (5% of cases) *(84)*, but not in *ML-1 (83)*. *TP53* (on 17p) is the most frequently studied gene in ESC, and nearly all cases have some genetic alteration in or near the gene, including mutation in more than three quarters of those studied from one high-risk region of China *(85)*. Numerous other candidate loss-of-function genes have been studied for mutations in ESC, including *APC* (5q), *CDKN2A* (also known as p16, on 9p), *RB1* (13q), and *DCC* (18q), with either no or only rare positive findings except for *CDKN2A*, which is often mutated *(86)*.

Gain-of-function changes (usually amplifications) have also been seen in ESC for *MYC*, *EGFR*, *INT-2 HST-1*, and *Cyclin D1 (86)*. Taken together, the temporal sequence proposed by Montesano, et al. *(86)* suggests that there are early events (*TP53* mutations), intermediate events (3p and 9q allelic loss), and late events (*CDKN2A* mutations, allelic loss at multiple sites, and amplification of *Cyclin D1* and *EGFR*) in ESC. Analysis of DNA, RNA, or protein abnormalities reflective of these events, therefore, all become potential molecular markers that might be useful in future ESC chemoprevention trials. With the advent of expression array analyses and their application to ESC *(87)*, the list of potential molecular abnormalities associated with this malignancy will no doubt rapidly expand.

3.2. Squamous Dysplasia

Histologic precursor lesions represent strong candidate biomarkers because they are thought to occur along the progression pathway from normal epithelium to invasive cancer. In low-risk populations, squamous dysplasia (including carcinoma *in situ*) is the accepted histologic precursor of ESC, based on its established association with cancer in other target organs lined by squamous epithelium (such as the cervix and the metaplastic bronchus) and its common adjacency to invasive ESC in esophagectomy specimens *(88)*. In high-risk populations, squamous dysplasia is also accepted as a precursor lesion of ESC *(89–92)*. In addition, other histologic lesions, including chronic esophagitis, atrophy, and basal cell hyperplasia, have been proposed as potential intermediate biomarkers, based primarily on ecologic comparisons of their prevalence rates in high- vs low-risk populations *(89,91,93)*. These ecologic comparisons, however, have not always been consistent *(94)*. The only two prospective studies followed biopsied patients over time, finding that squamous dysplasia alone was significantly associated with incident ESC *(90,92)*. Moreover, ESC risks increased with advancing dysplasia grade *(92)*. Thus, squamous dysplasia is currently the only confirmed histologic precursor lesion of ESC in both high- and low-risk populations.

One fortunate attribute of esophageal squamous dysplasia is that it can usually be visualized endoscopically following application of Lugol's iodine solution (dysplastic lesions appear unstained). In one study of 225 patients from a high-risk population, this technique identified 63% of mild, 93% of moderate, and 96% of severe dysplasias *(95)*. The high sensitivity of Lugol-unstained areas for squamous dysplasia affords an excellent opportunity to perform longitudinal assessment of nonmanipulated precursor lesions in the context of ESC chemoprevention trials.

3.3. Proliferation and Apoptosis

Alterations in cell proliferation and cell death are important factors in carcinogenesis. Estimates of proliferation and apoptosis have been applied to many biomarker studies of neoplastic development in the squamous esophagus, including evaluations of normal epithelium, noninvasive lesions, and invasive ESCs. These markers have been used primarily to evaluate prognosis, likelihood of treatment response, or potential chemopreventive benefit(s). Several studies have observed a positive correlation between proliferation index and histologic progression *(96–100)*. One study further reported that apoptotic index correlates with squamous carcinogenesis *(100)*. However, clinical trials have yielded mixed results regarding the utility of these potential intermediate biomarkers *(101–107)*. Most notably, two intervention trials measuring proliferation from esophageal biopsy specimens found no significant change among the active- vs placebo-treated

groups after short-term supplementation with calcium *(91)* or multivitamins *(108)*, respectively.

3.4. DNA Methylation

Normal growth control mechanisms can be dysregulated through epigenetic alterations to cellular DNA. Promoter hypermethylation of the *CDKN2A, FHIT*, and E-cadherin genes has been observed in various ESC cell lines *(109–111)*. Tissue-based studies have further confirmed or identified hypermethylation of E-cadherin, *CDKN2A, NMES1*, and the HLA class I genes in tumor specimens vs normal mucosa from ESC patients *(111–113)*. In one small case series, *CDKN2A* promoter hypermethylation was detected in both tissue- and serum-derived DNA from a subset of ESC patients *(114)*. Although less thoroughly investigated to date, hypomethylated DNA also appears to be a risk marker for some target organ malignancies *(115–117)*. Thus, it seems plausible that endogenous or exogenous factors affecting methyl group bioavailability might be important modifiers of ESC risk. Indeed, higher folate intake was associated with a statistically significant 42% risk reduction in a US-based case-control study *(118)*. Further, among Chinese cases and controls, polymorphisms in the methylenetetrahydrofolate reductase gene (which encodes a key folate-metabolizing enzyme) reportedly influenced ESC risk *(119)*. Emerging data in this area of research may facilitate the design of future chemoprevention trials at multiple levels, including selection of novel risk, compliance, and/or effect biomarkers.

4. CANDIDATE AGENTS

Many diverse compounds have demonstrated potential ESC chemopreventive effects in cell culture experiments, animal model studies, and epidemiologic investigations. Relatively fewer data are available from randomized, controlled trials. Detailed discussions for several of the most promising candidate agents are presented below. Factors used to determine these candidates include reported degree of preliminary efficacy, consistency of results across studies, and observed safety profile.

4.1. Selenium

Selenium is necessary for the appropriate functioning of critical cellular enzymes, such as glutathione peroxidase. Existing laboratory data suggest that selenium may afford cancer prevention through multiple mechanisms, including decreased carcinogen activation, reduced proliferation, and increased apoptosis *(120)*.

Most animal studies have shown no beneficial effect from selenium supplementation on esophageal carcinogenesis (incidence of adenocarcinoma was actually increased in one rodent model) *(120–125)*. However, in a recent case-cohort study from Linxian, China, Mark et al. reported that ESC risk was reduced by 44% (RR = 0.56; 95% CI = 0.44–0.71) among subjects in the highest vs lowest serum selenium quartiles *(126)*.

To date, three large randomized, double-blind intervention trials have been completed that administered selenium alone or in combination with other nutritional agents and then assessed esophageal cancer endpoints, either in the primary or secondary analyses. In the US Nutritional Prevention of Cancer Study (n=1312), treatment with 200 μg/d of high-selenium yeast for a mean of 4.5 years was associated with 67% fewer incident esophageal cancers (RR = 0.33; 95% CI = 0.03–1.84), but too few cases (n = 8) were observed to allow for stratification by histologic subtype or to afford precise risk estimation *(127)*. Two other Phase III intervention trials have been performed in Linxian, China. In the General Population Trial (n = 29,584), after 5.25 yr, asymptomatic adults randomly assigned to receive selenium (50 μg/d), β-carotene (15 mg/d) and α-tocopherol (30 mg/d) had essentially the same ESC mortality rate as participants who did not receive these micronutrients (RR = 0.96; 95% CI = 0.78–1.18) *(128)*. Among a subset of trial participants who underwent end-of-trial endoscopy, prevalent ESCs were somewhat reduced (OR = 0.58; 95% CI = 0.19–1.76), but this finding was not statistically significant *(129)*. In the Dysplasia Trial conducted in this same geographic region, subjects with esophageal dysplasia diagnosed by balloon cytology at baseline (n = 3,318) were randomly assigned to receive a nutritional supplement (26 vitamins and minerals, including selenium at 50 μg/d) vs placebo. Subjects in the active-treated group had minimally reduced overall ESC incidence (RR = 0.94; 95% CI = 0.73–1.20) and mortality (RR = 0.84; 95% CI = 0.54–1.29) rates *(130)*. However, stratified analysis based on the initial degree of cytologic atypia revealed a 25% reduction in ESC mortality (RR = 0.75; 95% CI = 0.44–1.31) associated with the active agent among subjects who had low-grade dysplasia at baseline (Philip R. Taylor, National Cancer Institute, personal communication). Of note, because data from the Dysplasia Trial cannot be analyzed for individual micronutrients, the results observed in this study may not be directly attributable to selenium.

The inconclusive results regarding selenium's potential effect on ESC in China may be related to suboptimal dosing. As noted above, subjects in the United States Nutritional Prevention of Cancer study received 200 μg/d of selenium, a fourfold dose increase relative to the two Linxian intervention trials. More recently, a pilot study of selenium (200 μg/d) and celecoxib (200 mg twice per day) among Linxian residents with histologically mild or moderate esophageal squamous dysplasia was reported in abstract form. Using a 2×2 factorial design and a 10-mo intervention, the investigators found that selenium was associated with a statistically significant improvement in disease course among subjects with mild dyplasia at baseline (no appreciable chemopreventive effects were observed with celecoxib) *(131)*.

4.2. Nonsteroidal Antiinflammatory Drugs and Cyclooxygenase-2 Inhibitors

Many nonsteroidal antiinflammatory drugs (NSAIDs) have been investigated for their efficacy at preventing neoplasia in multiple target organs, including the esophagus. NSAIDs and their derivatives, the selective cyclooxygenase-2 (COX-2) inhibitors, can induce apoptosis in both ESC and adenocarcinoma cell lines *(132,133)*. Among laboratory animals, indomethacin has shown greater chemopreventive effects on upper gastrointestinal tract neoplasms than sulindac or piroxicam *(134–139)*. With respect to observational data, Gridley et al. initially described a modest, non-statistically significant increase in esophageal cancer risk (standardized incidence ratio (SIR) = 1.32; 95% CI = 0.7–2.4) among a Swedish cohort of rheumatoid arthritis patients, who presumably may have been regular NSAID users *(140)*. Thun et al. later reported a 41% reduction in esophageal cancer mortality (adjusted RR = 0.59; 95% CI = 0.34–1.03) associated with regular aspirin use, defined as ≥16 doses/month, in the American Cancer Society cohort *(141)*. More strikingly, Funkhouser and Sharp reported a 90% reduction in esophageal cancer incidence among occasional aspirin users in the National Health and Nutrition Examination Survey and the National Epidemiologic Follow-up Studies (rate ratio = 0.10; 95% CI = 0.01–0.76) *(142)*. However, this latter result was based on a loosely defined NSAID exposure variable and an admittedly small number of observed esophageal cancer cases (n = 15). The strongest epidemiologic data come from a well-designed, case-control study by Farrow and colleagues *(143)*, wherein the investigators distinguished not only between histologic subtypes of esophageal cancer, but also between users of aspirin and nonaspirin NSAIDs. After adjusting for known risk factors, decreased incidences for ESC were observed among both aspirin users (OR = 0.49; 95% CI = 0.28–0.87) and nonaspirin NSAID users (OR = 0.33; 95% CI = 0.13–0.84).

One concern for incorporating NSAIDs into chemoprevention trials has been their relatively high rate of associated adverse events. Potentially serious complications that include hemorrhagic peptic ulcers and nephrotoxicity reportedly occur in up to 3% of patients who take traditional NSAIDs regularly (144). The estimated cost associated with NSAID-related complications in the United States exceeds $2 billion annually (145). Newer agents, such as the COX-2 inhibitors, appear to retain the chemopreventive properties of traditional NSAIDs with a lower frequency of untoward effects. The only clinical trial data reported to date regarding NSAIDs or their derivatives as potential ESC chemopreventive agents are from the aforementioned 2×2 factorial pilot study of selenomethionine and celecoxib in Linxian, China (see Section 4.1) (131). As noted above, celecoxib administration for 10 mo at an intermediate dose (200 mg twice per day) had no appreciable chemopreventive effects among subjects with histologically mild or moderate dyplasia at baseline.

4.3. Retinoids

Retinoids, the derivatives and synthetic analogs of vitamin A, appear to afford cancer chemopreventive benefits through mechanisms mediated by the activation of at least six nuclear receptors (146). Retinoids have been reported to reduce the risk of several premalignant aerodigestive tract lesions, including oral leukoplakia, laryngeal papillomatosis, and bronchial metaplasia, as well as squamous carcinomas in other target organs such as the skin and uterine cervix (147). However, the potential effects of retinoids on ESC remain indeterminate. Preclinical studies have shown favorable effects in both cell culture and animal model systems (148 151). Primary analyses from a 13.5-mo randomized intervention trial of 610 Chinese subjects showed no difference in the prevalence of histologic esophageal lesions (esophagitis, atrophy, dysplasia, or cancer) among those taking retinol (15 mg), riboflavin (200 mg), and zinc (50 mg) once per week vs those receiving placebo (152). Yet, based on secondary analyses, subjects with large increases in blood retinol, riboflavin, and zinc levels were more likely to have histologically normal esophageal mucosa at the end of the trial (153). Lin and colleagues noted an impressive 43.2% reduction in "cancerization rate" (not further defined) with escalating 4-ethoxycarbophenylretinamide doses (maximum 100 mg/d), given to more than 500 subjects with marked

esophageal dysplasia for a period of 5 yr (154). These results must be interpreted with caution, however, since eligibility criteria and outcome measures were based solely on nonstandard cytologic criteria rather than histology, and bioavailability of the nonstandardized intervention agent is unknown.

In the Linxian General Population Intervention Trial, combined effects of retinol (5,000 IU/d of natural vitamin A as palmitate) and zinc (22.5 mg/d) minimally influenced overall mortality (RR = 1.0; 95% CI = 0.92–1.09), cancer mortality (RR = 0.97; 95% CI = 0.85–1.12), and esophageal cancer mortality (RR = 0.93; 95% CI = 0.76–1.15) (128). In the associated end-of-trial endoscopy survey, no beneficial effects on the prevalence of esophageal dysplasia (OR = 1.12; 95% CI = 0.57–2.20) or ESC (OR = 1.02; 95% CI = 0.36–2.91) were observed in this treatment group (129). Subjects in the Dysplasia Trial who received the multinutrient supplement (including 10,000 IU of vitamin A as acetate as well as 25 other vitamins and minerals) experienced slight overall reductions in ESC incidence (OR = 0.94; 95% CI = 0.73–1.20) and mortality (OR = 0.84; 95% CI = 0.54–1.29) (130). However, as noted above (see Section 4.1), these results were not statistically significant and cannot be attributed to any single agent.

The available evidence pertaining to ESC chemoprevention with retinoids can be interpreted as mildly encouraging. Newer synthetic retinoids may have improved safety profiles (155), which would enhance their appeal for long-term use in generally healthy populations. Development of novel retinoid delivery systems with enhanced topical application and agents that may affect downstream targets of activated retinoid receptors represent additional areas of ongoing investigation.

4.4. Curcumin

Difcruloylmethane, or curcumin, is a dietary phytopolyphenol found in turmeric, curry, and mustard. This compound has a wide spectrum of biological effects, including antithrombosis, antimutagenesis, and antioxidation (156). In addition, curcumin has both antiinflammatory and antiangiogenic properties (157–159), which may be more relevant to its potential role as a cancer chemopreventive agent. Among carcinogen-induced rats, the tumor-inhibitory effects of curcumin seem to be maintained when the agent is given either at the time of initiation or during the post-initiation phase (160). Due to the relatively recent recognition of curcumin's anticancer potential, human observational and interventional data are currently limited. In two Phase I clinical trials reported to date, curcumin has been well tolerated at doses up to 8000 mg/d among patients with premalignant and malignant gastrointestinal lesions *(161, 162)*. Thus, further investigation of curcumin as an ESC chemopreventive agent appears warranted.

4.5. Diflouromethylornithine

Diflouromethylornithine (DFMO) irreversibly inhibits ornithine decarboxylase, which appears to be a critical enzyme for neoplasia initiation and progression. The chemopreventive effects of DFMO are thought to result from the depletion of cellular polyamine concentrations, with consequent decelerations in DNA replication, protein synthesis, and cell growth *(163,164)*. Supportive experimental data for DFMO chemoprevention include decreased proliferation and increased apoptosis among zinc-deficient rodents at risk for esophageal cancer *(165,166)*. In humans, DFMO has been investigated as a chemopreventive agent for colorectal cancer *(167–169)*, as well as non-esophageal squamous cancers *(170–172)*. Overall, the results from these preliminary trials have been encouraging. Additional studies are under way to explore the effects of DFMO on esophageal adenocarcinogenesis and to clarify the safety profile of this compound.

4.6. Protease Inhibitors

Dysregulated proteolysis may be an important factor in carcinogenesis *(173–175)*. Bowman-Birk inhibitors (BBIs), which constitute a large family of serine protease inhibitors, have received considerable attention in the context of oropharyngeal cancer prevention. Although the molecular and cellular mechanisms of these compounds remain poorly understood, BBIs have demonstrated some impressive in vivo and in vitro cancer protective effects, including the ability to inactivate initiated oral cancer cells *(176)*. BBI administration to *N*-nitrosomethylbenzylamine-treated rats was associated with a 45% reduction in esophageal papillomas and carcinomas compared to placebo-treated animals *(177)*. Among subjects with oral leukoplakia, minimal toxicities have been observed in Phase I and II clinical trials *(178)*. Further exploration of BBIs, as well as other agents in this class such as the matrix metalloproteinase inhibitors, appears to hold promise for ESC chemoprevention.

4.7. Vitamin E

Vitamin E is the generic name for a group of eight naturally occurring substances that exhibit the biologic activity of α-tocopherol. Vitamin E is an essential nutrient that functions as an antioxidant in the human body

to protect cells and other body components from free-radical attack *(179)*. As the body's primary fat-soluble antioxidant, vitamin E is present in lipids (particularly cell membranes and low-density lipoproteins). In addition to its antioxidant and free-radical scavenging properties, vitamin E has a number of known or presumed functions that may play a role in disrupting carcinogenesis: stimulation of the immune system *(180)*; inhibition of the formation of cancer-causing nitrosamines *(181)*; prevention of carcinogen activation and acceleration of carcinogen metabolism *(182)*; inhibition of proliferation, arachidonic acid metabolism, and ornithine decarboxylase activity *(183–185)*; induction of apoptosis *(186)*; reduction in hormone levels *(187)*; physicochemical stabilization of membranes *(188)*; and effects on cell signaling *(189)*.

Numerous rodent chemical carcinogenesis studies have shown vitamin E inhibition of cancer at various organ sites, including the squamous esophagus *(190–192)*. Case-control studies consistently show a significant association between high intake of vitamin E and/or vitamin E supplements and lower risk of ESC *(118,193–196)*. The more informative and appropriate prospective studies relating vitamin E status to ESC are limited to two published reports and one unpublished study. One of the published cohort studies *(197)* suggested a protective effect of high serum levels of vitamin E for upper gastrointestinal tract cancers combined (87 total cases, including 76 stomach and 11 esophagus), while the other published cohort study found no association between serum vitamin E levels and esophageal cancer (28 cases) *(198)*. Unpublished data from a study of 590 ESC cases, using the same cohort and study design described by Mark et al. *(126)*, show a strong inverse association between serum α-tocopherol levels and ESC risk (RR = 0.63 for the highest vs lowest quartiles of serum α-tocopherol; *p* trend = 0.008) (Dr. Philip R. Taylor, National Cancer Institute, unpublished results).

Vitamin E supplementation has been tested as an ESC chemopreventive agent in Linxian, China, using the approach described above for other antioxidants (*see* Section 4.1) *(128,130)*. However, the doses of vitamin E used in the Linxian trials were relatively low (30 mg/d in the General Population Trial; 60 mg/d in the Dysplasia Trial). While the overall results for ESC suggested protection, they were not statistically significant. In the Dysplasia Trial, however, the multivitamin-supplemented group had a significant 23% increase in reversion to normal cytology *(199)*. Thus, further exploration of vitamin E to prevent or reverse ESC may be rewarding.

4.8. Other Nutritional Compounds

Although existing data are more limited, a number of other nutritional agents may be of potential benefit in ESC chemoprevention. Examples include ascorbic acid, folate, riboflavin, zinc, and molybdenum. Evidence for biologically plausible mechanisms of action exist for each of these nutrients. Specifically, ascorbic acid inhibits nitrosation *(200)*; folate deficiency is thought to disrupt DNA synthesis and impair DNA repair *(201)*; riboflavin status influences a number of cellular processes that may be involved in carcinogenesis, including epithelial integrity and flavin, prostaglandin, and glutathione metabolism *(202)*; zinc deficiency enhances nitrosamine formation and increases cell proliferation *(203)*; molybdenum is a cofactor in nitrate reductase and low soil levels may increase nitrite and nitrate levels in plant foods *(27)*. Animal studies have shown possible protection against ESC from each of these nutrients *(121,204,205)*. Low dietary intakes of vitamin C, folate, riboflavin, and zinc have been associated with increased esophageal cancer risk in one or more case-control studies, as recently reviewed *(206)*.

Reported results from randomized, placebo-controlled clinical trials testing the efficacy of these additional nutrients are limited to three trials from Linxian, China *(128,130,152)*, all of which tested a combination of nutritional supplements rather than single candidate agents. In the 13.5-mo trial of retinol, riboflavin, and zinc reported by Munoz et al., no effect from the intervention was observed with regard to a histologic endpoint (defined as the combination of esophagitis with or without atrophy and dysplasia) *(152)*. Results from the Dysplasia Trial have been described earlier in this chapter (*see* Section 4.1). To reiterate, the intervention group received a combination of 26 vitamins and minerals, which included 180 mg/d of vitamin C, 800 μg/d of folate, 5.2 mg/d of riboflavin, 45 mg/d of zinc, and 30 μg/d of molybdenum. ESC mortality was reduced by 16% and ESC incidence was reduced by 6% in the intervention group, but neither difference was statistically significant *(130)*. In the larger General Population Trial, ESC deaths increased 5% in the vitamin C plus molybdenum group, decreased 10% in the riboflavin (plus niacin) group, and decreased 7% in the zinc (with retinol) group. However, these results also did not achieve statistical significance *(128)*.

5. SUMMARY

On a global scale, ESC incidence rates continue to exceed esophageal adenocarcinoma incidence rates by a wide margin *(2)*. However, considerable geographic variation exists. Although early detection of precursor lesions appears feasible in some high-risk populations, maximally effective ESC screening programs have yet to be implemented. Based on a growing body of experimental, observational, and clinical trial data, chemoprevention appears to offer real promise as an alternate (or ideally complementary) prevention strategy. Further elucidation of the key environmental factors, common genetic alterations, and critical cellular events associated with esophageal squamous carcinogenesis should greatly facilitate the design and conduct of future ESC chemoprevention trials.

REFERENCES

1. Parkin DM. Global cancer statistics in the year 2000. *Lancet Oncol* 2001;2:533–543.
2. Vizcaino AP, Moreno V, Lambert R, Parkin DM. Time trends incidence of both major histologic types of esophageal carcinomas in selected countries, 1973–1995. *Int J Cancer* 2002;99:860–868.
3. Stoner GD, Gupta A. Etiology and chemoprevention of esophageal squamous cell carcinoma. *Carcinogenesis* 2001;22:1737–1746.
4. Li JY, Ershow AG, Chen ZJ, et al. A case-control study of cancer of the esophagus and gastric cardia in Linxian. *Int J Cancer* 1989;43:755–761.
5. Saidi F, Sepehr A, Fahimi S, et al. Oesophageal cancer among the Turkomans of northeast Iran. *Br J Cancer* 2000;83:1249–1254.
6. Mehrotra ML, Lal H, Pant GC, et al. Oesophageal carcinoma in India. Some epidemiologic and morphologic considerations. *Trop Geogr Med* 1977;29:353–358.
7. Sumeruk R, Segal I, Te Winkel W, van der Merwe CF. Oesophageal cancer in three regions of South Africa. *S Afr Med J* 1992;81:91–93.
8. Castellsague X, Munoz N, De Stefani E, et al. Influence of mate drinking, hot beverages and diet on esophageal cancer risk in South America. *Int J Cancer* 2000;88:658–664.
9. Brown LM, Hoover R, Silverman D, et al. Excess incidence of squamous cell esophageal cancer among US Black men: role of social class and other risk factors. *Am J Epidemiol* 2001;153:114–122.
10. Vizcaino AP, Parkin DM, Skinner ME. Risk factors associated with oesophageal cancer in Bulawayo, Zimbabwe. *Br J Cancer* 1995;72:769–773.
11. Ahmed WU, Qureshi H, Alam E, et al. Oesophageal carcinoma in Karachi. *J Pak Med Assoc* 1992;42:133–135.
12. Tuyns AJ, Pequignot G, Jensen OM. Esophageal cancer in Ille-et-Vilaine in relation to levels of alcohol and tobacco consumption. Risks are multiplying. *Bull Cancer* 1977;64:45–60.
13. Tuyns AJ. Oesophageal cancer in non-smoking drinkers and in non-drinking smokers. *Int J Cancer* 1983;32:443–444.
14. Castellsague X, Munoz N, De Stefani E, et al. Independent and joint effects of tobacco smoking and alcohol drinking on the risk of esophageal cancer in men and women. *Int J Cancer* 1999;82:657–664.

15. Brown LM, Hoover RN, Greenberg RS, et al. Are racial differences in squamous cell esophageal cancer explained by alcohol and tobacco use? *J Natl Cancer Inst* 1994;86: 1340–1345.

16. Lagergren J, Bergstrom R, Lindgren A, Nyren O. The role of tobacco, snuff and alcohol use in the aetiology of cancer of the oesophagus and gastric cardia. *Int J Cancer* 2000;85: 340–346.

17. Cheng KK, Duffy SW, Day NE, et al. Stopping drinking and risk of oesophageal cancer. *Br Med J* 1995;310:1094–1097.

18. Castellsague X, Munoz N, De Stefani E, et al. Smoking and drinking cessation and risk of esophageal cancer (Spain). *Cancer Causes Control* 2000;11:813–818.

19. Cook-Mozaffari PJ, Azordegan F, Day NE, et al. Oesophageal cancer studies in the Caspian Littoral of Iran: results of a case-control study. *Br J Cancer* 1979;39: 293–309.

20. Wang YP, Han XY, Su W, et al. Esophageal cancer in Shanxi Province, People's Republic of China: a case-control study in high and moderate risk areas. *Cancer Causes Control* 1992;3:107–113.

21. Yu Y, Taylor PR, Li JY, et al. Retrospective cohort study of risk-factors for esophageal cancer in Linxian, People's Republic of China. *Cancer Causes Control* 1993;4: 195–202.

22. Hewer T, Rose E, Ghadirian P, et al. Ingested mutagens from opium and tobacco pyrolysis products and cancer of the oesophagus. *Lancet* 1978;2:494–496.

23. Roth MJ, Strickland KL, Wang GQ, et al. High levels of carcinogenic polycyclic aromatic hydrocarbons present within food from Linxian, China may contribute to that region's high incidence of oesophageal cancer. *Eur J Cancer* 1998;34: 757–758.

24. Lu SH, Ohshima H, Fu HM, et al. Urinary excretion of *N*-nitrosamino acids and nitrate by inhabitants of high- and low-risk areas for esophageal cancer in Northern China: endogenous formation of nitrosoproline and its inhibition by vitamin C. *Cancer Res* 1986;46:1485–1491.

25. Cheng KK, Day NE, Duffy SW, et al. Pickled vegetables in the aetiology of oesophageal cancer in Hong Kong Chinese. *Lancet* 1992;339:1314–1318.

26. Gao YT, McLaughlin JK, Gridley G, et al. Risk factors for esophageal cancer in Shanghai, China. II. Role of diet and nutrients. *Int J Cancer* 1994;58:197–202.

27. Yang CS. Research on esophageal cancer in China: a review. *Cancer Res* 1980;40:2633–2644.

28. Li JY. Epidemiology of esophageal cancer in China. *Natl Cancer Inst Monogr* 1982;62:113–120.

29. Toxins derived from Fusarium moniliforme: fumonisins B1 and B2 and Fusarin C. IARC Monographs on the evaluation of the carcinogenic risks to humans: some naturally occurring substances: food items and constituents, heterocyclic aromatic amines and mycotoxins. Vol. 56. Lyon, France: IARC Monogr 1993:445–466.

30. Marasas WF. Fumonisins: their implications for human and animal health. *Nat Toxins* 1995;3:193–198; discussion 221.

31. Abnet CC, Qiao YL, Mark SD, et al. Prospective study of tooth loss and incident esophageal and gastric cancers in China. *Cancer Causes Control* 2001;12:847–854.

32. Abnet CC, Borkowf CB, Qiao YL, et al. Sphingolipids as biomarkers of fumonisin exposure and risk of esophageal squamous cell carcinoma in China. *Cancer Causes Control* 2001;12:821–828.

33. De Jong UW, Breslow N, Hong JG, et al. Aetiological factors in oesophageal cancer in Singapore Chinese. *Int J Cancer* 1974;13:291–303.

34. Ghadirian P. Thermal irritation and esophageal cancer in northern Iran. *Cancer* 1987;60:1909–1914.

35. Hu J, Nyren O, Wolk A, et al. Risk factors for oesophageal cancer in northeast China. *Int J Cancer* 1994;57:38–46.

36. Terry P, Lagergren J, Hansen H, et al. Fruit and vegetable consumption in the prevention of oesophageal and cardia cancers. *Eur J Cancer Prev* 2001;10:365–369.

37. O'Neill C, Pan Q, Clarke G, et al. Silica fragments from millet bran in mucosa surrounding oesophageal tumours in patients in northern China. *Lancet* 1982;1:1202–1206.

38. Steinmetz KA, Potter JD. Vegetables, fruit, and cancer. I. Epidemiology. *Cancer Causes Control* 1991;2:325–357.

39. Brown LM, Swanson CA, Gridley G, et al. Dietary factors and the risk of squamous cell esophageal cancer among black and white men in the United States. *Cancer Causes Control* 1998;9:467–474.

40. De Stefani E, Brennan P, Boffetta P, et al. Vegetables, fruits, related dietary antioxidants, and risk of squamous cell carcinoma of the esophagus: a case-control study in Uruguay. *Nutr Cancer* 2000;38:23–29.

41. Syrjanen KJ. Histological changes identical to those of condylomatous lesions found in esophageal squamous cell carcinomas. *Arch Geschwulstforsch* 1982;52:283–292.

42. Dillner J, Knekt P, Schiller JT, Hakulinen T. Prospective seroepidemiological evidence that human papillomavirus type 16 infection is a risk factor for oesophageal squamous cell carcinoma. *Br Med J* 1995;311:1346.

43. Han C, Qiao G, Hubbert NL, et al. Serologic association between human papillomavirus type 16 infection and esophageal cancer in Shaanxi Province, China. *J Natl Cancer Inst* 1996;88:1467–1471.

44. Bjorge T, Hakulinen T, Engeland A, et al. A prospective, sero-epidemiological study of the role of human papillomavirus in esophageal cancer in Norway. *Cancer Res* 1997;57:3989–3992.

45. Lagergren J, Wang Z, Bergstrom R, et al. Human papillomavirus infection and esophageal cancer: a nationwide sero-epidemiologic case-control study in Sweden. *J Natl Cancer Inst* 1999;91:156–162.

46. Chen B, Yin H, Dhurandhar N. Detection of human papillomavirus DNA in esophageal squamous cell carcinomas by the polymerase chain reaction using general consensus primers. *Hum Pathol* 1994;25:920–923.

47. He D, Zhang DK, Lam KY, et al. Prevalence of HPV infection in esophageal squamous cell carcinoma in Chinese patients and its relationship to the p53 gene mutation. *Int J Cancer* 1997;72:959–964.

48. Chang F, Syrjanen S, Shen Q, et al. Evaluation of HPV, CMV, HSV and EBV in esophageal squamous cell carcinomas from a high-incidence area of China. *Anticancer Res* 2000;20:3935–3940.

49. Suzuk L, Noffsinger AE, Hui YZ, Fenoglio-Preiser CM. Detection of human papillomavirus in esophageal squamous cell carcinoma. *Cancer* 1996;78:704–710.

50. Turner JR, Shen LH, Crum CP, et al. Low prevalence of human papillomavirus infection in esophageal squamous cell carcinomas from North America: analysis by a highly sensitive and specific polymerase chain reaction-based approach. *Hum Pathol* 1997; 8:174–178.

51. Kok TC, Nooter K, Tjong AHSP, et al. No evidence of known types of human papillomavirus in squamous cell

cancer of the oesophagus in a low-risk area. Rotterdam Oesophageal Tumour Study Group. *Eur J Cancer* 1997;33:1865–1868.

52. Syrjanen KJ. HPV infections and oesophageal cancer. *J Clin Pathol* 2002;55:721–728.

53. Jenkins TD, Nakagawa H, Rustgi AK. The association of Epstein-Barr virus DNA with esophageal squamous cell carcinoma. *Oncogene* 1996;13:1809–1813.

54. Henrik Siman J, Forsgren A, Berglund G, Floren CH. *Helicobacter pylori* infection is associated with a decreased risk of developing oesophageal neoplasms. *Helicobacter* 2001;6:310–316.

55. Cucino C, Sonnenberg A. Occupational mortality from squamous cell carcinoma of the esophagus in the United States during 1991–1996. *Dig Dis Sci* 2002;47:568–572.

56. Gustavsson P, Jakobsson R, Johansson H, et al. Occupational exposures and squamous cell carcinoma of the oral cavity, pharynx, larynx, and oesophagus: a case-control study in Sweden. *Occup Environ Med* 1998;55:393–400.

57. Parent ME, Siemiatycki J, Fritschi L. Workplace exposures and oesophageal cancer. *Occup Environ Med* 2000;57:325–334.

58. Scholl B, Reis ED, Zouhair A, et al. Esophageal cancer as second primary tumor after breast cancer radiotherapy. *Am J Surg* 2001;182:476–480.

59. Csikos M, Horvath O, Petri A, et al. Late malignant transformation of chronic corrosive oesophageal strictures. *Langenbecks Arch Chir* 1985;365:231–238.

60. Isolauri J, Markkula H. Lye ingestion and carcinoma of the esophagus. *Acta Chir Scand* 1989;155:269–271.

61. Mayberry JF. Epidemiology and demographics of achalasia. *Gastrointest Endosc Clin N Am* 2001;11:235–248.

62. Ribeiro U Jr, Posner MC, Safatle-Ribeiro AV, Reynolds JC. Risk factors for squamous cell carcinoma of the oesophagus. *Br J Surg* 1996;83:1174–1185.

63. Dunaway PM, Wong RK. Risk and surveillance intervals for squamous cell carcinoma in achalasia. *Gastrointest Endosc Clin N Am* 2001;11:425–434.

64. Ciclitira PJ, King AL, Fraser JS. AGA technical review on celiac sprue. American Gastroenterological Association. *Gastroenterology* 2001;120:1526–1540.

65. Wright DH. The major complications of coeliac disease. *Baillieres Clin Gastroenterol* 1995;9:351–369.

66. Harper PS, Harper RM, Howel-Evans AW. Carcinoma of the oesophagus with tylosis. *Q J Med* 1970;39:317–333.

67. Ratnavel RC, Griffiths WA. The inherited palmoplantar keratodermas. *Br J Dermatol* 1997;137:485–490.

68. Risk JM, Evans KE, Jones J, et al. Characterization of a 500 kb region on 17q25 and the exclusion of candidate genes as the familial tylosis oesophageal cancer (TOC) locus. *Oncogene* 2002;21:6395–6402.

69. von Brevern M, Hollstein MC, Risk JM, et al. Loss of heterozygosity in sporadic oesophageal tumors in the tylosis oesophageal cancer (TOC) gene region of chromosome 17q. *Oncogene* 1998;17:2101–2105.

70. Iwaya T, Maesawa C, Ogasawara S, Tamura G. Tylosis esophageal cancer locus on chromosome 17q25.1 is commonly deleted in sporadic human esophageal cancer. *Gastroenterology* 1998;114:1206–1210.

71. Hoffman RM, Jaffe PE. Plummer-Vinson syndrome. A case report and literature review. *Arch Intern Med* 1995;155:2008–2011.

72. Messmann H. Squamous cell cancer of the oesophagus. *Best Pract Res Clin Gastroenterol* 2001;15:249–265.

73. Chen TS, Chen PS. Rise and fall of the Plummer-Vinson syndrome. *J Gastroenterol Hepatol* 1994;9:654–658.

74. Hu N, Dawsey SM, Wu M, Taylor PR. Family history of oesophageal cancer in Shanxi Province, China. *Eur J Cancer* 1991;27:1336.

75. Guo W, Blot WJ, Li JY, et al. A nested case-control study of oesophageal and stomach cancers in the Linxian nutrition intervention trial. *Int J Epidemiol* 1994;23:444–450.

76. Li G, He L. A survey of the familial aggregation of esophageal cancer in Yangcheng county, Shanxi Province. In *Genes and Disease* Proceedings of the First Sino-American Human Genetics Workshop. Wu M, Neberg D, eds. Science Press, Beijing, 1986; pp. 43–47.

77. Hu N, Dawsey SM, Wu M, et al. Familial aggregation of oesophageal cancer in Yangcheng County, Shanxi Province, China. *Int J Epidemiol* 1992;21:877–882.

78. Wu M, Hu N, Wang X. Genetic factors in the epidemiology of esophageal cancer and the strategy of its prevention in high-incidence areas of North China. In *Genetic Epidemiology for Cancer.* Lynch H, Hirayama T, eds. CRC Press, Boca Raton, FL, 1989; pp. 187–200.

79. Carter CL, Hu N, Wu M, et al. Segregation analysis of esophageal cancer in 221 high-risk Chinese families. *J Natl Cancer Inst* 1992;84:771–776.

80. Emmert-Buck MR, Lubensky IA, Dong Q, et al. Localization of the multiple endocrine neoplasia type I (MEN1) gene based on tumor loss of heterozygosity analysis. *Cancer Res* 1997;57:1855–1858.

81. Hu N, Roth MJ, Polymeropolous M, et al. Identification of novel regions of allelic loss from a genomewide scan of esophageal squamous-cell carcinoma in a high-risk Chinese population. *Genes Chromosomes Cancer* 2000;27:217–228.

82. Hu N, Li G, Li WJ, et al. Infrequent mutation in the BRCA2 gene in esophageal squamous cell carcinoma. *Clin Cancer Res* 2002;8:1121–1126.

83. Lo HS, Hu N, Gere S, et al. Identification of somatic mutations of the RNF6 gene in human esophageal squamous cell carcinoma. *Cancer Res* 2002;62:4191–4193.

84. Li W, Hu N, Su H, et al. Allelic loss on chromosome 13q14 and mutation in deleted in cancer 1 gene in esophageal squamous cell carcinoma. *Oncogene* 2003:16;22:314–318.

85. Hu N, Huang J, Emmert-Buck MR, et al. Frequent inactivation of the TP53 gene in esophageal squamous cell carcinoma from a high-risk population in China. *Clin Cancer Res* 2001;7:883–891.

86. Montesano R, Hollstein M, Hainaut P. Genetic alterations in esophageal cancer and their relevance to etiology and pathogenesis: a review. *Int J Cancer* 1996;69:225–235.

87. Selaru FM, Zou T, Xu Y, et al. Global gene expression profiling in Barrett's esophagus and esophageal cancer: a comparative analysis using cDNA microarrays. *Oncogene* 2002;21:475–478.

88. Ohta H, Nakazawa S, Segawa K, Yoshino J. Distribution of epithelial dysplasia in the cancerous esophagus. *Scand J Gastroenterol* 1986;21:392–398.

89. Munoz N, Crespi M, Grassi A, et al. Precursor lesions of oesophageal cancer in high-risk populations in Iran and China. *Lancet* 1982;1:876–879.

90. Qiu SL, Yang GR. Precursor lesions of esophageal cancer in high-risk populations in Henan Province, China. *Cancer* 1988;62:551–557.

91. Wang LD, Qiu SL, Yang GR, et al. A randomized double-blind intervention study on the effect of calcium supplementation on

esophageal precancerous lesions in a high-risk population in China. *Cancer Epidemiol Biomarkers Prev* 1993;2:71–78.

92. Dawsey SM, Lewin KJ, Wang GQ, et al. Squamous esophageal histology and subsequent risk of squamous cell carcinoma of the esophagus. A prospective follow-up study from Linxian, China. *Cancer* 1994;74:1686–1692.

93. Crespi M, Munoz N, Grassi A, et al. Precursor lesions of oesophageal cancer in a low-risk population in China: comparison with high-risk populations. *Int J Cancer* 1984;34: 599–602.

94. Dawsey SM, Lewin KJ. Histologic precursors of squamous esophageal cancer. *Pathol Annu* 1995;30:209–226.

95. Dawsey SM, Fleischer DE, Wang GQ, et al. Mucosal iodine staining improves endoscopic visualization of squamous dysplasia and squamous cell carcinoma of the esophagus in Linxian, China. *Cancer* 1998;83:220–231.

96. Wang LD, Lipkin M, Qui SL, et al. Labeling index and labeling distribution of cells in esophageal epithelium of individuals at increased risk for esophageal cancer in Huixian, China. *Cancer Res* 1990;50:2651–2653.

97. Liu FS, Dawsey SM, Wang GQ, et al. Correlation of epithelial proliferation and squamous esophageal histology in 1185 biopsies from Linxian, China. *Int J Cancer* 1993;55:577–579.

98. Wang LD, Zhou Q, Yang CS. Esophageal and gastric cardia epithelial cell proliferation in northern Chinese subjects living in a high-incidence area. *J Cell Biochem Suppl* 1997; 8–29:159–165.

99. Kuwano H, Saeki H, Kawaguchi H, et al. Proliferative activity of cancer cells in front and center areas of carcinoma in situ and invasive sites of esophageal squamous-cell carcinoma. *Int J Cancer* 1998;78:149–152.

100. Wang LD, Zhou Q, Yang WC, Yang CS. Apoptosis and cell proliferation in esophageal precancerous and cancerous lesions: study of a high-risk population in northern China. *Anticancer Res* 1999;19:369–374.

101. Youssef EM, Matsuda T, Takada N, et al. Prognostic significance of the MIB-1 proliferation index for patients with squamous cell carcinoma of the esophagus. *Cancer* 1995;76:358–366.

102. Sarbia M, Bittinger F, Porschen R, et al. The prognostic significance of tumour cell proliferation in squamous cell carcinomas of the oesophagus. *Br J Cancer* 1996;74:1012–1016.

103. Shibakita M, Tachibana M, Dhar DK, et al. Spontaneous apoptosis in advanced esophageal carcinoma: its relation to Fas expression. *Clin Cancer Res* 2000;6:4755–4759.

104. Imdahl A, Jenkner J, Ihling C, et al. Is MIB-1 proliferation index a predictor for response to neoadjuvant therapy in patients with esophageal cancer? *Am J Surg* 2000;179: 514–520.

105. Shibata H, Matsubara O. Apoptosis as an independent prognostic indicator in squamous cell carcinoma of the esophagus. *Pathol Int* 2001;51:498–503.

106. Rees M, Stahl M, Klump B, et al. The prognostic significance of proliferative activity, apoptosis and expression of DNA topoisomerase II alpha in multimodally-treated oesophageal squamous cell carcinoma. *Anticancer Res* 2001;21:3637–3642.

107. Ikeguchi M, Maeta M, Kaibara N. Bax expression as a prognostic marker of postoperative chemoradiotherapy for patients with esophageal cancer. *Int J Mol Med* 2001;7: 413–417.

108. Rao M, Liu FS, Dawsey SM, et al. Effects of vitamin/mineral supplementation on the proliferation of esophageal squamous

epithelium in Linxian, China. *Cancer Epidemiol Biomarkers Prev* 1994;3:277–279.

109. Maesawa C, Tamura G, Nishizuka S, et al. Inactivation of the CDKN2 gene by homozygous deletion and de novo methylation is associated with advanced stage esophageal squamous cell carcinoma. *Cancer Res* 1996;56: 3875–3878.

110. Tanaka H, Shimada Y, Harada H, et al. Methylation of the 5′ CpG island of the FHIT gene is closely associated with transcriptional inactivation in esophageal squamous cell carcinomas. *Cancer Res* 1998;58:3429–3434.

111. Si HX, Tsao SW, Lam KY, et al. E-cadherin expression is commonly downregulated by CpG island hypermethylation in esophageal carcinoma cells. *Cancer Lett* 2001;173:71–78.

112. Xing EP, Nie Y, Song Y, et al. Mechanisms of inactivation of p14ARF, p15INK4b, and p16INK4a genes in human esophageal squamous cell carcinoma. *Clin Cancer Res* 1999;5:2704–2713.

113. Zhou J, Wang H, Lu A, et al. A novel gene, NMES1, downregulated in human esophageal squamous cell carcinoma. *Int J Cancer* 2002;101:311–316.

114. Hibi K, Taguchi M, Nakayama H, et al. Molecular detection of p16 promoter methylation in the serum of patients with esophageal squamous cell carcinoma. *Clin Cancer Res* 2001;7:3135–3138.

115. Ehrlich M. DNA methylation in cancer: too much, but also too little. *Oncogene* 2002;21:5400–5413.

116. Scelfo RA, Schwienbacher C, Veronese A, et al. Loss of methylation at chromosome 11p15.5 is common in human adult tumors. *Oncogene* 2002;21:2564–2572.

117. Schulz WA, Elo JP, Florl AR, et al. Genomewide DNA hypomethylation is associated with alterations on chromosome 8 in prostate carcinoma. *Genes Chromosomes Cancer* 2002;35:58–65.

118. Mayne ST, Risch HA, Dubrow R, et al. Nutrient intake and risk of subtypes of esophageal and gastric cancer. *Cancer Epidemiol Biomarkers Prev* 2001;10:1055–1062.

119. Song C, Xing D, Tan W, et al. Methylenetetrahydrofolate reductase polymorphisms increase risk of esophageal squamous cell carcinoma in a Chinese population. *Cancer Res* 2001;61:3272–3275.

120. Kim YS, Milner J. Molecular targets for selenium in cancer prevention. *Nutr Cancer* 2001;40:50–54.

121. van Rensburg SJ, Hall JM, Gathercole PS. Inhibition of esophageal carcinogenesis in corn-fed rats by riboflavin, nicotinic acid, selenium, molybdenum, zinc, and magnesium. *Nutr Cancer* 1986;8:163–170.

122. Bogden JD, Chung HR, Kemp FW, et al. Effect of selenium and molybdenum on methylbenzylnitrosamine-induced esophageal lesions and tissue trace metals in the rat. *J Nutr* 1986;116:2432–2442.

123. Lijinsky W, Milner JA, Kovatch RM, Thomas BJ. Lack of effect of selenium on induction of tumors of esophagus and bladder in rats by two nitrosamines. *Toxicol Ind Health* 1989;5:63–72.

124. Hu G, Han C, Wild CP, et al. Lack of effects of selenium on N-nitrosomethylbenzylamine-induced tumorigenesis, DNA methylation, and oncogene expression in rats and mice. *Nutr Cancer* 1992;18:287–295.

125. Chen X, Mikhail SS, Ding YW, et al. Effects of vitamin E and selenium supplementation on esophageal adenocarcinogenesis in a surgical model with rats. *Carcinogenesis* 2000;21:1531–1536.

126. Mark SD, Qiao YL, Dawsey SM, et al. Prospective study of serum selenium levels and incident esophageal and gastric cancers. *J Natl Cancer Inst* 2000;92:1753–1763.

127. Clark LC, Combs GF Jr, Turnbull BW, et al. Effects of selenium supplementation for cancer prevention in patients with carcinoma of the skin. A randomized controlled trial. Nutritional Prevention of Cancer Study Group. *JAMA* 1996;276:1957–1963.

128. Blot WJ, Li JY, Taylor PR, et al. Nutrition intervention trials in Linxian, China: supplementation with specific vitamin/mineral combinations, cancer incidence, and disease-specific mortality in the general population. *J Natl Cancer Inst* 1993;85:1483–1492.

129. Wang GQ, Dawsey SM, Li JY, et al. Effects of vitamin/mineral supplementation on the prevalence of histological dysplasia and early cancer of the esophagus and stomach: results from the General Population Trial in Linxian, China. *Cancer Epidemiol Biomarkers Prev* 1994;3: 161–166.

130. Li JY, Taylor PR, Li B, et al. Nutrition intervention trials in Linxian, China: multiple vitamin/mineral supplementation, cancer incidence, and disease-specific mortality among adults with esophageal dysplasia. *J Natl Cancer Inst* 1993; 85:1492–1498.

131. Limburg P, Wei W, Ahnen D, et al. Chemoprevention of esophageal squamous cancer: Randomized, placebo-controlled trial in a high-risk population. *Gastroenterol* 2002;122:A71.

132. Shureiqi I, Xu X, Chen D, et al. Nonsteroidal anti-inflammatory drugs induce apoptosis in esophageal cancer cells by restoring 15-lipoxygenase-1 expression. *Cancer Res* 2001; 61:4879–4884.

133. Souza RF, Shewmake K, Beer DG, et al. Selective inhibition of cyclooxygenase-2 suppresses growth and induces apoptosis in human esophageal adenocarcinoma cells. *Cancer Res* 2000;60:5767–5772.

134. Rubio CA. Antitumoral activity of indomethacin on experimental esophageal tumors. *J Natl Cancer Inst* 1984;72: 705–707.

135. Rubio CA. Further studies on the therapeutic effect of indomethacin on esophageal tumors. *Cancer* 1986;58: 1029–1031.

136. Tanaka T, Kojima T, Yoshimi N, et al. Inhibitory effect of the non-steroidal anti-inflammatory drug, indomethacin on the naturally occurring carcinogen, 1-hydroxyanthraquinone in male ACI/N rats. *Carcinogenesis* 1991;12:1949–1952.

137. Shibata MA, Hirose M, Masuda A, et al. Modification of BHA forestomach carcinogenesis in rats: inhibition by diethylmaleate or indomethacin and enhancement by a retinoid. *Carcinogenesis* 1993;14:1265–1269.

138. Siglin JC, Barch DH, Stoner GD. Effects of dietary phenethyl isothiocyanate, ellagic acid, sulindac and calcium on the induction and progression of N-nitrosomethylbenzylamine-induced esophageal carcinogenesis in rats. *Carcinogenesis* 1995;16:1101–1106.

139. Carlton PS, Gopalakrishnan R, Gupta A, et al. Piroxicam is an ineffective inhibitor of N-nitrosomethylbenzylamine-induced tumorigenesis in the rat esophagus. *Cancer Res* 2002;62:4376–4382.

140. Gridley G, McLaughlin JK, Ekbom A, et al. Incidence of cancer among patients with rheumatoid arthritis. *J Natl Cancer Inst* 1993;85:307–311.

141. Thun MJ, Namboodiri MM, Calle EE, et al. Aspirin use and risk of fatal cancer. *Cancer Res* 1993;53:1322–1327.

142. Funkhouser EM, Sharp GB. Aspirin and reduced risk of esophageal carcinoma. *Cancer* 1995;76:1116–1119.

143. Farrow DC, Vaughan TL, Hansten PD, et al. Use of aspirin and other nonsteroidal anti-inflammatory drugs and risk of esophageal and gastric cancer. *Cancer Epidemiol Biomarkers Prev* 1998;7:97–102.

144. Trujillo MA, Garewal HS, Sampliner RE. Nonsteroidal antiinflammatory agents in chemoprevention of colorectal cancer. At what cost? *Dig Dis Sci* 1994;39:2260–2266.

145. Wolfe MM, Lichtenstein DR, Singh G. Gastrointestinal toxicity of nonsteroidal antiinflammatory drugs. *N Engl J Med* 1999;340:1888–1899.

146. Lippman SM, Lotan R. Advances in the development of retinoids as chemopreventive agents. *J Nutr* 2000;130: 479S–482S.

147. Singh DK, Lippman SM. Cancer chemoprevention. Part 1: Retinoids and carotenoids and other classic antioxidants. *Oncology* (Huntingt) 1998;12:1643–53, 1657–8; discussion 1659–1660.

148. Muller A, Nakagawa H, Rustgi AK. Retinoic acid and N-(4-hydroxy-phenyl) retinamide suppress growth of esophageal squamous carcinoma cell lines. *Cancer Lett* 1997;113: 95–101.

149. Liu G, Wu M, Levi G, Ferrari N. Inhibition of cancer cell growth by all-trans retinoic acid and its analog N-(4-hydroxyphenyl) retinamide: a possible mechanism of action via regulation of retinoid receptors expression. *Int J Cancer* 1998;78:248–254.

150. Koreeda T, Yamanaka E, Yamamichi K, et al. Inhibitory effect of retinoid on esophageal carcinogenesis in rats induced by N-nitroso-N-methylbutylamine in relation to cellular retinoic acid-binding protein. *Anticancer Res* 1999;19:4139–4143.

151. Wan X, Duncan MD, Nass P, Harmon JW. Synthetic retinoid CD437 induces apoptosis of esophageal squamous HET-1A cells through the caspase-3-dependent pathway. *Anticancer Res* 2001;21:2657–2663.

152. Munoz N, Wahrendorf J, Bang LJ, et al. No effect of riboflavine, retinol, and zinc on prevalence of precancerous lesions of oesophagus. Randomised double-blind intervention study in high-risk population of China. *Lancet* 1985;2:111–114.

153. Wahrendorf J, Munoz N, Lu JB, et al. Blood, retinol and zinc riboflavin status in relation to precancerous lesions of the esophagus: findings from a vitamin intervention trial in the People's Republic of China. *Cancer Res* 1988;48: 2280–2283.

154. Lin P, Zhang J, Rong Z, et al. Studies on medicamentous inhibitory therapy for esophageal precancerous lesions—3- and 5-year inhibitory effects of antitumor-B, retinamide and riboflavin. *Proc Chin Acad Med Sci Peking Union Med Coll* 1990;5:121–129.

155. Camerini T, Mariani L, De Palo G, et al. Safety of the synthetic retinoid fenretinide: long-term results from a controlled clinical trial for the prevention of contralateral breast cancer. *J Clin Oncol* 2001;19:1664–1670.

156. Lin J, Huang T, Shih C, Lin J. Molecular mechanisms of action of curcumin. In *Food Phtyochemicals for Cancer Prevention, II. Teas, Spices, and Herbs.* Ho C, Dsama T, Huang M, Rosen R, eds. American Chemical Society, Washington, DC, 1994; pp. 196–203.

157. Gururaj A, Belakavadi M, Venkatesh D, et al. Molecular mechanisms of anti-angiogenic effect of curcumin. *Biochem Biophys Res Commun* 2002;297:934.

158. Surh YJ. Anti-tumor promoting potential of selected spice ingredients with antioxidative and anti-inflammatory activities: a short review. *Food Chem Toxicol* 2002;40:1091–1097.

159. Surh YJ, Chun KS, Cha HH, et al. Molecular mechanisms underlying chemopreventive activities of anti-inflammatory phytochemicals: down-regulation of COX-2 and iNOS through suppression of NF-kappa B activation. *Mutat Res* 2001;480–481:243–268.

160. Ushida J, Sugie S, Kawabata K, et al. Chemopreventive effect of curcumin on N-nitrosomethylbenzylamine-induced esophageal carcinogenesis in rats. *Jpn J Cancer Res* 2000;91: 893–898.

161. Cheng AL, Hsu CH, Lin JK, et al. Phase I clinical trial of curcumin, a chemopreventive agent, in patients with high-risk or pre-malignant lesions. *Anticancer Res* 2001;21: 2895–2900.

162. Sharma RA, McLelland HR, Hill KA, et al. Pharmacodynamic and pharmacokinetic study of oral Curcuma extract in patients with colorectal cancer. *Clin Cancer Res* 2001;7:1894–1900.

163. Meyskens FL Jr, Gerner EW. Development of difluoromethylornithine (DFMO) as a chemoprevention agent. *Clin Cancer Res* 1999;5:945–951.

164. Pegg AE, Shantz LM, Coleman CS. Ornithine decarboxylase as a target for chemoprevention. *J Cell Biochem Suppl* 1995;22:132–138.

165. Fong LY, Pegg AE, Magee PN. Alpha-difluoromethylornithine inhibits N-nitrosomethylbenzylamine-induced esophageal carcinogenesis in zinc-deficient rats: effects on esophageal cell proliferation and apoptosis. *Cancer Res* 1998;58:5380–5388.

166. Fong LY, Nguyen VT, Pegg AE, Magee PN. Alpha-difluoromethylornithine induction of apoptosis: a mechanism which reverses pre-established cell proliferation and cancer initiation in esophageal carcinogenesis in zinc-deficient rats. *Cancer Epidemiol Biomarkers Prev* 2001;10: 191–199.

167. Love RR, Jacoby R, Newton MA, et al. A randomized, placebo-controlled trial of low-dose alpha-difluoromethylornithine in individuals at risk for colorectal cancer. *Cancer Epidemiol Biomarkers Prev* 1998;7:989–992.

168. Meyskens FL Jr, Gerner EW, Emerson S, et al. Effect of alpha-difluoromethylornithine on rectal mucosal levels of polyamines in a randomized, double-blinded trial for colon cancer prevention. *J Natl Cancer Inst* 1998;90:1212–1218.

169. Meyskens FL Jr, Emerson SS, Pelot D, et al. Dose de-escalation chemoprevention trial of alpha-difluoromethylornithine in patients with colon polyps. *J Natl Cancer Inst* 1994;6: 1122–1130.

170. Mitchell MF, Tortolero-Luna G, Lee JJ, et al. Phase I dose de-escalation trial of alpha-difluoromethylornithine in patients with grade 3 cervical intraepithelial neoplasia. *Clin Cancer Res* 1998;4:303–310.

171. Alberts DS, Dorr RT, Einspahr JG, et al. Chemoprevention of human actinic keratoses by topical 2-(difluoromethyl)-dl-ornithine. *Cancer Epidemiol Biomarkers Prev* 2000;9: 1281–1286.

172. Einspahr JG, Nelson MA, Saboda K, et al. Modulation of biologic endpoints by topical difluoromethylornithine (DFMO), in subjects at high-risk for nonmelanoma skin cancer. *Clin Cancer Res* 2002;8:149–155.

173. Noel A, Gilles C, Bajou K, et al. Emerging roles for proteinases in cancer. *Invasion Metastasis* 1997;17:221–239.

174. Kennedy AR. Prevention of carcinogenesis by protease inhibitors. *Cancer Res* 1994;54:1999s–2005s.

175. Lippman SM, Matrisian LM. Protease inhibitors in oral carcinogenesis and chemoprevention. *Clin Cancer Res* 2000;6: 4599–4603.

176. Kennedy AR, Billings PC, Maki PA, Newberne P. Effects of various preparations of dietary protease inhibitors on oral carcinogenesis in hamsters induced by DMBA. *Nutr Cancer* 1993;19:191–200.

177. von Hofe E, Newberne PM, Kennedy AR. Inhibition of N-nitrosomethylbenzylamine-induced esophageal neoplasms by the Bowman-Birk protease inhibitor. *Carcinogenesis* 1991;12:2147–2150.

178. Meyskens FL Jr. Development of Bowman-Birk inhibitor for chemoprevention of oral head and neck cancer. *Ann NY Acad Sci* 2001;952:116–123.

179. Dietery reference intakes for vitamin C, vitamin E, selenium, and carotenoids. Institute of Medicine. Panel on Dietary Antioxidants and Related Compounds. National Academy Press, Washington, DC, 2000; pp. 186–283.

180. Tengerdy RP. Effect of vitamin E on immune function. In *Vitamin E—A Comprehensive Treatise*. Machlin LJ, ed. Marcel Dekker, New York, 1980; pp. 429–444.

181. Ohshima H, Bartsch H. Quantitative estimation of endogenous nitrosation in humans by monitoring N-nitrosoproline excreted in the urine. *Cancer Res* 1981;41:3658–3662.

182. McCay PB, King MM. Vitamin E: its role as a biologic free radical scavenger and its relationship to the microsomal mixed-function oxidase system. In *Vitamin E—A Comprehensive Treatise*. Macklin LJ, ed. Marcel Dekker, New York; 1980; pp. 289–317.

183. Prasad KN, Edwards-Prasad J. Effects of tocopherol (vitamin E) acid succinate on morphological alterations and growth inhibition in melanoma cells in culture. *Cancer Res* 1982;42:550–555.

184. Chan AC. Vitamin E and the arachidonic acid cascade. In *Vitamin E—Its Usefulness in Health and in Curing Diseases*. Mino M, Nakamura H, Diplock AT, Kayden HJ, eds. Japan Scientific Societies Press, New York, 1993; pp. 197–207.

185. Perchellet JP, Abney NL, Thomas RM, et al. Effects of combined treatments with selenium, glutathione, and vitamin E on glutathione peroxidase activity, ornithine decarboxylase induction, and complete and multistage carcinogenesis in mouse skin. *Cancer Res* 1987;47:477–485.

186. Zhang D, Okada S, Yu Y, et al. Vitamin E inhibits apoptosis, DNA modification, and cancer incidence induced by iron-mediated peroxidation in Wistar rat kidney. *Cancer Res* 1997;57:2410–2414.

187. Hartman TJ, Dorgan JF, Virtamo J, et al. Association between serum alpha-tocopherol and serum androgens and estrogens in older men. *Nutr Cancer* 1999;35:10–15.

188. Lucy JA. Structural interactions between vitamin E and polyunsaturated phospholipids. In *Tocopherol, Oxygen and Biomembranes*. de Duve C, Hayaisi O, eds. Elsevier, Amsterdam, 1980; pp. 109–120.

189. Leibold E, Schwarz LR. Inhibition of intercellular communication in rat hepatocytes by phenobarbital, 1,1,1-trichloro-2,2-bis(p-chlorophenyl)ethane (DDT) and gammahexachlorocyclohexane (lindane): modification by antioxidants and inhibitors of cyclo-oxygenase. *Carcinogenesis* 1993;14:2377–2382.

190. Knekt P. Role of vitamin E in the prophylaxis of cancer. *Ann Med* 1991;23:3–12.

191. Odeleye OE, Eskelson CD, Mufti SI, Watson RR. Vitamin E protection against nitrosamine-induced esophageal tumor incidence in mice immunocompromised by retroviral infection. *Carcinogenesis* 1992;13:1811–1816.

192. Odeleye OE, Eskelson CD, Mufti SI, Watson RR. Vitamin E inhibition of lipid peroxidation and ethanol-mediated promotion of esophageal tumorigenesis. *Nutr Cancer* 1992;17: 223–234.

193. Barone J, Taioli E, Hebert JR, Wynder EL. Vitamin supplement use and risk for oral and esophageal cancer. *Nutr Cancer* 1992;18:31–41.

194. Launoy G, Milan C, Day NE, et al. Diet and squamous-cell cancer of the oesophagus: a French multicentre case-control study. *Int J Cancer* 1998;76:7–12.

195. Terry P, Lagergren J, Ye W, et al. Antioxidants and cancers of the esophagus and gastric cardia. *Int J Cancer* 2000;87: 750–754.

196. Bollschweiler E, Wolfgarten E, Nowroth T, et al. Vitamin intake and risk of subtypes of esophageal cancer in Germany. *J Cancer Res Clin Oncol* 2002;128:575–580.

197. Knekt P, Aromaa A, Maatela J, et al. Serum vitamin E, serum selenium and the risk of gastrointestinal cancer. *Int J Cancer* 1988;42:846–850.

198. Nomura AM, Ziegler RG, Stemmermann GN, et al. Serum micronutrients and upper aerodigestive tract cancer. *Cancer Epidemiol Biomarkers Prev* 1997;6:407–412.

199. Mark SD, Liu SF, Li JY, et al. The effect of vitamin and mineral supplementation on esophageal cytology: results from the Linxian Dysplasia Trial. *Int J Cancer* 1994;57:162–166.

200. Bartsch H, Pignatelli B, Calmels S, Ohshima H. Inhibition of nitrosation. *Basic Life Sci* 1993;61:27–44.

201. Choi SW, Mason JB. Folate and carcinogenesis: an integrated scheme. *J Nutr* 2000;130:129–132.

202. Rivlin RS. Riboflavin. *Adv Exp Med Biol* 1986;206:349–355.

203. Fong LY, Magee PN. Dietary zinc deficiency enhances esophageal cell proliferation and N-nitrosomethylbenzylamine (NMBA)-induced esophageal tumor incidence in C57BL/6 mouse. *Cancer Lett* 1999;143:63–69.

204. Balansky RM, Blagoeva PM, Mircheva ZI, De Flora S. Modulation of diethylnitrosamine carcinogenesis in rat liver and oesophagus. *J Cell Biochem* 1994;56:449–454.

205. Rogers AE. Reduction of N-nitrosodiethylamine carcinogenesis in rats by lipotrope or amino acid supplementation of a marginally deficient diet. *Cancer Res* 1977;37: 194–199.

206. Food, nutrition and the prevention of cancer: a global perspective. Oesophagus. American Institute for Cancer Research, Washington, DC; 1997; pp. 118–129.

HEAD AND NECK

28 Chemoprevention of Upper Aerodigestive Tract Cancer

Clinical Trials and Future Directions

Fadlo R. Khuri, MD, Edward S. Kim, MD, and Waun Ki Hong, MD

CONTENTS

1. INTRODUCTION

Head and neck cancer is a major cause of cancer-related deaths *(1)*. In the United States alone, head and neck cancer is the fifth most common cancer, with approximately 45,400 cases anticipated for the year 2002 and approx 12,600 deaths. We expect that more than 600,000 cases of head and neck cancer will have been diagnosed worldwide in the year 2002 *(2)*. The complexity of head and neck cancer treatment relates to substantial progress in surgery, concomitant chemoradiation therapy, and intensity-modulated radiotherapy over the past few decades. At least six active chemotherapeutic agents are available for this disease, but the 5-yr survival rate has improved only slightly since the 1960s. The overwhelming functional consequences of this disease, its effect on daily life (including problems with speech, swallowing, and profound cosmetic defects), and the subsequent loss of self-esteem and social status make it a particularly serious illness. Further, patients fortunate enough to be cured of head and neck cancer often succumb to a second smoking-related cancer. In addition, metachronous primary cancers in this high-risk group continue to confound care providers. Some studies indicate that these cancers are major determinants of overall prognosis in patients definitively treated for early-stage disease *(3)*.

Vikram *(3)* showed that second primary tumors largely determine survival among patients with advanced head and neck cancer who did not experience primary tumor recurrence within the first 2 yr. Since then, Cooper et al. *(4)* have assessed the impact of second malignancies in patients who had prior head and neck cancer, reviewing the database for those who were treated on various Radiation Therapy Oncology Group (RTOG) protocols. Despite improvements in local control, the development of second malignancies was found to be largely responsible for the failure to

From: Cancer Chemoprevention, Volume 2: Strategies for Cancer Chemoprevention
Edited by: G. J. Kelloff, E. T. Hawk, and C. C. Sigman © Humana Press Inc., Totowa, NJ

Adjuvant High-Dose 13cRA Trial in Head and Neck Cancer

Time to Development of Second Primary Tumors (SPT)

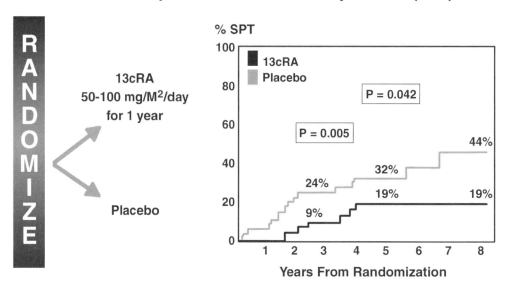

Fig. 1. One hundred two (102) patients definitively treated for head and neck squamous cell cancer to either adjuvant 13-*cis*-retinoic acid (50–100 mg/m²/d) or placebo for 1 yr. The patients randomized to the retinoid had a significantly lower incidence of second cancers. (From ref. *40.*)

improve overall survival; similar results were described by Licciardello et al. *(5)*.

Epithelial cancers therefore remain a major domestic and international health problem. Notwithstanding improvements achieved through the use of multidisciplinary cancer therapy programs, overall mortality from these epithelial malignancies, including head and neck cancer, has improved only slightly. Epithelial carcinogenesis is a multistep process in which a series of genetic events leads to a progressively dysplastic cellular appearance, dysregulated cell growth, and finally, to overt carcinoma *(6)*. Cancer prevention efforts in general have focused on reducing incidence of preventable cancers and on smoking cessation. Despite national and international efforts to discourage smoking and enhance smoking cessation efforts, there are still more than 46 million current and 46 million former smokers in the US *(7)*. Recent studies from the Harvard University Hospitals *(8)* and the University of Texas M. D. Anderson Cancer Center *(9)* demonstrate that approx 50% of lung cancers diagnosed in a given year occur in individuals who have quit smoking for at least 1 yr and are therefore defined as former smokers. These troubling data indicate that smoking-related aerodigestive

tract cancers continue to occur even in individuals who have successfully undertaken the difficult step of smoking cessation.

Head and neck squamous cell cancer (HNSCC) differs from non-small-cell lung cancer (NSCLC) in its epidemiology; it is associated not only with tobacco use but also with alcohol use. Several studies have indicated this synergistic relationship between tobacco and alcohol use in terms of cancer development in the upper aerodigestive tract. Data thus far indicate that the molecular underpinnings of the link between cigarette smoke and cancer causation are becoming increasingly well understood. Denissenko et al. *(10)* demonstrated that distribution of benzo[*a*]-pyrene diol epoxide (BPDE) adducts is nonrandom along axons of the p53 gene in BPDE-treated HeLa cells and bronchial epithelial cells, and that these adducts map to the guanine positions in codons 157, 248, and 273 of the p53 gene. Strong and selective adduct formation at these sites only, the major mutational hot spots in lung cancer, offered further proof of targeted adduct formation rather than phenotypic selection in the p53 mutational spectrum of lung cancer. These results reinforce a direct molecular link between a defined chemical carcinogen found in tobacco and development of human lung cancers (and possibly head and neck cancers).

2. MULTISTEP CARCINOGENESIS AND FIELD CANCERIZATION

In 1976, Knudson *(11)* hypothesized that retinoblastoma involved a two-hit carcinogenic process. Subsequent work by multiple investigators revealed that epithelial cancers, including HNSCC, are the end product of a complex, multistep carcinogenic process that involves at least 20 separate genetic events *(12)*. The possibility that this process might be blocked, reversed, or inhibited before cells and tissues reach the cancer end stage has been the impetus behind chemoprevention research.

Multiple molecular studies of premalignant tissue, particularly studies of loss of heterozygosity (LOH), provide strong evidence for the concept of multistep carcinogenesis. Van der Riet et al. *(13)* found a high rate of LOH at the human chromosomal locus *9p21* in squamous dysplasia and carcinoma *in situ* lesions. This LOH rate and location were similar to those found in invasive carcinomas. Mao et al. *(14)* subsequently found LOH at the chromosomal loci *9p21* and *3p14* in 19 of 37 oral leukoplakia samples examined (51%). Seven of 19 patients (37%) with LOH at one or both of these loci later developed SCC, whereas only 1 of 18 non-LOH patients (6%) developed head and neck cancers. These studies suggest the importance of clonal genetic alterations that occur at an early or premalignant stage of carcinogenesis and ultimately lead to frank neoplasia.

Further evidence for the multistep process of head and neck carcinogenesis cancer comes from studies of genetic alterations that demonstrate chromosomal abnormalities (polysomies), not only in tumor cells, but also in histologically defined premalignant lesions, such as oral leukoplakias and nonmalignant epithelial tissue adjacent to tumors. Hung et al. *(15)* observed highly specific allelic deletions in the short arm of chromosome 3 that occured at the earliest stage increment (i.e., hyperplasia) in the pathogenesis of lung and head and neck cancers; these deletions were found in cells scattered throughout the respiratory tract.

Much of this work follows the early research by Slaughter et al. *(16)*, who proposed the concept of field cancerization to explain development of second primary tumors (SPTs) of diffuse cancers associated with oral cancer in 1953. These diffuse carcinogenesis

fingerprints described by Slaughter et al. in the oral cavity and by Auerbach et al. in the lung *(17,18)* sought to explain field carcinogenesis as an extensive, multifocal developmental process of both premalignant and malignant lesions scattered outside of the entire carcinogen-scarred epithelial region. The classic example of field carcinogenesis, based on work by Auerbach and Slaughter, is tobacco-induced injury to the upper aerodigestive tract and lungs that ultimately leads to the possibility of multiple metachronous or synchronous primary cancers.

3. LONGITUDINAL STUDIES OF SECOND PRIMARY TUMORS

Several longitudinal studies show that patients treated for initial cancer constitute the individuals at the single highest risk for development of SPTs *(19,20)*. In fact, a recent survey of the SEER database showed that patients with prior laryngeal cancers had a lifetime risk for SPTs of 25–40% *(19)*. The high likelihood of SPTs after treatment of early HSNCC makes this disease an excellent model for the study of chemoprevention.

Controversy continues over the role of smoking in the development of SPTs. Most studies suggest that smoking cessation reduces risk for SPTs *(21–26)*. However, difficulties in collecting accurate data on factors related to smoking, and lack of biochemical confirmation through measurement of serum nicotine levels, have hindered a definitive conclusion in this regard. Nevertheless, some investigators continue to question the association between smoking and risk for second primary cancers *(20)*.

4. MOLECULAR DETERMINATION OF RECURRENCE VS SECOND PRIMARY TUMORS

To date, controversy persists regarding the clonal origin of metachronous or synchronous primary cancers. Bedi et al. *(27)* constructed a preliminary genetic progression model for HNSCC based on frequency of genetic alterations found in preneoplastic and neoplastic lesions from single biopsy specimens. To firmly establish the temporal order of established genetic events in HNSCC, they obtained serial biopsies from five patients with recurrent premalignant lesions at a single anatomic site over a period of time. By assaying these lesions using microsatellite analysis of minimal regions of loss on the 10 most frequently lost chromosomal arms in HNSCC, these investigators were able to demonstrate that three patients clearly had genetic progression with new lesions of LOH over time, correlating with histopathologic progression. They further identified one individual with lack of genetic progression associated with unchanged histopathologic morphology and another individual whose histopathologic progression was found in the absence of corresponding detectable genetic progression involving new LOH. These findings imply that many, if not most, of these tumors arise from a common clonal origin, despite presenting as apparently metachronous cancers. From the same group, Leong et al. *(28)* built on this work by evaluating paired tumors from 16 patients with HNSCC and a solitary lung SCC for LOH at chromosomal arms *3p* and *9p*. In most cases, a comparison of the genetic alterations clarified the relationship between the primary HNSCC and the lung tumor. Paired tumors from 10 patients were found to have concordant patterns of loss at all chromosomal loci, suggesting that these were clearly metastatically spread, whereas three paired tumors had discordant patterns at all assayed chromosomal loci, suggesting an independent tumor origin. These investigators concluded that most cases of second primary SCCs of the lung were most likely late metastases from the primary cancers, as opposed to metachronous independent SPTs.

Califano et al. *(29)* investigated the association between second esophageal SCCs and primary HNSCCs to better elucidate the clonal relationships. Their theory was that geographic limitations of clonal expansion had not been adequately explained. They therefore compared paired tumors from 16 HNSCC patients with a second SCC of the esophagus for patterns of LOH on chromosomal arms *3p*, *9p*, and *17p*. Losses at these loci are believed to occur early during neoplastic transformation of the aerodigestive tract, as had been shown previously by Califano et al. *(6)*. In 14 of the cases (87%), the paired tumors had discordant patterns of allelic loss, suggesting that the tumors were not clonally related. Conversely, two (13%) of the 16 paired tumors had identical genetic alterations, which suggests clonal expansion as the mechanism underlying tumor multiplicity. One clone may have spread from the hypopharynx into the cervical esophagus, and another may have spread from the tonsil to the distal esophagus. These authors concluded that most second primary esophageal cancers are truly independent neoplasms, in contrast to the solitary pulmonary nodules whose molecular features show them to be most likely metastases. However, the caveat is that a clonal population of neoplastic cells may be capable of traveling substantial distances to give rise to second tumors at different anatomic sites, as shown by these authors.

Khuri et al. *(30)* evaluated 53 samples from 38 patients in whom tissue was available for matched first and second events (recurrences or second or subsequent primary tumors). Evidence of clonality and interrelatedness between serial aerodigestive events was assessed by sequencing the p53 gene in serial tumors and studies of LOH and comparing them to the clinical outcomes in terms of the correlation between clinical and molecular events. Sequencing the p53 gene correlated highly with the clinical determination of second primary tumor events; in 17 of 18 second primaries with discordant p53 mutations, the clinical assessment was supported by the genomic sequence. LOH was generally more useful as a descriptor of the complexity of the carcinogen-damaged field and of the clonal heterogeneity process.

5. THE CONCEPT OF CHEMOPREVENTION

Primary therapy and relative rates of survival for patients with HNSCC are likely to continue to improve due to advances in the diagnostic and therapeutic modalities available for use in clinics. A direct consequence of this improvement will be that more patients could live long enough to develop SPTs, indicating the urgent need for measures to deter HNSCC. A vital part of this strategy is chemoprevention, a term coined initially by Sporn et al. *(31)* in 1976, and defined as the use of specific natural or synthetic chemical agents to reverse, suppress, or prevent premalignant lesions from progressing to invasive cancer. The concept is particularly applicable given the extent of smoking-induced injury documented initially by Slaughter et al. *(16)* and Auerbach et al. *(17,18)* and found throughout the epithelial tissue of the aerodigestive tract.

Much chemopreventive work has centered on using retinoids, synthetic or natural vitamin A derivatives, to reverse premalignant lesions and prevent second primary cancers in the head and neck area *(32–41)*. Wolbach and Howe *(42)* demonstrated that cattle and sheep deprived of vitamin A were far more likely to develop lung and upper aerodigestive tract cancer. Our improved understanding of retinoid biology is predicated on this seminal observation.

Retinoids have complex biological effects, including modulating differentiation, proliferation, apoptosis, and immune status in both normal and neoplastic tissues *(43,44)*. This complexity is a function of the diversity of retinoid ligands and the nuclear receptors that mediate their activity *(43,44)*. Different natural retinoids can activate selective retinoid receptors expressed in different cell types, therefore differentially regulating selective gene expression *(45,46)*. The two broad classes of nuclear retnoid receptors, retinoic acid receptors (RARs) and retinoid X receptors (RXRs), have three subclasses, α, β, and γ, each of which is further divided into multiple isoforms produced through differential promoter usage and alternative splicing of receptor transcripts *(45–48)*. Nuclear retinoid receptors function as either heterodimers or homodimers. RXRs can form homodimers or heterodimers by binding to RARs or a host of other receptors, all derivatives of the steroid hormone superfamily of receptors. RARs form only heterodimers and do so only with RXRs. Natural retinoids, such as retinyl palmitate, are nonselective, pan-receptor activators, meaning that they cause a wide spectrum of physiologic effects. Subtle differences in the structure of the cleft where retinoids bind to receptors have permitted development of receptor-specific synthetic retinoids *(48)*. Different receptors may mediate different effects, and this specificity or selectivity can have important clinical implications for enhancing anti-cancer efficacy and reducing toxic side effects.

Retinoids have undergone extensive development as chemopreventive agents. In addition to 13-*cis*-retinoic acid (13cRA), other retinoids tested in clinical trials of upper aerodigestive tract cancers include another retinoic acid stereoisomer, 9-*cis*-retinoic acid (9cRA), etretinate, 4-*N*-(4-hydroxyphenyl)retinamide (4-HPR or fenretinide), and bexarotene, an RXR-specific retinoid *(47,48)*. 4-HPR is unusual because it does not bind any of the nuclear retinoid receptors at physiologic doses of the compound, but is a potent in vitro inducer of apoptosis *(49)*. Mechanisms by which retinoids induce a chemopreventive effect in the upper aerodigestive tract are only partially understood. However, in vitro experiments appear to show that selective upregulation of RARβ *(50)* modulates squamous cell growth and differentiation. Better understanding of the interactions between selective ligands, and the interplay among various different retinoid receptors, is necessary to more selectively develop this class of compounds for a greater role in aerodigestive tract cancer chemoprevention and therapy.

6. EARLY INTERVENTIONAL CHEMOPREVENTION TRIALS IN ORAL PREMALIGNANT LESIONS

Several important randomized chemoprevention trials have been completed on oral premalignant lesions (OPLs), including both leukoplakia and erythroplakia. Small, hyperplastic leukoplakia lesions have a 30–40%

spontaneous regression rate and a <5% risk for malignant transformation *(51)*. Erythroleukoplakia and dysplastic leukoplakia lesions have a <5% rate of spontaneous regression and a 30–50% risk for progression to oral cancer *(51)*. This high-risk, diffuse, and multifocal disease accounts for 10–15% of all OPLs and is only somewhat treatable with local therapy involving surgery or radiation. Patients with OPLs often develop cancers at distant sites in the upper aerodigestive tract as well as in the oral cavity. Therefore, trials focusing on reversal of OPLs were among the first indicators of the respective efficacies of various compounds as chemopreventive agents for subsequent cancer prevention trials.

In the 1970s, several epidemiologic and interventional studies found that supplemental β-carotene and retinol could significantly reduce the frequency of oral micronuclei *(52)*. These fragments of extranuclear DNA may represent a nonspecific but quantifiable assessment of genetic damage in populations at high risk for oral cancer, including those who chew tobacco and betel nut. Several subsequent randomized trials have been conducted to investigate the effects of supplemental β-carotene, either alone or in combination with other agents, on oral leukoplakia regression. Five of these trials were nonrandomized studies that achieved response rates of 44–71% *(52)*. Results of these uncontrolled trials are tempered by the 30–40% spontaneous regression rate of leukoplakia and by different study response criteria in the absence of any readily apparent dose-response relationship *(52)*.

Multiple trials *(32–39,52)* of retinoids in OPLs have been conducted to date (Table 1). The results indicate that retinoids are far more effective in early to intermediate premalignancy chemoprevention *(32–39)* than in reversing advanced premalignant lesions of the larynx or oral cavity. The initial randomized trial in 1986 by Hong et al. *(32)*, which used high-dose 13cRA at 1–2 mg/kg/d for 3 mo vs placebo, demonstrated a 67% clinical response rate for retinoid vs 10% for placebo ($p = 0.002$). Several randomized trials confirmed retinoid activity in reversal of premalignant lesions. Lippman et al. *(35)* followed a high-dose induction of 13cRA for 3 mo (1.5 mg/kg/d) by randomizing patients to 13cRA at a low dose (0.5 mg/kg/d) for 9 mo vs 9 mo of β-carotene at 30 mg/day. Results indicated that the low-dose daily retinoid was substantially more effective in maintaining initial response to 13cRA induction than was β-carotene (92% vs 45%; $p = 0.001$). However, subsequent follow-up to this trial has found no significant difference between the two arms *(36)* in incidence of SCC development.

Table 1
Selected Completed Chemoprevention Trials in Oral Premalignancy Involving Retinoids and/or β-Carotene
and/or α-Tocopherol

Investigator(s)	Year	Agent(s)	Patients (N)	Results
Hong et al. (32)	1986	13cRA at 1–2 mg/kg/d for 3 mo vs placebo	44	67% response (13cRA) vs 10% response (placebo) ($p = 0.0002$)
Stich et al. (33)	1988	β-carotene + retinol (100,000 IU/wk) (180 mg/wk) vs placebo	103	27.5% vs 14.8% vs 3.0% ($p < 0.001$)
Stich et al. (34)	1988	Vitamin A (200,000 IU/wk) orally for 6 mo vs placebo	64	57.1% complete remission (vitamin A) vs 30% (controls) ($p < 0.01$)
Han et al. (37)	1990	4-HCR (40 mg/d) vs placebo	61	87% complete remission vs 17% ($p < 0.01$)
Lippman et al. (35)	1993	13cRA (1.5 mg/kg/d) for 3 mo followed by 13cRA (0.5 mg/kg/d) for 9 mo vs β-carotene (30 mg/d) for 9 mo	70	Initial response 55% to high-dose in 13cRA; continued response or stable disease 92% in 13cRA maintenance vs 45% β-carotene ($p < 0.001$)
Chiesa et al. (38)	1993,1994	4-HPR (200 mg/d) for 52 wk vs placebo	153	Failure in 6% (4-HPR) vs 305 (placebo) ($p < 0.05$)
Papadimitrakopoulou et al. (39)	1999	13cRA (50 mg/m^2/d), α-interferon (3 million IU/m^2 3×/wk), α-tocopherol 1200 IU/d)	36	7/14 (50%) pathologic CR rate in advanced laryngeal premalignant lesions vs 0/7 (0%) pathologic CR rate in advanced oral cavity premalignant lesions ($p = 0.02$)

13cRA, 13-*cis*-retinoic acid; 4-HCR, 4(hydroxycarbophenyl)retinamide; 4-HPR, 4-*N*-(4-hydroyphenyl)retinamide.

Papadimitrakopoulou et al. (39) demonstrated significant differential efficacy for a biochemoprevention combination of α-interferon (3 million IU/m2 three times per week SC) with 13cRA (50 mg/m2/d orally) and α-tocopherol (1200 IU daily orally) in reversal of advanced premalignant lesions of the larynx as opposed to those in the oral cavity. Durable complete responses were seen in approx 50% of 36 evaluable laryngeal premalignancy patients with advanced premalignant lesions of the larynx and oral cavity, defined as either moderate or severe dysplasia or carcinoma *in situ*. Several patients experienced durable complete responses for several months after discontinuation of therapy. On the other hand, none of 12 patients with oral cavity premalignant lesions had a durable complete response, and partial responses were generally transient, with disease progression not uncommon. These striking differences between the efficacy of this regimen in treating laryngeal and oral cavity premalignant lesions has led to the launch of a randomized trial of the same combination in advanced premalignant lesions of the larynx, in which patients with either moderate to severe dysplasia or carcinoma *in situ* of the larynx are treated for 1 yr with the 13cRA, α-interferon, and α-tocopherol combination, followed by randomization to either 4-HPR or placebo. The long-term results of this trial are likely to help further define the efficacy of this more aggressive therapeutic approach to advanced premalignant lesions of the larynx (Papadimitrakopoulou et al., personal communication). Further biological studies have indicated that this regimen appears quite effective in causing a complete phenotypic reversion; however, reversal of genetic abnormalities that underlie carcinogenic progression is rare (53).

These trials showed clearly that although retinoids are able to reverse early to intermediate premalignant lesions, this effect was transient, with the premalignant lesions reverting to their pretherapy histology within 3–6 mo after discontinuation of therapy. Further trials have also indicated that chemoprevention combining a retinoid and interferon has a great deal of promise, particularly because the regimen was reasonably well tolerated, with very few grade 4 toxicities seen by the National Cancer Institute (NCI) Common Toxicity Criteria *(39,53)*.

7. SECOND PRIMARY TUMOR PREVENTION STUDIES

7.1. First-Generation Trials

As previously indicated, several longitudinal studies found that patients treated for initial cancer constitute those at the single highest risk for SPT development. The recent SEER database, showing high numbers of second cancers in patients with a previous history of laryngeal cancer followed for many years, indicates the urgent need to develop effective chemopreventive strategies. The high likelihood of SPTs after treatment of early HNSCC makes this disease an excellent model for the study of chemoprevention. The most pivotal study in this area, a randomized, double-blinded, placebo-controlled trial of high-dose 13cRA as adjuvant therapy after curative surgery and/or radiation therapy for primary HNSCC, was conducted by Hong et al. *(40)*. A total of 103 patients were randomly assigned to either high-dose 13cRA (50–100 mg/m²/d) or placebo for 12 mo. After a median follow-up of 32 mo, SPTs developed in significantly fewer 13cRA-treated patients (4%) than in patients receiving placebo (24%) ($p = 0.005$). Of the 14 SPTs that occurred at the time of initial analysis, 13 (93%) were located in the tobacco smoke-exposed fields of the upper aerodigestive tract, lungs, and esophagus. Substantial toxicity of high-dose 13cRA caused one-third of the retinoid-treated patients to require dose reduction or discontinuation of therapy, and no impact was seen on recurrence rates or overall survival. Benner et al. *(54)* reported the second primary data further over a median follow-up period of 4.5 yr. Retinoid-treated patients continued to have significantly fewer total SPTs: seven (14%) in the 13cRA arm and 16 (31%) in the placebo arm ($p = 0.042$). The difference was considerably more striking when only SPTs from the tobacco-damaged fields of the upper aerodigestive tract and lungs were evaluated. Here, smoking-related SPTs occurred in 3 of 49 13cRA-treated patients and in 13 of 51 assessable patients who received placebo ($p = 0.008$). These provocative results suggested that the chemopreventive effects of 13cRA persisted for approx 2 yr after completion of therapy but then disappeared, as demonstrated by the fact that the SPT rates in both arms are equivalent from the 3-yr point onward (Table 2).

Bolla et al. *(41)* used etretinate, an alternative synthetic retinoid, to prevent SPTs in patients with prior SCCs of the oral cavity or oral pharynx. Patients were randomly assigned to either retinoid (50 mg/d for 1 mo, followed by 25 mg/d for 24 mo) or placebo. No SPT reduction was seen in the retinoid arm with a median follow-up of 41 mo. The two study arms were equivalent, both in occurrence of SPTs and relapse of initial cancer. This trial confirmed the high rate of head and neck SPTs seen in the earlier trial of Hong and coworkers *(40,54)*. SPTs occurred in 57 of the 316 (18%) patients enrolled, with 45 (79%) of these SPTs in the upper aerodigestive tract, lungs, or esophagus (Table 2).

Pastorino et al. *(55)* conducted a study using a natural vitamin A analog, retinol palmitate (300,000 IU/d for 12 mo), to prevent SPTs in patients previously treated for primary stage I NSCLC. This natural vitamin A analog was well tolerated, with more than 80% patient compliance. Eighteen patients in the retinol palmitate group developed SPTs, compared with 29 patients in the control arm at the time of reporting *(55)*. A reduction in tobacco-related SPTs was observed; only 13 smoking-related SPTs occurred in the retinol palmitate arm vs 25 SPTs for patients in the control arm. The timely development of a tobacco-related SPT statistically significantly favored the retinoid arm ($p = 0.045$). However, published data from Pastorino et al. indicate that there are no significant differences between the two arms at 8 yr in terms of SPT development (Pastorino et al., personal communication) (Table 2).

Thus, these first-generation SPT prevention trials yielded something of a mixed message. The trials of Hong et al. *(40)* and Pastorino et al. *(55)* indicated that retinoids were able to prevent SPTs in two different aerodigestive primary sites (HNSCC and NSCLC) but that this protection lasted only for approx 2–3 yr after discontinuation of therapy. The Bolla trial *(41)* using a different synthetic retinoid was negative, but yielded confirmatory data on the high incidence of aerodigestive tract SPTs found in HNSCC.

Another important aspect of these trials was their demonstration that high doses of retinoids, particularly 13cRA, were difficult to administer over an extended period of time in this patient population, because approx

Table 2
Randomized Chemoprevention Trials Involving Retinoids and/or β-Carotene in Patients With Aerodigestive
Tumors to Prevent Second Primary Tumors

Investigator(s)	Year population	Patient	Patients (N)	Median follow-up (mo)	Agent(s)	Results
Hong et al. (40)	1990		103	54	13cRA (50–100 mg/m^2) for 12 mo vs placebo	At 3 yr, 14% SPTs vs 24% ($p = 0.005$)
Benner et al. (54)	1994	HNSCC	103	54	13cRA (50–100 mg/m^2) for 12 mo vs placebo	At 4½ yr, 14% SPTs vs 31% ($p = 0.042$)
Pastorino et al. (55)	1993	NSCLC	307	46	Retinyl palmitate (300,000 IU) for 12 mo vs placebo	8.5% SPTs vs 18.8% SPTs ($p = 0.05$)
Bolla et al. (41)	1994	HNSCC	316	41	Etretinate (50 mg/d) for 1 mo followed by 25 mg/d for 24 mo vs placebo	No difference (25% in both groups)
EUROSCAN (56)	2000	HNSCC/ NSCLC	2,592	49	1. Retinyl palmitate (300,000 IU/d for 1 yr) followed by 150,000 IU for a 2nd year 2. N-acetylcysteine 600 mg/d for 2 yr 3. Both 4. Neither	No difference in SPT rate, event-free survival, or overall survival among any of the four arms
Intergroup (57)	2001	NSCLC	1,483	42	13cRA 30 mg/d for 36 mo vs placebo	No difference in SPT rate, event-free survival, or overall survival; patients randomized to 13cRA who continued to smoke had higher recurrence of primary tumors

HNSCC, head and neck squamous cell carcinoma; NSCLC, non-small-cell lung cancer; 13cRA, 13-*cis*-retinoic acid; SPT, second primary tumor.

30–40% of patients in the Hong trial *(40,54)* required significant dose reductions from their baseline 13cRA dose. This was markedly more striking than dose reductions required for placebo and was in keeping with the earlier toxicity of retinoids seen in the leukoplakia trials.

7.2. Second-Generation SPT Prevention Studies

Three large trials for prevention of second primary head and neck cancer were launched on the basis of promising initial data of Pastorino and Hong. The EUROSCAN trial *(56)* was a multi-institutional trial conducted by the European Organization for Research and Treatment of Cancer (EORTC). From June 19, 1994

through July 19, 1998, a total of 2592 patients (60% with stage I, II, or III HNSCC and 40% with stage I or II NSCLC) were randomly assigned to receive one of four treatment arms. The 2 × 2 factorial schema randomized patients to either retinyl palmitate (300,000 IU daily for 1 yr followed by 150,000 IU for a second year), N-acetylcysteine (600 mg/d for 2 yr), both compounds, or no intervention at all. After a median follow-up of 49 mo, events (recurrence, SPT, or death) were reported for 916 patients. No statistically significant difference was observed in overall survival or event-free survival between patients who received retinyl palmitate and those who did not *(56)*. Similarly, no difference was

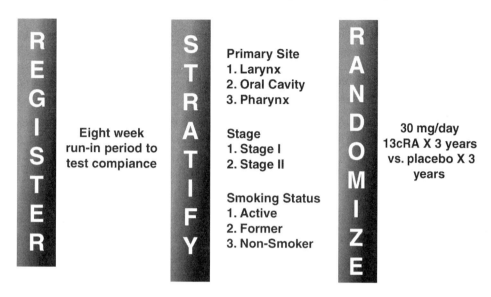

RTOG 91-15: Chemoprevention Trial to Prevent Second Primary Tumors with Low-Dose 13cRA in Head and Neck Cancer (HNSP Trial)

Fig. 2. Schema of the recently completed trial randomizing patients definitively treated for stage I or II HNSCC to either low-dose 13-*cis*-retinoic acid (30 mg/d) or placebo for 3 yr. The final analysis of this trial is anticipated for late 2002 or early 2003.

seen in overall survival or event-free survival by patients who received *N*-acetylcysteine and patients who did not *(56)*. Surprisingly, a lower incidence of SPTs was seen in the no-intervention arm, but the difference was not statistically significant. This led the investigators to conclude that the 2-yr supplementation of retinyl palmitate and *N*-acetylcysteine had no benefit in terms of survival, event-free survival, or SPT incidence for patients with either head and neck or lung cancer (Table 2).

US Intergroup NCI-91-0001, a randomized, double-blind study using low-dose 13cRA after surgery for stage I NSCLC, completed accrual in April 1997 with 1486 participants *(57)*. Study objectives were to evaluate efficacy of 13cRA in reducing SPT incidence in patients after complete resection of stage I NSCLC, to look at the qualitative and quantitative toxicity of low-dose 13cRA, and to compare overall survival rates of patients receiving 13cRA with those receiving placebo. This study, like the EUROSCAN study *(56)*, was launched based on the positive studies of Pastorino et al. *(55)* and Hong et al. *(40)* and in the belief that retinoid reversal of common carcinogenic injuries induced by tobacco was likely to yield positive results in the lung. Randomization of 1304 patients was completed in June 1997. Patients were required to have undergone complete resection of primary stage I NSCLC (postoperative

T1 or T2, N0 M0) 6 wk to 3 yr before enrollment. After a median follow-up of 3.5 yr, no statistically significant differences were seen between the placebo and the 13cRA arm with respect to time to SPT, recurrence, or mortality *(57)*. Isotretinoin (13cRA) treatment did not improve the overall rate of SPTs, recurrences, or mortality in stage I NSCLC. Secondary multivariate and subset analyses suggested that isotretinoin was harmful in current smokers and beneficial in never-smokers *(57)* (Table 2). Large trials, such as the EUROSCAN and US Intergroup, will better define new avenues for future chemopreventive treatment. An Eastern Cooperative Oncology Group (ECOG) trial is now studying the effects of daily selenium supplementation in patients with stage I NSCLC.

Perhaps most ambitious and extensive has been a large follow-up SPT prevention study developed in cooperation by the M. D. Anderson Cancer Center with its affiliated Community Clinical Oncology Program (CCOP) and RTOG *(58)* (Fig. 2). This randomized, double-blind trial, launched in 1991, studied the effect of low-dose 13cRA to prevent SPTs in patients definitively treated for stage I or II HNSCC for up to 3 yr before participation (T1, N0 M0 or T2, N0 M0). Patients received 30 mg/day of 13cRA or a placebo (similar to the lung Intergroup trial) for 3 yr and were followed for an additional 4 yr. The study completed accrual in July 1999 with 1189 eligible and evaluable patients randomized of 1384 patients registered effective September 1999. SPT incidence according to prior tumor stage as well as related to smoking status (current, former, never) has been reported. The annual primary tumor recurrence rate was 2.8% across the study and the annual SPT occurrence rate was 5.1%. Stage II HNSCC had a higher rate of SPT development than did stage I. In addition, active smokers had a significantly higher recurrence rate than former or never smokers (4.3% vs 3.3% vs 1.9%).

This study demonstrated prospectively for the first time the impact of active smoking status in SPT development. The SPT rate was significantly higher in smokers vs nonactive smokers ($p = 0.018$) and was marginally significant between former and never-smokers ($p = 0.11$). The site of SPT also differed by the primary index tumor. Patients with primary laryngeal cancers were most likely to develop SPT in either the lung or larynx, whereas patients with oral cavity primaries were most likely to develop second primaries in either the oral cavity or lung. Finally, patients with an index primary tumor of the pharynx developed SPTs in the lung, oral cavity, pharynx, or esophagus. Compared to previous trials, SPTs occurred more frequently than expected at the index primary sites of the oral upper aerodigestive tract. The lower dose of 13cRA was well tolerated, with few grade 3 toxicities. This trial was to be unblinded and analyzed in late 2002 (58).

8. INTERMEDIATE BIOMARKERS IN PREMALIGNANCY TRIALS

Studies completed to date, both in OPLs and in SPTs, have contributed a wealth of scientific knowledge to the medical community. Lotan and coworkers showed that upregulation of RARβ correlated with the likelihood of improvement in the premalignant lesions when samples obtained from the trials of Lippman et al. (35,59) were assayed. Xu et al. (60,61) have shown that RARβ is gradually lost in both head and neck and lung carcinogenesis. Assaying samples of patients treated with 13cRA for oral leukoplakia in the trial by Lippman et al. (35), Lotan demonstrated that RARβ was upregulated in individuals whose leukoplakia responded to 13cRA, whereas it was less likely to improve in individuals who were resistant to the retinoid (59). On the other hand, Lippman, Shin and coworkers studied the relationship between the p53 protein, as detected by immunohistochemistry, and the carcinogenic process. They demonstrated not only that p53 overexpression increased during progression from oral premalignant lesions to invasive cancer (62) but also that lesions with high p53 expression were very likely to be resistant to upregulation by 13cRA and correlated with lack of induction of RARβ expression (63). These investigators (64) also showed that overexpression of p53 protein by immunohistochemistry correlates with a high likelihood of SPTs and death from primary tumor relapse; ultimately this could lead to development of a molecular model of HNSCC to guide our therapy. Furthermore, Mao et al. (53) showed that molecular genetic abnormalities underlying histologic expressions of premalignancy do not appear to completely resolve in patients with advanced dysplastic lesions of the larynx who obtain a complete clinical and histologic response to biochemopreventive therapy, thereby implying the existence of an underlying genetic "scar" that may lead to development of cancer.

9. NOVEL AGENTS IN CHEMOPREVENTION

Several investigators have explored novel agents tested for cancer chemoprevention. For example, farnesyl transferase inhibitors, which affect the *ras* gene signaling pathway by preventing post-translational modification of RAS necessary for oncogenic RAS signaling and transformation, have been shown to have activity, both alone and in combination with cytotoxic agents, in advanced aerodigestive tract cancers (65–67). Similarly, molecules targeting epidermal growth factor receptor (EGFR), which is a critical growth factor for HNSCC and upregulated or overexpressed in 90–100% of HNSCCs (68–70), represent an equally attractive approach. Several agents in a class of compounds that inhibit the tyrosine kinase receptor of EGFR, such as ZD-1839 (gefitinib) (71,72) and OSI-774 (etorlinib) (73), have demonstrated activity in refractory NSCLC and HNSCC. These molecules are also being developed for future chemoprevention trials in aerodigestive tract malignancies. Given their anticancer activity and tolerability in treating advanced disease, these compounds could be deployed in the upper aerodigestive tract to reverse premalignant lesions and prevent SPTs.

With the progress to date in upper aerodigestive tract chemoprevention, and increasing specificity of these molecules, we predict that chemopreventive approaches targeting selective abnormalities in the carcinogenic pathway of the upper aerodigestive tract will lead to improvements not only in the incidence of SPTs but ultimately in the survival and quality of life of patients afflicted with these devastating diseases.

REFERENCES

1. Greenlee RT, Hill-Harmon MB, Murray T, Thun M. Cancer statistics, 2001. *CA Cancer J Clin* 2001;51:15–36.

2. Clayman GL, Lippman SM, Laramore GE, Hong WK. Head and neck cancer. In *Cancer Medicine*. Holland JF, Bast RC, Morton DL, et al., eds. Williams & Wilkins, Baltimore, 1997; pp. 1645–1710.

3. Vikram B. Changing patterns of failure in advanced head and neck cancer. *Arch Otolaryngol* 1984;110:564–565.

4. Cooper JS, Pajak TK, Rubin P, et al. Second malignancies in patients who have head and neck cancer: incidence, effect on survival and implications based on the RTOG experience. *Int J Radiat Oncol Biol Phys* 1989;17:449–456.

5. Licciardello JT, Spitz MR, Hong WK. Multiple primary cancers in patients with cancer of the head and neck: second cancer of the head and neck, esophagus and lung. *Int J Radiat Oncol Biol Phys* 1989;17:467–476.

6. Califano J, van der Riet P, Westra W, et al. Genetic progression model for head and neck cancer: implications for field cancerization. *Cancer Res* 1996;56:2488–2492.

7. Bergen AW, Caporaso N. Cigarette smoking. *J Natl Cancer Inst* 1999;91:1365–1375.

8. Dominioni L, Strauss GM, Imperatori A, et al. Screening for lung cancer. *Chest Surg Clin N Am* 2000;10:729–736.

9. Kurie JM, Spitz MR, Hong WK. Lung cancer chemoprevention: targeting former rather than current smokers. *Cancer Prev International* 1995;2:55–58.

10. Denissenko MF, Pao A, Tang M, Pfeifer GP. Preferential formation of benzo[a]pyrene adducts at lung cancer mutational hotspots in P53. *Science* 1996;274:430–432.

11. Knudson AG Jr. Mutation and cancer: statistical study of retinoblastoma. *Proc Natl Acad Sci USA* 1976;6:820–824.

12. Carey TE, Frank CJ, Raval JR, et al. Identifying genetic changes associated with tumor progression in squamous cell carcinoma. *Acta Otolaryngol (Stockh)* 1997;529:229–232.

13. van der Riet P, Nawroz H, Hruban RH, et al. Frequent loss of chromosome 9p21-22 early in head and neck cancer progression. *Cancer Res* 1994;54:1156–1158.

14. Mao L, Lee JS, Fan YH, et al. Frequent microsatellite alterations at chromosome 9p21 and 3p14 in oral premalignant lesions and their value in cancer risk assessment. *Nat Med* 1996;2:682–685.

15. Hung J, Kishimoto Y, Sujio K, et al. Allele-specific chromosome 3p deletions occur at an early stage in the pathogenesis of lung carcinoma [published erratum appears in *JAMA* 1995;273:1908]. JAMA 1995;273:558–563.

16. Slaughter DP, Southwick HW, Smejkal W. Field cancerization in oral stratified squamous epithelium: clinical implications of multicentric origin. *Cancer* 1953;6:963–968.

17. Auerbach O, Gere JB, Forman JB, et al. Changes in bronchial epithelium in relation to smoking and cancer of the lungs: a report of progress. *N Engl J Med* 1957;256:97–104.

18. Auerbach O, Hammond EC, Garfinkel L. Changes in bronchial epithelium in relation to cigarette smoking, 1955–1960 vs 1970–1977. *N Engl J Med* 1979;300:381–385.

19. Gao X, Fisher SG, Mohideen N, et al. Second primary cancers in patients with laryngeal cancer: a population-based study [Abstract]. *Proc Am Soc Clin Oncol* 2000;19:414a.

20. Tucker MA, Murray N, Shaw EG, et al. Second primary cancers related to smoking and treatment of small-cell lung cancer. *J Natl Cancer Inst* 1997;89:1782–1788.

21. Russo A, Crosignani P, Berrino F. Tobacco smoking, alcohol drinking and dietary factors as determinants of new primaries among male laryngeal cancer patients: a case-cohort study. *Tumori* 1996;82:519–525.

22. Kurokawa R, DiRenzo J, Boehm M, et al. Regulation of retinoid signaling by receptor polarity and allosteric control of ligand binding. *Nature* 1994;371:528–531.

23. Van Leeuwen FE, Klokman WJ, Stovall M, et al. Roles of radiotherapy and smoking in lung cancer following Hodgkin's disease. *J Natl Cancer Inst* 1995;87:1530–1537.

24. Richardson GE, Tucker MA, Venzon DJ, et al. Smoking cessation after successful treatment of small-cell lung cancer is associated with fewer smoking-related second primary cancers. *Ann Intern Med* 1993;119:383–390.

25. Silverman S Jr, Gorsky M, Greenspan D. Tobacco usage in patients with head and neck carcinomas: a follow-up study on habit changes and second primary oral/oropharyngeal cancers. *J Am Dent Assoc* 1983;106:33–35.

26. Castigliano SG. Influence of continued smoking on the incidence of second primary cancers involving mouth, pharynx, and larynx. *J Am Dent Assoc* 1968;77:580–585.

27. Bedi GC, Westra WH, Gabrielson E, et al. Multiple head and neck tumors: evidence for a common clonal origin. *Cancer Res* 1996;56:2484–2487.

28. Leong PP, Rezai B, Koch WM, et al. Distinguishing second primary tumors from lung metastases in patients with head and neck squamous cell carcinoma. *J Natl Cancer Inst* 1998;90:972–977.

29. Califano J, Leong PL, Koch WM, et al. Second esophageal tumors in patients with head and neck squamous cell carcinoma: an assessment of clonal relationships. *Clin Cancer Res* 1999;5:1862–1867.

30. Khuri FR, Rodriguez M, Lee JJ, et al. Comprehensive analysis of clinical and molecular determinants of second events in the randomized retinoid head and neck second primary tumor prevention trial. *Proc Am Assoc Cancer Res* 2002; abst. 2553.

31. Sporn MB, Dunlop NM, Newton DL, Smith JM. Prevention of chemical carcinogenesis by vitamin A and its synthetic analogs (retinoids). *Fed Proc* 1976;35:1332–1338.

32. Hong W, Endicott J, Itri LM, et al. 13-cis retinoic acid in the treatment of oral leukoplakia. *N Engl J Med* 1986;315:1501–1505.

33. Zaridze D, Evstifeeva T, Boyle P. Chemoprevention of oral leukoplakia and chronic esophagitis in an area of high incidence of oral and esophageal cancer. Ann Epidemiol 1993;3:225–234.

34. Stich HF, Rosin MP, Hornby P, et al. Remission of oral leukoplakias and micronuclei in tobacco/betel quid chewers treated with β-carotene and with β-carotene plus vitamin A. *Int J Cancer* 1988;42:195–199.

35. Lippman SM, Batsakis JG, Toth BB, et al. Comparison of low-dose isotretinoin with beta-carotene to prevent oral carcinogenesis. *N Engl J Med* 1993;328:15–20.

36. Papadimitrakopoulou VA, Hong WK, Lee JS, et al. Low-dose isotretinoin versus β-carotene to prevent oral carcinogenesis: long-term follow-up. J *Natl Cancer Inst* 1997;89:257–258.

37. Han J, Jiao L, Lu Y, et al. Evaluation of N-4-(hydroxycarbophenyl) retinamide as a cancer prevention agent and as a cancer chemotherapeutic agent. *In Vivo* 1990;4:153–160.

38. Chiesa F, Tradati N, Marazza M, et al. Prevention of local relapses and new localisations of oral leukoplakias with the synthetic retinoid fenretinide (4-HPR): preliminary results. *Eur J Cancer B Oral Oncol* 1992;28B:97–102.

39. Papadimitrakopoulou VA, Clayman GL, Shin DM, et al. Biochemoprevention for dysplastic lesions of the upper aerodigestive tract. *Arch Otolaryngol Head Neck Surg* 1999;125:1083–1089.

40. Hong WK, Lippman SM, Itri LM, et al. Prevention of second primary tumors with isotretinoin in squamous-cell carcinoma of the head and neck. *N Engl J Med* 1990;323:795–801.

41. Bolla M, Lefur R, Ton Van J, et al. Prevention of second primary tumours with etretinate in squamous cell carcinoma of the oral cavity and oropharynx. Results of a multicentric double-blind randomized study. *Eur J Cancer* 1994;30A:767–772.

42. Wolbach SB, Howe PR. Tissue changes following deprivation of fat soluble A vitamin. *J Exp Med* 1925;42:753.

43. Mangelsdorf DJ, Umesono K, Evans RM. The retinoid receptors. In *The Retinoids*. Sporn MB, Roberts AB, Goodman DS, eds. Raven Press, New York, 1994; pp. 319–349.

44. Chambon P. The retinoid signaling pathway: molecular and genetic analyses. *Semin Cell Biol* 1994;5:115–125.

45. Leid M, Kastner P, Chambon P. Multiplicity generates diversity in the retinoic acid signaling pathways. *Trends Biochem Sci* 1992;17:427–433.

46. Blaner WS. Biochemistry and pharmacology of retinoids. In *Retinoids in Oncology*. Hong WK, Lotan R, eds. Marcel Dekker, New York, 1993; pp. 1–42.

47. Boehm MF, Zhang L. Synthesis and structure-activity relationships of novel retinoid X receptor-selective retinoids. *J Med Chem* 1994;37:2930–2941.

48. Khuri FR, Rigas JR, Figlin RA, et al. Multi-institutional phase I/II trial of oral bexarotene in combination with cisplatin and vinorelbine in previously untreated patients with advanced non-small-cell lung cancer. *J Clin Oncol* 2001;19: 2626–2637.

49. Oridate N, Lotan D, Xu XC, et al. Differential induction of apoptosis by all-trans-retinoic acid and N-(4-hydroxyphenyl) retinamide in human head and neck squamous cell carcinoma cell lines. *Clin Cancer Res* 1996;2:855–863.

50. Xu XC, Zile MH, Lippman SM, et al. Anti-retinoic acid (RA) antibody binding to human premalignant oral lesions, which occurs less frequently than binding to normal tissue, increases after 13-cis-RA treatment in vivo and is related to RA receptor beta expression. *Cancer Res* 1995;55:5507–5511.

51. Silverman S, Gorsky M, Lozada F. Oral leukoplakia and malignant transformation: a follow-up study of 257 patients. *Cancer* 1984;53:563–568.

52. Stich HR, Rosin MP, Hornby P, et al. Remission of oral leukoplakias and micronuclei in tobacco/betel quid chewers treated with beta-carotene and with beta-carotene plus vitamin A. *Int J Cancer* 1988;42:195–199.

53. Mao L, El-Naggar AK, Papadimitrakopoulou VA, et al. Molecular paradox of complete phenotypic response of advanced head and neck premalignancies to biochemoprevention. *J Natl Cancer Inst* 1998;90:1545–1551.

54. Benner SE, Pajak TF, Lippman SM, et al. Prevention of second primary tumors with isotretinoin in patients with squamous cell carcinoma of the head and neck: long-term follow-up. *J Natl Cancer Inst* 1994;86:140–141.

55. Pastorino U, Infante M, Maioli M, et al. Adjuvant treatment of stage I lung cancer with high-dose vitamin A. *J Clin Oncol* 1993;11:1216–1222.

56. Van Zandwijk N, Dalesio O, Pastorino U, et al. EUROSCAN, a randomized trial of vitamin A and N-acetylcysteine in patients with head and neck cancer or lung cancer. *J Natl Cancer Inst* 2000;92:977–986.

57. Lippman SM, Lee JJ, Karp DD, et al. Randomized phase III intergroup trial of isotretinoin to prevent second primary tumors in stage I non-small-cell lung cancer. *J Natl Cancer Inst* 2001;93:605–618.

58. Khuri FR, Kim ES, Lee JJ, et al. The impact of smoking status, disease stage, and index tumor site on second primary tumor incidence and tumor recurrence in the head and neck retinoid chemoprevention trial. *Cancer Epidemiol Biomarkers Prev* 2001;10:823–829.

59. Lotan R, Xu XC, Lippman SM, et al. Suppression of retinoic acid receptor-beta in premalignant oral lesions and its upregulation by isotretinoin. N Engl J Med 1995;332: 1405–1410.

60. Xu XC, Ro JY, Lee JS, et al. Differential expression of nuclear retinoid receptors in normal, premalignant, and malignant head and neck tissues. *Cancer Res* 1994;54:3580–3587.

61. Xu XC, Sozzi G, Lee JS, et al. Suppression of retinoic acid receptor β in non-small-cell lung cancer in vivo: implications for lung cancer development. *J Natl Cancer Inst* 1997;89:624–629.

62. Lippman SM, Shin DM, Lee JJ, et al. p53 and retinoid chemoprevention of oral carcinogenesis. *Cancer Res* 1995;55:16–19.

63. Shin DM, Xu XC, Lippman SM, et al. Accumulation of p53 protein and retinoic acid receptor beta in retinoid chemoprevention. *Clin Cancer Res* 1997;3:875–880.

64. Shin DM, Lee JS, Lippman SM, et al. p53 expression: predicting recurrence and second primary tumors in head and neck squamous cell carcinoma. *J Natl Cancer Inst* 1996;88: 519–529.

65. Adjei AA. Blocking oncogenic Ras signaling for cancer therapy. *J Natl Cancer Inst* 2001;93:1062–1074.

66. Kies MS, Clayman GL, El-Naggar AK, et al. Induction therapy with SCH66336, a farnesyltransferase inhibitor, in squamous cell carcinoma (SCC) of the head and neck [Abstract]. *Proc Am Soc Clin Oncol* 2001;20:225a.

67. Khuri FR, Glisson BS, Meyers ML, et al. Phase I study of farnesyl transferase inhibitor (FTI) SCH66336 with paclitaxel in solid tumors: dose finding, pharmacokinetics, efficacy/safety [Abstract]. *Proc Am Soc Clin Oncol* 2000;19:205a.

68. Gullick WJ. Prevalence of aberrant expression of the epidermal growth factor receptor in human cancers. *Br Med Bull* 1991;47:87–98.

69. Grandis JR, Melhem MF, Barnes EL, et al. Quantitative immunohistochemical analysis of transforming growth factor-alpha and epidermal growth factor receptor in patients with squamous cell carcinoma of the head and neck. *Cancer* 1996;78:1284–1292.

70. Modjtahedi H, Affleck K, Stubberfield C, et al. EGFR blockade by tyrosine kinase inhibitor or monoclonal antibody inhibits growth, directs terminal differentiation and induces apoptosis in human squamous cell carcinoma HN5. *Int J Oncol* 1998;13:335–342.

71. Baselga J, Averbuch SD. ZD1839 ('Iressa") as an anti-cancer agent. *Drugs* 2000;60:33–40.

72. Sirotnak FM, Zakowiski MF, Miller VA, et al. Efficacy of cytotoxic agents against human tumor xenografts is markedly enhanced by coadministration of ZD1839 (Iressa), an inhibitor of EGFR tyrosine kinase. *Clin Cancer Res* 2000;6: 4885–4892.

73. Bonomi P. Erlotinib : a new therapeutic approach for non-small cell lung cancer. *Expert Opin Investig Drugs* 2003;12: 1395–1402.

29 Chemoprevention of Oral Cancer

Risk Assessment, Plausible Intervention, and Monitoring

Jon Sudbø, DDS, MD, PhD, *Steinar Aamdal,* MD, PhD,
Albrecht Reith, MD, PhD, MIAC, *and Asle Sudbø,* MSc, PhD

CONTENTS

1. INTRODUCTION TO ORAL CANCER AND PRECANCER

Oral squamous cell carcinoma (OSCC) afflicts an estimated 500,000 patients annually worldwide *(1,2)*. Oral carcinoma incidence is increasing in developing countries *(1,3)*, substantially among younger people *(4–6)*. Of note, patients with oral cavity cancer have an increased risk of acquiring a second primary cancer in other parts of the upper aerodigestive tract, such as the bronchial tree and esophagus *(7)*.

In developing countries with limited public health system resources, head and neck cancer may account for as much as 50% of all cancers *(5)*. Treating patients who have oral precancers with cancer-preventive agents is a possible low-cost approach to an important

global health problem that, in Western countries, has proven difficult to control by cost-intensive surgery, radiotherapy, and chemotherapy *(8)*. Current treatments and chemoprevention have not significantly improved the poor 5-yr survival rate of patients with OSCC, perhaps because intervention comes too late *(2)*. Increasing incidence of head and neck cancers even among the young *(9,10)* emphasizes the importance of early identification of oral leukoplakia, white patches that will develop into carcinomas *(11–17)*.

2. FIELD CANCERIZATION

The concept of multiclonal "field cancerization" is supported by patients with oral cancers who present with multiple primary tumors or secondary tumors *(18–20)*. Multifocal dysplastic lesions could arise from

From: Cancer Chemoprevention, Volume 2: Strategies for Cancer Chemoprevention
Edited by: G. J. Kelloff, E. T. Hawk, and C. C. Sigman © Humana Press Inc., Totowa, NJ

a single site as a result of lateral intraepithelial migration or intraoral dispersion and, with additional genetic changes, acquire a growth advantage (21–23). The clonal origin of multiple premalignant or malignant lesions in the same patient is supported by recent cytogenetic findings (24). Either a polyclonal or a monoclonal hypothesized origin of multiple oral cancers is consistent with the finding that aneuploidy in only one of several biopsy specimens obtained simultaneously or successively from the same patient can be used to predict subsequent carcinoma occurrence (25,26).

3. RISK FACTORS

Leukoplakia of the oral cavity is frequently encountered, and has a well-documented potential to develop into OSCC (27–29) with a poor 5-yr survival rate (30,31). Tobacco and alcohol are recognized as principal etiological factors in development of OSCC (14) and possible carcinogenic mechanisms have been proposed (32). Ogden and Wight found that tobacco use does not seem to have a confounding effect on the observation that DNA content is a significant prognostic marker in oral leukoplakia. Reliable data on alcohol consumption are difficult to establish (33); for almost half the patients in this retrospective study, such information was not available. A confounding effect of alcohol consumption on our results can therefore not be ruled out, although we demonstrate that DNA content is a significant prognostic factor independent of tobacco use. Carcinoma development in response to environmental factors may also be modified by the presence of susceptibility-conferring genotypes (34–36) with a relation to sporadic cancers that is, however, incompletely understood (37). In addition, genetic events may not be limited to rare, highly penetrant mutations that confer increased cancer risk, but could include more prevalent polymorphisms carrying a much lower risk for acquiring cancer (38). Accordingly, of the large number of risk-factor-exposed patients presenting with oral leukoplakia, only some will progress to carcinoma. Knowledge of patient exposure to risk factors still leaves the clinician challenged to identify those in particular need of preventive counseling or active treatment.

4. INSUFFICIENCY OF CONVENTIONAL TYPING AND GRADING IN DIAGNOSTIC HISTOPATHOLOGY

Adequate reproducibility in description of tissue architecture is still a challenge to diagnostic pathology, because systems for typing and grading cancerous and precancerous lesions can be clinically useful only if they are reproducible between separate observers (39). In addition, parameters considered in histological assessment should be biologically meaningful, i.e., should reflect the malignant potential of lesions (40–42).

Leukoplakia of the oral mucous membrane has well-documented potential to develop into OSCC. In this respect, the histological finding of dysplasia is of particular prognostic importance (27–29,41). Approximately one of 10 leukoplakias is histologically classified as dysplasia. However, no current marker exists that reliably predicts the clinical outcome of dysplastic leukoplakia (43). With current therapeutic options, it is too late for cure in the majority of patients with clinical manifestation of OSCC. The challenge therefore is to identify those leukoplakias with the potential to develop into OSCC, which accordingly demand particular attention.

Several published studies demonstrate a low intra- and interobserverver agreement in subjective grading of oral preneoplastic lesions. Approaches to improve the prognostic value of histological grading have been investigated, e.g., by simplifying grading systems that have proved superior to the Broders' grading, WHO, and UICC classification (Fig. 1) (44,45). Studies on the prognostic impact of grading generally have included a standard tutorial and prediagnostic calibration of participating pathologists. This, however, is most likely an exception in most situations of diagnostic pathology, particularly in routine settings. The consequence of these diagnostic shortcomings is to make reliable prognostication of oral preneoplastic lesions difficult, which not only makes treatment planning inefficient but also has implications on testing chemopreventive agents in trials (46). It is significant that even in lesions regarded as nonmalignant (e.g., hyperplasia, edema, or hyperkeratosis), we found gross quantitative aberrations in DNA content, and predicted subsequent carcinoma occurrence (47). This is in keeping with previous findings by Califano and coworkers (48), who used microsatellite analysis to identify possible sites of origin of unknown primary head and neck SCC.

5. IMPROVING PROGNOSTIC IMPACT BY ASSESSING GROSS GENOMIC ABERRATIONS

Genetic instability (aneuploidy) was one of the first characteristics postulated to underlie neoplasia (49).

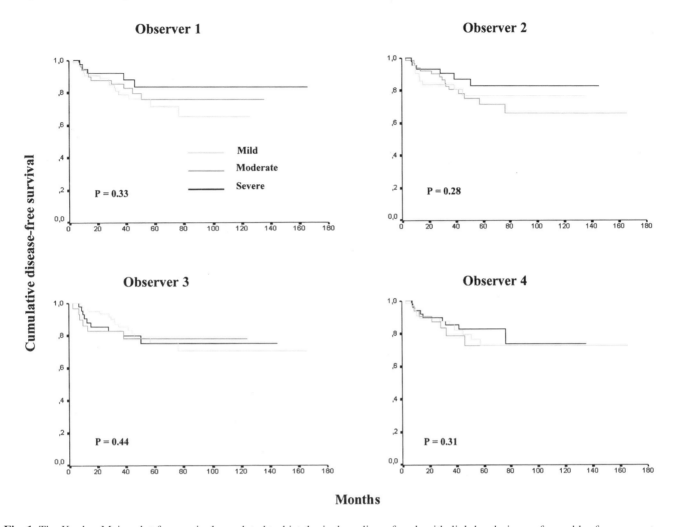

Fig. 1. The Kaplan-Meier plot for survival as related to histological grading of oral epithelial dysplasias performed by four separate pathologists (Observers 1–4). Total of evaluated cases is 150, representing leukoplakia histologically typed as dysplasia and not associated with previous or simultaneous carcinoma *in situ* or manifest carcinoma. The prognostic value of histological grading is not significant (*p*-values in the range 0.28–0.44). There are no significant differences in the gradings of the four pathologists (*p* = 0.39). From *(41)* by permission of the Pathological Society of Great Britain and Ireland.

Introduction of the mutation theory of cancer caused these findings of Boveri to be lost until recently. Several studies indicate that mutations in genes controlling chromosome segregation during mitosis and centrosome abnormalities play a critical role in causing chromosome instability in cancer *(50–54)*. Chromosomal aberrations consistent with impaired fidelity of chromosome segregation during mitotis have been shown to occur exclusively in aneuploid tumor cell lines *(55)*. These observations point to a key role of aberrant DNA content in carcinogenesis.

Previous efforts of investigators studying large-scale genomic status as a prognostic marker in oral preneoplastic lesions *(56–59)* either employed low-resolution image cytometric systems, investigated few cases, included manifest carcinomas, or stated no follow-up

time. In one study, interobserver agreement among experienced but uncalibrated pathologists grading oral dysplasias was quantified. In addition, results showing the prognostic value of subjective histological grading of dysplasias were compared to results obtained by assessing large-scale genomic status using high-resolution image cytometry (ICM) of the same lesions (Fig. 2) *(41)*. This study employed a simplified grading scheme for oral epithelial dysplasias according to the guidelines given by WHO.

Using kappa statistics, we were able to determine a very moderate interobserver agreement among pathologists when grading oral dysplasias, even among pathologists with special training in assessing oral mucous membrane lesions (Fig. 1). Kappa values in 150 cases assessed by histological grading and,

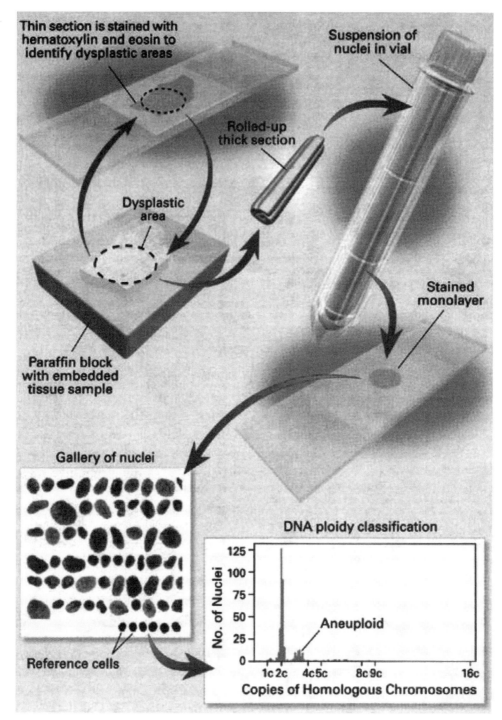

Fig. 2. Steps in Preparation of a Monolayer. First, paraffin-embedded blocks of biopsy specimens are sectioned and stained with hematoxylin and eosin. Stained sections identify dysplastic areas, and uninvolved areas are trimmed off. Two sections with a thickness of 50 μm—one of which is shown rolled up here—are deparaffinized and rehydrated before being enzymatically digested to yield a suspension of nuclei. The suspension is then centrifuged, and the pellet is resuspended and then placed on a slide to form a monolayer. After staining with Feulgen's stain and periodic acid-Schiff stain, nuclei are viewed under a microscope and images are collected in a computerized folder, or "gallery," for each patient. At least 300 nuclei of dysplastic epithelial cells are analyzed together with nuclei from reference cells (lymphocytes). Slides with cell nuclei are then viewed with a transmission light microscope equipped with a digital camera. The amount of light transmitted is registered digitally by the camera and stored in the computer; it is inversely proportional to the amount of DNA in the nuclei. The final classification of DNA ploidy is made from the DNA histogram that is generated from information in the gallery. In the histogram, results for reference-cell nuclei are shown in red and results for epithelial cells are shown in green. The y axis shows the number of epithelial-cell nuclei, and the x axis shows nuclear DNA content according to the number of copies (c) of homologous chromosomes. The diploid (2c) peak (in green) is the first column to the right of the reference cells (in red). From ref. *26* with permission from Massachusetts Medical Society.

using ICM, by large-scale genomic status were in the range of 0.21–0.33 when three diagnostic groups were considered (mild, moderate, and severe dysplasia), and in the range of 0.27–0.34 when only two diagnostic groups (favorable and poor) were considered. There was no significant correlation between histological findings of the four pathologists and measurements of large-scale genomic status in 150 cases of oral dysplastic leukoplakias.

These findings clearly demonstrate that the assessment of large-scale genomic status is superior to traditional histological assessment as a prognostic marker. Contrasting results by other authors, who demonstrated that DNA analysis by ICM may be a useful adjunct to histopathological evaluation, fall short in that resolution of the ICM system employed was considerably lower and numbers of cases investigated were limited. Furthermore, invasive carcinomas have been included in the analysis. Conceivably, the grading of frank carcinomas may not be subject to the same degree of interobserver variability as grading of dysplastic lesions. Our results were supported by the larger number of cases we considered and by using a high-resolution ICM system to sample a larger number of cells for evaluation (>300) than any previous study.

Molecular markers for predicting clinical behavior of premalignant oral lesions, such as expression of tumor suppressor genes, markers of protein synthesis and cell proliferation, adhesion molecules, loss of heterozygosity or allelic imbalance, and biological markers in chemopreventive trials, have been investigated. However, the prevailing lack of molecular prognostic markers in oral precancers has been recognized (43). This may be the consequence of using single gene probes, a shortcoming that may in principle be overcome by the use of composite molecular markers. Such a composite marker, the gross estimation of nuclear DNA content (DNA ploidy), has been shown to have considerable prognostic impact on clinical outcome in premalignant lesions of the head and neck. It is significant that the point-value genetic mutations underlying chromosomal imbalances are beginning to be revealed, and resulting DNA aneuploidy—reflecting genetic instability—may itself induce further genetic changes, as discussed later. Therefore, gross aberrations in DNA content of cells should be viewed as more than proxy variables that manifest themselves secondary to the carcinogenic process. Analysis of DNA content of cells, e.g., in cancerous or precancerous lesions, is no more laborious, time-consuming, or costly than the many molecular and immunohistochemical analyses commonly performed in pathology laboratories, nor does it require sophisticated equipment. Well-established protocols for such analyses exist, and have been published in consensus reports (60–63).

The value of DNA content as a prognostic marker may lie in its being a harbinger of a multitude of early and significant events in cancer development (55). Its specificity and sensitivity as a prognostic marker of oral cancer (85% and 97%, respectively) found in our study on cyclooxygenase (COX)-2 and DNA content confirms previous findings by us in a different group of patients (26). That COX-2 expression was a significant prognostic marker only in patients whose premalignant lesions had gross genomic aberrations (GGA) could reflect a cancer-promoting effect of COX-2 in early-stage malignant transformation. Subsequent clonal expansions, which may be reflected in GGA, could render pathways other than COX-2 activity equally important for the propagation of disease (64).

6. RISK ASSESSMENT IN ORAL LEUKOPLAKIAS

Accurate prognostication in patients with oral leukoplakia would ensure that they receive appropriate treatment necessary to prevent occurrence and dissemination of malignant disease (2). Furthermore, identifying patients with particularly aggressive leukoplakia may translate into more efficient primary preventive measures toward such well-known risk factors as tobacco and alcohol (46).

Approximately 10% of oral leukoplakias are histologically classified as dysplasias, and of these, a substantial part (15–20%) reportedly develop into carcinomas (27). However, histological assessment of oral dysplasias is of limited prognostic value (44,65), and therapeutic intervention is considered only in cases with histologically proven transition to carcinoma *in situ* or carcinoma. In order to investigate the prognostic value of large-scale genomic aberrations, we analyzed DNA content in a number of putatively premalignant lesions of the oral cavity (Fig. 3).

Our results support the practice of watchful waiting with respect to patients who have oral leukoplakia with normal (diploid) DNA content. By contrast, lesions with an abnormal (aneuploid) DNA content should be treated as true carcinomas. We found that the rate of malignant transformation of oral leukoplakia was substantial (24%), even though we excluded high-risk groups. We did not include patients with previous or concomitant erythroplakia, because erythroplakia carries a high risk of cancer (at least 90%) (32). We also

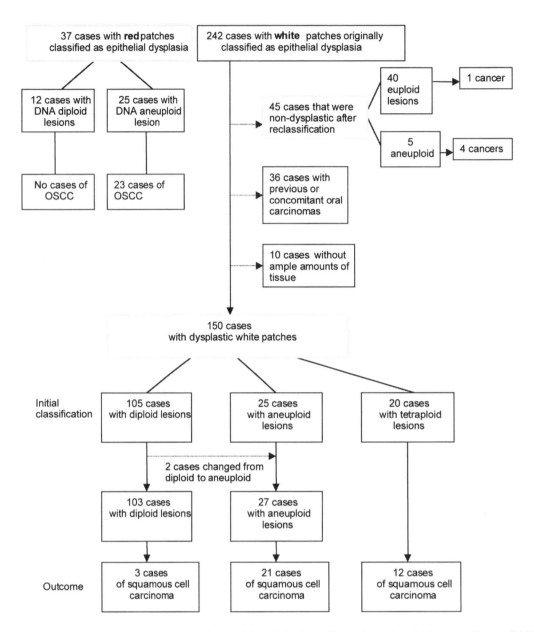

Fig. 3. Selection, classification, and outcome of patients with oral leukoplakia and erythroplakia according to DNA analysis of lesion content.

excluded patients with previous or concomitant tumors of the upper aerodigestive tract, because multiple lesions may arise as a result of the migration of transformed cells through the aerodigestive tract (Fig. 3). Thirty-six *(36)* patients who had already been diagnosed with oral carcinoma or carcinoma *in situ* were also excluded, as such patients are prone to a second carcinoma. We did include patients in whom leukoplakia was completely excised at time of diagnosis or during follow-up. At least some of these excisions could represent curative measures. Thus, of 27 patients with aneuploid lesions, six who did not develop carcinoma during follow-up may have been cured by exci-

sional biopsy. If so, the positive predictive value of 84% for aneuploidy with respect to carcinoma development and the rate of malignant transformation of 24% are underestimates. No correlation was found between histological grading and DNA content of lesions (Figs. 4 and 5).

7. RISK ASSESSMENT IN ORAL ERYTHROPLAKIAS

Oral erythroplakias are less common than leukoplakias. However, their rate of malignant transformation is considerably higher than that of oral leukoplakias.

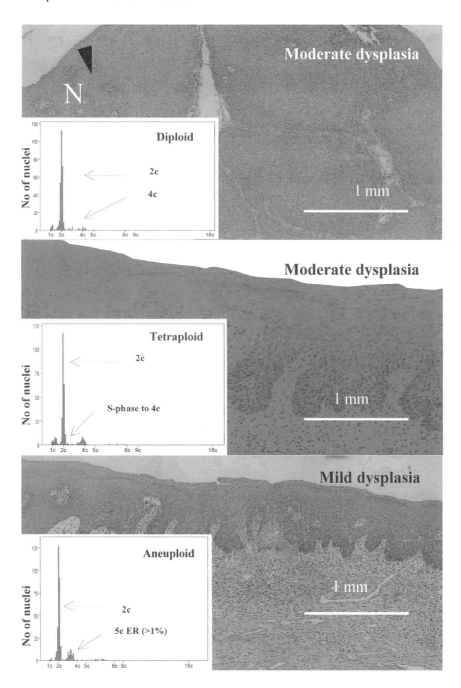

Fig. 4. DNA ploidy (insets) and histologic findings in two patients with moderate dysplasia (*top* and *center*) and one patient with mild dysplasia (*bottom*) (hematoxylin and eosin). In each histogram, *c* denotes copy or copies, and red columns to the left of the 2c (diploid) peak are internal controls. In the histogram shown inset in center panel, "S phase to 4c" indicates cells in synthesis phase that are about to double their DNA content. From ref. *26* with permission from Massachusetts Medical Society.

Therefore, it is reasonable to assume that they must represent a different biological process than oral leukoplakias. We therefore separately assessed the prognostic value of DNA content in oral erythroplakias that were histologically typed as dysplasias.

The limited number of subjects included in this study may also limit the extent to which general conclusions may be drawn. Nevertheless, although our results pertain to a small cohort of patients, the data are not only highly significant but are also consistent with previous oral leukoplakia findings by us *(26,47)*.

Though less common than leukoplakia, erythroplakia is biologically different with a higher malignant transformation rate, giving rise to a substantial fraction

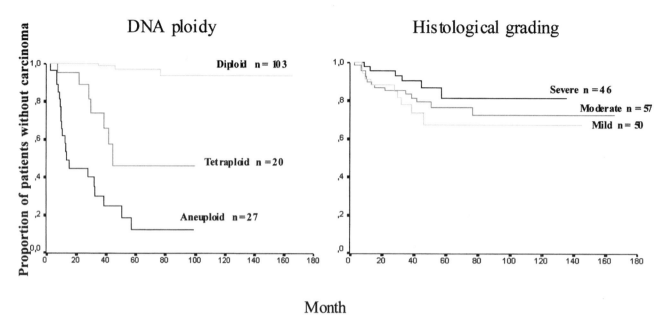

Fig. 5. Kaplan–Meier analysis of cumulative probability of survival free of OSCC, according to DNA ploidy (*left*) and histologic grade (*right*) of initial dysplastic lesions. From ref. *26* with permission from Massachusetts Medical Society.

of oral carcinoma *(66)*. Accordingly, a large fraction of lesions clinically defined as erythroplakias will histologically be verified as carcinomas *in situ*, or as frank carcinomas. Only a limited number of these red lesions will be histologically verified as dysplastic, and therefore premalignant. Taking this into account, the analysis of 57 dysplastic erythroplakias in 37 patients with a follow-up of more than 7 yr may be seen as a considerable effort. In short, we feel that our results are sufficiently significant to warrant similar investigations on the prognostic impact of GGA in other epithelial linings.

The present study represents an extension of previous work by our group restricted to leukoplakia only *(26,47)*. We demonstrate that it is also possible to predict the occurrence of carcinoma from erythroplakia. Several lines of evidence indicate a key role of GGA in malignant transformation *(67)*, and from our findings we further conjecture that GGA could apply as a predictor of subsequent cancers from a wide range of precancers. The clinical value of an early and reliable identification of the risk profile in individuals with precancers is underlined by the existance of established protocols for treatment with anticancer agents *(68)*. The finding that the majority of lesions with aberrant DNA content were identified at initial visits underscores the early and incentive role of GGA such as DNA aneuploidy in carcinogenesis *(67)*.

Patients with head and neck cancers are at increased risk of a second primary cancer in other locations of the upper aerodigestive tract *(18,69,70)*. Our studies have found no such association to other cancers of the upper aerodigestive tract *(26,47,64)*. However, the number of patients we have followed over a long period is limited (>300), and inferences from our data therefore must be drawn with caution. Furthermore, an extension of the follow-up time would possibly reveal an increased risk of a second primary cancer in the study group. Because of our limited number of patients, and because none of them developed carcinoma during the 10-yr follow-up period, our data do not allow us to draw any conclusions regarding a possible correlation between DNA content of the investigated lesions and subsequent occurence of carcinomas in other regions of the upper aerodigestive tract. Although initial lesions had been completely excised in all cases, with histologically confirmed free margins, we found a high rate of progression to malignant disease, indicating that malignant transformation of the oral mucous membranes is a multilocalized process, which could occur either through field cancerization or through clonal expansion by intraepithelial migration of agressive cell clones *(71,72)*. Thus, our results indicate that total excision of one or more visible lesions in the oral mucosa should not be viewed as a curative measure; treatment with systemically acting anticancer agents may be warranted.

It has been argued that the oral mucosa may be viewed as a surrogate marker site for other imminent malignancies of the upper aerodigestive tract *(73)*. In this perspective, the most promising treatment options for premalignant lesions of the oral cavity would be systemic agents with an established biological effect on oral mucosa epithelial cells.

As aberrant gross genomic content appears to be the cumulative expression of a series of pathological molecular events, it could be a predictive marker in a wider range of precancers. This marker could serve as a tool for tailoring preventive measures in precancerous epithelia outside the oral cavity at a disease stage where treatment achieves better rates of cure than in manifest carcinomas. Ultimately, the long-term effect of such a strategy should be evaluated through a prospective randomized trial, with incidence rates of new carcinomas as the endpoint.

8. COMPARATIVE GENOMIC HYBRIDIZATION AND CENTROSOMES

The application of comparative genomic hybridization (CGH) for identifying DNA copy number changes has revealed a surprisingly tumor type-specific pattern of chromosomal copy number changes in virtually all human carcinomas. This finding suggests that mechanisms controlling the fidelity of proper chromosome segregation during mitosis play an important role in the development of aneuploid tumors *(54)*. Colorectal carcinomas are an ideal model system for studying such processes because these tumors can be divided into two classes, those with a diploid genome and those that contain gross alterations in their nuclear DNA content (aneuploidy) *(54)*. Indeed, comparison of diploid and aneuploid colorectal carcinoma cell lines revealed a different pattern of genome instability, and further studies indicated that mutations of mitotic checkpoints contribute to frequent chromosome segregation errors *(74)*.

It is tempting to speculate that cellular structures involved in chromosome segregation at mitosis could contribute to chromosomal gains and losses. In its role as cellular organizer of the spindle apparatus responsible for physical separation of sister chromatids during mitosis, the centrosome is a candidate worthy of further study.

9. CHEMOPREVENTION

One promising approach to the difficult problem of reducing upper aerodigestive tract cancer incidence is intervention with preventive measures in high-risk individuals at a precancerous stage of disease *(75)*. The process of malignant transformation in the oral cavity particularly lends itself to chemopreventive measures, as premalignant lesions are easy to detect and tools exist for reliable risk assessment in this group of lesions.

Efficient chemopreventive intervention requires the identification of high-risk individuals and a plausible chemopreventive agent *(46)*. Individuals with aberrant DNA content in precancerous oral leukoplakia represent a subgroup of patients with considerably increased cancer risk *(26,76)*. COX-2 inhibition has been linked to cancer prevention through several mechanisms, such as inhibition of angiogenesis and local tumor invasion, or promotion of apoptosis *(77–81)*. Selective inhibitors of COX-2 (coxibs) have been shown to reduce the burden of premalignant lesions in the large bowel of patients with nearly 100% lifetime risk of acquiring a cancer (i.e., those with familial adenomatous polyposis, or FAP) *(82)*.

10. SURROGATE ENDPOINTS FROM MATHEMATICAL MODELING OF TISSUE ARCHITECTURE

Chemopreventive trials aim to prevent disease from occurring in the distant future, so monitoring treatment effect by measuring endpoints such as incidence rates of manifest cancer is not always feasible. Establishing surrogate endpoint biomarkers to monitor treatment effects at a much earlier stage is therefore an attractive approach. Using histopathological examination to monitor treatment effects on tissue architecture has been done in oral precancers *(68,83)*, but histological grading of oral epithelial dysplasia is notoriously unreliable (Fig. 1) *(44)*. Reduced consistency in histological grading inevitably reduces the prognostic value of such procedures. However, these limitations may be overcome by a strict quantitative assessment of tissue architecture *(84–86)*.

10.1. Graph Theory-Based Methods to Establish Intermediate Biomarkers

By employing graphs such as the Voronoi diagram (VD) (Fig. 6) and its subgraphs, the Delaunay triangulation (DT), minimum spanning tree (MST), Ulam tree (UT), and Gabriel graph (GG), the structural manifestations of cellular interactions in tissues may be quantified. In pilot studies *(84,86)*, we investigated reproducibility and prognostic impact of computing structural features that take into consideration the shape of individual structural entities (polygons, triangulations, arborizations), particularly derived from the VD; clusterings, particularly from the GG; and order or randomness in the distribution of pointlike seeds, particularly derived from the UT and MST. These graphs were chosen because a vast literature

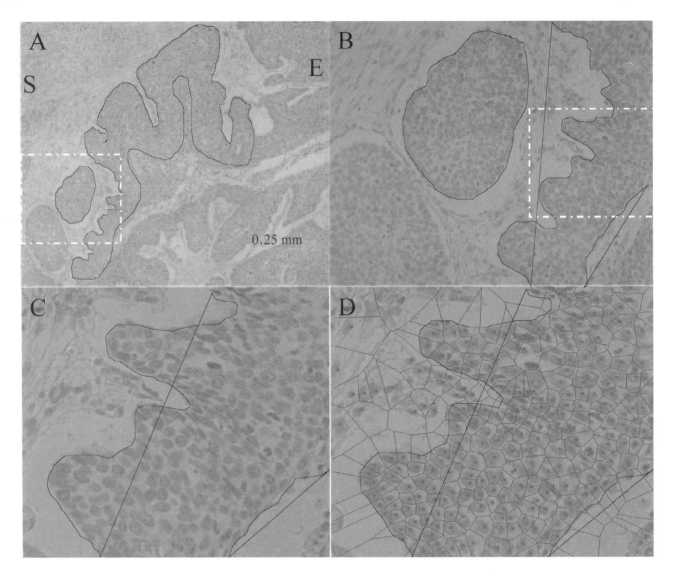

Fig. 6. Space partitioning of tissue sections for architectural analysis. **A**, selected area of interest with windows of analysis defined by the closed contours (black lines). **B**, detail corresponding to the delineated square in panel A. **C**, detail from an area to be analyzed, with tissue partitioned according to Voronoi diagram (VD) in panel D. Areas of interest (inside closed contours defined by black lines) were digitally defined according to an algorithm developed at our department. From ref. *85* with permission from US and Canadian Academy of Pathology.

points to these graphs as structures containing the most biological meaningful structural information. Using methods derived from graph theory, assessment of tissue architecture becomes highly reproducible.

Gray-level images were acquired from hematoxylin-eosin (HE)-stained sections by a charge coupled device (CCD) camera mounted on a microscope, and the geometrical centers of cell nuclei were computed. The resulting two-dimensional swarm of pointlike seeds distributed in a flat plane was the basis for construction of the VD and its subgraphs (Fig. 6). From the polygons, triangulations, and arborizations thus obtained, a number of structural features may be computed as numerical values. Comparison of groups (normal vs cancerous oral mucosa, cervical, and prostate carcinomas with good and poor prognosis) demonstrated that some structural features developed (average Delaunay edge length, DEL-av and ELH-av) are able to distinguish structurally between normal and cancerous oral mucosa and between good and poor outcome groups (Fig. 7) *(85)*.

10.2. Future Possibilities for Computing Tissue Architecture

Another approach to identifying pathological structures is the study of correlation functions between cell

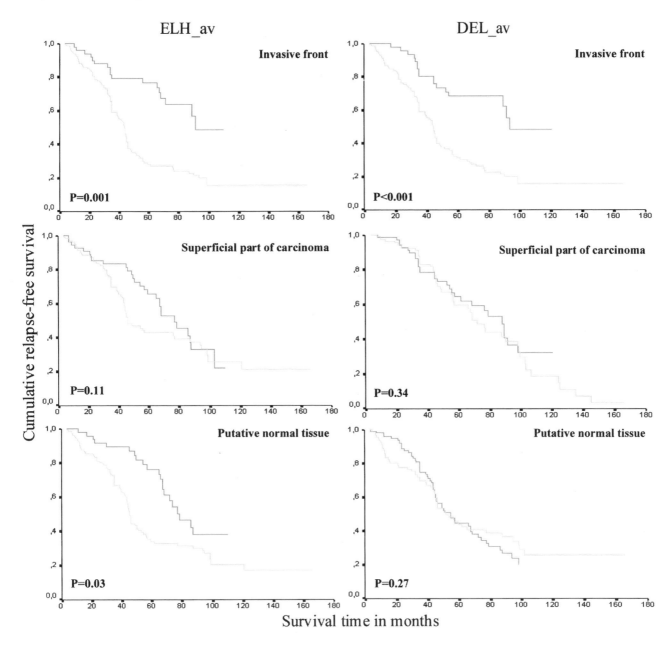

Fig. 7. Survival curves for ELH_av and DEL_av. For both structural features, significant prognostic information is demonstrated in the invasive front of the carcinomas. Interestingly, for the structural feature ELH_av, significant prognostic information was contained in putatively normal oral mucosa adjacent to carcinomas. From ref. *85* with permission from US and Canadian Academy of Pathology.

densities at various points in the tissue sample *(87)*. Since cancer development is a macroscopic phenomenon, the long-distance behavior of such correlation functions is of interest. Correlation functions have the advantage of yielding detailed quantitative information on large-scale structures of the tissue, and can be constructed systematically.

We study an ensemble of tissue samples from a particular individual, assuming that the tissue is essentially isotropic in three dimensions and that representative information is available from two-dimensional sections. The local density of cells at two points (r,r′) is denoted by (∂(r) ∂(r′)). The correlation between them is a function only of the separation r–r′. The pair-correlation function for this quantity is given by Γ (r–r′) =<∂ (r)∂(r′)> − <∂(r)> . <∂(r′)>. Here <..>denotes a double-average as follows: We first perform an average over all (r,r′) at fixed separation in a given sample. Then an averaging over all samples is carried out. We expect Γ (r–r′)to have the following asymptotic form for large separations: $\Gamma(r-r') = \Delta\exp(-|r-r'|/\varepsilon)$. The important quantity is the characteristic length, the correlation length ε of the sample. The idea is that in normal tissue, the correlation length should have a characteristic value for a given tissue type. If we extract this value from a correlation function computed for individual samples (tissue slices), there should be a characteristic variation in the correlation length from sample to sample, defining a distribution function for the correlation length.

Finding the correlation length is facilitated by Fourier transformation of the correlation function on a PC. This Fourier transform has a simple analytical form from which the correlation length can be found *(87)*.

11. COX-2 IN ORAL CARCINOGENESIS

Increased amounts of COX-2 are commonly found in premalignant tissues and cancers *(88–93)*. COX-2 influences several processes important to cancer development, such as apoptosis, angiogenesis, and invasiveness, although the relative importance of each of these effects in tumorigenesis is uncertain. The upregulation of COX-2 in malignancies probably reflects the influence of oncogenes, growth factors, and tumor promoters, which are known inducers of COX-2 *(94)*. Ample evidence suggests that COX-2 is mechanistically linked to development of malignancies. Thus, transgenic mice have been bred that specifically overexpress COX-2 in mammary glands. Among these, multiparous female mice had a high frequency of mammary gland hyperplasia, dysplasia, and metastatic tumors *(95)*. Such observations lend credit to the idea that increased levels of COX-2 promote malignant transformation of cells. The inducibility of COX-2 is explained, at least in part, by numerous *cis*-acting elements in the 5′-flanking region of the COX gene, such as at *NFκB*, *NF-IL6*, and *CRE* sites *(96)*. Increased stability of COX-2 mRNA also contributes to COX-2 induction *(97)*. When COX-2 is overexpressed in precancerous lesions, the levels of etheno-adducts are also increased, possibly as a result of increased oxidative stress *(98–100)*. Etheno-adducts may bind to DNA and give rise to permanent mutations in tissues if DNA repair mechanisms do not make complete DNA repairs during cell cycles *(98,99,101)*. Permanent mutations by this mechanism occur in head and neck cancers *(102)*. DNA damage restricted to certain human genes may lead to aneuploidy *(103)*, which has been found to be a driving force in several human malignancies *(67,98)*.

Chemopreventive studies have shown apparently contradictory results as to whether nonsteroidal anti-inflammatory drugs (NSAIDs) prevent progression from precancer to cancer in high-risk individuals. Thus, 400-mg doses of celecoxib, a selective inhibitor of COX-2, twice a day for 6 mo significantly reduced the polyp-burden in FAP patients *(104)*. In a primary preventive study, Giardiello and coworkers recently demonstrated that standard doses of sulindac did not prevent adenoma development in young persons genotypically affected with FAP but phenotypically unaffected *(105)*. However, the study was statistically powered to demonstrate a large effect from sulindac. This is an understandable objective for persons with FAP, who carry a 100% lifetime risk of colorectal cancer, but a smaller effect may be clinically meaningful for persons with sporadic cancers *(106)*. Therefore, COX-2 continues to be an attractive therapeutic target for chemopreventive measures in patients at high risk of oral cancer.

To see if individuals at considerably increased risk of oral cancer are candidates for treatment with coxibs, levels of COX-2 expression in healthy, premalignant, and cancerous oral mucosa were compared to the occurrence of a genetic risk marker of oral cancer. COX-2 gene product was detected immunohistochemically in 30 healthy persons, in 22 patients with dysplastic lesions without previous or concomitant carcinomas, and in 29 patients with oral carcinomas. In this study, COX-2 expression was compared to DNA content as a genetic risk marker of oral cancer.

COX-2 expression was found in one case of healthy oral mucosa (3%). All specimens from healthy mucosa had a normal DNA content. Of 22 patients with dysplastic lesions, nine (41%) expressed COX-2, and all nine had aberrant (aneuploid) DNA content. Carcinomas developed in six of seven patients whose lesions expressed COX-2 with aberrant DNA content and who were followed for 5 yr or more (85%). In 29 patients with oral carcinomas, COX-2 expression was observed in 26 (88%), and aneuploidy was observed in 25 (94%).

COX-2 was upregulated from healthy to premalignant to cancerous oral mucosa. In patients with premalignancies, COX-2 was exclusively expressed in a subgroup identified by aberrant DNA content as having considerably increased risk of cancer (Table 1, Fig. 8). These findings emphasize the need to determine whether coxibs can reduce oral cancer risk in patients with high-risk precancerous lesions.

Since COX-2 is not a specific marker of malignancy, treating all patients having COX-2-containing lesions

Table 1
Distribution of Cyclooxygenase-2 Expression and DNA Content Among Individuals With Healthy, Premalignant and Cancerous Oral Mucosa

	COX-2-positive biopsies			COX-2-negative biopsies		
	Aneuploid (high-risk)	Tetraploid	Diploid	Aneuploid (high-risk)	Tetraploid	Diploid
Healthy oral mucosa	0	0	1	0	0	29
Precancers	9	0	0	0	1	12
Carcinoma	24	2	0	1	1	1

with a coxib could lead to overtreatment. In contrast, our data indicate that including only patients with concomitant aneuploid and COX-2-expressing lesions would not lead to undertreatment. Further studies would have to show that patients whose aneuploid lesions lack COX-2 activity are not candidates for treatment with a coxib. Nevertheless, our findings emphasize the need to determine whether treating patients at high risk of oral carcinomas with coxibs can reduce the risk of cancer. Recently, the apoptosis-inducing activity of celecoxib was dissociated from its COX-2 inhibitory activity by structural modification of the molecule (107). This may provide the basis for developing new classes of apoptosis-inducing agents. These findings indicate that the apoptosis-inducing effect is important in preventing cancers, and may also explain why the antitumor dose-response curve of celecoxib exceeds that observed for pain relief.

12. COMBINATION CHEMOPREVENTION

Recent trials have shown that combinations of chemopreventive drugs may also hold exceptional promise for preventing the development of tumors (108). NSAIDs used in combination with epidermal growth factor receptor (EGFR) inhibitors lead to a 95% reduction in frequency of polyp formation in *Min* mice, even in doses in which neither the NSAID nor EGFR inhibitor would prevent disease on its own (109). Retinoids reverse potentially malignant lesions and inhibit development of second primary cancers in patients with head and neck cancer (68). Furthermore, there is a significant increase in retinoic acid receptor immunopositivity in OSCCs compared to normal tissue (110). Phase III trials have documented that retinoids can reverse malignant development in the oral mucosa (68), but these agents have adverse

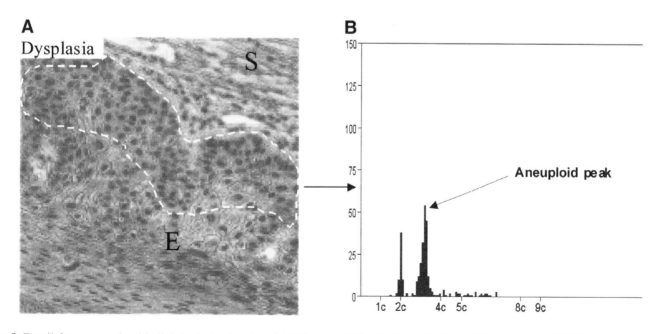

Fig. 8. Detail from an oral epithelial dyplasia showing COX-2 upregulation in the epithelium. Measurement of DNA content of cell nuclei from the demarcated area (basalomost layers) reveals GGA (DNA ploidy) in the cells.

effects that limit their long-term use for cancer prevention in asymptomatic individuals *(68,111,112)*. One effect of retinoids is to inhibit COX-2. Thus, a recent study *(113)* demonstrated EGF-mediated induction of COX-2 in OSCC and suppression of this upregulation by retinoids. A synergistic effect of retinoids and COX-2 inhibitors therefore seems reasonable. Whether a combination of coxibs, retinoids, or other inhibitors of the EGF pathway could be used as cancer-preventive drugs in doses that would not give significant side effects must be settled by undertaking a dose-ranging study.

13. CONCLUSION

Reliable risk assessment is possible in oral putatively premalignant lesions. High-risk oral premalignant lesions seem to have the particular property of expressing increased levels of COX-2, making them attractive targets for chemopreventive intervention using coxibs. Strict quantitative assessment of tissue architecture is a possible approach to monitoring treatment effects through surrogate endpoint biomarkers. Randomized trials to investigate the effect of coxibs on oral cancer from oral leukoplakias are under way.

REFERENCES

1. Pisani P, Parkin DM, Bray F, Ferlay J. Erratum: Estimates of the worldwide mortality from 25 cancers in 1990. *Int J Cancer* 1999;83:18–29. *Int J Cancer* 1999;83:870–873.
2. Silverman SJ, Gorsky M. Epidemiologic and demographic update in oral cancer: California and national data—1973 to 1985. *J Am Dent Assoc* 1990;120:495–499.
3. Lipkin A, Miller RH, Woodson GE. Squamous cell carcinoma of the oral cavity, pharynx, and larynx in young adults. *Laryngoscope* 1985;95:790–793.
4. Macfarlane GJ, Boyle P, Scully C. Rising mortality from cancer of the tongue in young Scottish males. *Lancet* 1987;2:912.
5. Macfarlane GJ, Boyle P, Evstifeeva TV, et al. Rising trends of oral cancer mortality among males worldwide: the return of an old public health problem. *Cancer Causes Control* 1994;5:259–265.
6. Macfarlane GJ, Evstifeeva TV, Robertson C, et al. Trends of oral cancer mortality among females worldwide. *Cancer Causes Control* 1994;5:255–258.
7. Kopelovich L, Henson DE, Gazdar AF, et al. Surrogate anatomic/functional sites for evaluating cancer risk: an extension of the field effect [editorial]. *Clin Cancer Res* 1999;5:3899–3905.
8. Landis SH, Murray T, Bolden S, Wingo PA. Cancer statistics, 1999. *CA Cancer J Clin* 1999;49:8–31, 1.
9. Shemen LJ, Klotz J, Schottenfeld D, Strong EW. Increase of tongue cancer in young men [letter]. *JAMA* 1984;252:1857.
10. Friedlander PL, Schantz SP, Shaha AR, et al. Squamous cell carcinoma of the tongue in young patients: a matched-pair analysis. *Head Neck* 1998;20:363–368.
11. Callery CD, Spiro RH, Strong EW. Changing trends in the management of squamous carcinoma of the tongue. *Am J Surg* 1984;148:449–454.
12. de Vries N, van Zandwijk N, Pastorino U. Chemoprevention in the management of oral cancer: EUROSCAN and other studies. *Eur J Cancer B Oral Oncol* 1992;28B:153–157.
13. Kelloff GJ, Boone CW, Steele VK, et al. Development of chemopreventive agents for lung and upper aerodigestive tract cancers. *J Cell Biochem Suppl* 1993;17F:2–17.
14. Schantz SP, Ostroff JS. Novel approaches to the prevention of head and neck cancer. *Proc Soc Exp Biol Med* 1997;216:275–282.
15. Kelloff GJ, Sigman CC, Greenwald P. Cancer chemoprevention: progress and promise. *Eur J Cancer* 1999;35:1755–1762.
16. Kelloff GJ, Crowell JA, Steele VE, et al. Progress in cancer chemoprevention. *Ann NY Acad Sci* 1999;889:1–13.
17. Greenlee RT, Murray T, Bolden S, Wingo PA. Cancer statistics, 2000. *CA Cancer J Clin* 2000;50:7–33.
18. Licciardello JT, Spitz MR, Hong WK. Multiple primary cancer in patients with cancer of the head and neck: Second cancer of the head and neck, oesophagus and lung. *Int J Radiat Oncol Biol Phys* 1989;17:467–476.
19. Hays GL, Lippman SM, Flaitz CM, et al. Co-carcinogenesis and field cancerization: oral lesions offer first signs. *J Am Dent Assoc* 1995;126:47–51.
20. Scholes AG, Woolgar JA, Boyle MA, et al. Synchronous oral carcinomas: independent or common clonal origin? *Cancer Res* 1998;58:2003–2006.
21. Califano J, Westra WH, Meininger G, et al. Genetic progression and clonal relationship of recurrent premalignant head and neck lesions. *Clin Cancer Res* 2000;6:347–352.
22. Bishop JM. The molecular genetics of cancer. *Science* 1987;235:305–311.
23. Cooper JS, Pajak TF, Rubin P, et al. Second malignancies in patients who have head and neck cancer: incidence, effect on survival and implications based on the RTOG experience. *Int J Radiat Oncol Biol Phys* 1989;17:449–456.
24. Weber RG, Scheer M, Born IA, et al. Recurrent chromosomal imbalances detected in biopsy material from oral premalignant and malignant lesions by combined tissue microdissection, universal DNA amplification, and comparative genomic hybridization. *Am J Pathol* 1998;153:295–303.
25. Sudbø J, Kildal W, Johannessen AC, et al. Gross genomic aberrations in precancers: clinical implications of a long-term follow-up study in oral erythroplakias. *J Clin Oncol* 2002;20:456–462.
26. Sudbø J, Kildal W, Risberg B, et al. DNA content as a prognostic marker in patients with oral leukoplakias. *N Engl J Med* 2001;344:1270–1278.
27. Waldron CA, Shafer WG. Leukoplakia revisited. A clinicopathologic study 3256 oral leukoplakias. *Cancer* 1975;36:1386–1392.
28. Bouquot JE, Gorlin RJ. Leukoplakia, lichen planus, and other oral keratoses in 23,616 white Americans over the age of 35 years. *Oral Surg Oral Med Oral Pathol* 1986;61:373–381.
29. Silverman SJ, Gorsky M, Lozada F. Oral leukoplakia and malignant transformation. A follow-up study of 257 patients. *Cancer* 1984;53:563–568.

30. Silverman SJ, Gorsky M. Epidemiologic and demographic update in oral cancer: California and national data—1973 to 1985. *J Am Dent Assoc* 1990;120:495–499.

31. Brunin F, Mosseri V, Jaulerry C, et al. Cancer of the base of the tongue: past and future. *Head Neck* 1999;21:751–759.

32. Wight AJ, Ogden GR. Possible mechanisms by which alcohol may influence the development of oral cancer—a review. *Oral Oncol* 1998;34:441–447.

33. Ogden GR, Wight AJ. Aetiology of oral cancer: alcohol. *Br J Oral Maxillofac Surg* 1998;36:247–251.

34. Schantz SP, Zhang ZF, Spitz MS, et al. Genetic susceptibility to head and neck cancer: interaction between nutrition and mutagen sensitivity. *Laryngoscope* 1997;107:765–781.

35. Cloos J, Spitz MR, Schantz SP, et al. Genetic susceptibility to head and neck squamous cell carcinoma. *J Natl Cancer Inst* 1996;88:530–535.

36. Schantz SP, Spitz MR, Hsu TC. Mutagen sensitivity in patients with head and neck cancers: a biologic marker for risk of multiple primary malignancies. *J Natl Cancer Inst* 1990;82:1773–1775.

37. Lichtenstein P, Holm NV, Verkasalo PK, et al. Environmental and heritable factors in the causation of cancer—analyses of cohorts of twins from Sweden, Denmark, and Finland [see comments]. *N Engl J Med* 2000;343:78–85.

38. Hoover RN. Cancer—nature, nurture, or both [editorial; comment]. *N Engl J Med* 2000;343:135–136.

39. Wasson JH, Sox HC, Neff RK, Goldman L. Clinical prediction rules. Applications and methodological standards. *N Engl J Med* 1985;313:793–799.

40. Kayser K, Schlegel W. Pattern recognition in histo-pathology: basic considerations. *Methods Inf Med* 1982;21:15–22.

41. Sudbφ J, Bryne M, Johannessen A, Reith A. Comparison of histological grading and large scale genomic status (DNA ploidy) as prognostic tools in oral dysplasia. *J Pathol* 2001; 194:946–955.

42. Heppner GH. Cancer cell societies and tumor progression. *Stem Cells* 1993;11:199–203.

43. Warnakulasuriya S. Lack of molecular markers to predict malignant potential of oral precancer [editorial; comment]. *J Pathol* 2000;190:407–409.

44. Karabulut A, Reibel J, Therkildsen MH, et al. Observer variability in the histologic assessment of oral premalignant lesions. *J Oral Pathol Med* 1995;24:198–200.

45. Sudbφ J, Bryne M, Johannessen AC, et al. Comparison of histological grading and large scale genomic status (DNA ploidy) as prognostic tools in oral dysplasia. *J Pathol* 2001;194:303–310.

46. Lee JJ, Hong WK, Hittelman WN, et al. Predicting cancer development in oral leukoplakia: ten years of translational research. *Clin Cancer Res* 2000;6:1702–1710.

47. Sudbφ J, Ried T, Bryne M, et al. Abnormal DNA content predicts the occurence of carcinomas in non-dysplastic oral white patches. *Oral Oncol* 2001;37:558–565.

48. Califano J, Westra WH, Koch W, et al. Unknown primary head and neck squamous cell carcinoma: molecular identification of the site of origin. *J Natl Cancer Inst* 1999;91:599–604.

49. Boveri T. *Zur Frage der Entstehung maligner Tumoren.* Gustav Fischer, Jena, 1914.

50. Saunders WS, Shuster M, Huang X, et al. Chromosomal instability and cytoskeletal defects in oral cancer cells. *Proc Natl Acad Sci USA* 2000;97:303–308.

51. Gardner RD, Burke DJ. The spindle checkpoint: two transitions, two pathways. *Trends Cell Biol* 2000;10:154–158.

52. Ried T, Heselmeyer-Haddad K, Blegen H, et al. Genomic changes defining the genesis, progression, and malignancy potential in solid human tumors: a phenotype/genotype correlation. *Genes Chromosomes Cancer* 1999;25:195–204.

53. Cahill DP, da Costa LT, Carson-Walter EB, et al. Characterization of MAD2B and other mitotic spindle checkpoint genes. *Genomics* 1999;58:181–187.

54. Lengauer C, Kinzler KW, Vogelstein B. Genetic instabilities in human cancers. *Nature* 1998;396:643–649.

55. Ghadimi BM, Sackett DL, Difilippantonio MJ, et al. Centrosome amplification and instability occurs exclusively in aneuploid, but not in diploid colorectal cancer cell lines, and correlates with numerical chromosomal aberrations. *Genes Chromosom Cancer* 2000;27:183–190.

56. Seoane J, Asenjo JA, Bascones A, et al. Flow cytometric DNA ploidy analysis of oral cancer comparison with histologic grading. *Oral Oncol* 1999;35:266–272.

57. Hogmo A, Munck-Wikland E, Kuylenstierna R, et al. Nuclear DNA content and p53 immunostaining in metachronous preneoplastic lesions and subsequent carcinomas of the oral cavity. *Head Neck* 1996;18:433–440.

58. Abdel-Salam M, Mayall BH, Chew K, Silverman S. Which oral white lesions will become malignant? An image cytometric study. *Oral Surg Oral Med Oral Pathol* 1990;69: 345–350.

59. Abdel-Salam M, Mayall BH, Chew K, et al. Prediction of malignant transformation in oral epithelial lesions by image cytometry. *Cancer* 1988;62:1981–1987.

60. Bocking A, Giroud F, Reith A. Consensus report of the ESACP task force on standardization of diagnostic DNA image cytometry. European Society for Analytical Cellular Pathology. *Anal Cell Pathol* 1995;8:67–74.

61. Giroud F, Haroske G, Reith A, Bocking A. 1997 ESACP consensus report on diagnostic DNA image cytometry. Part II: Specific recommendations for quality assurance. European Society for Analytical Cellular Pathology. *Anal Cell Pathol* 1998;17:201–208.

62. Haroske G, Giroud F, Reith A, Bocking A. 1997 ESACP consensus report on diagnostic DNA image cytometry. Part I: basic considerations and recommendations for preparation, measurement and interpretation. European Society for Analytical Cellular Pathology. *Anal Cell Pathol* 1998;17: 189–200.

63. Haroske G, Baak JP, Danielsen H, et al. Fourth updated ESACP consensus report on diagnostic DNA image cytometry. *Anal Cell Pathol* 2001;23:89–95.

64. Sudbφ J, Kildal W, Johannessen AC, et al. Gross genomic aberrations in precancers: clinical implications of a long-term follow-up study in oral erythroplakias. *J Clin Oncol* 2002;20:456–462.

65. Sudbφ J. Pathology in disgrace? *J Pathol* 2002;196:244–245.

66. Bouquot JE. Oral leukoplakia and erythroplakia: a review and update. *Pract Periodontics Aesthet Dent* 1994;6:9–17.

67. Sen S. Aneuploidy and cancer. *Curr Opin Oncol* 2000;12: 82–88.

68. Lotan R, Xu XC, Lippman SM, et al. Suppression of retinoic acid receptor-beta in premalignant oral lesions and its up-regulation by isotretinoin. *N Engl J Med* 1995;332: 1405–1410.

69. Lippman SM, Hong WK. Second malignant tumors in head and neck squamous cell carcinoma: the overshadowing threat for patients with early-stage disease. *Int J Radiat Oncol Biol Phys* 1989;17:691–614.

70. Vokes EE, Weichselbaum RR, Lippman SM, Hong WK. Head and neck cancer. *N Engl J Med* 1993;328:184–194.

71. Slaughter DP, Southwick HW, Smejkal W. Field canceriza-tion in oral stratified squamous epithelium: clinical implica-tions of multicentric origin. *Cancer* 1953;6:963–968.

72. van Oijen MG, Slootweg PJ. Oral field cancerization: carcino-gen-induced independent events or micrometastatic deposits? *Cancer Epidemiol Biomarkers Prev* 2000;9:249–256.

73. Zeng Q, Smith DC, Suscovich TJ, et al. Determination of intermediate biomarker expression levels by quantitative reverse transcription-polymerase chain reaction in oral mucosa of cancer patients treated with liarozole. *Clin Cancer Res* 2000;6:2245–2251.

74. Michel LS, Liberal V, Chatterjee A, et al. MAD2 haplo-insufficiency causes premature anaphase and chromosome instability in mammalian cells. *Nature* 2001;409:355–359.

75. Gupta PC, Mehta FS, Pindborg JJ, et al. Intervention study for primary prevention of oral cancer among 36,000 Indian tobacco users. *Lancet* 1986;1:1235–1239.

76. Lippman SM, Hong WK. Molecular markers of the risk of oral cancer [editorial]. *N Engl J Med* 2001;344:1323–1326.

77. Li M, Wu X, Xu XC. Induction of apoptosis by cyclo-oxy-genase-2 inhibitor NS398 through a cytochrome C-dependent pathway in esophageal cancer cells. *Int J Cancer* 2001; 93:218–223.

78. Chen WS, Wei SJ, Liu JM, et al. Tumor invasiveness and liver metastasis of colon cancer cells correlated with cyclooxyge-nase-2 (COX-2) expression and inhibited by a COX-2-selec-tive inhibitor, etodolac. *Int J Cancer* 2001;91: 894–899.

79. Taketo MM. Cyclooxygenase-2 inhibitors in tumorigenesis (Part II). *J Natl Cancer Inst* 1998;90:1609–1620.

80. van Rees BP, Ristimaki A. Cyclooxygenase-2 in carcinogen-esis of the gastrointestinal tract. *Scand J Gastroenterol* 2001; 36:897–903.

81. Williams CS, Mann M, DuBois RN. The role of cyclooxyge-nases in inflammation, cancer, and development. *Oncogene* 1999;18:7908–7916.

82. Steinbach G, Lynch PM, Phillips RK, et al. The effect of celecoxib, a cyclooxygenase-2 inhibitor, in familial adeno-matous polyposis. *N Engl J Med* 2000;342:1946–1952.

83. Hong WK, Endicott J, Itri LM, et al. 13-*cis*-retinoic acid in the treatment of oral leukoplakia. *N Engl J Med* 1986;315: 1501–1505.

84. Sudbø J, Marcelpoil R, Reith A. New algorithms based on the Voronoi Diagram applied in a pilot study on normal mucosa and carcinomas. *Anal Cell Pathol* 2000;21:71–86.

85. Sudbø J, Bankfalvi A, Bryne M, et al. Prognostic value of graph theory-based tissue architecture analysis in carcinomas of the tongue. *Lab Invest* 2000;80:1881–1889.

86. Sudbø J, Marcelpoil R, Reith A. Caveats: numerical require-ments in graph theory based quantitation of tissue architec-ture. *Anal Cell Pathol* 2000;21:59–69.

87. Chaikin PM, Lubensky TC. *Principles of Condensed Matter Physics*. Cambridge University Press, Cambridge; 1995.

88. Chan G, Boyle JO, Yang EK, et al. Cyclooxygenase-2 expression is up-regulated in squamous cell carcinoma of the head and neck. *Cancer Res* 1999;59:991–994.

89. Ristimaki A, Honkanen N, Jankala H, et al. Expression of cyclooxygenase-2 in human gastric carcinoma. *Cancer Res* 1997;57:1276–1280.

90. Ristimaki A, Nieminen O, Saukkonen K, et al. Expression of cyclooxygenase-2 in human transitional cell carcinoma of the urinary bladder. *Am J Pathol* 2001;158:849–853.

91. Zimmermann KC, Sarbia M, Weber AA, et al. Cyclooxygenase-2 expression in human esophageal carcinoma. *Cancer Res* 1999; 59:198–204.

92. Wilson KT, Fu S, Ramanujam KS, Meltzer SJ. Increased expression of inducible nitric oxide synthase and cyclooxy-genase-2 in Barrett's esophagus and associated adenocarci-nomas. *Cancer Res* 1998;58:2929–2934.

93. Eberhart CE, Coffey RJ, Radhika A, et al. Up-regulation of cyclooxygenase 2 gene expression in human colorectal ade-nomas and adenocarcinomas. *Gastroenterology* 1994;107: 1183–1188.

94. Dannenberg AJ, Altorki NK, Boyle JO, et al. Cyclo-oxyge-nase 2: a pharmacological target for the prevention of cancer. *Lancet Oncol* 2001;2:544–551.

95. Liu CH, Chang SH, Narko K, et al. Overexpression of cyclooxygenase-2 is sufficient to induce tumorigenesis in transgenic mice. *J Biol Chem* 2001;276:18,563–18,569.

96. Inoue H, Yokoyama C, Hara S, et al. Transcriptional regula-tion of human prostaglandin-endoperoxide synthase-2 gene by lipopolysaccharide and phorbol ester in vascular endothe-lial cells. Involvement of both nuclear factor for interleukin-6 expression site and cAMP response element. *J Biol Chem* 1995;270:24,965–24,971.

97. Sheng H, Shao J, Dixon DA, et al. Transforming growth fac-tor-beta1 enhances Ha-ras-induced expression of cyclooxy-genase-2 in intestinal epithelial cells via stabilization of mRNA. *J Biol Chem* 2000;275:6628–6635.

98. Bartsch H. Studies on biomarkers in cancer etiology and pre-vention: a summary and challenge of 20 years of interdisci-plinary research. *Mutat Res* 2000;462:255–279.

99. Nair J, Barbin A, Velic I, Bartsch H. Etheno DNA-base adducts from endogenous reactive species. *Mutat Res* 1999; 424:59–69.

100. Bartsch H, Nair J. Ultrasensitive and specific detection methods for exocylic DNA adducts: markers for lipid per-oxidation and oxidative stress. *Toxicology* 2000;153: 105–114.

101. Bartsch H, Nair J. Exocyclic DNA adducts as secondary markers for oxidative stress: applications in human cancer etiology and risk assessment. *Adv Exp Med Biol* 2001;500: 675–686.

102. Schmezer P, Rupprecht T, Tisch M, et al. Laryngeal mucosa of head and neck cancer patients shows increased DNA damage as detected by single cell microgel electrophoresis. *Toxicology* 2000;144:149–154.

103. Oberley TD. Oxidative damage and cancer. *Am J Pathol* 2002;160:403–408.

104. Steinbach G, Lynch PM, Phillips RK, et al. The effect of celecoxib, a cyclooxygenase-2 inhibitor, in familial adeno-matous polyposis. *N Engl J Med* 2000;342:1946–1952.

105. Giardiello FM, Yang WK, Hylind LM, et al. Primary chemo-prevention of familial adenomatous polyposis with sulindac. *N Engl J Med* 2002;346:1054–1059.

106. Chau I, Cunningham D. Cyxlooxygenase inhibition in cancer—a blind alley or a new therapeutic reality? *N Engl J Med* 2002;346:1085–1086.

107. Song X, Lin P-O, Johnson AL, et al. Cyclooxygenase-2, player or spectator in cyclooxygenase-2 inhibitor-induced apoptosis in prostate cancer cells. *J Natl Cancer Inst* 2002;94:585–591.

108. Chan TA. Nonsteroidal anti-inflammatory drugs, apoptosis, and colon-cancer prevention. *Lancet Oncol* 2002;3: 166–174.

109. Torrance CJ, Jackson PE, Montgomery E, et al. Combinatorial chemoprevention of intestinal neoplasia. *Nat Med* 2000;6:1024–1028.

110. Chakravarti N, Mathur M, Bahadur S, et al. Expression of RARalpha and RARbeta in human oral potentially malignant and neoplastic lesions. *Int J Cancer* 2001;91:27–31.

111. Lippman SM, Heyman RA, Kurie JM, et al. Retinoids and chemoprevention: clinical and basic studies. *J Cell Biochem Suppl* 1995;22:1–10.

112. Lippman SM, Spitz MR, Huber MH, Hong WK. Strategies for chemoprevention study of premalignancy and second primary tumors in the head and neck. *Curr Opin Oncol* 1995;7: 234–241.

113. Mestre JR, Subbaramaiah K, Sacks PG, et al. Retinoids suppress epidermal growth factor-induced transcription of cyclooxygenase-2 in human oral squamous carcinoma cells. *Cancer Res* 1997;57:2890–2895.

SKIN

30 Strategies in Skin Cancer Chemoprevention

*M. Suzanne Stratton, PhD, Steven P. Stratton, PhD,
James Ranger-Moore, Janine G. Einspahr, MS,
G. Tim Bowden, PhD, and David S. Alberts, MD*

1. INTRODUCTION

Formal studies of skin cancer began more than 200 yr ago. The first skin tumor model to appear in the literature was reported by London surgeon Percivall Pott in 1775 *(1)*. His account of scrotal cancer in chimney sweeps is considered the historical beginning of cancer research, as he delved beyond treatment into the etiology of the disease *(2)*. Pott's discovery of the linkage between scrotal carcinoma and soot exposure was the first evidence of a cancer cause, and launched research leading to the discovery of chemical carcinogens and their mechanisms of action.

The National Institutes of Health estimate that $56.4 billion in direct medical costs was spent on cancer in 2001 *(3)*. Skin cancer is by far the most common type of cancer, with a significant impact on morbidity, health, and health care economics. While skin cancer mortality is relatively low compared to that from other cancers, its contribution to total direct medical cancer costs is not insignificant. The annual direct cost of treating melanoma was estimated to be $563 million in the United States in 1997 *(4)*. For nonmelanoma skin cancers (NMSC), the total annual cost of care from 1992 through 1995 was estimated to be $426 million in the Medicare population alone *(5)*.

US estimates indicated that skin cancers would comprise 46% of all diagnosed malignancies in 2002 *(3,6)*. According to past American Cancer Society projections, recent incidence of NMSC has hovered near 1 million cases per year. Estimated new cases have risen from 0.9 million in 1997 *(7)* to 1.3 million new cases in 2000 *(8)*; 1 million new cases were expected in 2001 *(9)*. These estimates are probably lower than the actual number of cases, since many skin cancers are treated or removed in clinics without being reported to cancer registries. In spite of the tremendous number of NMSC cases, mortality of this disease is relatively low. Death rates are less than 1.5 per 100,000 *(10)*; however, morbidity can be dramatic due to excision of lesions in cosmetically sensitive areas *(11,12)*.

Melanoma accounts for 2.3% of new cancer cases (including NMSC) in the US. Approximately 53,600 new cases and 7400 deaths due to melanoma were estimated for 2002 *(6)*. Incidence and mortality rate increases are among the largest of all cancers *(13)*. Increased risk of melanoma is thought to be related to frequency of severe sunburn at an early age, as well as altered patterns of ultraviolet (UV) radiation exposure, skin type, and abnormal melanocytic nevi *(14–16)*. Melanoma can be cured by surgical excision if it is detected early. However, melanoma with distant

From: Cancer Chemoprevention, Volume 2: Strategies for Cancer Chemoprevention
Edited by: G. J. Kelloff, E. T. Hawk, and C. C. Sigman © Humana Press Inc., Totowa, NJ

metastasis is incurable, with a median survival of 4 to 8 mo. No adjuvant chemotherapeutic regimen has significantly improved overall survival in this patient population *(17,18)*. Because of the increasing incidence and burden of skin cancer and inadequacies in current melanoma treatment, effective chemoprevention strategies need to be developed.

1.1. Types of Skin Cancer

Melanoma originates from pigment producing cells (melanocytes) within the epidermis. Unlike keratinocytes, melanocytes are neural in origin and have a very limited proliferative capacity. These cells serve a photoprotective role in skin by producing UV-absorbing pigments on exposure to UV radiation. The mechanisms by which UV radiation can cause malignant transformation of melanocytes are poorly understood, and the relationship between UV radiation and melanoma incidence is much less well defined than the relationship between UV radiation and NMSC. While associated with exposure to sunlight, melanoma is thought to be more related to severe sunburns or patterns of exposure rather than to chronic exposure (reviewed in ref. *14*). Worldwide, melanoma incidence in white-skinned people is inversely associated with latitude. The highest rates occur in Australia, followed by the US and northern Europe *(19)*.

Almost all NMSC are keratinocytic and originate in the epidermis. Approximately 80% are basal cell carcinoma (BCC) *(20)*. These neoplasms, originally described by Jacob in 1827 *(21)*, appear to originate from basal cells of the epidermis and occasionally those of the infundibular and outer root sheath of hair follicles *(11)*. These slow-growing tumors are locally invasive and rarely metastasize. However, morbidity can be high as these tumors are often disfiguring and located in facial areas. Squamous cell carcinoma (SCC), the other major form of NMSC, originates in the keratinizing cells of the epidermis. These tumors are generally more aggressive than BCC, and have a much higher potential for metastasizing *(22,23)*. Mortality from NMSC is mainly due to SCC, with 1200–1500 deaths reported each year in the US *(12)*. The death rate of SCC is approximately equivalent to that of Hodgkin's disease and acute lymphocytic leukemia *(9)*.

1.2. Risk Factors

The most important risk factors in the development of NMSC are chronic exposure to UV radiation in sunlight *(24)* and fair skin that is susceptible to sunburns. UV radiation acts as a complete carcinogen, participating in all three phases of carcinogenesis, including initiation *(25,26)*, promotion *(27)*, and progression *(28)* (Fig. 1). Other risk factors include frequency of exposure, age, immune status, male gender, and DNA repair disorders such as xeroderma pigmentosum *(20)*. A history of BCC or SCC significantly increases the risk of melanoma *(29–31)*. Interestingly, it has only recently been shown that a history of prior cutaneous melanoma appears to significantly increase the risk of both BCC and SCC *(32)*. The association between UV exposure and cancer is strong for SCC, but less well defined for BCC, as approximately one-third of all BCCs originate in anatomical sites receiving minimal UV exposure *(11)*. Skin temperature may also be a factor, as cultured immortalized human keratinocytes have been shown to spontaneously convert to a tumorigenic phenotype when incubated at elevated temperature *(33)*. Skin temperature may also play a role in the genesis of melanoma *(34)*. Spurious oxidation of cellular biomolecules due to UV radiation exposure likely contributes to both aging and skin carcinogenesis. Continued increases in NMSC incidence are expected as the population ages and larger amounts of UV radiation reach the earth's surface due to depletion of the ozone layer *(35)*.

Skin is obviously a target organ for the damaging effects of ionizing radiation. Strong evidence from studies of atomic bomb survivors and radiation therapy patients suggests that skin exposure to high doses of ionizing radiation, especially at a young age, can cause BCC, but the evidence is weak for SCC and melanoma *(36,37)*. The relationship between protracted low-dose exposure of ionizing radiation and skin cancer risk is less clear. Interactions with host factors such as age, gender, tobacco use, chemotherapy, and the like may vary widely and are difficult to measure, thus limiting extrapolations *(38)*.

Inherent or induced alterations in normal immunity, such as UV radiation-induced immune suppression *(39,40)*, appear to have a strong relationship to skin cancer risk. The link between immune function and cancer is intensely studied, but still poorly understood. Solid organ transplant recipients are at extremely high risk for SCC. A comprehensive study of 5356 transplant recipients in Sweden showed that these patients experienced a 100-fold increase in relative risk of NMSC, almost exclusively in sun-exposed areas *(41)*. Increased frequency of SCC in these patients, especially in individuals with chronic actinic damage, is presumably due to long-term immunosuppressive therapy *(42)*, although nonimmune mechanisms and direct effects of immunosuppressive drugs may play a role *(43)*. Some evidence indicates

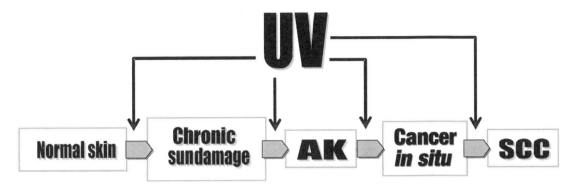

Fig. 1. The multi-step model of UVB-induced human skin carcinogenesis. UVB is a complete carcinogen that can play a role in every stage in the process of skin cancer development.

that human papilloma virus (HPV) infection may also increase NMSC risk, although the relationship is not clear *(44)*. The combination of lowered immune function and HPV infection may be involved in the development of NMSC and precursor lesions in these patients *(45)*, especially in the transplant setting *(46)*.

Fas and Fas ligand (FasL), immune system-regulated apoptosis effectors involved in photoimmune suppression *(47)*, are key players in regulating sunburn cell formation and keratinocyte homeostasis in response to DNA damage produced by UV exposure. Hill et al. have shown that UV-induced apoptotic sunburn cell formation is significantly decreased in the skin of FasL-deficient mice as compared to wild-type. Skin from these mice was shown to contain significantly higher levels of mutated p53, indicating that cells with high levels of DNA damage were present, thus pointing to a mechanism for accumulation of cells with high neoplastic risk *(48)*.

Inflammatory cytokines such as tumor necrosis factor α (TNFα) also play a role *(49)*. UV-irradiated cells have been shown to upregulate TNFα in response to DNA damage *(50)*, and p53 overexpression may repress TNFα *(51)*. The role of TNFα in skin carcinogenesis was recently explored by Moore et al. *(52)*, who showed that TNFα knockout mice were highly resistant to chemically induced skin papillomas and inflammatory cell infiltration of the skin compared to wild-type. However, no differences were seen in late-stage tumors, indicating that keratinocyte production of TNFα may contribute to skin tumor promotion in DNA-damaged cells. Thus, TNFα is an interesting potential target for skin cancer chemoprevention strategies.

1.3. Clinical Precancerous Lesions

Several precancerous lesions can form prior to development of epidermal malignancies. These include

Bowen's disease (SCC *in situ*), as well as radiation, tar, arsenical, thermal, and scar keratoses. Actinic keratosis (AK, also known as solar or senile keratosis), caused by UV radiation exposure, is the most common precancerous skin lesion *(53)*. AK results from proliferation of neoplastic keratinocytes in the epidermis. Clinically, AKs appear as rough, scaly papules on chronically sun-exposed areas such as the face, ears, scalp, forehead, forearms, and hands *(54)*. Histologically, AKs are characterized by dysplasia of keratinocytes with loss of cellular polarity and nuclear atypia. Cytologically, AK is indistinguishable from SCC *(55)*. AK treatment has been approved for Medicare reimbursement in the US.

AK is an extremely common lesion, especially in older Caucasian populations. US AK patients made an estimated 3.7 million physician office visits per year in 1993 and 1994 *(56)*. In spite of these epidemic proportions of AK, little comprehensive epidemiological data exist on AK incidence in North American populations. These data are difficult to collect due to variability in diagnosis and treatment, and lack of reporting. Based on limited available data, the best estimates for current prevalence of AK range from 5% to 14% in the US *(57)*. In high-risk groups, prevalence may be as high as 26% *(58)*. In Australia, where skin cancer incidence is highest, prevalence of AK ranges from 40%–60% in the adult population *(59)*. Those with high risk of developing AKs have skin types that burn easily and tan poorly. AKs may spontaneously regress following reduction in UV exposure, and reappear on resumption. Eventually lesions will become permanent *(60)*.

Shared risk factors, histological continuum, and the presence of similar molecular/genetic alterations are all evidence that AK is the premalignant precursor of SCC, but not BCC *(20)*. Approximately 40–50% of Australians aged 40 or older have at least one AK (average of six to eight), and incidence increases with age *(20,61,62)*. Other studies from Australia and the US have reported AKs in 11–26% of the adult population *(20)*. Few AKs progress to SCC *(62)*, but presence of AK serves as a major risk factor for increased NMSC risk. In a 5-yr longitudinal study, 60% of SCCs arose from a preexisting AK while a 10-yr follow-up of AK patients found a 6–10% rate of malignant progression to SCC or one per 1000 per year in individual lesions *(63)*. A study from Arizona in individuals with 10 or more AKs reported a cumulative probability of 14% for developing SCC within 5 yr *(64)*.

A new classification system proposed by Cockerell et al. *(65)* would replace the term AK with KIN (keratinocytic intraepidermal neoplasia), based on the system used to describe cervical intraepithelial neoplasia; it more closely reflects nomenclature and grading used in other types of intraepithelial neoplasia. An objective classification system for KIN would provide defined features for establishing treatment recommendations and speeding new clinical trial designs and drug approvals.

Research on melanoma precursors offers the largest opportunity for affecting skin cancer mortality with chemoprevention. Relatively few clinical studies in this area have focused on dysplastic nevi (DN) as a target *(66–68)*. DN are atypical moles characterized by abnormalities in size, color, shape, and/or frequency. Presence of DN is considered to be a risk factor for melanoma *(69)*, especially in the familial melanoma setting *(70)*. DN are considered by many to be a melanoma precursor *(71)*. Diagnosis of mild or moderate DN is difficult due to subjective histological criteria *(70,72)*. As more definitive histopathological techniques are established, new strategies will be developed to differentiate and identify melanoma precursor lesions and target their relevant molecular pathways.

2. MOLECULAR TARGETS FOR CANCER CHEMOPREVENTION

Ideally, a successful skin cancer chemopreventive agent would have little or no toxicity and would act specifically against damaged cells without affecting normal cells. Development of new agents is based on data from epidemiologic studies as well as in vitro and in vivo animal studies. Identification of mutations or specific components of signal transduction pathways may be the key to developing agents with well-characterized and very specific mechanisms of action.

2.1. UV-Induced Mitogen-Activated Protein Kinase Signal Transduction

UV radiation, in addition to causing erythema in skin, has been shown to upregulate the local inflammatory response in humans and rodent models. UVB-induced inflammation is characterized by an accumulation of immune cells within the dermal layer and induction of vascular endothelial adhesion molecules *(73)*. Production of inflammatory cytokines including interleukin 1α (IL-1α), IL-6, IL-8, and TNFα has been implicated in mediation of UVB-induced inflammation in the epidermis *(73)*. Genes that encode these cytokines contain nuclear factor-κB (NFκB) binding elements within their promoter regions *(74)*, implicating this proinflammatory *(75)* and redox-regulated *(76,77)* transcription factor in their transcriptional regulation.

UV radiation can be involved in the initiation phase of carcinogenesis by causing DNA mutations such as the CC → TT transitions that are considered a signature of UV-induced lesions *(78,79)*. However, the tumor-promoting effects of UV have been linked to alterations in mitogen-activated protein kinase (MAPK) signal transduction pathways *(80,81)*. These signaling pathways are directly involved with regulation of transcription factors, and therefore control genes that mediate cell proliferation *(82–84)*, differentiation *(85,86)*, and tumorigenesis *(87–91)*. The MAPK family of enzymes represent a critical link between signal transduction processes at the plasma membrane level and final nuclear events. These signaling cascades have been shown to be involved in regulation of cell proliferation and differentiation in human epidermis (reviewed in *92,93*).

Transcription factor activator protein-1 (AP-1) is upregulated in response to UV-induced MAPK signaling in human keratinocytes in vitro *(94)*, in mouse skin in vivo *(95–97)*, and in human skin in vivo *(98)*. AP-1 has been shown to play a role in both UV-induced and chemically induced tumor promotion in skin carcinogenesis models. Young et al. demonstrated that 12-*O*-tetradecanoylphorbol-13-acetate (TPA)-induced tumor promotion was inhibited in a transgenic mouse model that expressed a dominant mutant AP-1 component, c-Jun, in the epidermis, indicating that AP-1 is required for TPA promotion and may be required for UV-mediated tumor promotion *(99)*.

UVB can regulate MAPK signaling through activation of acidic sphingomyelinases and subsequent activation of various atypical protein kinase C (PKC)

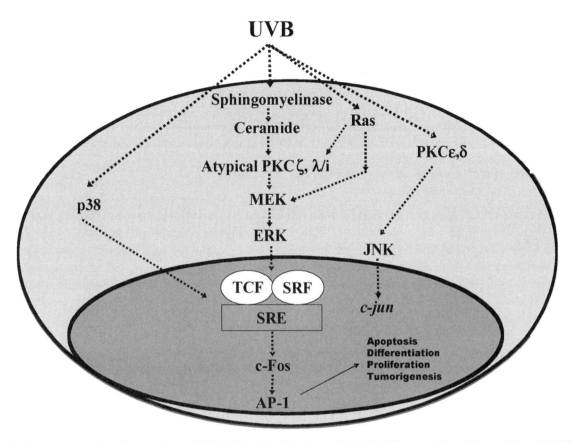

Fig. 2. UVB-induced MAPK signaling pathways. UVB elicits signaling through the MAPK cascade involving activity of ERK, JNK, and p38. Acidic sphingomyelinases activate ceramide and downstream atypical PKCs (PKC-z or PKC-l/i), which phosphorylate and activate MEK, followed by ERK. Ternary complex factor (TCF) undergoes phosphorylation and activation by ERK. Once activated, TCF then binds with serum response factor (SRF) to a serum response element (SRE) harbored within the promoter regions of target genes. Activation of the UVB-induced MAPK signaling pathway results in expression of c-Fos and AP-1 activation. UVB has also been shown to activate PKCε and PKCδ, which results in activation of JNK and c-Jun. UVB also can elicit signaling through p38 and ras. Downstream cellular responses of UVB-induced signal transduction include cell proliferation, apoptosis, and tumorigenesis.

by ceramide as illustrated in Fig. 2. MAPK/extracellular signal-regulated kinase (ERK)-kinase (MEK) then undergoes phosphorylation by atypical PKCs, followed by additional phosphorylation by ternary complex factor (TCF) *(100)*. Huang et al. demonstrated that UV-induced AP-1 activation is mediated by the atypical PKC isoform PKCς. Furthermore, activation of MAPK family members and AP-1 transcriptional activation occur through activation of ERKs, but not the c-Jun N-terminal kinases (JNKs) or p38 *(100)*.

The UV-induced signaling pathway through MEK and ERK ultimately results in transcription of an important member of the AP-1 family of proteins, c-Fos. UVB-induced c-Fos expression is mediated by binding of transcription factors to specific sequences within the promoter regions of the c-*fos* gene. The MAPK signaling pathways that regulate transcription

of AP-1 can regulate cellular responses, including cell proliferation and apoptosis *(101–104)*.

Also of interest, Peus et al. have demonstrated that UVB is involved in activation of the epidermal growth factor receptor (EGFR), ERK, and p38 signaling pathways. A specific EGFR inhibitor significantly decreased UVB-induced phosphorylation of EGFR and of ERK1 and 2. Furthermore, pretreatment with the EGFR inhibitor prior to UV irradiation significantly decreased production of reactive oxygen species and apoptosis *(105)*.

2.2. UVB and p53 Function

The many effects of UVB on cellular signal transduction are areas of intense study. UVB irradiation has a direct effect on p53 function by inducing phosphorylation at serine 15, which results in stabilization of p53 protein. This interferes with the binding and function of MDM2, a negative regulator of p53 transcription. ERKs and p38 kinase also appear to have a direct role in regulating the function of the p53 protein. She et al. *(106)* demonstrated that the phosphorylation of p53 is mediated by both ERKs and p38 kinase, which have a direct role in UVB-induced phosphorylation of p53 at serine 15 in vivo.

2.3. UVB and Cyclooxygenase (COX)-2 Signaling

Another affect of UV radiation in skin is increased prostanoid production and upregulation of COX-2 *(107,108)*. Chen et al. *(109)* showed that UVB irradiation of human keratinocytes in culture resulted in a strong induction of COX-2 protein between 2 and 12 h post-irradiation. They also showed for the first time that activation of stress-activated MAPK p38 was required for UVB-induced COX-2 gene expression. This group *(110)* demonstrated that the cyclic AMP (cAMP)-responsive element near the TATA box of the COX-2 gene was essential for both basal and UVB-induced COX-2 transcription. They also found that one signaling pathway for UVB induction of COX-2 involves activation of p38, subsequent phosphorylation of CRE binding protein (CREB)/activating transcription factor (ATF)-1, and activation of the COX-2 CRE through enhanced binding of phosphorylated CREB/ATF-1. Another UVB-initiated signaling pathway leading to COX-2 transcriptional activation discovered by this group was inactivation of glycogen synthase kinase-3β through UVB-mediated activation of Akt *(111)*. When human subjects were irradiated on sun-protected skin with up to four times their minimal erythemal dose, upregulation of COX-2 protein expression was observed at 24 h post-irradiation *(107)*. Expression of prostaglandin E_2 (PGE_2) has been shown to be increased in AK and in SCC *(112)*. COX-2 expression in normal epidermis is low and restricted to regions of differentiated epidermis. In contrast, overexpression of COX-2 in mouse and human skin carcinogenesis contributes to development of skin cancer *(113)*. Fischer et al. demonstrated that UV-induced carcinogenesis in a hairless mouse model could be inhibited by indomethacin, a nonselective COX inhibitor, and by the selective COX-2 inhibitor celecoxib *(114)*. These data suggest that COX-2 may be a successful target for skin cancer chemoprevention strategies.

2.4. Model Systems

Recent years have seen rapid advancement in the study of new therapeutic and chemopreventive agents

for skin cancer. Development of new models has contributed to this progress. Advances in vitro have been put to use in vivo. Previously, an understanding of skin cancer was based on clinical and microscopic observation. Now, new and more powerful molecular biological tools have increased our understanding and fostered development of new in vitro and in vivo models to explain how physical and biochemical carcinogens can induce neoplastic transformation in skin.

Advances in development of skin tumor models have occurred mainly in studies of mouse skin. Skin cancer models were some of the earliest ever developed to study chemically and physically induced carcinogenesis. One of the earliest experiments using skin cancer as a model system involved repeated topical application of croton oil following a single carcinogen application to mouse skin *(115)*. This type of two-stage carcinogenesis model is one of the most widely used for studying carcinogens and neoplasia development, and for testing new agents in human cancer. Carcinogenesis in mouse skin has advanced dramatically from the days of painting carcinogens and promoters onto the backs of mice. In the post-genome era, genetically modified strains of transgenic mutants and genetic knockouts are being used to identify the genetic events involved in multistep carcinogenesis (reviewed in *116*). Most in vivo skin cancer models involve artificially induced tumors using topically applied carcinogens or UV light. Skin tumors are unique in that they are easily observable and easily measured. They can also be induced in animal models in their native tissue, as opposed to xenografts commonly used for other tumor types.

Mouse skin is by far the most commonly used in vivo NMSC tumor model, and provides an excellent background for UV-induced skin tumors. The hairless albino SKH-1 mouse is exceptionally well suited for these studies. These mice are immune-competent and remain hairless into adulthood *(117)*. Chronic administration of UVB radiation results in the formation of papillomas at early stages *(96)* and ultimately SCC *(118)*. Jansen et al. *(119)* have developed a novel murine model of highly metastatic SCC using FVB/N transgenic mice that overexpress epitope-tagged PKC-ε protein in the epidermis. These animals develop invasive carcinomas at 15–20 wk following chemically induced carcinogenesis initiated with 7,12-dimethylbenz[a]anthracene (DMBA) followed by promotion with TPA. The utility of this model in UV-induced skin tumor formation remains to be investigated. In contrast to animal models of SCC, animal models of BCC have been lacking; however, Aszterbaum et al. *(120,121)* have recently reported a new mouse model of UV-induced BCC based on abnormalities in the hedgehog signaling pathway. These mice contain a heterozygous allele in the PTCH gene (ptc1+/−) resulting in primordial follicular neoplasms that shift in their histological features to closely resemble human BCC.

Multiple animal models of melanoma have been reported, but these typically bear little resemblance to human melanomas (reviewed in ref. *122*). Animal models include fish, opossum, rodent, guinea pig, and swine. Historically, only swine melanoma models have been shown to produce tumors histologically similar to human. Fortunately, recent advances in the development of transgenic mice have resulted in several murine models of malignant melanoma (reviewed in ref. *123*). Powell et al. have reported the development of a transgenic mouse strain that expresses a mutated human Ha-*ras* gene driven by a tyrosinase promoter. These animals all expressed metastatic melanoma following exposure to topical DMBA weekly for 16 wk *(124)*. Interestingly, crosses resulting in an albino phenotype *(125)* developed melanomas upon chronic exposure to UV radiation. Another model of UV-induced murine melanoma has been developed by Noonan et al. *(126)*. This transgenic model utilizes a metallothionein-gene promoter driving a hepatocyte growth factor/scatter factor (c-*met* receptor tyrosine kinase ligand) gene based on an albino inbred FVB background. Presence of the transgene results in deposition of melanocytes in both dermis and epidermis, more closely resembling human skin. A single acute exposure of the neonates to an erythemal dose of UV radiation resulted in formation of invasive melanomas in 80% of the animals by 400 d. In contrast to previously reported in vivo melanoma models, these tumors bore a striking histological resemblance to human melanomas in terms of junctional activity between the dermis and epidermis.

3. SURROGATE ENDPOINT BIOMARKERS IN SKIN CANCER

Chemoprevention clinical trials using cancer development as the primary endpoint can be very costly due to large sample size and long follow-up period. Use of surrogate endpoint biomarkers (SEBs) as endpoint measurements in clinical trials helps circumvent some of these issues because an SEB can be a biologic event that occurs subsequent to UV exposure but long before development of skin cancer. An SEB is an intermediate endpoint but should be an event occurring along the pathway of carcinogenesis. It can be considered valid if

a given risk factor, such as UV exposure, causes a similar change in the occurrence of both the intermediate endpoint and skin cancer incidence. Examples of SEBs include development of a premalignant lesion, such as AK, or a measurement of cellular and molecular characteristics of a cell such as proliferation or apoptosis. Clinical studies that employ SEBs as cancer surrogates are quicker, smaller, and less expensive than studies that use malignancy as the endpoint *(127,128)*.

3.1. Proliferating Cell Nuclear Antigen, p53, and Apoptosis

Expression levels of genes that are dysregulated during skin carcinogenesis are also used as quantitative endpoint biomarkers for skin cancer. Such biomarkers include proliferating cell nuclear antigen (PCNA), which is expressed at low amounts constitutively in nongrowing cells and is synthesized at a greater range in the S-phase of proliferating cells *(129)*, and tumor suppressor gene p53, which is necessary for maintenance of genomic integrity through its ability to block DNA replication in response to UV-induced DNA damage.

Studies have shown that expression levels of p53 in AK and SCC are highly variable, ranging from 0% to 60% in AK and 15% to 69% in SCC *(130–132)*. Furthermore, there often is discrepancy between presence of mutations in the p53 gene and expression of p53 protein *(27,133,134)*. Einspahr et al. examined frequency of p53 mutations and p53 protein expression in normal-appearing skin, in AK lesions, in normal-appearing skin adjacent to AK lesions (sun-damaged skin), and in SCC lesions. They showed an increase in frequency of p53 mutation incidence in AK lesions (62.5%) compared to normal skin (14.3%) and sun-damaged skin (38.5%) *(135)*. Variations in biomarker expression have also been observed in BCC compared to normal skin. Kazantscva et al. demonstrated that PCNA was overexpressed in recurrent (but not primary) BCC *(136)*. Similarly, PCNA expression was found to progressively and significantly increase between normal-appearing skin, skin adjacent to an AK, AK, and SCC lesions *(135)*.

In continually renewing tissues like skin, there is a homeostatic relationship between cell proliferation and cell death. Disruption of this balance can lead to loss of growth control, thereby contributing to the process of tumorigenesis. Apoptosis, a unique form of cell death characterized by distinct morphologic and ultrastructural changes *(137)*, is a potential histological SEB that plays an essential role in carcinogenesis. In addition, certain chemopreventive or chemotherapeutic agents may act to induce apoptosis as a mechanism of action. Einspahr et al. *(135)* reported that the number of apoptotic cells is significantly increased in AK and SCC compared to normal skin.

Use of SEBs in skin tumor models is a new area that requires further research to validate the SEBs. It will be important to show that a SEB varies between the stages of skin carcinogenesis. Encouragingly, PCNA, p53 expression, apoptosis, and p53 mutations have all been shown to be significantly different in human skin biopsy samples composed of normal-appearing skin, sun-damaged skin, and AK *(138,139)*. Since there is differential expression between the various stages of skin carcinogenesis with these SEBs, there is potential for modulation by an intervention. Development of SEBs in skin tumor models may enhance our ability to design meaningful chemoprevention strategies using intermediate endpoints. Ultimately, a lack of specificity to the skin carcinogenesis process may limit the utility of these SEBs in the setting of chemopreventive clinical trials.

3.2. Morphometric Imaging of Nuclear Chromatin (Karyometric Analysis)

At the University of Arizona, imaging techniques have been developed that can detect and objectively quantify subtle alterations in nuclear chromatin patterns not detected by standard histopathological examination. This technique has exhibited high precision and reproducibility in detecting subtle nuclear changes *(140,141)*.

Nuclear images from normal reference tissue and abnormal tissue are segmented and digitized, and information on 93 karyometric features is extracted from the digitized images. Global karyometric features include total nuclear area, average pixel optical density (OD), and variance of pixel OD values, among others. Features of intermediate complexity are derived directly from pixel characteristics, such as the histogram of pixel OD values. Features of greater complexity contain information on relationships between pixel characteristics, such as the frequency with which pixels in a given OD range border pixels in some other (or the same) OD range, yielding the co-occurrence matrix, or the relative frequency of pixel run lengths measured at a given OD range, yielding a run-length matrix.

Information contained in these 93 features allows detection of nuclear changes that reliably map onto progression curves for a wide variety of cancers, including skin cancer. Discriminant function analysis utilizing appropriate karyometric features reveals steadily increasing deviations from normal tissue as pathological gradation worsens.

Karyometric analysis is a promising approach for assessing efficacy of chemopreventive agents because it is extremely sensitive to early nuclear changes. It can be used to assess reversibility of nuclear damage in response to interventions; it provides a means for assessing the statistical significance of such changes, and it is relatively non-specific with respect to particular pathways for carcinogenesis. This latter property results from the use of spatial and statistical information from the entire nucleus. While this means that karyometric analysis is not useful in pinpointing specific pathways involved in a particular case or population, it is highly likely to detect the resulting nuclear changes regardless of the pathway involved.

In studies conducted at the Arizona Cancer Center, karyometric analyses of nuclei in the suprabasal and basal cell layers of sun-damaged skin were conducted on shave biopsy specimens collected from 10 patients *(140)*. Biopsies from sun-damaged areas were collected before and after treatment with α-difluoromethylornithine (DFMO) or placebo. Average nuclear abnormality scores were obtained for each subject by averaging deviations from the reference group across all 93 karyometric features, while discriminant function scores were developed using a subset of karyometric features that proved useful in discriminating between sun-damaged and normal (inner arm) skin samples. Assessing subjects along these measures showed that DFMO treatment was effective in reducing the level of nuclear abnormality seen in the biopsies. The improvement in nuclear abnormality was statistically significant in eight of 10 cases *(140)*. These and other analyses currently in progress at the Arizona Cancer Center suggest that karyometric features may prove to be valuable SEBs for skin cancer chemoprevention studies.

4. CLINICAL DEVELOPMENT OF CHEMOPREVENTIVE AGENTS

Over the past two decades, significant efforts have been made in the US to heighten awareness about skin cancer. The American Academy of Dermatology currently recommends daily use of sunscreens with a sun protection factor (SPF) of 15 or greater *(142)*. Additional recommendations include protective apparel choices and activity-planning strategies to avoid peak sun hours. Minimizing sun exposure by use of sunscreens and protective clothing may reduce skin cancer risk; however, for many reasons, these primary preventive measures have had limited success *(143)*. Several large clinical studies have shown that regular use of sunscreen reduces incidence of some NMSC. Studies conducted by Naylor et al. suggested that regular use of sunscreen significantly reduced AK incidence in a high-risk population *(144)*. Also, a more recent study conducted in Queensland, Australia, found that regular use of sunscreen had a preventive effect on SCC, but not BCC *(145)*. However, studies conducted by Harvey et al. on 1304 men and women 60 yr of age or older in New South Wales indicated that regular use of sunscreen and protective clothing had no effect on incidence of AK or SCC *(146)*.

Some data suggest that sunscreen use may be associated with an increased risk of melanoma. Studies conducted by Wolf et al. *(147)* reported that common sunscreens did not protect against UV radiation enhancement of melanoma incidence in a xenograft model of mouse melanoma. Garland et al. *(148,149)* hypothesize that increased incidence of melanoma in countries where chemical sunscreens have been highly promoted may be due to an increase in sun exposure times, although this remains controversial *(150)*.

Given the limited success of primary prevention strategies, development of successful secondary chemoprevention strategies may prove important in reducing skin cancer incidence. Ultimately, chemoprevention and primary prevention strategies could be used in combination. Many studies have indicated that most SCCs in sun-exposed areas arise from preexisting AKs. Therefore, AK lesions are considered to be a precursor to SCC *(151–153)*. Thus, one of the most promising strategies for chemoprevention of NMSC is treatment of AK *(154)*. Several chemopreventive agents are currently undergoing clinical development for eradication of clinically apparent AK.

4.1. Current Treatments for AK

One of the mainstays of AK treatment is local destruction of the lesion using cryotherapy or curettage with electrodessication. However, local destructive therapies are not feasible in patients with numerous AKs in areas of severely sun-damaged skin *(155)*. Standard approaches for treating sun-damaged areas with multiple AKs include topical application of the DNA synthesis inhibitor 5-fluorouracil *(156,157)*, an uncomfortable treatment that results in significant inflammation and painful erosions *(158)*. Other topical therapies include destructive chemical peels containing trichloroacetic or α-hydroxy acids, and photodynamic therapy with aminolevulinic acid *(159)*.

Topical diclofenac sodium in a hyaluronan complex (Solaraze) was recently approved in the US, Canada and Europe for treatment of AK. Diclofenac, a nonsteroidal antiinflammatory drug, interferes with arachidonic acid metabolism via inhibition of COX enzymes *(160,161)*. Early studies with topical diclofenac were encouraging and led to its evaluation for treating AK. Clinical studies demonstrated that 3% diclofenac in 2.5% hyaluronan gel was effective and well tolerated. In 1997, Rivers and McLean reported the results of a clinical trial evaluating the safety and efficacy of this formulation in an open-label study in patients with AK. The duration of treatment was 33–176 d. Thirty days following discontinuation of treatment, 22 of 27 patients (81%) experienced complete remission of the treated lesions and 4 of 27 (15%) showed significant clinical improvement. Although 7 of 24 patients (24%) experienced local irritation, the treatment was well tolerated overall *(162)*. Subsequently, a larger, randomized, placebo-controlled study confirmed that this formulation was effective in treating AK *(163)*. In this double-blind study, 96 patients with five or more AKs in a defined treatment area were treated for 90 d with either Solaraze or a vehicle containing 2.5% hyaluronan alone. At 30 d post-study, 50% of the patients in the diclofenac treatment group (vs 20% in the control group) reported complete resolution of AK present in the defined treatment area at the beginning of the study ($p < 0.001$). It is interesting that 20% of the control group reported complete resolution of AK, indicating that hyaluronan may contribute to the activity of diclofenac.

4.2. Retinoids

Vitamin A and its analogs (retinoids) have been shown to inhibit development of tumors in several epithelial models of carcinogenesis *(164–167)*. The mechanism by which vitamin A and vitamin A analogs elicit a chemopreventive effect is therefore the subject of intense study. Retinoids, the most well-studied chemoprevention agents, play a role in a number of biological processes including cell proliferation, differentiation, and apoptosis during embryogenesis *(168)*. Six human nuclear retinoic acid receptors (RARs) have been characterized; RARs and retinoid x receptors (RXR), each of which has three isoforms (α, β, γ) encoded by different genes. RARs bind to corresponding response elements in the DNA sequence of the genes they regulate. These receptors are the molecular targets of retinoid-specific drug development. Variation in tissue expression patterns, ligand specificity, functional redundancy, and the ability to regulate other signal transduction pathways (i.e., AP-1) all contribute to the complexity of RAR signaling *(169,170)*. An advantageous feature of retinoids is their effectiveness when administered systemically or topically, before or after carcinogen exposure. The effects are reversible when retinoids are discontinued *(164,165)*.

In the 1970s, Sporn et al. demonstrated that retinoids could prevent chemically induced skin carcinogenesis in animal models *(171)*. Since then, retinoids have undergone intense clinical development. In the mid-1980s, two randomized clinical trials were initiated examining the effect of retinol in SCC and BCC incidence. In a Phase III double-blind, placebo-controlled, randomized clinical study in 2297 patients with moderate to severe AK, moderate-risk subjects with a history of 10 or more AKs and no more than two prior skin cancers were enrolled in the SKICAP-AK trial and randomized to 25,000 IU retinol or placebo daily for 5yr. Daily retinol in this study was associated with a 32% reduction in risk of developing SCC of the skin, but had no effect on BCC incidence *(64)*. This effect was significantly more pronounced in patients with eight or more freckles or moles, suggesting that retinol was especially protective in subjects at higher risk. In a concurrent trial in high-risk subjects, 719 patients with at least four prior skin cancers were randomized to receive oral retinol (25,000 IU), isotretinoin (13-*cis*-retinoic acid, 5–10 mg) or placebo daily for 3yr in the SKICAP-S/B trial *(170)*. However, neither retinol nor isotretinoin was effective in reducing or delaying the occurrence of new SCC or BCC in this extremely high-risk population *(172)*. In a 2-yr Phase II trial, Kraemer et al. reported that isotretinoin prevented development of NMSC in patients with xeroderma pigmentosum *(173)*.

4.3. COX-2 Inhibitors

COX-2 overexpression has been documented in UV-exposed human skin cells. Buckman et al. demonstrated that in vitro exposure of human keratinocytes to UVB caused a significant increase in PGE_2 expression. Furthermore, COX-2 was upregulated in UV-exposed human skin in vivo *(107,174)*. In cultured human keratinocytes, UVB-induced COX-2 activity was completely blocked by indomethacin, a nonselective COX inhibitor, as well as by SC58125, a COX-2-selective inhibitor *(174)*. Using immunohistochemical analyses, Kogoura et al. demonstrated that four of 16 BCCs expressed COX-2. In Bowen's disease, the intensity of positive staining for COX-2 was even higher than that

in BCC; 11 of 15 SCCs were shown to express COX-2. Interestingly, the pattern of staining was heterogeneous, with more intense staining in the center of the tumor loci. In metastatic SCC tumors, the percentage of COX-2-positive tumor cells and their staining intensity was low compared with both Bowen's disease and SCC, suggesting that COX-2 may play a role in the early stages of SCC carcinogenesis *(175)*.

Currently, several ongoing NCI-sponsored clinical studies are examining COX-2 inhibition and skin cancer in high-risk populations. One randomized, double-blind, placebo-controlled Phase II study at the Herbert Irving Comprehensive Cancer Center (New York, NY) is evaluating the ability of celecoxib to inhibit UV-induced erythema in individuals with Fitzpatrick Type I–IV skin. This study is also examining effects of celecoxib on biomarkers of cutaneous carcinogenesis in these subjects. Another randomized, double-blind, placebo-controlled study being conducted at the University of California San Francisco Cancer Center and the Herbert Irving Comprehensive Cancer Center is testing celecoxib for chemopreventive activity against BCC in patients with basal cell nevus syndrome. Participants in this study are required to have at least five prior histologically confirmed BCCs, at least four of them within 12 months prior to study entry. Celecoxib is also being tested in a Phase II/III randomized, double-blind, placebo-controlled clinical trial for preventing development of new AK in patients with existing AK, at the University of Alabama at Birmingham Comprehensive Cancer Center. In addition to examining the safety profile of celecoxib in these subjects, this study will also examine the ability of celecoxib to induce regression of AK and alter potential SEBs in AK, sun-exposed skin, and non-sun-exposed skin. Biomarkers will be correlated with clinical outcome in these patients.

Reports examining COX-2 and skin carcinogenesis illustrate the need to evaluate the potential efficacy of COX-2 selective inhibitors as chemopreventive and chemotherapeutic agents for UV-induced skin cancers. Future research should combine in vitro techniques, transgenic knockout or overexpression mouse models, and human translational and clinical studies to define the role of COX-2 in UVB-induced skin carcinogenesis.

4.4. DFMO

Another chemopreventive strategy under investigation in clinical trials is the inhibition of polyamines, a family of ubiquitous polycations essential for normal cellular proliferation, differentiation, and apoptosis

(176,177). The polyamine-synthesizing enzyme ornithine decarboxylase (ODC) and polyamines, such as spermidine, are upregulated in rodent and human premalignant and malignant tumors *(178)*. DFMO, an irreversible inhibitor of ODC (the first step in polyamine synthesis) has been shown to block tumorigenesis in UV-induced skin carcinogenesis models. Oral administration of DFMO after UVB-induced tumor formation was shown to inhibit development of new UVB-induced mouse skin tumors and cause regression of established UV-induced tumors *(179,180)*. Since polyamines are known to play a role in cell proliferation, mechanisms for DFMO may also include reduction in the rate of tumor cell growth *(181,182)*. Other potential mechanisms for chemopreventive activity of DFMO may include inhibition of tumor invasion through upregulation of metalloproteinases *(183)*, suppression of angiogenesis *(184)*, and inhibition of DNA repair following DNA-damaging agents *(185,186)*.

At the Arizona Cancer Center, a clinical trial tested a topical formulation of DFMO (10% w/w bid) applied for 6 mo in 42 subjects who had at least 10 AK on their dorsal forearms *(187)*. A significant (23.5%) reduction was seen in AK number. The level of spermidine, a polyamine known to be involved in cell proliferation, was also significantly reduced. Since DFMO inhibits polyamine synthesis, measures of polyamine levels in the skin were included as an index of biological activity. p53 protein expression was also used as an indication of drug effect, since mutations in the p53 gene and overexpression of p53 protein are considered early events in development of AK and SCC. Data showed that DFMO significantly inhibited expression of p53 (26% reduction) without affecting cell proliferation. In this study, nuclear karyometric analyses, high-resolution images of nuclei from the suprabasal and basal cell layers of sun-damaged skin, were also recorded. DFMO treatment was effective overall in reducing the degree of nuclear abnormality seen in the biopsies; eight of ten cases treated with DFMO saw significant improvement. No significant change was observed with placebo *(140)*.

Another randomized, double-blind, placebo-controlled, Phase II study is being conducted at the Arizona Cancer Center to examine the effect of DFMO with or without triamcinolone as a chemopreventive strategy in patients with moderate to heavy AK. This study will examine whether this intervention can reverse existing AK, and if triamcinolone can reduce local skin irritation caused by topical application of DFMO. For this study, participants are required to have at least three AK on each forearm.

4.5. Epigallocatechin-3-Gallate (EGCG)

Green tea polyphenols have been reported to have antimutagenic and antitumor activities *(188–190)*. Mechanisms by which EGCG may elicit a chemopreventive effect are currently the subject of intense study. EGCG, the most abundant green tea polyphenol, is known to have antioxidant activity *(191)*. EGCG has also been shown to induce the signaling pathways involved in apoptosis *(192,193)*, inhibit the activity of topoisomerase II *(194)*, inhibit angiogenesis by blocking expression of vascular endothelial growth factor *(195)*, and inhibit UVB-induced activation of AP-1 through blocking p38 MAPK-mediated expression of c-*fos* *(81,97)*. In vitro studies have shown that EGCG can inhibit growth of human tumor cell lines, including melanoma *(189)*. EGCG has also been shown to have antitumor activity in skin cancer animal models *(196,197)*. Several studies examining potential chemopreventive mechanisms have shown that green and black tea polyphenols can block UVB-induced activation of several signal transduction pathways associated with skin carcinogenesis *(81,97,198)*. At the Arizona Cancer Center, a topical formulation of EGCG ointment is currently undergoing clinical evaluation in a randomized, double-blind, placebo-controlled, Phase IIa trial. In this study, subjects receive twice-daily administration of topical EGCG or placebo for 28 d, randomized in double-blind fashion to the right or left lower dorsal forearm and hand; patients are monitored for dermal and systemic toxicities. Skin punch biopsies taken at end of study will be evaluated for histopathological differences. Concurrently, the SPF of EGCG ointment is being evaluated on non-sun exposed buttock skin using a solar simulator.

4.6. Other Chemopreventive Agents with Potential

Several other agents currently in preclinical and clinical development also show promise for skin cancer chemoprevention. The immune modifier imiquimod (Aldara), approved for treatment of external genital and perianal condyloma acuminata, is being evaluated in trials of AK and BCC *(199,200)*. Curcumin (diferuloylmethane), a naturally occurring yellow pigment in turmeric and curry isolated from the rhizomes of the plant *Curcuma longa* Linn, has been shown to block both the initiation and promotion stages of tumorigenesis in DMBA/TPA mouse skin carcinogenesis models in vivo *(201,202)*. Furthermore, curcumin has been shown to inhibit TPA-induced increases in epidermal DNA synthesis *(203)*, ODC mRNA levels *(201,204)*, hyperplasia *(205)*, and AP-1 signaling *(206)* in various animal models.

The cytokine IL-12 is also being studied preclinically for chemopreventive activity in NMSC. Oshikawa et al. demonstrated that local delivery of a plasmid construct constitutively expressing IL-12 to a primary SCC tumor in a mouse model blocked formation of metastatic lesions *(207)*. IL-12 has also been shown to suppress UV-mediated apoptosis in human keratinocytes and induce DNA repair mechanisms, resulting in fewer UV-specific DNA lesions *(208)*.

Perillyl alcohol, a monoterpene derived from citrus peel, has been shown to inhibit UVB-induced mouse skin carcinogenesis *(96)*. Perillyl alcohol has multiple activities including the ability to inhibit Ras farnesylation. Barthelman et al. *(96)* found that perillyl alcohol inhibits UVB-induced AP-1 activation in cultured human keratinocytes and in mouse skin. Perillyl alcohol inhibition of Ras localization to the plasma membrane could block UVB-mediated activation of atypical PKCs (*see* Fig. 2).

5. CONCLUSION

Increases in skin cancer incidence have had a dramatic effect on quality of life and health care economics. Significant progress has been made characterizing mechanisms that mediate the process of skin cancer development and progression. Insight into UV-induced signaling pathways is providing an array of new molecular targets. Further research is needed to design safe and selective new agents to target these pathways for prevention of early damage and treatment of early neoplastic lesions such as AK. Identification and validation of new specific SEBs will allow practical testing of new chemopreventive agents in a clinical setting. Despite the challenges involved in developing these agents, investigators in this area remain committed to the production of new prevention strategies.

REFERENCES

1. Pott P. Chirurgical observations relative to the cataract, the polypus of the nose, the cancer of the scrotum, the different kinds of ruptures and the mortification of the toes and feet. Hawes, Clarke, & Collins, London, 1775.
2. Potter M. Percivall Pott's contribution to cancer research. In Urbach F, ed. *The First International Conference on the Biology of Cutaneous Cancer.* US Govt Printing Office, Washington DC, 1962; pp. 1–13.
3. *Cancer Facts & Figures 2002.* American Cancer Society, New York, 2002.
4. Kanzler MH. An estimate of the annual direct cost of treating cutaneous melanoma. *J Am Acad Dermatol* 1999;41: 281–283.
5. Chen JG, Fleischer AB Jr, Smith ED, et al. Cost of non-melanoma skin cancer treatment in the United States. *Dermatol Surg* 2001;27:1035–1038.
6. Jemal A, Thomas A, Murray T, Thun M. Cancer statistics, 2002. *CA Cancer J Clin* 2002; 52:23–47.
7. Parker SL, Tong T, Bolden S, Wingo PA. Cancer statistics, 1997. *CA Cancer J Clin* 1997;47:5–27.
8. Greenlee RT, Murray T, Bolden S, Wingo PA. Cancer statistics, 2000. *CA Cancer J Clin* 2000; 50:7–33.
9. Greenlee RT, Hill-Harmon MB, Murray T, Thun M. Cancer statistics, 2001. CA Cancer J Clin 2001; 51:15–36.
10. Lee JAH. Epidemiology of cancers of the skin. In *Cancer of the Skin.* Friedman RJ, Rigel DS, Kopf AW, et al., eds. W.B. Saunders, Philadelphia,1991; pp. 14–24.
11. Lang PG Jr, Maize JC. Basal cell carcinoma. In *Cancer of the Skin.* Friedman RJ, Rigel DS, Kopf AW, et al., eds. W.B. Saunders, Philadelphia, 1991; pp. 35–73.
12. Demetrius RW, Randle HW. High-risk nonmelanoma skin cancers. *Dermatol Surg* 1998;4:1272–1294.
13. Hall HI, Miller DR, Rogers JD, Bewerse B. Update on the incidence and mortality from melanoma in the United States. *J Am Acad Dermatol* 1999;40:35–42.
14. Gilchrest BA, Eller MS, Geller AC, Yaar M. The pathogenesis of melanoma induced by ultraviolet radiation. *N Engl J Med* 1999;340:1341–1348.
15. Masback A, Westerdahl J, Ingvar C, et al. Clinical and histopathological characteristics in relation to aetiological risk factors in cutaneous melanoma: a population-based study. *Melanoma Res* 1999;9:189–197.
16. Naldi L, Lorenzo IG, Parazzini F, et al. Pigmentary traits, modalities of sun reaction, history of sunburns, and melanocytic nevi as risk factors for cutaneous malignant melanoma in the Italian population: results of a collaborative case-control study. *Cancer* 2000;88:2703–2710.
17. Retsas S. Adjuvant therapy of malignant melanoma: is there a choice? *Crit Rev Oncol Hematol* 2001;40:187–193.
18. Lens MB, Dawes M. Interferon alfa therapy for malignant melanoma: a systematic review of randomized controlled trials. *J Clin Oncol* 2002;20:1818–1825.
19. MacKie RM. Incidence, risk factors and prevention of melanoma. *Eur J Cancer* 1998;34:S3–S6.
20. Salasche SJ. Epidemiology of actinic keratoses and squamous cell carcinoma. *J Am Acad Dermatol* 2000;42: S4–S7.
21. Jacob A. Observations respecting an ulcer of peculiar character, which attacks the eyelids and other parts of the face. *Dublin Hosp Rep Commun Med Surg* 1827;4:232–239.
22. Kwa RE, Campana K, Moy RL. Biology of cutaneous squamous cell carcinoma. *J Am Acad Dermatol* 1992;26:1–26.
23. Moller RF, Reymann F, Hou-Jensen K. Metastases in dermatological patients with squamous cell carcinoma. *Arch Dermatol* 1979;115:703–705.
24. Grossman D, Leffell DJ. The molecular basis of non-melanoma skin cancer: new understanding. *Arch Dermatol* 1997;133:1263–1270.
25. Gjersvik PJ. Etiology of non-melanoma skin cancer. *Tidsskr Nor Laegeforen* 2001;121:2052–2056.

26. Pathak MA. Ultraviolet radiation and the development of non-melanoma and melanoma skin cancer: clinical and experimental evidence. *Skin Pharmacol* 1991;4 Suppl 1:85–94.

27. Brash DE, Ziegler A, Jonason AS, et al. Sunlight and sunburn in human skin cancer: p53, apoptosis, and tumor promotion. *J Investig Dermatol Symp Proc* 1996;1:136–142.

28. Nishigori C. UV-induced DNA damage in carcinogenesis and its repair. *J Dermatol Sci* 2000;23:S41–S44.

29. Marghoob AA, Slade J, Salopek TG, et al. Basal cell and squamous cell carcinomas are important risk factors for cutaneous malignant melanoma. Screening implications. *Cancer* 1995;75:707–714.

30. Schottenfeld D. Basal-cell carcinoma of the skin: a harbinger of cutaneous and noncutaneous multiple primary cancer. *Ann Intern Med* 1996;125:852–854.

31. Frisch M, Hjalgrim H, Olsen JH, Melbye M. Risk for subsequent cancer after diagnosis of basal-cell carcinoma. A population-based, epidemiologic study. *Ann Intern Med* 1996;125:815–821.

32. Kroumpouzos G, Konstadoulakis MM, Cabral H, Karakousis CP. Risk of basal cell and squamous cell carcinoma in persons with prior cutaneous melanoma. *Dermatol Surg* 2000; 26:547–550.

33. Boukamp P, Popp S, Bleuel K, et al. Tumorigenic conversion of immortal human skin keratinocytes (HaCaT) by elevated temperature. *Oncogene* 1999;18:5638–5645.

34. Christophers AJ. Melanoma is not caused by sunlight. *Mutat Res* 1998;422:113–117.

35. Fears TR, Scotto J. Estimating increases in skin cancer morbidity due to increases in ultraviolet radiation exposure. *Cancer Invest* 1983;1:119–126.

36. Karagas MR, McDonald JA, Greenberg ER, et al. Risk of basal cell and squamous cell skin cancers after ionizing radiation therapy. For The Skin Cancer Prevention Study Group. *J Natl Cancer Inst* 1996;88:1848–1853.

37. Ron E, Preston DL, Kishikawa M, et al. Skin tumor risk among atomic-bomb survivors in Japan. *Cancer Causes Control* 1998;9:393–401.

38. Ron E. Ionizing radiation and cancer risk: evidence from epidemiology. *Radiat Res* 1998;150:S30–S41.

39. Ullrich SE. Photoimmune suppression and photocarcinogenesis. *Front Biosci* 2002;7:d684–703;d684–d703.

40. Matsumura Y, Ananthaswamy HN. Molecular mechanisms of photocarcinogenesis. *Front Biosci* 2002;7:d765–d783.

41. Lindelof B, Sigurgeirsson B, Gabel H, Stern RS. Incidence of skin cancer in 5356 patients following organ transplantation. *Br J Dermatol* 2000;143:513–519.

42. DiGiovanna JJ. Posttransplantation skin cancer: scope of the problem, management, and role for systemic retinoid chemoprevention. *Transplant Proc* 1998;30:2771–2778.

43. Hojo M, Morimoto T, Maluccio M, et al. Cyclosporine induces cancer progression by a cell-autonomous mechanism. *Nature* 1999;397:530–534.

44. Harwood CA, McGregor JM, Proby CM, Breuer J. Human papillomavirus and the development of non-melanoma skin cancer. *J Clin Pathol* 1999;52:249–253.

45. Jenson AB, Geyer S, Sundberg JP, Ghim S. Human papillomavirus and skin cancer. *J Investig Dermatol Symp Proc* 2001;6:203–206.

46. Bouwes Bavinck JN, Feltkamp M, Struijk L, ter Scheggett J. Human papillomavirus infection and skin cancer risk in organ transplant recipients. *J Investig Dermatol Symp Proc* 2001;6:207–211.

47. Hill LL, Shreedhar VK, Kripke ML, Owen-Schaub LB. A critical role for Fas ligand in the active suppression of systemic immune responses by ultraviolet radiation. *J Exp Med* 1999;189:1285–1294.

48. Hill LL, Ouhtit A, Loughlin SM, et al. Fas ligand: a sensor for DNA damage critical in skin cancer etiology. *Science* 1999;285:898–900.

49. Amerio P, Toto P, Feliciani C, et al. Rethinking the role of tumour necrosis factor-alpha in ultraviolet (UV) B-induced immunosuppression: altered immune response in UV-irradiated TNFR1R2 gene-targeted mutant mice. *Br J Dermatol* 2001;144:952–957.

50. Kibitel J, Hejmadi V, Alas L, et al. UV-DNA damage in mouse and human cells induces the expression of tumor necrosis factor alpha. *Photochem Photobiol* 1998;67: 541–546.

51. Yarosh D, Both D, Kibitel J, et al. Regulation of TNFalpha production and release in human and mouse keratinocytes and mouse skin after UV-B irradiation. *Photodermatol Photoimmunol Photomed* 2000;16:263–270.

52. Moore RJ, Owens DM, Stamp G, et al. Mice deficient in tumor necrosis factor-alpha are resistant to skin carcinogenesis. *Nat Med* 1999;5:828–831.

53. Stratton SP, Dorr RT, Alberts DS. The state-of-the-art in chemoprevention of skin cancer. *Eur J Cancer* 2000;36: 1292–1297.

54. Kuflik AS, Schwartz RA. Actinic keratosis and squamous cell carcinoma. *Am Fam Physician* 1994;49:817–820.

55. Dinehart SM, Nelson-Adesokan P, Cockerell C, et al. Metastatic cutaneous squamous cell carcinoma derived from actinic keratosis. *Cancer* 1997;79:920–923.

56. Smith ES, Feldman SR, Fleischer AB Jr, et al. Characteristics of office-based visits for skin cancer. Dermatologists have more experience than other physicians in managing malignant and premalignant skin conditions. *Dermatol Surg* 1998;24:981–985.

57. Johnson MT, Roberts J. Skin conditions and related need for medical care among persons 1–74 years. United States, 1971–1974. *Vital Health Stat* 1978;11:1–72.

58. Zagula-Mally ZW, Rosenberg EW, Kashgarian M. Frequency of skin cancer and solar keratoses in a rural southern county as determined by population sampling. *Cancer* 1974;34:345–349.

59. Frost CA, Green AC. Epidemiology of solar keratoses. *Br J Dermatol* 1994;131:455–464.

60. Sober AJ, Burstein JM. Precursors to skin cancer. *Cancer* 1995;75:645–650.

61. Fitzgerald DA. Cancer precursors. *Semin Cutan Med Surg* 1998;17:108–113.

62. Marks R, Rennie G, Selwood TS. Malignant transformation of solar keratoses to squamous cell carcinoma. *Lancet* 1988;1:795–797.

63. Dodson JM, DeSpain J, Hewett JE, Clark DP. Malignant potential of actinic keratoses and the controversy over treatment. A patient-oriented perspective. *Arch Dermatol* 1991; 127:1029–1031.

64. Moon TE, Levine N, Cartmel B, et al. Effect of retinol in preventing squamous cell skin cancer in moderate-risk subjects: a randomized, double-blind, controlled trial. Southwest Skin Cancer Prevention Study Group. *Cancer Epidemiol Biomarkers Prev* 1997;6:949–956.

65. Cockerell CJ. Histopathology of incipient intraepidermal squamous cell carcinoma ("actinic keratosis"). *J Am Acad Dermatol* 2000;42:S11–S17.

66. Halpern AC, Schuchter LM, Elder DE, et al. Effects of topical tretinoin on dysplastic nevi. *J Clin Oncol* 1994;12:1028–1035.

67. Stam-Posthuma JJ, Vink J, le Cessie S, et al. Effect of topical tretinoin under occlusion on atypical naevi. *Melanoma Res* 1998;8:539–548.

68. Meyskens FL Jr, Edwards L, Levine NS. Role of topical tretinoin in melanoma and dysplastic nevi. *J Am Acad Dermatol* 1986;15:822–825.

69. Tucker MA, Halpern A, Holly EA, et al. Clinically recognized dysplastic nevi. A central risk factor for cutaneous melanoma. *JAMA* 1997;277:1439–1444.

70. Kanzler MH, Mraz-Gernhard S. Primary cutaneous malignant melanoma and its precursor lesions: diagnostic and therapeutic overview. *J Am Acad Dermatol* 2001;45:260–276.

71. Marras S, Faa G, Dettori T, et al. Chromosomal changes in dysplastic nevi. *Cancer Genet Cytogenet* 1999;113:177–179.

72. Pozo L, Naase M, Cerio R, et al. Critical analysis of histologic criteria for grading atypical (dysplastic) melanocytic nevi. *Am J Clin Pathol* 2001;115:194–204.

73. Strickland I, Rhodes LE, Flanagan BF, Friedmann PS. TNF-alpha and IL-8 are upregulated in the epidermis of normal human skin after UVB exposure: correlation with neutrophil accumulation and E- selectin expression. *J Invest Dermatol* 1997;108:763–768.

74. Saliou C, Rimbach G, Moini H, et al. Solar ultraviolet-induced erythema in human skin and nuclear factor- kappa-B-dependent gene expression in keratinocytes are modulated by a French maritime pine bark extract. *Free Radic Biol Med* 2001;30:154–160.

75. Huang C, Mattjus P, Ma WY, et al. Involvement of nuclear factor of activated T cells activation in UV response. Evidence from cell culture and transgenic mice. *J Biol Chem* 2000;275:9143–9149.

76. Kulms D, Poppelmann B, Schwarz T. Ultraviolet radiation-induced interleukin 6 release in HeLa cells is mediated via membrane events in a DNA damage-independent way. *J Biol Chem* 2000;275:15,060–15,066.

77. Fisher GJ, Datta SC, Talwar HS, et al. Molecular basis of sun-induced premature skin ageing and retinoid antagonism. *Nature* 1996;379:335–339.

78. Dumaz N, Stary A, Soussi T, et al. Can we predict solar ultraviolet radiation as the causal event in human tumours by analysing the mutation spectra of the p53 gene? *Mutat Res* 1994;307:375–386.

79. Yuan J, Yeasky TM, Rhee MC, Glazer PM. Frequent T:A--> G:C transversions in X-irradiated mouse cells. Carcinogenesis 1995;16:83–88.

80. Chen YR, Tan TH. Inhibition of the c-Jun N-terminal kinase (JNK) signaling pathway by curcumin. *Oncogene* 1998;17:173–178.

81. Chen W, Dong Z, Valcic S, et al. Inhibition of ultraviolet B-induced c-fos gene expression and p38 mitogen-activated protein kinase activation by (−)-epigallocatechin gallate in a human keratinocyte cell line. *Mol Carcinog* 1999;24:79–84.

82. Perugini RA, McDade TP, Vittimberga FJ Jr, Callery MP. Pancreatic cancer cell proliferation is phosphatidylinositol 3-kinase dependent. *J Surg Res* 2000;90:39–44.

83. Tsang DK, Crowe DL. The mitogen activated protein kinase pathway is required for proliferation but not invasion of human squamous cell carcinoma lines. *Int J Oncol* 1999;15:519–523.

84. Sah JF, Eckert RL, Chandraratna RA, Rorke EA. Retinoids suppress epidermal growth factor-associated cell proliferation by inhibiting epidermal growth factor receptor-dependent ERK1/2 activation. *J Biol Chem* 2002;277:9728–9735.

85. Ding Q, Wang Q, Evers BM. Alterations of MAPK activities associated with intestinal cell differentiation. *Biochem Biophys Res Commun* 2001;284:282–288.

86. Aliaga JC, Deschenes C, Beaulieu JF, et al. Requirement of the MAP kinase cascade for cell cycle progression and differentiation of human intestinal cells. *Am J Physiol* 1999;277:631–641.

87. Oka H, Chatani Y, Hoshino R, et al. Constitutive activation of mitogen-activated protein (MAP) kinases in human renal cell carcinoma. *Cancer Res* 1995;55:4182–4187.

88. Attar BM, Atten MJ, Holian O. MAPK activity is down-regulated in human colon adenocarcinoma: correlation with PKC activity. *Anticancer Res* 1996;16:395–399.

89. Eggstein S, Franke M, Kutschka I, et al. Expression and activity of mitogen activated protein kinases in human colorectal carcinoma. *Gut* 1999;44:834–838.

90. Mishima K, Yamada E, Masui K, et al. Overexpression of the ERK/MAP kinases in oral squamous cell carcinoma. *Mod Pathol* 1998;11:886–891.

91. Chen N, Nomura M, She QB, et al. Suppression of skin tumorigenesis in c-Jun NH(2)-terminal kinase-2- deficient mice. *Cancer Res* 2001;61:3908–3912.

92. Chen YR, Tan TH. The c-Jun N-terminal kinase pathway and apoptotic signaling. *Int J Oncol* 2000;16:651–662.

93. Geilen CC, Wieprecht M, Orfanos CE. The mitogen-activated protein kinases system (MAP kinase cascade): its role in skin signal transduction. A review. *J Dermatol Sci* 1996;12:255–262.

94. Chen W, Borchers AH, Dong Z, et al. UVB irradiation-induced activator protein-1 activation correlates with increased c-fos gene expression in a human keratinocyte cell line. *J Biol Chem* 1998;273:32,176–32,181.

95. Huang C, Ma WY, Hanenberger D, et al. Inhibition of ultraviolet B-induced activator protein-1 (AP-1) activity by aspirin in AP-1-luciferase transgenic mice. *J Biol Chem* 1997;272:26,325–26,331.

96. Barthelman M, Chen W, Gensler HL, et al. Inhibitory effects of perillyl alcohol on UVB-induced murine skin cancer and AP-1 transactivation. *Cancer Res* 1998;58:711–716.

97. Barthelman M, Bair WB3, Stickland KK, et al. (−)-Epigallo-catechin-3-gallate inhibition of ultraviolet B- induced AP-1 activity. *Carcinogenesis* 1998;19:2201–2204.

98. Fisher GJ, Voorhees JJ. Molecular mechanisms of photoaging and its prevention by retinoic acid: ultraviolet irradiation induces MAP kinase signal transduction cascades that induce Ap-1-regulated matrix metalloproteinases that degrade human skin in vivo. *J Investig Dermatol Symp Proc* 1998;3:61–68.

99. Young MR, Li JJ, Rincon M, et al. Transgenic mice demonstrate AP-1 (activator protein-1) transactivation is required for tumor promotion. *Proc Natl Acad Sci USA* 1999;96:9827–9832.

100. Huang C, Li J, Chen N, et al. Inhibition of atypical PKC blocks ultraviolet-induced AP-1 activation by specifically inhibiting ERKs activation. *Mol Carcinog* 2000;27:65–75.

101. Shaulian E, Karin M. AP-1 in cell proliferation and survival. *Oncogene* 2001;20:2390–2400.
102. Hsu TC, Young MR, Cmarik J, Colburn NH. Activator protein 1 (AP-1)-and nuclear factor kappaB (NF-kappaB)- dependent transcriptional events in carcinogenesis. *Free Radic Biol Med* 2000;28:1338–1348.
103. Blumberg PM. Complexities of the protein kinase C pathway. *Mol Carcinog* 1991;4:339–344.
104. Fisher GJ, Talwar HS, Lin J, et al. Retinoic acid inhibits induction of c-Jun protein by ultraviolet radiation that occurs subsequent to activation of mitogen-activated protein kinase pathways in human skin in vivo. *J Clin Invest* 1998;101: 1432–1440.
105. Meves A, Stock SN, Beyerle A, et al. H(2)O(2) mediates oxidative stress-induced epidermal growth factor receptor phosphorylation. *Toxicol Lett* 2001;122:205–214.
106. She QB, Chen N, Dong Z. ERKs and p38 kinase phosphorylate p53 protein at serine 15 in response to UV radiation. *J Biol Chem* 2000;275:20,444–20,449.
107. Buckman SY, Gresham A, Hale P, et al. COX-2 expression is induced by UVB exposure in human skin: implications for the development of skin cancer. *Carcinogenesis* 1998;19: 723–729.
108. Athar M, An KP, Morel KD, et al. Ultraviolet B(UVB)-induced cox-2 expression in murine skin: an immunohistochemical study. *Biochem Biophys Res Commun* 2001;280: 1042–1047.
109. Chen W, Tang Q, Gonzales MS, Bowden GT. Role of p38 MAP kinases and ERK in mediating ultraviolet-B induced cyclooxygenase-2 gene expression in human keratinocytes. *Oncogene* 2001;20:3921–3926.
110. Tang Q, Chen W, Gonzales MS, et al. Role of cyclic AMP responsive element in the UVB induction of cyclooxygenase-2 transcription in human keratinocytes. *Oncogene* 2001;20:5164–5172.
111. Tang Q, Gonzales M, Inoue H, Bowden GT. Roles of Akt and glycogen synthase kinase 3beta in the ultraviolet B induction of cyclooxygenase-2 transcription in human keratinocytes. *Cancer Res* 2001;61:4329–4332.
112. Muller-Decker K, Reinerth G, Krieg P, et al. Prostaglandin-H-synthase isozyme expression in normal and neoplastic human skin. *Int J Cancer* 1999;82:648–656.
113. Higashi Y, Kanekura T, Kanzaki T. Enhanced expression of cyclooxygenase (COX)-2 in human skin epidermal cancer cells: evidence for growth suppression by inhibiting COX-2 expression. *Int J Cancer* 2000;86:667–671.
114. Fischer SM, Lo HH, Gordon GB, et al. Chemopreventive activity of celecoxib, a specific cyclooxygenase- 2 inhibitor, and indomethacin against ultraviolet light-induced skin carcinogenesis. *Mol Carcinog* 1999;25:231–240.
115. Berenblum L, Shubik P. The role of croton oil application associated with a single painting of a carcinogen in tumour induction of the mouse's skin. *Br J Cancer* 1947;1: 379–391.
116. Wu X, Pandolfi PP. Mouse models for multistep tumorigenesis. *Trends Cell Biol* 2001;11:S2–S9.
117. de Gruijl FR, Forbes PD. UV-induced skin cancer in a hairless mouse model. *Bioessays* 1995;17:651–660.
118. Das M, Bickers DR, Santella RM, Mukhtar H. Altered patterns of cutaneous xenobiotic metabolism in UVB-induced squamous cell carcinoma in SKH-1 hairless mice. *J Invest Dermatol* 1985;84:532–536.
119. Jansen AP, Verwiebe EG, Dreckschmidt NE, et al. Protein kinase C-epsilon transgenic mice: a unique model for

metastatic squamous cell carcinoma. *Cancer Res* 2001;61: 808–812.
120. Aszterbaum M, Epstein J, Oro A, et al. Ultraviolet and ionizing radiation enhance the growth of BCCs and trichoblastomas in patched heterozygous knockout mice. *Nat Med* 1999;5: 1285–1291.
121. Hebert JL, Khugyani F, Athar M, et al. Chemoprevention of basal cell carcinomas in the ptc1+/– mouse—green and black tea. *Skin Pharmacol Appl Skin Physiol* 2001;14: 358–362.
122. Kusewitt DF, Ley RD. Animal models of melanoma. *Cancer Surv* 1996;26:35–70.
123. Tietze MK, Chin L. Murine models of malignant melanoma. *Mol Med Today* 2000;6:408–410.
124. Powell MB, Gause PR, Hyman P, et al. Induction of melanoma in TPras transgenic mice. *Carcinogenesis* 1999; 20:1747–1753.
125. Powell MB, Hyman P, Bell OD, et al. Hyperpigmentation and melanocytic hyperplasia in transgenic mice expressing the human T24 Ha-ras gene regulated by a mouse tyrosinase promoter. *Mol Carcinog* 1995;12:82–90.
126. Noonan FP, Recio JA, Takayama H, et al. Neonatal sunburn and melanoma in mice. *Nature* 2001;413:271–272.
127. Schatzkin A, Freedman L, Schiffman M. An epidemiologic perspective on biomarkers. *J Intern Med* 1993;233:75–79.
128. Schatzkin A, Freedman LS, Schiffman MH, Dawsey SM. Validation of intermediate end points in cancer research. *J Natl Cancer Inst* 1990;82:1746–1752.
129. Schurtenberger P, Egelhaaf SU, Hindges R, et al. The solution structure of functionally active human proliferating cell nuclear antigen determined by small-angle neutron scattering. *J Mol Biol* 1998;275:123–132.
130. Einspahr J, Alberts DS, Aickin M, et al. Expression of p53 protein in actinic keratosis, adjacent, normal- appearing, and non-sun-exposed human skin. *Cancer Epidemiol Biomarkers Prev* 1997;6:583–587.
131. Nelson MA, Einspahr JG, Alberts DS, et al. Analysis of the p53 gene in human precancerous actinic keratosis lesions and squamous cell cancers. *Cancer Lett* 1994;85:23–29.
132. Taguchi M, Tsuchida T, Ikeda S, Sekiya T. Alterations of p53 gene and Ha-ras gene are independent events in solar keratosis and squamous cell carcinoma. *Pathol Int* 1998;48: 689–694.
133. Moles JP, Moyret C, Guillot B, et al. p53 gene mutations in human epithelial skin cancers. *Oncogene* 1993;8:583–588.
134. Pierceall WE, Mukhopadhyay T, Goldberg LH, Ananthaswamy HN. Mutations in the p53 tumor suppressor gene in human cutaneous squamous cell carcinomas. *Mol Carcinog* 1991;4:445–449.
135. Einspahr JG, Alberts DS, Warneke JA, et al. Relationship of p53 mutations to epidermal cell proliferation and apoptosis in human UV-induced skin carcinogenesis. *Neoplasia* 1999;1:468–475.
136. Kazantseva IA, Khlebnikova AN, Babaev VR. Immunohistochemical study of primary and recurrent basal cell and metatypical carcinomas of the skin. *Am J Dermatopathol* 1996;18:35–42.
137. Kerr JF, Wyllie AH, Currie AR. Apoptosis: a basic biological phenomenon with wide-ranging implications in tissue kinetics. *Br J Cancer* 1972;26:239–257.
138. Einspahr J, Alberts D, Xie T, et al. Comparison of proliferating cell nuclear antigen versus the more standard measures of rectal mucosal proliferation rates in subjects with a history of

colorectal cancer and normal age-matched controls. *Cancer Epidemiol Biomarkers Prev* 1995;4:359–366.

139. Einspahr JG, Alberts DS, Gapstur SM, et al. Surrogate endpoint biomarkers as measures of colon cancer risk and their use in cancer chemoprevention trials. *Cancer Epidemiol Biomarkers Prev* 1997;6:37–48.

140. Bozzo P, Alberts DS, Vaught L, et al. Measurement of chemopreventive efficacy in skin biopsies. *Anal Quant Cytol Histol* 2001;23:300–312.

141. Bozzo PD, Vaught LC, Alberts DS, et al. Nuclear morphometry in solar keratosis. *Anal Quant Cytol Histol* 1998;20: 21–28.

142. Scherschun L, Lim HW. Photoprotection by sunscreens. *Am J Clin Dermatol* 2001;2:131–134.

143. Baade PD, Balanda KP, Lowe JB. Changes in skin protection behaviors, attitudes, and sunburn: in a population with the highest incidence of skin cancer in the world. *Cancer Detect Prev* 1996;20:566–575.

144. Naylor MF, Boyd A, Smith DW, et al. High sun protection factor sunscreens in the suppression of actinic neoplasia. *Arch Dermatol* 1995;131:170–175.

145. Green A, Williams G, Neale R, et al. Daily sunscreen application and betacarotene supplementation in prevention of basal-cell and squamous-cell carcinomas of the skin: a randomised controlled trial. *Lancet* 1999;354:723–729.

146. Harvey I, Frankel S, Marks R, et al. Non-melanoma skin cancer and solar keratoses II analytical results of the South Wales Skin Cancer Study. *Br J Cancer* 1996;74:1308–1312.

147. Wolf P, Donawho CK, Kripke ML. Effect of sunscreens on UV radiation-induced enhancement of melanoma growth in mice. *J Natl Cancer Inst* 1994;86:99–105.

148. Garland CF, Garland FC, Gorham ED. Rising trends in melanoma. An hypothesis concerning sunscreen effectiveness. *Ann Epidemiol* 1993;3:103–110.

149. Garland CF, Garland FC, Gorham ED. Re: Effect of sunscreens on UV radiation-induced enhancement of melanoma growth in mice [letter; comment]. *J Natl Cancer Inst* 1994; 86:798–800.

150. Graham S, Marshall J, Haughey B, et al. An inquiry into the epidemiology of melanoma. *Am J Epidemiol* 1985;122: 606–619.

151. Schwarze HP, Loche F, Gorguet MC, et al. Invasive cutaneous squamous cell carcinoma associated with actinic keratosis: a case with orbital invasion and meningeal infiltration. *Dermatol Surg* 1999;25:587–589.

152. Lober BA, Lober CW. Actinic keratosis is squamous cell carcinoma. *South Med J* 2000;93:650–655.

153. Cohn BA. From sunlight to actinic keratosis to squamous cell carcinoma. *J Am Acad Dermatol* 2000;42:143–144.

154. O'Shaughnessy JA, Kelloff GJ, Gordon GB, et al. Treatment and prevention of intraepithelial neoplasia: an important target for accelerated new agent development. *Clin Cancer Res* 2002;8:314–346.

155. Jeffes EW III, Tang EH. Actinic keratosis. Current treatment options. *Am J Clin Dermatol* 2000;1:167–179.

156. Warnock GR, Fuller RP Jr, Pelleu GB Jr. Evaluation of 5-fluorouracil in the treatment of actinic keratosis of the lip. *Oral Surg Oral Med Oral Pathol* 1981;52:501–505.

157. Hodge SJ, Schrodt GR, Owen LG. Effect of topical 5-fluorouracil treatment on actinic keratosis: a light and electron microscopic study. *J Cutan Pathol* 1974;1:238–248.

158. Epstein E. Does intermittent "pulse" topical 5-fluorouracil therapy allow destruction of actinic keratoses without sig-

nificant inflammation? *J Am Acad Dermatol* 1998;38: 77–80.

159. Callen JP, Bickers DR, Moy RL. Actinic keratoses. *J Am Acad Dermatol* 1997;36:650–653.

160. Ku EC, Lee W, Kothari HV, et al. The effects of diclofenac sodium on arachidonic acid metabolism. *Semin Arthritis Rheum* 1985;15:36–41.

161. Ku EC, Lee W, Kothari HV, Scholer DW. Effect of diclofenac sodium on the arachidonic acid cascade. *Am J Med* 1986;80:18–23.

162. Rivers JK, McLean DI. An open study to assess the efficacy and safety of topical 3% diclofenac in a 2.5% hyaluronic acid gel for the treatment of actinic keratoses. *Arch Dermatol* 1997;133:1239–1242.

163. Wolf JE Jr, Taylor JR, Tschen E, Kang S. Topical 3.0% diclofenac in 2.5% hyaluronan gel in the treatment of actinic keratoses. *Int J Dermatol* 2001;40:709–713.

164. Lippman SM, Lotan R. Advances in the development of retinoids as chemopreventive agents. *J Nutr* 2000;130: 479S–482S.

165. Evans TR, Kaye SB. Retinoids: present role and future potential. *Br J Cancer* 1999;80:1–8.

166. Lotan R. Retinoids in cancer chemoprevention. *FASEB J* 1996;10:1031–1039.

167. Goodman DS. Vitamin A and retinoids in health and disease. *N Engl J Med* 1984;310:1023–1031.

168. Niles RM. Recent advances in the use of vitamin A (retinoids) in the prevention and treatment of cancer. *Nutrition* 2000;16:1084–1089.

169. DiSepio D, Sutter M, Johnson AT, et al. Identification of the AP1-antagonism domain of retinoic acid receptors. *Mol Cell Biol Res Commun* 1999;1:7–13.

170. Levine N. Role of retinoids in skin cancer treatment and prevention. *J Am Acad Dermatol* 1998;39:62–66.

171. Sporn MB, Dunlop NM, Newton DL, Smith JM. Prevention of chemical carcinogenesis by vitamin A and its synthetic analogs (retinoids). *Fed Proc* 1976;35:1332–1338.

172. Moon TE, Levine N, Cartmel B, Bangert JL. Retinoids in prevention of skin cancer. *Cancer Lett* 1997;114:203–205.

173. Kraemer KH, DiGiovanna JJ, Moshell AN, et al. Prevention of skin cancer in xeroderma pigmentosum with the use of oral isotretinoin. *N Engl J Med* 1988;318:1633–1637.

174. Fosslien E. Molecular pathology of cyclooxygenase-2 in neoplasia. *Ann Clin Lab Sci* 2000;30:3–21.

175. Kagoura M, Toyoda M, Matsui C, Morohashi M. Immunohistochemical expression of cyclooxygenase-2 in skin cancers. *J Cutan Pathol* 2001;28:298–302.

176. Sheftel VO. Health-related properties of polyamines. *Gig Sanit* 1991;4:29–31.

177. Farriol M, Segovia T, Venereo Y, Orta X. Importance of the polyamines: review of the literature. *Nutr Hosp* 1999;14: 101–113.

178. Peralta Soler A, Gilliard G, Megosh L, et al. Polyamines regulate expression of the neoplastic phenotype in mouse skin. *Cancer Res* 1998;58:1654–1659.

179. Gensler HL. Prevention by alpha-difluoromethylornithine of skin carcinogenesis and immunosuppression induced by ultraviolet irradiation. *J Cancer Res Clin Oncol* 1991;117: 345–350.

180. Fischer SM, Lee M, Lubet RA. Difluoromethylornithine is effective as both a preventive and therapeutic agent against the development of UV carcinogenesis in SKH hairless mice. *Carcinogenesis* 2001;22:83–88.

181. Igarashi K. Role of polyamines in cell proliferation and differentiation. *Seikagaku* 1993;65:86–104.

182. Quemener V, Moulinoux JP, Girre L. The effect of modification of the intracellular distribution of polyamines on the proliferation of hepatocytes treated with 2-methyl-9-hydroxyellipticine. *J Nat Prod* 1985;48:376–389.

183. Wallon UM, Shassetz LR, Cress AE, et al. Polyamine-dependent expression of the matrix metalloproteinase matrilysin in a human colon cancer-derived cell line. *Mol Carcinog* 1994;11:138–144.

184. Takahashi Y, Mai M, Nishioka K. alpha-difluoromethylornithine induces apoptosis as well as anti-angiogenesis in the inhibition of tumor growth and metastasis in a human gastric cancer model. *Int J Cancer* 2000;85:243–247.

185. Snyder RD, Bhatt S. Alterations in repair of alkylating agent-induced DNA damage in polyamine-depleted human cells. *Cancer Lett* 1993;72:83–90.

186. Snyder RD, Schroeder KK. Radiosensitivity of polyamine-depleted HeLa cells and modulation by the aminothiol WR-1065. *Radiat Res* 1994;137:67–75.

187. Alberts DS, Dorr RT, Einspahr JG, et al. Chemoprevention of human actinic keratoses by topical 2-(difluoromethyl)-dl-ornithine. *Cancer Epidemiol Biomarkers Prev* 2000; 9:1 281–1286.

188. Ishino A, Kusama K, Watanabe S, Sakagami H. Inhibition of epigallocatechin gallate-induced apoptosis by CoCl2 in human oral tumor cell lines. *Anticancer Res* 1999;19: 5197–5201.

189. Valcic S, Timmermann BN, Alberts DS, et al. Inhibitory effect of six green tea catechins and caffeine on the growth of four selected human tumor cell lines. *Anticancer Drugs* 1996;7:461–468.

190. Yamane T, Takahashi T, Kuwata K, et al. Inhibition of *N*-methyl-*N*'-nitro-*N*-nitrosoguanidine-induced carcinogenesis by (−)-epigallocatechin gallate in the rat glandular stomach. *Cancer Res* 1995;55:2081–2084.

191. Salah N, Miller NJ, Paganga G, et al. Polyphenolic flavanols as scavengers of aqueous phase radicals and as chain-breaking antioxidants. *Arch Biochem Biophys* 1995; 322:339–346.

192. Islam S, Islam N, Kermode T, et al. Involvement of caspase-3 in epigallocatechin-3-gallate-mediated apoptosis of human chondrosarcoma cells. *Biochem Biophys Res Commun* 2000; 270:793–797.

193. Hibasami H, Achiwa Y, Fujikawa T, Komiya T. Induction of programmed cell death (apoptosis) in human lymphoid leukemia cells by catechin compounds. *Anticancer Res* 1996; 16:1943–1946.

194. Suzuki K, Yahara S, Hashimoto F, Uyeda M. Inhibitory activities of (-)-epigallocatechin-3-O-gallate against topoisomerases I and II. *Biol Pharm Bull* 2001;24:1088–1090.

195. Jung YD, Kim MS, Shin BA, et al. EGCG, a major component of green tea, inhibits tumour growth by inhibiting VEGF induction in human colon carcinoma cells. *Br J Cancer* 2001;84: 844–850.

196. Gensler HL, Timmermann BN, Valcic S, et al. Prevention of photocarcinogenesis by topical administration of pure epigallocatechin gallate isolated from green tea. *Nutr Cancer* 1996;26:325–335.

197. Katiyar SK, Elmets CA. Green tea polyphenolic antioxidants and skin photoprotection (Review). *Int J Oncol* 2001;18: 1307–1313.

198. Nomura M, Ma WY, Huang C, et al. Inhibition of ultraviolet B-induced AP-1 activation by theaflavins from black tea. *Mol Carcinog* 2000;28:148–155.

199. Stockfleth E, Meyer T, Benninghoff B, Christophers E. Successful treatment of actinic keratosis with imiquimod cream 5%: a report of six cases. *Br J Dermatol* 2001;144: 1050–1053.

200. Marks R, Gebauer K, Shumack S, et al. Imiquimod 5% cream in the treatment of superficial basal cell carcinoma: Results of a multicenter 6-week dose-response trial. *J Am Acad Dermatol* 2001;44:807–813.

201. Huang MT, Ma W, Lu YP, et al. Effects of curcumin, demethoxycurcumin, bisdemethoxycurcumin and tetrahydrocurcumin on 12-O-tetradecanoylphorbol-13-acetate-induced tumor promotion. *Carcinogenesis* 1995;16:2493–2497.

202. Limtrakul P, Lipigorngoson S, Namwong O, et al. Inhibitory effect of dietary curcumin on skin carcinogenesis in mice. *Cancer Lett* 1997;116:197–203.

203. Pendurthi UR, Rao LV. Suppression of transcription factor Egr-1 by curcumin. *Thromb Res* 2000;97:179–189.

204. Ishizaki C, Oguro T, Yoshida T, et al. Enhancing effect of ultraviolet A on ornithine decarboxylase induction and dermatitis evoked by 12-o-tetradecanoylphorbol-13-acetate and its inhibition by curcumin in mouse skin. *Dermatology* 1996;193:311–317.

205. Chuang SE, Cheng AL, Lin JK, Kuo ML. Inhibition by curcumin of diethylnitrosamine-induced hepatic hyperplasia, inflammation, cellular gene products and cell-cycle- related proteins in rats. *Food Chem Toxicol* 2000;38:991–995.

206. Xu YX, Pindolia KR, Janakiraman N, et al. Curcumin inhibits IL1 alpha and TNF-alpha induction of AP-1 and NF-kB DNA-binding activity in bone marrow stromal cells. *Hematopathol Mol Hematol* 1997;11:49–62.

207. Oshikawa K, Rakhmilevich AL, Shi F, et al. Interleukin 12 gene transfer into skin distant from the tumor site elicits antimetastatic effects equivalent to local gene transfer. *Hum Gene Ther* 2001;12:149–160.

208. Schwarz A, Stander S, Berneburg M, et al. Interleukin-12 suppresses ultraviolet radiation-induced apoptosis by inducing DNA repair. *Nat Cell Biol* 2002;4:26–31.

31 Opportunities and Challenges for Skin Cancer Chemoprevention

Jaye L. Viner, MD, MPH, Ernest T. Hawk, MD, MPH, Ellen Richmond, MS, RN, Howard Higley, PhD, DABT, and Asad Umar, PhD, DVM

CONTENTS

1. INTRODUCTION

The cumulative personal, functional, and cosmetic burdens of skin cancer are compounded by massive health care expenditures *(1,2)*. Nonmelanoma skin cancer (NMSC) treatment in the Medicare population alone amounts to $426 million annually *(3)*, and malignant melanoma, or melanoma skin cancer (MSC) has been estimated to cost approx $1 billion annually *(4)*. Although these estimates are based on different populations and disease categories, they provide a measure of the vast direct and indirect costs of skin cancer screening, biopsy, and treatment. Despite this heavy toll, skin cancer remains a relatively underexplored area of chemoprevention research, perhaps illustrating the medical paradox that "rare conditions are intensively studied, while common conditions are often overlooked"*(2)*.

Skin cancer chemoprevention might complement traditional management by reducing the number of preneoplastic lesions and the morbidity associated with their identification and treatment, as well as their malignant potential. This chapter discusses challenges and opportunities for developing preventive interventions against skin cancer.

2. SKIN CANCER

Skin cancers account for more than 40% of all cancers diagnosed in the United States, and rates have increased dramatically over the last two decades. An estimated 1.3 million new cases of NMSC are reported annually, making it the most commonly diagnosed cancer in Caucasian populations *(5,6)*. These reports underestimate the true incidence, because many population-based cancer registries do not capture NMSC, and eradication techniques often preclude pathologic diagnosis. Despite these uncertainties, an estimated 40–50% of the US population will develop at least one NMSC by age 65 *(7,8)*, and 5-yr recurrence rates may be as high as 50%, depending on specifics of the index lesion *(9)*. Data on MSC are more comprehensive than those obtained for NMSC. The US National Cancer Institute (NCI) Surveillance, Epidemiology, and End Results (SEER) database from 1973 to 1995 shows 4%

annual increases in incidence (from 5.7 to 13.3 per 100,000) and 1.3% annual increases in mortality (from 1.6 to 2.2 per 100,000) (8). Because increases have been observed in both advanced and localized disease (10,11), enhanced detection alone is unlikely to account for this trend. MSC typically afflicts adults in their mid-40s to early 50s, and has become one of the foremost causes of cancer death among young adults. As a result, associated losses—in terms of potential life years and income—aggravate the serious impact of this disease (4).

2.1. Characteristics of Skin Cancers

Skin cancer is classified as NMSC or MSC depending on the cell of origin. NMSC consists chiefly of basal cell (BCC, ~80%) and squamous cell carcinomas (SCC, ~16%). BCC, the most common malignancy worldwide, has a sluggish growth pattern and rarely metastasizes from the basal layer keratinocytes in which it originates (12). In contrast, SCC derives from more superficial keratinocytes, and has greater risk for metastatic spread and higher mortality rates than BCC.

MSC derives from melanocytes located in the basal layer of the epidermis. Although a small fraction of skin cancers are MSC (~4%), this subset has the highest potential for metastasis, and consequently poses the greatest health threat. Indeed, the incidence rate for higher stage melanoma is comparable to the case fatality rate despite aggressive treatment. The relative public health impacts of NMSC and MSC are evident from the American Cancer Society 2002 incidence and mortality estimates of 1.3 million new cases and 2200 deaths from NMSC (6) vs 53,600 new cases and 7400 deaths from MSC (5). Solar ultraviolet (UV) radiation is the major modifiable risk factor in NMSC and MSC development, and exposures of greatest consequence are thought to occur in childhood and adolescence.

3. SKIN CARCINOGENESIS AND CANCER PREVENTION

Skin carcinogenesis involves a complex interplay between environmental insults and susceptible genes, and has been divided into three phases: initiation, promotion, and progression. It is generally accepted that independent insults enable cells to advance through these stages, and that the earliest steps of cancer initiation involve mutation of a single gene. Once initiated, cells are then susceptible to additional mutations. Several endogenous (e.g., DNA repair, oxygen radicals) and exogenous (e.g., UV light) factors have been shown to exacerbate genetic instability

through induction of reactive oxygen species, such as superoxide anion radicals, singlet oxygen, hydrogen peroxides, and organic free radicals. In the healthy state, endogenous mechanisms guard against genotoxic injury; however, damage leading to significant molecular alteration may overwhelm cellular defenses. A hypothesized role for oxidative stress in skin carcinogenesis has been studied in mouse models using antioxidants such as vitamins A, C, and E and green tea polyphenols, as reviewed elsewhere (13,14).

Specific changes are propagated at different rates and times within and across biologic strata (e.g., genetic, cellular, tissue), typically in sun-exposed skin (15,16). Precursor lesions, intermediates in the malignant transformation of epithelium (17–19), arise from the mutation of key genes that regulate cellular proliferation and apoptosis. Compared to multiple aberrations of late carcinogenesis, these relatively homogeneous changes of early disease present promising opportunities for detecting preneoplasia and developing molecularly targeted interventions. Invasive NMSC arises from precursor lesions, which include dysplastic nevi and actinic keratoses (AK). These hallmarks of carcinogenesis may be simultaneously used as molecular markers of cancer risk, targets for intervention, and measures of preventive response (16).

3.1. Risk Factors

Solar UV radiation accounts for most cases of NMSC, distantly followed by human papilloma virus (HPV) infection (20,21); chronic inflammatory skin conditions such as radiodermatitis (22); chemical carcinogens (23); impaired immune function (24) including congenital immune deficiencies, AIDS (25), and chronic immune suppression (26,27); and genetic susceptibilities such as fair skin phenotype (28), xeroderma pigmentosum (XP) (29), and basal cell nevus syndrome (30).

Predisposition to UV-induced neoplasia is a multifactorial trait that involves fair skin coloration and DNA repair capacity, as well as mole type and number (17). Host risk factors specific for SCC include faircolored skin, hair, and eyes, and inability to tan (28). MSC-specific risk factors are a matter of some debate, but include genetic traits associated with fair skin phenotype and UV exposure, which may account for at least two-thirds of cases (31–33). Twin studies have shown an almost complete lack of concordance for skin cancer development, confirming that environmental exposures are the key determinants of invasive disease (34).

3.2. Photocarcinogenesis

Photocarcinogenesis is a relatively recent concept. Indeed, observations in the mid-1800s associating skin cancer with outdoor exposure were not epidemiologically confirmed until the following century *(35)*. UV radiation has since been shown to initiate and promote cancer in sun-exposed skin through point mutations, oncogene activation, tumor suppressor gene inactivation, cellular proliferation, immunosuppression, and inflammation. Latency to malignant transformation allows time to use this array of markers as measures of risk, disease progression, and response to chemopreventive interventions *(36,37)*.

The UV spectrum spans wavelengths from 200 to 400 nm, which fall just short of visible light (400–700 nm). UV radiation is divided into UVA (320–400), UVB (280–320), and UVC (200–280). Only UVA and UVB penetrate to the earth's surface in biologically relevant amounts, with UVA accounting for 95% of solar UV radiation at the equator, whereas UVB accounts for 5%. Stratospheric ozone absorbs variable amounts of UV radiation—more UVB than UVA—depending on latitude, season, time of day, cloud cover, and air pollution levels. Despite relatively lower quantities and less penetration into the skin, UVB is more reactive and accounts for most sun-induced skin cancers and sunburns. Other adverse effects of UVA and UVB include age-associated skin changes such as wrinkling, telangiectasia, dyspigmentation, and coarse texture *(31)*.

Normal epidermis contains several molecules with absorption spectra within the UV range, including nucleic acids, aromatic amino acids (proteins), and melanin precursors. Photochemical reactions occurring in these absorbing biomolecules alter skin architecture, largely through erythema effects *(17)*. UVB is absorbed mostly in the epidermis, where it induces DNA adducts, strand breaks, and crosslinks. UV absorption by nucleotides leads to photoproduct formation of two main types: cyclobutane dimers between adjacent thymine or cytosine residues, and less commonly, pyrimidine (6–4) photoproducts *(38)*. Both lesions frequently occur in runs of tandem pyrimidines and are considered "hot spots" of UV-induced mutations. Cyclobutane dimers likely contribute to the majority of UV-induced mutations in mammalian cells as the (6–4) photoproducts are repaired much more quickly. Longer-wavelength UVA penetrates into the dermis where it can be absorbed by fibroblasts, induce reactive oxygen species, and further compromise mitochondrial

(mt) function through induction of mtDNA mutations and altered apoptosis *(39)*. UVA may also indirectly propagate oxidative damage through photosensitization reactions, which damage fibroblasts as well as vascular endothelium *(40)*.

NMSC incidence is proportionally related to proximity to the equator, with a doubling of SCC incidence for each 8–10-degree decrease in latitude. Based on UV gradients associated with skin cancer development, and allowing for latency to disease, ozone depletion by as little as 1% would be expected to increase skin cancer risk *(35,41,42)*. This is consistent with increased rates of skin cancer in recent decades that coincide with a 2% loss of stratospheric ozone, the earth's shield against harmful UV radiation *(31,43)*, and 4% increases in bioactive solar radiation *(10)*. Whether these increased rates arise from higher cumulative and/or intermittent UV exposure (e.g., through recreational activities and revealing attire), longer lifespans, depletion of the ozone layer, or the interplay of these factors remains a subject of debate *(44–46)*. Sporadic MSC is generally thought to arise from severe sunburns associated with intermittent rather than chronic solar exposure. DNA repair capacity may serve as a marker of risk for UV-induced skin cancer; and genetic susceptibility to skin cancer may be assessed through polymorphisms of DNA repair genes, particularly single-nucleotide polymorphisms.

3.3. UV Radiation and Immunosurveillance

Harmful effects of UV radiation include downregulation of immune responses to tumor antigens, partially due to reduced local production of interleukin-10 (IL-10) and tumor necrosis factor (TNF) α *(47)*. This accounts for high rates of skin cancers in solid organ recipients, who undergo immunosuppression in order to prevent transplant rejection. Skin carcinogenesis decelerates when immunosuppressive therapy is stopped, confirming the critical role of proper immune function *(48)*.

Experimental data further support the notion that immunosurveillance protects against development of malignant skin neoplasms. For example, studies have shown that UVB irradiation may alter cell-mediated immune response, thereby producing an environment conducive to skin carcinogenesis *(49)*. UV-induced immunosuppression has been clinically studied in healthy volunteers, in whom erythemal UV doses were shown to impair contact hypersensitivity reactions. Applying a high sun-protection factor (SPF) sunscreen prevented this effect, possibly by preserving epidermal Langerhans cell (LC) function at irradiated sites *(50,51)*.

3.4. Photoprotection

Few studies have investigated the effect of sunscreen in high-risk populations with skin cancer. One small study of 37 participants *(52)* and another larger study of 588 participants *(53)* showed that regular application of high SPF broad-spectrum sunscreen significantly reduced the total number of AK (generally regarded as *in situ* SCC), the most common precursor to NMSC, over intermediate and long terms (2 yr and 6 mo, respectively). Interestingly, the shorter-term study showed reductions in both AK incidence and prevalence, and dose-response effects were observed for both of these endpoints. Importantly, positive effects of higher dose sunscreen were observed with regard to AK regression and incidence *(53)*.

Exposure to the sun's UV rays appears to be the most important modifiable risk factor for skin cancer. Even so, 70% of American adults do not protect themselves and inconsistently protect their children from solar radiation *(54)*. Incidence rates for skin cancer are increasing and will likely to continue to do so, underscoring the importance of screening coupled with behavioral/preventive interventions against skin carcinogenesis in vulnerable populations.

3.5. Limits of Photoprotection

Many genes are involved in the nucleotide excision repair pathway and any compromise in their activity may increase skin cancer risk. The critical role of DNA repair capacity with regard to hereditary cancer syndromes, XP, and sporadic cancers such as BCC involves nucleotide excision, which removes the sequellae of DNA damage, such as UV-induced photoproducts, bulky adducts, cross-links, and oxidative damage *(38,55)*. Nucleotide excision repair defects account for the 1000-fold increased risk of sunlight-induced skin cancers in patients with XP. Photoprotection alone is unlikely to suffice for high-risk cohorts in whom disease is aggressive and multifocal. In such cases, the potential benefits of systemic interventions are likely to outweigh toxicities. This may be the case with systemic retinoids (13-*cis*-retinoic acid or acitretin) that reduce the number of skin cancers in very high-risk patients such as those with XP, or in solid organ transplant recipients *(56–58)*.

3.6. Enhancement of DNA Repair

A novel therapeutic intervention in UV-induced skin carcinogenesis provides nucleotide excision DNA repair enzymes directly to damaged or deficient skin. Bacteriophage T4 endonuclease V (T4N5) is a DNA repair enzyme with specificity for repairing cyclobutane pyrimidine dimers (CPD), the primary UVB photoproduct *(59,60)*. More than 25 yr ago, exogenous application of this enzyme to XP fibroblasts in culture was shown to enhance unscheduled DNA synthesis *(61)*. T4N5 is now available encapsulated in a pH-sensitive liposome *(62–70)*, and is known to deliver active enzyme into the nuclei of epidermal keratinocytes when topically applied *(62,65)*. Topical application of T4N5 not only increased CPD repair but also delayed increases in epidermal p53 protein accumulation *(68)*.

The chemopreventive potential of a lotion containing T4N5 liposomes in skin carcinogenesis has been demonstrated in both UV-irradiated mice and XP patients. In a series of experiments, T4N5 liposome lotion was highly effective in reducing skin tumor development in SKH-1 mice when applied three times weekly for 30 wk immediately after regular UV exposure *(66,67)*. It also prevented UV-induced systemic suppression of contact hypersensitivity and delayed-type hypersensitivity *(63)*, reduced sunburn cell formation locally, and maintained LC density, morphology, and antigen-presenting cell function *(64)*. Furthermore, in the mouse model, it prevented upregulation of immunosuppressive cytokines IL-10 and TNF-α *(62)*. A clinical trial of T4N5 liposome lotion in XP patients found decreased incidence of both AKs and BCC *(70)*. In humans, no allergic response has been reported after repeated application. IgG antibodies to T4N5 were not detectable in serum, and no serious adverse events occurred after 12 mo of daily use *(70)*. A phase study of T4N5 liposome lotion in immunosuppressed organ transplant recipients with a history of skin cancer is underway.

4. MARKERS OF SKIN CARCINOGENESIS AND CANCER PROGRESSION

Interest in using molecular and cellular markers as probes for early disease dates back to discovery of carcinoembryonic antigen (CEA) *(71)*, SV40 *(72)*, and major histocompatibility human leukocyte antigen (HLA) *(73)* in the 1970s. Early detection science has subsequently made considerable progress, moving from "one tumor, one gene" analysis to complete molecular profiles *(73–75)*. Technologic advances in molecular diagnosis and new statistical/analytic algorithms are hastening the emergence of tools that may detect key determinants of neoplasia. It is expected that profiling techniques that embed various biomarkers in dermatopathologic assessments will optimize the informative yield of each biopsy.

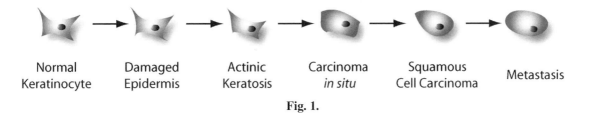

Normal Keratinocyte → Damaged Epidermis → Actinic Keratosis → Carcinoma *in situ* → Squamous Cell Carcinoma → Metastasis

Fig. 1.

Genetic and epigenetic aberrations contribute to the emergence of clones lacking normal cell cycle controls. These aberrations spawn cellular and molecular abnormalities that may culminate in invasive cancer. Genetic and molecular changes that may serve as biomarkers of risk and molecular targets of preventive intervention are discussed below, along with challenges to their development for clinical applications.

4.1. Actinic Keratoses

AKs, also termed solar keratoses, are rough, scaly, hyperpigmented plaques characterized by atypical keratinocyte maturation. AKs typically occur on sun-exposed skin on the face, neck, trunk, and upper extremities *(76)*. AKs that penetrate the papillary or reticular dermis are redefined as SCC *(77,78)*. Shared histologic/genetic features and risk factors point to AK as the earliest clinically identifiable SCC precursor, strengthening the case for reclassification of AK as intraepithelial neoplasia (IEN) *(79)*. Invasive NMSC arises from precursor lesions such as dysplasia and AK (Fig. 1).

Population-based estimates are incomplete for NMSC, and even spottier for AK. Like skin cancer, AK primarily occurs in older, lightly pigmented Caucasians. In susceptible populations, AK prevalence may be as high as 35% among men and 10% among women *(80–82)*. AK prevalence, incidence, and natural history data have been obtained in Australian populations, which have the world's highest skin cancer rates. In one study of 1040 subjects over age 40, 59% had AKs at baseline, and 60% developed new lesions over the 12-mo observation period *(83)*. By contrast, only 19% of study participants without AKs at baseline developed lesions during the same timeframe. Of note, incident AKs developed at sites of preexisting lesions, and as well as in ostensibly normal skin; 26% of all untreated lesions spontaneously regressed within 12 mo. Emerging molecular characterizations may provide important clues for discriminating the small subset (<20%) of AKs that will progress to SCC and require intervention from those that will not *(84–86)*.

Risk factors commonly shared by AK and SCC include older age, fair skin phenotype with a tendency to sunburn, impaired immune (e.g., solid organ transplant recipients on chronic immunosuppressive therapy) or DNA repair function (e.g., XP), oncogenic viral infections (e.g., HPV) in certain solid organ transplant recipients, and high cumulative sun exposure. In particular, prolonged UVB exposure is thought to initiate and promote the process through which AK invades underlying dermis and progresses to SCC *(87)*. Published estimates of the proportion of AKs that progress to SCC generally range from <0.1–10%, but may be as high as 25% in hyper-susceptible populations *(86,88,89)*. Individuals with heavy AK burdens (i.e., exceeding 10 lesions) have a 14% cumulative 5-yr probability of neoplastic transformation *(90)*. AK rarely develops into BCC, and appears to be unrelated to MSC. Regression of prevalent AK or reductions in incident AK have become primary or secondary endpoints in most NMSC chemoprevention trials, as reviewed elsewhere *(14,36,91–101)*.

Exogenous insults such as UV radiation and immunosuppression confer resistance to apoptosis; without these sustained selection pressures, mutant clones regress spontaneously. Even so, AK that regress with cessation of modifiable risk factors tend to recur upon re-exposure *(53)*. AK on the eye (actinic conjunctivitis) and lip (actinic cheilitis) are promptly eradicated owing to greater propensity for malignant transformation and metastatic spread. By contrast, current management of AK arising elsewhere is controversial, owing to high spontaneous regression rates *(83)*. It is impossible to distinguish AK from SCC without histological confirmation. Because AKs have malignant potential and because patients object to their cosmetic appearance, they are typically eradicated using any of several approved technologies such as excision, cryosurgery, curettage with or without electrodessication, laser surgery, or chemoexfoliation, as well as by topical compounds including 5-fluorouracil (Efudex), sodium diclofenac (Solaraze), imiquimod (Aldara), and aminolevulinic acid (ALA) hydrochloric acid (HCl) (Levulan Kerastick) in conjunction with photodynamic therapy.

4.2. Photoadducts

UV induces DNA damage by covalently cross-linking adjacent pyrimidines, thereby producing dimers (e.g., C to T or CC to TT base substitutions at dipyrimine sites) in susceptible epidermal keratinocytes *(102,103)*. In contrast to invasive cancers, amino acid substitutions in AK are spread evenly across the gene. These mutations are considered hallmarks of UV-induced DNA damage to tumor suppressor genes, and are evident in more than 90% of mutations in SCC *in situ*, which is considered an intermediate between AK and invasive SCC.

4.3. Mutations of p53

One major and early target for chemoprevention is the p53 tumor-suppressor gene located on chromosome 17p13, which encodes for a transcription factor that induces expression of regulatory components necessary for apoptosis. Insults such as severe sunburn are thought to induce p53-dependent apoptosis, which results in sloughing and eventual elimination of damaged cells. When keratinocytes sustain p53 damage at an early developmental stage, they lose the capacity to induce apoptotic response, and upon additional hits by other carcinogenic insults have the potential to progress toward neoplasia. It has been shown that induction of p53 in epidermal keratinocytes leads to G_1 cell cycle arrest and allows for DNA repair. Based on this observation, cells may tolerate UV radiation up to some threshold, beyond which DNA is so damaged that mutations start to accumulate more rapidly. From this point on it becomes increasingly likely that a key regulatory gene, such as p53, will become critically damaged. Patients with multiple AK typically have p53 mutations at different loci that vary from lesion to lesion, suggesting that each AK records a distinct UV photon-absorption event. Mutations in the p53 gene have also been found by immunohistochemistry in epidermal cells adjacent to AKs. Expansion of these p53-mutated cells is evident in cone-shaped clones, the apices of which concentrate at the dermal epidermal junction *(104)*. p53 mutations have been found in more than 90% of human SCC, of which 74% were localized to sun-exposed skin, compared to 5% in unexposed skin *(105)*. This finding further implicates solar exposure as a causative agent in NMSC pathogenesis.

4.4. Mutations of p16^INK4a

AK and SCC development may also involve dysregulation of the p16^INK4a tumor suppressor, which is encoded by the *CDKN2A* gene. This tumor suppressor inhibits pRB phosphorylation, thereby stalling progression beyond the G_1 phase of the cell cycle. Although inactivation of p16^INK4a is a frequent finding in SCC, genetic alterations in the p16^INK4a region are relatively rare in AK lesions. AK cells tend to express p16^INK4a, whereas most SCCs do not. This finding suggests that yet-to-be identified molecular events in AK with mutated p53 trigger progression to SCC through inactivation of the p16^INK4a tumor suppressor. Further supporting this hypothesis is the finding that highly dysplastic areas within AK lack p16^INK4a positive cells, perhaps indicating that these keratinocytes have already progressed to SCC. Also, p16^INK4a-positive and -negative cells are often found in the same AK. This may account for observed differences in p16^INK4a that may be statistically insignificant by loss of heterozygosity (LOH) analysis, but significant by immunohistochemistry (which distinguishes p16^INK4a-negative SCC areas from still-positive regions within the same AK lesion) *(106,107)*. Increased expression of matrix metalloproteinases has been reported as yet another early event that may contribute to AK development and progression *(108)*.

4.5. Proliferating Cell Nuclear Antigen

Epidermal cell proliferation, quantified by proliferating cell nuclear antigen (PCNA), is a commonly analyzed skin cancer marker *(85)*. There is a significant gradient of mean PCNA across basal and suprabasal layers, with progressively higher concentrations moving from nonexposed skin to AK with the highest proliferation index. Hence, skin PCNA levels may serve as an indirect dosimeter of UV-induced damage. In conjunction with histologic atypia, PCNA is being evaluated as a candidate biomarker for skin cancer in a variety of skin cancer chemoprevention studies.

4.6. Apoptosis Mediators (p53 and Fas)

Apoptosis triggered by activation of p53 or other proteins such as Fas, a defense mechanism against UV-induced carcinogenesis, is under investigation in experimental systems. Though the dynamics in patients with sun-induced lesions are largely unknown, a recent report showed Fas upregulation in chronically sun-exposed keratinocytes. However, continued solar exposure significantly downregulates this defense mechanism, in a manner proportional to the degree of dysplasia *(109)*. This suggests that Fas may play an important role in controlling sun-induced damage *(109)*.

Other novel biomarkers have been identified from the sera of patients with preneoplastic as well as advanced cancerous lesions. For example, circulating anti-p53 antibodies in patients with various cancers have strongly correlated with the cancers' p53 mutational status. However, prospective study of anti-p53 antibody prevalence in skin cancer patients detected anti-p53 antibodies in only 2.9% of patients, most of whom had the more aggressive disease type (i.e., 8% SCC vs 1.5% BCC) *(110)*. In addition, these low serum levels of anti-p53 antibody contrasted markedly with high rates of p53 mutations in the tumors. Based on these data, it has been hypothesized that tissue-specific effects or humoral factors unique to cutaneous malignancy may thwart the use of this serum-based detection method for skin cancer *(110)*.

4.7. β-Catenin/E-Cadherin

The Reverse E-catenin/E-cadherin complex plays a crucial role in controlling epithelial differentiation. Abnormal expression of the β-catenin/E-cadherin complex is seen in SCC and some AK, suggesting that these changes may be relevant to neoplastic progression *(111)*. In addition, abnormal expression of β-catenin correlated with high proliferation and high tumor grade in NMSC *(111)*. In aggregate, these preliminary data suggest a role for β-catenin as a marker of skin carcinogenesis.

4.8. Nucleotide Excision Repair

Many genes essential for genomic integrity are also crucial for cell viability. In the absence of inactivating mutations, certain DNA repair genes have been linked to increased cancer susceptibility in several organs. The critical role of DNA repair capacity with regard to hereditary cancer syndromes (e.g., XP) and sporadic cancer (BCC) was initially reported by Kraemer et al. *(42)* and Wei et al. *(112)*, respectively. The nucleotide excision repair pathway is critical for removing UV-induced photoproducts, bulky adducts, cross-links, and oxidative damage *(113)*. XP is the classic example of deranged nucleotide excision repair, characterized by a 1000-fold increased risk of sunlight-induced skin cancer. Interindividual variability in DNA repair capacity and diminished capacity to repair UV-induced photoproducts and benzo[*a*]pyrene diol epoxide-induced adducts in peripheral lymphocytes are also significant predictors of sun-induced skin cancer risk *(112)*.

DNA repair capacity may serve as a risk marker for UV-induced skin cancer. Genetic susceptibility to skin cancer may be assessed through polymorphisms of DNA repair genes, in particular single-nucleotide polymorphisms. Many genes are involved in the nucleotide excision repair pathway and if compromised, skin cancer risk may increase. For example, as described above, known polymorphisms of *XPC*, *XPD/ERCC2*, and *XRCC1* might compromise overall nucleotide excision repair capacity *(114)*. Mutations in *XPC* and *XPD* result in defective NER and XP phenotypes, the functional significance of which have yet to be determined. Understanding the effects these polymorphisms exert on protein function will be a first step toward understanding their association with complex diseases such as cancer. Variations in DNA repair capacity associated with skin neoplasia share many features of cancer susceptibility biomarkers, in that proteins encoded by variant alleles exhibit reductions in function, rather than complete nonfunction, and may give rise to skin cancers.

4.9. Inflammation

Inflammatory response has been proposed as a key determinant of progression from AK to SCC, perhaps via production of active oxygen species that induce genetic damage. In addition, cytokines and chemokine products of the inflammatory process may promote tumor cell growth and neovascularization. It has been suggested that inflammation may be a protective mechanism that induces AK regression, and that neoplastic transformation may result from a failure of this response *(115)*. Based on inflammatory response, AKs have been subclassified as asymptomatic AKs (AAKs) in dysplastic lesions lacking signs of inflammation *(116)*, and as inflammatory AKs (IAKs) in erythematous, tender lesions. It has been reported that approximately half of clinical IAK are SCC and the rest are AK, suggesting a continuum of carcinogenic stages between AK and SCC development.

5. ANIMAL MODELS OF SKIN CARCINOGENESIS

Skin tumorigenesis can be induced in these experimental systems using genotoxic agents such as 7,12-dimethylbenz[*a*]anthracene (DMBA) or UV light. Chronic irritants such as erythema, wounding, or phorbol esters promote neoplastic progression and development of lesions with p53 mutations or H-*ras* point mutations found in human NMSC. Animal models of multistage skin carcinogenesis are valuable tools for modeling and mimicking human disease, and provide insights into neoplastic mechanisms operative in skin and other epithelial tissues.

Animal models of AK include human skin maintained in severe combined immunodeficient (SCID) mice, in which lesions are induced by exposure to UVB (280–320 nm) light *(117)*. The hairless albino mouse (SKh/SK-1) is another model for studying UV-induced SCC *(118)*. The role of UV radiation has been well established in these mice with SCC occurrence peaking around 300 nm; however, UV radiation's role in AK induction is less well characterized *(119)*. Confirming the role of *p53* in skin cancer development, p53 knockout mice show a greatly increased sensitivity to AK and SCC induction by UV radiation.

To date, animal models have not been predictive of human melanomagenesis. For example, most animal models do not duplicate the conditions for melanoma development prior to diagnosis. Moreover, tumor antigens are likely to induce some measure of immune tolerance in humans. Incomplete understanding of mechanisms underlying immune-mediated tumor regression accounts for uncertainties regarding the type, magnitude and potency of immune response(s) necessary for tumor regression. Although melanoma research has been hampered by a paucity of relevant animal models, it has made great strides within the last decade *(120–122)*. Insights gleaned from melanoma vaccine therapy trials, coupled with a large and growing body of preclinical data in animal tumor models, are likely to accelerate advancement of tumor antigen vaccines in various stages of clinical testing for prevention research.

6. SKIN CANCER SCREENING

Mortality from skin cancer is preventable through early detection and the eradication of worrisome precursor lesions such as dysplastic nevi and AK. In even the most lethal variant MSC, 90% of lesions are detectable at curable stages with the naked eye. Melanoma lesions less than 1.4 mm in thickness have lower than 10% likelihood of recurrence, whereas the 5-yr case fatality exceeds 70% for those that are at least 3.6 mm *(123)*. Because skin is serially examined with various intents by patients, their contacts, primary health care providers, and/or dermatologists, it achieves more consistent and frequent screening than any other organ *(124)*. This ease of detection enables self-referral for formal skin evaluation, biopsy, and diagnosis on the basis of lesions defined as problematic by the patients, which accounts in part for broadly available treatment techniques that are readily reimbursed by third-party payers.

Skin cancer screening is a powerful tool for risk assessment and diagnosis, long before disease is likely to attain lethal potential. When accompanied by appropriate surgical or medical interventions, so-called secondary prevention may achieve clinical benefits such as reductions in skin cancer incidence, disease stage at diagnosis, and disease-associated mortality rates *(125)*. Despite interexaminer disagreement regarding lesional pathology *(126,127)* and common overdiagnosis in screening settings, population-based, case-control, and nonrandomized studies show that a 3-min visual inspection can identify (and allow for intervention against) early cutaneous malignancy. An audit of a skin cancer screening and educational campaign in western Scotland showed increased skin cancer incidence, percentage of thin tumors, and 5-yr survival after implementation of the program *(128)*. Another study conducted in 1987–1989 evaluated skin self-examination (SSE) among 650 newly diagnosed melanoma cases and 549 age- and gender-matched controls, all of whom were Caucasian residents of Connecticut *(129)*. SSE performed by 15% of study subjects was associated with a marginally reduced risk of incident melanoma with an odds ratio (OR) of 0.66 (95% CI = 0.44–0.99). SSE was also associated with reductions in incident melanoma during the 5-yr post-study follow-up, during which 110 fatal cases of melanoma were diagnosed. Based on these data, the investigators estimated that 63% reductions in disease-specific mortality were achievable with monthly SSE. Furthermore, they projected risk reductions in advanced melanoma, with an unadjusted risk ratio of 0.58 (95% CI = 0.31–1.11) *(129)*. These preliminary data justify further inquiries into SSE's potential as a practical, low-cost method for reducing skin cancer incidence, disease progression, and mortality *(130)*. Early detection efforts may account for recently improved survival trends among melanoma patients *(5)*. Even so, SSE and comparable measures alone are unlikely to provide adequate protection for certain groups at high risk for skin cancer, as discussed below.

6.1. Limits of Early Detection

Early melanoma growth is characterized by a prolonged horizontal growth phase characterized by subepidermal centrifugal expansion without invasion into the dermal layer. This horizontal growth phase coupled with 100% curability prior to invasion into the basement membrane makes screening an appealing approach. Nevertheless, the sensitivity and specificity of visual examinations vary widely depending on examiner skill *(127,131)*, and mortality reductions from serial screening have yet to be shown in prospective, randomized studies. Moreover, this approach will not suffice for certain high-risk cohorts in whom disease is aggressive, multifocal, and possibly confounded by morphologic/diagnostic uncertainty *(132–134)*. Such high-risk cohorts include certain highly penetrant genetic syndromes, e.g., XP *(70,135)* and familial atypical multiple-mole melanoma (FAMMM) *(136)*. These patients may benefit from adjunctive interventions that simultaneously improve the clinical yield of screening, increase latency to disease, reduce skin cancer-associated morbidity and mortality, limit the frequency and extent of deforming surgeries/excisions, and/or reduce cancer risk in multiple organs. Depending on the clinical context, such adjuncts might include single agents or agent combinations shown to be effective against skin carcinogens.

7. IMMUNOPREVENTION OF MELANOMA

Ecologic and behavioral trends discussed above suggest a strong need for preventive interventions that blunt the impact of skin carcinogenesis in vulnerable populations. Primary prevention against skin cancer in the general population would involve minimization of UV exposure starting in infancy. Secondary prevention would include skin cancer screening to detect subclinical disease in at-risk populations, using ablative techniques possibly in conjunction with chemo- or immunoprevention. Finally, tertiary prevention would reduce disease and/or therapy-induced morbidity and mortality in individuals diagnosed with skin cancer. The most immediate and obvious application of immunopreventive approaches would be in the higher-risk contexts of tertiary and secondary prevention, where the gradient of benefit:risk favors more aggressive approaches to disease management. As a result, the value of vaccine-based interventions will likely be proven first in genetically predisposed cohorts and individuals with completely resected preneoplastic (or neoplastic) lesions.

Antigens common to melanoma, a highly immunogenic tumor, appear early in melanomagenesis. Consequently, interest in vaccine-based prevention of MSC is growing *(137–140)*. Substantial basic and clinical research has focused on therapeutic and preventive applications of cancer vaccines and other forms of immunotherapy intended to induce antigen-specific antitumor immune responses. Interest in this area increased substantially as a result of clinical studies demonstrating the antitumor activity of IL-2, manifested as durable complete responses in approx 5–10% of patients with metastatic melanoma and renal cell carcinoma. Extrapolating from mechanistic studies in animal models, the antitumor activity of IL-2 in patients was attributed to induction or expansion of cell-mediated immune responses, although the full spectrum of biologic activities with which IL-2 mediates tumor regression have yet to be completely characterized. Although the toxicity of IL-2 likely precludes its use for chemoprevention, early data suggest the potential of cell-mediated immune responses to prevent and regress established neoplasms. These data provided a rationale for cancer antigen immunization that achieves broader and more potent antitumor immune responses, potentially with lower toxicity. Clinical antitumor activity has also been observed with passively transferred antibodies against tumor-associated antigens, implying that immunizations that induce serologic responses to cancer antigens might also prove a promising research area.

7.1. Opportunities for Vaccine Development

Emerging insights into molecular events involved with antigen presentation and T-cell activation are generating increased interest in vaccines for MSC treatment and secondary prevention. A variety of techniques have been developed to transfer genes directly into tumor cells in order to bypass the need to define specific tumor antigens. In animal models, some of these approaches have been shown to enhance the immunogenicity and antitumor activity of tumor cell vaccines, providing a mechanistic rationale for trials testing gene-modified autologous or allogeneic vaccines. In early clinical testing, autologous granulocyte-macrophage colony-stimulating factor (GM-CSF) transfected tumor cell vaccines have been reported to induce T-cell infiltrates in metastatic MSC lesions, suggesting clinically relevant biological activity that merits further exploration in the context of prevention. Moreover, several older vaccines consisting of autologous or allogeneic cancer cells admixed with nonspecific immune adjuvants have shown therapeutic efficacy as postsurgical adjuvants, including cases of tumor regression in certain patients with metastatic disease *(141,142)*. Although most of these data were obtained in uncontrolled or small randomized treatment studies, they provide clinical support for testing immunopreventives in the context of high-risk disease where the risk:benefit ratio favors intervention rather than watchful waiting. By this reasoning, immunologic assays in therapeutic vaccine studies with negative or null results may provide important clues about utility of various immune responses as endpoints for investigational studies of candidate vaccines for prevention.

7.2. Biomarkers of Immune Response

Several factors complicate vaccine development for melanoma immunoprevention, including the need to identify biological markers to serve as endpoints for cancer vaccine trials and regulatory approval. Furthermore, innate or acquired immune tolerance to tumor antigens, tumor expression of immunosuppressive molecules and cytokines, loss of tumor antigen expression, and/or baseline immune competence have only been partially characterized in preclinical and clinical settings. These factors will play a major role in selecting the appropriate disease (or risk) state to design trials leading to regulatory approval of melanoma immunoprevention agents. Ultimately, regulatory approval of chemopreventives—including vaccines —for prevention of melanoma and other cancers will facilitate greater certainty and precision in terms of agent and cohort prioritization, and provide direction for the development of other promising agents.

Also impeding vaccine development are uncertainties relating to monitoring immune responses to tumor antigens at baseline and in response to active immunization. Immune and biologic monitoring of early vaccine studies should provide adequate guidance for determining whether or not a particular vaccine should progress into more advanced clinical testing. However, lack of standardized immunologic assays and limitations of available techniques preclude comparisons between different vaccine approaches, and may also hamper efforts to evaluate meaningful modulations of immunologic activity. Melanomagenesis is a dynamic process, and monitoring immunologic status may prove exceedingly complex, depending on the risk status of each patient. As a result, prospects for immunoprevention of melanoma will likely improve with advances in biological and immunological monitoring technologies.

Pharmaceutical companies have been reluctant to engage in vaccine research for cancer treatment and prevention, largely owing to the high cost of vaccine development, liability issues, and the greater bottom-line appeal of approaches that use small molecules and antibody-based interventions. Other challenges include difficulty in obtaining and combining reagents from different pharmaceutical sponsors, and funding for coordinated trials of expensive and technically difficult approaches, such as immunization with dendritic cells or adoptive transfer of expanded antigen-specific T-cell clones.

8. CONVERGENCE OF CANCER PREVENTION AND TREATMENT

Arguably the skin is a model target in which to prove cancer chemopreventive concepts owing to its accessibility for serial assessments, albeit often with cosmetic intent. The same features that commend skin as a theoretical model, however, complicate practical investigations into epidemiologic trends, skin cancer risk assessment, and industrial/academic motivation to develop preventive interventions, as discussed above. Ambivalence as to whether and when ostensibly healthy at-risk individuals might benefit from early interventions that prevent downstream consequences of skin carcinogenesis explains, in part, why skin cancer prevention has yet to attain academic and industrial investment on a par with cancer treatment (1,4).

Conceptual boundaries between cancer therapy and prevention are eroding as new molecular, immunologic, and imaging technologies permit earlier disease detection and intervention. Molecular targets that are shared by early neoplasia and invasive disease provide opportunities to apply agents developed with therapeutic intent for cancer prevention. Skin cancer prevention research has already demonstrated this principle by translating observations of AK regression in colorectal cancer patients treated with systemic 5-fluorouracil into a topical formulation approved in 1970 for the management of AK (Efudex 5% cream). Further clinical research demonstrating reduction in early neoplasia and markers of disease risk, together with cancer-associated morbidity and mortality, will confirm the efficacy of agents that both treat and prevent cancers of the skin and other organs.

REFERENCES

1. Housman TS, Feldman SR, Williford PM, et al. Skin cancer is among the most costly of all cancers to treat for the Medicare population. *J Am Acad Dermatol* 2003;48:425–429.
2. Leman JA, McHenry PM. Basal cell carcinoma: still an enigma. *Arch Dermatol* 2001;137:1239–1240.
3. Chen JG, Fleischer AB, Jr., Smith ED, et al. Cost of non-melanoma skin cancer treatment in the United States. *Dermatol Surg* 2001;27:1035–1038.
4. Tsao H, Rogers GS, Sober AJ. An estimate of the annual direct cost of treating cutaneous melanoma. *J Am Acad Dermatol* 1998;38:669–680.

5. American Cancer Society CRIMSC, http://www.cancer.org/docroot/CRI/CRI_2_1x.asp?dt=39.

6. American Cancer Society CRINSC, http://www.cancer.org.docroot/lrn/lrn_0.asp.

7. Weinstock MA. Overview of ultraviolet radiation and cancer: what is the link? How are we doing? *Environ Health Perspect* 1995;103 Suppl 8:251–254.

8. Reis LAG, Kosary CL, Hankey BF, et al., eds. *SEER Cancer Statistics Review*, 1973–95. National Cancer Institute, Bethesda, MD, 1998.

9. Marcil I, Stern RS. Risk of developing a subsequent non-melanoma skin cancer in patients with a history of non-melanoma skin cancer: a critical review of the literature and meta-analysis. *Arch Dermatol* 2000;136:1524–1530.

10. Dennis LK. Analysis of the melanoma epidemic, both apparent and real: data from the 1973 through 1994 surveillance, epidemiology, and end results program registry. *Arch Dermatol* 1999;135:275–280.

11. Devesa SS, Blot WJ, Stone BJ, et al. Recent cancer trends in the United States. *J Natl Cancer Inst* 1995;87:175–182.

12. Miller DL, Weinstock MA. Nonmelanoma skin cancer in the United States: incidence. *J Am Acad Dermatol* 1994;30(5 Pt 1):774–778.

13. Lupulescu A. The role of vitamins A, beta-carotene, E and C in cancer cell biology. *Int J Vitam Nutr Res* 1994;64:3–14.

14. Stratton SP, Dorr RT, Alberts DS. The state-of-the-art in chemoprevention of skin cancer. *Eur J Cancer* 2000;36(10):1292–1297.

15. Kelloff GJ, Boone CW, Crowell JA, et al. Risk biomarkers and current strategies for cancer chemoprevention. *J Cell Biochem Suppl* 1996;25:1–14.

16. Hawk E, Viner JL, Lawrence JA. Biomarkers as surrogates for cancer development. *Curr Oncol Rep* 2000;2:242–250.

17. Brash DE, Ponten J. Skin precancer. *Cancer Surv* 1998;32:69–113.

18. Berwick M, Halpern A. Melanoma epidemiology. *Curr Opin Oncol* 1997;9:178–182.

19. Marks R. Epidemiology of non-melanoma skin cancer and solar keratoses in Australia: a tale of self-immolation in Elysian fields. *Australas J Dermatol* 1997;38 Suppl 1: S26–S29.

20. Mueller N. Overview of the epidemiology of malignancy in immune deficiency. *J Acquir Immune Defic Syndr* 1999;21 Suppl 1:S5–S10.

21. Bouwes Bavinck JN, Hardie DR, Green A, et al. The risk of skin cancer in renal transplant recipients in Queensland, Australia. A follow-up study. *Transplantation* 1996;61:715–721.

22. Corona R. Epidemiology of nonmelanoma skin cancer: a review. *Ann Ist Super Sanita* 1996;32:37–42.

23. Yuspa SH. Cutaneous chemical carcinogenesis. *J Am Acad Dermatol* 1986;15(5 Pt 1):1031–1044.

24. Elmets CA, Bergstresser PR. Ultraviolet radiation effects on immune processes. *Photochem Photobiol* 1982;36: 715–719.

25. Lyter DW, Bryant J, Thackeray R, et al. Incidence of human immunodeficiency virus-related and nonrelated malignancies in a large cohort of homosexual men. *J Clin Oncol* 1995; 13:2540–2546.

26. Penn I. Post-transplant malignancy: the role of immunosuppression. *Drug Saf* 2000;23:101–113.

27. Euvrard S, Kanitakis J, Pouteil-Noble C, et al. Skin cancers in organ transplant recipients. *Ann Transplant* 1997;2:28–32.

28. Tanenbaum L, Parrish JA, Haynes HA, et al. Prolonged ultraviolet light-induced erythema and the cutaneous carcinoma phenotype. *J Invest Dermatol* 1976;67:513–517.

29. Kraemer KH, Slor H. Xeroderma pigmentosum. *Clin Dermatol* 1985;3:33–69.

30. Lacour JP. Carcinogenesis of basal cell carcinomas: genetics and molecular mechanisms. *Br J Dermatol* 2002;146 Suppl 61:17–19.

31. Lim HW, Cooper K. The health impact of solar radiation and prevention strategies: Report of the Environment Council, American Academy of Dermatology. *J Am Acad Dermatol* 1999;41:81–99.

32. Khlat M, Vail A, Parkin M, Green A. Mortality from melanoma in migrants to Australia: variation by age at arrival and duration of stay. *Am J Epidemiol* 1992;135:1103–1113.

33. Armstrong BK, Kricker A. How much melanoma is caused by sun exposure? *Melanoma Res* 1993;3:395–401.

34. Milan T, Verkasalo PK, Kaprio J, et al. Malignant skin cancers in the Finnish Twin Cohort: a population-based study, 1976–97. *Br J Dermatol* 2002;147:509–512.

35. Urbach F. Ultraviolet radiation carcinogenesis. *J Dermatol Surg Oncol* 1983;9:597–599.

36. Einspahr JG, Nelson MA, Saboda K, et al. Modulation of biologic endpoints by topical difluoromethylornithine (DFMO), in subjects at high-risk for nonmelanoma skin cancer. *Clin Cancer Res* 2002;8:149–155.

37. Dore JF, Pedeux R, Boniol M, et al. Intermediate-effect biomarkers in prevention of skin cancer. *IARC Sci Publ* 2001; 154:81–91.

38. Queille S, Drougard C, Sarasin A, Daya-Grosjean L. Effects of XPD mutations on ultraviolet-induced apoptosis in relation to skin cancer-proneness in repair-deficient syndromes. *J Invest Dermatol* 2001;117:1162–1170.

39. Tada-Oikawa S, Oikawa S, Kawanishi S. Role of ultraviolet A-induced oxidative DNA damage in apoptosis via loss of mitochondrial membrane potential and caspase-3 activation. *Biochem Biophys Res Commun* 1998;247:693–696.

40. Wang SQ, Setlow R, Berwick M, et al. Ultraviolet A and melanoma: a review. *J Am Acad Dermatol* 2001;44:837–846.

41. Fitzpatrick TB. The skin cancer cascade: from ozone depletion to melanoma—some definitions and some new interpretation, 1996. *J Dermatol* 1996;23:816–820.

42. Kraemer KH, Lee MM, Andrews AD, Lambert WC. The role of sunlight and DNA repair in melanoma and nonmelanoma skin cancer. The xeroderma pigmentosum paradigm. *Arch Dermatol* 1994;130:1018–1021.

43. Bentham G, Aase A. Incidence of malignant melanoma of the skin in Norway, 1955–1989: associations with solar ultraviolet radiation, income and holidays abroad. *Int J Epidemiol* 1996;25:1132–1138.

44. Quinn AG. Ultraviolet radiation and skin carcinogenesis. *Br J Hosp Med* 1997;58:261–264.

45. Vitaliano PP, Urbach F. The relative importance of risk factors in nonmelanoma carcinoma. *Arch Dermatol* 1980;116: 454–456.

46. Urbach F. Potential effects of altered solar ultraviolet radiation on human skin cancer. *Photochem Photobiol* 1989; 50:507–513.

47. Streilein JW, Taylor JR, Vincek V, et al. Immune surveillance and sunlight-induced skin cancer. *Immunol Today* 1994;15: 174–179.

48. Otley CC, Coldiron BM, Stasko T, Goldman GD. Decreased skin cancer after cessation of therapy with transplant-associated immunosuppressants. *Arch Dermatol* 2001;137:459–463.

49. Kripke ML. Immunological unresponsiveness induced by ultraviolet radiation. *Immunol Rev* 1984;80:87–102.

50. Whitmore SE, Morison WL. Ultraviolet-induced suppression of the primary allergic reaction. Four times the minimal erythema dose of ultraviolet B administered 24 hours prior to sensitization. *Photodermatol Photoimmunol Photomed* 1995; 11:159–162.

51. Serre I, Cano JP, Picot MC, et al. Immunosuppression induced by acute solar-simulated ultraviolet exposure in humans: prevention by a sunscreen with a sun protection factor of 15 and high UVA protection. *J Am Acad Dermatol* 1997;37(2 Pt 1):187–194.

52. Naylor MF, Boyd A, Smith DW, et al. High sun protection factor sunscreens in the suppression of actinic neoplasia. *Arch Dermatol* 1995;131:170–175.

53. Thompson SC, Jolley D, Marks R. Reduction of solar keratoses by regular sunscreen use. *N Engl J Med* 1993;329:1147–1151.

54. Martin SC, Jacobsen PB, Lucas DJ, et al. Predicting children's sunscreen use: application of the theories of reasoned action and planned behavior. *Prev Med* 1999;29: 37–44.

55. Kraemer KH, Levy DD, Parris CN, et al. Xeroderma pigmentosum and related disorders: examining the linkage between defective DNA repair and cancer. *J Invest Dermatol* 1994;103(5 Suppl):96S–101S.

56. Kraemer KH, DiGiovanna JJ, Peck GL. Chemoprevention of skin cancer in xeroderma pigmentosum. *J Dermatol* 1992;19:715–718.

57. Bavinck JN, Tieben LM, Van der Woude FJ, et al. Prevention of skin cancer and reduction of keratotic skin lesions during acitretin therapy in renal transplant recipients: a double-blind, placebo-controlled study. *J Clin Oncol* 1995;13: 1933–1938.

58. DiGiovanna JJ. Posttransplantation skin cancer: scope of the problem, management, and role for systemic retinoid chemoprevention. *Transplant Proc* 1998;30:2771–2775; discussion 6–8.

59. Grossman D, Leffell DJ. The molecular basis of nonmelanoma skin cancer: new understanding. *Arch Dermatol* 1997;133:1263–1270.

60. Livneh Z, Cohen-Fix O, Skaliter R, Elizur T. Replication of damaged DNA and the molecular mechanism of ultraviolet light mutagenesis. *Crit Rev Biochem Mol Biol* 1993;28:465–513.

61. Tanaka K, Sekiguchi M, Okada Y. Restoration of ultraviolet-induced unscheduled DNA synthesis of xeroderma pigmentosum cells by the concomitant treatment with bacteriophage T4 endonuclease V and HVJ (Sendai virus). *Proc Natl Acad Sci USA* 1975;72:4071–4075.

62. Wolf P, Maier H, Mullegger RR, et al. Topical treatment with liposomes containing T4 endonuclease V protects human skin in vivo from ultraviolet-induced upregulation of interleukin-10 and tumor necrosis factor-alpha. *J Invest Dermatol* 2000;114:149–156.

63. Kripke ML, Cox PA, Alas LG, Yarosh DB. Pyrimidine dimers in DNA initiate systemic immunosuppression in UV-irradiated mice. *Proc Natl Acad Sci USA* 1992;89: 7516–7520.

64. Wolf P, Cox P, Yarosh DB, Kripke ML. Sunscreens and T4N5 liposomes differ in their ability to protect against ultraviolet-induced sunburn cell formation, alterations of dendritic epidermal cells, and local suppression of contact hypersensitivity. *J Invest Dermatol* 1995;104:287–292.

65. Yarosh D, Bucana C, Cox P, et al. Localization of liposomes containing a DNA repair enzyme in murine skin. *J Invest Dermatol* 1994;103:461–468.

66. Yarosh D, Klein J, Kibitel J, et al. Enzyme therapy of xeroderma pigmentosum: safety and efficacy testing of T4N5 liposome lotion containing a prokaryotic DNA repair enzyme. *Photodermatol Photoimmunol Photomed* 1996;12: 122–130.

67. Yarosh D, Alas LG, Yee V, et al. Pyrimidine dimer removal enhanced by DNA repair liposomes reduces the incidence of UV skin cancer in mice. *Cancer Res* 1992;52: 4227–4231.

68. Bito T, Ueda M, Nagano T, et al. Reduction of ultraviolet-induced skin cancer in mice by topical application of DNA excision repair enzymes. *Photodermatol Photoimmunol Photomed* 1995;11:9–13.

69. Yarosh DB, O'Connor A, Alas L, et al. Photoprotection by topical DNA repair enzymes: molecular correlates of clinical studies. *Photochem Photobiol* 1999;69:136–140.

70. Yarosh D, Klein J, O'Connor A, et al. Effect of topically applied T4 endonuclease V in liposomes on skin cancer in xeroderma pigmentosum: a randomised study. Xeroderma Pigmentosum Study Group. *Lancet* 2001;357:926–929.

71. Galambos JT. Carcinoembryonic antigen and neoplastic disease. *South Med J* 1973;66:1216–1217.

72. Lynch HT, Thomas RJ, Gurgis HA, Lynch J. Clues to cancer risk: biologic markers. *Am Fam Physician* 1975;11:153–158.

73. Petrakis NL, King MC. Genetic markers and cancer epidemiology. *Cancer* 1977;39(4 Suppl):1861–1866.

74. Hanash S, Brichory F, Beer D. A proteomic approach to the identification of lung cancer markers. *Dis Markers* 2001;17:295–300.

75. Jones MB, Krutzsch H, Shu H, et al. Proteomic analysis and identification of new biomarkers and therapeutic targets for invasive ovarian cancer. *Proteomics* 2002;2:76–84.

76. Marks R. Solar keratoses. *Br J Dermatol* 1990;122 Suppl 35:49–54.

77. Cockerell CJ. Histopathology of incipient intraepidermal squamous cell carcinoma ("actinic keratosis"). *J Am Acad Dermatol* 2000;42(1 Pt 2):11–17.

78. Yantsos VA, Conrad N, Zabawski E, Cockerell CJ. Incipient intraepidermal cutaneous squamous cell carcinoma: a proposal for reclassifying and grading solar (actinic) keratoses. *Semin Cutan Med Surg* 1999;18:3–14.

79. O'Shaughnessy JA, Kelloff GJ, Gordon GB, et al. Treatment and prevention of intraepithelial neoplasia: an important target for accelerated new agent development. *Clin Cancer Res* 2002;8:314–346.

80. Gupta AK, Cooper EA, Feldman SR, Fleischer AB, Jr. A survey of office visits for actinic keratosis as reported by NAMCS, 1990–1999. National Ambulatory Medical Care Survey. *Cutis* 2002;70(2 Suppl):8–13.

81. Memon AA, Tomenson JA, Bothwell J, Friedmann PS. Prevalence of solar damage and actinic keratosis in a Merseyside population. *Br J Dermatol* 2000;142: 1154–1159.

82. Strickland PT, Vitasa BC, West SK, et al. Quantitative carcinogenesis in man: solar ultraviolet B dose dependence of skin cancer in Maryland watermen. *J Natl Cancer Inst* 1989;81:1910–1913.

83. Marks R. Premalignant disease of the epidermis. The Parkes Weber lecture 1985. *J R Coll Physicians Lond* 1986;20:116–121.

84. Bozzo P, Alberts DS, Vaught L, et al. Measurement of chemopreventive efficacy in skin biopsies. *Anal Quant Cytol Histol* 2001;23:300–312.

85. Einspahr J, Alberts DS, Aickin M, et al. Evaluation of proliferating cell nuclear antigen as a surrogate end point biomarker in actinic keratosis and adjacent, normal-appearing, and non-sun-exposed human skin samples. *Cancer Epidemiol Biomarkers Prev* 1996;5:343–348.

86. Salasche SJ. Epidemiology of actinic keratoses and squamous cell carcinoma. *J Am Acad Dermatol* 2000;42(1 Pt 2):4–7.

87. Mittelbronn MA, Mullins DL, Ramos-Caro FA, Flowers FP. Frequency of pre-existing actinic keratosis in cutaneous squamous cell carcinoma. *Int J Dermatol* 1998;37: 677–681.

88. Ramsay HM, Fryer AA, Hawley CM, et al. Non-melanoma skin cancer risk in the Queensland renal transplant population. *Br J Dermatol* 2002;147:950–956.

89. Jemec GB, Holm EA. Nonmelanoma skin cancer in organ transplant patients. *Transplantation* 2003;75:253–257.

90. Moon TE, Levine N, Cartmel B, et al. Effect of retinol in preventing squamous cell skin cancer in moderate-risk subjects: a randomized, double-blind, controlled trial. Southwest Skin Cancer Prevention Study Group. *Cancer Epidemiol Biomarkers Prev* 1997;6:949–956.

91. Stratton SP. Prevention of non-melanoma skin cancer. *Curr Oncol Rep* 2001;3:295–300.

92. Katiyar SK, Mukhtar H. Tea antioxidants in cancer chemoprevention. *J Cell Biochem Suppl* 1997;27:59–67.

93. Bickers DR, Athar M. Novel approaches to chemoprevention of skin cancer. *J Dermatol* 2000;27:691–695.

94. DiGiovanna JJ. Retinoid chemoprevention in patients at high risk for skin cancer. *Med Pediatr Oncol* 2001;36:564–567.

95. Moon TE, Levine N, Cartmel B, Bangert JL. Retinoids in prevention of skin cancer. *Cancer Lett* 1997;114:203–205.

96. Einspahr JG, Stratton SP, Bowden GT, Alberts DS. Chemoprevention of human skin cancer. *Crit Rev Oncol Hematol* 2002;41:269–285.

97. Kraemer KH, DiGiovanna JJ, Moshell AN, et al. Prevention of skin cancer in xeroderma pigmentosum with the use of oral isotretinoin. *N Engl J Med* 1988;318:1633–1637.

98. Pentland AP. Cyclooxygenase inhibitors for skin cancer prevention: are they beneficial enough? *Arch Dermatol* 2002;138:823–824.

99. Carbone PP, Douglas JA, Larson PO, et al. Phase I chemoprevention study of piroxicam and alpha-difluoromethylornithine. *Cancer Epidemiol Biomarkers Prev* 1998;7: 907–912.

100. Carbone PP, Pirsch JD, Thomas JP, et al. Phase I chemoprevention study of difluoromethylornithine in subjects with organ transplants. *Cancer Epidemiol Biomarkers Prev* 2001; 10:657–661.

101. Meyskens FL, Jr., Gilmartin E, Alberts DS, et al. Activity of isotretinoin against squamous cell cancers and preneoplastic lesions. *Cancer Treat Rep* 1982;66:1315–1319.

102. Brash DE, Rudolph JA, Simon JA, et al. A role for sunlight in skin cancer: UV-induced p53 mutations in squamous cell carcinoma. *Proc Natl Acad Sci USA* 1991;88:10,124–10,128.

103. Bergstresser PR, Elmets CA, Takashima A, Mukhtar H. Photocarcinogenesis. *Photodermatol Photoimmunol Photomed* 1996;11:181–184.

104. Dumaz N, van Kranen HJ, de Vries A, et al. The role of UV-B light in skin carcinogenesis through the analysis of p53 mutations in squamous cell carcinomas of hairless mice. *Carcinogenesis* 1997;18:897–904.

105. Ziegler A, Jonason AS, Leffell DJ, et al. Sunburn and p53 in the onset of skin cancer. *Nature* 1994;372:773–776.

106. Kubo Y, Urano Y, Matsumoto K, et al. Mutations of the INK4a locus in squamous cell carcinomas of human skin. *Biochem Biophys Res Commun* 1997;232:38–41.

107. Linardopoulos S, Street AJ, Quelle DE, et al. Deletion and altered regulation of p16INK4a and p15INK4b in undifferentiated mouse skin tumors. *Cancer Res* 1995;55:5168–5172.

108. Tsukifuji R, Tagawa K, Hatamochi A, Shinkai H. Expression of matrix metalloproteinase-1, -2 and -3 in squamous cell carcinoma and actinic keratosis. *Br J Cancer* 1999;80: 1087–1091.

109. Filipowicz E, Adegboyega P, Sanchez RL, Gatalica Z. Expression of CD95 (Fas) in sun-exposed human skin and cutaneous carcinomas. *Cancer* 2002;94:814–819.

110. Moch C, Moysan A, Lubin R, et al. Divergence between the high rate of p53 mutations in skin carcinomas and the low prevalence of anti-p53 antibodies. *Br J Cancer* 2001;85: 1883–1886.

111. Papadavid E, Pignatelli M, Zakynthinos S, et al. Abnormal immunoreactivity of the E-cadherin/catenin (alpha-, beta-, and gamma-) complex in premalignant and malignant nonmelanocytic skin tumours. *J Pathol* 2002;196:154–162.

112. Wei Q, Matanoski GM, Farmer ER, et al. DNA repair and aging in basal cell carcinoma: a molecular epidemiology study. *Proc Natl Acad Sci USA* 1993;90:1614–1618.

113. Sancar A. DNA repair in humans. *Annu Rev Genet* 1995;29:69–105.

114. Qiao Y, Spitz MR, Shen H, et al. Modulation of repair of ultraviolet damage in the host-cell reactivation assay by polymorphic XPC and XPD/ERCC2 genotypes. *Carcinogenesis* 2002;23:295–299.

115. Viac J, Chardonnet Y, Euvrard S, et al. Langerhans cells, inflammation markers and human papillomavirus infections in benign and malignant epithelial tumors from transplant recipients. *J Dermatol* 1992;19:67–77.

116. Berhane T, Halliday GM, Cooke B, Barnetson RS. Inflammation is associated with progression of actinic keratoses to squamous cell carcinomas in humans. *Br J Dermatol* 2002;146:810–815.

117. Nomura T, Nakajima H, Hongyo T, et al. Induction of cancer, actinic keratosis, and specific p53 mutations by UVB light in human skin maintained in severe combined immunodeficient mice. *Cancer Res* 1997;57:2081–2084.

118. de Gruijl FR, Sterenborg HJ, Forbes PD, et al. Wavelength dependence of skin cancer induction by ultraviolet irradiation of albino hairless mice. *Cancer Res* 1993;53:53–60.

119. Soehnge H, Ouhtit A, Ananthaswamy ON. Mechanisms of induction of skin cancer by UV radiation. *Front Biosci* 1997;2:D538–D551.

120. Chin L. Modeling malignant melanoma in mice: pathogenesis and maintenance. *Oncogene* 1999;18:5304–5310.

121. Chin L, Pomerantz J, DePinho RA. The INK4a/ARF tumor suppressor: one gene—two products–two pathways. *Trends Biochem Sci* 1998;23:291–296.

122. Otsuka T, Takayama H, Sharp R, et al. c-Met autocrine activation induces development of malignant melanoma and acquisition of the metastatic phenotype. *Cancer Res* 1998;58:5157–5167.

123. Schuchter L, Schultz DJ, Synnestvedt M, et al. A prognostic model for predicting 10-year survival in patients with primary melanoma. The Pigmented Lesion Group. *Ann Intern Med* 1996;125:369–375.

124. Weinstock MA. Early detection of melanoma. *JAMA* 2000;284:886–889.

125. Parker C. Skin lesions in transplant patients. *Dermatol Clin* 1990;8:313–325.

126. Veenhuizen KC, De Wit PE, Mooi WJ, et al. Quality assessment by expert opinion in melanoma pathology: experience of the pathology panel of the Dutch Melanoma Working Party. *J Pathol* 1997;182:266–272.

127. Weinstock MA, Bingham SF, Cole GW, et al. Reliability of counting actinic keratoses before and after brief consensus discussion: the VA topical tretinoin chemoprevention (VATTC) trial. *Arch Dermatol* 2001;137:1055–1058.

128. MacKie RM, Hole D. Audit of public education campaign to encourage earlier detection of malignant melanoma. *Br Med J* 1992;304:1012–1015.

129. Berwick M, Begg CB, Fine JA, et al. Screening for cutaneous melanoma by skin self-examination. *J Natl Cancer Inst* 1996;88:17–23.

130. Cristofolini M, Bianchi R, Boi S, et al. Analysis of the cost-effectiveness ratio of the health campaign for the early diagnosis of cutaneous melanoma in Trentino, Italy. *Cancer* 1993;71:370374.

131. Helfand M, Mahon SM, Eden KB, et al. Screening for skin cancer. *Am J Prev Med* 2001;20(3 Suppl):47–58.

132. Berg D, Otley CC. Skin cancer in organ transplant recipients: Epidemiology, pathogenesis, and management. *J Am Acad Dermatol* 2002;47:1–17.

133. Stockfleth E, Ulrich C, Meyer T, Christophers E. Epithelial malignancies in organ transplant patients: clinical presentation and new methods of treatment. *Recent Results Cancer Res* 2002;160:251–258.

134. Euvrard S, Kanitakis J, Claudy A. Skin cancers after organ transplantation. *N Engl J Med* 2003;348:1681–1691.

135. Robbins JH, Kraemer KH, Lutzner MA, et al. Xeroderma pigmentosum. An inherited diseases with sun sensitivity, multiple cutaneous neoplasms, and abnormal DNA repair. *Ann Intern Med* 1974;80:221–248.

136. Lynch HT, Fusaro RM, Pester J, Lynch JF. Familial atypical multiple mole melanoma (FAMMM) syndrome: genetic heterogeneity and malignant melanoma. *Br J Cancer* 1980;42:58–70.

137. Lollini PL, Forni G. Antitumor vaccines: is it possible to prevent a tumor? *Cancer Immunol Immunother* 2002;51:409–16.

138. Lollini PL, Forni G. Cancer immunoprevention: tracking down persistent tumor antigens. *Trends Immunol* 2003;24:62–66.

139. Finn OJ, Forni G. Prophylactic cancer vaccines. *Curr Opin Immunol* 2002;14:172–177.

140. Forni G, Lollini PL, Musiani P, Colombo MP. Immunoprevention of cancer: is the time ripe? *Cancer Res* 2000;60:2571–2575.

141. Hsueh EC, Gupta RK, Qi K, Morton DL. Correlation of specific immune responses with survival in melanoma patients with distant metastases receiving polyvalent melanoma cell vaccine. *J Clin Oncol* 1998;16:2913–2920.

142. DiFronzo LA, Gupta RK, Essner R, et al. Enhanced humoral immune response correlates with improved disease-free and overall survival in American Joint Committee on Cancer stage II melanoma patients receiving adjuvant polyvalent vaccine. *J Clin Oncol* 2002;20: 3242–3248.

CERVIX

32 Progress in Developing Effective Chemoprevention Agents for Cervical Neoplasia

Ronald D. Alvarez, MD, William E. Grizzle, MD, PhD, Heidi L. Weiss, PhD, Clinton J. Grubbs, PhD, and Amit Oza, MD

CONTENTS

1. INTRODUCTION

Chemoprevention refers to the use of micronutrients or pharmaceutical agents to prevent or delay the development of cancer in healthy populations. Agents employed in chemopreventive trials should prevent or reverse the initiation, promotion, or progression processes involved with carcinogenesis. Chemoprevention strategies would therefore be best employed in patients with normal or premalignant lesions who are at high risk of developing a malignancy.

For several reasons, the cervix serves as an excellent organ site for development of effective chemoprevention strategies. First, cervical neoplasia is a worldwide health problem and one of the leading causes of cancer mortality in women, particularly women in developing countries. Second, human papilloma virus (HPV) has been identified as the primary carcinogen in this disease context, and a well-defined premalignant phase of cervical neoplasia is known to exist. Finally, available effective screening strategies (Papanicolaou [Pap] smear, HPV typing) identify patients at high risk for

developing cervical cancer, and the cervix is readily assessable and easily evaluated by conventional methodologies such as colposcopy, biopsy, and large-loop excision of the transformation zone (LLETZ). For these reasons, investigating chemopreventive agents in cervical neoplasia has been an active area of study. This chapter will review the progress of chemoprevention research in cervical neoplasia and identify potential opportunities in this field.

2. CERVICAL NEOPLASIA CHEMOPREVENTION DRUG DEVELOPMENT AND PRECLINICAL TESTING

2.1. Cervical Neoplasia Model Systems for Preclinical Chemopreventive Agent Validation

Since the human cervix is readily visualized and easy to biopsy, information about chemopreventive agents and biomarkers in cervical neoplasia have largely been derived from prospective clinical studies in

From: Cancer Chemoprevention, Volume 2: Strategies for Cancer Chemoprevention
Edited by: G. J. Kelloff, E. T. Hawk, and C. C. Sigman © Humana Press Inc., Totowa, NJ

women with cervical dysplasia. This easy accessibility to the cervix may in part account for the lack of interest or progress in developing preclinical models for cervical neoplasia. Problems associated with evaluating chemopreventive agents in humans, however, are many. Common use of supplemental vitamins and minerals by the public makes intervention studies evaluating nutrients for cervical cancer prevention difficult to perform. Also, unacceptable toxicity can occur with systemically administered chemopreventive agents. Thus, preclinical models of cervical cancer are needed to overcome commonly encountered biases and difficulties in assessing the efficacy of new chemopreventive agents in human subjects.

Cell lines can be used to evaluate such agents, but must be cautiously interpreted due to lack of differentiation between nonspecific toxicity and cancer-preventing effects. In addition, using already established cancers to investigate chemopreventive agents may erroneously over- or underestimate the agents' activity in normal or dysplastic tissues. To address this issue, investigators have developed animal models to evaluate the efficacy of chemopreventive agents, which differ from animal models used to evaluate chemotherapeutic agents in that preneoplasia or early cancerous lesions are the targets.

The following criteria should be used when establishing a cancer model to screen potentially large numbers of chemopreventive agents. Cancers should develop only in the organ of interest; they should be histologically, biochemically, and genetically similar to human cancer; and they should have short latency periods (6–8 mo or less). Also, the cancer model should be highly reproducible and require a minimal number of carcinogen treatments so that time of cancer initiation is known, and the animals used in the model should be inexpensive and easy to obtain. The National Cancer Institute (NCI) has typically used chemically induced rodent models such as the methylnitrosourea-induced mammary model *(1)*, the azoxymethane-induced colon model *(2)*, and the *N*-butyl-*N*-(4-hydroxybutyl) nitrosamine-induced urinary bladder model *(3)* for these studies. Only one chemically induced model of cervical cancer has been reported, used only sporadically. Murphy's string method employed a cotton thread dipped in a molten mixture of beeswax and 3-methycholanthrene (3-MCA) to determine the efficacy of various nutrients including retinoic acid, butylated hydroxyanisole, and garlic *(4,5)*.

Attempts have been made to develop orthotopic and transgenic models of cervical cancer for evaluating

potential chemopreventive agents. Tewari et al. recently reported successful subcutaneous implantation of normal and dysplastic human cervical tissues in severe combined immunodeficient (SCID) mice *(6)*. These xenografted models retained constitutive characteristics of transplanted epithelium and were proposed as potential models to study HPV-mediated human disease. Arbeit et al. reported that administration of estradiol to transgenic mice expressing HPV16 oncogenes under control of the human keratin-14 promoter induced squamous carcinomas specifically in the vagina and cervix *(7)*. This model has been used to investigate the efficacy of chemopreventive agents for cervical neoplasia *(8,9)*. Animal models hold considerable promise in understanding the basic mechanisms involved in cervical carcinogenesis and in identifying effective chemopreventive agents; however, the ultimate utility of these models awaits further verification.

2.2. Identifying Effective Chemoprevention Strategies for Cervical Neoplasia

Although beyond the scope of this review, molecular and cellular processes involved in transforming normal cervical epithelium to a malignant phenotype are being further elucidated. It is clear that HPV plays a significant role in malignant transformation of cervical epithelium. The interaction of HPV with cervical epithelium, however, is complex, affected by both exogenous (i.e., tobacco exposure, sexually transmitted diseases) and endogenous (i.e., hormonal and immunologic) factors. The processes downstream to HPV infection may lead to uncontrolled cellular proliferation and malignant behavior. Heretofore, prototypical classes of drugs have been investigated in the context of cervical neoplasia with the intent to inhibit mutagenesis, induce cellular apoptosis, or control cellular proliferation in a noncervical tissue-specific fashion. As processes involved with malignant transformation of the cervical epithelium are further clarified, more cervical tissue-specific agents may be developed and investigated as potential chemopreventive strategies.

3. ISSUES IN DESIGN AND IMPLEMENTATION OF CHEMOPREVENTION TRIALS IN CERVICAL NEOPLASIA

3.1. Chemoprevention Trial Design

Clinical development and validation of chemopreventive agents are carried out primarily in Phase I, II, and III trials *(10)*. Phase I trials of typical anticancer pharmaceuticals seek to identify the maximum tolerated dose (MTD) of an agent using a dose-escalating trial schema. In contrast, Phase I trials of chemopreventive agents seek to evaluate safety and pharmacokinetics of a particular agent using a dose-deescalating trial design. Phase I trials attempt to identify a well-tolerated dose that meets minimum effectiveness criteria. Serum, urine, or other tissue sample evidence of drug presence, drug metabolites, or expected biomarker alteration often form the basis for defining drug effectiveness in Phase I trials. Phase IIA trials are designed to assess potential efficacy of new agents and new biomarkers; Phase IIB studies are generally randomized, double-blind, and placebo-controlled, emphasizing the importance of intermediate biomarkers highly correlated to cancer incidence that may serve as surrogate endpoints for reducing cancer incidence. Large randomized, double-blind, placebo-controlled Phase III trials demonstrate a chemopreventive agent's effect on cancer incidence as their primary endpoint. Trial designs such as these have been used to study various cancer chemopreventive agents, including those for cervical cancer.

3.2. Logistic Considerations in Implementing Cervical Neoplasia Chemoprevention Trials

When designing a trial analyzing a chemoprevention agent in cervical neoplasia, issues regarding recruitment and retention must be addressed (11). The patient population often originates from a large colposcopy clinic, generally lacks insurance coverage, may be transient, and often faces barriers that preclude enrollment or compliance with prescribed treatment in chemoprevention trials. These barriers may include language and communication limitations, travel constraints, work and child care barriers, the inability to commit to long-term or multiple-visit trials, low tolerance of side effects, and in some instances, mistrust of established health systems. To address these barriers, investigators must configure a clinical trial staff capable of providing continuity of care and fostering a trusting relationship with patients. In addition, every effort should be made to construct the trial to be efficient and convenient to the participant. Financial incentives often provide the participant with resources for transportation, child care, or compensation for time lost from work. While these issues are germane to chemoprevention trials in many organ sites, they are especially relevant in the context of cervical dysplasia, which is easily treated in an outpatient setting.

A prerequisite in chemoprevention trials is that trial design and the agent selected for evaluation ensure patient safety. By definition, trial participants are only at risk of developing cancer; they do not have established cancer, and if they did, current invasive treatment modalities are generally highly effective.

4. CERVICAL NEOPLASIA CHEMOPREVENTION CLINICAL TRIALS

4.1. Micronutrient Chemoprevention Trials for Cervical Dysplasia (Table 1)

Given preliminary evidence linking folate deficiency to cytologic changes in the cervical epithelium that mimic dysplasia, Butterworth et al. initiated a prospective study. Forty-seven women with mild or moderate dysplasia diagnosed by cervical smear were randomized to folic acid (10 mg) or placebo (ascorbic acid, 10 mg) daily for 3 mo under double-blind conditions (12). All patients underwent colposcopy, Pap smear, and biopsy performed at end of treatment. Results of this study, reported in 1982, demonstrated that mean biopsy scores (correlating to the degree of dysplastic changes) from folate-supplemented patients were significantly better than those from patients who received placebo (2.28 vs 2.92, $p < 0.05$). Final vs initial cytology scores were also significantly better in supplemented subjects (1.95 vs 2.32, $p < 0.05$), but unchanged in the placebo group (2.27 vs 2.30). This preliminary study was the basis for a larger trial reported by Butterworth et al. in 1992 (13,14). In this second trial, 235 patients with a Pap smear suggestive of cervical intraepithelial neoplasia (CIN) 1/2 and a visible dysplastic lesion on colposcopic examination were randomly assigned to receive either folic acid (10 mg) or placebo (ascorbic acid, 10 mg) daily for a total of 6 mo. Although patients with lower red blood cell folate levels had a higher risk of HPV infection, no significant differences were noted between folate-supplemented and placebo-supplemented subjects regarding dysplasia status, biopsy results, or prevalence of HPV type 16 infection.

In 1995, Childers et al. reported similar results in a Southwest Oncology Group trial investigating the utility of folic acid as a chemopreventive agent for cervical dysplasia (15). In this multi-institutional trial, 331 women with biopsy-proven koilocytic atypia, CIN 1, or CIN 2 were randomized to receive oral folic acid (5 mg) or placebo (inert tablet) daily for 6 mo following a 1-mo run-in placebo period. In spite of a significant rise in serum folate levels at three and six months in the folate-supplemented group, there was no significant difference in Pap smear results or colposcopic picture between the two treatment groups.

Table 1
Micronutrient Chemoprevention Trials for Cervical Dysplasia

Author, year	Number of patients	Agent/dose	Placebo/dose	Disease	Efficacy
Butterworth, 1982	47	Folate/10 mg	Ascorbic acid/10 mg	CIN 1/2	Yes
Butterworth, 1992	235	Folate/10 mg	Ascorbic acid/10 mg	CIN 1/2	No
Childers, 1995	331	Folate/5 mg	Inert tablet	HPV/CIN 1/2	No
de Vet, 1991	278	β-carotene/10 mg	Inert tablet	CIN 1–3	No
Manetta, 1996	30	β-carotene/30 mg	None	CIN 1/2	Yes
Fairley, 1996	117	β-carotene/30 mg	Lecithin/ 400 mg	Atypia — CIN 2	No
Romney, 1997	98	β-carotene/30 mg	Lactose	CIN 1–3	No
Mackerras, 1999	141	β-carotene/30 mg +/– vitamin C/500 mg	Inert tablet	Atypia — CIN 1	No
Bell, 2000	30	Indole-3-carbinol/ 200 or 400 mg	Inert tablet	CIN 2/3	Yes
Keefe, 2001	124	β-carotene/30 mg	Inert tablet	CIN 2/3	No

Epidemiologic studies have demonstrated an association of low β-carotene levels and CIN. de Vet et al. randomized 137 patients with CIN 1–3 to receive 10 mg of β-carotene daily for 3 mo and 141 patients to receive placebo (16). No effect of β-carotene on regression percentages was observed: odds ratio (OR) = 0.68 (95% CI = 0.28–1.60). Manetta et al. reported the results of a Phase II trial in which 30 patients with documented CIN 1 or 2 were treated with 30 mg of β-carotene daily for 6 mo (17). Cytology, colposcopy, and/or biopsies were performed at 3, 6, and 12 mo after initiation of therapy. Response rates were reported to be 60%, 70% and 33% at 3, 6, and 12 mo, respectively. Based on these results, a prospective randomized trial that included a control arm was conducted; Keefe et al. reported the results of this randomized double-blind trial of oral β-carotene in 2001 (18). Patients with CIN 2/3 were randomized to receive 30 mg of β-carotene or placebo for a total of 24 mo. Patients were evaluated by Pap smear and colposcopic evaluation every 3 mo and by biopsy at 6 and 24 mo. Seventy-eight of the initial 124 patients completed the study. The overall response rate at 6 mo was 41% for the β-carotene group and 52% in the placebo group; the response rate at 24 mo was 25% for the β-carotene group and 38% for the placebo group (p = NS). Other studies have also failed to demonstrate significant regression difference in β-carotene-treated patients compared to controls (19–21).

Recently, Bell et al. reported the results of a randomized Phase II trial of indole-3-carbinol (I3C) (22). The efficacy of I3C, a component of cruciferous vegetables, has been demonstrated in treating HPV-induced lesions of the larynx. Thirty patients with biopsy-proven CIN 2/3 were randomized to receive either 200 or 400 mg I3C or placebo orally daily for 12 wk. None of the 10 patients randomized to placebo had regression of CIN. In contrast, four of eight patients (50%) randomized to the 200 mg/d arm and four of nine patients (44%) randomized to the 400 mg/d arm had complete regression of CIN. The protective effect of I3C was demonstrated by a relative risk of 0.50 (95% CI = 0.25–0.99, p = 0.023) for the 200 mg/d arm and 0.55 (95% CI = 0.31–0.99, p = 0.032) for the 400 mg/d arm. A randomized trial by the Gynecologic Oncology Group has been proposed to further investigate the efficacy of I3C.

4.2. Retinoic Acid Chemoprevention Trials for Cervical Dysplasia (Table 2)

Vitamin A and its natural and synthetic derivatives (retinoids) prevent progression of normal epithelial cells to a malignant phenotype via several mechanisms. Based on this information and preliminary animal efficacy studies, in 1982 Surwit et al. reported results of a Phase I/II trial of β-all-trans-retinoic acid (ATRA) delivered via collagen sponge/diaphragm insert in 18 patients with CIN 2/3 (23). Patients underwent four consecutive daily applications of β-ATRA (0.05% liquid, 0.1% liquid, 0.2% liquid, or 0.1% cream) placed on a collagen sponge in an individually fitted diaphragm. All patients had conization performed 4 wk later. Colposcopic evaluation prior to conization demonstrated a reduction in lesion size in 10 of 18 patients (55%); two

Table 2
Retinoic Acid Chemoprevention Trials for Cervical Dysplasia

Author, year	Number of patients	Agent/dose	Placebo/dose	Disease	Efficacy
Surwit, 1982	18	Topical ATRA/0.05%–0.2%	None	CIN 2/3	Yes
Meyskns, 1983	35	Topical ATRA/0.05%–0.484%	None	CIN 1/2	Yes
Romney,1985	50	Topical retinyl acetate gel/3–18 mg	Inert vehicle	CIN 1/2	Not reported
Weiner, 1986	36	Topical ATRA/0.05%–0.484%	None	CIN 1–3	Yes
Meyskns, 1994	301	Topical ATRA/0.372%	Inert vehicle	CIN 2/3	Yes (CIN 2)
Follen, 2001	36	4-HPR/200 mg	Yes	CIN 2/3	No
Alvarez, 2002	104	9-cis retinoic acid 25/50 mg	Inert vehicle	CIN 2/3	No

patients had complete resolution of disease upon histologic evaluation of the cone specimen.

A subsequent Phase I trial, reported by Meyskens et al. in 1983, employed 1 mL of β-ATRA delivered daily for four consecutive days in a collagen sponge and cervical cap in 35 patients with biopsy evidence of CIN 1/2 *(24)*. The dose of β-ATRA was escalated from a starting concentration of 0.05%; MTD was determined to be a concentration of 0.372%. Colposcopic appearance of the dysplastic lesion improved by 50% or more in 23 of 27 evaluable patients. Cytology improved in nine of 25 evaluable patients, and biopsy results improved in seven of 22 evaluable patients.

In 1985, Romney et al. published the results of a Phase I/II trial of retinyl acetate gel applied to the cervix and vagina of 50 patients with biopsy evidence of CIN 1/2 *(25)*. Retinyl acetate gel was self administered for a 7-d treatment course over three successive menstrual cycles; the dose ranged from 0–18 mg per 6 g of an inert vehicle. Although no dose-limiting effects were noted, all patients treated at the 18-mg dose experienced "significant" discomfort; it was concluded that the 9-mg dose should be employed in future trials. No efficacy data was reported.

In 1986, Weiner et al. reported the results of a Phase I trial of ATRA at concentrations ranging from 0.05% to 0.484% delivered via collagen sponge in a cervical cap in 36 patients with biopsy evidence of CIN 1–3 *(26)*. Patients were treated with four consecutive 24-h applications and then followed for response at 3-mo intervals with Pap smear, colposcopy, and selected biopsies. Complete resolution of disease was seen in 12 of 36 patients (33%). Of the 12, 4 had mild dysplasia, 6 had moderate dysplasia, and 2 had severe dysplasia. A dose-response noted as complete regression was seen in only 2 of 14 patients (14%) treated with concentrations of 0.05%–0.1167%, but 10 of 22 patients (45%) treated

with concentrations of 0.1583%–0.484% were noted to have a complete response ($p < 0.05$).

In 1994, Meyskens et al. reported the results of a randomized Phase II trial of ATRA delivered via collagen sponge and cervical cap to 301 patients with CIN 2/3 *(27)*. Patients were treated with 1.0 mL ATRA (0.372%) or placebo for four consecutive days at study entry and then for two consecutive days at months 3 and 6. At 15 mo (9 mo after maintenance treatment), all patients were evaluated for response by Pap smear, colposcopy, and biopsy. Patients who missed their 15-mo follow-up were evaluated at the 21-or 27-mo follow-up. The complete histologic regression rate was 47% in patients with CIN 2 treated with ATRA compared to 27% in patients treated with placebo ($p < 0.041$). No differences were noted between the two treatment arms in patients with CIN 3 (25% ATRA vs 31% placebo).

Follen et al. reported the results of a randomized trial of 4-hydroxy-phenylretinamide (4-HPR) in patients with high-grade cervical dysplasia *(28)*. 4-HPR, a novel synthetic retinoid, exerts potent apoptotic activity via nonretinoid receptor pathways. For this trial, patients with CIN 2/3 were randomized to receive 200 mg of 4-HPR vs placebo daily for 12 mo. Patients were evaluated by biopsy at 6 mo and by biopsy or loop at 12 mo. At 6 mo, 20 evaluable patients in the 4-HPR arm had a 25% response rate and 16 evaluable patients in the placebo arm had a 44% response rate ($p = NS$). At 12 mo, 14 evaluable patients in the 4-HPR arm had a 14% response rate and 16 evaluable patients in the placebo arm had a 50% response rate ($p = 0.04$). No significant toxicity was experienced.

Alvarez et al. recently reported the randomized double-blind trial results of the pan-retinoid receptor agonist 9-*cis*-retinoic acid (9-*cis*-RA) in patients with histologic evidence of CIN 2/3 *(29)*. Patients were randomized to receive either high (50 mg) or low (25 mg)

Table 3
Polyamine Synthesis Inhibitor Chemoprevention Trials for Cervical Dysplasia

Author, year	Number of patients	Agent/dose	Placebo	Disease	Efficacy
Mitchell,1998	30	DFMO/1.0–0.06 g/m²/d	None	CIN 3	Yes

doses of 9-*cis*-RA or placebo daily for 12 wk. Compliance and side effects were monitored at various time points during therapy. At completion of therapy, all patients underwent a loop procedure. Histology of pretreatment biopsies was compared to that of loop specimens. Headache was the most common clinical side effect, and was experienced more frequently (74%) in the high-dose 9-*cis*-RA group. Among 104 patients evaluable for efficacy, no statistical difference was found in rate of regression among placebo (32%), low-dose 9-cis-RA (32%), and high-dose 9-*cis*-RA (36%) groups (p = NS).

4.3. Polyamine Synthesis Inhibitor Chemoprevention Trials for Cervical Dysplasia (Table 3)

Polyamines are organic polycations known to play a role in various epithelial cell functions. α-Difluoromethylornithine (DFMO), a specific suicide inhibitor of ornithine decarboxylase (a key enzyme in polyamine biosynthesis), has shown antitumor activity in several animal models of cancer. Given this background, Mitchell et al. conducted a dose de-escalating Phase I trial of DFMO in patients with cervical dysplasia *(30)*. Thirty patients with biopsy-proven CIN 3 were assigned to one of five DFMO doses (1.0, 0.5, 0.25, 0.125, or 0.06 g/m²) given daily for 31 d. At completion of therapy, all patients underwent a loop procedure. Partial response (defined as downstaging of CIN 3 to CIN 1 or 2) occurred in 10 patients and a complete response (defined as resolution of CIN) in five patients.

5. EVALUATION OF SURROGATE ENDPOINT BIOMARKERS IN CERVICAL NEOPLASIA CHEMOPREVENTION TRIALS

5.1. Choosing Appropriate SEBs for Cervical Neoplasia Chemoprevention Trials

Excellent reviews have been published describing in detail potential surrogate endpoint biomarkers (SEBs) for application in the context of cervical cancer chemoprevention trials *(31,32)*. SEBs are used as intermediate indicators of a reduction in cancer incidence and should be easily measurable, differentially expressed in normal and abnormal tissues, appear at a well-defined

stage of carcinogenesis, associated with reasonable sensitivity, specificity, and accuracy, and modulated with a chemoprevention agent. Recommended SEBs generally fall into the broad categories of quantitative cytologic and histopathologic markers, proliferation markers, regulation markers, differentiation markers, general genomic instability markers, and tissue maintenance markers. Strong rationale exists for evaluating use of these markers as SEBs in cervical tissues. Most markers are applicable to various organ sites; some, such as the presence of HPV and HPV viral load, are more applicable to investigation in cervical tissues. Nevertheless, much remains to be done to validate these markers for use in cervical cancer chemoprevention trials. SEBs based on a molecular target or its downstream effects may be used as markers of tissue activity or responsiveness following intervention with a chemopreventive agent.

5.2. Issues Regarding Tissue Sample and Analysis in Cervical Neoplasia Clinical Trials

Selecting an area for biopsy requires consideration of lesion size, residual abnormality for assessing chemopreventive activity, and need for future biopsy. A biopsy that leaves little or no disease would render the patient inevaluable for any chemopreventive strategy. Colposcopic photographs before and after biopsy would be valuable in this context for objective assessment of response (spontaneous or induced).

5.3. Results of SEB Studies in Cervical Dysplasia Chemoprevention Trials (Table 4)

Comerci et al. reported on the effect of β-carotene with respect to induction of transforming growth factor (TGF)-β1 in 10 patients with CIN 2 treated in an unpublished randomized trial *(33)*. After treatment with β-carotene, a marked increase in TGF-β1 immunoreactivity was noted in all three epithelial layers (p = 0.003) and within the surrounding stromal cells (p = 0.024). No difference in degree of TGF-β1 immunoreactivity was noted between four patients whose disease regressed vs six patients who had stable disease.

Several publications have detailed the results of SEB analyses conducted in conjunction with a Phase I trial

Table 4
Assessment of Surrogate Endpoint Biomakers in Cervical Chemoprevention Trials

Author, year	Agent/placebo	Number of patients	SEB	Effect
Comerci, 1997	β–carotene/yes	10	TGF-β1	Increase in epithelium and stroma after therapy
Boiko, 1997	DFMO/No	25	Mean normalized summed absorbance ($\sigma\ OD_n$)	Reduction in responders
Poulin, 1999	DFMO/No	30	Morphometric index	Reduction in responders
Boiko, 1998	DFMO/No	22	EGFR	Downregulation away from basal layer in responders

of DFMO in patients with CIN 3 [30]. Preliminary image morphometric analysis of DFMO-treated patients detected a lower posttreatment mean nuclear grade in 12 of 14 samples ($p < 0.05$) and a decrease in the standard deviation of their nuclear grade distributions ($p < 0.01$) [34,35]. These findings were noted despite no histopathologic differences being observed. Subsequent studies by Boiko et al. demonstrated that, although both responders and nonresponders had an overall significant decrease in σOD_n, the responders' values dropped more than the nonresponders' values after DFMO treatment ($p = 0.02$) [36]. In a subsequent publication, Poulin et al. reported that the morphometric index specifically and consistently decreased in patients who responded to DFMO and was unchanged in patients who did not respond to DFMO treatment [37]. Last, Boiko et al. demonstrated that although overall levels of epidermal growth factor receptor (EGFR) expression were not modulated in DFMO-treated patients, responders showed a prominent downregulation of EGFR expression away from the basal layer [38]. Pretreatment EGFR expression levels were predictive for DFMO response.

5.4. Assessing HPV Status in Cervical Neoplasia Chemoprevention Trials (Table 5)

Given the role of HPV in cervical carcinogenesis, it would seem logical to consider the presence or absence of HPV and perhaps HPV viral load as potential biomarkers for chemoprevention trials. Indeed, two studies have done so. Fairley et al., using hybrid capture technology, noted no significant difference in HPV presence in β-carotene-treated vs placebo-treated atypia/CIN 1–2 patients [19]. Using polymerase chain reaction and Southern blot hybridization techniques, Romney et al. demonstrated resolution of HPV infection in CIN 1–3 patients with low oncogenic risk HPV types, but no

effect of β-carotene on HPV clearance [20]. No study has quantitated viral load as an endpoint.

6. PROSPECTS FOR FUTURE CERVICAL NEOPLASIA CHEMOPREVENTION TRIALS

6.1. Issues Regarding Trial Design for Investigating Chemoprevention Agents in Cervical Neoplasia

Recent commentary by Follen et al. points out flaws in the design of most published chemoprevention trials in cervical neoplasia [32]. Lack of a placebo-controlled group, underestimating spontaneous regression rates in biopsied CIN patients, inadequate sample size, lack of predefined endpoints, and utilizing Pap smears or colposcopic evaluations as endpoints, all contribute to making many trials uninformative. Given the natural regression rate of CIN and its response to relatively easy-to-administer therapies, Follen et al. propose that a chemoprevention agent should achieve a 40%–50% benefit over a placebo effect. These important insights need to be incorporated into future chemoprevention trial design.

6.2. Design of Chemopreventive Trials

Clinical trials must be designed with a realistic chance of demonstrating the chemopreventive agent's efficacy or lack thereof. The trial design has to recognize and account for the dynamic nature of changes in cervical mucosa, and the possibility of spontaneous or biopsy-induced regression. Therefore, trials must be of sufficient size to allow for this statistically. Phase I and IIA trials that explore potential for activity have to define up front if the trial endpoints are response or surrogate, and how changes in these will be interpreted statistically. Phase I/IIA trials are exploratory, dose-finding, and assess whether sufficient activity with

Table 5
Assessment of HPV in Cervical Chemoprevention Trials

Author, year	Agent/placebo	Number of patients	HPV assessment	Effect
Fairley, 1997	β-carotene/yes	117	Hybrid capture	None
Romney, 1997	β-carotene/yes	98	PCR, Southern blot	None

"acceptable" toxicity justifies larger-scale trials. Demonstration of appropriate activity over placebo controls is essential in well-designed Phase IIB and large randomized Phase III studies.

6.3. Potential Chemopreventive Strategies for Cervical Neoplasia

We are in the era of molecular targeting, where recognition of molecular aberrations in a neoplastic cell can potentially be exploited therapeutically. A note of caution is necessary here, however, as simply demonstrating a targetable molecular aberration is not sufficient to start clinical trials. Molecular changes may have clinical significance and be etiologically causative, or may be bystander effects. In addition, as has been emphasized, serious toxicity, even infrequently, is unacceptable in this patient population. Therefore the prerequisites are scientific rationale, availability of targeted therapy, and safety.

Several potential pathways can be targeted in cervical neoplasia. Some of these, such as modulating effects on the EGFR pathway, have not been previously studied. Also, variations of looking at old targets with new agents can be useful—for example, exploring the retinoid pathway or angiogenesis with cyclooxygenase (COX)-2 inhibitors. Although rationale, targets, or therapeutic agents may be neatly arranged into different mechanistic groups, there is considerable overlap and cross-talk within cells, with multiple pathways being affected.

The EGFR is a transmembrane glycoprotein; once activated by a growth stimulus, it starts a signal transduction cascade of biochemical and physiological changes that culminate in DNA synthesis and cell division. There are compelling data that dysregulation of the EGFR signal transduction pathway plays a critical role in the process of tumor formation, growth, and metastasis. Oncogenic properties of EGFR may, at least in part, be mediated by stimulation of tumor angiogenesis through upregulating potent angiogenesis growth factors such as vascular endothelial growth factor (VEGF) or vascular permeability factor (VPF). These genetic changes may cooperate with epigenetic/environmental effects such as hypoxia to maximally stimulate VEGF/VPF expression (Fig. 1) (39).

In cervical cancer, HPV16 and E6/E7 oncoproteins may affect transcriptional regulation of EGFR by increasing EGFR promoter activity (40). EGFR is overexpressed in 30–60% of cancers of the cervix (41). Although EGFR expression and serum EGFR are not predictive for survival, EGFR activation may influence progression and resistance in vitro (41).

Selective COX-2 inhibitors such as refecoxib or celecoxib have generated interest. COX-2 is an inducible enzyme required in converting prostaglandins (PGs) from arachidonic acid. Overexpression of COX-2 has been linked to promotion of tumorigenesis, resistance to apoptosis, and abnormal cell cycle regulation. COX-2 is inducible by oncogenes ras and scr, interleukin (IL)-1, hypoxia, benzo[a]pyrene, ultraviolet light, EGF, TGF-β, and tumor necrosis factor α. COX-2 synthesizes prostaglandin E2 (PGE2), which stimulates bcl-2 and inhibits apoptosis, and induces IL-6, which enhances haptoglobin synthesis. Data in the literature show a link between COX-2 activity and hypoxia-induced angiogenesis in cancer. Angiogenesis, a complex process with a number of regulatory factors at work, is required for both tumor growth and metastasis. It has been studied as a potential area of cancer therapy since Folkman's work in the 1970s (42). Additionally, early studies show promising activity using COX-2 inhibitors for secondary chemoprevention in familial adenomatous polyposis (43).

Little is known about COX-2 expression in gynecological malignancies. Increased expression of COX-2 was described in high-grade squamous intraepethelial lesions (HSIL) and invasive carcinoma of the cervix (44). By immunoblot analysis, COX-2 was detected in 12 of 13 cases of cervical cancer but was undetectable in normal cervical tissue (45). Immunohistochemistry revealed COX-2 in malignant epithelial cells. The mechanism by which COX-2 is upregulated in cervical cancer is unknown. The link in between the EGF pathway and COX-2 was investigated. Treatment with EGF markedly induced COX-2 protein, COX-2 mRNA, and stimulated COX-2 promoter activity. COX-2 induction

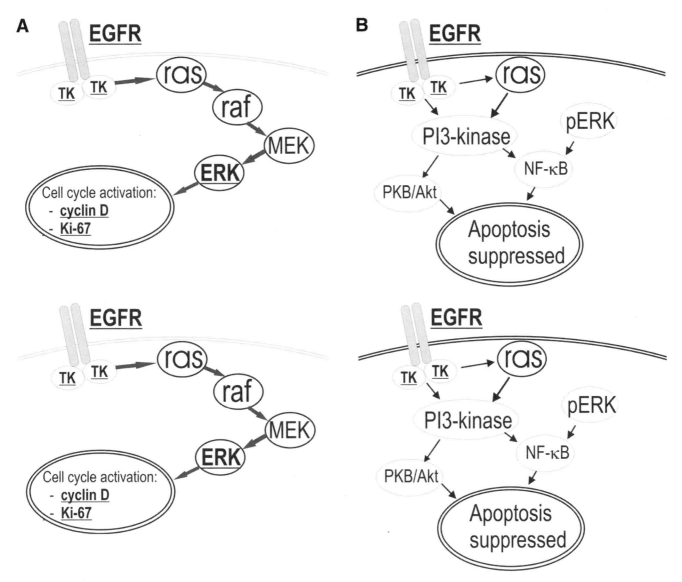

Fig. 1. (A) Ras/raf/ERK pathway: Potentially, this pathway can promote tumor growth both by stimulating cell cycle activation and by suppressing apoptosis. Inhibition of ras/raf/ERK signaling may contribute to cutaneous toxicity seen with EGFR inhibitors. **(B)** Anti-apoptotic pathways: Several mechanisms are proposed for suppression of apoptosis via EGFR signaling, including activation of the ras/raf/ERK pathway demonstrated here.

by EGF is suppressed by inhibitors of tyrosine kinase activity, phosphatidylinositol 3-kinase, mitogen-activated protein kinase (MAPK) kinase, and p38 MAPK. Moreover, overexpressing dominant-negative forms of extracellular signal-regulated kinase 1, c-Jun NH2-terminal kinase, p38, and c-Jun blocks EGF-mediated induction of COX-2 promoter activity. These findings suggest that deregulation of the EGF receptor signaling pathway may lead to enhanced COX-2 expression in cervical cancer. Ryu et al. studied stage IB cervical cancer patients treated with primary surgery, and found significantly increased COX-2 expression with lymph node or parametrial involvement (46). They suggested that COX-2 expression in these patients may downregulate apoptotic processes and enhance tumor invasion and metastasis.

Several of these potential strategies are being explored in Phase II clinical trials in patients with cervical neoplasia. The increasing characterization of molecular abnormalities leading to malignant transformation will hopefully allow implementation of screening strategies and simple therapies that will make a significant difference to invasive cervical cancer incidence in the future.

REFERENCES

1. Lubet RA, Steele VE, DeCoster R, et al. Chemopreventive effects of the aromatase inhibitor vorozole (R83842) in the methylnitrosourea-induced mammary cancer model. *Carcinogenesis* 1998;19:1345–1351.

2. Reddy BS, Hirose Y, Lubet R, et al. Chemoprevention of colon cancer by specific cyclooxygenase-2 inhibitor, celecoxib, administered during different stages of carcinogenesis. *Cancer Res* 2000;60:293–297.

3. Grubbs CJ, Lubet RA, Koki AT, et al. Celecoxib inhibits *N*-butyl-*N*-(4-hydroxybutyl)-nitrosamine induced urinary bladder cancers in male B6D2F1 mice and female Fischer-344 rats. *Cancer Res* 2000;60:5599–5602.

4. Manoharan K, Rao AR. Inhibitory actions of retinoic acid and butylated hydroxyanisole on cervical carcinogenesis induced by 3-methylcholanthrene in mouse. *Indian J Exp Biol* 1984;22:195–198.

5. Hussain SP, Jannu LN, Rao AR. Chemopreventive actions of garlic on methylcholanthrene-induced carcinogenesis in the uterine cervix of mice. *Cancer Lett* 1990;49:175–180.

6. Tewari KS, Taylor JA, Liao SY, et al. Development and assessment of a general theory of cervical carcinogenesis utilizing a severe combined immunodeficiency murine-human zenograft model. *Gynecol Oncol* 2000;77:137–148.

7. Arbeit JM, Howley PM, Hanahan D. Chronic estrogen-induced cervical and vaginal squamous carcinogenesis in human papillomavirus type 16 transgenic mice. *Proc Natl Acad Sci USA* 1996;93:2930–2935.

8. Jin L, Qi M, Chen DZ, et al. Indole-3-carbinol prevents cervical cancer in human papilloma virus type 16 (HPV16) transgenic mice. *Cancer Res* 1999;59:3991–3997.

9. Arbeit JM, Riley RR, Huey B, et al. Difluoromethylornithine chemoprevention of epidermal carcinogenesis in K14-HPV16 transgenic mice. *Cancer Res* 1999;59:3610–3620.

10. Mitchell MF, Hittelman WN, Lotan R, et al. Chemoprevention trials in the cervix: design, feasibility, and recruitment. *Cancer* 1995;76:104–112.

11. Ruffin MT, Baron J. Recruiting subjects in cancer prevention and control studies. *J Cell Biochem Suppl* 2000;34:80–83.

12. Butterworth CE Jr, Hatch KD, Gore H, et al. Improvement in cervical dysplasia associated with folic acid therapy in users of oral contraceptives. *Am J Clin Nutr* 1982;35:73–82.

13. Butterworth CE Jr, Hatch KD, Soong SJ, et al. Oral folic acid supplementation for cervical dysplasia: a clinical intervention trial. *Am J Obstet Gynecol* 1992;166:803–809.

14. Butterworth CE Jr, Hatch KD, Macaluso M, et al. Folate deficiency and cervical dysplasia. *JAMA* 1992;267:528–533.

15. Childers JM, Chu J, Voigt LF, et al. Chemoprevention of cervical cancer with folic acid: a Phase III Southwest Oncology Group Intergroup study. *Cancer Epidemiol Biomarks Prev* 1995;4:155–159.

16. de Vet HC, Knipschild PG, Wilebrad D, et al. The effect of beta-carotene on the regression and progression of cervical dysplasia: a clinical experiment. *J Clin Epidemiol* 1991;44:273–283.

17. Manetta A, Schubbert T, Chapman J, et al. beta-Carotene treatment of cervical intraepithelial neoplasia: a phase II study. *Cancer Epidemiol Biomarkers Prev* 1006;5:929–932.

18. Keefe KA, Schell MJ, Brewer C, et al. A randomized, double blind, Phase III trial using oral b-carotene supplementation for women with high-grade cervical intraepithelial neoplasia. *Cancer Epidemiol Biomarkers Prev* 2001;10:1029–1035.

19. Fairley CK, Tabrizi SN, Chen S, et al. Randomized double-blind trial of beta-carotene and vitamin C in women with minor cervical abnormalities. *Int J Gynecol Cancer* 1996;6:225–230.

20. Romney SL, Ho GY, Palan PR, et al. Effects of beta-carotene and other factors on outcome of cervical dysplasia and human papilloma virus infection. *Gynecol Oncol* 1997;65:483–492.

21. Mackerras D, Irwig L, Simpson JM, et al. Randomized double-blind trial of beta-carotene and vitamin C in women with minor cervical abnormalities. *Br J Cancer* 1999;79:1448–1453.

22. Bell MC, Crowley-Nowick P, Bradlow HL, et al. Placebo-controlled trial of indole-3-carbinol in the treatment of CIN. *Gynecol Oncol* 2000;78:123–129.

23. Surwit EA, Graham V, Droegemueller W, et al. Evaluation of topically applied trans-retinoic acid in the treatment of cervical intraepithelial lesions. *Am J Obstet Gynecol* 1982;143:821–823.

24. Meyskens FL Jr, Graham V, Chvapil M, et al. A Phase I trial of beta-all-trans-retinoic acid delivered via a collagen sponge and a cervical cap for mild or moderate intraepithelial cervical neoplasia. *J Natl Cancer Inst* 1983;71:921–925.

25. Romney SL, Dwyer A, Slagle S, et al. Chemoprevention of cervix cancer: Phase I–II: a feasibility study involving the topical vaginal administration of retinyl acetate gel. *Gynecol Oncol* 1985;20:109–119.

26. Weiner SA, Surwit EA, Graham VE, Meyskens FL Jr. A Phase I trial of topically applied trans-retinoic acid in cervical dysplasia-clinical efficacy. *Invest New Drugs* 1986;4:241–244.

27. Meyskens FL Jr, Surwit E, Moon TE, et al. Enhancement of regression of cervical intraepithelial neoplasia II (moderate dysplasia) with topically applied all-*trans*-retinoic acid: a randomized trial. *J Natl Cancer Inst* 1994;86:539–543.

28. Follen M, Atkinson EN, Schottenfeld D, et al. A randomized clinical trial of 4-hydroxyphenylretinamide for high-grade squamous intraepithelial lesions of the cervix. *Clin Cancer Res* 2001;7:3356–3365.

29. Alvarez RD, Conner MG, Weiss HL, et al. The efficacy of 9-*cis* retinoic acid as a chemopreventive agent for cervical dysplasia: results of a randomized double blind clinical trial. *Cancer Epidemiol Biomarkers Prev* 2003;12:114–119.

30. Mitchell MF, Tortolero-Luna G, Lee JJ, et al. Phase I dose de-escalation trial of alpha-difluoromethylornithine in patients with grade 3 cervical intraepithelial neoplasia. *Clin Cancer Res* 1998;4:303–310.

31. Mitchell MF, Hittelman WN, Lotan R, et al. Chemoprevention trials and surrogate end point biomarkers in the cervix. *Cancer* 1995;76:1956–1977.

32. Follen M, Schotenfeld D. Surrogate endpoint biomarkers and their modulation in cervical chemoprevention trials. *Cancer* 2001;91:1758–1776.

33. Comerci JT Jr, Runowicz CD, Fields AL, et al. Induction of transforming growth factor beta-1 in cervical intraepithelial neoplasia in vivo after treatment with beta-carotene. *Clin Cancer Res* 1997;3:157–160.

34. Bacus JW. Cervical cell recognition and morphometric grading by image analysis. *J Cell Biochem* 1995;23:33–42.

35. Bacus JW, Boone CW, Bacus JV, et al. Image morphometric nuclear grading of intraepithelial neoplastic lesions with applications to cancer chemoprevention trials. *Cancer Epidemiol Biomarkers Prev* 1999;8:1087–1094.

36. Boiko IV, Mitchell MF, Pandey DK, et al. DNA image cyto-metric measurement as a surrogate end point biomarker in a phase I trial of alpha-difluoromethylornithine for cervical intraepithelial neoplasia. *Cancer Epidemiol Biomarkers Prev* 1997;6:849–855.

37. Poulin N, Boiko I, MacAulay C, et al. Nuclear morphometry as an intermediate endpoint biomarker in chemoprevention of cervical carcinoma using alpha-difluoromethylornithine. *Cytometry* 1999;38:214–223.

38. Boiko IV, Mitchell MF, Hu W, et al. Epidermal growth factor receptor expression in cervical intraepithelial neoplasia and its modulation during an alpha-difluoromethylornithine chemoprevention trial. *Clin Cancer Res* 1998;4:1383–1391.

39. Petit AM, Rak J, Hung MC, et al. Neutralizing antibodies against epidermal growth factor and ErbB-2/neu receptor tyrosine kinases down-regulate vascular endothelial growth factor production by tumor cells in vitro and in vivo: angio-genic implications for signal transduction therapy of solid tumors. *Am J Pathol* 1997;151:1523–1530.

40. Sizemore N, Choo CK, Eckert RL, Rorke EA. Transcriptional regulation of the EGF receptor promoter by HPV16 and retinoic acid in human ectocervical epithelial cells. *Exp Cell Res* 1998;244:349–356.

41. Donato NJ, Perez M, Kang H, et al. EGF receptor and p21WAF1 expression are reciprocally altered as ME-180 cervical carcinoma cells progress from high to low cisplatin sensitivity. *Clin Cancer Res* 2000;6:193–202.

42. Folkman, J. Tumor angiogenesis: therapeutic implications. N Engl J Med 1971;285:1182–1186.

43. Steinbach G, Lynch PM, Phillips RK, et al. The effect of celecoxib, a cyclooxygenase-2 inhibitor, in familial adeno-matous polyposis. *N Engl J Med* 2000;342:1946–1952.

44. Sukumvanich P, Cost M, Deal K, et al. Cyclooxygenase-2 expression in normal cervical epithelium and cervical neo-plasia. *Gynecol Oncol* 2001;80:290–291.

45. Kulkarni S, Rader JS, Zhang F, et al. Cyclooxygenase-2 is overexpressed in human cervical cancer. *Clin Cancer Res* 2001;7:429–434.

46. Ryu HS, Chang KH, Yang HW, et al. High cyclooxygenase-2 expression in stage IB cervical cancer with lymph node metastasis or parametrial invasion. *Gynecol Oncol* 2000;76: 320–325.

33 Immunoprevention of Cervical Cancer

John T. Schiller, PhD, *and Douglas R. Lowy,* MD

CONTENTS

1. INTRODUCTION

Cervical cytological screening, as first proposed by Papanicolaou, is one of the most successful cancer prevention strategies ever devised *(1)*. Nevertheless, cervical cancer is the second or third most frequent cancer and cause of cancer deaths in women *(2)*. This paradox has arisen because many of the world's women either do not have access to an effective screening program or do not properly comply with an existing program *(1)*. The problem of access is particularly acute in developing countries, where the high cost of screening limits access to only the wealthiest subset of women *(3)*. Consequently, cervical cancer is the leading cause of cancer death in many developing countries *(2)*. Countries with effective screening programs spend a substantial amount of health care financial resources on them. The cost of screening and follow-up of abnormal Papanicolaou (Pap) smears was recently estimated to cost more than $5 billion annually in the United States alone (National HPV & Cervical Cancer Prevention Resource Center; http://www.ashastd.org/hpvccrc/background.html). Thus cervical cancer prevention strategies that are both more accessible and acceptable to women need to be developed.

Infection with certain types of sexually transmitted human papillomaviruses (HPVs) is the central cause of cervical cancer, providing an opportunity to implement new approaches to cervical cancer prevention *(4)*. One approach is to screen directly for high-risk HPV infec-

tions of the cervix *(5,6)*. This strategy is based on the finding that 99% of cervical cancers are HPV DNA positive *(7)*, and that persistent cervical HPV DNA is the major risk factor for progression to cervical neoplasia *(8–10)*. Detection of high-risk HPV DNA has been extensively evaluated as a substitute for or adjunct to cervical cytologic screening. HPV DNA-based screening strategies appear to have higher sensitivity and greater reproducibility relative to Pap screening, although they generally have lower specificity for neoplastic disease, especially in younger women *(6,11,12)*. Because of the effort needed to train competent cytologists and the limited number of samples that a cytologist can process daily, it also may be easier to introduce an effective HPV DNA-based program in settings that currently lack comprehensive screening programs. However, it is unclear whether HPV DNA screening can be made affordable to women in the lowest resource settings that are at highest risk of cervical cancer *(3)*. In addition, since HPV DNA testing would require collection of a cervical specimen, it is unlikely to increase compliance among women who choose not to participate in Pap screening programs.

The causal link between HPV infection and cervical cancer also raises the possibility that cervical cancer could be prevented with an antiviral vaccine. Vaccines against other viral diseases are among the most effective and inexpensive public health intervention measures *(13)*, leading to eradication of smallpox and control of polio, rubella, and several other viral infections. It is widely believed that vaccines against the major HPV

From: Cancer Chemoprevention, Volume 2: Strategies for Cancer Chemoprevention
Edited by: G. J. Kelloff, E. T. Hawk, and C. C. Sigman © Humana Press Inc., Totowa, NJ

types that cause cervical cancer offer the best hope for cervical cancer prevention in developing countries (*see* http://www.who.int/vaccines-documents/DocsPDF99/ www9914.pdf for a World Health Organization report). Effective HPV vaccines could reduce incidence, cost and morbidity associated with prevention programs in developed countries as well.

Two distinct classes of vaccines could be used to prevent cervical cancer *(14)*. The first type would prevent HPVs from infecting the cervix. Antibodies are believed to be the main immune effectors of immunoprophylaxis for other viral vaccines *(15)*. Vaccine-induced antibodies to virion surface epitopes bind the virions and prevent them from infecting target cells in a process called virus neutralization. Since it takes years to decades for primary HPV infection to progress to cancer, it should be possible to prevent cervical cancer by inducing regression of established HPV-induced lesions before they undergo malignant progression *(16)*. Immune effector mechanisms for therapeutic vaccines are largely cell-mediated responses rather than antibody-dependent. It is very unlikely that viral antibodies will induce regression of HPV lesions, since HPVs are nonenveloped viruses that assemble in the nucleus, and HPV infection does not appear to expose sufficient numbers of intact viral proteins on the cell surface to serve as targets for antibody-mediated effector mechanisms. Both prophylactic and therapeutic HPV vaccines are under active development for cervical cancer prevention *(17)*. In addition, some strategies attempt to generate both neutralizing antibodies and cell-mediated responses to non-virion HPV proteins, thereby generating combined prophylactic/therapeutic vaccines.

2. PROPHYLACTIC VACCINES

Most currently licensed viral vaccines are based on live attenuated virus strains or inactivated virus preparations *(13)*. These approaches are not reasonable for developing prophylactic HPV vaccines. As papillomaviruses cannot be efficiently grown in cultured cells *(18)*, the viruses cannot be mass-produced, even if they could be attenuated. Also, HPVs that cause cervical cancer encode oncogenes in their genomes *(19)*. The theoretical possibility of vaccine-induced carcinogenesis would preclude using a live or inactivated virus vaccine that contained the viral genome in healthy young people, the probable target group for a prophylactic vaccine.

2.1. Preclinical Studies

Early studies in animal models made it clear that neutralizing antibodies to papillomaviruses primarily recognized conformation-dependent epitopes on the virion surface. Although intact virions were excellent inducers of neutralizing antibodies, subunit vaccines based on denatured forms of the L1 major virion protein, or peptides thereof, were not *(20,21)*. However, approx 10 yr ago, papillomavirus L1s were found to assemble into virus-like particles (VLPs) if they were expressed from a strong heterologous promoter in the absence of all other viral gene products *(22)*. VLPs retain the structural features and high immunogenicity of authentic virions, but are noninfectious since they are composed of a single viral protein and contain no viral genes. HPV VLPs have been produced in mammalian and insect cells, yeast, and even to a limited extent in bacteria *(23–27)*. Prophylactic vaccine candidates now in clinical trials are based on L1 VLPs.

Papillomavirus infections are species-restricted, and experimental inoculation of HPVs does not induce productive infection or disease in any animal model *(28)*. Therefore, prophylactic vaccine studies have involved VLPs from animal papillomaviruses and their corresponding host species. Unfortunately, no domestic mouse papillomavirus has been isolated. This has limited using the best-characterized immune response model in prophylactic papillomavirus vaccine studies. Prevention of experimental papillomavirus infection after VLP vaccination has been demonstrated in rabbit, dog, and cow models using L1 VLPs and challenge virus of cottontail rabbit papillomavirus, canine oral papillomavirus, and bovine papillomavirus type 4, respectively *(29–32)*. Low-microgram doses of VLPs produced excellent protection against high-dose challenge with the homologous virus type in each experimental model, and adjuvant was not required. However, no protection was seen after vaccination with a heterologous VLP type. Protection could be passively transferred to naive animals via serum, indicating that neutralizing antibodies alone can prevent infection.

A number of studies have addressed the question of whether antibodies (raised in mice or rabbits) against VLPs of one HPV type will neutralize other HPV types in in vitro infectivity assays. The question of cross-protection is important because more than a dozen HPV types have been found repeatedly in cervical cancers. Cross-protective responses could greatly simplify vaccine development and manufacture. Unfortunately, cross-neutralizing antibodies were infrequently detected. Limited cross-neutralization was detected for some closely related types (e.g., HPV16/HPV31 and HPV18/HPV45), but the cross-neutralizing titers were always much lower than titers against the homologous type *(33–37)*. It therefore seems most likely that protection from VLP vaccines will be type-specific in people. However, types 16 and 18 are found in 70% of cervical cancers worldwide and these types, plus types 31 and 45, are found in more than 80% *(38)*. Therefore, a multivalent vaccine containing a limited number of VLP types could potentially prevent most cervical cancer. Two other HPVs, types 6 and 11, are found in most external genital warts, but are rarely found in cancers *(38,39)*.

2.2. Clinical Studies

Based on encouraging results of animal studies described above, several early-phase clinical trials of HPV L1 VLP vaccines were conducted. Three trials in healthy individuals have been published and the results of several others have been discussed at scientific meetings *(40–42)*. These trials consistently found that after three intramuscular injections, HPV VLPs were highly immunogenic and had low reactogenicity in people. One study, in which three 50-μg doses of HPV16 VLPs were administered without adjuvant, reported that vaccinees attained vaccine-specific serum IgG titers 40-fold greater than those generated by natural infection *(40)*. Vaccine-induced serum titers in humans were equal to those that gave excellent protection from virus challenge in animal models. However, no animal models involved natural sexual transmission of the papillomavirus to the female genital tract. Therefore, the relevance of this observation to protection in women is uncertain. An HPV6 VLP vaccine was also highly immunogenic and well tolerated in individuals with preexisting genital warts *(43)*.

HPV infections involved in cervical carcinogenesis are confined to genital tract epithelia and do not induce viremias *(44)*. Therefore, local genital tract mucosal antibodies, not serum antibodies, would be the mediators of protection from infection. However, serum neutralizing antibody levels are indirectly relevant to protection, because cervical mucus secretions in women contain large amounts of IgG, much of which is apparently transudated from the serum *(45)*. An unpublished clinical study, which supports previous studies in monkeys *(46)*, found substantial levels of VLP-specific IgG in the cervical secretions of women after intramuscular VLP vaccination (see http://www.IPVSoc.org for 19th International Papillomavirus Conference Abstract No. O52). Whether these titers of transudated antibodies will be sufficient to protect against sexual transmission of the virus can only be answered in upcoming efficacy trials.

Three large randomized placebo-controlled efficacy trials of HPV VLPs are in planning and initial recruitment stages *(47)*. Several thousand young women per study arm, mostly or entirely genital HPV DNA-negative, will be vaccinated and followed over the course of several years for the appearance of genital tract HPV infection as measured by sensitive DNA-based assays *(12)* and HPV-induced cervical neoplasia. The National Cancer Institute (NCI) will conduct an HPV16, and HPV18 VLP vaccine trial in Costa Rica in collaboration with the Costa Rican government *(48)* in the province of Guantecaste, the site of a long-term NCI-sponsored natural history study of HPV and cervical cancer. Current indications are that GlaxoSmithKline is planning a multicenter trial of a bivalent HPV16/18 VLP vaccine. Merck appears to be entering a multicenter trial of a tetravalent vaccine containing VLPs of types 6, 11, 16, and 18. The Merck vaccine could therefore potentially prevent two distinct genital HPV-related diseases, cervical cancer, and genital warts. Vaccine for NCI and GlaxoSmithKline trials is produced in L1 recombinant baculovirus-expressing insect cells, and the Merck vaccine is derived from L1-expressing yeast. All will be administered in three intramuscular injections in alum-based adjuvants.

Appropriate endpoints for the above efficacy trials are currently being debated. For ethical reasons, cervical cancer, the ultimate endpoint of interest, cannot be used in trials with active follow-up. Also, it generally takes decades for primary infections to progress to cervical cancer *(16)*. High-grade cervical dysplasia, designated histologically as cervical intraepithelial neoplasia grade 3 (CIN 3) and cytologically as high-grade squamous intraepithelial neoplasia, may be a preferred surrogate endpoint. It is widely accepted as the immediate precursor to cervical cancer and is itself a treatable disease. Current standard of care dictates removal of high-grade lesions; ablative treatment of the lesion is generally effective and well tolerated *(49)*. However, only a small percentage of incident infections by oncogenic HPVs progress to high-grade dysplasia, generally taking years to do so *(16)*. Using high-grade dysplasia as a primary endpoint would necessitate a large long-term trial, which could delay implementation of an effective vaccine. Because follow-up of vaccinees will be expensive, it could overtax the resources needed for conducting efficacy trials. Also, during the trials, standard of care could evolve to the point where it would be considered inappropriate to follow low-grade dysplasias that contain oncogenic HPVs. Practical considerations suggest that low-grade cervical dysplasia, a frequent and relatively rapid outcome of persistent oncogenic

HPV infection, would be the preferred clinical endpoint. However, most low-grade dysplasias regress spontaneously and are not generally considered to need treatment *(16)*. In addition, intralaboratory consistency of this diagnosis can be problematic *(50)*. Finally, there is controversy in the literature over what percentage of high-grade cervical dysplasias may develop de novo without going through a detectable low-grade intermediate *(51)*. Using the intermediate position of CIN 2 and CIN 3 (i.e., intermediate and advanced cervical dysplasias) as a clinical endpoint has also been suggested (http://www.fda.gov/ohrms/dockets/ac/01/transcripts/3805t2_02.pdf). This could decrease trial size and length compared with using CIN 3 as an endpoint. However, there is disagreement over whether CIN 2 is a biologically distinct entity, and if so, what criteria distinguish it from CIN 1 and CIN 3.

Persistent cervical HPV DNA is also being considered as a virologic endpoint for efficacy trials. In contrast to histologic or cytologic endpoints, standardized assays have been developed to reliably measure type-specific HPV DNA with a minimum of intralaboratory variation *(12)*. Also, persistent HPV DNA of an oncogenic HPV type is the strongest predictor of progression to high-grade cervical dysplasia *(8–10)*. However, the length of time that distinguishes low-risk transient infections from persistent infections with a high probability of progression is not precisely known *(52)*. For practical purposes, infection by the same type for at least 1 yr will be operationally defined as persistent in the NCI trial. It is likely that most if not all trials will assess protection from incident infection by the types included in the vaccine, as measured in a PCR-based assay for genital tract HPV DNA. The trials may be stopped if substantial protection from incident infection is not found, as it is unlikely that an L1 VLP vaccine would protect against cervical cancer if it did not provide protection from initial viral infection.

2.3. Implementation Issues

It may seem premature to consider issues involving distribution of a vaccine that has not yet been proven to work. Nevertheless, several issues should be carefully considered at this point to ensure the broadest and most rapid implementation if or when a successful vaccine becomes available. Some issues arise from vaccination programs that seek to protect against a sexually transmitted disease (STD). Prospective studies indicate that high-risk HPV infections are often acquired soon after initiating sexual activity *(53)*.

Since there is no indication that an L1 VLP vaccine will induce regression of established papillomavirus-induced lesions *(29)*, it will be necessary to vaccinate adolescents or preadolescents before the onset of sexual activity. There is currently no established program of pediatric clinic visits by young people that would be compatible with a series of three vaccinations within a 6-mo interval. It is uncertain what percentage of parents would be sufficiently motivated to take their children to a clinic for the vaccination series. It is unclear how much disincentive it would be to parents that the vaccine targets an STD. Emphasizing the anticancer aspects of the program rather than the anti-STD ones may be advantageous. But this possibility needs to be more rigorously assessed.

Should boys as well as girls be vaccinated? It seems reasonable to expect that, on a population basis, an STD vaccine will more effectively prevent cervical infections in women if genital infection is prevented in both sexes. However, many uncertainties remain *(54)*. First, transmission dynamics for genital HPV infections are poorly understood. It is possible that maximum coverage in women may be more effective than partial coverage of both sexes for reducing prevalence rates in both men and women. Second, it is unclear whether a vaccine that is effective in preventing HPV infection in women will be equally effective in men. The natural history of genital HPV infection in men is less well understood than in women. It is possible that women will be protected because their genital mucosa are bathed in transudated IgG, but this may not be the case for infection sites of the male genitalia that are critical for transmission *(45)*. No large-scale vaccine trials of men appear to be planned.

A third major implementation issue is access to vaccine in low-resource settings. Most cervical cancer deaths occur in underdeveloped countries or among poorer women in industrialized countries *(2)*. Unfortunately, current vaccine candidates have less than ideal characteristics for distribution to women most in need of them. The vaccines must be purified from cultured cells, making them expensive to produce. A vaccine that will likely require refrigeration and three separate injections will be expensive to distribute. Last, the target population of preadolescents is especially difficult to reach through current public health programs in developing countries. If HPV VLP-based vaccines are successful, it may be important to begin development of alternative vaccine candidates that are much less expensive to produce and distribute but can induce equally safe and protective immune

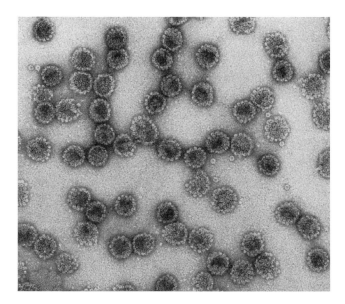

Fig. 1. Transmission electron micrograph of HPV 16L1 virus-like particles generated from recombinant baculovirus infected cells. Orginal magnification was × 36,000

responses to VLPs. Among several possibilities is a vaccine based on oral or upper respiratory tract administration of live bacteria expressing VLPs. Using HPV16 L1 recombinant *Salmonella typhimurium*, this strategy was successful in generating HPV16 neutralizing antibodies in mice *(27)* *(see* Fig. 1). Translation for human use would require generation of a recombinant strain of *Salmonella*, or some other mucosatropic bacteria, with a suitable combination of safety, immunogenicity, and capacity for VLP production. An alternative possibility would be to vaccinate via ingestion of crude yeast or plant extracts containing VLPs. Supporting this approach is the finding that purified VLPs are immunogenic after oral delivery in mice *(55)*. Generating consistently high-titer antibody responses after oral delivery of a sub-unit vaccine may require coexpression of a mucosal adjuvant. An L1 DNA vaccine would be easily generated and inexpensive to produce *(56)*. However, it would remain relatively expensive to deliver if injection was required.

3. THERAPEUTIC VACCINES

Vaccines to induce regression of HPV-induced pre-malignant lesions would be prophylactic with respect to cervical cancer. However, they would normally be considered therapeutic vaccines, since they would treat, rather than prevent, virus infection. Premalignant cervical lesions are attractive targets for tumor

immunotherapy for several reasons. First, they are routinely identified in Pap screening programs, which provide potential vaccinees for trials and eventually for wider implementation of a therapeutic vaccination program. Second, HPV-induced dysplasias generally take many years to progress to cervical cancer. This provides a long window of opportunity in which to attempt immunotherapeutic intervention. Third, the status of the lesion in response to immunotherapy can be monitored in a simple and noninvasive way by colposcopy. Fourth, there are well-established and effective ablative therapies for HPV-induced cervical dysplasias *(49)*. Therefore, women who fail immunotherapy would not be placed at undue risk of malignant progression. Fifth, viral oncogenes E6 and E7 are attractive tumor antigen targets for immunotherapy, as they are uniformly retained and expressed throughout the course of disease *(57)*. Introduced exogenously by viral infection, they are not subject to mechanisms of embryologic T cell tolerance relevant to self-tumor antigens being targeted for other cancers. However, because they are potentially oncogenic, vaccination strategies involving transfer of wild-type E6 or E7 genes will probably be unacceptable. This problem can be overcome by gene shuffling approaches in which overlapping oligonucleotides of the target gene, potentially representing all class I and II peptides, are randomly arranged *(58)*.

3.1. Studies in Animal Models

Because there is no animal challenge model that produces cervical neoplasia, studies of papillomavirus immunotherapy have taken two directions. First is an extensive series of mouse studies involving transplantable tumors expressing E6 and/or E7 of HPV16 or HPV18. Many immunotherapeutic strategies developed in recent years involving peptide, whole protein, naked DNA, viral-vectored, bacteria-vectored, or cell-based strategies for generating cell-mediated immunity (CMI) have been attempted using E6 or E7 as the target antigen (Table 1). It is beyond the scope of this review to detail the individual strategies, which are well covered in a number of reviews *(see 59,60)*. To summarize, many of these approaches were able to specifically prevent outgrowth of E6/E7-expressing tumor cells after subcutaneous challenge. A more limited set was also shown to induce regression of pre-established tumors. Relative effectiveness is difficult to judge, since most assays were semiquantitative, with few head-to-head comparisons of distinct approaches. In any event, the relevance of these results to HPV-induced neoplasia developing *in situ* at

Table 1
Therapeutic HPV Vaccine Studies in Mouse Tumor Models

Vaccine	References
Peptide	
Mouse class I specific 16 E7	*89*
Human class I specific 16 E7	*90*
Protein	
GST-16 E7	*91*
Mycobacterium bovis Hsp65–16 E7	*92*
16 L2-E6–E7	*93*
Cell-Based	
Dendritic Cells: 16 E7 peptide	*94*
Dendritic Cells: 16 E7 protein	*95*
Dendritic Cells: 16 E7 gene	*96,97*
E6/E7 Tumor Cells+IL-2 gene	*98*
E6/E7 Tumor Cells+IL-12 gene	*99*
Naked DNA	
Mutated 16 E7	*100*
Sig-Lamp1–16 E7	*101*
M. bovis Hsp70–16 E7	*102*
"Shuffled" 16 E7	*103*
Calreticulin- 16 E7	*104*
Viral vectors	
Vaccinia: 16 E6/E7	*105,106*
Adenovirus: 16 E7 peptides	*107*
Adenovirus: 16 E6 + E7	*108*
AAV: 16 E7 peptide	*109*
Bacterial vectors	
Streptococcus gordonii: 16 E7	*110*
M. bovis: 16 E7	*111*
Listeria: 16 E7	*112*

the cervix remains unclear. In a potentially more relevant mouse model of cervical carcinogenesis, HPV16 E6/E7 transgenic mice develop cervical neoplasia in response to estrogen treatment *(61)*. However, E6 and E7 in the transgenic mice are self rather than foreign antigens and are expressed throughout the tissue rather than focally as is the case after virus infection. Therefore, this is likely to be a stringent model for testing immunotherapy, and it has not yet been exploited in vaccine studies.

The second group of perhaps more biologically relevant studies involved attempts to induce regression of papillomas experimentally induced by corresponding animal papillomavirus. The most extensively studied model is cottontail rabbit papilloma virus (CRPV)-induced cutaneous papillomas of domestic

rabbits *(28)*. A number of studies have demonstrated protection from experimental virus challenge after vaccine-induced CMI to nonstructural (also called early) viral proteins. Good protection from DNA vaccination required either co-injection of multiple early genes or injection of the GM-CSF gene to potentiate immune responses to a single viral early protein *(62,63)*. It has been difficult to clearly demonstrate regression of well-established lesions with defined vaccines, despite the eventual spontaneous regression of a vast majority of papillomas in humans and experimental animals, almost certainly through CMI mechanisms. Vaccine-induced papilloma regression in rabbits was demonstrated 40 yr ago after injection of crude wart extracts *(64)*. However, it was only recently reported that gene gun vaccination of a combination of CRPV E1, E2, E6, and E7 DNA suppressed outgrowth of preestablished papillomas in most vaccinated rabbits, although they were not completely eradicated. Interestingly, progression to carcinoma was prevented in most rabbits *(65)*. A combination of the intralesional injection of the antiviral cidofovir and the above vaccine did induce regression of papillomas and prevent recurrences in the majority of rabbits *(66)*.

3.2. Clinical Studies

A number of clinical trials of HPV therapeutic vaccines, some involving cancer patients, have been completed. Vaccines based on HPV16 E7 peptides or HPV16 and 18 E6 and E7 expressed from recombinant vaccinia were tested *(67,68)*. Both types of vaccines generated detectable CMI to the viral proteins in some patients. Not unexpectedly, however, clinical responses were infrequently observed. Patients with high-grade cancers often have cancer- and/or therapy-induced general immunosuppression. Also, cervical cancer cells usually have defects in class I antigen presentation that can make them refractory to CD8 positive T cell-mediated cytotoxicity responses *(69–71)*. While the latter observation suggests that immunotherapy of cancers may be difficult, it is somewhat encouraging from the point of view of developing immunotherapies against premalignant lesions. Frequent loss of antigen presentation in advanced lesions implies that CMI is normally effective at some point during tumor development and that only those lesions that escape class I presentation have a good chance of progressing to cancers.

In contrast to cervical cancer patients, the immune status of women with premalignant cervical lesions is generally normal. Whether many high-grade premalignant lesions already have defects in viral antigen presentation *(72,73)* or induce a state of specific immune tolerance to the viral antigens *(74)* are important questions currently being investigated. Low-grade dysplasias are less likely to have defects in antigen presentation because they are genetically more stable than high-grade lesions. However, most low-grade dysplasias regress spontaneously and are not normally treated, whereas high-grade lesions tend to persist and are surgically treated *(53,75)*. Therefore, high-grade dysplasias are preferred targets for immunotherapy trials of HPV-induced premalignant disease. Two early-phase trials have been reported. One involved vaccination of patients with HPV16-positive high-grade cervical or vulvar dysplasias with an HPV16 E7 peptide vaccine *(76)*. The other trial involved vaccination of cervical and anal dysplasia patients with *Mycobacteria* heat shock protein 65-HPV16 E7 fusion proteins (see http://www.stressgen.com/publications/art13.htm for a summary of the unpublished results). In both studies, measurable cell-mediated responses were generated in most patients, and clinical responses, as indicated by regression or downgrading of lesions, were noted in a subset of vaccinees. Larger trials involving these vaccines and other vaccine strategies are likely to follow.

4. PROPHYLACTIC/THERAPEUTIC VACCINES

A vaccine that could prevent initial infection as well as induce regression of existing genital HPV-induced neoplasias is preferable *(14)*. Strictly therapeutic vaccines would be of limited use in low-resource settings, unless they were active against advanced cancers. This is because premalignant lesions and low-grade cervical cancers are not routinely diagnosed in poor women *(3)*. A strictly prophylactic vaccine would offer nothing to the millions of sexually active women with prevalent HPV infections who are most motivated to use an HPV vaccine. A combined prophylactic/therapeutic vaccine could be used in mass immunization campaigns involving both preadolescents and adults. Such an approach would also be expected to have the greatest and most immediate impact on transmission rates, thereby rapidly reducing both HPV prevalence and cervical cancer incidence in a population.

At least three possibilities exist for a combined prophylactic/therapeutic vaccine. First, as noted above, vaccination with combinations of early proteins or genes not only prevents the initial appearance of papillomas, but also induces regression of established lesions in the CRPV-rabbit model. It is possible that the

strategy of inducing CMI against early viral proteins would also be successful in preventing genital HPV neoplastic disease, if not infection. However, no successful viral vaccines are based solely on generating CMI responses.

Unfortunately, it is unlikely that L1 VLP vaccines will eliminate established lesions, despite their ability to induce potent cell-mediated responses and neutralize antibodies. This is because L1 is not detectably expressed in basal epithelial cells of the stratified squamous epithelium in which viral infection is normally maintained *(44)*. It is only expressed in the overlying terminally differentiated cells, shortly before the cells are sloughed off. This expression pattern has presumably evolved to avoid immune surveillance of the virion proteins *(14)*. So while L1 VLPs can induce potent antitumor responses against mouse tumors that have artificially been made to express L1 *(77)*, these types of responses will probably not benefit vaccinees with preexisting infections. A second possibility would combine L1 VLPs with a vaccine based on an E6/E7 protein or gene. This approach has not been critically evaluated in animal studies. Disinclination to test this approach may be due in part to the obvious increase in manufacturing complexity inherent in a mixed vaccine strategy. However, it is interesting to note that papillomavirus VLPs can induce phenotypic maturation of dendritic cells as antigen-presenting cells and thereby promote CMI responses *(78,79)*. It is therefore possible that they would act as an effective adjuvant for generating CMI to co-administered antigens.

The third approach for a combined prophylactic/therapeutic vaccine is to incorporate viral early polypeptides or genes into VLPs. Chimeric VLPs are generated from recombinant proteins composed of a papillomavirus virion protein fused to a target polypeptide. L1 chimeric VLPs were generated by fusion of up to 50 amino acids of E7 to the C-terminus of L1 *(80,81)*. L1/L2 chimeric VLPs were generated by coexpressing wild-type L1 with a recombinant L2 containing the entire 100 amino acids of E7 *(82)*. L2 is the minor papillomavirus virion protein and will coassemble with L1 into VLPs when coexpressed in the same cell *(24)*. Several studies have demonstrated that low-dose vaccination using chimeric VLPs without adjuvant induces potent CMI against transplantable tumors in mice *(81,82)*. Of potentially critical importance for a combined prophylactic/therapeutic vaccine, chimeric VLPs can fully retain the ability to generate neutralizing antibodies *(82,83)*. It is likely that the ability to strongly interact with dendritic cells and induce their phenotypic activation as antigen-presenting cells is largely responsible for the ability of chimeric VLPs to induce strong antitumor responses against that inserted polypeptide *(78,79)*. Based on these results, chimeric VLPs are currently the leading candidate for a combined vaccine. HPV16L1-E7 chimeric VLPs are being tested in a therapeutic trial of high-grade cervical dysplasia *(59)*.

A variation on chimeric VLPs is use of pseudovirions, which incorporate the target antigen, e.g., E7, into the VLPs as a DNA molecule rather than a polypeptide. In the pseudovirion vaccine strategy, the VLP acts as a gene delivery vehicle, as well as an adjuvant and inducer of neutralizing antibody. Several studies have demonstrated in vitro gene transfer via HPV pseudovirions *(34,84–86)*. However, only one study of pseudovirion vaccination has been reported *(87)*. It is encouraging that cytotoxic T cell responses could be detected after oral delivery of a relatively low dose of pseudovirions in mice. The pseudovirions were generated by disassembling VLPs in a test tube followed by reassembly in the presence of target DNA. Unfortunately, inability to generate large numbers of HPV pseudovirions by a scalable process limits investigation of this strategy in animal models and translation of this potentially attractive approach to human trials.

5. CONCLUSIONS

Vaccines to prevent genital tract infection by oncogenic HPVs and to treat premalignant lesions induced by these viruses are under active investigation. The first generation of prophylactic and therapeutic HPV vaccines is likely to undergo comprehensive clinical evaluation in the immediate future. Within the next 5 yr, we should have a good indication of whether these vaccines will effectively prevent cervical cancer, although definitive proof may take decades. There certainly are reasons to be optimistic, based on studies with animal papillomaviruses, early-phase clinical trials, and the success of a hepatitis B VLP vaccine in preventing hepatocellular carcinoma *(88)*. However, neither animal papillomavirus models nor HBV disease mimic HPV-induced cervical carcinogenesis, so the outcome of the trials remains quite uncertain.

It is unlikely that any current vaccine candidates, even if very effective, would obviate the need for effective cervical cancer screening programs in the future. Prophylactic vaccines will almost certainly be type-restricted, and first-generation vaccines will target at most 70–80% of cancer-causing HPV types. Also, women with prevalent HPV-induced neoplasia at the time of vaccination are not likely to be helped. Therapeutic vaccines would be effective only in conjunction with screening programs to identify women with premalignant lesions. Consequently, health care providers would need to continue promoting cervical cancer screening programs and convincing women to use them. Otherwise, we could be left with the paradoxical situation in which widespread introduction of an effective HPV vaccine in countries that currently have effective cervical cancer screening programs would increase cervical cancer rates by leading women to believe they no longer needed screening, rather than decrease cancer.

REFERENCES

1. Schneider V, Henry MR, Jimenez-Ayala M, et al. Cervical cancer screening, screening errors and reporting. *Acta Cytol* 2001;45:493–498.
2. Parkin DM, Bray F, Ferlay J, Pisani P. Estimating the world cancer burden: Globocan 2000. *Int J Cancer* 2001;94: 153–156.
3. Sankaranarayanan R, Budukh AM, Rajkumar R. Effective screening programmes for cervical cancer in low- and middle-income developing countries. *Bull WHO* 2001; 79:954–962.
4. Bosch FX, Lorincz A, Munoz N, et al. The causal relation between human papillomavirus and cervical cancer. *J Clin Pathol* 2002;55:244–265.
5. Schiffman M, Hildesheim A, Herrero R, Bratti C. Human papillomavirus testing as a screening tool for cervical cancer. *JAMA* 2000;283:2525–2526.
6. Kulasingam SL, Koutsky LA. Will new human papillomavirus diagnostics improve cervical cancer control efforts? *Curr Infect Dis Rep* 2001;3:169–182.
7. Walboomers JM, Jacobs MC, Manos MM, et al. Human papillomavirus is a necessary cause of invasive cervical cancer worldwide. *J Pathol* 1999;189:12–19.
8. Ho GY, Bierman R, Beardsley L, et al. Natural history of cervicovaginal papillomavirus infection in young women. *N Engl J Med* 1998;338:423–428.
9. Nobbenhuis MA, Walboomers JM, Helmerhorst TJ, et al. Relation of human papillomavirus status to cervical lesions and consequences for cervical-cancer screening: a prospective study. *Lancet* 1999;354:20–25.
10. Liaw KL, Hildesheim A, Burk RD, et al. A prospective study of human papillomavirus (HPV) type 16 DNA detection by polymerase chain reaction and its association with acquisition and persistence of other HPV types. *J Infect Dis* 2001; 183:8–15.
11. Cuzick J, Sasieni P, Davies P, et al. A systematic review of the role of human papilloma virus (HPV) testing within a cervical screening programme: summary and conclusions. *Br J Cancer* 2000;83:561–565.
12. Davies P, Kornegay J, Iftner T. Current methods of testing for human papillomavirus. *Best Pract Res Clin Obstet Gynaecol* 2001;15:677–700.
13. Ulmer JB, Liu MA. Ethical issues for vaccines and immunization. *Nat Rev Immunol* 2002;2:291–296.
14. Stern PL, Brown M, Stacey SN, et al. Natural HPV immunity and vaccination strategies. *J Clin Virol* 2000;19:57–66.

15. Robbins JB, Schneerson R, Szu SC. Hypothesis: serum IgG antibody is sufficient to confer protection against infectious diseases by inactivating the inoculum. *J Infect Dis* 1995;171: 1387–1398.

16. Schiffman MH, Burk RD. Human papillomaviruses. In: *Viral Infections in Humans.* Evans AS, Kaslow R, eds. Plenum Medical Book Company, New York, 1997; pp. 983–1023.

17. Frazer I. Strategies for immuoprophylaxis and immunotherapy of papillomaviruses. *Clin Dermatol* 1997;15:285–297.

18. Hagensee M, Galloway D. Growing human papillomaviruses and virus-like particles in the laboratory. *Papillomavirus Rep* 1993;4:121–124.

19. zur Hausen H. Immortalization of human cells and their malignant conversion by high risk human papillomavirus genotypes. *Semin Cancer Biol* 1999;9:405–411.

20. Jarrett WFH, O'Neill BW, Gaukroger JM, et al. Studies on vaccination against papillomaviruses: the immunity after infection and vaccination with bovine papillomaviruses of different types. *Vet Rec* 1990;126:473–475.

21. Jin XW, Cowsert L, Marshall D, et al. Bovine serological response to a recombinant BPV-1 major capsid protein vaccine. *Intervirology* 1990;31:345–354.

22. Kirnbauer R, Booy F, Cheng N, et al. Papillomavirus L1 major capsid protein self-assembles into virus-like particles that are highly immunogenic. *Proc Natl Acad Sci USA* 1992;89:12180–12184.

23. Hagensee ME, Yaegashi N, Galloway DA. Self-assembly of human papillomavirus type 1 capsids by expression of the L1 protein alone or by coexpression of the L1 and L2 capsid proteins. *J Virol* 1993;67:315–322.

24. Kirnbauer R, Taub J, Greenstone H, et al. Efficient self-assembly of human papillomavirus type 16 L1 and L1-L2 into virus-like particles. *J Virol* 1993;67:6929–6936.

25. Sasagawa T, Pushko P, Steers G, et al. Synthesis and assembly of virus-like particles of human papillomaviruses type 6 and type 16 in fission yeast Schizosaccharomyces pombe. *Virology* 1995;206:126–135.

26. Hofmann KJ, Neeper MP, Markus HZ, et al. Sequence conservation within the major capsid protein of human papillomavirus (HPV) type 18 and formation of HPV-18 virus-like particles in Saccharomyces cerevisiae. *J Gen Virol* 1996; 77:465–468.

27. Nardelli-Haefliger D, Roden RBS, Benyacoub J, et al. Human papillomavirus type 16 virus-like particles expressed in attenuated Salmonella typhimurium elicit mucosal and systemic neutralizing antibodies in mice. *Infect Immun* 1997,65:3328–3336.

28. Brandsma JL. Animal models of human-papillomavirus-associated oncogenesis. *Intervirology* 1994;37:189–200.

29. Breitburd F, Kirnbauer R, Hubbert NL, et al. Immunization with virus-like particles from cottontail rabbit papillomavirus (CRPV) can protect against experimental CRPV infection. *J Virol* 1995;69:3959–3963.

30. Christensen ND, Reed CA, Cladel NM, et al. Immunization with virus-like particles induces long-term protection of rabbits against challenge with cottontail rabbit papillomaviruses. *J Virol* 1996;70:960–965.

31. Suzich JA, Ghim S, Palmer-Hill FJ, et al. Systemic immunization with papillomavirus L1 protein completely prevents the development of viral mucosal papillomas. *Proc Natl Acad Sci USA* 1995;92:11553–11557.

32. Kirnbauer R, Chandrachud L, O'Neil B, et al. Virus-like particles of Bovine Papillomavirus type 4 in prophylactic and therapeutic immunization. *Virology* 1996;219:37–44.

33. Roden RBS, Hubbert NL, Kirnbauer R, et al. Assessment of the serological relatedness of genital human papillomaviruses by hemagglutination inhibition. *J Virol* 1996;70:3298–3301.

34. Roden RBS, Greenstone HL, Kirnbauer R, et al. In vitro generation and type-specific neutralization of a human papillomavirus type 16 virion pseudotype. *J Virol* 1996;70: 5875–5883.

35. White WI, Wilson SD, Bonnez W, et al. In vitro infection and type-restricted antibody-mediated neutralization of authentic human papillomavirus type 16. *J Virol* 1998;72:959–964.

36. Christensen ND, Kirnbauer R, Schiller JT, et al. Human papillomavirus types 6 and 11 have antigenically distinct strongly immunogenic conformationally dependent neutralizing epitopes. *Virology* 1994;205:329–335.

37. Touze A, Dupuy C, Mahe D, et al. Production of recombinant virus-like particles from human papillomavirus types 6 and 11, and study of serological reactivities between HPV 6, 11, 16 and 45 by ELISA: implications for papillomavirus prevention and detection. *FEMS Microbiol Lett* 1998;160:111–118.

38. Bosch FX, Manos MM, Munoz N, et al. Prevalence of human papillomavirus in cervical cancer: a worldwide prospective. *J Nat Cancer Inst* 1995;87:796–802.

39. Greer CE, Wheeler CM, Lander MB, et al. Human papillomavirus (HPV) type distribution and serological response to HPV 6 virus-like particle in patients with genital warts. *J Clin Microbiol* 1995;33:2058–2063.

40. Harro CD, Pang YY, Roden RB, et al. Safety and immunogenicity trial in adult volunteers of a human papillomavirus 16 L1 virus-like particle vaccine. *J Natl Cancer Inst* 2001;93: 284–292.

41. Evans TG, Bonnez W, Rose RC, et al. A Phase I study of a recombinant viruslike particle vaccine against human papillomavirus type 11 in healthy adult volunteers. *J Infect Dis* 2001;183:1485–1493.

42. Brown DR, Bryan JT, Schroeder JM, et al. Neutralization of human papillomavirus type II (HPV-II) by serum from women vaccinated with yeast-derived HPV-11 L1 virus-like particles: correlation with competitive radioimmunoassay titer. *J Infect Dis* 2001;184:1183–1186.

43. Zhang LF, Zhou J, Chen S, et al. HPV6b virus like particles are potent immunogens without adjuvant in man. *Vaccine* 2000;18:1051–1058.

44. Stubenrauch F, Laimins LA. Human papillomavirus life cycle: active and latent phases. *Semin Cancer Biol* 1999;9:379–386.

45. Mestecky J, Russell MW. Induction of mucosal immune responses in the human genital tract. FEMS *Immunol Med Microbiol* 2000;27:351–355.

46. Lowe RS, Brown DR, Bryan JT, et al. Human papillomavirus type 11 (HPV11) neutralizing antibodies in the serum and genital mucosal secretions of African green monkeys immunized with HPV-11 virus-like particles expressed in yeast. *J Infect Dis* 1997;176:1141–1145.

47. Connett H. HPV vaccine moves into late stage trials. *Nat Med* 2001;7:388.

48. Schiller JT, Hildesheim A. Developing HPV virus-like particle vaccines to prevent cervical cancer: a progress report. *J Clin Virol* 2000;19:67–74.

49. Montz FJ. Management of high-grade cervical intraepithelial neoplasia and low- grade squamous intraepithelial lesion and potential complications. *Clin Obstet Gynecol* 2000;43: 394–409.

50. Stoler MH, Schiffman M. Interobserver reproducibility of cervical cytologic and histologic interpretations: realistic

estimates from the ASCUS-LSIL Triage Study. *JAMA* 2001;285:1500–1505.

51. Kiviat NB, Koutsky LA. Do our current cervical cancer control strategies still make sense? *J Natl Cancer Inst* 1996;88:317–318.

52. Einstein MH, Burk RD. Persistent human papillomavirus infection: definitions and clinical implications. *Papillomavirus Rep* 2001;12:119–123.

53. Koutsky L. Epidemiology of genital human papillomavirus infection. *Am J Med* 1997;102:3–8.

54. Garnett GP, Waddell HC. Public health paradoxes and the epidemiological impact of an HPV vaccine. *J Clin Virol* 2000;19:101–111.

55. Rose RC, Lane C, Wilson S, et al. Oral vaccination of mice with human papillomavirus virus-like particles induces systemic virus-neutralizing antibodies. *Vaccine* 1999;17: 2129–2135.

56. Donnelly JJ, Martinez D, Jansen KU, et al. Protection against papillomavirus with a polynucleotide vaccine. *J Infect Dis* 1996;173:314–320.

57. zur Hausen H. Papillomaviruses in human cancers. *Proc Assoc Am Physicians* 1999;111:581–587.

58. Osen W, Peiler T, Ohlschlager P, et al. A DNA vaccine based on a shuffled E7 oncogene of the human papillomavirus type 16 (HPV 16) induces E7-specific cytotoxic T cells but lacks transforming activity. *Vaccine* 2001;19:4276–4286.

59. Gissmann L, Osen W, Muller M, Jochmus I. Therapeutic vaccines for human papillomaviruses. *Intervirology* 2001;44: 167–175.

60. Da Silva DM, Eiben GL, Fausch SC, et al. Cervical cancer vaccines: emerging concepts and developments. *J Cell Physiol* 2001;186:169–182.

61. Arbeit JM, Howley PM, Hanahan D. Chronic estrogen-induced cervical and vaginal squamous carcinogenesis in human papillomavirus type 16 transgenic mice. *Proc Natl Acad Sci USA* 1996;93:2930–2935.

62. Leachman SA, Tigelaar RE, Shlyankevich M, et al. Granulocyte-macrophage colony-stimulating factor priming plus papillomavirus E6 DNA vaccination: effects on papilloma formation and regression in the cottontail rabbit papillomavirus–rabbit model. *J Virol* 2000;74:8700–8708.

63. Han R, Reed CA, Cladel NM, Christensen ND. Immunization of rabbits with cottontail rabbit papillomavirus E1 and E2 genes: protective immunity induced by gene gun-mediated intracutaneous delivery but not by intramuscular injection. *Vaccine* 2000;18:2937–2944.

64. Evans CA, Gorman LR, Ito Y, Weiser RS. Antitumor immunity in the Shope papilloma-carcinoma complex of rabbits. Papilloma regression induced by homologous and autologous tissue vaccines. *J Natl Cancer Inst* 1962;29: 277–285.

65. Han R, Cladel NM, Reed CA, et al. DNA vaccination prevents and/or delays carcinoma development of papillomavirus-induced skin papillomas on rabbits. *J Virol* 2000; 74:9712–9716.

66. Christensen ND, Han R, Cladel NM, Pickel MD. Combination treatment with intralesional cidofovir and viral-DNA vaccination cures large cottontail rabbit papillomavirus-induced papillomas and reduces recurrences. *Antimicrob Agents Chemother* 2001;45:1201–1209.

67. Borysiewicz LK, Fiander A, Nimako M, et al. A recombinant vaccinia virus encoding human papillomavirus types 16 and 18, E6 and E7 proteins as immunotherapy for cervical cancer. *Lancet* 1996;347:1523–1527.

68. Adams M, Borysiewicz L, Fiander A, et al. Clinical studies of human papilloma vaccines in pre-invasive and invasive cancer. *Vaccine* 2001;19:2549–2556.

69. Connor ME, Stern PL. Loss of MHC class-1 expression in cervical carcinomas. *Int J Cancer* 1990;46:1029–1034.

70. Brady CS, Bartholomew JS, Burt DJ, et al. Multiple mechanisms underlie HLA dysregulation in cervical cancer. *Tissue Antigens* 2000;55:401–411.

71. Evans M, Borysiewicz LK, Evans AS, et al. Antigen processing defects in cervical carcinomas limit the presentation of a CTL epitope from human papillomavirus 16 E6. *J Immunol* 2001;167:5420–5428.

72. Bontkes HJ, Walboomers JM, Meijer CJ, et al. Specific HLA class I down-regulation is an early event in cervical dysplasia associated with clinical progression. *Lancet* 1998;351: 187–188.

73. Abdel-Hady ES, Martin-Hirsch P, Duggan-Keen M, et al. Immunological and viral factors associated with the response of vulval intraepithelial neoplasia to photodynamic therapy. *Cancer Res* 2001;61:192–196.

74. Doan T, Herd K, Street M, et al. Human papillomavirus type 16 E7 oncoprotein expressed in peripheral epithelium tolerizes E7-directed cytotoxic T-lymphocyte precursors restricted through human (and mouse) major histocompatibility complex class I alleles. *J Virol* 1999;73:6166–6170.

75. Schiffman MH, Brinton LA. The epidemiology of cervical carcinogenesis. *Cancer* 1995;76:1888–1901.

76. Muderspach L, Wilczynski S, Roman L, et al. A Phase I trial of a human papillomavirus (HPV) peptide vaccine for women with high-grade cervical and vulvar intraepithelial neoplasia who are HPV 16 positive. *Clin Cancer Res* 2000;6:3406–3416.

77. De Bruijn MLH, Greenstone HL, Vermeulen H, et al. L1-specific protection from tumor challenge elicited by HPV16 virus-like particles. *Virology* 1998;250:371–376.

78. Lenz P, Day PM, Pang YS, et al. Papillomavirus-like particles induce acute activation of dendritic cells. *J Immunol* 2001;166:5346–5355.

79. Rudolf MP, Fausch SC, Da Silva DM, Kast WM. Human dendritic cells are activated by chimeric human papillomavirus type-16 virus-like particles and induce epitope-specific human T cell responses in vitro. *J Immunol* 2001;166:5917–5924.

80. Muller M, Zhou J, Reed TD, et al. Chimeric papillomavirus-like particles. *Virology* 1997;234:93–111.

81. Peng S, Frazer IH, Fernando GJ, Zhou J. Papillomavirus virus-like particles can deliver defined CTL epitopes to the MHC class I pathway. Virology 1998;240:147–157.

82. Greenstone HL, Nieland JD, de Visser KE, et al. Chimeric papillomavirus virus-like particles elicit antitumor immunity against the E7 oncoprotein in an HPV16 tumor model. *Proc Natl Acad Sci USA* 1998;95:1800–1805.

83. Jochmus I, Schafer K, Faath S, et al. Chimeric virus-like particles of the human papillomavirus type 16 (HPV 16) as a prophylactic and therapeutic vaccine. *Arch Med Res* 1999;30:269–274.

84. Unckell F, Streeck RE, Sapp M. Generation and neutralization of pseudovirions of human papillomavirus type 33. *J Virol* 1997;71:2934–2939.

85. Touze A, Coursaget P. In vitro gene transfer using human papillomavirus-like particles. *Nucleic Acids Res* 1998;26: 1317–1323.

86. Rossi JL, Gissmann L, Jansen K, Muller M. Assembly of human papillomavirus type 16 pseudovirions in Saccharomyces cerevisiae. *Hum Gene Ther* 2000;11:1165–1176.

87. Shi W, Liu J, Huang Y, Qiao L. Papillomavirus pseudovirus: a novel vaccine to induce mucosal and systemic cytotoxic T-lymphocyte responses. *J Virol* 2001;75:10139–10148.

88. Huang K, Lin S. Nationwide vaccination: a success story in Taiwan. *Vaccine* 2000;18:S35–S38.

89. Feltkamp MC, Smits HL, Vierboom MP, et al. Vaccination with cytotoxic T lymphocyte epitope-containing peptide protects against a tumor induced by human papillomavirus type 16-transformed cells. *Eur J Immunol* 1993;23:2242–2249.

90. Ressing ME, Sette A, Brandt RM, et al. Human CTL epitopes encoded by human papillomavirus type 16 E6 and E7 identified through in vivo and in vitro immunogenicity studies of HLA-A*0201-binding peptides. *J Immunol* 1995;154:5934–5943.

91. Fernando GJ, Murray B, Zhou J, Frazer IH. Expression, purification and immunological characterization of the transforming protein E7, from cervical cancer-associated human papillomavirus type 16. *Clin Exp Immunol* 1999;115:397-403.

92. Chu NR, Wu HB, Wu T, et al. Immunotherapy of a human papillomavirus (HPV) type 16 E7-expressing tumour by administration of fusion protein comprising Mycobacterium bovis bacille Calmette-Guerin (BCG) hsp65 and HPV16 E7. *Clin Exp Immunol* 2000;121:216–225.

93. van der Burg SH, Kwappenberg KM, O'Neill T, et al. Preclinical safety and efficacy of TA-CIN, a recombinant HPV16 L2E6E7 fusion protein vaccine, in homologous and heterologous prime-boost regimens. *Vaccine* 2001;19: 3652–3660.

94. Mayordomo JI, Zorina T, Storkus WJ, et al. Bone marrow-derived dendritic cells pulsed with synthetic tumour peptides elicit protective and therapeutic antitumour immunity. *Nat Med* 1995;1:1297–302.

95. De Bruijn ML, Schuurhuis DH, Vierboom MP, et al. Immunization with human papillomavirus type 16 (HPV16) oncoprotein-loaded dendritic cells as well as protein in adjuvant induces MHC class I-restricted protection to HPV16-induced tumor cells. *Cancer Res* 1998;58:724–731.

96. Tuting T, DeLeo AB, Lotze MT, Storkus WJ. Genetically modified bone marrow-derived dendritic cells expressing tumor-associated viral or "self" antigens induce antitumor immunity in vivo. *Eur J Immunol* 1997;27:2702–2707.

97. Wang TL, Ling M, Shih IM, et al. Intramuscular administration of E7-transfected dendritic cells generates the most potent E7-specific anti-tumor immunity. *Gene Ther* 2000;7:726–733.

98. Bubenik J, Simova J, Hajkova R, et al. Interleukin 2 gene therapy of residual disease in mice carrying tumours induced by HPV 16. *Int J Oncol* 1999;14:593–597.

99. Hallez S, Detremmerie O, Giannouli C, et al. Interleukin-12-secreting human papillomavirus type 16-transformed cells provide a potent cancer vaccine that generates E7-directed immunity. *Int J Cancer* 1999;81:428–437.

100. Shi W, Bu P, Liu J, et al. Human papillomavirus type 16 E7 DNA vaccine: mutation in the open reading frame of E7 enhances specific cytotoxic T-lymphocyte induction and antitumor activity. *J Virol* 1999;73:7877–7881.

101. Ji H, Wang TL, Chen CH, et al. Targeting human papillomavirus type 16 E7 to the endosomal/lysosomal compartment enhances the antitumor immunity of DNA vaccines against murine human papillomavirus type 16 E7-expressing tumors. *Hum Gene Ther* 1999;10:2727–2740.

102. Chen CH, Wang TL, Hung CF, et al. Enhancement of DNA vaccine potency by linkage of antigen gene to an HSP70 gene. *Cancer Res* 2000;60:1035–1042.

103. Osen W, Peiler T, Ohlschlager P, et al. A DNA vaccine based on a shuffled E7 oncogene of the human papillomavirus type 16 (HPV 16) induces E7-specific cytotoxic T cells but lacks transforming activity. *Vaccine* 2001;19: 4276–4286.

104. Cheng WF, Hung CF, Chai CY, et al. Tumor-specific immunity and antiangiogenesis generated by a DNA vaccine encoding calreticulin linked to a tumor antigen. *J Clin Invest* 2001;108:669–678.

105. Chen L, Thomas EK, Hu SL, et al. Human papillomavirus type 16 nucleoprotein E7 is a tumor rejection antigen. *Proc Natl Acad Sci USA* 1991;88:110–114.

106. Meneguzzi G, Cerni C, Kieny MP, Lathes R. Immunization against human papillomavirus type 16 tumor cells with recombinant vaccinia virus expressing E6 and E7. *Virology* 1991;181:62–69.

107. Toes RE, Hoeben RC, van der Voort EI, et al. Protective anti-tumor immunity induced by vaccination with recombinant adenoviruses encoding multiple tumor-associated cytotoxic T lymphocyte epitopes in a string-of-beads fashion. *Proc Natl Acad Sci USA* 1997;94:14660–14665.

108. He Z, Wlazlo AP, Kowalczyk DW, et al. Viral recombinant vaccines to the E6 and E7 antigens of HPV-16. *Virology* 2000;270:146–161.

109. Liu DW, Tsao YP, Kung JT, et al. Recombinant adeno-associated virus expressing human papillomavirus type 16 E7 peptide DNA fused with heat shock protein DNA as a potential vaccine for cervical cancer. *J Virol* 2000;74: 2888–2894.

110. Di Fabio S, Medaglini D, Rush CM, et al. Vaginal immunization of Cynomolgus monkeys with Streptococcus gordonii expressing HIV-1 and HPV 16 antigens. *Vaccine* 1998;16:485–492.

111. Jabbar IA, Fernando GJ, Saunders N, et al. Immune responses induced by BCG recombinant for human papillomavirus L1 and E7 proteins. *Vaccine* 2000;18:2444–2453.

112. Gunn GR, Zubair A, Peters C, et al. Two Listeria monocytogenes vaccine vectors that express different molecular forms of human papilloma virus-16 (HPV-16) E7 induce qualitatively different t cell immunity that correlates with their ability to induce regression of established tumors immortalized by HPV-16. *J Immunol* 2001;167: 6471–6479.

ENDOMETRIUM

34 Objective Biomarkers in Endometrioid-Type Endometrial Carcinogenesis

Jan P. A. Baak, MD, PhD, FRCPath, FIAC(Hon), DrHC(Antwerp),
George L. Mutter, MD, Anita Steinbakk, Luly Taddele, MD,
Bianca van Diermen, MA, Tove Helliesen MD,
Paul J. van Diest, MD, PhD, Renee Verheijen, MD, PhD,
Peter J. Kenemans, MD, PhD, Curt Burger, MD, PhD,
Kjell Løvslett, MD, Bent Fiane, MD,
and Kjell-Henning Kjellevold, MD

CONTENTS

1. INTRODUCTION

Endometrial hyperplasia (EH) is a common disease. An estimated 180,000–200,000 new cases occur annually in the Western world; approx 39,200 new cases and 6600 deaths were expected in the United States in 2002 *(1)*. About 8–20% of all EH is associated with subsequent endometrial cancer of the endometrioid type. Major problems in treating EH include poor diagnostic reproducibility and inaccurate prediction of cancer progression. This has resulted in enormous overtreatment. The World Health Organization (WHO)'s 1994 histologic classification is widely used but is not reproducible, does not adequately predict the risk of cancer progression, and lacks a molecular and cell biology basis. Computerized morphometric analysis has identified a multivariate combination of architectural and nuclear features, called the DS, which is reproducible, fits with therapeutic options, and accurately predicts cancer outcome. Cases with DS ≥ 1 have a negligible progression risk (0.3%), contrasting with a 37% progression risk for those with DS < 1 found in a large multicenter study with more than 18 yr of follow-up. Moreover, molecular-genetic studies have found a

From: Cancer Chemoprevention, Volume 2: Strategies for Cancer Chemoprevention
Edited by: G. J. Kelloff, E. T. Hawk, and C. C. Sigman © Humana Press Inc., Totowa, NJ

Table 1
Functional, Diagnostic and Therapeutic Aspects of EIN

EIN nomenclature	Topography	Functional category	Treatment	
Benign endometrial hyperplasia	Diffuse	Estrogen effect	Hormonal therapy	
EIN	Focal, later diffuse	Precancer	Hormonal or surgical	
Carcinoma	Focal, later diffuse	Cancer	Surgical, stage-based	

strong correlation between clonality and DS; monoclonal cases nearly always have DS < 0; cases with DS ≥ 1 are mostly polyclonal. This has resulted in a new classification, endometrial intraepithelial neoplasia (EIN), which does not mimic subjective WHO hyperplasia diagnoses but rather uses new criteria for prognostic prediction of cancer endpoints. Moreover, high-risk EIN-DS lesions often show clonal inactivation of the phosphatase and tensin homologue (PTEN) tumor-supressor gene by immunohistochemistry. Based on EIN-DS, patients can now be reproducibly assigned with high accuracy to high- and low-risk categories, permitting appropriate management. EIN-DS application is easy, can be done on standard histologic sections, and has reasonable cost. EIN-DS thus can be assessed in any pathology laboratory, but sections can also be sent to reference laboratories for measurement if necessary.

DS and its component features have quantitatively defined histopathologic changes that occur during endometrial carcinogenesis. These morphologic changes coincide with acquisition of genetic damage that confers a proliferative advantage over normal cells, resulting in clonal expansion to a localizing lesion. Progression through additional intermediate phases culminates in endometrioid-type endometrial cancer.

EH offers an early opportunity for preventive intervention. Patients with EH are on average 10 yr younger than those with endometrial cancer, but this age varies widely depending on degree of severity of hyperplasia and grade of cancer differentiation. Approximately 180,000 hysterectomies are performed annually in the US based on a diagnosis of EH (2). This is alarming in that diagnoses of atypical EH, the subset of EH that most commonly precipitates hysterectomy, are confirmed by a second pathologist in only half of cases (3,4). This reality has driven a need for improved diagnostic procedures with validated prognostic significance.

Many new systems have been proposed over the past decades, but often they lacked a biological, genetic, or prognostic foundation. This chapter will give an overview of new developments in EH classification. Moreover, objective prognostic markers for early-stage endometrial cancer will be discussed. Also, changes in therapy as a result of EIN-DS will be shown.

2. ENDOMETRIAL HYPERPLASIA

The WHO 1994 classification for EH, based on clinical outcomes of 170 cases, achieved widespread implementation and clarification of terminology (5). However, later studies have shown that the WHO 1994 classification is not reproducible (4,6,7) and its prognostic value is limited (8). The subgroup of complex atypical hyperplasia (CAH) has the worst prognosis, but incidence of CAH is relatively low, and even CAH cancer progression rates are not higher than 29% (5,9). This means that preventive hysterectomy in CAH as usually applied is overtreatment in as many as (100 − 29 =) 71% of all patients.

Although WHO classification delineates four subgroups (simple, complex, simple atypical, and CAH), in practice these do not match with available therapeutic options (observe or treat surgically or hormonally with intent to ablate lesion). As a result, many gynecologists often use atypia as an indication to perform hysterectomy, although reproducibility of atypia diagnosis is poor. This has led to both over- and undertreatment of many patients. Finally, since the WHO classification was formulated, many scientific advances have altered our perception of the pathogenesis and presentation of premalignant endometrial disease, with direct diagnostic implications.

3. EIN: A DIFFERENT CONCEPT

The new classification is not just another change in nomenclature, but is based on integrated morphologic, genetic, molecular, cell biology, and prognostic morphometric studies (10,11). Three disease categories of EIN are defined: benign hyperplasia (a hormone-dependent diffuse lesion); EIN (a precancerous lesion that is a monoclonal and neoplastic localized proliferation); and cancer. Table 1 summarizes each category's nomenclature, topography, functional category, and treatment. Each category combines a pathogenetic

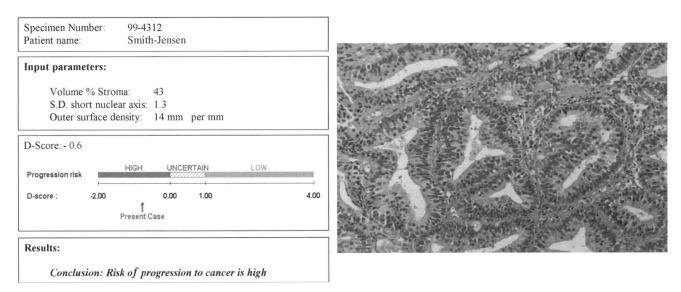

Specimen Number: 99-4312
Patient name: Smith-Jensen

Input parameters:

Volume % Stroma: 43
S.D. short nuclear axis: 1.3
Outer surface density: 14 mm per mm

D-Score: - 0.6

Progression risk   HIGH   UNCERTAIN   LOW

D-score: -2.00   0.00   1.00   4.00
↑
Present Case

Results:

Conclusion: Risk of progression to cancer is high

Fig. 1. Diagram used in our laboratory to routinely present the DS to the requesting clinician.

mechanism with histologic appearance and biological behavior. Diagnosis and treatment are based on these fundamental aspects.

Central to the concept of EIN is achieving a high degree of clinical prognostic relevance with objective quantitative diagnostic markers. Fundamental properties of premalignant endometrial disease such as monoclonal growth and frequent genetic inactivation of tumor supressor genes like PTEN have been confirmed as features of EIN *(12)*. The prognostic foundation is a unique combination of reproducible morphometrical features combined in DS, developed in the early 1980s not to mimic the subjective existing WHO hyperplasia classification system, but as a prognostic test *(13)*. Essential features of DS, selected using multivariate regression analysis from a large group of other features, include architecture-related (volume percentage stroma [VPS] and outer surface density of the glands [OSD]) and those of cytologic nature, i.e., nuclear size variation and standard deviation of the shortest nuclear axis (SDSNA). The prognostic value of localization of nuclei in the superficial layers of the epithelium and DNA ploidy is overshadowed by DS and has no additional prognostic value *(14)*. Three clinical outcome studies in the US, the Netherlands, and Norway confirmed the prognostic value of DS in predicting cancer risk *(8,14,15)*. Moreover, a recent 10-yr prospective routine multicenter study has shown that prognostic value of DS for cancer association/progression is maintained during long-term follow-up, where its prognostic value exceeds that of WHO classification *(16)*. Figure 1 shows a typical diagram that we use routinely

to report results of morphometric DS analysis to the requesting specialist.

An EH grading by four expert gynecopathologists comparing WHO diagnostic criteria with DS showed that DS correlated more strongly to clonality than WHO diagnoses; DS also was more reproducible than the WHO score *(17)*. Nearly all cases with DS ≥ 1 are polyclonal, whereas many (but not all) cases with DS < 1 are monoclonal. Some apparent polyclonal cases with DS < 1 can be attributed to technical error in clonality assessment, where contaminating polyclonal normal tissues obscured the monoclonal nature of the tested samples.

p53 mutations are thought to play an important role in tumorigenesis of endometrial cancers of the serous papillary type *(18)*. In contrast, PTEN tumor suppressor gene is hormonally regulated in the normal endometrium and mutated in EIN; functional inactivation of PTEN results in upregulation of proliferation *(19–21)*. Its role in endometrioid-type endometrial carcinogenesis has been confirmed in an animal model *(22)*. A recently developed PTEN monoclonal antibody (6h2.1, Cascade Biosciences, Winchester, MA) allows routine immunohistochemical evaluation of PTEN in processed paraffin-embedded tissues. Although 83% of endometrioid-type endometrial cancers preceded by a precursor lesion are PTEN-negative, those of the serous papillary type are not *(21,23)*. Moreover, 60% of EIN lesions and 56% of unopposed estrogen-induced hyperplasias showed PTEN-negative glands (Fig. 2). Finally, isolated PTEN-negative glands also occur in routine curettings of proliferative endometrium *(24,25)*. These data confirm that PTEN inactivation is a specific feature

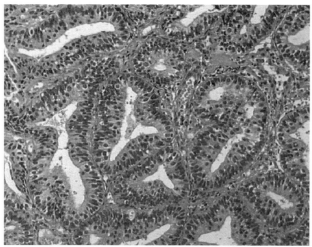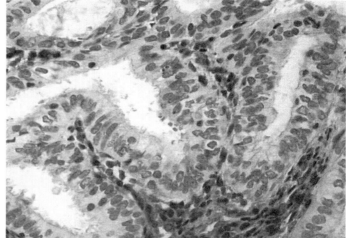

Fig. 2. Example of an EIN, which was a complex endometrial hyperplasia without atypia according to the WHO classification. This diagnosis usually results in conservative watchful follow-up. However, the DS in this case was −0.6, interpreted and reported to the gynecologist as high risk of cancer progression. Because of this, a hysterectomy was performed after 3.5 mo, which revealed unequivocal well-differentiated endometrioid adenocarcinoma infiltrating into the myometrium up to 50% of the wall thickness. **(Left)** Curettage, × 200. Complex glands with little intervening stroma, but no nuclear atypia. Because of the DS = −0.6 (as confirmed by repeat assessments), the case was an EIN with a high cancer risk. **(Right)** PTEN negative glands, stroma strongly positive.

of the endometrioid endometrial cancer subtype *(25)*, occurring so early in carcinogenesis that it may precede onset of any discernable histological changes. Significantly, loss of PTEN function is maintained in EIN, where lesions with DS < 1 show clonal loss of PTEN protein in a geographic distribution corresponding to that of the hematoxylin-eosin-stained lesion. It is important to note that one-third of EIN lesions with DS < 1 maintain normal PTEN function (Table 2); thus, PTEN stains alone will miss this fraction of high-risk lesions. The cancer progression risk of PTEN negativity in EH thus remains to be assessed. Furthermore, one-third of histologically normal endometria will contain isolated PTEN-null glands, so loss of PTEN function in this pattern is not necessarily associated with heightened cancer risk.

Thus, EINs are those hyperplasia cases with a DS < 1. These are truly neoplastic lesions; if left alone, a large fraction become invasive cancer in time. In contrast, hyperplasias with DS > 1 are nonprogressive lesions,

which should be regarded as harmless sequelae of an abnormal hormonal state and treated accordingly.

Using EIN criteria to rediagnose EHs that were originally classified using WHO criteria yields an EIN fraction of 8% of simple hyperplasia, 41% of complex hyperplasia (CH), and 60% of atypical hyperplasia (AH) (simple and complex) *(26)*. On the other hand, 59% of CH and 21% of CAH are benign lesions according to EIN classification. The atypia-cancer association is so deeply rooted that AH for some gynecologists and pathologists is synonymous with high cancer risk. This is a dangerous oversimplification, given the low cancer risk of AH, poor reproducibility of atypia assessments, and high cancer-predictive value of noncytologic (architectural) features. Balanced assessment of architectural with cytologic features in diagnosis of EIN, a significant change from previous practice, will require reeducation of pathologists and clinicians alike.

4. PROGNOSTIC VALUE OF EIN

The EIN-DS classification is reproducible *(17)*, as shown by multicenter evaluations on hundreds of cases *(8,16)*. Long-term prospective multicenter routine application of the EIN-DS has shown that it is prognostically superior to WHO criteria *(13)*. A recent international survival analysis of 477 cases with up to 18 yr follow-up has again shown the overriding prognostic value of DS-based EIN *(26)*. Table 3 summarizes different prognostic criteria of EIN-DS as found in different studies.

Table 2
DS and PTEN Correlate to a Certain Degree but are Not Completely in Agreement

DS	PTEN-Positive	PTEN-negative	Total
>1 (low risk)	18	3	21
<1 (high risk)	5	9	14
Total	23	12	35

Table 3
Sensitivity, Specificity, Positive and Negative Predictive Values of EIN-DS in Different Studies

Study	Sensitivity	Specificity	Positive PV[a]	Negative PV[b]	Number of patients
Delft 1988	100	63	40	100	39
Philadelphia 1996	100	71	67	100	54
Tromsø 2000	100	78	58	100	68
Multicenter Prospective Study AJSP 2001	100	82	38	100	132
Average	100	74	51	100	293[b]

[a]PV, Predictive value.

[b]Total number of patients.

5. DIAGNOSING EIN

EIN diagnosis is often made easily (10,11,23). The most important diagnostic features for EIN include lesion size of at least 1 mm in diameter; DS < 1, or alternatively a VPS in the relevant diagnostic area less than 55% of the endometrium as a whole (i.e., stromal compartment smaller than glandular compartment); and cytology differing between architecturally crowded focus and background.

Diagnostic mimics should be diagnosed separately from EIN, although EIN must also be diagnosed if it coexists with any of these discrete conditions (for example, EIN within an endometrial polyp). Such mimics include carcinoma on the basis of mazelike, cribriform, or solid growth patterns; basal endometrium, endometrial polyps, regenerative endometrium, and hyper-secretory endometrium (secretory hyperplasia, Arias-Stella); and artifacts (e.g., gland telescoping or otherwise distorted glands). Table 4 summarizes these diagnostic difficulties.

Practical EIN diagnosis procedure includes a number of steps. First, exclude possible mimics and confirm possible EIN or EH. Assess whether the lesion is localized or changes are global throughout the endometrial compartment. If focal, apply diagnostic criteria to that area. Localizing EIN lesions must have coordinate changes in cytology and architecture relative to the background pattern. Absence of cytologic changes in an area of architecturally crowded glands may be due to artifactual displacement of glands, or random proximity of irregularly distributed benign glands. If the maximal diameter of the cytologically demarcated lesion is smaller than 1 mm, classify the lesion as benign hyperplasia. If greater than 1 mm, assess VPS. VPS < 55% is more strongly correlated to genetic monoclonality than is nuclear atypia. Any EH case

with more than two-thirds of the section occupied by stroma as judged subjectively is benign. Any case with less than one-third VPS is neoplastic and thus EIN (cancer has already been excluded at the start). If one-third < VPS < two-thirds, VPS cannot be assessed accurately and reproducibly by subjective conventional light-microscopy alone. In these cases, with VPS subjectively certainly or possibly under 66%, apply computerized morphometrical analysis (CMA) to find a reliable EIN diagnosis by means of DS. CMA of glands can be done on a standard histological hematoxylin-eosin stained section and takes approx 5–10 min per case.

Individual DS values can be calculated with the following formula (13):

$$DS = + 0.6229 + 0.0439 \times VPS - 3.9934 \times \ln(SDSNA) - 0.1592 \times OSD$$

Table 4
Histological EIN Criteria. All Criteria Must be Fulfilled to Diagnose EIN

EIN Criterion	Comments
Architecture	Area of glands exceeds that of stroma (VPS < 55%); DS < 1
Cytology	Cytology differs between architecturally crowded focus and background
Diameter >1mm	Maximum linear dimension of the lesion exceeds 1 mm
Exclude mimics[a]	Benign conditions with overlapping criteria: basalis, secretory, polyps, repair, etc.
Exclude cancer[a]	Carcinoma if mazelike glands, solid areas, or significant cribriforming

[a]These patterns should not be confused with EIN, but EIN may coexist with them, in which case it should be separately diagnosed. For more details, see also www.endometrium.org (25).

The value of DS can vary from -4 to $+4$. Cases with DS < 1 have a high likelihood to progress; if DS > 1, no progression has been observed with long-term follow-up (up to 18 yr) when the election of the diagnostic area and measurements are done properly.

6. EIN CASE REPORT

A 49-year-old woman suffered from postmenopausal bleeding. Vaginal ultrasonography showed a double-layered endometrial thickness of 6 mm. After Pipelle biopsy, an experienced surgical pathologist classified the endometrial lesion according to the WHO criteria as CH without atypia. This diagnosis was independently confirmed by four experienced surgical pathologists. CMA showed a DS of -0.6. The final diagnosis was EIN, with hysterectomy recommended. Performed 3.5 mo later, the hysterectomy showed a grade 1 (well differentiated) diffuse endometrioid carcinoma with infiltration into the upper half of the myometrium. Figure 2 shows microscopic details of the biopsy and hysterectomy.

7. TREATMENT OF EIN AND BENIGN HYPERPLASIAS

EH with a DS > 1 (benign hyperplasias) should be treated symptomatically using hormonal therapies. If symptoms persist, follow-up surveillance by repeat endometrial sampling is advised. It is critical that follow-up biopsies not be obtained while the patient is receiving active hormonal therapy. Withdrawal of exogenous hormones and completion of a withdrawal bleed is thus advised before rebiopsy. Usually waiting 3 to 6 wk after hormone discontinuation is adequate. Surveillance ultrasonography and/or hysteroscopy may be performed if desired by the individual clinician, but there is no clear necessity for this during follow-up.

EIN cases with DS < 1 require treatment. In most cases this will be hysterectomy. A hysterectomy may not be appropriate if the patient is a poor surgical risk, desires maintenance of fertility despite known cancer risks, or refuses hysterectomy for other reasons. In these cases, it is especially important to rule out a coexisting carcinoma before undertaking hormonal therapy.

The clinician and pathologist must consider sampling adequacy. If the sample is scanty, or thought not to be representative for any reason, a repeat biopsy to further exclude carcinoma should be considered. Ultrasonography and/or hysteroscopy may be chosen by some clinicians as supplemental evaluations to exclude carcinoma.

Once the clinician has done everything possible to exclude a coexisting carcinoma, and the patient is informed of the risks and benefits, a course of progesterone therapy can be undertaken. Adequacy of hormonally induced EIN involution can be documented after completion of hormonal therapy by a minimum of two successive lesion-free endometrial biopsies separated by at least 6 mo. As above, follow-up biopsies are invalid if obtained while the patient is still taking progestins, as this may mask persistent EIN.

These procedures are specified in the therapeutic decision scheme shown in Fig. 3 *(13)*, developed by leading oncological gynecologists to prevent unnecessary overtreatment while improving quality of life. It has been adopted in a number of hospitals in the Netherlands and Norway.

8. IMPLEMENTATION OF EIN-DS CMA

Implementation of routine EIN-DS CMA in two general surgical pathology laboratories took less than 3 mo. Daily routine application has discovered high-risk EIN cases (DS < 1) that would have been undertreated by virtue of their simple or complex (non-atypical) hyperplasia diagnoses according to the WHO criteria. Hysterectomy immediately following an EIN diagnosis can reveal intramucosal or superficially invasive carcinoma (see the case study above). Thus, the EIN-DS classification detects high-risk cases at a very early stage and can be truly cancer preventive. Correspondingly, overtreatment of misdiagnosed atypical endometrial hyperplasias has been prevented.

9. DS PITFALLS

Many errors can result in incorrect DS values or lack of reproducibility: inclusion of mimics; too small a measurement area (< 1 mm); too large a measurement area that includes nondiagnostic tissue; incorrect measurement; incorrect definition of tissue compartments; measuring the wrong area; performing measurements on selected areas and nuclei instead of randomly selected areas; not selecting nuclei at random with point sampling; other measurement deviations; erroneous calibration of the system; use of an objective lens with insufficient power; and incorrect calculations.

10. COST-BENEFIT ANALYSIS

If the therapeutic scheme indicated above is followed throughout the Netherlands (16 million inhabitants), it could save more than US $9 million per year by pre-

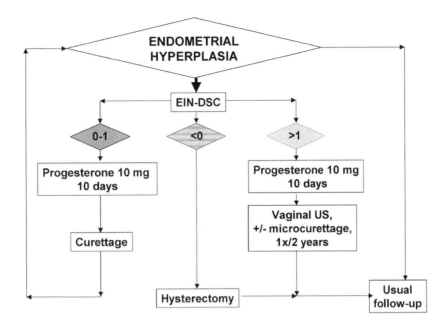

Fig. 3. Therapeutic decision scheme for endometrial hyperplasias based on the EIN-DS technology.

venting 2000 unnecessary hysterectomies, based on our previous work *(9,13)* and incidence figures from our current practices *(16,26)*. Approximately 5000 new cases of EH are diagnosed per year in the Netherlands, the majority treated with hysterectomy. Of these, 65% (or 3250) with a DS > 1 (benign hyperplasia in the EIN nomenclature) have a negligible cancer risk and do not require hysterectomy. Conservatively, at least 2000 EH hysterectomies can be prevented (but 3000 is perhaps a more realistic figure). Cost of one hysterectomy for the national health care system, not including cost for the patient (hospital days, operation, etc.) is approximately $6000. Cost of the surveillance scheme described above for one woman over 5 yr is approximately $1500. Prevention of 2000 unnecessary hysterectomies (low estimation) per year by DS therefore will save 2000 × ($6000 – $1500 = $4500) or $9 million. Nationwide use of DS assessment will cost approx $250,000 (5000 x $50 per case). Hence, the net benefit to the Netherlands of nationwide computerized morphometrical analysis application in all EH could be well over $9 million per year. In a country such as the US (population 250 million), annual savings of $125 million may be possible, not including prevention of direct patient costs, disease absence, and immaterial losses.

11. CONCLUSIONS

EIN classification, based on morphological, genetic, molecular, and prognostic morphometrical data, is reproducible; its prognostic value regarding cancer progression exceeds that of WHO criteria. In selected diagnostic cases, CMA is important for reliable EIN classification. DS-supported EIN classification can discover high-risk lesions that would otherwise go undetected. Implementation and daily use is patient-friendly and meets with easy acceptance by clinicians, pathologists, and technicians when the background is well understood. Overall application of EIN/DS classification and the therapeutic decision scheme results in a better quality of life and is highly cost-effective.

REFERENCES

1. American Cancer Society. *Cancer Facts and Figures—2002.* American Cancer Society, Atlanta, 2002.
2. Lepine LA, Hillis SD, Marchbanks PA, et al. Hysterectomy surveillance—United States, 1980–1993. *Mor Mortal Wkly Rep CDC Surveill Summ* 1997;46:1–15.
3. Winkler B, Alvarez S, Richart R, Crum C. Pitfalls in the diagnosis of endometrial neoplasia. *Obstet Gynecol* 1984;64:185–194.
4. Kendall BS, Ronnett BM, Isacson C, et al. Reproducibility of the diagnosis of endometrial hyperplasia, atypical hyperplasia, and well-differentiated carcinoma. *Am J Surg Pathol* 1998;22:1012–1019.
5. Kurman RJ, Kaminski PF, Norris HJ. The behavior of endometrial hyperplasia. A long-term study of "untreated " hyperplasia in 170 patients. *Cancer* 1985;56:403–412.
6. Skov BG, Broholm H, Engel U, et al. Comparison of the reproducibility of the WHO classifications of 1975 and 1994 of endometrial hyperplasia. *Int J Gynecol Pathol* 1997; 16:33–37.
7. Bergeron C, Nogales FF, Masseroli M, et al. Multicentric European study testing the reproducibility of the WHO classification of endometrial hyperplasia with a proposal of a

simplified working classification for biopsy and curettage specimens. *Am J Surg Pathol* 1999;23:1102–1108.

8   Dunton CJ, Baak JPA, Palazzo JP, et al. Use of computerized morphometric analyses of endometrial hyperplasias in the prediction of coexistent cancer. *Am J Obstet Gynecol* 1996;174:1518–1521.

9. Baak JPA, Wisse-Brekelmans ECM, Fleege JC, et al. Assessment of the risk on endometrial cancer hyperplasia, by means of morphological and morphometrical features. *Pathol Res Pract* 1992;188:856–859.

10. Mutter GL. Commentary. Endometrial Intraepithelial Neoplasia (EIN): will it bring order to chaos? Endometrial Collaborative Group. *Gynecol Oncol* 2000;76:287–290.

11. Mutter GL, Nogales F, Kurman R, et al. Endometrial cancer. In *WHO Classification of Tumors: Pathology and Genetics, Tumors of the Breast and Female Genital Organs.* Tavassoli FA, Stratton MR, eds. IARC Press, Lyon, France, 2002.

12. Mutter GL, Lin MC, Fitzgerald JT, et al. Altered PTEN expression as a diagnostic marker for the earliest endometrial precancers. *J Natl Cancer Inst* 2000;92:924–930.

13. Baak JPA, Nauta JJP, Wisse-Brekelmans ECM, Bezemer PD. Architectural and nuclear morphometrical features together are more important prognosticators in endometrial hyperplasia than nuclear features alone. *J Pathol* 1988; 154:335–341.

14. Baak JPA, Kuik DJ, Bezemer PD. The additional prognostic value of morphometric nuclear arrangement and DNA-ploidy to other morphometric and stereologic features in endometrial hyperplasias. *Int J Gynecol Cancer* 1994;4:289–297.

15. Orbø A, Baak JPA, Kleivan I, et al. Computerized morphometrical analysis in endometrial hyperplasia for the prediction of cancer development. A long term population based retrospective study from northern Norway. *J Clin Pathol* 2000;53:697–703.

16. Baak JPA, Ørbo A, van Diest PJ, et al. Prospective multicenter evaluation of the morphometric D-Score for prediction of the outcome of endometrial hyperplasias. *Am J Surg Pathol* 2001;25:930–935.

17. Mutter GL, Baak JPA, Crum PC, et al. Endometrial precancer diagnosis by histopathology, clonal analysis and computerized morphometry. *J Pathol* 2000;190:462–469.

18. Sherman ME, Bur ME, Kurman RJ. p53 in endometrial cancer and its putative precursors: evidence for diverse pathways of tumorigenesis. *Hum Pathol* 1995;26:1268–1274.

19. Mutter GL. PTEN, a protean tumor suppressor. *Am J Pathol* 2001;158:1895–1898.

20. Mutter GL. Histopathology of genetically defined endometrial precancers. Review. *Int J Gynecol Pathol* 2000;19:301–309.

21. Mutter GL. Diagnosis of premalignant endometrial disease. *J Clin Pathol* 2002;55:326–331.

22. Stambolic V, Tsao MS, Macpherson D, et al. High incidence of breast and endometrial neoplasia resembling human Cowden syndrome in pten ± mice. Cancer Res 2000;60:3605–3611.

23. Mutter G, Nogales F, Kurman R, et al. Endometrial cancer. In *WHO Classification of Tumors: Pathology and Genetics, Tumors of the Breast and Female Genital Organs.* Tavassoli FA, Stratton MR, eds. IARC Press, Lyon, France, 2002.

24. Mutter GL, Ince TA, Baak JPA, et al. Molecular identification of latent precancers in histologically normal endometrium. *Cancer Res* 2001;61:4311–4314.

25. Mutter GL. EIN Central [On Line]. http://www.endometrium.org, updated 2004.

26. Baak JPA, Mutter GL, Diest PJ, et al. Evaluation of cancer progression risks of the WHO94 and EIN classifications for endometrial hyperplasias. A meta-analysis of 477 cases with long follow-up. 2004, in preparation.

OVARY

35 Epithelial Ovarian Cancer

Kristin K. Zorn, MD, *Ginger J. Gardner,* MD,
and Michael J. Birrer, MD, PhD

CONTENTS

1. INTRODUCTION

Epithelial ovarian cancer has the highest mortality rate of all gynecologic cancers *(1)*. The majority of patients are diagnosed with advanced-stage disease and consequently have a poor prognosis *(1)*. Despite progress in surgical approaches and chemotherapeutic regimens for ovarian cancer during the last several decades, 5-yr survival rates remain essentially unchanged at 30% *(2)*. Due to the difficulty in treating advanced-stage ovarian carcinoma, increased attention is now focused on preventing this devastating disease. This chapter discusses problems that have hindered chemoprevention efforts as well as some recent advances that may provide solutions.

2. CHEMOPREVENTION TRIAL DESIGN

In general, chemoprevention trials present more design challenges than do treatment trials. Since long-term observation of a large number of subjects is required to evaluate effects of potential agents, prevention trials are lengthy and expensive *(3)*. In addition, trials aimed at prevention of epithelial ovarian cancer pose particular difficulties. Assessment of potential preventive agents, for instance, has been hampered by lack of an animal model for spontaneous epithelial ovarian cancer *(2,4)*. Further, the relative rarity of

ovarian cancer, lack of effective screening techniques, and relative inaccessibility of the ovary for monitoring studies make human trials especially challenging to conduct *(5)*.

3. ANIMAL MODELS

Development of an animal model for epithelial ovarian cancer is critical for preclinical evaluation of potential chemopreventive agents. Researchers have explored several possibilities, including murine, avian, and primate models. Unfortunately, each has significant drawbacks that limit applicability to human ovarian cancer at this time (Table 1).

Numerous attempts have been made to create a murine model *(6–10)*. The advantages of such a model include widespread familiarity with and access to rodents, the relatively low cost of their use, and their rapid development of tumors. The major disadvantage is that spontaneous ovarian cancer is rare in rodents. Chemical agents such as 7,12-dimethylbenz[*a*]anthracene are therefore used to induce ovarian cancer. However, the resulting tumors frequently are of stromal rather than epithelial origin and are usually highly immunogenic *(4,6,7)*. Alternatively, immunocompromised rodents are injected with ovarian cancer cell lines to induce tumors, but these malignancies may poorly mimic tumors in immunocompetent hosts *(10,11)*.

From: Cancer Chemoprevention, Volume 2: Strategies for Cancer Chemoprevention
Edited by: G. J. Kelloff, E. T. Hawk, and C. C. Sigman © Humana Press Inc., Totowa, NJ

Table 1
Summary of Animal Models for Epithelial Ovarian Cancer

Model	Advantages	Disadvantages
Murine	Low cost Familiar model Rapid tumor development	Rare spontaneous EOC Tumor induction limits applicability by producing stromal or immunogenic tumors or by requiring immunocompromised host
Avian	Spontaneous EOC	Tumor development requires years High cost Must distinguish oviductal from ovarian tumors
Nonhuman primate	Most similar to human physiology	Rare spontaneous EOC High cost Used only to study OSE function, not EOC, to date

EOC, epithelial ovarian cancer; OSE, ovarian surface epithelium.

A recent study by Rose et al. addresses some of these concerns. They describe a model using intraperitoneal injections of NuTu-19, a cell line derived from rat ovarian surface epithelium (OSE) following spontaneous transformation, in immunocompetent Fischer 244 rats (6). Importantly, tumors that arose were papillary serous epithelial ovarian cancers, consistent with the pathology in most human cases. As an additional advantage, these tumors were weakly immunogenic, similar to human tumors (6).

Other researchers have focused on an avian model because chickens are one of the few animals with a high rate of spontaneous epithelial ovarian cancer (12). Fredrickson reported the development of malignant ovarian adenocarcinomas in 24% of 466 hens ranging in age from 2 to 7 yr (13). The rate increased with age, reaching 50% by 6 yr. Rodriguez-Burford et al recently noted a 4% rate of spontaneous epithelial ovarian cancer at 2 yr in another avian study (4). In addition, immunohistochemical staining of the cancers suggested an epithelial origin. Positive staining was seen with cytokeratin AE1/AE3, pan cytokeratin, epidermal growth factor receptor (EGFR), Lewis Y, carcinoembryonic antigen (CEA), Tag 72, and erbB-2. The tumors, however, did not express CA-125, Ki-67, Muc1, or Muc2, which is unlike human ovarian cancer. In addition, tumors of oviductal origin metastatic to the ovary, which are common in hens, were not distinguished from tumors originating in the ovary in this study (4). The avian model has the distinct advantage of condensing a 28-d ovulation process in humans to 28 ho in hens, facilitating study of the potential role of incessant ovulation in ovarian cancer pathogenesis (4). In light of a 4% cancer rate at 2 yr, however, the process still requires too many years to accumulate significant

numbers of ovarian cancer cases, adding to the length and expense of trials using this model.

A nonhuman primate model has been described to study the function of OSE, not ovarian cancer per se. Rodriguez et al. used macaques to evaluate the effects of hormonal agents on apoptosis in OSE (14,15). Similarly, Brewer and colleagues evaluated macaques in a pilot study that examined the effect of fenretinide and oral contraceptives on intermediary biomarkers for ovarian cancer (11). The model provides a close approximation of human reproductive physiology that is useful for mechanistic studies such as these. Large-scale studies, however, are limited by the cost of primate subjects. Because spontaneous ovarian cancers are rare in primates, the model has been only used to evaluate intermediate markers to date.

Since no animal model currently demonstrates development of a reasonably high rate of spontaneous epithelial ovarian cancer in a relatively short time period, ongoing research efforts to develop an appropriate model are critical to the field of chemoprevention. An important recent advance reported by Bao et al. is the isolation of ovarian-specific promoter (OSP)-1, a retrovirus-like element that drives gene expression specifically in cells of OSE lineage (2,16). Such a promoter should further efforts to create a transgenic model for ovarian cancer. Specifically, development of a transgenic murine model will likely be the next major advance in this area.

4. HUMAN TRIALS

4.1. High-Risk Population

Another critical requirement for successful chemoprevention trials is identification of a high-risk population.

The advantage of studying such a population is that adequate power to detect an effect of preventive agents can be achieved with a smaller sample size and shorter follow-up period (3). Over the past decade, genes responsible for currently recognized hereditary ovarian cancer syndromes have been identified, providing a pool of potential subjects for such studies. Together, breast and ovarian cancer syndrome and hereditary nonpolyposis colorectal cancer (HNPCC) syndrome account for approximately 10% of all ovarian cancer (17).

Germline mutations in the BRCA-1 and BRCA-2 genes account for the increased risk of malignancy in breast and ovarian cancer syndrome. Estimates for the fraction of familial ovarian cancer attributable to these mutations vary. BRCA-1 is thought to account for anywhere from 40 to 90%, while BRCA-2 accounts for 10 to 30% (3,17–19). Similarly, assessments of lifetime ovarian cancer risk for women who carry the mutations are still being defined; currently they range from 16 to 60% for BRCA-1 and 10 to 27% for BRCA-2 (3,17–19). Regardless of the specific percentage, comparison to the general population's ovarian cancer rate of 1% emphasizes the high-risk nature of this population.

HNPCC syndrome accounts for the remaining 10 to 30% of recognized hereditary ovarian cancer (17). Mutations identified to date in HNPCC families, including hMSH2, hMLH1, and hPMS2, are involved in the DNA mismatch repair pathway (17). Carriers are estimated to have a 9–12% lifetime risk of ovarian cancer (20,21). This pool of potential subjects is generally highly motivated to enroll in chemoprevention trials and to remain compliant with a given preventive therapy to identify methods that reduce cancer risk for themselves and their families (3). Given that BRCA-1/2 mutation frequency is estimated to approach 2.5% in Ashkenazi Jews, approx 30,000 women in Israel alone are carriers who potentially could participate in these types of studies (3,22).

However, several issues must be addressed regarding studies in high-risk populations such as those with BRCA-1/2 or HNPCC. One caveat concerns the applicability of results to the general population. For instance, BRCA-1/2-related breast tumors have a higher likelihood of being estrogen receptor (ER)-negative than sporadic tumors (23). As tamoxifen appears to be less effective in preventing ER-negative tumors, results of breast chemoprevention trials involving selective ER modulators (SERMs) such as tamoxifen have been affected by differing proportions of BRCA

mutation carriers in their study populations (3,18). Ovarian tumors arising in the HNPCC study population are more likely to be well- or moderately differentiated Stage I or II tumors than those occurring in the general population; these differences cannot completely be explained by increased screening in HNPCC patients (24). Ongoing research into the mechanisms of carcinogenesis in familial vs sporadic ovarian cancer should provide further insight into this issue.

A second concern regarding trials based on genetically predisposed populations is the earlier onset of disease. Mutation carriers frequently develop ovarian cancer in their 30s and 40s, while sporadic cases occur more commonly after menopause (3,24). The implication for chemopreventive efforts in BRCA and HNPCC is that women must begin treatment during their 20s and 30s, while fertility is still an issue. This may limit trial participation to women who have completed childbearing or who do not desire fertility.

A third caveat when designing trials for preventing ovarian cancer is that populations harboring a BRCA or HNPCC mutation are also at increased risk for many other malignancies, most notably breast, endometrial, and colon cancer. The impact of ovarian cancer prevention therapies on these other diseases must be considered (25); for instance, hormonal agents such as progestins and SERMs have differing effects on breast, uterine, and ovarian tissues.

Finally, the design of any trial evaluating chemopreventive effects in ovarian cancer must recognize the role that gynecologic surgery plays in reducing ovarian cancer risk. Epidemiological evidence suggests that bilateral tubal ligation, hysterectomy without oophorectomy, and bilateral salpingoophorectomy (BSO) protect against ovarian cancer (26–29). Some experts recommend prophylactic BSO for high-risk patients who have completed childbearing (1,21). Clearly, participation of women who have undergone prophylactic BSO in ovarian cancer chemoprevention trials should be limited to analysis of primary peritoneal cancer risk, while participation of those who have had other gynecologic procedures may require stratification in the data analysis.

4.2. Surrogate Markers

Similar to the lack of an appropriate animal model, our limited understanding of ovarian cancer pathogenesis impedes development of effective chemopreventive agents. Identifying precursor lesions would allow interventions to be tested on progression from premalignant state to frank cancer. Trials utilizing a surrogate endpoint, like those involving high-risk groups, are shorter and less expensive to conduct *(3)*.

Despite success in pinpointing precursor lesions in cervical, uterine, and colorectal malignancies, little progress has been made in identifying premalignant conditions in the ovary. Early interest in OSE dysplasia, particularly when located in an inclusion cyst, was generated by observing that dysplastic areas have been identified adjacent to frank cancer and inclusion cysts on the contralateral ovary *(30)*. In addition, features of malignancy such as CA-125 production and p53 mutation are more common in inclusion cysts than in OSE *(5,12)*. Incessant ovulation was proposed by Fathalla to play a role in development of dysplasia and inclusion cysts by disrupting OSE, causing proliferation that predisposes to mutation *(31)*. Inclusion cysts, however, have been documented in women of all ages, including fetuses, and only rarely contain dysplasia *(5)*. Moreover, in the majority of ovarian cancers, no transition area from normal to dysplastic to malignant epithelium can be identified.

Borderline ovarian tumors have been proposed as intermediate lesions between benign tumors and ovarian cancer. Mounting evidence, however, points to serous borderline lesions as a distinct entity rather than a step in the progression to malignancy. Serous borderline tumors have a low frequency of p53 mutation, minimal loss of heterozygosity (LOH), and microsatellite instability (MSI). In contrast, invasive serous ovarian cancer is characterized by frequent p53 mutation, LOH on multiple chromosomes, and lack of MSI *(30,32–34)*. Additionally, a higher rate of *ras* mutation is found in borderline lesions than in either cystadenomas or carcinoma *(33)*. Mucinous neoplasms, on the other hand, appear to have a genetic profile that is common to both borderline and invasive lesions but distinct from serous tumors. Specifically, *ras* mutation and LOH patterns are similar in borderline and invasive mucinous cancers *(34)*. Further, transitions between benign and malignant areas are found in 80% of mucinous lesions but only 8% of serous ones *(30)*. Together, these data suggest that while some borderline mucinous tumors may progress to invasion, this rarely occurs in serous tumors.

While a precursor lesion is difficult to identify in most cases of ovarian cancer, a subset of tumors clearly arise from endometriosis. At least 28% of endometrioid ovarian cancers and 49% of clear-cell cancers are associated with endometriosis, compared to 3–4% of mucinous and serous cancers *(30)*. Emerging genetic evidence now supports this long-observed epidemiologic association between endometriosis and ovarian cancer. Studies have documented LOH in endometriosis but not in normal endometrium *(35,36)*. Further, similar patterns of LOH are found in malignant lesions and adjacent endometriosis *(36)*. Specifically, LOH on chromosome 10q occurs at high rates in endometriomas, endometrioid cancers, and clear cell cancers; frequently, this LOH is accompanied by mutations in the tumor suppressor gene PTEN *(35,37,38)*. Still, despite genetic similarities between endometriosis and some types of ovarian cancer, we have yet to identify the factors that distinguish the rare endometriosis lesion that progresses to malignancy from the vast majority of lesions that remain benign. As understanding of those factors evolves, high-risk features of endometriosis may be identified, potentially allowing those patients to participate in chemoprevention trials.

While precursor lesions exist for some mucinous, endometrioid, and clear cell ovarian cancers, predicting which of these lesions will progress and by what mechanisms the transformation occurs is still difficult. Further, no premalignant state has been found for papillary serous ovarian cancer, the most common of the histologic subtypes.

4.3. Monitoring

Difficulties involved in monitoring the ovaries have complicated attempts to elucidate epithelial ovarian cancer pathogenesis and identify surrogate markers that can be used in prevention studies. Biopsy is hampered by the ovaries' location deep in the pelvis. Imaging via ultrasound and computed tomography is helpful for determining ovarian size and morphology but cannot distinguish more subtle lesions such as ovarian dysplasia or inclusion cysts. However, new modalities such as spectroscopy are being evaluated for their ability to monitor tissue architecture and biochemical composition noninvasively *(5,11,39)*. Optical spectroscopy can distinguish inclusion cysts, areas of apoptosis, and dysplasia in preliminary testing. In a recent study, fluorescence spectroscopy was used to assess cellular metabolism in monkey ovaries in response to treatment with oral contraceptives and fenretinide *(11)*.

Such imaging advances should partly address the current lack of an effective screening mechanism for epithelial ovarian cancer. Even in high-risk populations, traditional approaches to screening such as pelvic exam, ultrasound, and CA-125 are hampered by their poor ability to detect early-stage disease and to distinguish benign from malignant neoplasms. As Bell concludes in a recent review of prospective studies, "there is currently no reliable evidence that screening for ovarian cancer is effective in improving the length and quality of life of women with the disease" *(40)*. Screening may be improved by inclusion of novel tumor markers for epithelial ovarian cancer. A long list of potential markers has accumulated (Table 2); some, such as CASA, tetranectin, M-CSF, and OVX1, have been shown to increase the sensitivity and specificity of CA-125 in small studies *(41–46)*. These results, if confirmed in large-scale trials, may help identify a panel of markers to aid in ovarian cancer diagnosis.

Recently, discovery of new tumor markers has been facilitated by microarray technology, which allows for transcriptional profiling of tumors. The role that differentially expressed ovarian cancer genes play in pathogenesis can then be explored. Use of this technique can lead to identification of potential serum markers, as Mok et al. demonstrate in a recent study of prostasin *(47)*.

5. CHEMOPREVENTIVE AGENTS

5.1. Oral Contraceptive Pills

Even as the effort to define chemopreventive therapies in epithelial ovarian cancer continues, one agent has already emerged as an effective means of reducing epithelial ovarian cancer risk: oral contraceptive pills (OCPs). Abundant evidence supports a 50% reduction in epithelial ovarian cancer risk with 5 yr of OCP use and a 30% reduction with ever-use *(29)*. Reduced risk persists for at least 10 years after cessation of OCP use *(29,48)*.

The mechanisms by which OCPs decrease ovarian cancer risk remain unclear. Suggested mechanisms include ovulation suppression, lowering of basal and peak luteinizing hormone and follicle stimulating hormone levels, and progestin-mediated apoptosis of OSE *(49)*. As a result of the popularity of the incessant ovulation model of ovarian cancer pathogenesis, ovulation suppression has been the favored theory, but recent evaluations point to a reduction in ovarian cancer risk that exceeds the fraction of lifetime ovulations inhibited by OCP use *(14,49)*. In addition, women with a history of spontaneous multiple births are known to have higher levels of gonadotropins and more frequent double ovulations. Despite the fact that they should therefore be at an increased risk for ovarian cancer by both the incessant ovulation hypothesis and the elevated gonadotropin theory, these women in fact have a reduced risk *(50)*.

Observations such as these have directed increasing attention to the role of progestin in preventing ovarian cancer. High levels of progestin, similar to those found in pregnancy and with OCP use, inhibit OSE proliferation and induce apoptosis *(51,52)*. Further, Rodriguez and

colleagues' research in primates revealed an increase in OSE apoptosis with OCPs but an even greater increase with progestin treatment alone *(14)*. Additional research suggests that the progestin effect may be mediated by TGFβ, which previously has been shown to regulate normal OSE proliferation *(15,53)*. Progesterone receptor expression has also been shown to be downregulated in ovarian cancer cell lines compared with normal cells *(54)*, suggesting that transformation may involve loss of progesterone-induced TGFβ-mediated control of OSE proliferation and apoptosis.

The effect of OCPs on the high-risk BRCA1/2 population is being evaluated. Early evidence suggested that OCPs provide a protective effect in this population similar to that in the general population; that is, a 20% risk reduction was seen after 3 yr of use, 60% after 6 or more years of use *(55)*. A second study, however, showed that OCP use was protective only in BRCA-1/2 mutation noncarriers, whereas multiparity was protective in both noncarriers and carriers *(56)*. A recent case-control study included only women who harbor BRCA mutations and who had not undergone BSO. Ever-use of OCPs was associated with a 50% reduction in ovarian cancer risk *(57)*. As the impact of OCP use on breast cancer risk is still controversial, further research to clarify the protective effect of OCPs on ovarian cancer risk is needed to aid clinicians in making recommendations to BRCA-1/2 patients.

In response to evidence supporting the preventive effect of OCPs on ovarian and endometrial cancer on the one hand, and concerns about OCPs possibly increasing breast cancer risk on the other hand, Pike and Spicer suggest a combined hormonal therapy approach to address all these issues *(58)*. They propose a regimen of a gonadotropin-releasing hormone agonist (GnRHA) with add-back low-dose estrogen and intermittent progestin. Although the risk of breast cancer with low-dose estrogen is also controversial, the regimen would include GnRHA to induce ovulation suppression and low-dose add-back estrogen to relieve symptoms associated with hypoestrogenism such as bone mineral loss, vasomotor instability, and urogenital atrophy. The intermittent progestin dosing would prevent endometrial hyperplasia and potentially contribute to OSE apoptosis. It remains to be seen whether such a complicated regimen will be tolerated by most women, even if it proves to be effective.

5.2. Retinoids

Retinoids, the natural and synthetic analogs of vitamin A, represent another class of agents with potential

Table 2
Potential Tumor Markers for Epithelial Ovarian Cancer

Name	Description	References
CA 15-3	Cancer antigen. 15 Mucin-based assay[a].	98–107
CA 19-9	Cancer antigen. 19-9 Mucin-based assay[a].	99,101,106–114
CA 54/61	Cancer antigen. 54/61 Mucin-based assay[a].	99,106,111
CA 72-4 (TAG-72)	Cancer antigen or tumor-associated glycoprotein 72. Mucin-based assay[a].	99,101,102,104–107,109,111,113–118
CASA	Cancer-associated serum antigen. Mucin-based assay[a].	41,42,100,109,111,112,119–124
CEA	Carcinoembryonic antigen. Oncofetal antigen elevated in many conditions.	4,99,109,110,112,113,119,125–130
CYFRA 21-1	Soluble cytokeratin 19 fragment. Marker of epithelial differentiation.	112,131,132
GAT	Galactosyltransferase associated with tumor. Isoenzyme of normal galactosyltransferase.	133,134
HMFG 1 HMFG 2	Human milk fat globule protein 1 and 2. Mucin-based assays[a].	98,99,111,135
IAP	Immunosuppressive acidic protein. One of group of substances, which includes mucins, thought to play a role in immunosuppression in cancer.	6,127,136–140
IL-6	Interleukin 6. Multifunctional cytokine.	99,139,141–145
Kallikreins	Human kallikrein family of serine proteases. Includes hK3 (PSA), hK4, hK6, hK8, hK9, hK10 (NES1) hK11.	146–152
LASA (LSA)	Lipid-associated sialic acid. Assay for glycoprotein-bound sialic acid.	99,105,106,110,153–161
LPA	Lysophosphatidic acid. Lipid involved in growth regulation of ovarian cancer cells.	162,163
M-CSF (CSF-1)	Macrophage colony-stimulating factor. Cytokine produced by OSE.	43,44,99,106,139,164–166
MSA	Mammary serum antigen. Mucin-based assay[a].	42,111,119,135
NB70K	Ovarian tzumor-associated antigen.	99,135,159,160,167–174
OSA	Ovarian serum antigen. Mucin-based assay[a].	42,122
OVX1	Mucin-based assay[a].	43,44,99,106,120,130,164,175
PLAP	Placental-like alkaline phosphatase. Isoenzyme of alkaline phosphatase produced by tumor.	98,99,128,129,176–180
Pro-α C inhibin	Immunoreactive form of inhibin. Member of TGFβ family.	181–186
Prostasin	Serine protease originally identified in prostate.	47,187
SLX	Sialyl SSEA-1 antigen. Mucin-based assay[a].	111,133,188-191
TATI	Tumor-associated trypsin inhibitor. Polypeptide found in urine and serum of ovarian cancer patients.	101,112,125,192–195
Tetranectin	Plasminogen-binding plasma protein.	45,46,120,196
TPS	Tissue polypeptide-specific antigen on soluble cytokeratin 18 fragment. Proliferation marker closely related to tumor marker TPA.	41,99,112,113,128,129,197
UGF (UGP, beta-core fragment)	Urinary gonadotropin fragment or peptide. Mixture of chorionic gonadotropin, β subunit, and fragments.	99,153,154,160,194,198–204
VEGF	Vascular endothelial growth factor. Paracrine and autocrine role in angiogenesis.	205–208

[a]These assays recognize polymorphic epithelial mucin (MUC1), a glyoprotein that is secreted by epithelial cells after transformation. They differ in which antibody is used, thereby recognizing various epitopes of mucin (42,111).

application as chemopreventive agents for ovarian cancer. Toxicity associated with natural retinoids frequently limits their use; consequently, synthetic vitamin A analogs have been developed. Fenretinide has emerged as one of the most promising alternatives to natural retinoids. An Italian trial that evaluated fenretinide treatment in prevention of second primary breast malignancies provides preliminary evidence that fenretinide may be an effective agent to reduce ovarian carcinoma incidence in high-risk patients *(59,60)*. Although the number of ovarian cancer cases in this study was small, the finding was a secondary endpoint of the study, and fenretinide's protective effect did not persist after discontinuation of therapy, these clinical data generated interest in better defining fenretinide's activity in ovarian cancer. It has since been shown that fenretinide induces growth inhibition and induces apoptosis in ovarian cancer cell lines *(61,62)*. Further, fenretinide effectively improved survival in human ovarian cancer xenograft rodents *(63)*. More recently, Brewer et al. demonstrated that fenretinide in combination with OCPs results in a less tumorigenic fluorophore profile as assessed by fluorescence spectroscopy in rhesus monkeys *(11)*. Investigations are currently under way to delineate fenretinide's mechanism of activity in ovarian cancer cells while clinical trials are accruing to directly assess its use as a chemopreventive agent for ovarian cancer.

Retinoid derivatives containing heteroatoms in a cyclic ring, termed heteroarotentoids, are emerging as a class of compounds with structural similarity to fenretinide but a higher therapeutic index. In 1997, Benbrook et al. generated a series of heteroarotenoids and demonstrated anticancer activity in a cervical cancer cell line. Mice treated with these same compounds showed low in vivo toxicity *(64)*. In 2001, Benbrook examined the effect of heteroarotenoids in ovarian carcinoma using organotypic cultures, which represent in vivo conditions more accurately than in vitro monolayer cell growth. Heteroarotenoids effectively induced cellular differentiation, growth inhibition, and apoptosis in organotypic ovarian cancer cultures *(65)*.

Thus, data are accumulating to suggest that retinoids may be effective chemopreventive agents for ovarian cancer. While new retinoid derivatives such as heteroarotenoids are being characterized, the mechanism of fenretinide activity in ovarian cancer cells is still unclear. Larger clinical trials are required to effectively evaluate fenretinide as a chemopreventive agent.

5.3. Vitamin D

Ovarian cancer mortality has been shown to be inversely proportional to sunlight exposure, a primary source of vitamin D *(66)*. Receptors for 1,25-dihydroxyvitamin D_3 (calcitriol) are documented in ovarian cancer tumor specimens and cell lines *(67)*. Further, calcitriol causes a decrease in proto-oncogene c-*myc* expression and leads to ovarian cancer cell growth inhibition *(68)*. Vitamin D therefore requires further investigation, as it may represent a useful chemopreventive strategy for ovarian cancer.

5.4. Cyclooxygenase Inhibitors

Based on clinical and epidemiologic data, anti-inflammatory agents may be an effective option for ovarian cancer chemoprevention. Large epidemiologic cohorts have demonstrated that local inflammatory processes, including talc and/or asbestos exposures, endometriosis, and pelvic inflammatory disease, are risk factors for ovarian cancer. Conversely, factors reducing local inflammation such as tubal ligation and hysterectomy without oophorectomy appear to reduce ovarian cancer risk *(27–29)*. Based on these observations, Ness et al. proposed that as inflammation contributes to development of epithelial ovarian cancer *(26,69)*, anti-inflammatory agents might be effective in ovarian cancer chemoprevention. To date, several studies have examined a clinical cohort for an association between use of anti-inflammatory agents and decreased ovarian cancer risk. Initially, Tzonou et al. performed a hospital-based case-control study that included 189 epithelial ovarian cancer patients and 200 hospital visitor controls. This study suggested reduced risk of ovarian cancer with frequent use of primarily salicylate analgesics (RR=0.51, 95%; CI= 0.26–1.02) *(70)*. More recently, Rosenberg et al. found that regular long-term use of anti-inflammatory agents was inversely associated with risk of ovarian malignancy (OR=0.5, 95%; CI=0.3–0.8) when comparing analgesic use among 780 ovarian cancer patients, 2053 cancer controls, and 2570 noncancer controls *(71)*. In contrast, several case-control studies failed to show a statistical association between use of anti-inflammatory agents and ovarian cancer risk; however, they reported a decreased risk of ovarian cancer with acetaminophen, another over-the-counter analgesic *(72–74)*. To date, clinical investigations attempting to identify an association between ovarian cancer risk and anti-inflammatory drug use are controversial, as they are based solely on case-control experimental design with inherent selection and recall bias. Despite these limitations, epidemiologic studies and clinical data, taken together, suggest a putative role for anti-inflammatory agents in the prevention of ovarian cancer.

Table 3
Chemopreventive Agents

Agent	Potential mechanisms	Advantages
Oral contraceptive pills (OCPs)	Ovulation suppression Reduction of LH, FSH levels Progestin-mediated apoptosis	Frequently prescribed in the general population Substantial ovarian cancer risk reduction already shown in large clinical cohorts
Retinoids and heteroarotenoids	Alter expression and/or activate retinoid receptors Increase production of reactive oxygen species	Currently used in treatment of leukemia and head and neck
1,25-Dihydroxy vitamin D (Calcitriol)	Activate vitamin D receptors Decrease c-*myc* expression	A vitamin derivative frequently taken in the general population
COX-2 inhibitors	Reduce activity of COX-2 enzyme and thereby induce apoptosis and reduce angiogenesis	Currently used in the treatment of arthritis
PPARγ ligands	Activate transcription factor PPARγ and thereby affect target genes involved in cellular differentiation Increase production of reactive oxygen species	Currently used in the treatment of Type II DM

Molecular studies indicate that one group of antiinflammatory agents, Cyclooxygenase (COX)-2 inhibitors, represent a primary candidate for ovarian cancer chemoprevention. While COX-1 is ubiquitously expressed, COX-2 is an early response gene that generally maintains low-level expression until induced by growth factors and carcinogens *(75–78)*. Increased levels of COX-2 are frequently detected in epithelial cancers *(79–86)*. COX-2 overexpression has been reported to induce angiogenesis, reduce immune surveillance, and inhibit apoptosis in various malignancies *(87–90)*. Further, selective COX-2 inhibitors have been shown to reduce the rate of breast cancer in animal model systems *(91)*. In clinical trials, COX-2 inhibitors decrease incidence of colonic polyps, precursor lesions of colon cancer *(92)*. Preliminary work in our lab demonstrates that COX-2 is overexpressed in ovarian cancer specimens and in ovarian cancer cell lines. Notably, COX-2 inhibitors inhibit ovarian cancer cell growth and induce apoptosis. Thus, clinically available COX-2 inhibitors represent a promising chemopreventive candidate for several epithelial malignancies, including ovarian carcinoma.

5.5 Peroxisome Proliferator Activated Receptor (PPAR)γ Ligands

Peroxisome proliferator activated receptor (PPAR)γ ligands represent another clinically available class of compounds with potential application to ovarian cancer

chemoprevention. A nuclear steroid hormone receptor, PPARγ functions as a ligand-activated transcription factor *(93)*. PPARγ ligands promote differentiation of pre-adipocytes into metabolically active fat cells and are currently used in the treatment of Type II diabetes *(94,95)*. Current breast and colon cancer clinical trials include PPARγ ligands based on their demonstrated ability to reduce cellular proliferation and increase cellular differentiation *(96,97)*. Ongoing work in our lab demonstrates that PPARγ ligands induce growth inhibition and apoptosis in ovarian cancer cells.

Novel application of several clinically available agents (retinoids, COX-2 inhibitors, PPAR ligands, and calcitriol) (Table 3), potentially in combination with OCPs, offers exciting potential for reducing ovarian cancer mortality through chemoprevention.

6. CONCLUSION

In the past few years, ovarian cancer research has focused increasingly on disease prevention. Although significant gains have been made, major challenges remain. At this time, there is no optimal animal model of ovarian cancer development, clearly limiting study of ovarian cancer pathogenesis and preclinical development of novel chemopreventive agents. In addition, a high-risk patient population for sporadic ovarian cancer must be identified to test potential agents because of limitations in extrapolating data from the BRCA population to sporadic ovarian cancer cases. Further, while a large number of surrogate markers that could serve as preliminary study endpoints have been identified, very few have been assessed adequately by large prospective clinical trials. Thus, a number of paramount issues remain to be addressed in developing and testing agents for ovarian cancer chemoprevention before we reach our goal of substantially reducing ovarian cancer mortality.

REFERENCES

1. NIH consensus conference. Ovarian cancer. Screening, treatment, and follow-up. NIH Consensus Development Panel on Ovarian Cancer. *JAMA* 1995;273:491–497.
2. Selvakumaran M, Bao R, Crijns AP, et al. Ovarian epithelial cell lineage-specific gene expression using the promoter of a retrovirus-like element. *Cancer Res* 2001;61:1291–1295.
3. Levy-Lahad E, Krieger M, Gottfeld O, et al. BRCA1 and BRCA2 mutation carriers as potential candidates for chemoprevention trials. *J Cell Biochem Suppl* 2000;34:13–18.
4. Rodriguez-Burford C, Barnes MN, Berry W, et al. Immunohistochemical expression of molecular markers in an avian model: a potential model for preclinical evaluation of agents for ovarian cancer chemoprevention. *Gynecol Oncol* 2001;81:373–379.
5. Brewer MA, Mitchell MF, Bast RC. Prevention of ovarian cancer. *In Vivo* 1999;13:99–106.
6. Rose GS, Tocco LM, Granger GA, et al. Development and characterization of a clinically useful animal model of epithelial ovarian cancer in the Fischer 344 rat. *Am J Obstet Gynecol* 1996;175:593–599.
7. Sekiya S, Endoh N, Kikuchi Y, et al. In vivo and in vitro studies of experimental ovarian adenocarcinoma in rats. *Cancer Res* 1979;39:1108–1112.
8. Silva EG, Tornos C, Deavers M, et al. Induction of epithelial neoplasms in the ovaries of guinea pigs by estrogenic stimulation. *Gynecol Oncol* 1998;71:240–246.
9. Silva EG, Tornos C, Fritsche HA Jr, et al. The induction of benign epithelial neoplasms of the ovaries of guinea pigs by testosterone stimulation: a potential animal model. *Mod Pathol* 1997;10:879–883.
10. Walker W, Gallagher G. The development of a novel immunotherapy model of human ovarian cancer in human PBL-severe combined immunodeficient (SCID) mice. *Clin Exp Immunol* 1995;101:494–501.
11. Brewer M, Utzinger U, Satterfield W, et al. Biomarker modulation in a nonhuman rhesus primate model for ovarian cancer chemoprevention. *Cancer Epidemiol Biomarkers Prev* 2001;10:889–893.
12. Auersperg N, Wong AS, Choi KC, et al. Ovarian surface epithelium: biology, endocrinology, and pathology. *Endocr Rev* 2001;22:255–288.
13. Fredrickson TN. Ovarian tumors of the hen. *Environ Health Perspect* 1987;73:35–51.
14. Rodriguez GC, Walmer DK, Cline M, et al. Effect of progestin on the ovarian epithelium of macaques: cancer prevention through apoptosis? *J Soc Gynecol Investig* 1998;5:271–276.
15. Rodriguez GC, Nagarsheth NP, Lee KL, et al. Progestin-induced apoptosis in the macaque ovarian epithelium: differential regulation of transforming growth factor-beta. *J Natl Cancer Inst* 2002;94:50–60.
16. Bao R, Selvakumaran M, Hamilton TC. Targeted gene therapy of ovarian cancer using an ovarian-specific promoter. *Gynecol Oncol* 2002;84:228–234.
17. Boyd J. Molecular genetics of hereditary ovarian cancer. *Oncology (Huntingt)* 1998;12:399–406; discussion 409–410, 413.
18. Eeles RA, Powles TJ. Chemoprevention options for BRCA1 and BRCA2 mutation carriers. *J Clin Oncol* 2000;18: 93S–99S.
19. Kuschel B, Lux MP, Goecke TO, Beckmann MW. Prevention and therapy for BRCA1/2 mutation carriers and women at high risk for breast and ovarian cancer. *Eur J Cancer Prev* 2000;9:139–150.
20. Aarnio M, Sankila R, Pukkala E, et al. Cancer risk in mutation carriers of DNA-mismatch-repair genes. *Int J Cancer* 1999;81:214–218.
21. Lynch HT, Casey MJ, Lynch J, et al. Genetics and ovarian carcinoma. *Semin Oncol* 1998;25:265–280.
22. Struewing JP, Hartge P, Wacholder S, et al. The risk of cancer associated with specific mutations of BRCA1 and BRCA2 among Ashkenazi Jews. *N Engl J Med* 1997;336: 1401–1408.
23. Srivastava A, McKinnon W, Wood ME. Risk of breast and ovarian cancer in women with strong family histories. *Oncology (Huntingt)* 2001;15:889–902; discussion 902, 905–907, 911–913.
24. Watson P, Butzow R, Lynch HT, et al. The clinical features of ovarian cancer in hereditary nonpolyposis colorectal cancer. *Gynecol Oncol* 2001;82:223–228.
25. Nayfield SG. Ethical and scientific considerations for chemoprevention research in cohorts at genetic risk for breast cancer. *J Cell Biochem Suppl* 1996;25:123–130.
26. Ness RB, Grisso JA, Cottreau C, et al. Factors related to inflammation of the ovarian epithelium and risk of ovarian cancer. *Epidemiology* 2000;11:111–117.
27. Ness RB, Grisso J A, Vergona R, et al. Oral contraceptives, other methods of contraception, and risk reduction for ovarian cancer. *Epidemiology* 2001;12:307–312.
28. Green A, Purdie D, Bain C, et al. Tubal sterilisation, hysterectomy and decreased risk of ovarian cancer. Survey of Women's Health Study Group. *Int J Cancer* 1997;71: 948–951.
29. Riman T, Persson I, Nilsson S. Hormonal aspects of epithelial ovarian cancer: review of epidemiological evidence. *Clin Endocrinol (Oxf)* 1998;49:695–707.
30. Feeley KM, Wells M. Precursor lesions of ovarian epithelial malignancy. *Histopathology* 2001;38:87–95.
31. Fathalla MF. Incessant ovulation—a factor in ovarian neoplasia? *Lancet* 1971;2:163.
32. Gardner GJ, Birrer MJ. Ovarian tumors of low malignant potential: can molecular biology solve this enigma? *J Natl Cancer Inst* 2001;93:1122–1123.
33. Teneriello MG, Ebina M, Linnoila RI, et al. p53 and Ki-ras gene mutations in epithelial ovarian neoplasms. *Cancer Res* 1993;53:3103–3108.
34. Caduff RF, Svoboda-Newman SM, Ferguson AW, et al. Comparison of mutations of Ki-RAS and p53 immunoreactivity in borderline and malignant epithelial ovarian tumors. *Am J Surg Pathol* 1999;23:323–328.
35. Sato N, Tsunoda H, Nishida M, et al. Loss of heterozygosity on 10q23.3 and mutation of the tumor suppressor gene PTEN in benign endometrial cyst of the ovary: possible sequence progression from benign endometrial cyst to endometrioid

carcinoma and clear cell carcinoma of the ovary. *Cancer Res* 2000;60:7052–7056.

36. Thomas EJ, Campbell IG. Molecular genetic defects in endometriosis. *Gynecol Obstet Invest* 2000;50:44–50.

37. Obata K, Morland SJ, Watson RH, et al. Frequent PTEN/MMAC mutations in endometrioid but not serous or mucinous epithelial ovarian tumors. *Cancer Res* 1998;58: 2095–2097.

38. Obata K, Hoshiai H. Common genetic changes between endometriosis and ovarian cancer. *Gynecol Obstet Invest* 2000;50:39–43.

39. Brewer M, Utzinger U, Silva E, et al. Fluorescence spectroscopy for in vivo characterization of ovarian tissue. *Lasers Surg Med* 2001;29:128–135.

40. Bell R, Petticrew M, Sheldon T. The performance of screening tests for ovarian cancer: results of a systematic review. *Br J Obstet Gynaecol* 1998;105:1136–1147.

41. Devine PL, McGuckin MA, Quin RJ, Ward BG. Predictive value of the combination of serum markers, CA125, CASA and TPS in ovarian cancer. *Int J Gynecol Cancer* 1995;5: 170–178.

42. McGuckin MA, Ramm LE, Joy GJ, et al. Preoperative discrimination between ovarian carcinoma, non-ovarian gynecological malignancy and benign adnexal masses using serum levels of CA125 and the polymorphic epithelial mucin antigens CASA, OSA and MSA. *Int J Gynecol Cancer* 1992;2:119–128.

43. Woolas RP, Xu FJ, Jacobs IJ, et al. Elevation of multiple serum markers in patients with stage I ovarian cancer. *J Natl Cancer Inst* 1993;85:1748–1751.

44. van Haaften-Day C, Shen Y, Xu F, et al. OVX1, macrophage-colony stimulating factor, and CA-125-II as tumor markers for epithelial ovarian carcinoma: a critical appraisal. *Cancer* 2001;92:2837–2844.

45. Hogdall CK, Mogensen O, Tabor A, et al. The role of serum tetranectin, CA 125, and a combined index as tumor markers in women with pelvic tumors. *Gynecol Oncol* 1995;56: 22–28.

46. Hogdall CK, Hogdall EV, Hording U, et al. Plasma tetranectin and ovarian neoplasms. *Gynecol Oncol* 1991;43:103–107.

47. Mok SC, Chao J, Skates S, et al. Prostasin, a potential serum marker for ovarian cancer: identification through microarray technology. *J Natl Cancer Inst* 2001;93:1458–1464.

48. Siskind V, Green A, Bain C, Purdie D. Beyond ovulation: oral contraceptives and epithelial ovarian cancer. *Epidemiology* 2000;11:106–110.

49. Risch HA. Hormonal etiology of epithelial ovarian cancer, with a hypothesis concerning the role of androgens and progesterone. *J Natl Cancer Inst* 1998;90:1774–1786.

50. Whiteman DC, Murphy MF, Cook LS, et al. Multiple births and risk of epithelial ovarian cancer. *J Natl Cancer Inst* 2000;92:1172–1177.

51. Bu SZ, Yin DL, Ren XH, et al. Progesterone induces apoptosis and up-regulation of p53 expression in human ovarian carcinoma cell lines. *Cancer* 1997;79:1944–1950.

52. Syed V, Ulinski G, Mok SC, et al. Expression of gonadotropin receptor and growth responses to key reproductive hormones in normal and malignant human ovarian surface epithelial cells. *Cancer Res* 2001;61:6768–6776.

53. Berchuck A, Rodriguez G, Olt G, et al. Regulation of growth of normal ovarian epithelial cells and ovarian cancer cell lines by transforming growth factor-beta. *Am J Obstet Gynecol* 1992;166:676–684.

54. Lau KM, Mok SC, Ho SM. Expression of human estrogen receptor-alpha and -beta, progesterone receptor, and androgen receptor mRNA in normal and malignant ovarian epithelial cells. *Proc Natl Acad Sci USA* 1999;96:5722–5727.

55. Narod SA, Risch H, Moslehi R, et al. Oral contraceptives and the risk of hereditary ovarian cancer. Hereditary Ovarian Cancer Clinical Study Group. *N Engl J Med* 1998;339:424–428.

56. Modan B, Hartge P, Hirsh-Yechezkel G, et al. Parity, oral contraceptives, and the risk of ovarian cancer among carriers and noncarriers of a BRCA1 or BRCA2 mutation. *N Engl J Med* 2001;345:235–240.

57. Narod SA, Sun P, Risch HA. Ovarian cancer, oral contraceptives, and BRCA mutations. *N Engl J Med* 2001;345: 1706–1707.

58. Pike MC, Spicer DV. Hormonal contraception and chemoprevention of female cancers. *Endocr Relat Cancer* 2000;7:73–83.

59. De Palo G, Veronesi U, Camerini T, et al. Can fenretinide protect women against ovarian cancer? *J Natl Cancer Inst* 1995;87:146–147.

60. Veronesi U, De Palo G, Marubini E, et al. Randomized trial of fenretinide to prevent second breast malignancy in women with early breast cancer. *J Natl Cancer Inst* 1999;91: 1847–1856.

61. Sabichi AL, Hendricks DT, Bober MA, Birrer MJ. Retinoic acid receptor beta expression and growth inhibition of gynecologic cancer cells by the synthetic retinoid N-(4-hydroxyphenyl) retinamide. *J Natl Cancer Inst* 1998;90: 597–605.

62. Supino R, Crosti M, Clerici M, et al. Induction of apoptosis by fenretinide (4HPR) in human ovarian carcinoma cells and its association with retinoic acid receptor expression. *Int J Cancer* 1996;65:491–497.

63. Formelli F, Cleris L. Synthetic retinoid fenretinide is effective against a human ovarian carcinoma xenograft and potentiates cisplatin activity. *Cancer Res* 1993;53:5374–5376.

64. Benbrook DM, Madler MM, Spruce LW, et al. Biologically active heteroarotinoids exhibiting anticancer activity and decreased toxicity. *J Med Chem* 1997;40:3567–3583.

65. Guruswamy S, Lightfoot S, Gold MA, et al. Effects of retinoids on cancerous phenotype and apoptosis in organotypic cultures of ovarian carcinoma. *J Natl Cancer Inst* 2001;93:516–525.

66. Lefkowitz ES, Garland CF. Sunlight, vitamin D, and ovarian cancer mortality rates in US women. *Int J Epidemiol* 1994;23:1133–1136.

67. Ahonen MH, Zhuang YH, Aine R, et al. Androgen receptor and vitamin D receptor in human ovarian cancer: growth stimulation and inhibition by ligands. *Int J Cancer* 2000;86:40–46.

68. Saunders DE, Christensen C, Wappler NL, et al. Inhibition of c-myc in breast and ovarian carcinoma cells by 1,25-dihydroxyvitamin D3, retinoic acid and dexamethasone. *Anticancer Drugs* 1993;4:201–208.

69. Ness RB, Cottreau C. Possible role of ovarian epithelial inflammation in ovarian cancer. *J Natl Cancer Inst* 1999;91: 1459–1467.

70. Tzonou A, Polychronopoulou A, Hsieh CC, et al. Hair dyes, analgesics, tranquilizers and perineal talc application as risk factors for ovarian cancer. *Int J Cancer* 1993;55:408–410.

71. Rosenberg L, Palmer JR, Rao RS, et al. A case-control study of analgesic use and ovarian cancer. *Cancer Epidemiol Biomarkers Prev* 2000;9:933–937.

72. Cramer DW, Harlow BL, Titus-Ernstoff L, et al. Over-the-counter analgesics and risk of ovarian cancer. *Lancet* 1998; 351:104–107.

73. Moysich KB, Mettlin C, Piver MS, et al. Regular use of analgesic drugs and ovarian cancer risk. *Cancer Epidemiol Biomarkers Prev* 2001;10:903–906.

74. Rodriguez C, Henley SJ, Calle EE, Thun MJ. Paracetamol and risk of ovarian cancer mortality in a prospective study of women in the USA. *Lancet* 1998;352:1354–1355.

75. Smith WL, Garavito RM, DeWitt DL. Prostaglandin endoperoxide H synthases (cyclooxygenases)-1 and -2. *J Biol Chem* 1996;271:33,157–33,160.

76. Taketo MM. Cyclooxygenase-2 inhibitors in tumorigenesis (Part II). *J Natl Cancer Inst* 1998;90:1609–1620.

77. Taketo MM. Cyclooxygenase-2 inhibitors in tumorigenesis (part I). *J Natl Cancer Inst* 1998;90:1529–1536.

78. Williams CS, Mann M, DuBois RN. The role of cyclooxygenases in inflammation, cancer, and development. *Oncogene* 1999;18:7908–7916.

79. Ristimaki A, Honkanen N, Jankala H, et al. Expression of cyclooxygenase-2 in human gastric carcinoma. *Cancer Res* 1997;57:1276–1280.

80. Uefuji K, Ichikura T, Mochizuki H. Expression of cyclooxygenase-2 in human gastric adenomas and adenocarcinomas. *J Surg Oncol* 2001;76:26–30.

81. Chan G, Boyle JO, Yang EK, et al. Cyclooxygenase-2 expression is up-regulated in squamous cell carcinoma of the head and neck. *Cancer Res* 1999;59:991–994.

82. Ristimaki A, Nieminen O, Saukkonen K, et al. Expression of cyclooxygenase-2 in human transitional cell carcinoma of the urinary bladder. *Am J Pathol* 2001;158:849–853.

83. Shirahama T, Sakakura C. Overexpression of cyclooxygenase-2 in squamous cell carcinoma of the urinary bladder. *Clin Cancer Res* 2001;7:558–561.

84. Wolff H, Saukkonen K, Anttila S, et al. Expression of cyclooxygenase-2 in human lung carcinoma. *Cancer Res* 1998;58:4997–5001.

85. Tucker ON, Dannenberg AJ, Yang EK, et al. Cyclooxygenase-2 expression is up-regulated in human pancreatic cancer. *Cancer Res* 1999;59:987–990.

86. Hwang D, Scollard D, Byrne J, Levine E. Expression of cyclooxygenase-1 and cyclooxygenase-2 in human breast cancer. *J Natl Cancer Inst* 1998;90:455–460.

87. Tsujii M, Kawano S, DuBois RN. Cyclooxygenase-2 expression in human colon cancer cells increases metastatic potential. *Proc Natl Acad Sci USA* 1997;94:3336–3340.

88. Tsujii M, Kawano S, Tsuji S, et al. Cyclooxygenase regulates angiogenesis induced by colon cancer cells. *Cell* 1998; 93: 705–716.

89. Masferrer JL, Zweifel BS, Manning PT, et al. Selective inhibition of inducible cyclooxygenase 2 in vivo is antiinflammatory and nonulcerogenic. *Proc Natl Acad Sci USA* 1994; 91:3228–3232.

90. Tsujii M, DuBois RN. Alterations in cellular adhesion and apoptosis in epithelial cells overexpressing prostaglandin endoperoxide synthase 2. *Cell* 1995;83:493–501.

91. Harris RE, Alshafie GA, Abou-Issa H, Seibert K. Chemoprevention of breast cancer in rats by celecoxib, a cyclooxygenase 2 inhibitor. *Cancer Res* 2000;60:2101–2103.

92. Steinbach G, Lynch PM, Phillips RK, et al. The effect of celecoxib, a cyclooxygenase-2 inhibitor, in familial adenomatous polyposis. *N Engl J Med* 2000;342:1946–1952.

93. Murphy GJ, Holder JC. PPAR-gamma agonists: therapeutic role in diabetes, inflammation and cancer. *Trends Pharmacol Sci* 2000;21:469–474.

94. Adams M, Montague CT, Prins JB, et al. Activators of peroxisome proliferator-activated receptor gamma have depot-specific effects on human preadipocyte differentiation. *J Clin Invest* 1997;100:3149–3153.

95. Nolan JJ, Ludvik B, Beerdsen P, et al. Improvement in glucose tolerance and insulin resistance in obese subjects treated with troglitazone. *N Engl J Med* 1994;331:1188–1193.

96. Mueller E, Sarraf P, Tontonoz P, et al. Terminal differentiation of human breast cancer through PPAR gamma. *Mol Cell* 1998;1:465–470.

97. Sarraf P, Mueller E, Jones D, et al. Differentiation and reversal of malignant changes in colon cancer through PPARgamma. *Nat Med* 1998;4:1046–1052.

98. Bast RC Jr, Knauf S, Epenetos A, et al. Coordinate elevation of serum markers in ovarian cancer but not in benign disease. *Cancer* 1991;68:1758–1763.

99. Berek JS, Bast RC Jr. Ovarian cancer screening. The use of serial complementary tumor markers to improve sensitivity and specificity for early detection. *Cancer* 1995;76:2092–2096.

100. Devine PL, McGuckin MA, Quin RJ, Ward BG. Serum markers CASA and CA 15-3 in ovarian cancer: all MUC1 assays are not the same. *Tumour Biol* 1994;15:337–344.

101. Gadducci A, Ferdeghini M, Ceccarini T, et al. A comparative evaluation of the ability of serum CA 125, CA 19-9, CA 15-3, CA 50, CA 72-4 and TATI assays in reflecting the course of disease in patients with ovarian carcinoma. *Eur J Gynaecol Oncol* 1990;11:127–133.

102. Jacobs IJ, Rivera H, Oram DH, Bast RC Jr. Differential diagnosis of ovarian cancer with tumour markers CA 125, CA 15-3 and TAG 72.3. *Br J Obstet Gynaecol* 1993;100:1120–1124.

103. Scambia G, Benedetti Panici P, Baiocchi G, et al. CA 15-3 serum levels in ovarian cancer. *Oncology* 1988;45:263–267.

104. Soper JT, Hunter VJ, Daly L, et al. Preoperative serum tumor-associated antigen levels in women with pelvic masses. *Obstet Gynecol* 1990;75:249–254.

105. Zhang Z, Barnhill SD, Zhang H, et al. Combination of multiple serum markers using an artificial neural network to improve specificity in discriminating malignant from benign pelvic masses. *Gynecol Oncol* 1999;73:56–61.

106. Woolas RP, Conaway MR, Xu F, et al. Combinations of multiple serum markers are superior to individual assays for discriminating malignant from benign pelvic masses. *Gynecol Oncol* 1995;59:111–116.

107. Woolas RP, Oram DH, Jeyarajah AR, et al. Ovarian cancer identified through screening with serum markers but not by pelvic imaging. *Int J Gynecol Cancer* 1999;9:497–501.

108. Gocze PM, Szabo DG, Than GN, et al. Occurrence of CA 125 and CA 19-9 tumor-associated antigens in sera of patients with gynecologic, trophoblastic, and colorectal tumors. *Gynecol Obstet Invest* 1988;25:268–272.

109. Guadagni F, Roselli M, Cosimelli M, et al. CA 72-4 serum marker—a new tool in the management of carcinoma patients. *Cancer Invest* 1995;13:227–238.

110. Schwartz PE, Chambers SK, Chambers JT, et al. Circulating tumor markers in the monitoring of gynecologic malignancies. *Cancer* 1987;60:353–361.

111. Devine PL, McGuckin MA, Ward BG. Circulating mucins as tumor markers in ovarian cancer (review). *Anti Cancer Res* 1992;12:709–717.

112. Mazurek A, Niklinski J, Laudanski T, Pluygers E. Clinical tumour markers in ovarian cancer. *Eur J Cancer Prev* 1998; 7:23–35.

113. Tamakoshi K, Kikkawa F, Shibata K, et al. Clinical value of CA125, CA19-9, CEA, CA72-4, and TPA in borderline ovarian tumor. *Gynecol Oncol* 1996;62:67–72.

114. Wakahara F, Kikkawa F, Nawa A, et al. Diagnostic efficacy of tumor markers, sonography, and intraoperative frozen section for ovarian tumors. *Gynecol Obstet Invest* 2001;52:147–152.

115. Hasholzner U, Baumgartner L, Stieber P, et al. Clinical significance of the tumour markers CA 125 II and CA 72-4 in ovarian carcinoma. *Int J Cancer* 1996;69:329–334.

116. Negishi Y, Iwabuchi H, Sakunaga H, et al. Serum and tissue measurements of CA72-4 in ovarian cancer patients. *Gynecol Oncol* 1993;48:148–154.

117. Schutter EM, Sohn C, Kristen P, et al. Estimation of probability of malignancy using a logistic model combining physical examination, ultrasound, serum CA 125, and serum CA 72-4 in postmenopausal women with a pelvic mass: an international multicenter study. *Gynecol Oncol* 1998;69:56–63.

118. Scambia G, Benedetti Panici P, Perrone L, et al. Serum levels of tumour associated glycoprotein (TAG 72) in patients with gynaecological malignancies. *Br J Cancer* 1990;62:147–151.

119. Devine PL, McGuckin MA, Ramm LE, et al. Serum mucin antigens CASA and MSA in tumors of the breast, ovary, lung, pancreas, bladder, colon, and prostate. A blind trial with 420 patients. *Cancer* 1993;72:2007–2015.

120. Hogdall EV, Hogdall CK, Tingulstad S, et al. Predictive values of serum tumour markers tetranectin, OVX1, CASA and CA125 in patients with a pelvic mass. *Int J Cancer* 2000;89:519–523.

121. Kierkegaard O, Mogensen O, Mogensen B, Jakobsen A. Predictive and prognostic values of cancer-associated serum antigen (CASA) and cancer antigen 125 (CA 125) levels prior to second-look laparotomy for ovarian cancer. *Gynecol Oncol* 1995;59:251–254.

122. McGuckin MA, Layton GT, Bailey MJ, et al. Evaluation of two new assays for tumor-associated antigens, CASA and OSA, found in the serum of patients with epithelial ovarian carcinoma—comparison with CA125. *Gynecol Oncol* 1990;37:165–171.

123. Meisel M, Straube W, Weise J, Burkhardt B. A study of serum CASA and CA 125 levels in patients with ovarian carcinoma. *Arch Gynecol Obstet* 1995;256:9–15.

124. Ward BG, McGuckin MA, Ramm LE, et al. The management of ovarian carcinoma is improved by the use of cancer-associated serum antigen and CA 125 assays. *Cancer* 1993;71:430–438.

125. Halila H, Lehtovirta P, Stenman UH. Tumour-associated trypsin inhibitor (TATI) in ovarian cancer. *Br J Cancer* 1988;57:304–307.

126. Roman LD, Muderspach LI, Burnett AF, Morrow CP. Carcinoembryonic antigen in women with isolated pelvic masses. Clinical utility? *J Reprod Med* 1998;43:403–407.

127. Sawada M, Okudaira Y, Matsui Y, Shimizu Y. Immunosuppressive acidic protein in patients with ovarian cancer. *Cancer* 1983;52:2081–2085.

128. Tholander B, Taube A, Lindgren A, et al. Pretreatment serum levels of CA-125, carcinoembryonic antigen, tissue polypeptide antigen, and placental alkaline phosphatase in patients with ovarian carcinoma: influence of histological type, grade of differentiation, and clinical stage of disease. *Gynecol Oncol* 1990;39:26–33.

129. Tholander B, Taube A, Lindgren A, et al. Pretreatment serum levels of CA-125, carcinoembryonic antigen, tissue polypeptide antigen, and placental alkaline phosphatase, in patients

130. Xu FJ, Yu YH, Li BY, et al. Development of two new monoclonal antibodies reactive to a surface antigen present on human ovarian epithelial cancer cells. *Cancer Res* 1991;51:4012–4019.

with ovarian carcinoma, borderline tumors, or benign adnexal masses: relevance for differential diagnosis. *Gynecol Oncol* 1990;39:16–25.

131. Gadducci A, Ferdeghini M, Cosio S, et al. The clinical relevance of serum CYFRA 21-1 assay in patients with ovarian cancer. *Int J Gynecol Cancer* 2001;11:277–282.

132. Inaba N, Negishi Y, Fukasawa I, et al. Cytokeratin fragment 21-1 in gynecologic malignancy: comparison with cancer antigen 125 and squamous cell carcinoma-related antigen. *Tumour Biol* 1995;16:345–352.

133. Udagawa Y, Aoki D, Ito K, et al. Clinical characteristics of a newly developed ovarian tumour marker, galactosyltransferase associated with tumour (GAT). *Eur J Cancer* 1998;34:489–495.

134. Uemura M, Sakaguchi T, Uejima T, et al. Mouse monoclonal antibodies which recognize a human (beta 1-4)galactosyltransferase associated with tumor in body fluids. *Cancer Res* 1992;52:6153–6157.

135. Ward BG, McGuckin MA, Hurst TG, Khoo SK. Expression of multiple tumour markers in serum from patients with ovarian carcinoma and healthy women. *Aust NZ J Obstet Gynaecol* 1989;29:340–345.

136. Botti C, Seregni E, Ferrari L, et al. Immunosuppressive factors: role in cancer development and progression. *Int J Biol Markers* 1998;13:51–69.

137. Castelli M, Romano P, Atlante G, et al. Immunosuppressive acidic protein (IAP) and CA 125 assays in detection of human ovarian cancer: preliminary results. *Int J Biol Markers* 1987;2:187–190.

138. Castelli M, Battaglia F, Scambia G, et al. Immunosuppressive acidic protein and CA 125 levels in patients with ovarian cancer. *Oncology* 1991;48:13–17.

139. Foti E, Ferrandina G, Martucci R, et al. IL-6, M-CSF and IAP cytokines in ovarian cancer: simultaneous assessment of serum levels. *Oncology* 1999;57:211–215.

140. Scambia G, Foti E, Ferrandina G, et al. Prognostic role of immunosuppressive acidic protein in advanced ovarian cancer. *Am J Obstet Gynecol* 1996;175:1606–1610.

141. Maccio A, Lai P, Santona MC, et al. High serum levels of soluble IL-2 receptor, cytokines, and C reactive protein correlate with impairment of T cell response in patients with advanced epithelial ovarian cancer. *Gynecol Oncol* 1998;69:248–252.

142. Scambia G, Testa U, Panici PB, et al. Interleukin-6 serum levels in patients with gynecological tumors. *Int J Cancer* 1994;57:318–323.

143. Plante M, Rubin SC, Wong GY, et al. Interleukin-6 level in serum and ascites as a prognostic factor in patients with epithelial ovarian cancer. *Cancer* 1994;73:1882–1888.

144. Scambia G, Testa U, Benedetti Panici P, et al. Prognostic significance of interleukin 6 serum levels in patients with ovarian cancer. *Br J Cancer* 1995;71:354–356.

145. Tempfer C, Zeisler H, Sliutz G, et al. Serum evaluation of interleukin 6 in ovarian cancer patients. *Gynecol Oncol* 1997;66:27–30.

146. Diamandis EP, Yousef GM, Soosaipillai AR, Bunting P. Human kallikrein 6 (zyme/protease M/neurosin): a new serum biomarker of ovarian carcinoma. *Clin Biochem* 2000;33:579–583.

147. Diamandis EP, Okui A, Mitsui S, et al. Human kallikrein 11: a new biomarker of prostate and ovarian carcinoma. *Cancer Res* 2002;62:295–300.

148. Dong Y, Kaushal A, Bui L, et al. Human kallikrein 4 (KLK4) is highly expressed in serous ovarian carcinomas. *Clin Cancer Res* 2001;7:2363–2371.

149. Luo LY, Bunting P, Scorilas A, Diamandis EP. Human kallikrein 10: a novel tumor marker for ovarian carcinoma? *Clin Chim Acta* 2001;306:111–118.

150. Magklara A, Scorilas A, Katsaros D, et al. The human KLK8 (neuropsin/ovasin) gene: identification of two novel splice variants and its prognostic value in ovarian cancer. *Clin Cancer Res* 2001;7:806–811.

151. Obiezu CV, Scorilas A, Katsaros D, et al. Higher human kallikrein gene 4 (KLK4) expression indicates poor prognosis of ovarian cancer patients. *Clin Cancer Res* 2001;7: 2380–2386.

152. Yousef GM, Kyriakopoulou LG, Scorilas A, et al. Quantitative expression of the human kallikrein gene 9 (KLK9) in ovarian cancer: a new independent and favorable prognostic marker. *Cancer Res* 2001;61:7811–7818.

153. Cane P, Azen C, Lopez E, et al. Tumor marker trends in asymptomatic women at risk for ovarian cancer: relevance for ovarian cancer screening. *Gynecol Oncol* 1995;57: 240–245.

154. Cole LA, Schwartz PE, Wang YX. Urinary gonadotropin fragments (UGF) in cancers of the female reproductive system. I. Sensitivity and specificity, comparison with other markers. *Gynecol Oncol* 1988;31:82–90.

155. Patsner B, Mann WJ, Vissicchio M, Loesch M. Comparison of serum CA-125 and lipid-associated sialic acid (LASA-P) in monitoring patients with invasive ovarian adenocarcinoma. *Gynecol Oncol* 1988;30:98–103.

156. Schutter EM, Visser JJ, van Kamp GJ, et al. The utility of lipid-associated sialic acid (LASA or LSA) as a serum marker for malignancy. A review of the literature. *Tumour Biol* 1992;13:121–132.

157. Vardi JR, Tadros GH, Malhotra C, et al. Lipid associated sialic acid in plasma in patients with advanced carcinoma of the ovaries. *Surg Gynecol Obstet* 1989;168:296–301.

158. Dwivedi C, Dixit M, Hardy RE. Plasma lipid-bound sialic acid alterations in neoplastic diseases. *Experientia* 1990;46:91–94.

159. Petru E, Sevin BU, Averette HE, et al. Comparison of three tumor markers—CA-125, lipid-associated sialic acid (LSA), and NB/70K—in monitoring ovarian cancer. *Gynecol Oncol* 1990;38:181–186.

160. Schwartz PE, Chambers JT, Taylor KJ, et al. Early detection of ovarian cancer: preliminary results of the Yale Early Detection Program. *Yale J Biol Med* 1991;64:573–582.

161. Vardi JR, Tadros GH, Foemmel R, Shebes M. Plasma lipid-associated sialic acid and serum CA 125 as indicators of disease status with advanced ovarian cancer. *Obstet Gynecol* 1989;74:379–383.

162. Shen Z, Wu M, Elson P, et al. Fatty acid composition of lysophosphatidic acid and lysophosphatidylinositol in plasma from patients with ovarian cancer and other gynecological diseases. *Gynecol Oncol* 2001;83:25–30.

163. Xu Y, Shen Z, Wiper DW, et al. Lysophosphatidic acid as a potential biomarker for ovarian and other gynecologic cancers. *JAMA* 1998;280:719–723.

164. Bast RC Jr, Boyer CM, Xu FJ, et al. Molecular approaches to prevention and detection of epithelial ovarian cancer. *J Cell Biochem Suppl* 1995;23:219–222.

165. Suzuki M, Ohwada M, Sato I, Nagatomo M. Serum level of macrophage colony-stimulating factor as a marker for gynecologic malignancies. *Oncology* 1995;52:128–133.

166. Suzuki M, Ohwada M, Aida I, et al. Macrophage colony-stimulating factor as a tumor marker for epithelial ovarian cancer. *Obstet Gynecol* 1993;82:946–950.

167. Bizzari JP, Mackillop WJ, Buick RN. Cellular specificity of NB70K, a putative human ovarian tumor antigen. *Cancer Res* 1983;43:864–867.

168. Dembo AJ, Chang PL, Urbach GI. Clinical correlations of ovarian cancer antigen NB/70K: a preliminary report. *Obstet Gynecol* 1985;65:710–714.

169. Knauf S, Urbach GI. Identification, purification, and radioimmunoassay of NB/70K, a human ovarian tumor-associated antigen. *Cancer Res* 1981;41:1351–1357.

170. Knauf S, Taillon-Miller P, Helmkamp BF, et al. Selectivity for ovarian cancer of an improved serum radioimmunoassay for human ovarian tumor-associated antigen NB/70K. *Gynecol Oncol* 1984;17:349–355.

171. Knauf S, Kalwas J, Helmkamp BF, et al. Monoclonal antibodies against human ovarian tumor associated antigen NB/70K: preparation and use in a radioimmunoassay for measuring NB/70K in serum. *Cancer Immunol Immunother* 1986;21:217–225.

172. Knauf S, Bast RC Jr. Tumor antigen NB/70K and CA 125 levels in the blood of preoperative ovarian cancer patients and controls: a preliminary report of the use of the NB12123 and CA 125 radioimmunoassays alone and in combination. *Int J Biol Markers* 1988;3:75–81.

173. Knauf S. Clinical evaluation of ovarian tumor antigen NB/70K: monoclonal antibody assays for distinguishing ovarian cancer from other gynecologic disease. *Am J Obstet Gynecol* 1988;158:1067–1072.

174. Knauf S. Monoclonal antibody assays for measuring ovarian tumor antigen in blood. Detection of NB/70K in patients with ovarian cancer and nongynecologic diseases. *Cancer* 1988;62:922–925.

175. Xu FJ, Yu YH, Daly L, et al. OVX1 radioimmunoassay complements CA-125 for predicting the presence of residual ovarian carcinoma at second-look surgical surveillance procedures. *J Clin Oncol* 1993;11:1506–1510.

176. Ben-Arie A, Hagay Z, Ben-Hur H, et al. Elevated serum alkaline phosphatase may enable early diagnosis of ovarian cancer. *Eur J Obstet Gynecol Reprod Biol* 1999;86:69–71.

177. Fishman WH. Clinical and biological significance of an isozyme tumor marker–PLAP. *Clin Biochem* 1987;20: 387–392.

178. Fisken J, Leonard RC, Shaw G, et al. Serum placental-like alkaline phosphatase (PLAP): a novel combined enzyme linked immunoassay for monitoring ovarian cancer. *J Clin Pathol* 1989;42:40–45.

179. Muensch HA, Maslow WC, Azama F, et al. Placental-like alkaline phosphatase. Re-evaluation of the tumor marker with exclusion of smokers. *Cancer* 1986;58:1689–1694.

180. Vergote I, Onsrud M, Nustad K. Placental alkaline phosphatase as a tumor marker in ovarian cancer. *Obstet Gynecol* 1987;69:228–232.

181. Burger HG, Robertson DM, Cahir N, et al. Characterization of inhibin immunoreactivity in post-menopausal women with ovarian tumours. *Clin Endocrinol (Oxf)* 1996;44: 413–418.

182. Burger HG, Fuller PJ, Chu S, et al. The inhibins and ovarian cancer. *Mol Cell Endocrinol* 2001;180:145–148.

183. Lambert-Messerlian GM, Steinhoff M, Zheng W, et al. Multiple immunoreactive inhibin proteins in serum from postmenopausal women with epithelial ovarian cancer. *Gynecol Oncol* 1997;65:512–516.

184. Cooke I, O'Brien M, Charnock FM, et al. Inhibin as a marker for ovarian cancer. *Br J Cancer* 1995;71:1046–1050.

185. Lambert-Messerlian GM. Is inhibin a serum marker for ovarian cancer? *Eur J Endocrinol* 2000;142:331–333.

186. Robertson DM, Cahir N, Burger HG, et al. Combined inhibin and CA125 assays in the detection of ovarian cancer. *Clin Chem* 1999;45:651–658.

187. Mills GB, Bast RC Jr, Srivastava S. Future for ovarian cancer screening: novel markers from emerging technologies of transcriptional profiling and proteomics. *J Natl Cancer Inst* 2001;93:1437–1439.

188. Iwanari O, Miyako J, Date Y, et al. Differential diagnosis of ovarian cancer, benign ovarian tumor and endometriosis by a combination assay of serum sialyl SSEA-1 antigen and CA125 levels. *Gynecol Obstet Invest* 1990;29:71–74.

189. Iwanari O, Miyako J, Date Y, et al. Clinical evaluations of the tumor marker sialyl SSEA-1 antigen for clinical gynecological disease. *Gynecol Obstet Invest* 1990;29:214–218.

190. Kobayashi H, Kawashima Y. Clinical usefulness of serum sialyl SSEA-1 antigen levels in patients with epithelial ovarian cancer. Comparative effectiveness of sialyl SSEA-1 and CA 125. *Gynecol Obstet Invest* 1990;30:52–58.

191. Suzuki M, Ohwada M, Tamada T. Clinical value of sialyl SSEA-1 antigen in patients with ovarian cancer. *Gynecol Oncol* 1990;36:371–375.

192. Peters-Engl C, Medl M, Ogris E, Leodolter S. Tumor-associated trypsin inhibitor (TATI) and cancer antigen 125 (CA125) in patients with epithelial ovarian cancer. *Anti Cancer Res* 1995;15:2727–2730.

193. Medl M, Ogris E, Peters-Engl C, Leodolter S. TATI (tumour-associated trypsin inhibitor) as a marker of ovarian cancer. *Br J Cancer* 1995;71:1051–1054.

194. Vartiainen J, Lehtovirta P, Finne P, et al. Preoperative serum concentration of hCGbeta as a prognostic factor in ovarian cancer. *Int J Cancer* 2001;95:313–316.

195. Venesmaa P, Lehtovirta P, Stenman UH, et al. Tumour-associated trypsin inhibitor (TATI): comparison with CA125 as a preoperative prognostic indicator in advanced ovarian cancer. *Br J Cancer* 1994;70:1188–1190.

196. Hogdall CK, Christensen L, Clemmensen I. The prognostic value of tetranectin immunoreactivity and plasma tetranectin in patients with ovarian cancer. *Cancer* 1993;72:2415–2422.

197. Van Dalen A, Favier J, Baumgartner L, et al. Serum levels of CA 125 and TPS during treatment of ovarian cancer. *Anti Cancer Res* 2000;20:5107–5108.

198. Cole LA, Nam JH, Chambers JT, Schwartz PE. Urinary gonadotropin fragment, a new tumor marker. II. Differentiating a benign from a malignant pelvic mass. *Gynecol Oncol* 1990;36:391–394.

199. Cole LA, Nam JH. Urinary gonadotropin fragment (UGF) measurements in the diagnosis and management of ovarian cancer. *Yale J Biol Med* 1989;62:367–378.

200. Schutter EM, Mijatovic V, Kok A, et al. Urinary gonadotropin peptide (UGP) and serum CA 125 in gynaecologic practice, a clinical prospective study. *Anti Cancer Res* 1999;19:5551–5557.

201. Schwartz PE, Cracchiolo BM, Cole LA. Clinical applications of urinary gonadotropin peptides (UGP) in gynecologic oncology. *Anti Cancer Res* 1996;16:2135–2139.

202. Walker R, Crebbin V, Stern J, et al. Urinary gonadotropin peptide (UGP) as a marker of gynecologic malignancies. *Anti Cancer Res* 1994;14:1703–1709.

203. Wang YX, Schwartz PE, Chambers JT, Cole LA. Urinary gonadotropin fragments (UGF) in cancers of the female reproductive system. II. Initial serial studies. *Gynecol Oncol* 1988;31:91–102.

204. Okamoto T, Niu R, Matsuo K, et al. Human chorionic gonadotropin beta-core fragment is directly produced by cancer cells. *Life Sci* 2001;68:861–872.

205. Obermair A, Tempfer C, Hefler L, et al. Concentration of vascular endothelial growth factor (VEGF) in the serum of patients with suspected ovarian cancer. *Br J Cancer* 1998;77:1870–1874.

206. Oehler MK, Caffier H. Prognostic relevance of serum vascular endothelial growth factor in ovarian cancer. *Anti Cancer Res* 2000;20:5109–5112.

207. Hazelton DA, Hamilton TC. Vascular endothelial growth factor in ovarian cancer. *Curr Oncol Rep* 1999;1:59–63.

208. Tempfer C, Obermair A, Hefler L, et al. Vascular endothelial growth factor serum concentrations in ovarian cancer. *Obstet Gynecol* 1998;92:360–363.

PANCREAS

36 Strategies for Chemoprevention in Pancreatic Cancer

Chandrajit P. Raut, MD, David J. McConkey, PhD, and James L. Abbruzzese, MD

1. PANCREATIC CANCER: OVERVIEW

1.1. Statistics and Epidemiology

The incidence of pancreatic cancer has been increasing steadily. In 2002, 30,300 Americans were estimated to be diagnosed with this malignancy, and 29,700 died from it *(1)*.

Pancreatic cancer is the tenth leading cause of cancer in men and ninth leading cause in women, accounting for 2% of cancer cases in either gender. It is the fourth leading cause of cancer deaths in the United States, with 5% of all cancer deaths in men and 6% in women due to this malignancy *(2)*. At diagnosis, approx 40% of patients have metastatic disease and another 40–50% have locally advanced disease not amenable to surgical resection. Only 10–20% of patients can be considered candidates for curative resection *(3)*. Despite advances in surgical techniques and adjuvant therapy, survival has changed little in the last 20 yr *(4)*, with a 5-yr survival rate of 4% according to the American Cancer Society *(5)*.

Epidemiological studies have identified groups at increased risk for pancreatic risk (Table 1) *(6)*. High intake of fried foods, cigarette smoking, long-standing diabetes mellitus, chronic pancreatitis, and prior history of lung, head and neck, and bladder cancer confer a higher risk *(6)*. New Zealand Maoris, native Hawaiians, and African Americans are also at increased risk *(6)*.

1.2. Familial Pancreatic Cancer

An estimated 10% of patients with pancreatic cancer may have an inherited predisposition to this disease

(6,7). While genetic mutations have been identified as responsible for at least five syndromes linked with pancreatic cancer, most kindreds with familial aggregation do not have one of these syndromes *(7)*.

Several genetic syndromes associated with familial aggregation of pancreatic cancer have been characterized, including familial breast cancer with germline mutations in the *BRCA2* gene on chromosome 13q encoding a protein functioning in DNA repair *(8,9)*, familial atypical multiple-mole melanoma with germline mutations in the *p16* tumor suppressor gene on chromosome 9p *(10)*, Peutz-Jeghers syndrome with germline mutations in the *STK11/LKB1* gene on chromosome 19p encoding a serine/threonine kinase *(11,12)*, hereditary nonpolyposis colorectal cancer with germline mutations in one of the DNA mismatch repair genes (*hMLH1*, *hMSH2*) *(13,14)*, and hereditary pancreatitis with germline mutations in the *PRSS1* gene on chromosome 7q encoding cationic trypsinogen *(15,16)* (Table 2) *(7)*. Furthermore, kindreds with multiple endocrine neoplasia, Hippel-Lindau syndrome, and familial adenomatous polyposis (FAP) and Gardner's syndrome may also have an increased risk for pancreatic cancer *(6)*.

Genetic lesions associated with pancreatic adenocarcinoma include mutations of the K-*ras* (found in approx 90% of patients with pancreatic cancer), *p16* (80%), p53 (50%), and *DPC4* (50%) genes *(17,18)*. K-*ras* and *p16* mutations have also been detected in noninvasive intraductal lesions, which are considered neoplastic precursors of invasive pancreatic cancer *(19)*.

From: *Cancer Chemoprevention, Volume 2: Strategies for Cancer Chemoprevention*
Edited by: G. J. Kelloff, E. T. Hawk, and C. C. Sigman © Humana Press Inc., Totowa, NJ

Table 1
Groups With Increased Risk of Pancreatic Cancer

Increasing age (>45 yr)

New Zealand Maoris

Native Hawaiians

African Americans

High intake of fried foods

Cigarette smokers

Prior history of lung, head and neck, or bladder cancer

Long-standing diabetes mellitus

Chronic pancreatitis

Adapted from ref. *(6)* with permission.

Table 2
Risk of Pancreatic Cancer in Familial Syndromes

Individual	Gene	Chromosome	Relative risk	Risk by age 70 (%)
no history	—	—	1	<0.5
HNPCC	*hMLH1, hMSH2*	2,3	unknown	unknown
BRCA2	*Brca2*	13q	10	5
Familial pancreatic cancer	unknown	unknown	18[a]	9–10
FAMMM	*p16*	9p	20	10
Familial pancreatitis	*PRSS1*	7q	50	25–40
Peutz-Jeghers syndrome	*STK11*	10p	132	66

HNPCC = Hereditary nonpolyposis colorectal cancer.

FAMMM = familial atypical multiple mole melanoma.

[a]Prospective risk in an asymptomatic individual who has two first-degree relatives with pancreatic cancer.

[Adaped from ref. *(7)* with permission].

Based on the National Familial Pancreas Tumor Registry, pancreatic cancer risk and incidence are exceptionally high among at-risk first-degree relatives in familial pancreatic cancer kindreds in which at least three first-degree relatives have already been diagnosed with pancreatic cancer *(20)*. Recently, Hruban et al. *(7)* reported that kindreds with two first-degree relatives diagnosed with pancreatic cancer had an 18-fold increased risk of prospectively developing pancreatic cancer; with three first-degree relatives, the risk rose to a 57-fold increase. These kindreds are a reasonable high-risk group for pancreatic cancer screening and chemoprevention research *(20)*.

1.3. Precursors to Invasive Pancreatic Cancer

Epithelial proliferations in the small pancreatic ductules appear to be the histological precursors to invasive ductal adenocarcinoma of the pancreas (reviewed in *7*). A new unifying nomenclature, pancreatic intraepithelial neoplasia (PanIN), has been proposed to describe these lesions and their neoplastic nature *(21)*.

PanINs are found more frequently in pancreas specimens with cancer than those without, appear to progress to invasive pancreatic cancer, and manifest some of the same genetic alterations found in infiltrating carcinomas (reviewed in *7*). This progression from normal epithelium to high-grade intraepithelial neoplasia is associated with an accumulation of genetic mutations in several of the genes mentioned above (Fig. 1) *(22)*. Thus, these lesions could also provide potential targets for screening.

1.4. Screening

No effective strategies currently exist for screening the general population or even those at an increased risk of developing pancreatic cancer. However, several invasive and noninvasive techniques are under investigation. Potential techniques for screening include stool or blood analysis for K-*ras* mutations; noninvasive imaging via computed tomography, positron emission tomography, or magnetic resonance imaging; and endoscopic ultrasonography, endoscopic retrograde cholangiopancreatography

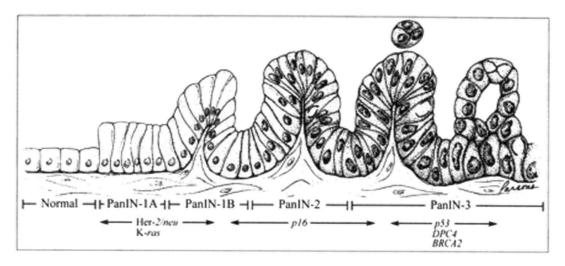

Fig. 1. This progression model for pancreatic cancer illustrates the association between increasingly abnormal epithelial architecture and the accumulation of abnormalities in genes implicated in malignancies (from *[22]* with permission. Artwork by Jennifer Parsons).

with brush or fluid cytology and K-*ras* mutation analysis, or Dreiling tube collection of pancreatic fluid for analysis. K-*ras* mutations can be detected in bile, stool, and blood in patients with advanced pancreatic cancer *(23,24)*. However, the sensitivity and specificity of these tests need to be further elaborated before any can be recommended for routine screening.

2. REPRESENTATIVE CLASSES OF CHEMOPREVENTIVE AGENTS

Chemopreventive agents by definition should slow the progression of, reverse, or inhibit carcinogenesis *(25)*. In turn, this should lower the risk of developing invasive or clinically significant disease. Strategies for chemoprevention may target processes or enzymes that appear to be upregulated in pancreatic neoplasia, such as cyclooxygenase (COX)-2 and farnesyl protein transferase. Other agents, such as retinoids and the various antioxidants, appear to have some chemopreventive properties, but their mechanisms of action need further elucidation. All these agents are discussed in detail below.

2.1. COX-2 Inhibitors

COX is a rate-limiting enzyme in prostaglandin synthesis. Two isoforms have been characterized. The COX-1 isoform is expressed constitutively in most tissues and produces prostaglandins regulating normal cellular processes *(26)*. The COX-2 isoform is not present under physiologic conditions, but is upregulated by cytokines, growth factors, and tumor promoters at sites of inflammation *(27–31)*. The COX-2 protein is involved in mechanisms such as promotion of angiogenesis *(32)*, inhibition of immunosurveillance *(33)*, and inhibition of apoptosis *(34)*.

COX-2 activation may play a role in carcinogenesis. Its impact in colorectal tumorigenesis was illustrated with the dramatic suppression of intestinal polyp formation in Apc$^{\Delta 716}$ knockout mice crossed with COX-2 knockout mice *(35)*. Upregulation of COX-2 has been detected in human colorectal *(28)*, gastric *(36)*, esophageal *(37)*, and lung *(38)* carcinomas. Thus, the COX-2 enzyme is an attractive target for chemopreventive strategies.

Aspirin and other nonsteroidal anti inflammatory drugs (NSAIDs), which inhibit both isoforms of the COX protein, reduce the incidence and mortality of colorectal cancer *(39–43)*. Treatment of colon carcinoma cells in vitro with the nonspecific COX inhibitors sulindac sulfide and indomethacin elevated levels of arachidonic acid, the precursor of prostaglandins, which stimulate conversion of sphingomyelin to ceramide, a potent inducer of apoptosis *(44)*. FAP patients treated with sulindac showed a significant decrease in both number and size of polyps *(45,46)*. However, NSAIDs can produce toxic side effects, including gastrointestinal mucosal injury and renal dysfunction due to inhibition of COX-1. This has led to the development of specific COX-2 inhibitors *(47)*. Selective inhibitors would appear to avoid some of the toxic side effects of nonspecific COX inhibitors while specifically targeting tissues in which COX-2 expression has been upregulated.

Kokawa et al. *(48)* studied COX-2 expression in human pancreatic cancer tissue specimens and immortalized pancreatic cancer cells lines. They demonstrated marked COX-2 expression in 57% (24/42) of pancreatic ductal adenocarcinomas, 58% (11/19) of intraductal papillary mucinous tumor (IPMT) adenomas, and 70% (7/10) of IPMT adenocarcinomas (defined by more than 5% of tumor cells clearly positive by immunohistochemical staining). Adjacent normal pancreatic tissue demonstrated no apparent expression. Although it is unclear whether COX-2 is expressed in the early stages of adenocarcinoma, its expression in noninvasive IPMT adenomas suggests it may play some early role in tumor progression. Consistent with previous reports in other organs, there was no significant correlation between COX-2 expression and any clinicopathologic factors, such as mean age, gender, tumor size and location, histologic type, lymphatic or venous invasion, lymph node metastases, and TNM stage. Furthermore, all four immortalized pancreatic cancer cell lines tested also expressed COX-2 protein. They all demonstrated dose-dependent growth inhibition following 72 h of treatment with aspirin and the NSAID etodolac. The inhibitory effect of aspirin, but not etodolac, on cell growth correlated with COX-2 expression; the two lines with stronger staining (MIAPaCa-2 and Panc-1) were inhibited at lower inhibitory concentrations (IC_{50}) of aspirin than those staining weakly (KP-2 and PNS-1). The IC_{50} for etodolac, a COX-2-specific inhibitor, was lower than that of aspirin, as previously shown in colon cancer cell lines *(49,50)*.

Molina et al. *(51)* demonstrated elevated levels of COX-2 mRNA and protein in human pancreatic adenocarcinoma and cell lines derived from such tumors. Immunohistochemistry demonstrated that cytoplasmic COX-2 protein expression was elevated in 67% (14/21) of tumors (in normal pancreatic tissue, COX-2 was detected only in islet cells, not acinar or ductal cells). Western blot assay detected COX-2 protein expression in three of five cell lines (BxPC-3, Capan-1, MDAPanc-3). Reverse-transcriptase PCR demonstrated increased levels of COX-2 mRNA in four of five cell lines, while the remaining line, Panc-1, expressed levels lower than normal pancreas. In contrast, Kokawa et al. *(48)* showed strong immunohistochemical staining of Panc-1 cells. Cell lines with the highest COX-2 levels were derived from moderately well- and well-differentiated carcinomas. Two NSAIDs, nonselective sulindac sulfide and COX-2-selective NS398, both produced a dose-dependent inhibition of cell proliferation in all pancreatic cell lines tested. This inhibition was independent of the level of COX-2 expression, suggesting that the inhibitory effect of both drugs may be mediated by pathways independent of the COX-2 enzyme. Both drugs also induced COX-2 expression in BxPC-3 cells; this was greater with the COX-2-specific inhibitor NS398 than with the nonspecific sulindac. The number of viable cells in the two highest concentrations of sulindac sulfide tested was reduced compared to the initial cell number, suggesting that this drug may induce apoptosis as well.

In summary, these in vitro studies suggest that the enzyme COX-2 is overexpressed in some, but not all, pancreatic cancers and in certain noninvasive pancreatic tumors. In normal pancreatic tissue, COX-2 is expressed only in islet cells. Its expression in neoplastic tissue does not correlate with any other clinicopathologic factors. Pancreatic cancer cell lines expressing COX-2 demonstrate growth inhibition when treated with NSAIDs; this inhibition depends on drug dose, but probably not on COX-2 expression level.

Little has been published testing the effects of COX inhibitors in in vivo models. The NSAIDs indomethacin and phenylbutazone have been shown to reduce pancreatic cancer development in a hamster model in which pancreatic tumors were induced by treatment with *N*-nitrosobis(2-oxopropyl)amine *(52)*. COX-2 inhibitors are currently being investigated in animal orthotopic models. Further work is necessary in this area to determine the effectiveness of these drugs and the appropriateness of this target.

2.2. Farnesyl Protein Transferase Inhibitors

Ras genes encode 21-kDa proteins that belong to a large superfamily of guanosine triphosphate (GTP)-binding proteins cycling between an active GTP-bound and an inactive guanosine diphosphate (GDP)-bound state (reviewed in *53*). Four human *ras* genes have been identified: H-*ras*, K-*ras*-4A, K-*ras*-4B, and N-*ras* *(54)*. Ras proteins connect signals generated at the plasma membrane with nuclear effectors, serving as crucial regulators of many physiological functions, including cell growth and differentiation. Oncogenic activity results most commonly from remaining in the active GTP-bound state *(54)*, thereby constitutively transmitting growth signals, and to a lesser extent from overexpression of the normal Ras proteins *(55)*. K-*ras* mutations are the most common genetic mutation in pancreatic cancer, occur in preinvasive lesions, and do not correlate with prognosis or tumor stage, suggesting that these mutations occur in the early stages of carcinogenesis

(56). Disruption of the *ras* signaling pathway could serve as a chemopreventive strategy *(53).*

One such strategy exploits the fact that Ras proteins require post-translational modification with a farnesyl moiety by the enzyme farnesyl protein transferase (FPT) for both normal and oncogenic activity *(57).* A strategy for developing Ras FPT inhibitors as chemopreventive agents is outlined by Kelloff et al. *(53).* Requirements for FPT inhibitors include specificity for the enzyme (as opposed to other post-translational transferases), the ability to specifically inhibit processing of mutant K-*ras*, high potency, selective activity in intact cells, activity in vivo, and lack of toxicity *(53).*

Two target substrates have been identified: farnesyl pyrophosphate (FPP), and the carboxy-terminal CAAX motif of Ras proteins (where C is cysteine, A is an aliphatic amino acid, and X is another amino acid). When a protein acceptor such as Ras is not available, FPP forms a stable noncovalent complex with FPT (or a similar tranferase). Thus FPP competitive inhibitors could bind FPT and prevent Ras farnesylation. Several potential competitive inhibitors, such as perillyl alcohol, *d*-limonene, and related metabolites, have demonstrated chemopreventive *(58)* and tumor-shrinking potential *(59).* Furthermore, isoprenoid compounds (farnesol, geraniol, and perillyl alcohol) suppress pancreatic tumor growth in animal models *(60).* Perillyl alcohol may also induce apoptosis; in vitro studies found an association between a perillyl-alcohol-induced increase in apoptosis and a two- to eightfold increase in expression of the pro-apoptotic protein Bak in pancreatic cancer cells, but not in nonmalignant cells *(61).*

The second potential strategy employs the CAAX tetrapeptide motif required for protein interaction with FPT. While structural activity analysis of tetrapeptides conforming to the CAAX consensus sequence suggests that they should serve as potent competitive inhibitors, they have been inactive in whole cells *(62).*

Potential toxicity to wild-type Ras inhibition remains a concern with the use of FPT inhibitors, though they appear to only inhibit the growth of transformed cells in vitro and in reported animal studies *(53).*Theoretical side effects notwithstanding, FPT inhibitors currently in clinical development (e.g., R115777, SCH66336) remain a particularly attractive target for chemopreventive strategies in pancreatic cancer due to the high incidence of K-*ras* mutation in pancreatic cancer. Additional studies, including the effects of chronic exposure to these agents, need to be undertaken.

2.3. Retinoids

Vitamin A, which consists of retinol, its fatty acid esters, and retinal, is required for growth and bone development, vision, reproduction, epithelial tissue differentiation, immune system integrity, and various biochemical reactions *(63).* Vitamin A and its analogs (retinoids) act by inhibiting proliferation *(64)* and inducing differentiation *(65).* Retinoid receptors, like steroid and hormone receptors, function directly as transcription factors, regulating specific genes *(66).* Two specific subfamilies of retinoid receptors, RAR and RXR, appear to be important in carcinogenesis. RAR expression is lost in some lung and head and neck cancers *(67).* Moreover, 9-*cis*-retinoic acid, which has a high affinity for RXR *(68),* has proven chemopreventive effects in rat mammary carcinogenesis *(69).* Differences in tissue distribution and ligand specificity suggest that these individual receptors could be targets for chemoprevention.

Vitamin A-deficient animals have an increased risk for developing carcinomas when exposed to chemical carcinogens *(70).* Low dietary and serum levels of preformed retinol and β-carotene have been associated with a number of different malignancies (reviewed in *25*). Synthetic compounds with vitamin A-like activity inhibit carcinogenesis induced in rat breast, skin, and bladder tumors *(71).* Studies of various retinoids on pancreatic cancer induced in rats demonstrated inhibition of carcinogenesis, but at the expense of toxicity from effective levels of the retinoids *(72–74).* Toxicities included growth failure in both sexes, testicular atrophy in males, and an increase in hepatocellular carcinomas in females *(73).* Curphey et al. *(75)* confirmed that the retinoid *N*-(2-hydroxyethyl)retinamide inhibited progression of pancreatic carcinogenesis in a dose-dependent fashion in rats induced with azaserine. The degree of inhibition seen with a lower dose of retinoid was comparable to previous studies. Toxicity in the form of major testicular atrophy previously noted by Longnecker et al. *(73)* with four different retinoids was not seen with *N*-(2-hydroxyethyl)retinamide. Furthermore, retinoid treatment in combination with selenium produced a significant inhibition of tumor growth that was greater than that observed with retinoid (or, for that matter, selenium) alone. Selenium is discussed in greater detail below.

Different tissue distributions of individual retinoid receptors in conjunction with their ligand specificity should help target specific organs for treatment with individual retinoids. However, toxicities at effective doses may make single-drug therapy prohibitive.

Combination therapy with other chemopreventive agents may further define the role for this class.

2.4. Antioxidants: Oltipraz

Dietary phenolic antioxidants have long been a focus of interest for their ability to protect against carcinogen-induced tumors when administered before or during carcinogen exposure (76). The antioxidant oltipraz (4-methyl-5-(α-pyrazinyl)-1,2-dithiole-3-thione) is a synthetic dithiolthione structurally similar to anticarcinogenic dithiolthiones found in *Cruciferae* vegetable oils (77). In animal studies, oltipraz administered by gavage prior to carcinogen treatment reduced the incidence of induced lung and fore-stomach cancers in mice treated with benzo[a]-pyrene (B[a]P), lung tumors in mice treated with uracil mustard or diethylnitrosamine (78), hepatocellular carcinomas in Fischer rats treated with aflatoxin (79), and colonic adenocarcinomas and preneoplastic lesions in rats treated with azoxymethane (AOM) (80). In studies sponsored by the National Cancer Institute, oltipraz was effective in inhibiting induced lung tumors in Syrian hamsters, colon tumors in mice, mammary tumors in rats, and bladder carcinomas in mice (81).

Clapper et al. (77) tested the effectiveness of oltipraz on hamster pancreatic tumors induced by *N*-nitrosobis(2-oxopropyl)amine. Oltipraz at 600 mg/kg reduced the incidence of pancreatic adenocarcinomas, but had no effect on the incidence of metastases. Lower-dose oltipraz at 300 mg/kg had no effect on primary tumors or metastases. Interestingly, dietary oltipraz at both doses reduced morbidity and mortality in tumor-bearing animals with metastatic disease.

Clearly, this class needs further characterization. Its effects on morbidity and mortality suggest a possible role in both chemoprevention and chemotherapy.

2.5. Antioxidants: Selenium

Selenium is a micronutrient whose only well-defined function in animals is as a constituent of the selenium-dependent form of glutathione peroxidase. It is incorporated into the active site of the enzyme as the substituted amino acid selenocysteine (82). This cytosolic enzyme reduces both hydrogen peroxide and organic hydroperoxides, functioning as a potential antioxidant. However, its chemopreventive activity may reside elsewhere, as serum and plasma enzyme activity can be detected. Furthermore, selenium may have chemopreventive properties independent of glutathione peroxidase; studies suggest it may inhibit both DNA (83) and protein synthesis (84).

Two animal studies have examined the effect of selenium in pancreatic cancer models, with contradictory results. Inhibition of development of pancreatic acinar cell adenocarcinomas induced in rats by azaserine was most pronounced in those supplemented with either selenium or β-carotene (85). However, a prior study by Curphey et al. (75) failed to demonstrate any effect of selenium alone on azaserine-induced pancreatic tumors in Lewis rats, although selenium combined with retinoid was more effective than retinoid alone, as discussed above. Thus, selenium is probably not effective as a single therapy, but could be an adjunct to chemopreventive treatment with other agents.

2.6. Antioxidants: β-Carotene

β-carotene is the most abundant of the carotenoids, found in dark green leafy vegetables, carrots, and yellow or red fruits and vegetables. Daily consumption of high levels reportedly diminishes the risk of development of lung, colon, stomach, prostate, and cervical cancer in humans (86,87).

The Alpha-Tocopherol Beta-Carotene Cancer Prevention Study randomized 29,133 male smokers aged 50–69 to one of four intervention groups: α-tocopherol, β-carotene, both, or placebo. Daily supplementation lasted 5–8 yr. Supplementation with either or both did not have a statistically significant effect on the rate of incidence of or mortality from pancreatic cancer. The rate of incidence of carcinoma of the pancreas was 25% lower among men receiving β-carotene supplements and 34% higher among men receiving α-tocopherol compared to those who did not, although the differences were not statistically significant (88). There were similar trends but again no statistically significant difference in mortality rate; those receiving β-carotene supplementation had 19% lower mortality, while those receiving α-tocopherol supplementation had 10% higher mortality. No known mechanisms explain what may be a potentially preventive effect of β-carotene against pancreatic carcinoma.

Majima et al. (89) induced pancreatic tumors in Syrian hamsters by treating with *N*-nitrosobis(2-oxopropyl)amine. They demonstrated a reduced number of pancreatic hyperplasias, carcinomas, and total ductal lesions after treatment with oral emulsions of either β- or palm carotene (the latter, derived from palm oil, contains 60% β-carotene). Oral administration of green tea polyphenols (GTP) at high doses also significantly decreased the numbers of hyperplasia and total ductal lesions. Palm carotene combined with lower doses of GTP similarly inhibited pancreatic lesion development;

α-carotene did not affect pancreatic carcinogenesis. These results suggest that combined administration of β- or palm carotene and GTP may be a viable chemopreventive strategy.

Appel et al. *(90)* reported that azaserine-treated rats administered a diet high in β-carotene developed fewer pancreatic tumors than controls. Similar results were seen with combinations of β-carotene and selenium, which reduced both multiplicity and incidence of pancreatic tumors, and with vitamin C, which reduced the multiplicity of tumors. However, this same group saw no effect with vitamin E. Whether these results are produced by a direct scavenging effect on active oxygen radicals or on active carcinogens remains unclear.

These animal studies suggest that β-carotene may have a chemopreventive effect. While the human trials show a trend toward decreased incidence of and lower mortality from pancreatic cancer, the results are not statistically significant.

2.7. Antioxidants: Vitamin E

Vitamin E, a lipid-soluble essential nutrient, is a major antioxidant in all cell membranes (reviewed in *91*). Naturally occurring substrates with vitamin E activity include α-, β-, γ-, and δ-tocopherol. By reacting with a variety of oxygen radicals and singlet oxygen, vitamin E prevents peroxidation of polyunsaturated membrane lipids. Although d-α-tocopherol inhibits carcinogenesis in a number of animal chemopreventive studies (reviewed in *91*), its antioxidant properties are not a sufficient explanation in some models. Also, the Alpha-Tocopherol Beta-Carotene Cancer Prevention Study in humans suggested a trend toward an increase in the incidence of pancreatic carcinoma as well as a higher rate of mortality in patients receiving α-tocopherol, although these trends were not statistically significant. Furthermore, the effectiveness of vitamin E at pharmacological doses remains to be seen.

2.8. Antioxidants: Tea

Tea, a beverage made from the leaves of *Camellia sinensis* of the family Theaceae, is the most widely consumed liquid in the world after water. Tea leaves are manufactured primarily as black (80% of tea consumed), green, and oolong. Specific chemopreventive mechanisms of action remain unclear, although several have been proposed. These include inhibition of lipid peroxidation and free-radical formation, inhibition of cellular proliferation, antiinflammatory changes including inhibition of interleukin (IL)-1 mRNA, and modulation of cytochrome P450 activity. Studies have shown that tea polyphenols exert antioxidant properties by protecting against oxidative DNA damage *(92)*.

Drinkers of green and black tea have lower risks of heart attacks and strokes *(93)*. Green tea exhibits health-promoting actions in cancers of the colon, pancreas, uterus, and rectum *(94)*. Black tea intake has been associated with reduced breast, colon, and ultraviolet-induced skin cancer in animal models *(95,96)*. Lyn-Cook et al. *(97)* demonstrated significant inhibition of cell growth in vitro in two human pancreatic cancer cell lines treated with black and green tea extracts (~90% growth inhibition), green tea phenols (GTP) (~90%) and its purified components epicatechin-3-gallate (ECG) and epigallocatechin-3-gallate (EGCG) (~95%), and black tea phenols (BTP) (approx 90%). Black and green tea extracts, GTP, and EGCG decreased expression of the K-*ras* gene as shown by reverse-transcriptase polymerase chain reaction. The mechanism of action of K-*ras* downregulation remains unclear. Furthermore, green and black tea extracts decreased expression of the multidrug-resistant gene *mdr-1*, although GTP and EGCG increased its expression. This suggests that other components of tea extracts mediate the inhibitory effect on *mdr-1*.

The precise mechanism of action of tea extracts remains ambiguous. Moreover, it is still unclear which tea component(s) are effective. Nevertheless, tea as a chemopreventive agent remains an intriguing possibility, particularly given its wide acceptance in daily life.

2.9. Antioxidants: Curcumin

The Rel/nuclear factor (NF)κB transcription factor controls expression of a variety of genes involved in diverse processes including immune response and lymphoid differentiation, embryonic development, and both oncogenesis and apoptosis *(98,99)*. RelA, a subunit of NFκB, is constitutively active in 67% of human pancreatic adenocarcinomas, but not in normal pancreatic tissues *(100)*. This activation may thus have a critical role in tumorigenesis. Curcumin is a potent antioxidant and cancer chemopreventive agent that inhibits activation of NFκB *(101,102)*. Wang et al. *(100)* demonstrated that curcumin completely inhibited the RelA-DNA binding activity in Panc-28 pancreatic cancer cells, but this failed to inhibit the growth of these cells. However, the curcumin-mediated RelA inhibition did appear to sensitize the Panc-28 cancer to paclitaxel-induced apoptosis.

The mechanisms of action of the antioxidants remain unclear, so it is difficult to determine their best applications. Some, notably β-carotene and tea polyphenols, appear more promising than others such as vitamin E. Selenium may not be effective on its own, but could potentiate the effects of other chemopreventive agents. Oltipraz and curcumin could play additional roles in chemoprevention.

3. CONCLUSIONS

The distinction between chemoprevention and chemotherapy is somewhat ambiguous; agents such as COX-2 inhibitors may inhibit angiogenesis as well as modulate an enzyme involved in early neoplastic transformation (6,32). Many chemopreventive agents, including antioxidants, may also have chemotherapeutic applications as well.

Chemopreventive strategies as applied to pancreatic cancer are still in their infancy. Target-specific agents, such as inhibitors of COX-2 and FPT, provide some degree of selectivity, and further work in developing these agents could have an impact on pancreatic cancer. Other recently studied targeted agents, such as the epidermal growth factor antagonists (103,104) may be applicable to a chemopreventive setting as well. The benefit of the other agents described above may not be realized until their mechanisms of action are more clearly elucidated.

In the meantime, more sophisticated screening strategies need to be developed. Even then, there is no guarantee that such tests will be applicable to patient cohorts beyond genetically defined high-risk patients and those in pancreatic cancer kindreds. These groups of high-risk individuals may be the most appropriate group for early chemoprevention efforts.

Until effective chemopreventive strategies can be identified, lifestyle modifications can play an important role. Even without developing the strategies described above, complete avoidance of tobacco could significantly reduce the risk of developing pancreatic cancer.

REFERENCES

1. Greenlee RT, Hill-Harmon MB, Murray T, Thun M. Cancer statistics, 2001. *CA Cancer J Clin* 2001;51:15–36.
2. Landis SH, Murray T, Bolden S, Wingo PA. Cancer Statistics, 1998. *CA Cancer J Clin* 1998;48:6–29.
3. Warshaw AL, Gu ZY, Whittenberg J, Waltman AC. Preoperative staging and assessment of respectability of pancreatic cancer. *Arch Surg* 1990;125:230–233.
4. Niederhuber JE, Brennan MF, Menck HR. The National Cancer Data Base report on pancreatic cancer. *Cancer* 1995;76:1671–1677.
5. Jemal A, Thomas A, Murray T, Thun M. Cancer Statistics, 2002. *CA Cancer J Clin* 2002;52:23–47.
6. Levin B. An overview of preventive strategies for pancreatic cancer. *Ann Oncol* 1999;10 Suppl 4:193–196.
7. Hruban RH, Canto MI, Yeo CJ. Prevention of pancreatic cancer and strategies for management of familial pancreatic cancer. *Dig Dis* 2001;19:76–84.
8. Goggins M, Schutte M, Lu J, et al. Germline *BRCA2* gene mutations in patients with apparently sporadic pancreatic carcinomas. *Cancer Res* 1996;56:5360–5364.
9. Abbott DW, Freeman ML, Holt JT. Double-strand break repair deficiency and radiation sensitivity in *BRCA2* mutant cancer cells. *J Natl Cancer Inst* 1998;90:978–985.
10. Goldstein AM, Fraser MC, Struewing JP, et al. Increased risk of pancreatic cancer in melanoma-prone kindreds with p16^{INK4} mutations. *N Engl J Med* 1995;333:970–974.
11. Bowlby LS. Pancreatic adenocarcinoma in an adolescent male with Peutz-Jeghers syndrome. *Hum Pathol* 1986; 17:97–99.
12. Hemminki A, Markie D, Tomlinson I, et al. A serin/threonine kinase gene defective in Peutz Jeghers syndrome. *Nature* 1998;391:184–187.
13. Lynch HT, Voorhees GJ, Lanspa S, et al. Pancreatic carcinoma and hereditary nonpolyposis colorectal cancer: a family study. *Br J Cancer* 1985;52:271–273.
14. Goggins M, Offerhaus GJ, Hilgers W, et al. Pancreatic adenocarcinomas with DNA replication errors (RER+) are associated with wild-type K-*ras* and characteristic histopathology. Poor differentiation, a syncytial growth pattern, and pushing borders suggest RER+. *Am J Pathol* 1998;152:1501–1507.
15. Finch MD, Howes N, Ellis L, et al. Hereditary pancreatitis and familial pancreatic cancer. *Digestion* 1997;58:564–569.
16. Whitcomb DC, Gorry MC, Preston RA, et al. Hereditary pancreatitis is caused by a mutation in the cationic trypsinogen gene. *Nat Genet* 1996;14:141–145.
17. Hahn SA, Kern SE. Molecular genetics of exocrine pancreatic neoplasms. *Surg Clin North Am* 1995;75:857–869.
18. Hahn SA, Schutte M, Hoque AT, et al. DPC4, a candidate tumor suppressor gene at human chromosome 18q21.1. *Science* 1996;271:350–353.
19. Moskaluk CA, Hruban RH, Kern SE. *P16* and K-*ras* gene mutations in the intraductal precursors of human pancreatic adenocarcinoma. *Cancer Res* 1997;57:2140–2143.
20. Tersmette AC, Petersen GM, Offerhaus GJ, et al. Increased risk of incident pancreatic cancer among first-degree relatives of patients with familial pancreatic cancer. *Clin Cancer Res* 2001;7:738–744.
21. Hruban RH, Adsay NV, Albores-Saavedra J, et al. Pancreatic intraepithelial neoplasia (PanIN): a new nomenclature and classification system for pancreatic duct lesions. *Am J Surg Pathol* 2001;25:579–586.
22. Hruban RH, Goggins M, Parsons J, Kern SE. Progression model for pancreatic cancer. *Clin Cancer Res* 2000;6: 2969–2972.
23. Abbruzzese JL, Evans DB, Raijman I, et al. Detection of mutated c-Ki-ras in the bile of patients with pancreatic cancer. *Anticancer Res* 1997;17:795–802.
24. Caldas C, Hahn SA, Hruban RH, et al. Detection of K-ras mutations in the stool of patients with pancreatic adenocarcinoma and pancreatic ductal hyperplasia. *Cancer Res* 1994;54:3568–3573.
25. Kelloff GJ. Perspectives on cancer chemoprevention research and drug development. *Adv Cancer Res* 2000;78:199–334.
26. O'Neill GP, Ford-Hutchinson AW. Expression of mRNA for cyclooxygenase-1 and cyclooxygenase-2 in human tissues. *FEBS Lett* 1993;330:156–160.

27. Maier JA, Hla T, Maciag H. Cyclooxygenase is an immediate-early gene induced by interleukin-1 in human endothelial cells. *J Biol Chem* 1990;265:10850–10858.

28. Eberhart EC, Coffey RJ, Radhika A, et al. Up-regulation of cyclooxygenase-2 gene expression in human colorectal adenomas and adenocarcinomas. *Gastroenterology* 1994;107:1183–1188.

29. Jones DA, Carlton DP, McIntyre TM, et al. Molecular cloning of human prostaglandin endoperoxide synthases type II and demonstration of expression in response to cytokines. *J Biol Chem* 1993;268:9049–9054.

30. Seibert K, Zhang Y, Leahy K, et al. Pharmacological and biochemical demonstration of the role of cyclooxygenase 2 in inflammation and pain. *Proc Natl Acad Sci USA* 1994;91:12,013–12,017.

31. Williams CS, DuBois RN. Prostaglandin endoperoxide synthase: why two isoforms? *Am J Physiol* 1996;270:393–400.

32. Tsujii M, Kawano S, Tsuji S, et al. Cyclooxygenase regulates angiogenesis induced by colon cancer cells. *Cell* 1998;93:705–716.

33. Huang M, Stolina M, Sharma S, et al. Non-small cell lung cancer cyclooxygenase-2-dependent regulation of cytokine balance in lymphocytes and macrophages: up-regulation of interleukin 10 and down-regulation of interleukin 12 production. *Cancer Res* 1998;58:1208–1216.

34. Tsujii M, DuBois RN. Alterations in cellular adhesion and apoptosis in epithelial cells overexpressing prostaglandin and endoperoxidase synthase 2. *Cell* 1995;83:493–501.

35. Oshima M, Dinchuk JE, Kargman SL, et al. Suppression of intestinal polyposis in APC delta716 knockout mice by inhibition of cyclooxygenase-2 (COX-2). *Cell* 1996;87:803–809.

36. Ristimaki A, Honkanen N, Jankala H, et al. Expression of cyclooxygenase-2 in human gastric cancinoma. *Cancer Res* 1997;57:1276–1280.

37. Wilson KT, Fu S, Ramanujam KS, Meltzer SJ. Increased expression of inducible nitric oxide synthase and cyclooxygenase-2 in Barrett's esophagus and associated adenocarcinomas. *Cancer Res* 1998;58:2929–2934.

38. Hida T, Yatabe Y, Achiwa H, et al. Increased expression of cyclooxygenase-2 occurs frequently in human lung cancers, specifically in adenocarcinomas. *Cancer Res* 1998;58:3761–3764.

39. Giovannucci E, Egan KM, Hunter DJ, et al. Aspirin and the risk of colorectal cancer in women. *N Engl J Med* 1995;333:609–614.

40. Greenberg ER, Baron JA, Freeman DHJ, et al. Reduced risk of large-bowel adenomas among aspirin users. The Polyp Prevention Study Group. *J Natl Cancer Inst* 1993;85:912–916.

41. Thun MJ, Namboodiri MM, Heath CWJ. Aspirin use and reduced risk of fatal colon cancer. *N Engl J Med* 1991;325:1593–1596.

42. Peleg II, Maibach HT, Brown SH, Wilcox CM. Aspirin and nonsteroidal anti-inflammatory drug use and the risk of subsequent colorectal cancer. *Arch Intern Med* 1994;154:394–399.

43. Giovannucci E, Rimm EB, Stampfer MJ, et al. Aspirin use and the risk for colorectal cancer and adenoma in male health professionals. *Ann Intern Med* 1994;121:241–246.

44. Chan TA, Morin PJ, Vogelstein B, Kinzler KW. Mechanisms underlying nonsteroidal anti-inflammatory drug-mediated apoptosis. *Proc Natl Acad Sci USA* 1998;95:681–686.

45. Giardielio FM, Hamilton SR, Krush AJ, et al. Treatment of colonic and rectal adenomas with sulindac in familial adenomatous polyposis. *N Engl J Med* 1993;328:1313–1316.

46. Spagnesi MT, Tonelli F, Dolara P, et al. Rectal proliferation and polyp occurrence in patients with familial adenomatous polyposis after sulindac treatment. *Gastroenterology* 1994;106: 362–366.

47. Liu X-H, Yao S, Kirschenbaum A, Levin AC. NS398, a selective cyclooxygenase inhibitor, induces apoptosis and down-regulates bcl-2 expression in LNCaP cells. *Cancer Res* 1998; 58:4245–4249.

48. Kokawa A, Kondo H, Gotoda T, et al. Increased expression of cyclooxygenase-2 in human pancreatic neoplasms and potential for chemoprevention by cyclooxygenase inhibitors. *Cancer* 2000;91:333–338.

49. Shiff SJ, Koutsos MI, Qiao L, Rigas B. Nonsteroidal anti-inflammatory drugs inhibit the proliferation of colon adenocarcinoma cells: effects on cell cycle and apoptosis. *Exp Cell Res* 1996;222:179–188.

50. Hara A, Yoshimi N, Niwa M, et al. Apoptosis induced by NS-398, a selective cyclooxygenase-2 inhibitor, in human colorectal cancer cell lines. *Jpn J Cancer Res* 1997;88:600–604.

51. Molina, MA, Sitja-Arnau M, Lemoine MG, et al. Increased cyclooxygenase-2 expression in human pancreatic carcinomas and cell lines: growth inhibition by nonsteroidal anti-inflammatory drugs. *Cancer Res* 1999;59:4356–4362.

52. Takahashi M, Furukawa F, Toyoda K, et al. Effects of various prostaglandin synthesis inhibitors on pancreatic carcinogenesis in hamsters after initiation with *N*-nitrosobis(2-oxopropyl)amine. *Carcinogenesis* 1990;11: 393–395.

53. Kelloff GJ, Lubet RA, Fay JR, et al. Farnesyl protein transferase inhibitors as potential cancer chemopreventives. *Cancer Epidemiol Biomarkers Prev* 1997;6:267–282.

54. Lowy DR, Willumsen BM. Function and regulation of *ras*. *Annu Rev Biochem* 1993;62:851–891.

55. Barbacid M. *ras* genes. *Annu Rev Biochem* 1987;56:779–827.

56. Motojima K, Urano T, Nagata Y, et al. Mutations in the Kirsten-*ras* oncogene are common but lack correlation with prognosis and tumor stage in human pancreatic cancer. *Am J Gastroenterol* 1991;86:1784–1788.

57. Khosravi-Far R, Cox AD, Kato K, Der CJ. Protein prenylation: key to *ras* function and cancer intervention? *Cell Growth Differ* 1992;3:461–469.

58. Stark MJ, Burke YD, McKinzie JH, et al. Chemotherapy of pancreatic cancer with the monoterpene perillyl alcohol. *Cancer Lett* 1995;96:15–21.

59. Haag JD, Cromwell PL, Gould MN. Enhanced inhibition of protein isoprenylation and tumor growth by perillyl alcohol, a hydroxylated analog of *d*-limonene. *Proc Am Assoc Cancer Res* 1992;33:524.

60. Burke YD, Stark MJ, Roach SL, et al. Inhibition of pancreatic cancer growth by the dietary isoprenoids farnesol and geraniol. *Lipids* 1997;32:151–156.

61. Stayrook KR, McKinzie JH, Burke YD, et al. Induction of the apoptosis promoting protein *Bak* by perillyl alcohol in pancreatic ductal adenocarcinoma relative to untransformed ductal epithelial cells. *Carcinogenesis* 1997;18: 1655–1658.

62. Gibbs JB, Oliff A, Kohl NE. Farnesyltransferase inhibitors: *Ras* research yields a potential cancer therapeutic. *Cell* 1994;77:175–178.

63. McEvoy GK, McQuarrie GM. *Drug Information*. American Society of Hospital Pharmacists, Bethesda, MD, 1986, pp. 2391–2393.

64. Verma AK. Vitamins and cancer prevention. In Laidlaw SA, Swendseid ME, eds. Contemporary Issues in Clinical Nutrition, vol. 14. Gladys Emerson-UCLA Clinical Nutrition Research Unit Symposium, Los Angeles, CA, Mary 2–3, 1989. Wiley-Liss, Inc. New York, 1991; 25–38.

65. Mehta PP, Bertram JS, Loewenstein WR. The actions of retinoids on cellular growth correlate with their actions on gap junctional communication. *J Cell Biol* 1989;108: 1053–1065.

66. Gudas LJ, Sporn MB, Roberts AB. Cellular biology and biochemistry of the retinoids. In *The Retinoids: Biology, Chemistry, and Medicine*, 2nd Ed. Sporn MB, Roberts, AB, Goodman DS, eds. Raven, New York, 1994; pp. 443–520.

67. Hong WK, Sporn MB. Recent advances in chemoprevention of cancer. *Science* 1997;278:1073–1077.

68. Heyman RA, Mangelsdorf DJ, Dyck JA, et al. 9-*cis* Retinoic acid is a high affinity ligand for the retinoid receptor. *Cell* 1992;68:397–406.

69. Gottardis MM, Lamph WW, Shalinsky DR, et al. The efficacy of 9-*cis* retinoic acid in experimental models of cancer. *Breast Cancer Res Treat* 1996;38:85–96.

70. Nettesheim P, Williams ML. The influence of vitamin A on the susceptibility of the rat lung to 3-methylcholanthrene. *Int J Cancer* 1976;17:351–357.

71. Sporn MB, Newton DL. Chemoprevention of cancer retinoids. *Fed Proc* 1979;38:2528–2534.

72. Longnecker DS, Curphey TJ, Kuhlmann ET, Roebuck BD. Inhibition of pancreatic carcinogenesis by retinoids in azaserine-treated rats. *Cancer Res* 1982;42:19–24.

73. Longnecker DS, Kuhlmann ET, Curphey TJ. Divergent effects of retinoids on pancreatic and liver carcinogenesis in azaserine-treated rats. *Cancer Res* 1983;43:3219–3225.

74. Roebuck BD, Baumgartner KJ, Thron CD, Longnecker DS. Inhibition by retinoids of the growth of azaserine-induced foci in the rat pancreas. *J Natl Cancer Inst* 1984;73:233–236.

75. Curphey TJ, Kuhlmann ET, Roebuck BD, Longnecker DS. Inhibition of pancreatic and liver carcinogenesis in rats by retinoid- and selenium-supplemented diets. *Pancreas* 1988;3:36–40.

76. Roebuck BD, MacMillan DL, Bush DM, Kensler TW. Modulation of azaserine-induced pancreatic foci by phenolic antioxidants in rats. *J Natl Cancer Inst* 1984;72:1405–1410.

77. Clapper ML, Wood M, Leahy K, et al. Chemopreventive activity of oltipraz against *N*-nitrosobis(2-oxopropyl)amine (BOP)-induced ductal pancreatic carcinoma development and effects on survival of Syrian golden hamsters. *Carcinogenesis* 1995;16:2159–2165.

78. Wattenberg LW, Bueding E. Inhibitory effects of 5-(2-pyrazinyl)-4-methyl-1,2-dithole-3-thione (oltipraz) on carcinogenesis induced by benzo(*a*)pyrene, diethylnitrosamine, and uracil mustard. *Carcinogenesis* 1986;7:1379–1381.

79. Roebuck BD, Liu Y-L, Rogers AR, et al. Protection against aflatoxin B1-induced hepatocarcinogenesis in F344 rats by 5-(2-pyrazinyl)-4-methyl-1,2-dithole-3-thione (oltipraz): predictive role for short-term molecular dosimetry. *Cancer Res* 1991;51:5501–5506.

80. Rao CG, Rivenson A, Katiwalla M, et al. Chemopreventive effect of oltipraz during different stages of experimental colon carcinogenesis induced by azoxymethane in male F344 rats. *Cancer Res* 1993;53:2502–2506.

81. Kensler TW, Groopman JD, Roebuck BD. Chemoprevention by oltipraz and other dithiolethiones. In *Cancer Chemoprevention*. Wattenberg L, Lipkin M, Boone CW, Kelloff GJ, eds. CRC Press, Boca Raton, FL, 1992; pp. 205–226.

82. Wendel A. In Jakoby WB, ed. *Enzymatic Basis of Detoxification*, vol. 1. Academic Press, New York, 1980; 33–353.

83. Arthur JR, Beckett GJ. New metabolic roles for selenium. *Proc Nutr Soc* 1994;53:615–624.

84. Kohrle J. Thyroid hormone deiodination in target tissues–a regulatory role for the trace element selenium? *Exp Clin Endocrinol* 1994;102:63–89.

85. Konishi Y, Tsutsumi M, Longnecker DS. Mechanistic analysis and chemoprevention of pancreatic carcinogenesis. *Pancreas* 1998;17:334–340.

86. Ziegler RG. Vegetables, fruits, and carotenoids and the risk of cancer. *Am J Clin Nutr* 1991;53:251s–259s.

87. Peto R, Doll R, Buckley JD, Sporn M. Can dietary beta-carotene materially reduce human cancer rates? *Nature* 1981;290:201–208.

88. Rautalahti MT, Virtamo JRK, Taylor PR, et al. The effects of supplementation with α-tocopherol and β-carotene on the incidence and mortality of carcinoma of the pancreas in a randomized controlled trial. *Cancer* 1999;86:37–42.

89. Majima T, Tsutsumi M, Nishino H, et al. Inhibitory effects of β-carotene, palm carotene, and green tea polyphenols on pancreatic carcinogenesis initiated by *N*-nitrosobis(2-oxopropyl)amine in Syrian golden hamsters. *Pancreas* 1998; 16:13–18.

90. Appel MJ, Roberts G, Wouterson RA. Inhibitory effects of micronutrients on pancreatic carcinogenesis in azaserine-treated rats. *Carcinogenesis* 1991;12:2157–2161.

91. Kelloff GJ, Crowell JA, Boone CW, et al. Clinical development plan: vitamin E. *J Cell Biochem Suppl* 1994;20:282–299.

92. Grinberg LN, Newmark H, Kitrossky N, et al. A. Protective effects of tea polyphenols against oxidative damage to red blood cells. *Biochem Pharmacol* 1997;54:973–978.

93. Hertog MGL, Sweetnam PM, Fehily AM, et al. Antioxidant flavonols and ischemic heart disease in a Welsh population of men: the Caerphilly Study. *Am J Clin Nutr* 1997;65: 1489–1494.

94. Bushman JL. Green tea and cancer in humans: a review of the literature. *Nutr Cancer* 1998;34:151–159.

95. Weisburger JH, Rivenson A, Garr K, Aliaga C. Tea, or tea and milk, inhibit mammary gland and colon carcinogenesis in rats. *Cancer Lett* 1997;114:323–327.

96. Wang ZY, Huang MT, Ferraro T, et al. Inhibitory effect of green tea in the drinking water on tumorigenesis by ultraviolet light and 12-*O*-tetradecanoylphorbol-13-acetate in the skin of SKH-1 mice. *Cancer Res* 1992;52:1162–1165.

97. Lyn-Cook BD, Rogers T, Yan Y, et al. Chemopreventive effects of tea extracts and various components on human pancreatic and prostate tumor cells in vitro. *Nutr Cancer* 1999;35: 80–86.

98. Verma IM, Stevenson JK, Schwarz EM, et al. Rel/NF-κB/IκB family: intimate tales of association and dissociation. *Genes Dev* 1995;9:2723–2735.

99. Baldwin A Jr. The NF-κB and IκB proteins: new discoveries and insights. *Annu Rev Immunol* 1996;14:681–694.

100. Wang W, Abbruzzese JL, Evans DB, et al. The nuclear factor-κB RelA transcription factor is constitutively activated in human pancreatic adenocarcinoma cells. *Clin Cancer Res* 1999;5:119–127.

101. Singh S, Aggarwal BB. Activation of transcription factor NFκB is suppressed by curcumin (diferuloylmethane). *J Biol Chem* 1995;270:24,995–25,000.

102. Korutla L, Kumar R. Inhibitory effect of curcumin on epidermal growth factor receptor kinase activity in A431 cells. *Biochem Biophys Acta* 1994;1224:597–600.

103. Bruns CJ, Solarzano CC, Harbisan MT, et al. Blockade of the epidermal growth factor receptor signaling by a novel tyrosine kinase inhibitor leads to apoptosis of endothelial cells and therapy of human pancreatic carcinoma. *Cancer Res* 2000;60:2926–2935.

104. Bruns CJ, Harbisan MT, Davis DW, et al. Epidermal growth factor receptor blockade with C225 plus gemcitabine results in regression of human pancreatic carcinoma growing orthotopically in nude mice by antiangiogenic mechanisms. *Clin Cancer Res* 2000;6:1936–1948.

LIVER

37 Clinical Strategies for Chemoprevention of Liver Cancer

Ziad Hassoun, MD, and Gregory J. Gores, MD

CONTENTS

INTRODUCTION
HCC EPIDEMIOLOGY, RISK FACTORS, AND PATHOGENESIS
CHEMOPREVENTION OF HCC
SUMMARY AND CONCLUSION
REFERENCES

1. INTRODUCTION

Primary liver cancer includes hepatocellular carcinoma (HCC), intrahepatic cholangiocarcinoma, hepatoblastoma, and other rare tumors of mesodermal origin such as angiosarcoma. The terms "primary liver cancer" and "hepatocellular carcinoma" are often used interchangeably in the literature. HCC accounts for 70–85% of primary liver cancers *(1)*, and although intrahepatic cholangiocarcinoma is rare, it accounts for 5–30% of all liver cancers *(2)*. Hepatoblastoma, a rare tumor that occurs only in children, represents approximately 1% of childhood cancers *(3)*. This chapter will focus on HCC; cholangiocarcinoma, hepatoblastoma, and primary malignancies of mesodermal origin that develop in the liver will not be addressed.

Cancer risk definition, both at individual and at population levels, is an important step in developing chemoprevention strategies. An adequate understanding of the pathogenic mechanisms involved is equally important for rational use of chemopreventive agents. We will, therefore, discuss pertinent aspects of HCC's epidemiology, risk factors, and pathogenesis at the beginning of the chapter.

2. HCC EPIDEMIOLOGY, RISK FACTORS, AND PATHOGENESIS

2.1. Epidemiology

HCC represents the fifth most common malignancy and the third most frequent cause of cancer death around the globe. More than 564,000 new cases were estimated to occur worldwide in 2000, accounting for 5.6% of all cancer cases. The incidence-to-mortality ratio is very close to 1, with more than 548,000 deaths worldwide in 2000 *(4)*. There is considerable geographic, ethnic, and gender variation in the incidence of HCC.

2.1.1. GEOGRAPHIC DIFFERENCES IN HCC INCIDENCE

The highest HCC incidence rates occur in eastern Asia. China accounted for more than 306,000 cases of HCC in 2000, representing 54% of total cases worldwide. Other regions of high incidence include middle Africa, some countries of western Africa, and southeastern Asia. Geographic areas of lowest HCC incidence are northern Europe, Australia, and New Zealand *(4)*. Geographic regions are usually categorized as having low incidence of HCC (<3 cases/100,000), intermediate incidence (3–30 cases/100,000), or high incidence (>30 cases/100,000) *(1)*.

2.1.2. ETHNIC DIFFERENCES IN HCC INCIDENCE

In the United States, high HCC incidence occurs among Native Americans, Pacific Islanders, African Americans, and Hispanics, while lower rates are observed among Caucasians. HCC incidence is highest among recent Asian immigrants and decreases significantly in subsequent US-born generations *(5)*.

2.1.3. GENDER DIFFERENCES IN HCC INCIDENCE

Worldwide, HCC male-to-female incidence ratio is 2.7:1. In general, the male:female ratio is highest in regions with highest HCC incidence rates *(4)*. Some

From: Cancer Chemoprevention, Volume 2: Strategies for Cancer Chemoprevention
Edited by: G. J. Kelloff, E. T. Hawk, and C. C. Sigman © Humana Press Inc., Totowa, NJ

evidence associates higher androgen levels with an increased risk of hepatitis B virus (HBV)-related HCC in men *(6)*.

2.2. Risk Factors

2.2.1. HBV

HBV is the most frequent underlying cause for HCC worldwide; more than half of HCC cases are attributed to chronic HBV infection. Epidemiological studies have shown that seropositivity for hepatitis B surface antigen (HBsAg) is associated with a 3–148-fold increased risk of developing HCC. There is also a significant positive correlation between prevalence of HBsAg seropositivity and HCC incidence, particularly in high-incidence regions *(5)*.

Between 70 and 90% of HBV-related HCCs develop in patients with cirrhosis *(1)*. In areas where HBV is endemic, it is frequently transmitted from mother to newborn (vertical transmission). Ninety percent of individuals who acquire HBV infection during the perinatal period will develop chronic hepatitis or become chronic carriers. On the other hand, in areas of low prevalence, HBV infection is usually acquired in late adolescence and early adulthood through sexual and parenteral routes (horizontal transmission). Less than 10% of exposed adults will become chronically infected, although males have a higher rate of chronicity than females following viral acquisition in adulthood *(7)*.

2.2.2. HEPATITIS C

The role of chronic hepatitis C virus (HCV) infection in the etiology of HCC is also well established. 25% of HCC cases worldwide are attributable to HCV. Besides, HCV is the dominant etiologic factor in areas with low to intermediate HCC incidence such as Europe and Japan *(5)*. In a meta-analysis of epidemiological studies, the odds ratio (OR) of HCC development was 17.3 in patients with positive hepatitis C serology. In this study, the OR was 22.5 in HBV-infected patients, and 165 in patients infected with both HBV and HCV, indicating a synergism between HBV and HCV infections in HCC development *(8)*.

Almost all HCV-related HCCs occur among patients with cirrhosis *(9)*. Persistent hepatitis and regeneration of liver cells increase the risk of HCC development. Heavy alcohol consumption accelerates the evolution toward cirrhosis *(10,11)* and increases the risk of HCC *(12–14)*.

2.2.3. AFLATOXIN

Aflatoxins, produced by the fungi *Aspergillus flavus* and *Aspergillus parasiticus*, are carcinogenic in many animal species. *A. flavus* is ubiquitous in nature and is most commonly found on certain grains and nuts. In developed countries, levels of aflatoxins in grains are monitored to prevent contamination of food. However, exposure to significant aflatoxin levels from contaminated food is common in most countries of Africa and some areas of China and southeast Asia. Among several types of aflatoxins, aflatoxin B_1(AFB$_1$) is the most prevalent and potent carcinogen. Epidemiological studies have demonstrated a positive correlation between dietary exposure to AFB$_1$ and HCC incidence *(15)*. The oncogenic potential of aflatoxins is significantly increased in the presence of concomitant HBV infection *(16–19)*, suggesting a strong interaction between these two risk factors.

Surrogate markers have been developed to assess aflatoxin exposure because an accurate measurement of individual exposure is problematic. These markers include urinary aflatoxin metabolites, aflatoxin-albumin adducts, and aflatoxin-DNA adducts. These biomarkers, validated and used in a number of epidemiological studies, have established the relationship between aflatoxin exposure and HCC incidence. They also appear to correlate well with measurements of dietary intake at the individual level, and to be associated with the risk of HCC development. Aflatoxin-albumin adducts provide a more stable biomarker than urinary metabolites, as the half-life of the conjugate is identical to that of albumin itself. Aflatoxin-DNA adducts are of major interest because they represent surrogate markers for damage to a critical macromolecular target. The major DNA adduct species, aflatoxin-N^7-guanine, is rapidly excised and excreted exclusively in urine, thus allowing its measurement *(20–22)*. In addition to their usefulness in assessing exposure to aflatoxin, these biomarkers can also be used as surrogate endpoints in intervention studies designed to reduce aflatoxin exposure or for chemoprevention studies (see below).

2.2.4. ALCOHOL AND CIRRHOSIS

Cirrhosis from any cause, including chronic alcohol abuse, increases the risk of HCC development. However, it is not clear whether alcohol per se is carcinogenic *(23)*. The magnitude of HCC risk differs according to the underlying etiology. HCV-related cirrhosis carries the greatest risk *(12)*, followed by HBV- and alcohol-related cirrhosis. The relative risk of HCC in patients with hereditary hemochromatosis may be as high as 200 *(24,25)*. Certain causes of cirrhosis, such as autoimmune hepatitis, carry a relatively low risk of HCC development *(26)*.

2.3. Pathogenesis

Carcinogenesis is a multistep process that can be divided schematically into three stages: initiation, promotion, and progression. Initiation results from exposure to a carcinogenic agent that causes genetic mutations. The principal targets of genetic damage are oncogenes, tumor suppressor genes, and genes regulating apoptosis. Promotion is a reversible process that facilitates expression of the initiated phenotype by stimulating cellular proliferation. During progression, multiple genetic mutations and karyotypic changes result in greater malignant potential (27,28).

Molecular steps in HCC development have not been fully elucidated yet. Multiple mutations of p53 and several other known or putative tumor-suppressor genes have been demonstrated in HCC (29,30). One p53 mutation, the so-called codon 249 "hot spot" (20,31), has been linked to aflatoxin exposure. Other chemical carcinogens have also been implicated in the pathogenesis of HCC, such as microcystin, a blue-green algal hepatotoxin that acts as a promoter in Chinese areas of high HCC prevalence (32,33). There is also evidence for an overexpression of certain oncogenes in HCC. Finally, a number of growth factors involved in cell signaling pathways have also played a role in hepatocarcinogenesis (30). A subset of molecular alterations may preferentially contribute to HBV- and HCV-induced carcinogenesis.

2.3.1. HEPATITIS B

HBV-induced hepatocarcinogenesis is multifactorial. Chronic liver injury caused by viral infection and host immune response results in inflammation, hepatocellular regeneration, and cirrhosis. DNA damage induced by cytokines or by reactive oxygen species leads to mutations. Progressive accumulation of mutations after years of persistent hepatitis ultimately results in malignant transformation (34,35).

However, there is evidence for a specific role for HBV in HCC development. HBV has a partially double-stranded circular DNA genome. HBV-DNA is integrated into the hepatocyte genome of more than 90% of patients with HCC. Sites of integration into host chromatin appear to be random. Integration of HBV-DNA has been shown to result in deletions, translocations, and gene amplification at the site of integration. In a number of cases, HBV integration occurs adjacent to or within a gene involved in cell growth or apoptotic pathways. However, integrated sequences appear to act more frequently via a trans-mechanism (36,37).

The HBV HBx gene, frequently present in integrated form, has been shown to interact with transcription factors, to activate signal transduction pathways, and to interfere with tumor suppression (particularly, to inhibit tumor suppressor protein p53 function), apoptosis, and DNA repair. Hepatitis B surface proteins may also play significant roles in hepatocarcinogenesis. The PreS and 5′ portion of the S gene, encoding for truncated surface antigen polypeptides, integrate into host DNA. These sequences alter the expression of many cellular genes important to HCC development (36,37).

2.3.2. HEPATITIS C

HCV is an RNA virus. There is no evidence of reverse transcription or integration of viral nucleic acid into DNA of infected cells. Precise molecular mechanisms of HCV-associated hepatic carcinogenesis are, therefore, currently unknown. Persistent liver damage appears to play a major role. In addition, the HCV core protein seems to be directly involved in hepatocarcinogenesis (38). It regulates transcription of cellular and viral promoters (39), interferes with transcription of tumor suppressor gene p53 (40), stimulates cellular proliferation via cell signaling activation (41,42), and inhibits apoptotic cell death (43,44). Other viral proteins may also have oncogenic potential. HCV envelope protein E2 and nonstructural protein NS5A appear to interfere with cell growth regulation via multiple mechanisms (45–47). The nonstructural protein NS3 may also be involved in cell transformation (48). Because we lack appropriate animal models of viral replication, our understanding of HCV-associated carcinogenesis is hindered. Transgenic animals expressing a single viral protein are difficult models given the artifacts that can arise from overexpression of a protein in the absence of other viral factors.

2.3.3. AFLATOXIN

AFB$_1$, a procarcinogen, is metabolized in the liver into two 8,9-epoxide isomers by hepatic microsomal cytochrome P450. Glutathione *S*-transferases (GSTs) and other phase 2 detoxification enzymes are responsible for the subsequent detoxification of this DNA-reactive metabolite (31). As a result of genetic polymorphism, interindividual differences in the biotransformation of dietary aflatoxins may result in differing susceptibility to aflatoxin-induced carcinogenesis (49–52). The 8,9-epoxide binds covalently to DNA, forming mutagenic adducts; there is a positive correlation between risk of tumor formation and levels of AFB$_1$-DNA adducts in the liver in animal models (31).

A specific mutation in the third base of codon 249 of the p53 gene has been demonstrated in populations

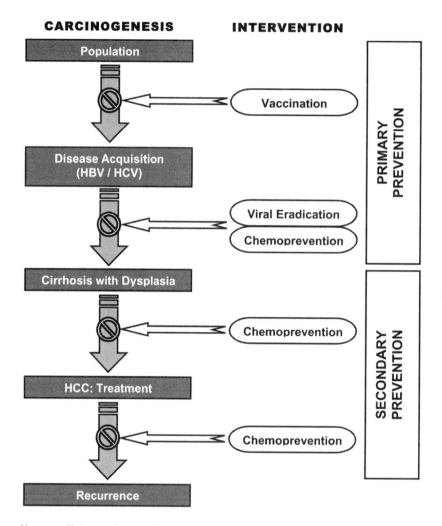

Fig. 1. Levels of prevention of hepatocellular carcinoma. HBV; hepatitis B virus; HCC; hepatocellular carcinoma; HCV; hepatitis C virus.

exposed to high levels of aflatoxin; this mutation is not found in areas with little exposure to aflatoxin. Codon 249 of p53 appears to be a preferential site for formation of AFB_1-DNA adducts. Furthermore, the frequency of codon 249 mutation parallels the level of aflatoxin exposure *(20,31)*. Thus, this mutation appears to be aflatoxin-specific and provides a "molecular fingerprint" of aflatoxin exposure.

The mechanism of the aforementioned synergistic interaction between HBV and aflatoxin in HCC development has not yet been elucidated. One possibility is that hepatocellular proliferation induced by viral infection favors the selective clonal development of cells mutated by AFB_1 *(20)*. Chronic liver injury secondary to HBV infection can also alter the expression of carcinogen-metabolizing enzymes (especially cytochrome P450) and consequently affect the extent to which aflatoxin metabolites bind to DNA. Experimental evidence

supports the latter hypothesis, but it has not been confirmed in human studies *(53)*.

3. CHEMOPREVENTION OF HCC

Disease prevention can be divided into three sequential levels. Primary prevention addresses healthy individuals, while secondary prevention targets patients in a preclinical stage of the disease. Tertiary prevention attempts to halt further deterioration or reduce complications after a disease has declared itself. Cancer chemoprevention, which attempts to arrest the initiation phase of carcinogenesis or progression of premalignant lesions, falls within the primary or secondary levels of prevention (Fig. 1).

In the US, survival of HCC patients has not changed significantly over the past 20 yr, despite improvements in HCC's early diagnosis and management. Most HCC

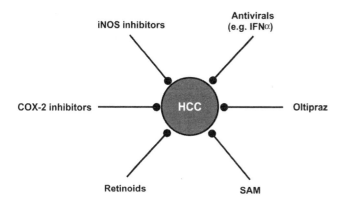

Fig. 2. Potential chemoprevention strategies for hepatocellular carcinoma. COX: cyclooxygenase; IFN; interferon; iNOS; inducible nitric oxide synthase; SAM-*S*-adenosylmethoinine.

patients still have advanced disease at the time of diagnosis. Fewer than 1% of patients diagnosed with HCC in the US between 1974 and 1996 underwent radical surgery *(54)*. Most patients have metastases or multifocal disease at time of diagnosis and are unsuitable candidates for resection. This underscores the importance of preventing this cancer.

In many instances, development of specific chemopreventive agents is hindered by the lack of a comprehensive understanding of HCC pathogenesis. Moreover, cancer prevention trials using cancer incidence or mortality as an endpoint require large sample sizes and prolonged duration of follow-up. Biomarkers developed as intermediate endpoints for many cancers offer a solution to these problems *(55)*. Unfortunately, such biomarkers are lacking for HCC, except for aflatoxin exposure *(22)*. In addition to biomarkers, markers of risk also hold promise for cancer chemoprevention. Several carcinogen-metabolizing enzymes have been studied as potential susceptibility markers of HCC development in various contexts, but none appears to have a clinically meaningful overall impact on hepatocarcinogenesis *(56)*. Preventive strategies for HCC differ according to the level of prevention and to the underlying risk factors (Fig. 2).

3.1. Primary Prevention

3.1.1. HEPATITIS B

Because HCC is closely associated with chronic hepatitis B, a preemptive strategy aiming at preventing HBV infection would be the most effective way to prevent HCC, especially in developing countries (Fig. 1). A safe and effective vaccine has been available for two decades *(57)*. Immunization programs in areas of high endemicity currently focus on universal vaccination

of newborns to prevent perinatal HBV transmission *(58,59)*. In areas of low prevalence, efforts are focused on vaccination of adolescents or high-risk groups *(59)*. Universal immunization of the total world population, a desirable goal, would be cost-effective while suppressing hepatitis B to clinical nonrelevance *(57)*. Routine immunization of infants has already decreased the prevalence of chronic HBV infection in endemic populations *(59)*. In Taiwan, a nationwide vaccination program implemented in 1984 has reduced the number of infected children by 85% *(60)* and HCC incidence in immunized children by 75% *(61)*.

In patients with chronic hepatitis B, the aim of treatment is termination of viral replication. Currently, the FDA has approved three agents to treat chronic hepatitis B, interferon alpha (IFNα) and lamivudine, and adefovir nucleoside analogs. Other antiviral agents have also shown promise in clinical trials. However, none of these agents effectively eradicates the virus *(7)*. IFNα suppresses HBV replication in approximately one-third of selected patients *(62)*. This is associated in most instances with long-term remission of liver disease, decreased rate of complications, and improved survival *(63–65)*.

IFNα is a cytokine that exhibits antiproliferative activity and controls apoptosis, in addition to its antiviral and immunomodulatory activities *(66)*. Long-term IFNα therapy was associated with a decrease in oncogenesis in a mouse model mimicking HBV-induced hepatocarcinogenesis *(67)*. In humans, sustained remission of chronic hepatitis B induced by IFNα treatment appears to be associated with a decreased incidence of HCC *(64,65)*. IFNα has been suggested to delay or prevent HCC in patients with HBV-related cirrhosis independent of its antiviral effect *(68)*. This issue has subsequently been examined in several nonrandomized or retrospective studies *(69–73)* and in a recent meta-analysis of these studies *(74)*. A significant reduction in the rate of HCC development was observed in IFN-treated patients in two Asian studies *(68,73)*. However, these studies are remarkable for their heterogeneity, which makes the reliability of conclusions drawn from individual trials questionable *(74)*. Moreover, neither of the studies was a randomized controlled trial. In the meta-analysis, consistent results were observed only when assessing data pooled from European reports; in this subgroup, no significant preventive effect on HCC was shown *(74)*.

The decrease in inflammatory activity that accompanies sustained virologic response to IFNα probably accounts for the observed reduction in cancer risk in these patients. However, the association between viral integration and carcinogenesis explains why treatment with antiviral agents is not sufficient to prevent HBV-related carcinogenesis, given that these agents do not eliminate the virus and may enhance viral integration. The evidence discussed above does not support a chemopreventive effect of IFNα independent of its antiviral activity in chronic hepatitis B.

3.1.2. HEPATITIS C

Currently, there is no effective vaccine to prevent the transmission of hepatitis C. Development of a successful vaccine will face many obstacles (75). Public health strategies such as counseling high-risk groups, screening blood donors, and widespread use of disposable syringes and needles can reduce the risk of HCV transmission (76).

70–80% of those infected with HCV develop chronic hepatitis C (CHC), a slow-progressing disease resulting in cirrhosis in approximately 20% of subjects after 10 to 20 yr (9,77). The annual incidence of HCC ranges from 3 to 10% in those with established cirrhosis (77). Interferon-based regimens currently represent the only therapies of proven benefit for CHC. Treatment with IFN alone results in a sustained virologic response (long-term eradication of viremia) in 15–25% of patients at best (78). A combination of IFNα and ribavirin is more effective and yields a sustained response rate around 40% (79). Conjugation of the IFN molecule to polyethyleneglycol (PEG) increases its blood circulation lifetime (80). The results of treatment with PEG-IFN appear roughly equivalent to those of IFNα plus ribavirin (81,82). Adding ribavirin to PEG-IFN generates even higher response rates (55–60%) (83,84). The latter combination will probably become the standard of care for the treatment of CHC. This sustained virologic response is accompanied by significant reduction in necroinflammatory activity and slowing (or even regression) of fibrosis (85–87). A similar although less marked effect is observed in nonresponders (87,88).

Since HCV-related HCC is primarily a complication of cirrhosis (9), halting or slowing down progression to cirrhosis can be expected to prevent or delay HCC development (Fig. 1). This issue was addressed in a number of studies (89–97) that all found a significant reduction in rate of HCC development in sustained responders to IFN treatment. In general, carcinogenesis rates in nonresponders did not appear to differ significantly from those of untreated controls, and results of transient responders were variable. However, these studies are either retrospective or noncontrolled;

observed benefit could be due to spurious associations. Prospective studies specifically designed to evaluate the effect of IFN treatment on HCC incidence are needed but difficult to perform. Since the interval between HCV acquisition and HCC development is estimated to be around 30 yr (9), the duration of follow-up required for such a study to yield meaningful results is correspondingly long. Furthermore, inclusion of an untreated control group can be ethically questionable (98).

Whether IFN treatment can likewise prevent the progression to HCC in patients with HCV-related cirrhosis is still controversial. Individual studies have yielded heterogeneous results. The number of randomized studies is small, but when data from controlled retrospective studies were also pooled in a recent meta-analysis (74), the results suggested a slight preventive effect of IFN on HCC development. The preventive effect was more evident among sustained responders, but was still significant in patients who did not achieve a sustained response. The same reservations mentioned above apply to these studies; results need confirmation before IFN treatment can be recommended in patients with HCV-related cirrhosis for prevention of HCC.

3.1.3. AFLATOXIN

Interventions against aflatoxin involve initiatives at the community level in developing countries to limit aflatoxin formation before and after crop harvest, using a variety of methods that include sorting, biocontrol, and chemical and physical methods for aflatoxin degradation. In addition, genetic engineering can select grains resistant to infestation by *Aspergillus* or that limit aflatoxin synthesis. At the individual level, dietary change to avoid intake of frequently contaminated foods may not be feasible (99). Biomarkers of aflatoxin exposure can be used to assess the efficacy of these interventions. Thus, primary prevention measures aiming at reducing aflatoxin intake should lead to a reduction in all biomarker levels (22).

Since primary prevention of aflatoxin exposure may not be economically feasible in many areas of the world, chemopreventive agents that block activation or enhance detoxification of AFB_1 have been investigated. Induction of phase 2 detoxification enzymes is indeed one of the major mechanisms of protection against chemical carcinogens. Experimental evidence indicates that this induction is sufficient for chemoprevention (100). Oltipraz, a substituted dithiolethione, appears to be one of the most promising inductors. Originally developed as an antischistosomal agent, oltipraz was

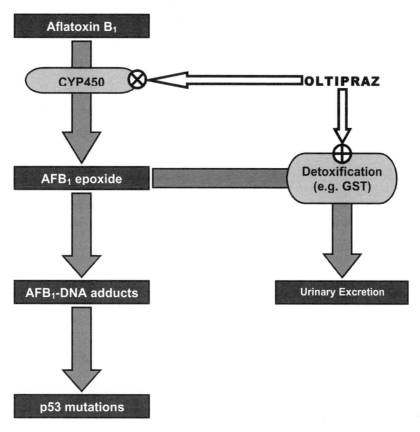

Fig. 3. Molecular mechanisms of chemoprevention with oltipraz. AFB_1 is metabolized in the liver by cytochrome P450 into a toxic epoxide that binds to DNA, forming mutagenic adducts. The epoxide is detoxified by GST and other phase 2 enzymes and subsequently eliminated. Oltipraz can inhibit phase 1 metabolism of AFB_1 and induce phase 2 detoxification enzymes. AFB_1; aflatoxin B_1; CYP450; cytochrome P450; GST; glutathione S-transferase.

discovered in animal experiments to be a potent inducer of several phase 2 detoxification enzymes, including GSTs, UDP-glucuronyl transferases, epoxide hydrolase, superoxide dismutase, and others. With different dose scheduling, oltipraz was also shown to inhibit cytochrome P450 activities *(101)* (Fig. 3). Subsequent studies demonstrated that oltipraz could inhibit experimental carcinogenesis, including AFB_1-induced hepatocarcinogenesis *(100)*. These experiments also showed reduced hepatic AFB-DNA adducts, serum AFB-albumin adducts, and urinary AFB-N^7-guanine in animals given oltipraz during aflatoxin administration *(21,101)*.

After Phase I dose-finding studies confirmed that oltipraz triggered phase 2 enzyme expression in humans *(100,101)*, a Phase II randomized, placebo-controlled, double-blind chemoprevention trial was conducted in 1995 in Qidong City, China *(102)*. Aflatoxin exposure, in addition to HBV infection, has been suggested to be responsible for the very high prevalence of HCC in this area. Serum aflatoxin-albumin adducts and urinary

aflatoxin metabolites were used as primary outcome measures in this trial. Individuals receiving 500 mg of oltipraz weekly for 8 wk had significantly reduced levels of serum aflatoxin-albumin adducts and a urinary metabolite of aflatoxin. In contrast, daily administration of 125 mg of oltipraz led to a significant increase in urinary excretion of a conjugated metabolite of AFB_1 *(103,104)*. These results indicate that sustained administration of low-dose oltipraz increased the extent of phase 2 conjugation of AFB_1, while intermittent administration of the high dose inhibited phase 1 activation of aflatoxin. A second phase 2 trial was conducted in Qidong in 1999 and 2000, where 250 or 500 mg of oltipraz were administered weekly over 1 year. This should serve as a foundation for a Phase III trial using HCC incidence as an endpoint *(101)*.

3.1.4. CHEMOPREVENTION WITH S-ADENOSYLMETHIONINE

S-adenosylmethionine (SAM) acts as a methyl donor in transmethylation reactions essential to cell structure and function *(105)*. DNA methylation plays an important role in the regulation of gene expression and hence in carcinogenesis *(106)*. Dietary methyl group deficiency, as well as various carcinogens, result in a decrease in intracellular SAM, and have been linked to experimental hepatocarcinogenesis through the hypomethylation of oncogenes *(106,107)*. The administration of SAM prevents development of preneoplastic and neoplastic liver lesions in experimental animals *(108–110)*. This is associated with a restoration of the SAM pool, DNA methylation, and inhibition of oncogene expression *(107)*. SAM also appears to be selectively pro-apoptotic in transformed cells as compared to normal hepatocytes *(111)*. If these results can be confirmed, SAM could become a very potent chemopreventive agent. Ongoing research is aimed at identifying phenotypic and genotypic aberrations in SAM metabolism that occur during the process of hepatocarcinogenesis *(112–114)*. Several trials are now in place using SAM as primary therapy for alcoholic liver disease *(115)*; a secondary assessment of HCC development in these studies should prove interesting and could justify larger chemoprevention studies.

3.1.5. Chemoprevention With Cyclooxygenase Inhibitors

Cyclooxygenases (COX) are key enzymes responsible for prostaglandin synthesis. Two isoenzymes have been identified. COX-1 is expressed constitutively, while COX-2 is an inducible form. A large body of evidence indicates that aspirin and other nonsteroidal anti-inflammatory drugs, well-known inhibitors of COX, have the potential to prevent colon cancer development. The recent discovery that overexpression of COX-2 is an early event in colon carcinogenesis and that selective COX-2 inhibitors had chemopreventive potential in animal models has triggered similar research in hepatocarcinogenesis *(116)*. Increased expression of COX-2 was indeed demonstrated in well-differentiated HCC, suggesting that this was an early event in tumor development *(117,118)*. Selective inhibitors of COX-2 suppressed the growth of HCC cell lines and induced apoptosis, though this appeared to be unrelated to COX-2 inhibition *(118,119)*. An epidemiologic assessment of the relationship between aspirin use and the occurrence of hepatocellular cancer in patients with cirrhosis due to HCV or HBV is needed now. Such population analysis proved useful in helping establish a plausible link between COX-2 and colon cancer. Several clinical trials are now under way

to evaluate the efficacy of COX-2 inhibitors in preventing colorectal cancer. These agents may have a role in the chemoprevention of HCC in the future.

3.1.6. Chemoprevention With Inhibitors of Inducible Nitric Oxide Synthase

The inducible form of nitric oxide synthase (iNOS) is frequently expressed in inflammation by both macrophages and epithelial cells. Presumably, pro-inflammatory cytokines present in the inflammatory milieu induce expression of this enzyme, a potent generator of nitric oxide (NO), which can have myriad effects. NO can nitrosylate proteins, resulting in loss of DNA repair and inhibition of normal apoptotic processes *(120)*. Furthermore, NO also directly induces oxidative DNA damage *(120)*. The combination of DNA damage, inability to repair damaged DNA, and failure of physiologic apoptosis would appear to be a very procarcinogenic process. NO is also an angiogenic agent expected to favor tumor progression *(120)*. Evidence suggesting a role for iNOS in carcinogenesis comes from several recent studies assessing colon carcinogenesis. Mice with defects in the APC gene are less susceptible to cancer if iNOS is inhibited *(121)*. Furthermore, iNOS inhibitors also decrease the incidence of colon cancers in azoxymethane-treated mice *(122)*. iNOS is strongly expressed in HCV-infected human liver tissue *(123)*. Thus, the role of iNOS inhibitors in hepatocarcinogenesis deserves further study.

3.2. Secondary Prevention

Malignant transformation in the liver is believed to proceed from adenomatous hyperplasia through dysplasia to early, well-differentiated hepatocellular carcinoma. The term "dysplastic nodule" has been coined to describe premalignant lesions. However, there is still confusion about their pathologic diagnosis *(124,125)*. For a molecular diagnosis to be possible, a better knowledge of the sequence of genetic mutations during the process of hepatocarcinogenesis is necessary *(126)*. Characterization of genetic alterations corresponding to these precancerous lesions and determination of the exact pathogenetic mechanisms involved in early steps of malignant transformation would open up new horizons for secondary chemoprevention of HCC. Increased understanding of metabolic and molecular aberrations that characterize preneoplastic lesions in experimental models may provide a basis for developing chemopreventive drugs *(127)*. Future prospects also include application of gene therapy strategies in secondary prevention of HCC. Strategies include replacement of tumor suppressor genes such as p53 and antisense techniques to inhibit oncogene expression or to reestablish apoptosis *(128–130)*.

3.2.1. HEPATITIS B

The woodchuck hepatitis virus (WHV) is a member of the *Hepadnaviridae* family, to which HBV belongs. Woodchucks infected with WHV represent an appropriate animal model for human HCC. Just as in humans, integrated WHV-DNA sequences have been found in most HCCs of woodchucks. *cis*-regulatory mechanisms play a much more important role in this model than in human HCC. In particular, viral integration into the *myc* family of proto-oncogenes appears to be a central event in WHV-mediated hepatocarcinogenesis *(131)*. Wang et al. transfected a woodchuck HCC cell line with N-*myc* antisense vectors, thus suppressing the expression of N-*myc*1 protein and preventing tumor development *(132)*. Similarly, suppression of HBx or surface protein expression or inhibition of cellular gene transactivation by these proteins may prevent the development of HBV-related HCC.

3.2.2. HEPATITIS C

After surgical resection or local ablation of HCC, the presence of active hepatitis C is a risk factor for tumor recurrence *(133,134)*. Long-term postoperative maintenance therapy with IFN appeared protective against this recurrence in two prospective, randomized, controlled trials *(135,136)*. However, the number of patients in these trials was too small and the duration of follow-up too short to allow any definitive conclusion to be drawn. Furthermore, the difference in carcinogenesis rates between IFN-treated and untreated patients was so dramatic in one study *(135)* as to arouse skepticism about an adequate matching of the two groups *(137)*. Finally, these studies did not distinguish between true recurrence and second primary tumors.

3.2.3. CHEMOPREVENTION WITH RETINOIDS

Retinoids, including vitamin A and its analogs, have been the subject of extensive research directed toward primary or secondary prevention of cancer. Their limited efficacy and/or their toxicity have so far prevented their widespread application in the clinical setting *(138)*.

Intrahepatic recurrence of HCC and development of second primary tumors after surgical resection or local ablation therapy are common causes of treatment failure and mortality *(30)*. Polyprenoic acid, an acyclic retinoid, has been shown to inhibit experimental hepa-

tocarcinogenesis *(139)*. In a prospective randomized controlled study conducted in Japan, polyprenoic acid appeared to significantly reduce incidence of second primary tumors after surgical resection or percutaneous ethanol ablation of HCC, without affecting disease recurrence incidence *(140)*. In this study, the distinction between second primary tumors and recurrent tumors was made according to clinical criteria, mainly time to tumor development. The 6-mo cut-off chosen in the study was arbitrary, and time is probably not an adequate criterion to make such a distinction. In a study using comparative genomic hybridization to establish a clonality relationship between primary and recurrent HCC, Chen et al. found that the time intervals from initial surgery to tumor "recurrence" did not differ significantly between true relapses and second primary tumors *(141)*. When recurrences and second primary tumors were added in the study from Muto et al. *(140)* and an adequate statistical test was used, no significant difference was found in the incidence of treatment failure between treated and untreated groups. Furthermore, Muto et al. subsequently reported a survival benefit in the treated group that was not apparent at the time of the initial report *(142)*. It is surprising that the survival advantage provided by a chemopreventive treatment of limited duration (12 mo) becomes apparent several years later, when the preneoplastic condition (cirrhosis) is still present.

In brief, retinoids offer the promise of chemoprevention through a variety of mechanisms *(138)*. Their potential role in the primary or secondary prevention of HCC needs further investigation.

4. SUMMARY AND CONCLUSION

Despite recent progress in diagnosis and treatment, HCC is still diagnosed at an advanced stage when prognosis is poor. Important efforts should therefore be directed toward developing chemoprevention strategies. The multiple stages of hepatocarcinogenesis offer several potential points for intervention. However, our understanding of this process remains sketchy. Moreover, intermediate biomarkers of hepatocarcinogenesis are lacking.

Universal vaccination against HBV has the potential to significantly reduce worldwide incidence of HCC. Treatment of chronic hepatitis B with IFN administered at a precirrhotic stage that successfully achieves virologic remission, appears to reduce the incidence of HBV-related HCC. Treatment of chronic hepatitis C with IFN, on the other hand, appears to have an impact on HCC incidence, whether administered to cirrhotic or noncirrhotic patients. These data, derived essentially from retrospective or noncontrolled studies, need prospective confirmation.

Oltipraz has become a paradigm of drug development for chemoprevention. It inhibits cytochrome P450 activity and induces phase 2 detoxification enzymes. It is tested for prevention of aflatoxin-induced hepatocarcinogenesis and should enter Phase III trials in the coming years. Nevertheless, other enzyme inductors are likely to become available in the meantime. They may be more potent and more readily available than oltipraz. Alternative strategies for chemoprevention could also be developed. For example, chlorophyllin inhibits aflatoxin adduct formation by adsorbing AFB_1.

As in many areas of therapeutics, using a combination of drugs for chemoprevention of HCC will probably prove more efficient than monotherapy. The choice of agents should be based on the complementarity of their mechanisms and possibly on their synergism, resulting in improved efficacy and reduced toxicity.

REFERENCES

1. Serag HB. Epidemiology of hepatocellular carcinoma. *Clin Liver Dis* 2001;5:87–107.
2. Colombari R, Tsui WM. Biliary tumors of the liver. *Semin Liver Dis* 1995;15:402–413.
3. Pappo AS, Rodriguez-Galindo C, Dome JS, Santana VM. Pediatric tumors. In *Clinical Oncology*, 2nd ed. Abeloff MD, Armitage JO, Lichter AS, Niederhuber JE, eds. Churchill Livingstone, New York, 2000: pp. 2346–2401.
4. Ferlay J, Bray F, Pisani P, Parkin DM. GLOBOCAN 2000: Cancer Incidence, Mortality and Prevalence Worldwide. Version 1.0. ed: IARC CancerBase No. 5. IARC Press, Lyon, 2001.
5. Bosch FX, Ribes J, Borras J. Epidemiology of primary liver cancer. *Semin Liver Dis* 1999;19:271–285.
6. Yu MW, Cheng SW, Lin MW, et al. Androgen-receptor gene CAG repeats, plasma testosterone levels, and risk of hepatitis B-related hepatocellular carcinoma. *J Natl Cancer Inst* 2000;92:2023–2028.
7. Lok AS, McMahon BJ. Chronic hepatitis B. *Hepatology* 2001;34:1225–1241.
8. Donato F, Boffetta P, Puoti M. A meta-analysis of epidemiological studies on the combined effect of hepatitis B and C virus infections in causing hepatocellular carcinoma. *Int J Cancer* 1998;75:347–354.
9. Alter HJ, Seeff LB. Recovery, persistence, and sequelae in hepatitis C virus infection: a perspective on long-term outcome. *Semin Liver Dis* 2000;20:17–35.
10. Poynard T, Bedossa P, Opolon P. Natural history of liver fibrosis progression in patients with chronic hepatitis C. The OBSVIRC, METAVIR, CLINIVIR, and DOSVIRC groups. *Lancet* 1997;349:825–832.
11. Harris DR, Gonin R, Alter HJ, et al. The relationship of acute transfusion-associated hepatitis to the development

12. Ikeda K, Saitoh S, Suzuki Y, et al. Disease progression and hepatocellular carcinogenesis in patients with chronic viral hepatitis: a prospective observation of 2215 patients. *J Hepatol* 1998;28:930–938.
13. Aizawa Y, Shibamoto Y, Takagi I, et al. Analysis of factors affecting the appearance of hepatocellular carcinoma in patients with chronic hepatitis C. A long term follow-up study after histologic diagnosis. *Cancer* 2000;89:53–59.
14. Colombo M. Hepatitis C virus and hepatocellular carcinoma. *Semin Liver Dis* 1999;19:263–269.
15. Jackson PE, Groopman JD. Aflatoxin and liver cancer. *Baillieres Best Pract Res Clin Gastroenterol* 1999;13:545–555.
16. Ross RK, Yuan JM, Yu MC, et al. Urinary aflatoxin biomarkers and risk of hepatocellular carcinoma. *Lancet* 1992;339:943–946.
17. Qian GS, Ross RK, Yu MC, et al. A follow-up study of urinary markers of aflatoxin exposure and liver cancer risk in Shanghai, People's Republic of China. *Cancer Epidemiol Biomarkers Prev* 1994;3:3–10.
18. Wang LY, Hatch M, Chen CJ, et al. Aflatoxin exposure and risk of hepatocellular carcinoma in Taiwan. *Int J Cancer* 1996;67:620–625.
19. Yu MW, Lien JP, Chiu YH, et al. Effect of aflatoxin metabolism and DNA adduct formation on hepatocellular carcinoma among chronic hepatitis B carriers in Taiwan. *J Hepatol* 1997;27:320–330.
20. Montesano R, Hainaut P, Wild CP. Hepatocellular carcinoma: from gene to public health. *J Natl Cancer Inst* 1997;89: 1844–1851.
21. Kensler TW, Groopman JD, Roebuck BD. Use of aflatoxin adducts as intermediate endpoints to assess the efficacy of chemopreventive interventions in animals and man. *Mutat Res* 1998;402:165–172.
22. Wild CP, Turner PC. Exposure biomarkers in chemoprevention studies of liver cancer. *IARC Sci Publ* 2001;154:215–222.
23. Di Bisceglie AM, Carithers RL Jr, Gores GJ. Hepatocellular carcinoma. *Hepatology* 1998;28:1161–1165.
24. Niederau C, Fischer R, Sonnenberg A, et al. Survival and causes of death in cirrhotic and in noncirrhotic patients with primary hemochromatosis. *N Engl J Med* 1985;313: 1256–1262.
25. Bradbear RA, Bain C, Siskind V, et al. Cohort study of internal malignancy in genetic hemochromatosis and other chronic nonalcoholic liver diseases. *J Natl Cancer Inst* 1985;75:81–84.
26. Park SZ, Nagorney DM, Czaja AJ. Hepatocellular carcinoma in autoimmune hepatitis. *Dig Dis Sci* 2000;45:1944–1948.
27. Norris J, King D. Carcinogenesis. In *Basic Science of Cancer*. Kruh GD, Tew KD, eds. Current Medicine, Inc., Philadelphia; 2000; pp. 154–167.
28. Perantoni AO. Carcinogenesis. In McKinnell RG, Parchment RE, Perantoni AO, Barry PG, eds. *The Biological Basis of Cancer*. Cambridge University Press, New York, 1998; pp. 79–114.
29. Ozturk M. Genetic aspects of hepatocellular carcinogenesis. *Semin Liver Dis* 1999;19:235–242.
30. Roberts LR, Gores GJ. Hepatocellular carcinoma. In Yamada T, Alpers DH, Kaplowitz N, et al., eds. *Textbook of Gastroenterology*, 4th ed. Lippincott Williams & Wilkins; Philadephia, 2003.
31. Wang JS, Groopman JD. DNA damage by mycotoxins. *Mutat Res* 1999;424:167–181.

of cirrhosis in the presence of alcohol abuse. *Ann Intern Med* 2001;134:120–124.

32. Ueno Y, Nagata S, Tsutsumi T, et al. Detection of microcystins, a blue-green algal hepatotoxin, in drinking water sampled in Haimen and Fusui, endemic areas of primary liver cancer in China, by highly sensitive immunoassay. *Carcinogenesis* 1996;17:1317–1321.

33. Sekijima M, Tsutsumi T, Yoshida T, et al. Enhancement of glutathione *S*-transferase placental-form positive liver cell foci development by microcystin-LR in aflatoxin B1-initiated rats. *Carcinogenesis* 1999;20:161–165.

34. Nakamoto Y, Guidotti LG, Kuhlen CV, et al. Immune pathogenesis of hepatocellular carcinoma. *J Exp Med* 1998;188: 341–350.

35. Chen PJ, Chen DS. Hepatitis B virus infection and hepatocellular carcinoma: molecular genetics and clinical perspectives. *Semin Liver Dis* 1999;19:253–262.

36. Feitelson MA. Hepatitis B virus in hepatocarcinogenesis. *J Cell Physiol* 1999;181:188–202.

37. Rabe C, Caselmann WH. Interaction of hepatitis B virus with cellular processes in liver carcinogenesis. *Crit Rev Clin Lab Sci* 2000;37:407–429.

38. Moriya K, Fujie H, Shintani Y, et al. The core protein of hepatitis C virus induces hepatocellular carcinoma in transgenic mice. *Nat Med* 1998;4:1065–1067.

39. Ray RB, Lagging LM, Meyer K, et al. Transcriptional regulation of cellular and viral promoters by the hepatitis C virus core protein. *Virus Res* 1995;37:209–220.

40. Ray RB, Steele R, Meyer K, Ray R. Transcriptional repression of p53 promoter by hepatitis C virus core protein. *J Biol Chem* 1997;272:10,983–10,986.

41. Kato N, Yoshida H, Kioko Ono-Nita S, et al. Activation of intracellular signaling by hepatitis B and C viruses: C-viral core is the most potent signal inducer. *Hepatology* 2000;32: 405–412.

42. Hayashi J, Aoki H, Kajino K, et al. Hepatitis C virus core protein activates the MAPK/ERK cascade synergistically with tumor promoter TPA, but not with epidermal growth factor or transforming growth factor alpha. *Hepatology* 2000;32:958–961.

43. Ray RB, Meyer K, Steele R, et al. Inhibition of tumor necrosis factor (TNF-alpha)-mediated apoptosis by hepatitis C virus core protein. *J Biol Chem* 1998;273:2256–2259.

44. Tai DI, Tsai SL, Chen YM, et al. Activation of nuclear factor kappaB in hepatitis C virus infection: implications for pathogenesis and hepatocarcinogenesis. *Hepatology* 2000;31:656–664.

45. Rehermann B. Interaction between the hepatitis C virus and the immune system. *Semin Liver Dis* 2000;20:127–141.

46. Ghosh AK, Steele R, Meyer K, et al. Hepatitis C virus NS5A protein modulates cell cycle regulatory genes and promotes cell growth. *J Gen Virol* 1999;80:1179–1183.

47. Ghosh AK, Majumder M, Steele R, et al. Hepatitis C virus NS5A protein modulates transcription through a novel cellular transcription factor SRCAP. *J Biol Chem* 2000;275: 7184–7188.

48. Sakamuro D, Furukawa T, Takegami T. Hepatitis C virus nonstructural protein NS3 transforms NIH 3T3 cells. *J Virol* 1995;69:3893–3896.

49. Chen CJ, Yu MW, Liaw YF, et al. Chronic hepatitis B carriers with null genotypes of glutathione *S*-transferase M1 and T1 polymorphisms who are exposed to aflatoxin are at increased risk of hepatocellular carcinoma. *Am J Hum Genet* 1996;59:128–134.

50. Omer RE, Verhoef L, Van't Veer P, et al. Peanut butter intake, GSTM1 genotype and hepatocellular carcinoma: a case-control study in Sudan. *Cancer Causes Control* 2001; 12:23–32.

51. Sun CA, Wang LY, Chen CJ, et al. Genetic polymorphisms of glutathione *S*-transferases M1 and T1 associated with susceptibility to aflatoxin-related hepatocarcinogenesis among chronic hepatitis B carriers: a nested case-control study in Taiwan. *Carcinogenesis* 2001;22:1289–1294.

52. Tiemersma EW, Omer RE, Bunschoten A, et al. Role of genetic polymorphism of glutathione-S-transferase T1 and microsomal epoxide hydrolase in aflatoxin-associated hepatocellular carcinoma. *Cancer Epidemiol Biomarkers Prev* 2001;10:785–791.

53. Sylla A, Diallo MS, Castegnaro J, Wild CP. Interactions between hepatitis B virus infection and exposure to aflatoxins in the development of hepatocellular carcinoma: a molecular epidemiological approach. *Mutat Res* 1999;428: 187–196.

54. El-Serag HB, Mason AC, Key C. Trends in survival of patients with hepatocellular carcinoma between 1977 and 1996 in the United States. *Hepatology* 2001;33:62–65.

55. Kelloff GJ, Sigman CC, Johnson KM, et al. Perspectives on surrogate end points in the development of drugs that reduce the risk of cancer. *Cancer Epidemiol Biomarkers Prev* 2000;9:127–137.

56. Blum HE. Hepatocellular carcinoma: susceptibility markers. *IARC Sci Publ* 2001;154:241–244.

57. Hilleman MR. Overview of the pathogenesis, prophylaxis and therapeusis of viral hepatitis B, with focus on reduction to practical applications. *Vaccine* 2001;19:1837–1848.

58. Kane M. Global programme for control of hepatitis B infection. *Vaccine* 1995;13:S47–49.

59. Kane MA. Status of hepatitis B immunization programmes in 1998. *Vaccine* 1998;16:S104–S108.

60. Chen HL, Chang MH, Ni YH, et al. Seroepidemiology of hepatitis B virus infection in children: ten years of mass vaccination in Taiwan. *JAMA* 1996;276:906–908.

61. Chang MH, Chen CJ, Lai MS, et al. Universal hepatitis B vaccination in Taiwan and the incidence of hepatocellular carcinoma in children. Taiwan Childhood Hepatoma Study Group. *N Engl J Med* 1997;336:1855–1859.

62. Wong DK, Cheung AM, O'Rourke K, et al. Effect of alpha-interferon treatment in patients with hepatitis Be antigen-positive chronic hepatitis B. A meta-analysis. *Ann Intern Med* 1993;119:312–323.

63. Niederau C, Heintges T, Lange S, et al. Long-term follow-up of HBeAg-positive patients treated with interferon alfa for chronic hepatitis B. *N Engl J Med* 1996;334:1422–1427.

64. Lin SM, Sheen IS, Chien RN, et al. Long-term beneficial effect of interferon therapy in patients with chronic hepatitis B virus infection. *Hepatology* 1999;29:971–975.

65. Papatheodoridis GV, Manesis E, Hadziyannis SJ. The long-term outcome of interferon-alpha treated and untreated patients with HBeAg-negative chronic hepatitis B. *J Hepatol* 2001;34:306–313.

66. Stark GR, Kerr IM, Williams BR, et al. How cells respond to interferons. *Annu Rev Biochem* 1998;67:227–264.

67. Merle P, Chevallier M, Levy R, et al. Preliminary results of interferon-alpha therapy on woodchuck hepatitis virus-induced hepatocarcinogenesis: possible benefit in female transgenic mice. *J Hepatol* 2001;34:562–569.

68. Oon CJ. Long-term survival following treatment of hepatocellular carcinoma in Singapore: evaluation of Wellferon in the prophylaxis of high-risk pre-cancerous conditions. *Cancer Chemother Pharmacol* 1992;31:S137–S142.

69. Mazzella G, Accogli E, Sottili S, et al. Alpha interferon treatment may prevent hepatocellular carcinoma in HCV- related liver cirrhosis. *J Hepatol* 1996;24:141–147.

70. Fattovich G, Giustina G, Realdi G, et al. Long-term outcome of hepatitis B e antigen-positive patients with compensated cirrhosis treated with interferon alfa. European Concerted Action on Viral Hepatitis (EUROHEP). *Hepatology* 1997;26:1338–1342.

71. Effect of interferon-alpha on progression of cirrhosis to hepatocellular carcinoma: a retrospective cohort study. International Interferon-alpha Hepatocellular Carcinoma Study Group. *Lancet* 1998;351:1535–1539.

72. Benvegnu L, Chemello L, Noventa F, et al. Retrospective analysis of the effect of interferon therapy on the clinical outcome of patients with viral cirrhosis. *Cancer* 1998;83:901–909.

73. Ikeda K, Saitoh S, Suzuki Y, et al. Interferon decreases hepatocellular carcinogenesis in patients with cirrhosis caused by the hepatitis B virus: a pilot study. *Cancer* 1998;82:827–835.

74. Camma C, Giunta M, Andreone P, Craxi A. Interferon and prevention of hepatocellular carcinoma in viral cirrhosis: an evidence-based approach. *J Hepatol* 2001;34:593–602.

75. Lechmann M, Liang TJ. Vaccine development for hepatitis C. Semin Liver Dis 2000;20:211–1226.

76. Lavanchy D. Hepatitis C: public health strategies. *J Hepatol* 1999;31:146–151.

77. Marcellin P. Hepatitis C: the clinical spectrum of the disease. *J Hepatol* 1999;31:9–16.

78. Hoofnagle JH, di Bisceglie AM. The treatment of chronic viral hepatitis. *N Engl J Med* 1997;336:347–356.

79. Heathcote J. Antiviral therapy for patients with chronic hepatitis C. *Semin Liver Dis* 2000;20:185–199.

80. Kozlowski A, Harris JM. Improvements in protein PEGylation: pegylated interferons for treatment of hepatitis C. *J Control Release* 2001;72:217–224.

81. Zeuzem S, Feinman SV, Rasenack J, et al. Peginterferon alfa-2a in patients with chronic hepatitis C. *N Engl J Med* 2000;343:1666–1672.

82. Lindsay KL, Trepo C, Heintges T, et al. A randomized, double-blind trial comparing pegylated interferon alfa-2b to interferon alfa-2b as initial treatment for chronic hepatitis C. *Hepatology* 2001;34:395–403.

83. Manns MP, McHutchison JG, Gordon SC, et al. Peginterferon alfa-2b plus ribavirin compared with interferon alfa-2b plus ribavirin for initial treatment of chronic hepatitis C: a randomised trial. *Lancet* 2001;358:958–965.

84. Gordon SC. Treatment of viral hepatitis—2001. *Ann Med* 2001;33:385–390.

85. Camma C, Giunta M, Linea C, Pagliaro L. The effect of interferon on the liver in chronic hepatitis C: a quantitative evaluation of histology by meta-analysis. *J Hepatol* 1997;26:1187–1199.

86. Poynard T, Moussalli J, Ratziu V, et al. Effect of interferon therapy on the natural history of hepatitis C virus-related cirrhosis and hepatocellular carcinoma. *Clin Liver Dis* 1999;3:869–881.

87. Poynard T, McHutchison J, Davis GL, et al. Impact of interferon alfa-2b and ribavirin on progression of liver fibrosis in patients with chronic hepatitis C. *Hepatology* 2000;32: 1131–1137.

88. Poynard T, Moussali J, Ratziu V, et al. Effects of interferon therapy in "non responder" patients with chronic hepatitis C. *J Hepatol* 1999;31:178–183.

89. Kuwana K, Ichida T, Kamimura T, et al. Risk factors and the effect of interferon therapy in the development of hepatocellular carcinoma: a multivariate analysis in 343 patients. *J Gastroenterol Hepatol* 1997;12:149–155.

90. Imai Y, Kawata S, Tamura S, et al. Relation of interferon therapy and hepatocellular carcinoma in patients with chronic hepatitis C. Osaka Hepatocellular Carcinoma Prevention Study Group. *Ann Intern Med* 1998;129:94–99.

91. Kasahara A, Hayashi N, Mochizuki K, et al. Risk factors for hepatocellular carcinoma and its incidence after interferon treatment in patients with chronic hepatitis C. Osaka Liver Disease Study Group. *Hepatology* 1998;27:1394–1402.

92. Camma C, Di Marco V, Lo Iacono O, et al. Long-term course of interferon-treated chronic hepatitis C. *J Hepatol* 1998;28: 531–537.

93. Yoshida H, Shiratori Y, Moriyama M, et al. Interferon therapy reduces the risk for hepatocellular carcinoma: national surveillance program of cirrhotic and noncirrhotic patients with chronic hepatitis C in Japan. IHIT Study Group. Inhibition of Hepatocarcinogenesis by Interferon Therapy. *Ann Intern Med* 1999;131:174–181.

94. Ikeda K, Saitoh S, Arase Y, et al. Effect of interferon therapy on hepatocellular carcinogenesis in patients with chronic hepatitis type C: a long-term observation study of 1,643 patients using statistical bias correction with proportional hazard analysis. *Hepatology* 1999;29:1124–1130.

95. Okanoue T, Itoh Y, Minami M, et al. Interferon therapy lowers the rate of progression to hepatocellular carcinoma in chronic hepatitis C but not significantly in an advanced stage: a retrospective study in 1148 patients. Viral Hepatitis Therapy Study Group. *J Hepatol* 1999;30:653–659.

96. Shindo M, Ken A, Okuno T. Varying incidence of cirrhosis and hepatocellular carcinoma in patients with chronic hepatitis C responding differently to interferon therapy. *Cancer* 1999;85:1943–1950.

97. Tanaka H, Tsukuma H, Kasahara A, et al. Effect of interferon therapy on the incidence of hepatocellular carcinoma and mortality of patients with chronic hepatitis C: a retrospective cohort study of 738 patients. *Int J Cancer* 2000;87:741–749.

98. Emanuel EJ, Miller FG. The ethics of placebo-controlled trials—a middle ground. *N Engl J Med* 2001;345:915–919.

99. Wild CP, Hall AJ. Primary prevention of hepatocellular carcinoma in developing countries. *Mutat Res* 2000;462: 381–393.

100. Kwak MK, Egner PA, Dolan PM, et al. Role of phase 2 enzyme induction in chemoprotection by dithiolethiones. *Mutat Res* 2001;480–481:305–315.

101. Kensler TW, Groopman JD, Sutter TR, et al. Development of cancer chemopreventive agents: oltipraz as a paradigm. *Chem Res Toxicol* 1999;12:113–126.

102. Jacobson LP, Zhang BC, Zhu YR, et al. Oltipraz chemoprevention trial in Qidong, People's Republic of China: study design and clinical outcomes. *Cancer Epidemiol Biomarkers Prev* 1997;6:257–265.

103. Kensler TW, He X, Otieno M, et al. Oltipraz chemoprevention trial in Qidong, People's Republic of China: modulation of serum aflatoxin albumin adduct biomarkers. *Cancer Epidemiol Biomarkers Prev* 1998;7:127–134.

104. Wang JS, Shen X, He X, et al. Protective alterations in phase 1 and 2 metabolism of aflatoxin B1 by oltipraz in res-

idents of Qidong, People's Republic of China. *J Natl Cancer Inst* 1999;91:347–354.

105. Mato JM, Alvarez L, Ortiz P, Pajares MA. S-adenosylmethionine synthesis: molecular mechanisms and clinical implications. *Pharmacol Ther* 1997;73:265–280.

106. Zingg JM, Jones PA. Genetic and epigenetic aspects of DNA methylation on genome expression, evolution, mutation and carcinogenesis. *Carcinogenesis* 1997;18:869–882.

107. Pascale RM, Simile MM, Feo F. Genomic abnormalities in hepatocarcinogenesis. Implications for a chemopreventive strategy. *Anticancer Res* 1993;13:1341–1356.

108. Pascale RM, Marras V, Simile MM, et al. Chemoprevention of rat liver carcinogenesis by *S*-adenosyl-L-methionine: a long-term study. *Cancer Res* 1992;52:4979–4986.

109. Gerbracht U, Eigenbrodt E, Simile MM, et al. Effect of S-adenosyl-L-methionine on the development of preneoplastic foci and the activity of some carbohydrate metabolizing enzymes in the liver, during experimental hepatocarcinogenesis. *Anticancer Res* 1993;13:1965–1972.

110. Pascale RM, Simile MM, De Miglio MR, et al. Chemoprevention by *S*-adenosyl-L-methionine of rat liver carcinogenesis initiated by 1,2-dimethylhydrazine and promoted by orotic acid. *Carcinogenesis* 1995;16: 427–430.

111. Ansorena E, Garcia-Trevijano ER, Martinez-Chantar ML, et al. *S*-adenosylmethionine and methylthioadenosine are anti-apoptotic in cultured rat hepatocytes but proapoptotic in human hepatoma cells. *Hepatology* 2002;35:274–280.

112. Cai J, Sun WM, Hwang JJ, Stain SC, Lu SC. Changes in *S*-adenosylmethionine synthetase in human liver cancer: molecular characterization and significance. *Hepatology* 1996;24:1090–1097.

113. Cai J, Mao Z, Hwang JJ, Lu SC. Differential expression of methionine adenosyltransferase genes influences the rate of growth of human hepatocellular carcinoma cells. *Cancer Res* 1998;58:1444–1450.

114. Yang H, Huang ZZ, Wang J, Lu SC. The role of c-Myb and Sp1 in the up-regulation of methionine adenosyltransferase 2A gene expression in human hepatocellular carcinoma. *Faseb J* 2001;15:1507–1516.

115. Mato JM, Camara J, Fernandez de Paz J, et al. *S*-Adenosylmethionine in alcoholic liver cirrhosis: a randomized, placebo-controlled, double-blind, multicenter clinical trial. *J Hepatol* 1999;30:1081–1089.

116. Vainio H. Is COX-2 inhibition a panacea for cancer prevention? *Int J Cancer* 2001;94:613–614.

117. Koga H, Sakisaka S, Ohishi M, et al. Expression of cyclooxygenase-2 in human hepatocellular carcinoma: relevance to tumor dedifferentiation. *Hepatology* 1999;29: 688–696.

118. Bae SH, Jung ES, Park YM, et al. Expression of cyclooxygenase-2 (COX-2) in hepatocellular carcinoma and growth inhibition of hepatoma cell lines by a COX-2 inhibitor, NS-398. *Clin Cancer Res* 2001;7:1410–1418.

119. Rahman MA, Dhar DK, Masunaga R, et al. Sulindac and exisulind exhibit a significant antiproliferative effect and induce apoptosis in human hepatocellular carcinoma cell lines. *Cancer Res* 2000;60:2085–2089.

120. Jaiswal M, LaRusso NF, Gores GJ. Nitric oxide in gastrointestinal epithelial cell carcinogenesis: linking inflammation to oncogenesis. *Am J Physiol Gastrointest Liver Physiol* 2001;281:G626–634.

121. Ahn B, Ohshima H. Suppression of intestinal polyposis in Apc(Min/+) mice by inhibiting nitric oxide production. *Cancer Res* 2001;61:8357–8360.

122. Rao CV, Indranie C, Simi B, et al. Chemopreventive properties of a selective inducible nitric oxide synthase inhibitor in colon carcinogenesis, administered alone or in combination with celecoxib, a selective cyclooxygenase-2 inhibitor. *Cancer Res* 2002;62:165–170.

123. Kane JM, 3rd, Shears LL, 2nd, Hierholzer C, et al. Chronic hepatitis C virus infection in humans: induction of hepatic nitric oxide synthase and proposed mechanisms for carcinogenesis. *J Surg Res* 1997;69:321–324.

124. Terasaki S, Kaneko S, Kobayashi K, et al. Histological features predicting malignant transformation of nonmalignant hepatocellular nodules: a prospective study. *Gastroenterology* 1998;115:1216–1222.

125. Kojiro M. Premalignant lesions of hepatocellular carcinoma: pathologic viewpoint. *J Hepatobiliary Pancreat Surg* 2000;7: 535–541.

126. Zondervan PE, Wink J, Alers JC, et al. Molecular cytogenetic evaluation of virus-associated and non-viral hepatocellular carcinoma: analysis of 26 carcinomas and 12 concurrent dysplasias. *J Pathol* 2000;192:207–215.

127. Bannasch P, Nehrbass D, Kopp-Schneider A. Significance of hepatic preneoplasia for cancer chemoprevention. *IARC Sci Publ* 2001;154:223–240.

128. Qian C, Drozdzik M, Caselmann WH, Prieto J. The potential of gene therapy in the treatment of hepatocellular carcinoma. *J Hepatol* 2000;32:344–351.

129. Baba M, Iishi H, Tatsuta M. In vivo electroporetic transfer of bcl-2 antisense oligonucleotide inhibits the development of hepatocellular carcinoma in rats. *Int J Cancer* 2000;85: 260–266.

130. Baba M, Iishi H, Tatsuta M. Transfer of bcl-xs plasmid is effective in preventing and inhibiting rat hepatocellular carcinoma induced by *N*-nitrosomorpholine. *Gene Therapy* 2001;8:1149–1156.

131. Tennant BC. Animal models of hepadnavirus-associated hepatocellular carcinoma. *Clin Liver Dis* 2001;5:43–68.

132. Wang HP, Zhang L, Dandri M, Rogler CE. Antisense down-regulation of N-myc1 in woodchuck hepatoma cells reverses the malignant phenotype. *J Virol* 1998;72:2192–2198.

133. Ko S, Nakajima Y, Kanehiro H, et al. Significant influence of accompanying chronic hepatitis status on recurrence of hepatocellular carcinoma after hepatectomy. Result of multivariate analysis. *Ann Surg* 1996;224:591–595.

134. Tung-Ping Poon R, Fan ST, Wong J. Risk factors, prevention, and management of postoperative recurrence after resection of hepatocellular carcinoma. *Ann Surg* 2000;232: 10–24.

135. Ikeda K, Arase Y, Saitoh S, et al. Interferon beta prevents recurrence of hepatocellular carcinoma after complete resection or ablation of the primary tumor-A prospective randomized study of hepatitis C virus-related liver cancer. *Hepatology* 2000;32:228–232.

136. Kubo S, Nishiguchi S, Hirohashi K, et al. Effects of long-term postoperative interferon-alpha therapy on intrahepatic recurrence after resection of hepatitis C virus-related hepatocellular carcinoma. A randomized, controlled trial. *Ann Intern Med* 2001;134:963–967.

137. Everson GT. Maintenance interferon for chronic hepatitis C: more issues than answers? *Hepatology* 2000;32: 436–438.

138. Hansen LA, Sigman CC, Andreola F, et al. Retinoids in chemoprevention and differentiation therapy. *Carcinogenesis* 2000;21:1271–1279.

139. Muto Y, Moriwaki H. Antitumor activity of vitamin A and its derivatives. *J Natl Cancer Inst* 1984;73:1389–1393.

140. Muto Y, Moriwaki H, Ninomiya M, et al. Prevention of second primary tumors by an acyclic retinoid, polyprenoic acid, in patients with hepatocellular carcinoma. Hepatoma Prevention Study Group. *N Engl J Med* 1996;334: 1561–1567.

141. Chen YJ, Yeh SH, Chen JT, et al. Chromosomal changes and clonality relationship between primary and recurrent hepatocellular carcinoma. *Gastroenterology* 2000;119: 431–440.

142. Muto Y, Moriwaki H, Saito A. Prevention of second primary tumors by an acyclic retinoid in patients with hepatocellular carcinoma. *N Engl J Med* 1999;340:1046–1047.

MULTIPLE MYELOMA

38 Chemoprevention

A New Paradigm for Managing Patients With Smoldering/Indolent Myeloma and High-Risk MGUS

John A. Lust, MD, PhD, and Kathleen A. Donovan, PhD

CONTENTS

1. INTRODUCTION

Cancer chemoprevention can be defined as pharmacologic intervention to suppress or reverse carcinogenesis and to prevent the development of invasive cancer. Multiple myeloma (MM) is an ideal disease for chemoprevention because its clinically benign precursor condition, monoclonal gammopathy of undetermined significance (MGUS), is easily identifiable. Preventing or delaying the transition from MGUS to myeloma with an effective chemopreventive agent would have a major impact on the treatment of high-risk MGUS patients. The molecular and cellular changes that occur in the clonal plasma cell during progression from MGUS to myeloma have not been clearly delineated. Defining these changes could make it possible to establish new surrogate endpoint biomarkers (SEBs) for use in clinical protocols to identify those patients who will progress from MGUS to MM.

2. CLINICAL MANIFESTATIONS OF MM AND MGUS

MM is recognized clinically by the proliferation of malignant plasma cells in bone marrow, detection of a serum or urine monoclonal protein, anemia, hypercalcemia, renal insufficiency, and lytic bone lesions (1). MGUS, characterized by a monoclonal protein (M protein) in the serum or urine without the other clinical features of MM (1,2), is more common than myeloma, occurring in 1% of the population over age 50 and 3% over age 70 (2). It is of great clinical importance to distinguish between patients with MGUS and MM because MGUS patients may be safely observed off chemotherapy. Unnecessary treatment can lead to acute leukemia or morbidity/mortality from chemotherapy. However, during long-term follow-up of 241 patients with MGUS, 59 patients (24.5%) went on to develop MM or a related plasma cell proliferative disorder (3).

From: Cancer Chemoprevention, Volume 2: Strategies for Cancer Chemoprevention
Edited by: G. J. Kelloff, E. T. Hawk, and C. C. Sigman © Humana Press Inc., Totowa, NJ

Table 1

Characteristic	MGUS	SMM	IMM	MM
Marrow plasma cells	<10%	≥10% OR	≥10% OR	≥10%
Serum M-spike	<3 g/dL	≥3 g/dL	≥3 g/dL	≥3 g/dL
Bence-Jones protein	<1 g/24 h	<1 g/24 h	<1 g/24 h	1 g/24 h
Anemia	Absent	May be present	May be present	Usually present
Hypercalcemia, renal insufficiency	Absent	Absent	Absent	May be present
Lytic bone lesions	Absent	Absent	A few may be present	Usually present
Requires chemotherapy	No	No	No	Yes

3. MGUS, MM, AND SMOLDERING AND INDOLENT MM

Specific criteria that serve as useful guidelines allow clinicians to differentiate between MM, MGUS, and other related plasma proliferative disorders. As shown in Table 1, patients with MGUS usually have fewer than 10% marrow plasma cells, a serum monoclonal protein <3 gm/dL, and no renal failure, lytic bone lesions, hypercalcemia, urinary Bence-Jones protein, or anemia. In contrast, patients with active myeloma will present with a marrow plasmacytosis of ≥10%, a serum monoclonal protein of ≥3 gm/dL, a 24-h urine monoclonal protein of ≥1 gm, and lytic bone lesions, and often have back pain, severe fatigue, pneumonia, or other bone pain (1). Between these extremes of the disease are two clinically intermediate stages, smoldering multiple myeloma (SMM) and indolent multiple myeloma (IMM). Patients with SMM are usually asymptomatic with marrow plasmacytosis ≥10% and/or serum monoclonal protein ≥3 gm/dL; lytic bone lesions are absent (4). Patients with IMM are similar to those with SMM, except that a small number of bone lesions may be present on bone survey studies. In contrast to MM patients, who receive chemotherapy, patients with MGUS, SMM, and IMM have stable disease and are followed off chemotherapy. However, patients who have MGUS ≥1.5 g/dL, SMM, or IMM are at high risk of eventually developing active MM, which requires chemotherapy (5–7). Such patients are candidates for novel therapeutic strategies to inhibit or prevent the development of active MM.

4. PROGRESSION OF HIGH-RISK MGUS, SMM, AND IMM TO ACTIVE MM

Kyle has shown that during long-term follow-up of 241 patients with MGUS, 59 patients (24.5%) went on to develop MM or a related plasma cell proliferative disorder (3). Of those who developed MM or a related plasma proliferative disorder, the majority remained stable for an extended period of time and then subsequently progressed to overt MM over a relatively short period. Of the 59 patients who progressed, 39 went on to develop MM. Serial serum studies were performed on 18 of these 39 patients. In these 18 who developed myeloma, the monoclonal protein remained stable for a median of 8 yr and then increased slowly over 1 to 4 yr in 11 patients or rapidly in less than 1 yr in seven patients (3). Based on these clinical observations, it is likely that genetic differences exist between MGUS and myeloma in which additional changes arise in the monoclonal plasma cells, leading to overt myeloma.

In a more recent analysis of 1395 patients with MGUS, Kyle et al. found that during follow-up MM, lymphoma with an IgM monoclonal protein, primary amyloidosis, macroglobulinemia, chronic lymphocytic leukemia, or plasmacytoma developed in 115 patients (8%) (5). The cumulative probability of progression to one of these disorders was 10% at 10 yr, 21% at 20 yr, and 26% at 25 yr. Only the concentration and type of monoclonal protein were independent predictors of progression. The presence of a monoclonal urinary light chain or a reduction in one or more uninvolved immunoglobulins was not a risk factor for progression. Patients with IgM or IgA monoclonal protein had an increased risk of progression to disease compared with patients who had an IgG monoclonal protein. The risk of progression to MM or a related disorder at 20 yr was 14% for an initial monoclonal protein value of 0.5 g/dL or less, 25% for an initial monoclonal protein value of 1.5 g/dL, 41% for an initial monoclonal protein value of 2.0 g/dL, 49% for an initial monoclonal protein value of 2.5 g/dL, and 64% for an initial monoclonal protein value of 3.0 g/dL (5).

For SMM and IMM, the risk of progression is even higher. In several studies, patients with indolent MM and one or more lytic bone lesions were found to have a short median time to progression of 8–10 months *(6,8,9)*. Weber et al. reported on 101 patients with Stage 1 asymptomatic MM (or SMM) out of a total of 695 consecutive, previously untreated patients with MM evaluated between October 1974 and October 1995 *(7)*. Patients with MGUS were excluded. Factors associated with disease progression included a serum monoclonal protein >3.0 g/dL, IgA heavy chain type, and Bence Jones protein excretion >50 mg/24 hr urine collection. Patients with at least two of these risk factors (high risk) had a median time to disease progression of 17 mo. In contrast, patients with none of the risk factors (low risk) had a median time to progression of 95 mo. Patients with one risk factor (intermediate risk) had a median time to progression of 39 mo and could be further subclassified based on MRI imaging of the thoracic and lumbar spine. Patients with abnormal MRI imaging had significantly earlier disease progression (median 21 mo) than those with a normal pattern (median 57 mo). Based on the above clinical observations, it is now possible to identify those patients with high-risk MGUS and SMM/IMM who are at high risk for disease progression. Since myeloma is incurable, these patients should be targeted for novel chemoprevention trials.

5. CURRENT TREATMENT OF MM

Chemotherapy is the initial treatment for symptomatic patients with active MM *(10–12)*. Patients who are candidates for peripheral blood stem cell harvest typically receive four cycles of vincristine, doxorubicin (Adriamycin), and dexamethasone (VAD) chemotherapy followed by peripheral blood stem cell harvest. Subsequently, myeloma patients either continue on standard chemotherapy such as vincristine, carmustine (BCNU), melphalan, cyclophosphamide, and prednisone (VBMCP), or proceed directly to transplant *(13,14)*. Patients who are not candidates for transplantation receive standard chemotherapy consisting of either melphalan and prednisone (MP) cycled every 4–6 wk or VBMCP *(15)*. Most recently, thalidomide has been shown to have activity in patients with recurrent myeloma *(16)*. Several protocols, at various institutions throughout the United States, are now using thalidomide as initial therapy for patients with active MM. Chemotherapy is usually continued until the patient has reached a plateau state, which is defined as a stable monoclonal protein in the serum and urine and no evidence of progression of myeloma. In most patients, chemotherapy plus analgesics can control the bone pain

characteristic of the disease. Radiation therapy is limited to patients who have disabling pain from a localized process. Patients with active myeloma who have extensive lytic bone disease also typically receive monthly pamidronate *(17,18)*. Supplemental erythropoietin is also useful in MM patients with symptomatic anemia *(19)*.

Survival duration of patients with MM ranges from a few months to many years; median survival is 2.5–3 yr *(15)*. With rare exceptions, even patients with transplantation eventually relapse and succumb to their disease *(13)*. Plasma cell labeling index, β 2-microglobulin, C-reactive protein, and soluble interleukin-6 receptor (IL-6R) have all been shown to be significant univariate prognostic factors *(20,21)*.

6. BIOLOGY OF MM: IL-6 IS MAJOR GROWTH FACTOR FOR MYELOMA CELLS

New therapeutic strategies needed for myeloma are likely to arise from a better understanding of disease biology. In normal B-cell ontogeny, IL-6 induces the terminal differentiation of B-cells into immunoglobulin-secreting plasma cells. Normal plasma cells produce antibody in response to IL-6, but do not proliferate. In contrast, IL-6 has been shown to be a central growth factor for myeloma cells *(22)*. That myeloma cells proliferate in response to IL-6 is a major difference distinguishing malignant from normal plasma cells and is of critical importance in disease pathogenesis.

Early work by Potter demonstrated that paraffin oil or pristane injected into BALB/c mice induced plasmacytomas *(23,24)*. Generation of the plasmacytomas was dependent on factors produced by the inflammatory cells. These cells were subsequently shown to produce IL-6, a potent growth factor for plasmacytomas *(24)*. Transgenic mice (C57BL/6) carrying the human IL-6 gene fused to a human immunoglobulin heavy chain enhancer developed a massive lethal plasmacytosis *(25,26)*. Most importantly, animal studies utilizing IL-6 knockout mice have shown that IL-6 is an essential requirement for the development of B lineage neoplasms *(27)*.

Kawano and colleagues demonstrated that IL-6 is an autocrine growth factor for human myeloma cells *(28)*. They have shown that myeloma cells freshly isolated from patients produce IL-6 and express its receptor. Exogenous IL-6 augments the in vitro growth of myeloma cells, and anti- IL-6 antibody inhibits their growth *(28)*. Schwab et al. demonstrated that myeloma cell line U266 expresses mRNA for both IL-6 and IL-6R. Proliferation of this cell line can be inhibited using anti- IL-6 antibody or anti-sense IL-6 oligonucleotides, further supporting the critical role of IL-6 in the growth of these cells *(29)*. Significantly elevated serum IL-6 levels have been detected in 3% of MGUS/SMM patients, 35% of overt myeloma patients, and 100% of a plasma cell leukemia group *(30)*. Using an anti-bromodeoxyuridine monoclonal antibody to specifically count myeloma cells in *S*-phase (i.e., the labeling index), the IL-6 responsiveness of myeloma cells in vitro correlates with their labeling index in vivo, and hence with severity of the disease *(31)*. An antibody to IL-6 administered in vivo dramatically decreased the labeling index of tumor cells in patients with aggressive multiple myeloma *(32)*. IL-6 has also been shown to protect myeloma cells against chemotherapy-induced apoptosis *(33)*.

Although it is clear that IL-6 expression plays a fundamental role in the growth of MM cells, the source of IL-6 expression is controversial. As discussed above, Kawano and colleagues demonstrated that IL-6 is an autocrine growth factor for human myeloma cells *(28)*. However, Klein et al. reported that high levels of IL-6 found in the bone marrow of patients with progressive MM are confined to the adherent cells of the bone marrow environment, and that IL-6 is not expressed by myeloma cells *(34)*. In addition, bone marrow monocytic and myeloid cells, but not myeloma cells, have been reported to express IL-6 mRNA *(35)*. Carter et al. found that human myeloma cells produce IL-1b that can induce IL-6 production by marrow stromal cells *(36)*. Together, these results suggest a paracrine rather than autocrine mechanism of myeloma cell growth by IL-6.

In addition to its role as the major growth factor for myeloma cells, IL-6 also protects myeloma cells from apoptosis and is essential for the terminal differentiation of normal B cells into antibody-secreting plasma cells *(33,37,38)*. Grigorieva et al. showed that marrow stromal cell IL-6 protects myeloma cells from dexamethasone-induced apoptosis. This protective effect could be abrogated by anti-IL-6 antibody *(33)*. Anti-IL-6 antibody also effectively inhibited pokeweed mitogen (PWM)-induced immunoglobulin production by normal mononuclear cells, but not PWM-induced proliferation *(38)*.

7. OTHER CYTOKINES INVOLVED IN MYELOMA CELL GROWTH

The IL-6 receptor consists of an 80-kD IL-6 binding molecule (gp80) and a 130-kD signal-transducing chain (gp130) *(39)*. gp130 also serves as the signal-transducing chain for leukemia inhibitory factor (LIF), oncostain M (OSM), ciliary neurotophic factor (CNTF), and IL-11 *(40)*. Therefore, all these factors have been shown to stimulate myeloma cell growth *(41,42)*. However, the observed responsiveness of most myeloma cells to these growth factors is variable when compared to IL-6 because the ligand-binding receptors for these cytokines are not as consistently expressed on myeloma cells as the IL-6 binding gp80 receptor *(43)*.

Other cytokines such as insulin-like growth factor I, IL-10, hepatocyte growth factor, and interferon-α have also been shown to stimulate myeloma cell line growth *(43–46)*. A recent report documented that myeloma cells produce vascular endothelial growth factor (VEGF). The authors postulated that myeloma cell VEGF can stimulate IL-6 from marrow stromal cells in a paracrine fashion, leading to myeloma cell growth *(47)*. In contrast, purified myeloma cells from patients have been shown to be unresponsive to cytokines such as GM-CSF, G-CSF, M-CSF, IL-2, or IL-4 *(48)*.

Studies on normal plasmablasts underscore the importance of IL-6 as a key growth factor for plasma cells. Anti-IL-6 antibodies prevented Ig secretion and cell differentiation of normal plasmablasts obtained from patients with reactive plasmacytoses by inducing apoptosis of the plasmablasts *(49)*. IL-6 may be the major growth factor for myeloma cells because it is an essential survival factor for normal plasmablasts.

8. ROLE OF IL-1β IN THE PATHOGENESIS OF MYELOMA

Aside from IL-6, myeloma cells have been observed to produce IL-1β, a cytokine with potent osteoclast activating factor (OAF) activity. Comparison of bone marrow plasma cells from patients with MGUS or MM has demonstrated that IL-1β mRNA was detectable in plasma cells from >95% of patients with MM but <25% of patients with MGUS, using either a combination of flow cytometry to enrich for plasma cells and reverse transcriptase/polymerase chain reaction (RT/PCR), or *in situ* hybridization (ISH) *(50,51)*. In contrast, IL-6 mRNA was undetectable in all MGUS patients and MM patients with a low labeling index, but present in the subgroup of myeloma patients with a high labeling index *(50)*. These results suggest that aberrant IL-1β production is an early event in the pathogenesis of MM and could help distinguish MGUS from MM better than IL-6.

Normal plasma cells do not produce IL-1β; however, IL-1β is detectable in culture supernatants from patients with MM (36). IL-1β has potent OAF activity and can induce the paracrine expression of IL-6 and several adhesion molecules such as ICAM-1, VCAM-1, and ELAM in other cellular systems (36,52–56). These biologic effects of IL-1β closely parallel several of the clinical features of human myeloma such as osteolytic bone lesions, IL-6-induced cell growth, and "homing" of myeloma cells to the bone marrow (1,57). The development of osteolytic lesions is an important clinical finding that clearly distinguishes MGUS from myeloma. Initially, two different groups had shown that bone- resorbing activity in supernatants of myeloma cell cultures was likely due to IL-1β and not to IL-1α, tumor necrosis factor (TNF), or lymphotoxin (56,58). More recently, Torcia and colleagues have clearly shown a critical role for IL-1β in the pathogenesis of bone disease (55). Using the fetal rat long-bone tissue culture assay, they demonstrated that OAF activity of culture supernatants from unfractionated bone marrow cells from myeloma patients correlated with IL-1β content (r = 0.949). Furthermore, OAF activity could be completely abolished by IL-1 receptor antagonist, sIL-1R type I or II, or neutralizing anti-IL-1β antibodies, but not by anti-IL-6 antibodies (55). These results demonstrate that OAF activity of myeloma cells from patients is predominantly related to IL-1β.

IL-6 has been shown to be a central growth factor for myeloma cells. Production of IL-1β by myeloma cells can induce paracrine generation of IL-6 by marrow stromal cells that in turn can stimulate myeloma cell proliferation. Carter et al. found that human myeloma cells are able to induce IL-6 production by marrow stromal cells. The stimulatory activity of the myeloma cells is mediated through endogenously released IL-1β, since antibodies to IL-1β completely abrogate the IL-6 production (36). In addition, IL-1β can act as an autocrine growth factor for myeloma cells in certain cases (59). The ability of IL-1R antagonist (IL-1Ra) to inhibit paracrine IL-6 production by bone marrow cultures from myeloma patients has been reported by Costes et al. (60). Using the bromodeoxyuridine method, they also demonstrated that IL-1Ra inhibited the percentage of myeloma cells in S-phase (60).

IL-1β has the ability to upregulate adhesion molecule expression and/or function. Murine plasmacytoma (B9) cells, transfected with an IL-1α cDNA and injected intravenously into syngeneic mice, "homed" to the bone marrow and produced metastatic bone lesions (61). (Unlike human cells, mouse cells produce and release

IL-1α, which is functionally homologous to human IL-1β.) By comparison, intravenous injection of autonomously-growing B-cell lines generated in vitro by retroviral insertion of an IL-6 cDNA did not result in bone marrow or bone metastases (61). Alterations in CD54 expression were identified between the parent line and the IL-1α transfected mouse plasmacytoma cells (62). In human disease, IL-1β activated bone marrow endothelial cells (BMEC), but not unstimulated BMEC, adhering to myeloma cells. This binding was inhibited by monoclonal antibodies against E-selectin (ELAM-1); however, antibodies to IL-1β were not tested. It is of note that transcription of endothelial-leukocyte adhesion molecule- 1 (ELAM-1 or CD62E), as well as vascular cell adhesion molecule-1 (VCAM-1 or CD 106) and intercellular adhesion molecule-1 (ICAM-1 or CD54) can be induced by IL-1β via a nuclear factor-kB (NFkB) intermediate. The positive regulatory domains required for maximal levels of cytokine induction have been defined in the promoters of all three genes; DNA binding studies reveal a requirement for NfkB (52).

The biologic effects of IL-1β closely parallel several clinical features of human myeloma. IL-1β has potent OAF activity, can increase the expression of adhesion molecules, and can induce paracrine IL-6 production. Increased production of adhesion molecules could explain why myeloma cells are found predominantly in the bone marrow. Subsequently, these "fixed" monoclonal plasma cells could now stimulate osteoclasts through production of IL-1β and paracrine generation of IL-6, resulting in osteolytic disease. Paracrine generation of IL-6 by marrow stromal cells may further support the growth and survival of myeloma cells.

9. STROMAL CELL IL-6 PRODUCTION DIFFERENTIATES MGUS FROM MM: IMPORTANCE OF IL-1β

The IL-1β bioassay uses IL-6 production by bone marrow stromal cells as a surrogate marker for IL-1β functional activity. After a 48-h culture with either recombinant IL-1β or supernatants harvested from unsorted bone marrow cell cultures obtained from patients with various plasma proliferative disorders, the amount of IL-6 produced by bone marrow stromal cells is quantitated by ELISA.

IL-6 results by ELISA from six representative patients with either MGUS, SMM, or myeloma are detailed in Fig. 1. Supernatants from two MGUS patients generated low levels of IL-6 not significantly different from the media control. In contrast, IL-6 levels measured in bone

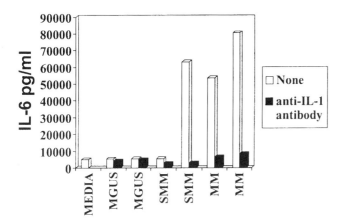

Fig. 1. Stromal cell co-cultures with patient's supernatants.

marrow supernatants from two myeloma patients were approximately 50–80 ng/mL, clearly distinguishable from those with MGUS. Both myeloma patients had bone lesions evident on X-ray. SMM patients appear to fall into two groups, those with high values similar to patients with myeloma and those with low values like patients with MGUS. We have observed that two of four patients with SMM and high IL-6 values have subsequently progressed to active myeloma within 2 yr. Finally, in three patients with elevated IL-6 levels, anti-IL-1β antibody is able to inhibit paracrine IL-6 production by the marrow stromal cells by approximately 90%. Our results demonstrate that stromal cell IL-6 production is induced predominantly by IL-1β in this model, is useful in differentiating patients with active myeloma from those with clinically benign disease, and may be helpful to identify patients at high risk who may benefit from novel chemoprevention trials.

10. CLINICAL STRATEGIES

Chemoprevention is a new paradigm for the management of patients with MGUS and SMM/IMM, since these patients are typically asymptomatic and the standard of care is currently observation. A chemoprevention trial investigating the activity of dehydroepiandrosterone (DHEA) or Biaxin (clarithromycin) in high-risk MGUS is ongoing at the Mayo Clinic. This trial was formulated based on evidence in the literature that DHEA can downregulate IL-6 and that Biaxin can downregulate IL-1β (63–65).

DHEA, an adrenal steroid, is a glucose phosphate dehydrogenase inhibitor with antiproliferative effects that may be a useful chemopreventive agent because of its capability of modulating multiple cytokines (63,64,66–68). Most notably, an age-associated

decline in DHEA and its sulfated derivative has been linked to increased IL-6 production (67), a critical factor necessary for generation of plasmacytomas in mice (24). As MGUS is more common with increasing age, exogenous DHEA may have an effect in preventing the progression of MGUS to MM by downregulation of IL-6.

Biaxin is a semisynthetic macrolide antimicrobial agent, differing from erythromycin by an O-methyl substitution at position 6 of the 14-membered lactone ring. Biaxin was shown in vitro by Northern analysis to suppress IL-1β expression in human nasal epithelial cells stimulated by *Haemophilus influenzae* endotoxin (HIE) (65). Furthermore, the electrophoretic mobility shift assay demonstrated that clarithromycin reduced DNA-binding activity of NFκB in both human nasal epithelial cells and fibroblasts stimulated by HIE or IL-1, respectively (65). No previous studies have been done on the use of Biaxin as a chemopreventive agent in myeloma. However, 30 patients with myeloma were treated empirically with Biaxin 500 mg BID for 1 to 2 mo with six complete responses and seven partial responses (69). Some patients received dexamethasone simultaneously, making it difficult to discern the effectiveness of Biaxin alone. However, these compelling clinical responses warrant further investigation in patients with plasma proliferative disorders.

In the Mayo study, eligible patients must have a new or preexisting diagnosis of MGUS and a monoclonal IgG or IgA M-protein of ≥1.5 g/dL. The trial is a three-arm double-blinded study comparing DHEA vs Biaxin vs placebo for 6 mo. During treatment, the following biomarkers are determined: nuclear pleomorphism index; ploidy; proliferative index; Thelper1/Thelper2 ratios; serum IL-6 and sIL-6R; adhesion molecule expression; FISH/cytogenetics; cytokine expression (IL-1β, IL-6, IL-6R); stromal cell IL-6 production; circulating monoclonal plasma cells; and plasma cell apoptosis. Since eligible patients must have a monoclonal protein >1.5 g/dL and are considered at high risk for progression to MM, it is anticipated that one or more of these biomarkers will be useful in identifying those who will progress from MGUS to myeloma. To date, no statement can be made about efficacy since the trial is blinded. However, toxicity has been minimal.

Based on clinical and experimental observations detailed above, several clinical strategies focused around the inhibition of paracrine IL-6 production may be proposed for chemoprevention in myeloma, since IL-6 plays a major role in myeloma cell growth and

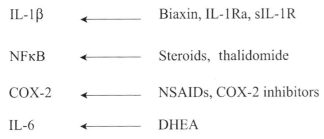

Fig. 2. Current potential chemoprevention agents in MM.

resistance to apoptosis (Fig. 2). The importance of this pathway is supported by combined clinical and experimental observations that dexamethasone and thalidomide both inhibit NFκB and that the combination of both agents is highly effective therapeutically in patients with active or relapsing myeloma (70–72).

Although not a formal chemoprevention study, between January 1987 and March 1993, 145 consecutive previously untreated patients with asymptomatic multiple myeloma (Stage 1) were randomized between treatment with melphalan and prednisone (MP) just after diagnosis and treatment only at disease progression (73). Response rate was similar in both groups but duration of response was shorter in patients who were treated at disease progression (48 vs 79 mo; $p = 0.044$). Survival was not influenced by MP treatment administered at diagnosis or at disease progression (64 vs 71 mo respectively). Survival was shorter for patients treated at disease progression than for those who had neither disease progression nor treatment (56 vs 92 mo; $p = 0.005$). Because patients treated at disease progression fared worse than those who had no disease progression and were untreated, biologic or other disease features must be found to identify these subgroups of stage 1 MM patients (73).

Our group conducted a clinical trial of thalidomide as initial therapy for 16 asymptomatic SMM or IMM patients (74). Thalidomide was given orally at a dose of 200 mg/d for 2 wk, and then increased as tolerated by 200 mg/d every 2 wk to a maximum dose of 800 mg/d. Six patients had a confirmed response to therapy with at least 50% or greater reduction in serum and urine monoclonal protein. When minor response (25–49%) decreases in monoclonal protein concentration were included, 11 of 16 patients (69%) responded to therapy. Major grade 3–4 toxicities included two patients with somnolence, and one patient each with syncope and neutropenia. Pretreatment microvessel density (MVD) was not a significant predictor of response to therapy (median MVD 4

and 12 in responders and nonresponders respectively, $p = 0.09$) (73). We concluded that thalidomide has significant activity in treating newly diagnosed SMM/IMM. However, we do not recommend treatment with thalidomide at this stage in all patients, since some patients with SMM/IMM can be stable for several months or years without any therapy. Additional randomized trials are needed to determine if thalidomide will delay progression to active multiple myeloma and whether other, less toxic therapies would yield similar results.

In animal models of myeloma, it has been shown that indomethacin added to drinking water is highly effective at inhibiting plasmacytomagenesis (75,76). Additional experiments have shown that inhibition of cyclooxygenase-2 (COX-2) by either a nonselective agent such as indomethacin or a selective COX-2 inhibitor can effectively inhibit IL-6 production in vitro or in vivo (77–79). A Phase II randomized, placebo-controlled trial of an NSAID for modulation of biomarkers in MGUS is planned.

Although many cytokines can stimulate IL-6 production, IL-1β appears to be a major cytokine responsible for paracrine production of IL-6 by marrow stromal cells in myeloma (36). IL-1β is expressed by the plasma cells of virtually all myeloma patients; however, it is not produced by normal plasma cells (50,51,57). Aberrant IL-1β produced by myeloma cells induces IL-6 by bone marrow stromal cells (Fig. 2), which in turn supports the growth and survival of myeloma cells (57). This paracrine model of IL-6 production suggests a rational therapeutic approach for high-risk MGUS and SMM/IMM, i.e., inhibit the IL-1β-induced IL-6 production with a potent IL-1β inhibitor. It is hypothesized that treatment with an IL-1β inhibitor will reduce plasma cell growth and ultimately slow or reverse further progression of the disease. Agents such as IL-1Ra have shown clinical activity in rheumatoid arthritis and have a favorable toxicity profile compared to steroids or thalidomide. The ability of IL-1Ra to inhibit paracrine IL-6 production by bone marrow cultures from myeloma patients has been reported in vitro by Costes et al. (60). Using the bromodeoxyuridine method, they also demonstrated that IL-1Ra inhibited the percentage of myeloma cells in S-phase (60). Based on the above observations, we have developed a Phase II clinical trial using IL-1Ra in patients with smoldering/indolent myeloma that do not require chemotherapy but are at high risk for progression to active disease.

11. SUMMARY

Chemoprevention is a new paradigm for management of patients with high-risk MGUS and SMM/IMM. MM is an ideal disease for chemoprevention because its precursor condition, MGUS, is easily identifiable by serum protein electrophoresis/immunoelectrophoresis of a blood sample and because myeloma is a universally fatal malignancy. As future trials are opened and completed, cohorts of patients will be identified, allowing for rapid testing of new agents. Clinical parameters such as the level and type of serum M-protein, the amount of Bence Jones protein, and possibly MRI of the spine as well as biomarkers such as IL-1β-induced IL-6 production, C-reactive protein, and the plasma cell labeling index are likely to be useful in distinguishing patients with clinically benign disease from those with active myeloma. Agents such as DHEA, Biaxin, NSAIDs, COX-2 inhibitors, and IL-1β inhibitors are currently being used or may be useful in future chemoprevention trials based on their favorable toxicity profile.

REFERENCES

1. Kyle RA, Lust JA. Monoclonal gammopathies of undetermined significance. *Semin Hematol* 1989;26:176–200.
2. Greipp PR, Lust JA. Pathogenetic relation between monoclonal gammopathies of undetermined significance and multiple myeloma. *Stem Cells* 1995;13:10–21.
3. Kyle RA. "Benign" monoclonal gammopathy—after 20 to 35 years of follow-up. *Mayo Clin Proc* 1993;68:26–36.
4. Kyle RA, Greipp PR. Smoldering multiple myeloma. *N Engl J Med* 1980;302:1347–1349.
5. Kyle RA, Therneau TM, Rajkumar SV, et al. A long-term study of prognosis in monoclonal gammopathy of undetermined significance. *N Engl J Med* 2002;346:564–569.
6. Dimopoulos MA, Moulopoulos A, Smith T, et al. Risk of disease progression in asymptomatic multiple myeloma. *Am J Med* 1993;94:57–61.
7. Weber DM, Dimopoulos MA, Moulopoulos LA, et al. Prognostic features of asymptomatic multiple myeloma. *Brit J Haematol* 1997;97:810–814.
8. Facon T, Menard JF, Michaux JL, et al. Prognostic factors in low tumour mass asymptomatic multiple myeloma: a report on 91 patients. The Groupe d'Etudes et de Recherche sur le Myelome (GERM). *Am J Hematol* 1995;48:71–75.
9. Wisloff F, Andersen P, Andersson TR, et al. Incidence and follow-up of asymptomatic multiple myeloma. The myeloma project of health region I in Norway. II. *Eur J Haematol* 1991;47:338–341.
10. Kyle RA. High-dose therapy in multiple myeloma and primary amyloidosis: an overview. *Semin Oncol* 1999;26:74–83.
11. Kyle RA. Newer approaches to the management of multiple myeloma. *Cancer* 1993;72:3489–3494.
12. Greipp PR, Witzig T. Biology and treatment of myeloma [see comments]. *Curr Opin Oncol* 1996;8:20–27.
13. Attal M, Harousseau JL, Stoppa AM, et al. A prospective, randomized trial of autologous bone marrow transplantation and chemotherapy in multiple myeloma. Intergroupe Francais du Myelome [see comments]. *N Engl J Med* 1996;335:91–97.
14. Alexanian R, Dimopoulos M. The treatment of multiple myeloma. *N Engl J Med* 1994;330:484–489.
15. Oken, MM, Harrington DP, Abramson N, et al. Comparison of melphalan and prednisone with vincristine, carmustine, melphalan, cyclophosphamide, and prednisone in the treatment of multiple myeloma: results of Eastern Cooperative Oncology Group Study E2479. *Cancer* 1997;79:1561–1567.
16. Singhal S, Mehta J, Desikan R, et al. Antitumor activity of thalidomide in refractory multiple myeloma [see comments] [published erratum appears in *N Engl J Med* 2000 Feb 3;342(5):364]. *N Engl J Med* 1999;341:1565–1571.
17. Berenson JR, Lichtenstein A, Porter L, et al. Efficacy of pamidronate in reducing skeletal events in patients with advanced multiple myeloma. Myeloma Aredia Study Group. *N Engl J Med* 1996;334:488–493.
18. Berenson JR, Lichtenstein A, Porter L, et al. Long-term pamidronate treatment of advanced multiple myeloma patients reduces skeletal events. Myeloma Aredia Study Group. *J Clin Oncol* 1998;16:593–602.
19. Garton JP, Gertz MA, Witzig TE, et al. Epoetin alfa for the treatment of the anemia of multiple myeloma. A prospective, randomized, placebo-controlled, double-blind trial. *Arch Int Med* 1995;155:2069–2074.
20. Greipp PR, Katzmann JA, O'Fallon WM, Kyle RA. Value of beta 2-microglobulin level and plasma cell labeling indices as prognostic factors in patients with newly diagnosed myeloma *Blood* 1988;72:219–223.
21. Greipp PR, Lust JA, O'Fallon WM, et al. Plasma cell labeling index and beta 2- microglobulin predict survival independent of thymidine kinase and C-reactive protein in multiple myeloma. *Blood* 1993;81:3382–3387.
22. Kishimoto T. The biology of interleukin-6. *Blood* 1989;74:1–10.
23. Potter M, Sklar MD, Rowe WP. Rapid viral induction of plasmacytomas in pristane-primed BALB-c mice. *Science* 1973;182:592–594.
24. Potter M. Perspectives on the origins of multiple myeloma and plasmacytomas in mice. *Hematol Oncol Clin North Am* 1992;6:211–223.
25. Potter M, Mushinski JF, Mushinski EB, et al. Avian v-myc replaces chromosomal translocation in murine plasmacytomagenesis. *Science* 1987;235:787–789.
26. Clynes R, Wax J, Stanton LW, et al. Rapid induction of IgM-secreting murine plasmacytomas by pristane and an immunoglobulin heavy-chain promoter/enhancer-driven c-myc/v-Ha-ras retrovirus. *Proc Natl Acad Sci USA* 1988;85:6067–6071.
27. Hilbert DM, Kopf M, Mock BA, et al. Interleukin 6 is essential for in vivo development of B lineage neoplasms. *J Exp Med* 1995;182:243–248.
28. Kawano M, Hirano T, Matsuda T, et al. Autocrine generation and requirement of BSF- 2/IL-6 for human multiple myelomas. *Nature* 1988;332:83–85.
29. Schwab G, Siegall CB, Aarden LA, et al. Characterization of an interleukin-6-mediated autocrine growth loop in the human multiple myeloma cell line, U266. *Blood* 1991;77:587–593.
30. Bataille R, Jourdan M, Zhang XG, Klein B. Serum levels of interleukin 6, a potent myeloma cell growth factor, as a reflect of disease severity in plasma cell dyscrasias. *J Clin Invest* 1989;84:2008–2011.

31. Zhang XG, Klein B, Bataille R. Interleukin-6 is a potent myeloma-cell growth factor in patients with aggressive multiple myeloma. *Blood* 1989;74:11–13.

32. Bataille R, Barlogie B, Lu ZY, et al. Biologic effects of anti-interleukin-6 murine monoclonal antibody in advanced multiple myeloma. *Blood* 1995;86:685–691.

33. Grigorieva I, Thomas X, Epstein J. The bone marrow stromal environment is a major factor in myeloma cell resistance to dexamethasone. *Exp Hematol* 1998;26:597–603.

34. Klein B, Zhang XG, Jourdan M, et al. Paracrine rather than autocrine regulation of myeloma-cell growth and differentiation by interleukin-6. *Blood* 1989;73:517–526.

35. Portier M, Rajzbaum G, Zhang XG, et al. In vivo interleukin 6 gene expression in the tumoral environment in multiple myeloma. *Eur J Immunol* 1991;21:1759–1762.

36. Carter A, Merchav S, Silvian-Draxler I, Tatarsky I. The role of interleukin-1 and tumour necrosis factor-alpha in human multiple myeloma. *Br J Haematol* 1990;74:424–431.

37. Lichtenstein A, Tu Y, Fady C, et al. Interleukin-6 inhibits apoptosis of malignant plasma cells. *Cell Immunol* 1995; 162:248–255.

38. Muraguchi A, Hirano T, Tang B, et al. The essential role of B cell stimulatory factor 2 (BSF-2/IL-6) for the terminal differentiation of B cells. *J Exp Med* 1988;167:332–344.

39. Kishimoto T, Akira S, Taga T. Interleukin-6 and its receptor: a paradigm for cytokines. *Science* 1992;258:593–597.

40. Hirano T, Matsuda T, Nakajima K. Signal transduction through gp130 that is shared among the receptors for the interleukin 6 related cytokine subfamily. *Stem Cells* 1994;12:262–277.

41. Westendorf JJ, Jelinek, DF. Growth regulatory pathways in myeloma. Evidence for autocrine oncostatin M expression. *J Immunol* 1996;157:3081–3088.

42. Zhang XG, Gu JJ, Lu ZY, et al. Ciliary neurotropic factor, interleukin 11, leukemia inhibitory factor, and oncostatin M are growth factors for human myeloma cell lines using the interleukin 6 signal transducer gp130. *J Exp Med* 1994; 179:1337–1342.

43. Jelinek DF. Mechanisms of myeloma cell growth control. *Hematol Oncol Clin North Am* 1999;13:1145–1157.

44. Lu ZY, Zhang XG, Rodriguez C, et al. Interleukin-10 is a proliferation factor but not a differentiation factor for human myeloma cells. *Blood* 1995;85:2521–2527.

45. Borset M, Hjorth-Hansen H, Seidel C, et al. Hepatocyte growth factor and its receptor c- met in multiple myeloma. *Blood* 1996;88:3998–4004.

46. Jelinek DF, Aagaard-Tillery KM, Arendt BK, et al. Differential human multiple myeloma cell line responsiveness to interferon-alpha. Analysis of transcription factor activation and interleukin 6 receptor expression. *J Clin Invest* 1997;99:447–456.

47. Dankbar B, Padro T, Leo R, et al. Vascular endothelial growth factor and interleukin-6 in paracrine tumor-stromal cell interactions in multiple myeloma. *Blood* 2000;95: 2630–2636.

48. Anderson KC, Jones RM, Morimoto C, et al. Response patterns of purified myeloma cells to hematopoietic growth factors. *Blood* 1989;73:1915–1924.

49. Jego G, Bataille R, Pellat-Deceunynck C. Interleukin-6 is a growth factor for nonmalignant human plasmablasts. *Blood* 2001;97:1817–1822.

50. Donovan KA, Lacy MQ, Kline MP, et al. Contrast in cytokine expression between patients with monoclonal gammopathy of undetermined significance or multiple myeloma. *Leukemia* 1998;12:593–600.

51. Lacy MQ, Donovan KA, Heimbach JK, et al. Comparison of interleukin-1 beta expression by in situ hybridization in monoclonal gammopathy of undetermined significance and multiple myeloma. *Blood* 1999;93:300–305.

52. Collins T, Read MA, Neish AS, et al. Transcriptional regulation of endothelial cell adhesion molecules: NF-kappa B and cytokine-inducible enhancers. *FASEB J* 1995;9:899–909.

53. Dustin ML, Rothlein R, Bhan AK, et al. Induction by IL 1 and interferon-gamma: tissue distribution, biochemistry, and function of a natural adherence molecule (ICAM-1). *J Immunol* 1986;137:245–254.

54. Terry RW, Kwee L, Levine JF, Labow MA. Cytokine induction of an alternatively spliced murine vascular cell adhesion molecule (VCAM) mRNA encoding a glycosylphosphatidylinositol- anchored VCAM protein. *Proc Natl Acad Sci USA* 1993;90:5919–5923.

55. Torcia M, Lucibello M, Vannier E, et al. Modulation of osteoclast-activating factor activity of multiple myeloma bone marrow cells by different interleukin-1 inhibitors. *Exp Hematol* 1996;24:868–874.

56. Yamamoto I, Kawano M, Sone T, et al. Production of interleukin 1 beta, a potent bone resorbing cytokine, by cultured human myeloma cells. *Cancer Res* 1989;49:4242–4246.

57. Lust JA, Donovan KA. The role of interleukin-1 beta in the pathogenesis of multiple myeloma. *Hematol Oncol Clin North Am* 1999;13:1117–1125.

58. Klein B, Lu ZY, Gaillard JP, et al. Inhibiting IL-6 in human multiple myeloma. *Curr Top Microbiol Immunol* 1992;182:237–244.

59. Nagata K, Tanaka Y, Oda S, et al. Interleukin 1 autocrine growth system in human multiple myeloma. *Jpn J Clin Oncol* 1991;21:22–29.

60. Costes V, Portier M, Lu ZY, et al. Interleukin-1 in multiple myeloma: producer cells and their role in the control of IL-6 production. *Br J Haematol* 1998;103:1152–1160.

61. Hawley TS, Lach B, Burns BF, et al. Expression of retrovirally transduced IL-1 alpha in IL-6-dependent B cells: a murine model of aggressive multiple myeloma. *Growth Factors* 1991;5:327–338.

62. Hawley RG, Wang MH, Fong AZ, Hawley TS. Association between ICAM-1 expression and metastatic capacity of murine B-cell hybridomas. *Clin Exp Metastasis* 1993;11:213–226.

63. Casson PR, Andersen RN, Herrod HG, et al. Oral dehydroepiandrosterone in physiologic doses modulates immune function in postmenopausal women. *Am J Obstet Gynecol* 1993;169:1536–1539.

64. Gordon GB, Shantz LM, Talalay P. Modulation of growth, differentiation and carcinogenesis by dehydroepiandrosterone. *Adv Enzyme Regul* 1987;26:355–382.

65. Miyanohara T, Ushikai M, Matsune S, et al. Effects of clarithromycin on cultured human nasal epithelial cells and fibroblasts. *Laryngoscope* 2000;110:126–131.

66. Daynes RA, Araneo BA. Natural regulators of T-cell lymphokine production in vivo. *J Immunother* 1992;12:174–179.

67. Daynes RA, Araneo BA, Ershler WB, et al. Altered regulation of IL-6 production with normal aging. Possible linkage to the age-associated decline in dehydroepiandrosterone and its sulfated derivative. *J Immunol* 1993;150:5219–5230.

68. Schwartz AG, Pashko LL. Cancer prevention with dehydroepiandrosterone and non- androgenic structural analogs. *J Cell Biochem Suppl* 1995;22:210–217.

69. Durie BGM, Villarete L, Farvard A, et al. Clarithromycin (Biaxin) as primary treatment for myeloma. *Blood* 1997;90 (10 Suppl 1 Part 1):p579a.

70. Brostjan C, Anrather J, Csizmadia V, et al. Glucocorticoid-mediated repression of NFkappaB activity in endothelial cells does not involve induction of IkappaBalpha synthesis. *J Biol Chem* 1996;271:19,612–19,616.

71. Sharma HW, Narayanan R. The NF-kappaB transcription factor in oncogenesis. *Anticancer Res* 1996;16:589–596.

72. Auphan N, DiDonato JA, Rosette C, et al. Immunosuppression by glucocorticoids: inhibition of NF-kappa B activity through induction of I kappa B synthesis. *Science* 1995;270:286–290.

73. Riccardi A, Mora O, Tinelli C, et al. Long-term survival of stage I multiple myeloma given chemotherapy just after diagnosis or at progression of the disease: a multicentre randomized study. Cooperative Group of Study and Treatment of Multiple Myeloma. *Br J Cancer* 2000;82:1254–1260.

74. Rajkumar SV, Dispenzieri A, Fonseca R, et al. Thalidomide for previously untreated indolent or smoldering multiple myeloma. *Leukemia* 2001;15:1274–1276.

75. Potter M, Wax JS, Anderson AO, Nordan RP. Inhibition of plasmacytoma development in BALB/c mice by indomethacin. *J Exp Med* 1985;161:996–1012.

76. Potter M, Wax J, Jones GM. Indomethacin is a potent inhibitor of pristane and plastic disc induced plasmacytomagenesis in a hypersusceptible BALB/c congenic strain. *Blood* 1997;90:260–269.

77. Hinson RM, Williams JA, Shacter E. Elevated interleukin 6 is induced by prostaglandin E2 in a murine model of inflammation: possible role of cyclooxygenase-2. *Proc Natl Acad Sci USA* 1996;93:4885–4890.

78. Shacter E, Arzadon GK, Williams J. Elevation of interleukin-6 in response to a chronic inflammatory stimulus in mice: inhibition by indomethacin. *Blood* 1992;80:194–202.

79. Tsuboi I, Tanaka H, Nakao M, et al. Nonsteroidal anti-inflammatory drugs differentially regulate cytokine production in human lymphocytes: up-regulation of TNF, IFN-gamma and IL-2, in contrast to down-regulation of IL-6 production. *Cytokine* 1995;7:372–379.

Index